Heart's Vortex

Intracardiac Blood Flow Phenomena

Ares Pasipoularides, MD, PhD, FACC

Consulting Professor of Surgery
Duke University School of Medicine
Durham, North Carolina, U.S.A.

Formerly, Director of Cardiac Function of the Duke/NSF Research Center for Emerging Cardiovascular Technologies, Duke University

Formerly, Director of Cardiovascular Research at Brooke Army Medical Center
Fort Sam Houston, San Antonio, Texas

PEOPLE'S MEDICAL PUBLISHING HOUSE
SHELTON, CONNECTICUT

People's Medical Publishing House-USA
2 Enterprise Drive, Suite 509
Shelton, CT 06484
Tel: 203-402-0646
Fax: 203-402-0854
E-mail: info@pmph-usa.com

PMPH-USA

09 10 11 12/PMPH/9 8 7 6 5 4 3 2

ISBN 978-1-60795-033-2
Printed in China by People's Medical Publishing House
Copyeditor/typesetter: Newgen; Cover designer: Mary McKeon; Cover art: Ares Pasipoularides, MD, PhD, FACC

Sales and Distribution

Canada
McGraw-Hill Ryerson Education
Customer Care
300 Water St
Whitby, Ontario L1N 9B6
Canada
Tel: 1-800-565-5758
Fax: 1-800-463-5885
www.mcgrawhill.ca

Foreign Rights
John Scott & Company
International Publisher's Agency
P.O. Box 878
Kimberton, PA 19442
USA
Tel: 610-827-1640
Fax: 610-827-1671

Japan
United Publishers Services Limited
1-32-5 Higashi-Shinagawa
Shinagawa-ku, Tokyo 140-0002
Japan
Tel: 03-5479-7251
Fax: 03-5479-7307
Email: kakimoto@ups.co.jp

United Kingdom, Europe, Middle East, Africa
McGraw Hill Education
Shoppenhangers Road
Maidenhead
Berkshire, SL6 2QL
England
Tel: 44-0-1628-502500
Fax: 44-0-1628-635895
www.mcgraw-hill.co.uk

Singapore, Thailand, Philippines, Indonesia, Vietnam, Pacific Rim, Korea
McGraw-Hill Education
60 Tuas Basin Link
Singapore 638775
Tel: 65-6863-1580
Fax: 65-6862-3354
www.mcgraw-hill.com.sg

Australia, New Zealand
Elsevier Australia
Tower 1, 475 Victoria Avenue
Chatswood NSW 2067
Australia
Tel: 0-9422-8553
Fax: 0-9422-8562
www.elsevier.com.au

Brazil
Tecmedd Importadora e Distribuidora
de Livros Ltda.
Avenida Maurilio Biagi 2850
City Ribeirao, Rebeirao, Preto SP
Brazil
CEP: 14021-000
Tel: 0800-992236
Fax: 16-3993-9000
Email: tecmedd@tecmedd.com.br

India, Bangladesh, Pakistan, Sri Lanka, Malaysia
CBS Publishers
4819/X1 Prahlad Street 24
Ansari Road, Darya, New Delhi-110002
India
Tel: 91-11-23266861/67
Fax: 91-11-23266818
Email:cbspubs@vsnl.com

People's Republic of China
PMPH
Bldg 3, 3rd District
Fangqunyuan, Fangzhuang
Beijing 100078
P.R. China
Tel: 8610-67653342
Fax: 8610-67691034
www.pmph.com

The image is more than an idea.
It is a vortex or cluster of fused ideas
and is endowed with energy.
—Ezra Pound

For, verily, art is embedded in nature;
whoever can draw her out, has her.
—Albrecht Dürer

To my wife, Jane Wright Pasipoularides,
who is the foundation of joy
for all I do.

Contents

Foreword

Concern for man and his fate must always form the chief interest of all technical endeavors. Never forget this in the midst of your diagrams and equations, and
Most of the fundamental ideas of science are essentially simple, and may, as a rule, be expressed in a language comprehensible to everyone.
——Albert Einstein

Perfection is achieved, not when there is nothing more to add, but when there is nothing left to take away.
——Antoine de Saint-Exupéry

We are what we repeatedly do; excellence, then, is not an act but a habit.
——Aristotle

THERE ARE CHALLENGES in academic medicine that are especially noteworthy. Dr. Donald Kennedy, President Emeritus of Stanford University, references these challenges in some of his writings where he describes the responsibilities of academicians as including teaching and mentoring, discovery and publication, among other obligations.[1] When I assumed the chair of surgery at Duke University's School of Medicine and Hospital several years ago, I was, of course, aware of the department's long and distinguished history in thoracic surgery, as well as its prowess in associated scientific investigation. Indeed, as a "card-carrying" surgeon-scientist with an abiding interest in and commitment to clinical and academic excellence, these characteristics of the department were major attractions for me to move to Durham, North Carolina.

Nevertheless, there is nothing quite like having the opportunity to meet, face-to-face, with some of the individuals responsible for Duke's historical successes. Dr. Ares Pasipoularides, one of our emeritus research professors, is one of those individuals. Within minutes of meeting him, the depth and breadth of his intellect and dedication to science are palpable. His desire to educate and to inform becomes apparent only a short while later. After only brief study, it becomes obvious that he does these things very well.

[1]Kennedy, D. *Academic Duty*. Cambridge, MA: Harvard University Press, 1997.

Cardiovascular disease remains a major cause of death for many of the world's people. Simultaneously, our ability to assess the heart, and the methods that can be used for this purpose, continue to expand and improve rapidly. High resolution digital imaging and associated computational assessments of flow and physiological function are now commonly available to clinicians and scientists. Whether directly caring for patients or researching the mechanisms of disease, one must be able to understand and assimilate the data obtained from measurements of changes in intracardiac blood flow induced by or associated with particular diseases because these are the final macroscopic biological correlates or "read-outs" of the underlying cellular or subcellular events that govern the heart's *raison d'être*. However, understanding these flow phenomena and their relationships is a fundamentally difficult task since the scientific and physiological underpinnings are quite complex and require an appropriate understanding of mathematics, fluid dynamics, computer modeling and simulation in the context of their relationship to the biological sciences. Explaining and teaching this information is at least an order of magnitude more difficult than understanding it, and the ability to do so is a rare talent, in my view.

When I had the opportunity to see a draft of what Ares and I affectionately describe as his "opus magnum," I first remembered the expectations that were enumerated by Dr. Kennedy. It was clear to me that Dr. Pasipoularides' book, *Heart's Vortex: Intracardiac Blood Flow Phenomena*, would be much more than just an encyclopedic source of information. It would be equally valuable as an illustration of a lifelong commitment to learning, insight, the joys inherent to scientific investigation and discovery, and a dedication to teaching and other experiences that could be shared with and enjoyed by students of the cardiovascular sciences of all ages, regardless of their backgrounds, preparation, or knowledge bases. As one begins to digest its contents, which are organized around well-referenced fundamentals of intracardiac flows as well as their visualization and measurement, one truly has the sense that an expert teacher is there with you, looking over your shoulder as you learn about cardiac hemodynamics—including its developmental history, theoretical frameworks, and practical applications. The loving attention to detail and the care taken in constructing the book is evident; it is a tangible projection of Dr. Kennedy's concepts of academic duty.

As I further studied the contents of Dr. Pasipoularides' book, I was reminded of another literary masterpiece, *The Visual Display of Quantitative Information* by Edward Tufte, which is another of my favorite books. One of Dr. Tufte's goals was to illustrate how complex ideas, concepts and data can be best presented visually – although this is not an easy task and certainly may not be straightforward! Indeed, in my opinion, his studies suggest that knowledge can often be most efficiently and effectively exchanged when crisp and clearly written, parsimonious text is complemented by informative figures, graphs, or other displays. Therein lies another strength of *Heart's Vortex*. Dr. Pasipoularides has provided the correct number of carefully designed figures to illustrate important principles that significantly increase the accessibility of the material that is presented. To my eye, they all, perhaps intuitively, reflect Dr. Tufte's highest principles.

I am honored to have been invited to write this Foreword to what I think will be an important contribution to the world's scientific literature. I believe it will be found to be a masterwork by a mastermind.

Danny O. Jacobs, M.D., M.P.H.
David C. Sabiston, Jr. Professor
Chair, Department of Surgery
Duke University School of Medicine
Duke University Hospital
Durham, North Carolina, U.S.A.

Prologue

Whosoever loveth instruction loveth knowledge

——Prov. xii 1

I do not intend to avoid digressions and episodes; that is part of every conversation; indeed of life itself.

——Alexander Herzen

Herzen, A. and D. Macdonald (1973). My past and thoughts: the memoirs of Alexander Herzen. New York, Knopf.

The men of experiment are like the ant, they only collect and use; the reasoners resemble spiders, who make cobwebs out of their own substance. But the bee takes a middle course: it gathers its material from the flowers of the garden and of the field, but transforms and digests it by a power of its own. Not unlike this is the true business of [natural] philosophy; for it neither relies solely or chiefly on the powers of the mind, nor does it take the matter which it gathers from natural history and mechanical experiments and lay it up in the memory whole, as it finds it, but lays it up in the understanding altered and digested. Therefore from a closer and purer league between these two faculties, the experimental and the rational (such as has never yet been made), much may be hoped.

——Sir Francis Bacon (1561–1626)

Novum Organum (1620), Book I, Aphorism XCV. From the translation of James Spedding, Robert Leslie Ellis, and Douglas Denon Heath in The Works (Vol. VIII), published in Boston by Taggard and Thompson, 1863.

TODAY, MEASUREMENTS OF 3-D cardiac chamber contours and flow patterns in humans and experimental animals can be routinely acquired non-invasively. High resolution digital imaging modalities, e.g., 3-D echo, Doppler, spiral CT and MRI, advances in computing, numerical simulations and scientific visualization, and sophisticated experimental flow models have expanded rapidly the information becoming available to cardiologists and researchers. The growing availability of such data adds a new dimension to the assessment of cardiac disease. The observable patterns can be looked upon as letters of an alphabet. To understand their meaning, the observer needs the ability to "read the script."

This book addresses this urgent need for proper understanding of the physiologic and clinical relevance of intracardiac flow patterns and flow-related variables, associated with cardiac pumping under normal and disease conditions. It will be useful in elucidating the generation and the (patho-) physiologic implications of flow effects that are noted in vivo, and will guide improved therapeutic interventions.

To help make sense of even the most difficult concepts, this book introduces physical and physiological ideas in a singular way: it is illustrated profusely with insightful, multi-panel drawings and schematics by the author, in addition to reproductions of high-fidelity fluid dynamic recordings at cardiac catheterization, and computer-generated intracardiac flow maps and flow variable plots. The primary emphasis is on using basic principles and approaches of fluid dynamics to better understand intracardiac blood flow phenomena, in both the normal and the abnormal (diseased) human heart.

To this end, results have been used not only from clinical and animal multisensor catheterization and angiography studies but also from a novel Functional imaging (FI) method. This FI method has been developed by the author and his co-workers at the Cardiac Surgical Research Lab at Duke University and the Duke/NSF Research Center for Emerging Cardiovascular Technologies. It evolved from our method of predetermined boundary motion (PBM) for the investigation of intracardiac blood flows by computational fluid dynamics (CFD) methodology. In both of these methods, the movement of the endocardial chamber boundary is determined independently of the flow, which is generated by and depends on it. Only the resulting flow field of the intraventricular blood must be computed, by incorporating the uncoupled wall motion into the CFD.

The FI method reveals detailed blood flow patterns in the hearts of individual experimental animals and human subjects. It uses information derived from digital imaging modalities that can provide dynamic 3-D cardiac chamber contours with high spatiotemporal resolution. The method combines geometric modeling of the cardiac chambers throughout the cardiac cycle with computational fluid dynamics. Instantaneous chamber geometry is derived directly from dynamic endocardial 3-D contours, which permits ventricular blood flow simulations on individual experimental animals or patients with normal or abnormal regional wall motion patterns.

Insight into a physical process can be improved if a pattern produced by or related to it is accessible to visual inspection. FI can extend our understanding of the ventricular ejection and filling processes and of dynamic patterns of intracardiac flows in previously unattainable ways. Global vortical flow patterns that are beautifully visualized by FI can be identified as the main flow feature associated with ventricular filling, and, as the title suggests, figure prominently in the book.

Through several decades, I have been engaged in clinical multisensor catheterization and noninvasive imaging research, in (patho-) physiologic and bioengineering animal and bench experiments, and in mathematical modeling and computational simulation studies of cardiac fluid dynamics and function. I have invested the years of firsthand research and teaching needed in order to develop a truly integrative and effective approach to communicating knowledge and difficult concepts to others, including undergraduate, graduate and medical students, postdoctoral fellows, residents and medical and surgical specialists.

An underlying theme of the book is to share with the reader the pleasures that come with successfully completing difficult research programs on intracardiac fluid dynamics and with constructing a number of new clinically relevant theories on cardiac function. Digital imaging and visualization as well as computational fluid dynamics are difficult subjects, regrettably beyond the reach of many interested people who are afraid of being inundated with equations. Nevertheless, these rapidly evolving tools have allowed fascinating discoveries that intrigue, interest strongly, and can be understood by the average clinician or investigator.

The book is not a mere compilation of the most up-to-date scientific data and relevant concepts. Rather, it is an integrated educational means to developing pluridisciplinary background, knowledge, and understanding. Such understanding allows an appreciation of the crucial, albeit heretofore generally unappreciated, importance of intracardiac blood flow phenomena in a host of multifaceted functional and morphogenetic[2] cardiac adaptations. These adaptations are physiologically and clinically relevant, since they can potentially bring about transitions to maladaptive disease states.

The book concentrates on cardiological and (patho-)physiological fluid dynamic concepts, many developed by the author, and is profusely illustrated with over 400 Figures and multipanel Diagrams, forming a vital part of the pedagogy and explaining the concepts. All these illustrations were prepared by the author, using Adobe CS [versions 1–4]™ and other graphic design software suites. I endorse heartily Ezra Pound's view that

The image is more than an idea.
It is a vortex or cluster of fused ideas
and is endowed with energy.

The book is organized in two parts. Part I provides comprehensive pedagogic background from many disciplines that are necessary for a deep and broad understanding and appreciation of intracardiac blood flow phenomena. Such indispensable background spans several chapters and covers necessary mathematics, a brief history of the evolution of ideas and methodological approaches that are relevant to cardiac fluid dynamics and imaging, a qualitative introduction to fluid dynamic stability theory, chapters on physics and fluid dynamics of unsteady blood flows and an intuitive introduction to various kinds of relevant vortical fluid motions.

An extensive and intensive grounding is provided in high-fidelity multisensor catheterization, and in angiocardiographic and conventional echocardiographic imaging modalities. An entire chapter is devoted to functional cardiac anatomy and myofiber histoarchitectonics and to their interactions with intracardiac blood flow. A unique and comprehensive presentation of the cardiac cycle in depth, both in health and in disease,

[2]Morphogenetic = giving rise to form; Gk $\mu o \rho \varphi \eta$ (morphe), form; $\gamma \epsilon \nu \eta \tau \iota \kappa o \nu$ (genetikon), giving rise to, bearing.

is then developed, along with the fluid dynamics of heart valve operation. Powerful new pathophysiological concepts that have, on the basis of fluid dynamic reasoning applied to physiological and clinical problems, been developed and published by the author in influential cardiology journals, are thoroughly explained and discussed. They include *complementarity and competitiveness* of the *intrinsic* and *extrinsic components* of the *systolic ventricular load*, the *convective deceleration component* of the *diastolic ventricular load*, the important *facilitative role* of the normal diastolic ventricular vortex for *filling, systolic*, and *diastolic ventriculoannular disproportion*, and more.

A gallery of human high-fidelity multisensor-catheter hemodynamics and fluid dynamics covering a variety of important normal and abnormal cardiac states follows. I look upon this gallery as a veritable National Treasure. I acquired the high-fidelity multisensor catheterization datasets that I utilized in its creation mostly during my tenure as Director of Cardiology Research at Brooke Army Medical Center, in San Antonio, TX. At the time, the Cardiac Catheterization Laboratories at BAMC were by far the most outstanding diagnostic and investigative catheterization labs in the world, performing over 1200 (!) high-fidelity multisensor catheterizations per year.

Part II. is devoted to pluridisciplinary approaches to the visualization of intracardiac blood flows. It begins with a Chapter on 3-D real-time and "live 3-D" echocardiography and Doppler echocardiography, CT tomographic scanning modalities, including multidetector spiral and helical dataset acquisitions, MRI and cardiac MRA, including phase-contrast velocity mapping (PCVM), etc. An entire chapter is then devoted to the understanding of postprocessing exploration techniques and the display of tomographic data, including *"slice-and-dice"* 3-D techniques and cine-MRI.

The course encompasses an intuitive introduction to CFD as it pertains to intracardiac blood flow simulations. This is followed—in separate chapters—by conceptually rich treatments of the CFD of ejection and of diastolic filling, presenting at some length the method of "PBM," developed at Duke University by the author and his collaborators. An entire chapter is devoted to fluid dynamic epigenetic factors in cardiogenesis and pre- and postnatal cardiac remodeling, and the book closes with Chapter 16, on Clinical and Basic Science Perspectives, and their implications for emerging research frontiers.

I am exceedingly gratified to have created this work as a single author, with a unified, single-person point of view, communicating with each grouping of my pluridisciplinary readers as *"one of them,"* notwithstanding their diverse backgrounds! There are about 1,500 pluridisciplinary bibliographic references cited in the text. The audience will encompass undergraduate and graduate/post-graduate levels of training in medical and related biomedical science and technology fields of study. It will include cardiologists, cardiovascular surgeons, and radiologists; medical physicists, fluid dynamicists, and biomedical engineers; physiologists and other medical scientists—including embryologists and geneticists interested in the role of flow-related forces in phenotypic expression; and zoologists and comparative physiologists.

Throughout the many years of writing and illustrating this book, I have felt like being there, *over-the-shoulder* of my readers, sparing no effort whatsoever to render their task of comprehending sometimes quite difficult concepts, and their implications, as tractable as humanly possible. In part as a consequence of this fact, the text is punctuated with many informative and explanatory footnotes, as well as numerous in-text referrals to insight-promoting figures and previous or subsequent book sections containing necessary background material, relevant explanations, or interesting clinical correlations.

The recognition of the unity of scientific inquiry is largely due to patient studies and research in diverse disciplines. Throughout my career, I have been struck by how the fertilization of one field by another makes new and important problems apparent; it also makes simpler solutions of old problems possible. Yet, very few biomedical scientists are adequately trained in mathematics and mechanics, and many others trained in quantitative methods have inadequate grounding in physiological and biomedical science theory. The book will serve a variety of audiences encompassing these extremes. The primary one is medical students and doctors seeking understanding and knowledge about clinically important intracardiac fluid flow phenomena. The range of medical professionals includes cardiologists, imaging specialists, cardiac surgeons and physiologists, at all levels of training and career development.

The book is certainly well-suited as both a supporting text and a reference book for university courses in biomedical engineering and physiological fluid dynamics, cardiac imaging, cardiovascular physiology, cardiology, physiology and biophysics, and fluid mechanics with an eye to pluridisciplinary applications. It also aims at the needs of biomedical engineers and technologists who are interested in learning about what people involved in clinically motivated studies of cardiovascular fluid mechanics have been up to.

A.P.
Durham and Asheville, North Carolina

Acknowledgments

Thanks to Jason Malley, Executive Editor, PMPH-USA, for his great insight and intuition and for his continued support and guidance, and to the tireless and expert Joanne Jay and her coworkers at Newgen North America's New York and India teams who did their utmost to support my quest for the highest possible quality of both the written and visual presentations.

To those who have contributed to this book indirectly, you will find acknowledgments and due thanks woven throughout the text. I employed this method purposely, hoping it would make your reading of the book more enjoyable and provocative, and my thanks and gratitude more profound and meaningful.

The resources and helpful, expert librarians at the Duke University and Medical Center Libraries, the North Carolina State University Libraries, the University of North Carolina Asheville Library, the University of Texas and Health Sciences Center at San Antonio Libraries, the Brooke Army Medical Center at San Antonio Library, the Trinity University at San Antonio Library, the Harvard University and School of Medicine (Countway) Libraries, the New England Primate Research Center Library, the Massachusetts General Hospital Library, the Barker Engineering Library at M.I.T., and the Brown University Libraries have proven invaluable, as have those of the Library of Congress and the National Library of Medicine of the U.S.A.

Part I

Fundamentals of Intracardiac Flows and Their Measurement

Chapter 1

Introduction

A man is not a dog to smell out each individual track, he is a man to see, and seeing, to analyze. He is a sight tracker with each of the other senses in adjunctive roles. Further, man is a scanner, not a mere looker. A single point has little meaning unless taken with other points and many points at different times are little better. He needs the whole field, the wide view.

——Professor F. M. N. Brown of the University of Notre Dame [9].

The real voyage of discovery consists not in seeking new landscapes, but in having new eyes.

——Marcel Proust (1871–1922), French novelist, in his autobiography [62].

PERHAPS BECAUSE OF OUR PAST AS HUNTERS AND GATHERERS, our visual perception is excellent at detecting and recognizing spatial patterns. We also very spontaneously compare them to one another. This is why, in the common language, we speak of "ripples" on *water* as well as on *sand* or we describe cortical cell "dendrites" (Gk. dendron = tree) as *tree*-like structures. Observation and interpretation of intricate spatiotemporal patterns are fundamental to many areas of medicine, yet in hemodynamics and ventricular dynamics, our historic interest has been more related to *temporal* patterns and in particular those of pulsatile waveform analyses. The fact that *spatial* patterns are everywhere in cardiovascular flows hardly needs amplification. From the rich color Doppler images of intracardiac blood flow, to the intriguing pictures from cardiac MRI studies illustrating intraventricular diastolic vortical motions, there is a wide range of spatial arrangements present. Nevertheless, because of an interest in nominal[1] "left ventricular," "right atrial," "aortic," and so on, pulses of pressure, flow, and volume, we have until recently managed to more often than not avoid confronting the challenges of spatial heterogeneity in intracardiac blood flow.

The last few decades however have heralded an explosion of interest in cardiac fluid dynamics, particularly in spatiotemporal patterns of intracardiac flow, which we will address in proper detail in Chapters 12–16. Two important areas of work are arguably the catalyst that brought the questions of intracardiac flow patterns to the forefront of the minds of clinicians, biomedical engineers, physiologists, cellular biologists, and embryologists. The first is the ready availability of high spatiotemporal resolution digital imaging modalities and the attendant analysis that is possible with these data, made all the easier by the ever decreasing cost of computing power and the availability of "off-the-shelf," low-cost simulation, and scientific visualization software. The second is the rise in awareness of the broader impact of normal and abnormal intracardiac flow patterns on, e.g., shear forces, which modulate important cellular processes, including morphogenesis, hyperplasia and myocardial remodeling, as well as factors involved in clotting activation and thrombosis.

Digital cardiac imaging is providing enormous amounts of spatiotemporal data to complement the temporal data traditionally measured, and we are eagerly looking to use this for predictive modeling of myocardial responses. In principle, we have the tools available to undertake this work and, already, impressive intracardiac blood flow models and color graphics are being generated. However, in many cases, the scientific understanding of these measurements is questionable. We need better ways to develop and assess spatiotemporal patterns of intracardiac flow, as well as to exploit properly and fully the information that is becoming available from new measurement methods, which often provide us with very different information to that which we are using today.

In the analysis of cardiac hemodynamic performance, two major viewpoints are possible; the first is derived from the traditional temporal approach, while the second encompasses detailed spatiotemporal phenomena and processes:

[1] Nominal values are those that we can obtain by ordinary means, such as a fluid-filled catheter connected to an external strain gauge for pressure measurements.

- a "black-box" approach—the overall relationships between input and output are examined to varying degrees of mechanistic resolution; and,
- a "glass-box," or "clear-box" approach—the spatiotemporal details of intracardiac blood flow phenomena are evaluated.

The vastly different levels of the spatial capabilities of these two limiting approaches must be considered when deciding how best to study specific aspects of cardiac function. This is a question of "horses for courses"—of choosing the appropriate tool for the job.

1.1 Processes

In approaching blood flow phenomena, it is usually advantageous to take processes rather than events as basic entities. I shall not attempt any rigorous definition of a *process*; rather I shall allude to examples and make some very informal remarks. The main difference between events and processes is that events are relatively *localized* in space and time, while processes have much greater temporal *duration*, and in many cases, much greater spatial *extent*. In space–time diagrams, events are represented by points, whereas processes are represented by lines. A ball colliding with a tree would count as an event; the ball, traveling from the kicker's foot to the tree, would constitute a process. The activation of an x-ray detector by an x-ray would be an event; the x-ray beam, traveling from its source through the body and emerging modified to activate the detector would be a process. Complex processes involve a large number of changing interacting variables. The basic problem in understanding complex systems [35] is that, as the number of interactions between variables increases, the complexity of the system increases exponentially and such complex systems become exceedingly difficult, or even impossible, to solve.

A complex process may include a large number of variables, as long as there are few interconnections between the variables [36]; when the number of interconnections (k) becomes large, $k > 5$, the system becomes unstable over time and is usually insoluble [78]. Complex multiple interactions can be reduced through the creation of higher-order theoretical concepts [43]. A higher-order concept (C) takes account of the effects of subordinate variables, but reduces the group to just one variable. In effect, the original interactions have been disposed of and the newly fashioned concept C can interact with new variables as a single variable.

Proceeding to an interesting example, a well-known example of a physical process is the *Brownian movement or motion*, the ceaseless, erratic, zigzag movement exhibited by minute particles of matter when suspended in a fluid.[2] The molecules of the liquid itself are similarly subjected to a movement of this kind, but it is not directly observable by microscope. This movement is due to the ceaseless "bombardment" of the solid particles by the molecules of the liquid, moving because of *thermal* agitation. The existence of

[2] It was first observed with a microscope by Robert Brown in 1827, on particles of a size of the order of the micrometer, i.e., sufficiently small to be pushed around to a substantial extent by the water molecules, but sufficiently large to be observable with his microscope.

the Brownian movement is thus closely related to and is a mark of the discontinuous (molecular, atomic) nature of matter. Einstein's approach [21] to Brownian movement is instructive: he identified the mean-square displacements of suspended particles, rather than their velocities, as suitable *observable* quantities. Previous investigators had tried to determine the "mean velocity of agitation" by following as nearly as possible the path of individual particles. Values so obtained were always a few microns per second for particles of the order of a micron.

But the particle trajectories are confused and complicated so often and so rapidly that it is impossible to follow them. Similarly, because of the large number of interconnections between the variables (i.e., the molecular velocities of the suspending medium) the apparent mean speed of a suspended particle during a given time varies in the wildest way in magnitude and direction, and does not tend to a limit as the time taken for an observation decreases. Neglecting, therefore, the true velocity, which cannot be measured, and disregarding the extremely intricate path followed by a particle during a given time, Einstein chose, as the magnitude characteristic of the process, the mean-square displacements of suspended particles; this displacement will clearly be longer, the more active the agitation. Thus, by neglecting the intricate path of suspended particles—reflecting the large number of interconnections between the molecular velocities of the liquid—and by introducing another concept, far more easily extracted by observation, Einstein opened a new promising way to study the complex system, and proved that the mean square of the horizontal displacement during time t increases in proportion to that time.

Physical processes can be investigated analytically, experimentally, via computer simulations, and by combined methods of attack. An example is provided by the direct modeling by random steps of the *diffusive* phenomena, which comprise the spontaneous movement and scattering of particles (atoms and molecules) of liquids, gases, and solids. Imagine placing a small drop of ink in a perfectly motionless—macroscopically—glass of water. Even without stirring, the particles of ink will be gradually spread out in the water. While being spread out, the drop of ink remains centered on its starting point. This physical process is what is called diffusion. It can be shown, by applying the random-walk[3] model to the process, that the average distance reached by the particles increases proportionally with the *square root* of time, in line with the analysis of Brownian movement that was outlined above.

An example of a process from molecular science relates to the theory of the size of *polymer* macromolecules, obtained by the sequencing of a great number, N, of small identical *monomers*, connected together by covalent chemical bonds (a macromolecular polymer chain can be visualized as a pearl necklace). It is notable that the geometry of such macromolecules is not linear; the chain can fold up in many ways to form a kind of *ball*. Naturally then the question arises of the polymer size, which depends in some way on the number N of monomers. Modeling the folding process as a simple random walk with

[3] The random-walk process may be envisioned by considering the following process: A person takes a step in a randomly chosen direction, then takes another step in a randomly chosen direction, and then takes another step in a randomly chosen direction, and so on until a total of N successive steps have been taken. This process is known as the random walk and it has been extremely useful to scientists in many fields who study stochastic (probabilistic) processes.

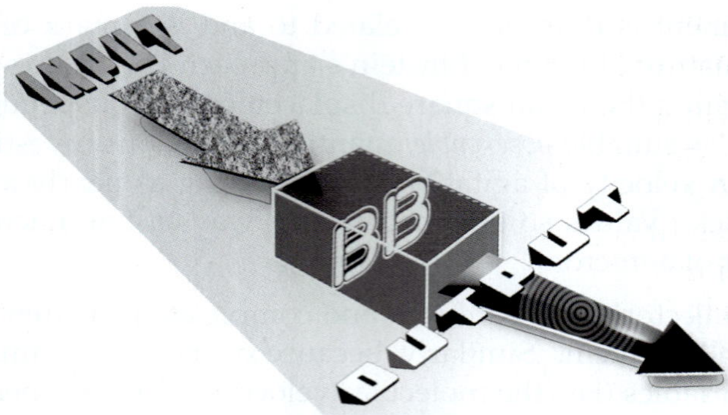

Figure 1.1: The system or process investigated is inside the black-box (BB) but all we are interested in is the input and output. We do not have to know *what* is inside the system or *how* it works. We can change the output by modifying either the input or the process itself.

3 dimensions, in which the successive monomers have random orientations completely *independent* from each other, the size of the molecule can be shown to increase as the square root of N. Taking account of steric constraints, it can be shown that the size of the molecule increases in parallel with N raised to the power *0.59* approximately (and not *0.5*, which is not much different).

1.2 The black-box approach

The time-honored method of scientific inquiry is to treat the system or the process that is being investigated as a black-box, as is depicted in Figure 1.1. Black-box models are applied when there are plenty of data available regarding the performance of a system of interest [7], but its functioning is unknown or very complex—there is not enough knowledge to create a mathematical model, the system is very nonlinear and dependent on operation point, or the analysis of the system is very time-consuming. The black-boxes are data-driven models, which do not explicitly model the physics of the system, but establish a mathematical relationship between a large number of input-output pairs measured from the system. Good quality data are essential for the approach. Input–output black-box data mapping can be modeled in terms of a mathematical function (linear or nonlinear model), which contains a number of parameters whose values are determined with the help of the data. In most cases, it is not necessary or, in view of measurement errors, meaningful to describe all the details of the measured data. The outputs will vary slightly due to errors. Because the model outputs are part of the equations for the statistical parameter estimates, these parameters must also be subject to uncertainties, and statistical methods are available to compute the variance of parameters.[4] A smooth func-

[4] For the regression model to be stable and statistically valid, the confidence intervals must be smaller (preferably, much smaller) in absolute value than the respective parameter values [20,66]. An unstable model

tion which describes the phenomenon reliably is of much more use in the estimation of physiological performance characteristics than an "exact" representation of the data.

The mathematical input–output relationship is an empirical model, which is computed statistically from clinical measurements or experimental time-series data. For systems evolving in space, the output may also be pictures. This opens the vast field of image processing, basically extending to two-dimensional (2-D) quasi-continuous arrays the viewpoint of one-dimensional (1-D), discrete time-series. The internal characteristics of the system are unknown but amenable to probing and analysis. One applies some appropriately selected input stimulus to the black-box and determines the output response to the specific stimulus. By varying the input and correlating with it the response, one deduces information about the most probable behavior of the box for a given magnitude of stimulus. One then speculates on models of the process that would reproduce, first qualitatively and then quantitatively, such a spectrum of responses. Then one proceeds to design critical tests for discriminating between the initially acceptable models. The classic experimental development of the Frank–Starling law of the heart, discussed in Chapter 3, on pp. 143 ff., and in Chapter 15, on pp. 836 ff., is a prime instance of its application in physiology.

The black-box approach is focused on parameters that can be measured to gain insights into normal and abnormal function from the observed input–output associations. For instance, the continuous biorheologic process of ejection results in a single assessment of a number, a measurable stroke volume (SV); this is merely a global concept that represents the difference between the end-diastolic (EDV) and end-systolic (ESV) chamber volumes. Both the SV and the ejection fraction (EF), derived immediately from it—$EF = \mathrm{SV}/\mathrm{EDV}$—transcend completely possibly crucial "details" of the ejection process that influence SV. One continuous act, the process of ejection, results in a single assessment of SV that depends on two instants in the cycle. However, the imposition of discrete steps on the overall act may reveal a wealth of additional descriptive detail. Having elected an incremental volume element represented by ΔV in a certain time increment Δt, the effective volumetric ejection velocity, or rate of change of chamber volume, is simply the ratio $\Delta V/\Delta t$—but the ratio taken is of *this* incremental volume to *this* time in the course of ejection. There are now as many assessments of speed as there are intervals Δt of time; and of these, there are, in principle, arbitrarily many.[5] An overall average value, the mean ejection flow rate, is obtained as the ratio of SV to ejection time.

Since the ventricle's function is to set the blood in motion, to evaluate its functional characteristics, one needs knowledge of stroke volume but also of the velocities and accelerations in the course of ejection. Looked at from this viewpoint a single ejection time index of ventricular function is almost inconceivable; any single index will give evidence of only one aspect of function related to either blood displacement, velocity, or acceleration. Which of these aspects is most important will depend on the problem at hand and on how subtle the changes evaluated are. The hemodynamic situation is best explained

may yield very inaccurate derivative values and absurd results for even a small range of extrapolation. For an unstable model, a small change in the data (e.g., by adding or removing just one data point) may lead to large changes in the parameter values.

[5]Similar considerations apply for the rate of change of ejection velocity, or volumetric acceleration of outflow.

by an analogy. Suppose that one cylinder of an automobile engine is dead and the problem is to discover the resulting performance defect. Clearly, the information given by the odometer would be useless for this problem, since the car could still be driven over a long distance. Input from the speedometer would probably not reveal the weakness, since the car might still cruise at 65 mph on the freeway. However, knowledge of acceleration will detect the weakness readily, because with one cylinder out, the pickup will certainly be impaired. From these simple considerations, we can expect that ventricular dysfunction (or hyperfunction) will best be revealed by estimates of acceleration during ejection. Since the simple "black-box" approach can readily provide such estimates, it is a useful tactic.

1.3 The glass-box approach

For the glass-box approach [22,63], the differential equations which describe the evolution and spatiotemporal characteristics of the intracardiac flow field are analyzed, using as inputs measurements obtained by emerging sophisticated imaging modalities. Medical imaging had conventionally been viewed as a way of viewing anatomical structures of the body. However, cardiac imaging has seen truly exciting advances in recent years. New imaging methods can now display cardiac anatomy and dynamic flow phenomena, and we can envision emerging important applications to a wide range of diagnostic and therapeutic procedures.

Not only can growing technological advances create new and better ways to extract dynamic information about intracardiac flows, but they also offer the promise of making some existing imaging tools more convenient and economical, thus increasing their clinical and research use. However, while exponential improvements in computing power have contributed to the development of today's biomedical imaging capabilities, they alone do not provide a sufficient springboard to enable the development of truly novel concepts of cardiac physiology and its derangements. That development will require continued training and research in fluid dynamic aspects of cardiac function and associated areas. Afterall, the optimal use of medical imaging and visualization obviously depends on what the user wants to see! Especially in the case of visualization, the questions of users often vary in a significant way. In turn, that depends on their appreciation of the flow phenomena that are there to recognize, understand, and incorporate in an integrated framework of cardiac function. New ideas in the field may well replace other already existing methods; in any event, they enrich the assortment of possible views of patient or experimental animal derived imaging data.

The imaging and numerical investigation of intracardiac flows in the glass-box approach is still at an early stage. However, the physiological, embryological, and clinical importance of this class of flows is not in question. This book has evolved over many years in order to introduce, develop, and integrate concepts and methods from several fields, which underlie a pluridisciplinary approach to intracardiac flow phenomena. It is aimed at context-setting for what the reader will encounter in the literature of intracardiac blood flow; i.e., on providing a mental structure in which to place findings in the biomedical engineering, physiological, and medical literature, as well as his or her own relevant clinical or experimental observations. Most models describing the flow within the human heart are derived from empirical observations in animals and also in human subjects undergoing diagnostic evaluation and follow-up studies. The available measurement techniques are, therefore, important and they have evolved in parallel with an increased understanding of intracardiac flow phenomena. With rapid developments in measurement methods and tools for analyses, we should have all the ingredients to give us new insights into interactive aspects of cardiac function.

Even so, just how do we go about it? Are the paradigms we develop able to use all or most of the information we have available? Needless to say, between the black- and glass-box views, as we defined them here, there exists in actual practice a *continuum* that admits different levels of exposure of any given system's detailed mechanisms and of the equations that govern its dynamic behavior, under any set of operating conditions.

1.4 Intracardiac flow phenomena

The term *phenomenon*[6] denotes an observable event. Phenomena make up the raw data of science in general and fluid dynamics and physiology in particular. One of the more serious hurdles in analyzing the flow of fluids is the bewildering range of phenomena which may occur in seemingly simple flow situations; and how, at times, very small changes in flow parameters produce drastic changes in flow patterns. Thus, when we open a water faucet, water comes out initially in a smooth "transparent" stream and remains so as the flow rate is increased. Then, suddenly, when a critical flow rate is exceeded, the smooth stream breaks up into an irregular one. Clearly, the mathematical models describing the behavior of the water stream in the two cases have to be quite different.

Many flow phenomena can be exploited by technology and medicine. *Intracardiac flow phenomena* refer to flow events and spatiotemporal flow patterns occurring according to biorheological laws, in both health and disease, within the cardiac chambers and the adjoining trunks of the great vessels. They have physiologic, clinical, embryological, and pathological interest, and are susceptible to scientific description and explanation. Their recognition and enhanced understanding, as a result of recent advances in imaging, are conducive to better evaluation of ventricular performance and adaptations, and to improved diagnosis and management of functional abnormalities and failure.

There are degrees to which we can observe and explain flow phenomena and their functional consequences, due to limitations in our knowledge of processes and/or our measurement and modeling methods. It is important to realize that the scale at which we take our measurements will also affect the extent to which we are able to observe and describe spatiotemporal patterns of intracardiac flow phenomena [24, 26, 27, 52, 55]. If we have only a few data points, we are unlikely to identify a meaningful pattern. With just a few measurements, we might he tempted to treat a distribution of intraventricular blood velocities as a random field. We must be confident that the measurements we are interpreting are capturing the nature of the underlying phenomena, and are not simply

[6] Exact transliteration from the Gk.

a function of our sampling extent or density (cf. Fig. 12.23 and the associated discussion on pp. 672 f.). Because we may not be able to sample densely enough to fully define the underlying patterns, we must exploit our understanding of large scale "coherent" (i.e., spatiotemporally correlated) motions and dominant processes and of their manifestations at different scales.

We generally formulate our understanding of processes in the form of models [53, 56, 57], which in turn need measurements for proper testing, and so we have a theme of observations, understanding and modeling linked in an iterative loop. Our models ought to seek enlightenment [52–54, 69], rather than imitation. We might then look for the essence of the intracardiac flow system under study, disregarding all aspects and processes that we think are not absolutely essential. The resulting set of essential processes will then define our model. The object is to reproduce the consequences of what we think are the essentials, and the only thing that can prevent us from achieving this is an inaccurate specification of the physics. What we can hope to get right is the interactions between processes. In the simulation model, this can sometimes get lost in the process of adjusting parameters to make the answer better—a process known as *fine-tuning*. In the enlightenment model one would aim to get the physics right in a parsimonious way, perhaps at the expense of a somewhat lower accuracy.

1.5 Dissipative structures and flow patterns

Nature presents us with countless events and objects that exhibit a high degree of order. They often organize themselves out of disorder and once formed they manifest varying degrees of stability against external and internal disturbances [10, 11]. Self-organizing phenomena are not limited to physiological systems; seasonal weather patterns, fluid flow systems, artistic work, etc., also display comparable characteristics. Physiological science strives to explain how Nature matches form to function at all levels of organization, from subcellular to intact organ-systems, and at the level of the organism as a whole.

Any effort to understand such self-organizing phenomena in a system must begin with understanding that the underlying processes do not happen in a static or quasistatic fashion. Rather, they occur under conditions that keep the system away from equilibrium, and they exhibit a stable order—either temporal, or spatial—instead of proceeding toward an equilibrium state.

In 1952, Alan Turing, a British mathematician and artificial intelligence pioneer, suggested [74] that the competition of chemical reactions and diffusion can bring about a rich variety of pattern forming instabilities (see Section 9.2.1, on p. 445 f.), which give rise to *Turing patterns* [44], so called in his honor. Turing was apparently the first to point out that if diffusion, autocatalysis, and autoinhibition are combined in a set of rate equations for two morphogens, a sinusoidal disturbance with a particular wavelength grows out of thermal noise, thus leading to the spontaneous appearance of an ordered spatial pattern [74]. The outcome of the pattern-generating reaction-diffusion mechanism depends on at least five parameters: initial synthesis rate of the activator, diffusion rates of the activator and of the inhibitor, and degradation rates of the activator and of the inhibitor. Apart from chemical systems, this mechanism is also relevant to pattern forming biological systems, which were Turing's main motivation, since he proposed these phenomena to explain the genesis of such biological patterns as a zebra's stripes. He demonstrated that the characteristic dimensions of the resulting stationary patterns are independent of the characteristic lengths in the system, a feature that is qualitatively different from the case of many hydrodynamic instabilities, for which the characteristic dimensions of the patterns are usually given by the geometry of the set-up. This is, for example, the case for Rayleigh–Bénard convection (see below) and for Taylor vortex flow (see Section 9.5.4, on pp. 463 ff.). Turing pattern-forming chemical reactions can, in turn, induce and interact with fluid motions because of the fluid density dependent gravity effects that they induce, via concentration or temperature gradients that they create. Technical obstacles placed Turing structures virtually beyond experimental reach for nearly four decades following his ground breaking 1952 *Royal Society* paper [74]. Eventually, experimental evidence for the existence of Turing structures, in comparatively simple chemical systems, emerged [14,42,45,51].

The solutions obtained by means of various mathematical and computational techniques will be described in Chapters 2, 4, 9, and 12–14, to many flow phenomena reveal rich features, including self-regulatory and self-organizing processes. In our study of intracardiac flow phenomena, particularly in Chapters 13–16, we will encounter flow events and processes that undergo self-regulatory and self-organizing evolution driven by causal organizing factors. We label such processes "patterns." By closely studying the characteristics of a pattern, we may arrive at a mathematical description of its dynamics.

1.5.1 Dissipative structures

A profound distinction between *equilibrium* and *dissipative* structures was introduced by Glansdorff and Prigogine [25,47]. Equilibrium structures may be formed and maintained through reversible transformations, implying no appreciable deviation from equilibrium. A crystal is a typical example of an equilibrium structure, and macroscopically its state corresponds to a static equilibrium. Dissipative structures, on the other hand, are formed and maintained through effects arising out of the exchange of energy [3], and possibly matter, under nonequilibrium conditions. Dissipative structures are maintained far away from thermodynamic equilibrium by fluxes of energy, and possibly matter. A critical distance from equilibrium, i.e., a minimum level of dissipation, is needed to maintain them [61], and in this situation "specific kinetic laws permit the construction and maintenance of a functional and structural order" [25].

Heat transfer from a wall to the fluid has stability consequences due to changes in buoyancy and, to a secondary extent, in viscosity. A recurring example of instability and an ensuing dissipative structure is that of the Rayleigh–Bénard cells in a thin layer of liquid, enclosed between two plates so that no free air gap forms, and heated slowly from below [4, 6, 38]. For small temperature gradients, i.e., near thermodynamic equilibrium, heat diffusion is sufficient to dissipate the thermal energy supplied, with the

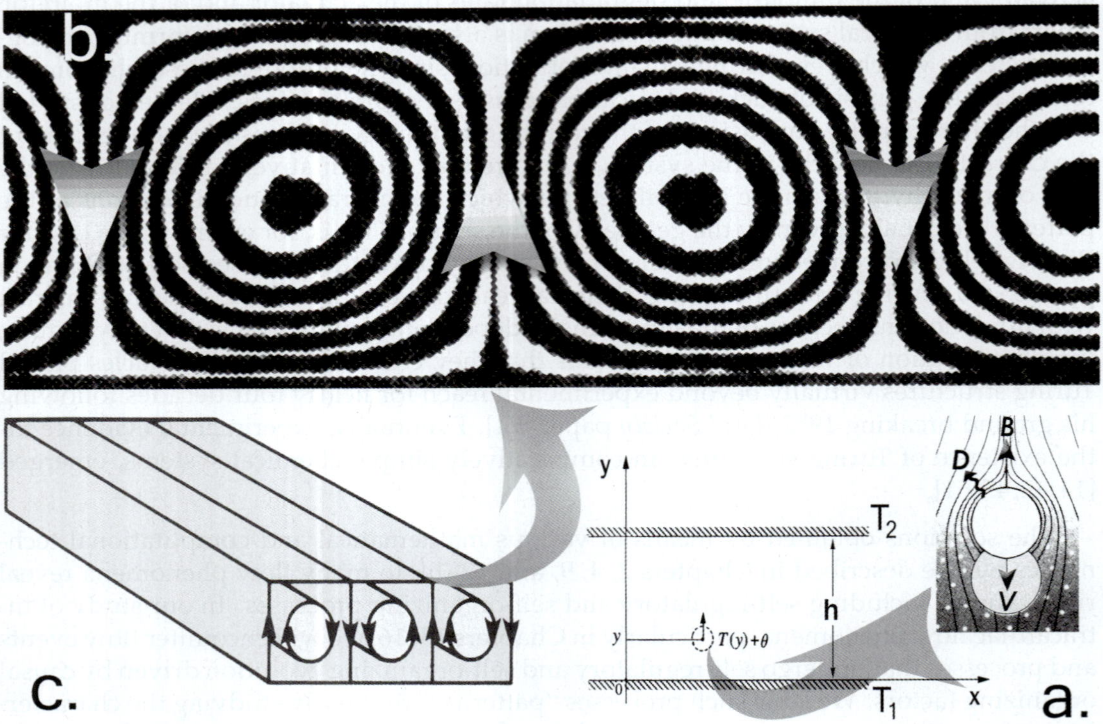

Figure 1.2: a. Rayleigh–Bénard instability in a thin layer of fluid between two flat surfaces heated from below, to produce a gradient of temperature and density ($T_1 > T_2$; $\rho_1 < \rho_2$). If some of the warmer fluid in the lower portion of the layer is displaced toward the upper part, it enters a region of greater density and is subjected to a buoyancy force, B, acting toward the top. B is opposed by a viscous force, V, and by heat diffusion, D, which tends to revert the temperature, $T + \theta$, of the rising particle to the temperature, T, of its surrounding fluid. In the same way, fluid displaced downward from the upper portion of the layer, is denser than the surrounding fluid and tends to descend further toward the bottom. b. Convection begins when B exceeds the dissipative effects of V and D; it gives rise to beautiful dissipative structures; first to the *Rayleigh–Bénard rolls*, shown in panels b. and c., and then—at higher Rayleigh numbers—to hexagonal *Rayleigh–Bénard cells*, and, eventually, turbulence.

liquid remaining macroscopically in a state of rest, albeit in a "top-heavy" arrangement engendered by the "adverse" temperature gradient. The temperature gradient acts as a controlling parameter of the dynamic behavior of the system. When the flow of energy into the liquid is raised, and with it the temperature gradient, the liquid—still below the boiling point—moves away from thermodynamic equilibrium. It becomes increasingly difficult for heat diffusion, by itself, to ensure the dissipation of the thermal energy supplied. Unexpectedly, another channel opens, in competition with the diffusive channel, through which the energy supplied may be dissipated: and abruptly, at the so-called *Rayleigh–Bénard instability*, a macroscopic collective motion is triggered.

A flow produced by such effects is called *buoyant convection*. The hottest parts of the liquid, those closest to the heat source, expand, and because of Archimedes's buoyancy tend to float, moving upward. Here they are cooled down, thus falling again toward the bottom. Thus, a process of heat transport by convection is established by a collective motion of liquid particles that is produced through the kinetic energy developed by the work of the buoyancy forces generated by the gradient. The circulatory movement is slowed down by two stabilizing processes: by heat diffusion, which aims at ironing out the temperature gradient, thus tending to cancel out the density gradient, and by the viscosity of the liquid, which causes any induced buoyant velocities to naturally tend to decay. The liquid layer stays at rest as long as dissipation dominates but convection develops when the destabilization is sufficient. The relative importance of the mutually opposed forces is assessed by the Rayleigh number. Convection begins when the buoyancy force exceeds the dissipative effects of viscous resistance and thermal diffusion, namely, when the Rayleigh number exceeds a critical level. Convection aims at restoring a stable density stratification, with heavy fluid at the bottom. Steady, stable roll-like *Rayleigh–Bénard vortices* are illustrated in Figure 1.2. With further increase of the Rayleigh number the rolls become unstable, and 3-D convection flows come into being. Best-known among the steady, 3-D flow configurations are hexagonal vortex cells—Bénard cells—that give the impression of honey combs when viewed from above in the presence of an appropriate marker, such as aluminum flakes. At still higher Rayleigh numbers, the flow regime becomes turbulent.

1.5.2 Flow patterns

We recognize any self-organizing flow event or phenomenon as a process involving dynamic interaction. The interaction embodies two mutually opposed actions: ordering and disordering effects. We can place the concept of "pattern" in a proper perspective by classifying such self-organizing flow events and observations in terms of the underlying ordering/disordering effects. The nature of interaction depends on the characteristics of the flow process, and energy exchanges and transformations among fluid particles are extremely important in dictating the nature of the evolving pattern. Depending on the relative importance (or strength) of the antagonistic influences, a flow system may—on the basis of a black-box approach (see Fig. 1.3)—be classified into the following three main classes:

(i) *Ordering effect* $\ll$ *Disordering effect*: The flow system eventually ends up in complete randomness, as is exemplified by established *homogeneous isotropic*, or nearly isotropic, *turbulence*, because the overall appearance of the flow seems not to change (in a statistical sense) under translations and rotations.[7] Fluid turbulence is a good example of a homogeneous phenomenon. There are many scales of motion present

[7]The compound term *homogeneous isotropic turbulence* was introduced by Lord Kelvin (1824–1907), in 1887 [23,37]—see also discussion and pertinent footnote on p. 125.

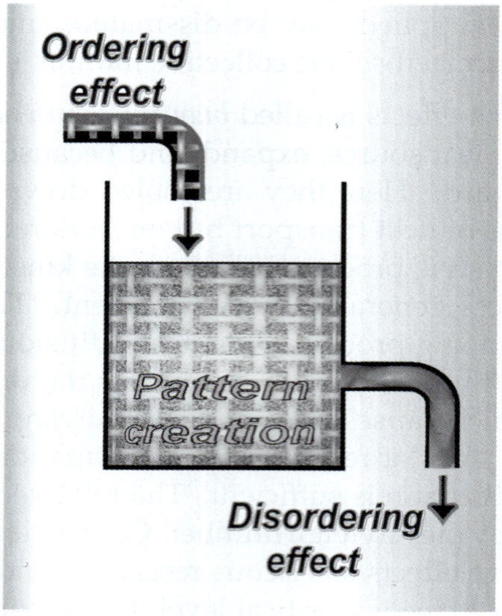

Figure 1.3: Tank black-box model of the generation of a dynamic coherent flow pattern. The tank level is determined by the applying rates of input and output, which correspond to ordering and disordering effects. This may be expressed in terms of a difference between "gain" and "loss"; that is, between an external destabilizing action and the system's dissipative reaction that tends to maintain it in the status quo. When the destabilizing action wins out, the critical fluctuation associated with one of the system's collective variables, instead of regressing, emerges as the order parameter, and the system organizes itself, quite abruptly, into a pattern according to a new structure.

at the same time and in the same region of space: the small scales of motion are embedded in the larger-scale eddies. On the other hand, a flow is inhomogeneous and exhibits discernible features and patterns if the different phenomena of interest are widely separated in space, or time.

(ii) *Ordering effect* $\approx$ *Disordering effect*: Order and disorder coexist heterogeneously, as exemplified by intermittent turbulence. *Intermittency* is a situation in which flow, usually considered turbulent globally, manifests several identifiably different and distinct states. Each of the states has a statistical probability of existing in a particular region of the flow field, but there is no predictable time of recurrence. An example of intermittency is an overall laminar flow with finite-sized turbulent "patches" convected along with it. The existence of intermittency indicates the presence of relatively narrow interfaces separating regions of fluid having distinctly different properties. Usually the system displaying intermittent turbulence is very sensitive to an additional disturbance—ordering or disordering. In some cases, a "disturbance" may then drive the system to either uniform order (laminar flow) or uniform disorder (established turbulence).

(iii) *Ordering effect* $\gg$ *Disordering effect*: The flowing fluid particles are set in formation by an ordering effect, as exemplified by large-scale coherent vortical motions. As a

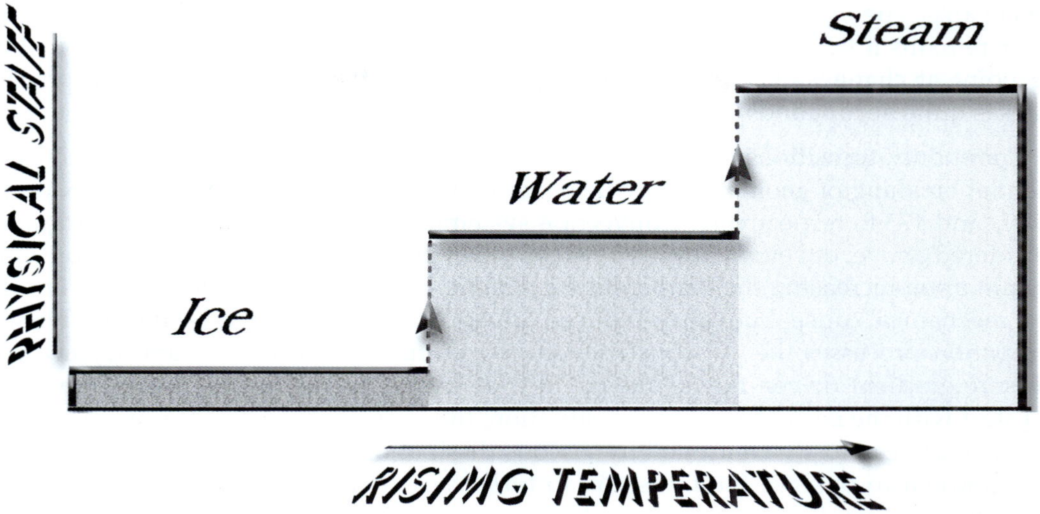

Figure 1.4: The chemical compound H_2O can exhibit not merely quantitative property changes, but also striking *qualitatively different* physical states as its temperature rises. This behavior displays a wonderfully nonlinear character, shifting *abruptly* from a solid to a liquid, and shifting *abruptly again* from a liquid to a gas.

result, the system exhibits a characteristic order, structurally and functionally, as a collective feature of the flow field. Such collective features can be very stable against disturbances, as long as the disturbances are not very strong. We characterize them as "flow patterns."[8]

It should be especially noted that the appearance and evolution of flow patterns are usually neither gradual nor continuous; rather, they come about abruptly once certain threshold values of flow-regime governing parameters are attained, or exceeded. A familiar example of this sort of nonlinear, abrupt, and striking transition patterns is found in the behavior of H_2O as a function of temperature (see Fig. 1.4).

At low temperatures, H_2O exhibits properties[9] of a crystallized solid, ice. Up to a point, increasing temperature has very little effect on this crystalline physical state. H_2O remains crystallized and solid. As temperature continues to rise, however, there is an abrupt and unexpected dramatic *qualitative change*. Ice becomes a liquid. This change is nonlinear. If the temperature is below the melting point, ice remains ice. If the temperature is held at the melting point, however, all the ice becomes water—not instantaneously, but without any further rise in temperature. Continuing to increase the temperature changes the behavior of this liquid very little, for another extensive range on the temperature

[8] In specific flow situations that we will examine in subsequent chapters, we have made an attempt at extracting laws that govern the characteristic behavior and the dynamics of such patterns.

[9] A property of a substance or a system is any observable characteristic of the substance or system. The properties of a substance or system characterize its state.

dimension. The water molecules move around more as they absorb heat, but the hot water remains a liquid up to another critical temperature. When H_2O reaches its boiling point, it changes character again, to a gas. Again the transition between physical states is quite abrupt and *qualitative*, rather than merely quantitative.

Commonly, transitions into different successive flow patterns are accompanied by sequential breaking of geometric flow-field symmetries—see Sections 9.5.4 and 9.6, on pp. 463 ff. and 473 f., respectively. Convection systems, such as the Rayleigh–Bénard model considered above, develop patterns by steps when progressively driven away from equilibrium upon increasing the temperature gradient. The physical problem is clearly ruled by a mechanical cause, buoyancy-induced advection[10], counteracted by thermodynamic dissipation processes, i.e., viscous friction and thermal diffusion. When dealing with pressure gradient driven flows, one could thus try to stay within the same framework and start with the *no-flow* equilibrium situation, then consider weakly out-of-equilibrium *laminar* regimes mostly controlled by viscous dissipation, and further increase the pressure gradient to observe the transition to *turbulence* after some cascade of instabilities. This approach can indeed be followed in some cases [44] but, in most strong pressure gradient flows, mechanical evolution largely preempts the relaxation trends of thermodynamic origin.

1.6 The continuum assumption

People have tried to understand space, time, motion, and the notion of "continuum" for thousands of years. This pursuit lead the Pythagoreans to the discovery of irrational numbers, to Zeno's paradoxes, to infinitesimal calculus, and many more intriguing ideas. What do we mean when we say "continuum?" Here is a description that was given by Albert Einstein [39]: "The surface of a marble table is spread out in front of me. I can get from any one point on this table to any other point by passing continuously from one point to a 'neighboring' one, and repeating this process a (large) number of times, or, in other words, by going from point to point without executing 'jumps.' I am sure the reader will appreciate with sufficient clearness what I mean here by 'neighbouring' and by 'jumps' (if he is not too pedantic). We express this property of the surface by describing the latter as a continuum."

The flow-governing equations arise in describing the flow characteristics of an infinitesimal fluid element using such a continuum assumption [15]. Imagine that we take a fluid sample volume large enough to include a sufficient number of constituents of a fluid medium so that it accurately represents the macroscopic density of the fluid within a flow region of interest. We call this sample volume a fluid parcel. The parcel must contain enough constituents of the fluid medium at hand to represent the average characteristics of the fluid at the center point of the parcel; at the same time, it must be small enough so that a parcel taken contiguous to it will have properties differing by only a small amount from the other parcel. Therefore, when modeling a fluid as a continuum,

[10]We use the terms advection/convection interchangeably to denote the macroscopic transport (or movement) of a fluid and its properties by the fluid's organized velocity field.

the averaging parcel size should be much smaller than the smallest length scales in which we are interested, so that we can consider the averaging parcel to be a "point."

If we consider the smallest parcel of a fluid having the gross properties of the fluid to be a material point, the properties of interest vary gradually from point to point in the fluid, as though the fluid were a continuum. Material lines, surfaces, and volumes are composed of material points. The preceding formulation is the *continuum* concept. Treating a fluid, including blood in intracardiac flow studies, as a continuum allows the use of very powerful tools, and it is therefore a very important concept. Once we assume that the fluid itself is continuous in its properties, we may describe these properties with continuous functions and apply differential equations in the analysis of flow processes. This allows us to utilize the rather considerable stock of mathematical tools involving continuous mathematical functions in its entirety in both the description and solution of fluids problems.

In particular, the continuum assumption of the Navier–Stokes equations, which govern flow of viscous fluids, is valid provided that the mean free path of the molecules is negligible compared to the characteristic dimensions of the problem, i.e., of the flow region in which the fluid is contained—a condition which requires a very high frequency of molecular collisions with the wall. If this condition is not sufficiently met, the fluid will not be under local thermodynamic equilibrium and the linear relationship between shear stress and rate of shear strain (Newton's law of viscosity, see Section 4.6, on pp. 190 f.) cannot be applied. Velocity profiles, boundary wall shear stresses, mass flow rates and pressure differences will then be influenced by noncontinuum effects, such as those applying in the study of rarefied gas dynamics [5].[11] Moreover, the conventional "no-slip" boundary condition imposed at a solid–fluid interface will begin to break down even before the linear stress-rate of shear strain relationship becomes invalid.

1.7 Properties of fluid media

We distinguish fluid media from solids based on their response to an applied static shear force [6]. If, e.g., we subject a solid bar to a torque, it twists. The restoring elastic stresses within a solid (below the yield limit) are proportional to the strains, and therefore, when subjected to the shear force of a torque, a solid distorts through a specific angle (equilibrium distortion) such that it develops internal stresses that just balance the applied torque. The magnitude of the distortion angle generally depends on the applied torque as well as on the elastic properties of the solid. When the torque is removed, the solid regains its prior configuration.

If, on the other hand, the torque is applied to a fluid, the behavior is entirely different. The fluid does not acquire an equilibrium distortion but continues to deform for as long as the torque acts [6]. We make use of this behavior to define a fluid. Thus, a fluid is a

[11] There are microscopic (molecular) models that recognize the particulate structure of the rarefied gas as a myriad of discrete molecules and provide information for the position, velocity, and state of every molecule at any instant.

medium that cannot be in equilibrium under the action of any shear force, no matter how small. Although a fluid does not resist a shear force by acquiring an equilibrium deformation, nonetheless it exhibits an equilibrium *velocity*. This equilibrium value increases with the applied shear force. This suggests that a fluid does resist a shear force, not by acquiring an equilibrium deformation but by acquiring an equilibrium rate of deformation. Thus, a fluid deforms continuously under the action of a shear force, but at a finite rate determined by the applied shear force and the fluid properties. When the torque is removed, the velocity of the fluid medium drops back to zero but it does not regain its prior configuration.

Clearly, the constitutive equations for fluids are markedly different from those for solids. There are substances, so-called "elastico-viscous fluids" or "visco-elastic solids," such as recently coagulated blood and mucous, which display behaviors intermediate between those characterizing solid and fluid media.

1.8 What is fluid flow?

In this Section, we define more precisely what we mean by "fluid flow," a phrase that we have been using and will be using repeatedly, and we consider how a fluid flow is like and unlike solid particle dynamics. In fact, the dynamics of fluid flows that we will consider in the succeeding chapters are straightforward applications of classical physics, built upon the familiar conservation laws [28, 52]—conservation of mass, linear and angular momentum, and energy, which will be developed in Chapters 2, 4 and 9. In this regard, the physics of fluid flow are no different from the physics of solid particle mechanics.

Consider a collection of an arbitrarily large number of solid particles as "point masses" moving under the influence of internal and external forces. We could conceive such point masses to make up an extended fluid medium. However, there are important differences. A fluid particle is in a literal sense pushed and pulled around by its surroundings (other fluid particles, or the flow-field boundaries) in a way that solid particles may not be. At the same time, a fluid particle may be quite dramatically stretched and strained and may become so intermingled with its fluid surroundings as to effectively lose its identity. It is this complete and intimate interaction between a fluid particle and its surroundings that characterizes fluid flows and that distinguishes fluid dynamics from solid particle dynamics. Thus, in a fluid mechanics problem, we have to solve for the fluid motion of the entire fluid domain at once; we generally cannot understand or predict the motion of one fluid parcel without understanding the overall fluid motion, i.e., obtaining the solution, over the entire flow domain.

For even the simplest problems, this often will be a huge task that can be approached in full only with the aid of a powerful computer, which is carefully programmed to follow the laws governing fluid motion. The systems of equations governing the evolution of intracardiac flow are nonlinear and are solved using numerical methods, which reflect the spatiotemporal scale of the underlying flow phenomena. The *rapid upstrokes* in

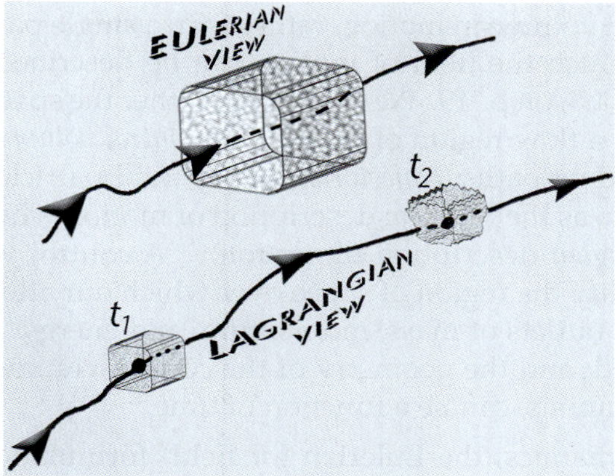

Figure 1.5: When we consider a continuous system such as the motion of blood in the heart we have a choice in the way that we set up the analysis. One option is to consider every quantity at a fixed location in space, and to specify how these quantities change with time. In that case the change of the properties with time is described by the partial time derivative $\partial/\partial t$. This is called an *Eulerian* description. As an alternative we may follow a certain property as it is being carried around by the flow. In that case, the change of this property with time is given by the *total* time derivative D/Dt (see Section 2.13, on pp. 65 f.). This is called a *Lagrangian* description. Which description is most convenient depends on the problem.

the normal ventricular ejection or early inflow (E-wave) waveforms produce large time derivatives of flow velocity (local acceleration), which require representation of the solution at high temporal resolution. Moreover, the *high spatial gradients* in flow velocity (convective acceleration) near the outflow and inflow valve orifices during ejection and rapid filling, similarly require representation of the solution at a high spatial resolution.

Approximate solutions of fluid flow often yield crucial insights, and many widely used techniques of applied mathematics were, in fact, developed to make useful approximate solutions of fluid flow. A convenient approach is to find solutions to simplified approximations to the flow situation under investigation, which are subsequently tested by comparisons with laboratory experiments and animal and clinical measurements. Although we discard a lot of detail in these simplified models, the combination of the variables in the resulting equations remains correct, and we can get approximate solutions that tell us how each variable depends on the others. They will not always be absolutely accurate, and sometimes we will have to conduct experiments to obtain one or two coefficients, but we can go a long way with this approach. One obvious point in favor of such an approximate analysis is that in intracardiac flows we do not know the "exact" values of all the variables anyway, so there is already a limit to how accurate we can be.

The challenges of intracardiac fluid dynamics stem mainly from the very complex three-dimensional (3-D) and highly time-dependent kinematics typifying intracardiac flow. By fluid flow, we mean the motion of fluid material throughout the entirety of the 3-D space defined by the walls of the flow domain. The phrase 'fluid flow' conjures up the mental image of the entire fluid volume in motion, rather than a single particle in isolation. There are two methods by which the field of motion can be described, which are pictorially distinguished in Figure 1.5, on p. 19. We can specify either the spatiotemporal distribution of the velocity through a flow region of interest, or *control volume*; or, we can specify the space- and time-dependent paths (*trajectories*) of the fluid particles within the flow field. The former is referred to as the *Eulerian* description of motion while the latter is endowed with the title of *Lagrangian* description of motion.[12] A control volume is an imaginary boundary used to identify the region of space over which our attention is focused, and to locate all the inlets and outlets of mass, momentum, and energy. In a control volume, all quantities are conserved, and the geometry of the control volume, on which we apply a set of conservation equations, can be a function of time.

In classical fluid dynamics, the Eulerian (or field) formulation is preferred because it is difficult to follow a fluid particle (which cannot be differentiated visually from its neighbors), and also because measurements are easier made at fixed locations. In contrast to this, the Lagrangian approach is usually preferred in the description of moving solids as, for example, in describing the motion of a projectile. Thus, if the fluid is in motion, a point fixed in space is occupied by different fluid particles at different instants of time. The time rate of change of a flow-field variable, which is measured by a sensor stationed at a fixed location, therefore, does not give the total rate of change of the variable "experienced" by any fluid particle. To measure this rate the sensor would have to, somehow, move with the fluid. The rates of change measured by probes at fixed locations represent the local rates of change as opposed to the total rates of change experienced by a flowing fluid particle. We denote the latter as the *material* or *substantial* rates of change.

The basic physical laws applicable in fluid mechanics are the same as those in the mechanics of solids. Newton's second law of motion is, indeed, applicable to any class of matter, irrespective of its physical state, representing as it does, equality between the rate of change of momentum and the forces acting on a body. When Newton's law is applied to fluids, the appropriate rate of change of momentum is the material or substantial rate of change and not the local one. This is so because the rate of change envisaged in Newton's law refers to a specific body of matter. Similarly, the principle of conservation of mass also applies to both solids and fluids, though in solid mechanics one is rarely, if ever, called upon to use it explicitly, unless the body is breaking up, or different parts are coalescing to form a composite body during motion or deformation. In the study of fluids, on the other hand, the principle of conservation of mass is used as an essential analytic aid because a distinct body of matter is not that readily identifiable.

1.9 Flow-mediated interactions of form and function

Cardiology has always been an integrative field, concerned as it is with elucidating how the *structure and function*[13] of myocardial cells and tissues explain quantitatively the com-

[12]It is believed however that Euler is actually responsible for both approaches [40].

[13]The philosophy based on the precept that form and function are intimately linked was developed by Aristotle. In modern times, it was pivotal in the work of the great French comparative anatomist Georges

plex behavior of the heart and its adaptations in health and disease. Today, there is an explosion of information obtained from the numerous imaging modalities currently used for clinical diagnosis (MRI, ultrafast CT, real-time 3-D echocardiography and Doppler color flow mapping, etc.). Parallel to it, is the burgeoning accumulation of data at the subcellular and molecular biology level that are difficult to interpret in relation to the function of the intact body and its organs, including the heart.

A surprise that emerged from the full sequence of the human genome in recent years is that humans possess a relatively small complement of roughly 30,000–40,000 protein-coding genes—barely twice the number for a worm or a fruit fly [75,76]. In fact, in humans, only about 15,000 are ever "expressed," that is, called upon to make something [29]. This presents us with a puzzle: how can we possibly be made with relatively such a limited amount of genetic information. Clearly, the genetic blueprints cannot specify all details of the assembly throughout our development and life. In view of these recent discoveries, it appears that the increased intricacy in the machinery that controls gene expression is an important reason why humans are more complex than "lowly" creatures, such as worms and flies.

The human body has 256 different kinds of cells, and it is inside those cells that the proteins are manufactured in response to some set of instructions or restrictions. What happens is a lot of local adjustment and adaptive self-organization, in which "environmental" factors enter into play [12]. Importantly, human genes can give rise to many related proteins, each potentially capable of performing a different function in our bodies, depending, in part, on "environmental" factors.[14]

The heart integrates structure and function across multiple spatial scales [33, 48, 70]. Great challenges revolve around developing the means of linking models across the spatial scales. A unique characteristic of myocardium is its ability to grow and remodel in response to changing environments; this is determined partly by genes and partly by the physical environment [18, 59]. There is emerging a need to ascertain not only the physiological functions of myocardial genes and proteins but also their endocardium-mediated modulations by mechanical "environmental factors." Mechanical stresses [31], or lack thereof, may act as important epigenetic factors[15] in cardiovascular development, adaptation, and disease. Different levels of mechanical factors such as strain, or fluid shear stress, or pressure may initiate or modulate signal transduction cascades and other cellular processes that underlie cardiac adaptations, remodeling, and transition to pathology, which may be reversible.

All cardiovascular diseases with aberrant growth and remodeling may be in the class of diseases with a mechanical etiology. This is so because it is now evident that local me-

Cuvier (1769–1832). It also has clear ties to the Natural Theology of the British naturalists of the nineteenth century, which argued that God had created a universe in which nature revealed its rules through its structures [1].

[14] A conservative estimate is that 30,000 human genes may produce up to *ten times* as many proteins in the human body.

[15] *Epigenetic factors* are genetic modifiers that influence cell behavior; examples include environmental effects and chemical modifications. Unlike mutations, epigenetic modifications of DNA are *potentially reversible* molecular events that cause changes in gene expression.

chanical stimuli are major controllers of growth and remodeling in cardiovascular tissues. In the vasculature, it appears that perturbed loading conditions heighten the turnover of cells (proliferation and apoptosis[16]) and matrix (synthesis and degradation), thus resulting in altered geometries, properties, and biologic function [32]. Just as comparable mechanisms appear to be operative in hypertension, aneurysms, and microgravity induced changes [50], it is likely that they are operative in cardiac disease too.

1.9.1 Murray's law

Consider blood flow in vessels: changes in blood flow elicit both acute and long-term compensatory responses that ultimately result in normalization of wall shear stress. In the short term, to quickly accommodate changes in blood flow, vessels either dilate or constrict, usually due to the local release of vasoactive peptides, including 'endothelial-derived relaxing factor,' whose discovery led eventually to the development of Viagra. In the case of *persistent* increases or decreases in flow, however, a different process evolves that includes adaptive remodeling of the vessel wall, characterized by the reorganization of cellular and extracellular components. Indeed, clinical findings imply that chronic changes in blood flow rates through large arteries induce corresponding adjustments of artery diameter; thus, vessels exposed to elevated flow, such as arteries feeding an arteriovenous fistula, or collateral vessels after arterial occlusion, tend to enlarge.

"Environmental" forces acting on a vessel due to blood flow can be resolved into two principal directions. One is perpendicular to the wall and represents intraluminal blood pressure; the other acts parallel to the wall to create a frictional force, and a corresponding shear stress, at the surface of the endothelium. In 1926, Murray presented his theory of optimal cardiovascular design, considering progressive vascular branching from the aorta to the arterioles and from the venules to the venae cavae. It determined the optimal sizes of blood vessels, based on principles of minimum power expenditure and constant wall shear stress in the vascular network, for a fixed investment in blood and vessel volume. Under ideal conditions, and if the volumetric flow rate of the blood is conserved within the vascular system and the flow is laminar, the optimal design was found to equalize the sum of all radii cubed across all branchings along the flow path. This result is "Murray's law" [46].

Where this law is obeyed, a functional relationship exists between the vessel radius and the volumetric flow rate ($\propto r^3$), the average and maximum linear velocities of flow ($\propto r$) and the velocity profile, the mean wall shear stress, which is constant ($\propto r^0$) throughout an optimum vascular system, the mean Reynolds number ($\propto r^2$), and the mean pressure gra-

[16] *Apoptosis* is a form of programmed cell death in multicellular organisms [41]. It involves a series of biochemical events leading to a characteristic cell morphology and death. In contrast to *necrosis*, which is a form of traumatic cell death resulting from acute cellular injury, apoptosis confers advantages during an organism's development and life cycle; e.g., the differentiation of fingers and toes in a developing human embryo comes about because cells between the fingers apoptose, bringing about digit separation. Between 50 billion and 70 billion cells die each day due to apoptosis in the average human adult; intensified apoptotic processes cause hypotrophy, such as in *ischemic damage*, whereas an impaired apoptosis results in excessive cell proliferation.

dient in individual vessels ($\propto r^{-1}$). In homogeneous, full-flow sets of vessels, approximate relationships can also be established [68] between the vessel radius and the conductance, the resistance, and the cross-sectional area of a set of vessels (family of components *in parallel*). The enhanced wall shear stress associated with an increased blood flow correlates with an *up-regulation*[17] of the production of nitric oxide, which is a powerful vasodilator that allows constituents within the arterial wall to turnover in a dilated state, thereby increasing the size of the lumen [31]. Similar mechanically stimulated developmental processes are operative in most other tissues.

Conversely, it has been found that if flow is experimentally reduced (increased) in a blood vessel, the inside diameter of the vessel decreases (increases) until it stabilizes at a new and "appropriate" size. These adjustments in diameter are just about what one would expect if the system were rearranging itself to keep the mean shear stress at the wall unchanged [60, 77]. It appears that the endothelial cells lining the blood vessels can quite literally sense changes in the mean shear stress, and thus the frictional forces exerted by the flowing blood on their surface. An increase in the mean flow rate through a vessel increases the velocity gradient and the shear at its walls. An increase in shear stress stimulates cell division, which would increase vessel diameter as appropriate to offset the faster flow velocity; this entails a direct effect of the flow shear on the synthesis of some intermediating chemical signal by the endothelial cells. Because of Murray's Law, endothelial cells can be given the same specific instruction wherever they might be located, a command initiating self-adjusting changes in vessel size when the flow velocity, and thus the mean shear stress, exceeds a specific value.

1.10 The morphogenetic role of endothelial fluid shear

Many receptors, present on the surface of endothelial cells, allow vessels to detect subtle changes in their physical environment, rendering them capable of a true autonomic regulation, which enables them to adapt to their mechanical environment. Moreover, inside the vascular cells, cytoskeletal proteins transmit and modulate mechanical forces. In addition to structural modifications, such forces may induce changes in the ionic composition of the cells, mediated by membrane ion channels, may stimulate various membrane receptors, and may induce complex biochemical cascades.

Blood vessels have *autocrine* and *paracrine* hormonal mechanisms[18] enabling them to respond immediately to local hemodynamic changes involving not only tangential stretch, which rises with distending pressure, but also shear stress, which increases in

[17] An *up-regulation* is an increase in the usual intensity of response associated with exposure of a cellular receptor to the same concentration of agonist agent; it can result from an increase in the *density* or the *absolute number* of a particular receptor.

[18] *Autocrine* signaling is a form of signaling in which a cell secretes a chemical messenger, the autocrine agent, that signals the same cell. *Paracrine* signaling is a form of cell signaling in which the target cell is *close to* (the Gk. word $\pi\alpha\rho\alpha$ = *para* conveys the meaning of "alongside of" or "next to") the signal releasing cell; for diverse possible reasons the signal chemical is not carried to other parts of the body—e.g., it is broken down too quickly.

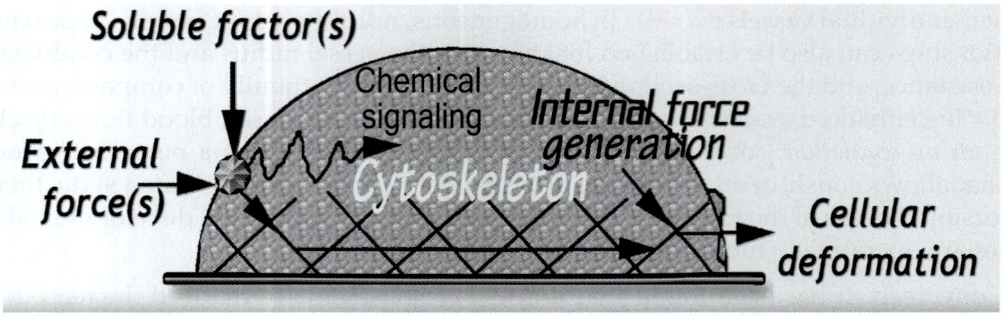

Figure 1.6: Schematic drawing of different factors influencing cell morphology. Both externally imposed forces (e.g., blood pressure, hydrodynamic shear stress, tensile and compressive stresses) and soluble substances can be transduced into cellular shape changes, through two cooperating pathways: *direct mechanical action* on the cell structure, intermediated by a spatial reorganization of the *cytoskeleton* [64], which comprises, e.g., actin microfilaments and microtubules, and *chemical signalling* which then can stimulate mechanisms of internal force generation.

intensity with flow velocity. Vascular tone is modified to compensate almost immediately for the changes and, ordinarily, this efficiently restores mechanical forces to normal levels. Sometimes, the variations in vasomotor tone do not suffice to compensate, and the gene expression, or *phenotype*, of the vascular cells is altered, causing local adaptive adjustments, which also tend to restore mechanical forces to physiological levels. Many intracellular mechanotransduction cascades are activated by flow-induced shear and initiate, via sequential phosphorylation pathways, the activation of transcription factors and subsequent gene expression. Vascular *remodeling* ensues.

The forces acting on the endothelial cells by the flowing blood, i.e., the fluid shear stress, are much weaker in magnitude than the wall stresses resisting the transmural pressure, but are powerful determinants of vascular diameter. Moreover, they can have important morphogenetic actions. Shear stress as a molding force was recognized over a century ago; the embryologist Thoma described the relationship between the diameter of an artery and its blood flow velocity [71]. Any sustained deviation from that relationship initiates processes of either growth or atrophy. Consider, for instance, occlusion of an artery causing the pressure distal to the lesion and in the interconnecting *in-parallel* vascular network to fall. A pressure gradient between the vascular regions that lie proximal and distal to the occlusion then develops. This augments the blood flow in the interconnecting vessels, and consequently, the endothelial fluid shear stress, which is linearly related to the velocity of flow but inversely related to the cube of the radius. As the endothelial fluid shear stress triggers vascular growth, it falls again in step with the larger radius, and the remodeling stops. This is probably the reason why collaterals are normally never as good as the artery which they have replaced.

Kamiya and Togawa [34] studied the remodeling of the dog carotid artery in response to increased flow produced by carotid to jugular anastomosis; they showed that the flow-loaded artery adapted completely by enlarging to the point where wall shear stress returned to physiological baseline values of about 15 dyn/cm^2. Similarly, Tronc et al. [73] found that wall shear stress levels in flow-loaded carotid arteries were abnormally high three days after an arteriovenous fistula but then decreased as the vessels remodeled, such that after 15 days they were no longer significantly different from their baseline values. There are numerous reports demonstrating the important morphogenetic power of fluid shear stress on arteries in experimental animals, but clinical application is difficult. An "experiment of nature" is the Bland–White–Garland syndrome, where one of the coronary arteries originates from the pulmonary artery [8]. This leads to ischemia after birth because one coronary artery operates under a low pressure and carries venous blood. Furthermore, collaterals between the right and left coronary artery are formed, which first alleviates ischemia but later creates a left-to-right shunt from the high pressure aorta via coronary artery and collaterals to the low pressure pulmonary artery. This results in ongoing growth of the collaterals and to more shunt flow, a vicious circle that leads again to ischemia and pulmonary hypertension. Above all, it shows the power of fluid shear stress as a morphogenetic factor.

In the clinical management of arterial flow insufficiency one should try to increase flow, which can be done with exercise (an accepted treatment in peripheral artery disease) or with drugs. However, vasodilatory drugs are not very specific and may cause hypotension, thereby reducing the fluid shear stress. Arteriovenous shunts applied to renal patients for hemodialysis usually lead to growth of the artery, and may require repeated operations. There is reason to expect that such adaptations to "external" (endocardial) shear forces associated with intracardiac flow phenomena [58] may be important in cardiac remodeling.

The preceding idea is in harmony with insightful concepts formulated by D'Arcy Wentworth Thompson (1860–1948), the Scottish zoologist, biomathematician and Greek scholar, who translated Aristotle's biological works, and authored *A glossary of Greek birds* and *A glossary of Greek fishes.* His masterwork, *On Growth and Form* [72], is a profound study of the shapes of living beings, elaborated based on the premise that "the form of an object is a 'diagram of forces,' and from it we can judge or deduce the forces that are acting, or have acted, upon it." Thompson thought of his fundamental physical forces as rivals of natural selection, because they are inescapable and immutable over time.

Since the first studies by Dewey et al. [17], examining the realignment of endothelial cells and their actin filaments caused by fluid shear, a host of other responses have been investigated, including the intracellular release of Ca^{++} ions and a variety of second messengers, and the shear-induced activation of various membrane receptor proteins. Because of the smallness of tissues and organs in the embryo and fetus and the rapidity of successive changes in their structure, function, and properties, there has been much more limited consideration of flow shear effects during development compared with studies during adulthood and aging. Fortunately, however, technological advances are nowadays allowing this important aspect of biofluid dynamics to be studied experimentally in animals. The need for such research is great. Recently, there has been a heightened interest in the relationships between blood flow and cardiac embryology and morphogenetic development. Evidence has been accumulating [30] that the creation of a normal heart involves intricate interactions between a genetic program, mechanical stimuli, and the cellular processes that link them, but the influence of factors such as blood flow [13] on heart development has been unclear. Capturing these structure–function relationships is an emerging challenge in clinical and investigative cardiology and basic research (cf. Fig. 1.6, on p. 24, and Chapter 15). In particular, the need to understand the role of fluid shear stress in endothelial cell function has led to a major new area of research of the cellular response to shear. In a common experimental approach, endothelial monolayers are grown in tissue culture and then put in flow chambers where their reaction to variable fluid shear levels and patterns can be examined under carefully controlled conditions. Interestingly, several gene products, whose expression and activation are influenced by flow in such cultured endothelial cell preparations, are also necessary for embryonic cardiac development [49,67]. As we will discuss in Chapter 15, emerging research challenges encompass linking physiological pre- and postnatal intracardiac blood flow phenomena to cognate medical science theory, relating to comparative physiology and embryology. At this juncture, it suffices to note that, during early embryonic development, reducing the shear stress that is normally exerted by the flowing blood on endothelial and adjacent cells causes the growing heart to develop abnormally.

Hove and his coworkers showed that intracardiac fluid forces are indeed essential for normal heart looping and for chamber and valve development in early embryonic stages [30]. In their elegant studies in zebrafish embryos, embryos with impaired cardiac flow demonstrated three dramatic phenotypes: first, their hearts did not form the bulbus cordis; secondly, they lacked heart looping, the normal process resulting in the repositioning of the ventricle and atrium from a cephalo-caudal into a side-by-side arrangement; finally, the walls of the inflow and outflow tracts collapsed and fused. Laminar and disturbed flows produce different shear stress patterns that, in turn, should have disparate effects on endothelial cells. Oscillatory shear stresses [52] induced by vortical motions [58] correlate with augmented cell proliferation [16]. Both the magnitude of shear stress and local fluctuations in shear stress may be important mechanosensory signals [16]. Such studies support the paradigm that alteration in fluid dynamic loading is a mechanism that can induce changes in cardiac function and structure. Evolving understanding of genetic factors relating to blood flow in the developing heart could eventually be used in early surgical correction of, or even genetic intervention in, prenatal heart disease. Moreover, the same responses to shear forces that normally shape the developing heart may also contribute to later abnormalities and disease processes.

1.11 Optimal use of medical imaging and flow visualization data

The ever-increasing power of imaging and instrumentation technologies and computers [2], enabling the generation and processing of vast amounts of diagnostic data, also creates the need for techniques that facilitate the visualization, analysis, and interpretation of

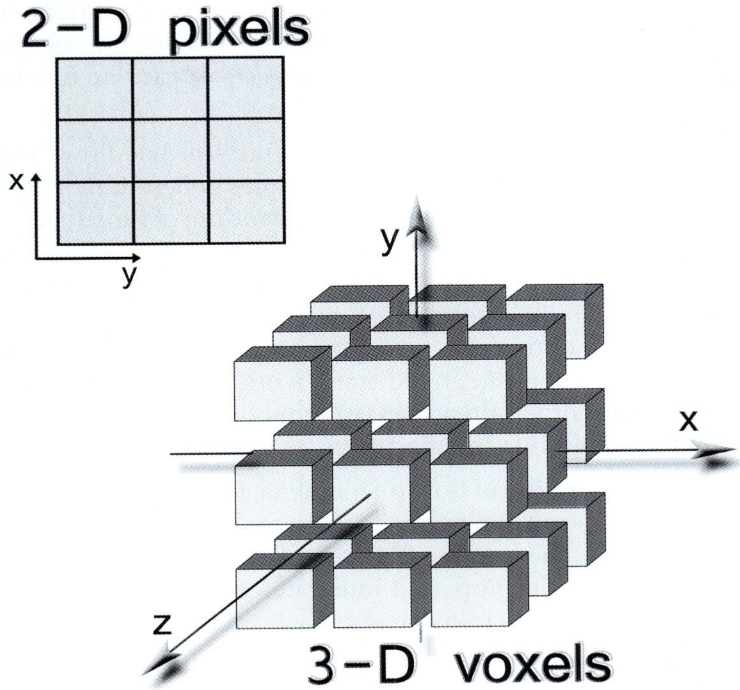

Figure 1.7: Individual picture elements or "pixels" of a 2-D matrix make up each digital 2-D image; individual volume elements or "voxels" of a 3-D matrix make up each digital 3-D image—here, individual voxels are shown separated from their neighbors, for better definition.

that data.[19] More and more, that imperative is being effectively answered by using the capability of computers to present data in graphical form. Medical imaging, which is discussed at length in Chapters 5, 10, and 11, had conventionally been viewed as a way of viewing anatomical structures of the body, in both 2-D and 3-D representations (see Fig. 1.7). However, cardiac imaging has seen truly exciting advances in recent years [19, 65]. New imaging methods can now display cardiac anatomy and dynamic flow phenomena, and we can envision emerging important applications to a wide range of diagnostic and therapeutic procedures.

Not only can growing technological advances create new and better ways to extract dynamic information about intracardiac flows, but they also offer the promise of making some existing imaging tools more convenient and economical, thus increasing their clinical and research use. However, while exponential improvements in computing power have contributed to the development of today's biomedical imaging capabilities, they

[19] *Scientific visualization* in this book means the application of graphic representations and supporting techniques that facilitate the visual communication of knowledge—that make computer images speak to us. *Visualization* means the bringing out and *seeing* of meaning in data. *Data* means any form of number created by or input to a computer.

alone do not provide a sufficient springboard to enable the development of truly novel concepts of cardiac physiology and its derangements. That development will require continued training and research in fluid dynamic aspects of cardiac function and in associated areas of applied mathematics.

Linking a knowledge of the fluid dynamics of intracardiac flows with a knowledge of medical imaging and scientific visualization enables generation of meaningful images and their insightful interpretation, fostering understanding of functional–structural correlations of physiologic and pathophysiologic interest. Afterall, the optimal use of medical imaging and visualization obviously depends on what the user wants to see! Especially in the case of visualization, the questions of users often vary in a significant way. That depends on their appreciation of the flow phenomena that are there to recognize, understand and incorporate in an integrated framework of cardiac function. New ideas in the field may well replace other already existing methods; in any event, they enrich the assortment of possible views into imaging data.

Building one's understanding of flow phenomena, to be able to exploit the information that is (and will be) coming from emerging imaging techniques, presents a major challenge for cardiologists and researchers of the 21st century. This book has evolved over many years in order to introduce, develop, and integrate concepts and methods from several fields, which underlie a pluridisciplinary approach to intracardiac flow phenomena. It is aimed at context-setting for what the reader will read in the literature of intracardiac blood flow phenomena, on providing a mental structure in which to place it, as well as his or her own, clinical or experimental, observations, and findings.

References and further reading

[1] Appel, T.A. Toby, A. The Cuvier-Geoffroy debate: French biology in the decades before Darwin. 1987, New York: Oxford University Press. 305 p., [16] p. of plates.

[2] Bankman, I.N. [Ed.] Handbook of medical imaging: processing and analysis. 2000, San Diego, CA, USA: Academic. xvi, 901 p., [64] p. of plates (some col.).

[3] Bejan, A. Entropy generation through heat and fluid flow. 1982, New York: Wiley. xiv, 248 p.

[4] Bejan, A. Convection heat transfer. 3rd ed. 2004, Hoboken, N.J.: Wiley. xxxi, 694 p.

[5] Bird, G.A. Molecular gas dynamics and the direct simulation of gas flows. 1994, Oxford [England], New York: Clarendon Press; Oxford University Press. xvii, 458 p.

[6] Bird, R.B., Stewart, W.E., Lightfoot, E.N. Transport phenomena. 2nd ed. 2002, New York: J. Wiley. xii, 895 p.

[7] Bishop, C.M. Neural networks for pattern recognition. 1995, Oxford [England], New York: Clarendon Press; Oxford University Press. xvii, 482 p.

[8] Bland, E.F., White, P.D., Garland, J. Congenital anomalies of the coronary arteries: report of an unusual case associated with cardiac hypertrophy. Am. Heart J. 8: 787–801, 1933.

[9] Brown, F.N.M., Nicolaides, J.D. See the wind blow. 1971, Notre Dame, Ind.: University of Notre Dame. 1 v. (various paging).

[10] Bushnell, D.M., Hefner, J.M. [Eds.] Viscous drag reduction in boundary layers (Progress in Astronautics and Aeronautics, Vol. 123) 1990, Washington, DC: American Institute of Aeronautics and Astronautics. xv, 517 p.

[11] Bushnell, D.M., Moore, K.J. Drag reduction in nature. Annu. Rev. Fluid Mech. 23: 65–79, 1991.

[12] Carroll, S.B. Endless forms most beautiful: the new science of evo devo and the making of the animal kingdom. 2005, New York: Norton. xi, 350 p.

[13] Cartwright, J.H., Piro, O., Tuval, I. Fluid-dynamical basis of the embryonic development of left-right asymmetry in vertebrates. Proc. Natl. Acad. Sci. USA 101: 7234–9, 2004.

[14] Castets, V., Duclos, E., Boissonade, J., Kepper, P. Experimental evidence of a sustained standing Turing type non-equilibrium chemical pattern. Phys. Rev. Lett. 64: 2953–6, 1990.

[15] Chevray, R., Mathieu J. Topics in fluid mechanics. 1993, Cambridge; New York, NY, USA: Cambridge University Press. xv, 320 p.

[16] Chiu, J.J., Wang, D.L., Chien, S., Skalak, R., Usami, S. Effects of disturbed flow on endothelial cells. J. Biomech. Eng. 120: 2–8, 1998.

[17] Dewey, C.F., Bussolari, S.R., Gimbrone, M.A., Jr., Davies, P.F. Dynamic response of vascular endothelial cells to fluid shear stress. J. Biomech. Eng. (ASME) 103: 177–85, 1981.

[18] DeWitt, T.J., Scheiner, S.M. [Eds.] Phenotypic plasticity: functional and conceptual approaches. 2004, Oxford; New York: Oxford University Press. xii, 247 p.

[19] Dilsizian, V., Pohost, G.M. [Eds.] Cardiac CT, PET, and MRI. 2006, Malden, Mass.: Blackwell. 272 p.

[20] Dupont, W.D. Statistical modeling for biomedical researchers: a simple introduction to the analysis of complex data. 2002, Cambridge, U.K.; New York, NY: Cambridge University Press. xvii, 386 p.

[21] Einstein, A., Furth, R. Cowper, A.D. Investigations on the theory of the Brownian movement. 1956, New York: Dover. 119 p.

[22] Elliot, P. Computer "glass boxes" as advanced organizers in mathematics instruction. Int. J. Math. Sci. Technol. Educ. 9: 79–87, 1978.

[23] Frisch, U., Kolmogorov, A.N. Turbulence: the legacy of A.N. Kolmogorov. 1995, Cambridge; New York: Cambridge University Press. xiii, 296 p.

[24] Georgiadis, J.G., Wang, M., Pasipoularides, A. Computational fluid dynamics of left ventricular ejection. Ann. Biomed. Eng. 20: 81–97, 1992.

[25] Glansdorff, P., Prigogine, I. Thermodynamic theory of structure, stability and fluctuations. 1971, London, New York: Wiley–Interscience. xxiii, 306 p.

[26] Hampton, T., Shim, Y., Straley, C., Pasipoularides, A. Finite element analysis of cardiac ejection dynamics: Ultrasonic implications. Am. Soc. Mech. Engin., Bioengin. Div. (ASME BED) Adv. Bioengin. 22: 371–4, 1992.

[27] Hampton, T., Shim, Y., Straley, C., Uppal, R., Smith, P.K., Glower, D., Pasipoularides, A. Computational fluid dynamics of ventricular ejection on the CRAY Y-MP. IEEE Proc. Comp. Cardiol. 19: 295–8, 1992.

[28] Holland, F.A., Bragg, R. Fluid flow for chemical engineers. 2nd ed. 1995, London: E. Arnold. (Elsevier). xv, 358 p.

[29] Hoog de, C.L., Mann, M. Proteomics. Ann. Rev. Genom. Hum. Genet. 5: 267–93, 2004.

[30] Hove, J.R., Koster, R.W., Forouhar, A.S., Acevedo-Bolton, G., Fraser, S.E., Gharib, M. Intracardiac fluid forces are an essential epigenetic factor for embryonic cardiogenesis. Nature 421: 172–7, 2003.

[31] Humphrey, J.D. Cardiovascular solid mechanics: cells, tissues, and organs. 2002, New York: Springer. xvi, 757 p.

[32] Humphrey, J.D., Rajagopal, K.R. A constrained mixture model of arterial adaptations to a sustained step change in blood flows. Biomech. Model Mechanobiol. 2: 107–26, 2003.

[33] Hunter, P., Nielsen, P. A strategy for integrative computational physiology. Physiology 20: 316–25, 2005.

[34] Kamiya A., Togawa T. Adaptive regulation of wall shear stress to flow change in the canine carotid artery. Am. J. Physiol. 239: H14–H21, 1980.

[35] Kauffman, S.A. The origins of order: self-organization and selection in evolution. 1993, New York: Oxford University Press. xviii, 709 p.

[36] Kauffman, S.A. At home in the universe: the search for laws of self-organization and complexity. 1995, New York: Oxford University Press. viii, 321 p.

[37] Kelvin, Lord (Sir W. Thomson). On the propagation of laminar motion through a turbulently moving inviscid fluid. Phil. Mag. 24: 342–53, 1887.

[38] Kessler, R. Nonlinear transition in three-dimensional convection. J. Fluid Mech. 174: 357–79, 1987.

[39] Knedler, J.W. Masterworks of science; digests of 13 great classics [Relativity: the special and general theory, by Albert Einstein]. 1947, Garden City, NY: Doubleday. ix, 637 p.

[40] Lamb, H. Hydrodynamics. 6th ed. 1993, Cambridge, UK: Cambridge University Press. xxv, 738 p.

[41] Lawen, A. Apoptosis—an introduction. BioEssays 25: 888–96, 2003.

[42] Lengyel, I., Epstein, I.R. Modeling of turing structures in the chlorite iodide malonic-acid starch reaction system. Science 251: 650–2, 1991.

[43] Leve, R. Informational acquisition and cognitive models. Complexity 9: 31–7, 2004.

[44] Manneville, P. Instabilities, chaos and turbulence: an introduction to nonlinear dynamics and complex systems. 2004, London; Hackensack, NJ: Imperial College Press; Distributed by World Scientific. xiv, 391 p.

[45] Míguez, D.G., Dolnik, M., Muñuzuri, A.P., Kramer, L. Effect of axial growth on Turing pattern formation. Phys. Rev. Lett. 96: 048304-1–4, 2006.

[46] Murray, C.D. The physiological principle of minimum work. I. The vascular system and the cost of blood volume. Proc. Natl. Acad. Sci. USA. 12: 207–14, 1926.

[47] Nicolis, G., Prigogine, I. Self-organization in nonequilibrium systems: from dissipative structures to order through fluctuations. 1977, New York: Wiley. xii, 491 p.

[48] Noble, D. Modeling the heart: from genes to cells to the whole organ. Science 295: 1678–82, 2002.

[49] Ohno, M., Cooke, J.P., Dzau, V.J., Gibbons, G.H. Fluid shear stress induces endothelial transforming growth factor beta-1 transcription and production. Modulation by potassium channel blockade. J. Clin. Invest. 95: 1363–9, 1995.

[50] Omens, J.H. Stress and strain as regulators of myocardial growth. Prog. Biophys. Molec. Biol. 69: 559–72, 1998.

[51] Ouyang, Q., Swinney, H.L. Transition from a uniform state to hexagonal and striped Turing patterns. Nature 352: 610–12, 1991.

[52] Pasipoularides, A. Clinical assessment of ventricular ejection dynamics with and without outflow obstruction. [Survey]. J. Am. Coll. Cardiol. 15: 859–82, 1990.

[53] Pasipoularides, A. Cardiac mechanics: basic and clinical contemporary research. Ann. Biomed. Eng. 20: 3–17, 1992.

[54] Pasipoularides, A. Complementarity and competitiveness of the intrinsic and extrinsic components of the total ventricular load: demonstration after valve replacement in aortic stenosis [Editorial]. Am. Heart J. 153: 4–6, 2007.

[55] Pasipoularides, A., Shu, M., Shah, A., Tucconi, A., Glower, D.D. RV instantaneous intraventricular diastolic pressure and velocity distributions in normal and volume overload awake dog disease models. Am. J. Physiol. Heart Circ. Physiol. 285: H1956–65, 2003.

[56] Pasipoularides, A.D., Shu, M., Shah, A., Glower, D.D. Right ventricular diastolic relaxation in conscious dog models of pressure overload, volume overload and ischemia. J. Thorac. Cardiovasc. Surg. 124: 964–72, 2002.

[57] Pasipoularides, A., Shu, M., Shah, A., Silvestry, S., Glower, D.D. Right ventricular diastolic function in canine models of pressure overload, volume overload and ischemia. Am. J. Physiol. Heart Circ. Physiol. 283: H2140–50, 2002.

[58] Pasipoularides, A., Shu, M., Shah, A., Womack, M.S., Glower, D.D. Diastolic right ventricular filling vortex in normal and volume overload states. Am. J. Physiol. Heart Circ. Physiol. 284: H1064–72, 2003.

[59] Pigliucci, M. Phenotypic plasticity: beyond nature and nurture. 2001, Baltimore: Johns Hopkins University Press. xvi, 328 p.

[60] Pries, A.R., Reglin, B., Secomb, T.W. Remodeling of blood vessels: responses of diameter and wall thickness to hemodynamic and metabolic stimuli. Hypertension 46:725–31, 2005.

[61] Prigogine, I., Stengers, I. La nouvelle alliance: métamorphose de la science. 1979, Paris: Gallimard. 302 p.

[62] Proust, M., Scott-Moncrieff, C.K. The sweet cheat gone: an autobiography. 1st Modern Library ed. 1948, New York: Modern Library. 4 p. l., 379 p.

[63] Resnick, M., Berg, R., Eisenberg, M. Beyond black boxes: bringing transparency and aesthetics back to scientific investigation. J. Learn. Sci. 9: 7–30, 2000.

[64] Revenu, C., Athman, R., Robine, S., Louvard, D. The co-workers of actin filaments: from cell structures to signals. Nat. Rev. Mol. Cell. Biol. 5: 635–46, 2004.

[65] Robb, R.A. Biomedical imaging, visualization, and analysis. 2000, New York, NY: Wiley–Liss. xvi, 339 p.

[66] Rosner, B. Fundamentals of biostatistics. 6th ed. 2006, Pacific Grove, CA: Duxbury. xix, 784 p.

[67] Shay-Salit, A., Shushy, M., Wolfovitz, E., Yahav, H., Breviario, F., Dejana, E., Resnick, N. VEGF receptor 2 and the adherens junction as a mechanical transducer in vascular endothelial cells. Proc. Natl. Acad. Sci. USA 99: 9462–7, 2002.

[68] Sherman, T.F. On connecting large vessels to small: the meaning of Murray's law. J. Gen. Physiol. 78: 431–53, 1981.

[69] Shim, Y., Hampton, T.G., Straley, C.A., Harrison, J.K., Spero, L.A., Bashore, T.M., Pasipoularides, A.D. Ejection load changes in aortic stenosis. Observations made after balloon aortic valvuloplasty. Circ. Res. 71: 1174–84, 1992.

[70] Smith, N.P., Mulquiney, P.J., Nash, M.P., Bradley, C.P., Nickerson, D.P., Hunter, P.J. Mathematical modelling of the heart: cell to organ. Chaos, Solitons and Fractals 13: 1613–21, 2002.

[71] Thoma, R. Untersuchungen über die Histogenese und Histomechanik des Gefässystems. 1893, Stuttgart, Germany: F. Enke.

[72] Thompson, D.A.W., On growth and form. 2d ed. 1963, Cambridge, UK: Cambridge University Press. 2 v. viii, 1116 p.

[73] Tronc, F., Mallat, Z., Lehoux, S., Wassef, M., Esposito, B., Tedgui, A. Role of matrix metalloproteinases in blood flow-induced arterial enlargement: interaction with NO. Arterioscler. Thromb. Vasc. Biol. 20: 120–6, 2000.

[74] Turing, A.M. The chemical basis of morphogenesis. [Reprinted from Phil. Trans. Roy. Soc. London, B237: 37–72, 1952.] Bull. Math. Biol. 52: 153–97, 1990.

[75] Venter, C., et al. The sequence of the human genome. Science 291: 1304–51, 2001.

[76] Venter, J.C. A life decoded: my genome, my life. 2007, New York: Viking. 390 p., [16] p. of plates.

[77] Vogel, S. Vital circuits: on pumps, pipes, and the workings of circulatory systems. 1993, New York: Oxford University Press. x, 315 p.

[78] Weinberger, E.D. Local properties of the NK model, a tuneably rugged energy landscape. Phys. Rev. A 44: 6399–413, 1991.

Chapter 2

Handy Mathematical Instruments of Thought

Ich behaupte aber, dass in jeder besonderen Naturlehre nur soviel eigentliche Wissenschaft angetroffen werden könne, als darin Mathematik anzutreffen ist. [In my view, there is only so much real science in each physical theory, as mathematics is found in it.]

——Immanuel Kant, in Metaphysische Anfangsgründe der Naturwissenschaft, Vorrede (1786) p. 470 [43].

When a somewhat lengthy calculation has conducted to us some simple and striking result, we are not satisfied until we have shown that we might have foreseen, if not the whole result, at least its most characteristic features. Why? Because the lengthy calculation might not be used again, while this is not true of the reasoning, often semiintuitive, which might have enabled us to foresee the result?

——Henri Poincaré (1854–1912), one of France's greatest theoretical scientists–mathematicians, in [72].

The next great awakening of human intellect may well produce a method of understanding the qualitative content of equations. Today we cannot. Today we cannot see that the water-flow equations contain such things as the barber pole structure of turbulence that one sees between rotating cylinders ...

——Richard Feynman, in Volume II, Section 41, p. 12 of [30].

A DESCRIPTION OF PHYSICAL EVENTS and their evolution can be formulated in ordinary prose and, before Newton's era, most scientific work was cast in that form. However, verbal discourse by itself can be unwieldy and unsuited to accurate descriptions and analysis of physical systems. In Mechanics, we must therefore use the language of Mathematics [37], and must represent the phenomena of nature by mathematical objects—such as geometric figures, vectors, functions, derivatives or integrals of functions, equations, and the like—which correspond to observations in some manner.

Mathematics lies at the heart of physics and engineering [10, 19, 33, 35, 46, 54, 63, 85]: each advance in physics has entailed the construction of a mathematical description of the phenomenon in question. Physicists, engineers, and applied mathematicians are accustomed to the combination of elegance, rigor, and utility that characterize mathematical models. They are familiar with the need to dip into their mathematical toolbox to select the technique of choice.

Advances in instrumentation, including multisensor cardiac catheterization technology and digital imaging modalities, basic hemodynamic and cardiac mechanics understanding, and computational and mathematical techniques are contributing to the growing significance of mathematical approaches in cardiac dynamics. There is a strong case for arguing that the new diagnostic instrumentation means an urgent need for sophisticated concepts from mathematics and modern fluid dynamics. It is perhaps unreasonable to expect the college physics and mathematics courses to be immediately applicable to emergent phenomena of intracardiac blood flow and sufficient for their understanding. Recent clinical as well as basic research in cardiology reflects this. In this chapter, we shall review some mathematical concepts that are very useful in the study and the understanding of intracardiac blood flows.

2.1 Ensemble averages

A set of observations forms an "ensemble" of events. The ensemble is a valuable concept in hemodynamics and cardiac mechanics. In everyday life, pulsatile dynamic phenomena are replicated many times every minute, so that we have an enormous number of copies, each possessing in the main the same physical characteristics of volume oscillations, pressure and flow pulsations, and so on. Since we are interested in the dynamics of the main pulsatile phenomena, it is not necessary for these replicas to have *exactly* the same time-courses of volume, pressure, and velocities. In other words, the replicas are allowed to differ at random to some small extent, while retaining the same general properties. Such a collection of replicated systems is called an ensemble.

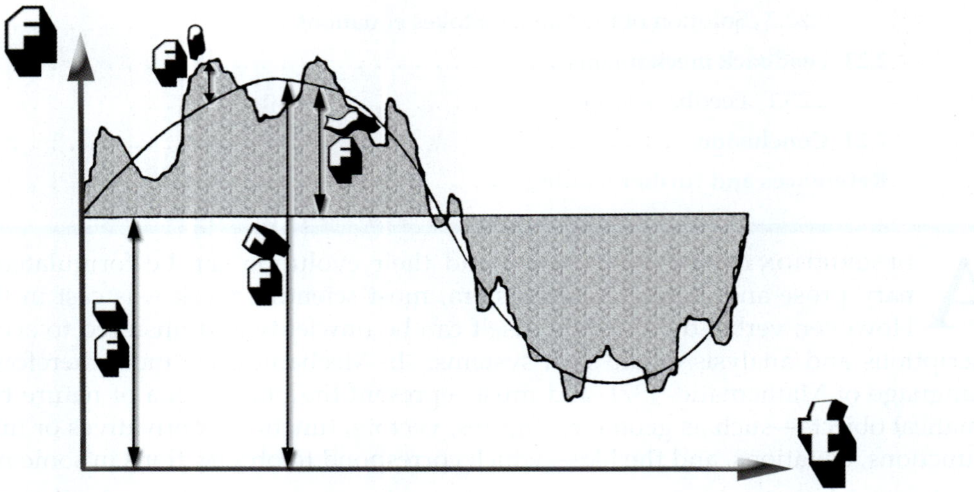

Figure 2.1: Ensemble average ($\hat{f}$), time-mean ($\bar{f}$), periodic fluctuation ($\tilde{f}$), and stochastic (random) fluctuation (f') values in a periodic pulsatile flow, $f(t)$.

Generally speaking, a *period* is an interval of time characterized by the occurrence of a certain condition or event. Any variable in a periodic system exactly repeats its past behavior after the passage of a fixed interval of time, equal to one period or integer multiple thereof—think of the position, velocity, and acceleration of a swinging pendulum. *Aperiodic* behavior occurs when no dynamic variable characterizing the system undergoes a completely regular repetition of values. Unstable aperiodic behavior is highly complex and never repeats itself; this produces a series of measurements that appear at random. Examples of behavior that is so complex as to be unstable and aperiodic are given by the image of the fluctuations of an unruly crowd, or those of a flag waving in the breeze. Behavior that is unstable yet periodic appears to be a contradiction in terms. However, history provides us with quite a few examples of just such a phenomenon. We can effectively chart broad patterns in the rise and fall of civilizations. We can see that these patterns are, broadly speaking, periodic. Nevertheless, events by no means repeat themselves exactly; in this stricter sense, history is aperiodic. Ensemble average analyses allow us to identify important aspects of dynamic system behavior.

Because of the way an ensemble of events is constructed, if a snapshot of all the replicas is taken at the same instant, they will be found to differ in the instantaneous values of their bulk properties. This phenomenon is what we techically denote as *fluctuation*. Thus, the true value of any particular bulk phenomenon must be calculated as an average over all the replicas. This is what is meant by an ensemble average, as is exemplified in Figures 2.1 and 2.2, and the instantaneous values are said to "fluctuate" about the mean value.[1]

[1]Details on specific techniques for the calculation of different kinds of ensemble averages of hemodynamic signals may be found in refs. [68] and [79].

In flows with periodic unsteadiness, an instantaneous quantity f can be separated into three components, as is sketched pictorially in Figure 2.1:

$$f = \bar{f} + \tilde{f} + f' = \hat{f} + f', \tag{2.1}$$

where, $\bar{f}$ is the time-mean value, $\hat{f}$ the ensemble average value, $\tilde{f}$ the periodic fluctuation, and f' a stochastic (random) fluctuation. Notice how the mean of $\hat{f}$ over any integral multiple of one period coincides with $\bar{f}$.

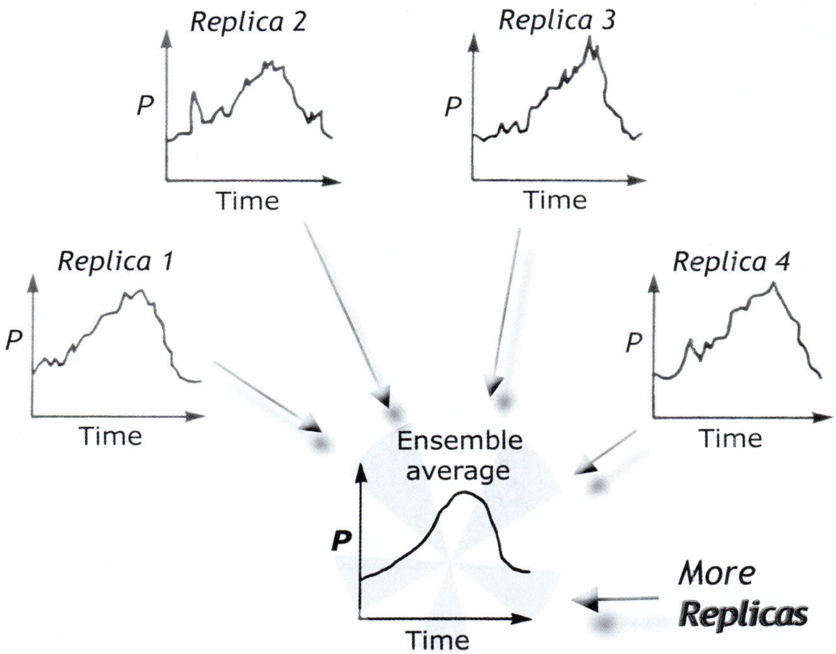

Figure 2.2: If a snapshot of all the replicas of a variable P that are encompassed in an ensemble is taken at the same instant, they differ in their instantaneous values. This is the phenomenon of fluctuation. The true value of P is an average taken over all the replicas, the ensemble average, and the instantaneous P values fluctuate about it.

For flows that do not change with time, in the sense that the gross boundary conditions are constant, we can define ordinary and familiar time averages. These are useful parameters for the description of such flows. For intracardiac pulsatile flows where the applying macroscopic boundary conditions change with time, time averages lose their dynamic usefulness—they reduce to mean blood pressure, mean cardiac output, and the like. Accordingly, we will take recourse to ensemble averages. In using an ensemble average in hemodynamics, we are making an implicit assumption that an ensemble average (which relates to many replicas of the system) is a representative average for the individual subject under a given physiologic condition. This assumption corresponds to the *ergodic hypothesis*.[2] Fortunately, it seems to be generally true, provided a sufficiently long time to yield a large number of pulses, or replicas, is taken in the average.

2.2 Vectors and scalars

The word vector comes from the Latin term vehere, to carry. Thus, in biomedical terminology, a vector is an agent such as a mosquito, which carries disease from one patient to the next. In mathematics, a vector is a quantity, such as velocity, that has both a magnitude and a direction associated with it. Position is also a vector, since an object's position must be defined relative to some other position, and in the difference between the two we have both a distance and a direction. On the other hand, quantities such as mass that cannot be expressed as having a direction are called scalars.

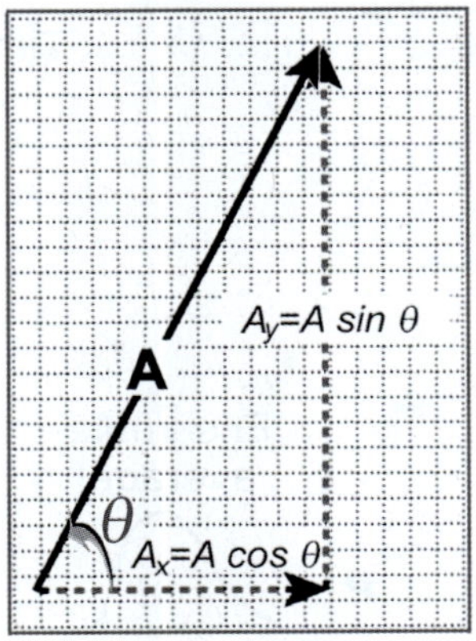

Figure 2.3: There are various ways of describing vectors on a plane. Number-pairs corresponding to the two end points of a vector may be used as a labeling device. The first number in a pair indicates the x-coordinate value and the second the y-coordinate value. The x-component of the vector is obtained as the algebraic difference between the x-coordinates of its two end points; the y-component, as the difference between their y-coordinates. Information about the magnitude, i.e., the length of the vector, and direction, i.e., the angle θ that it makes with the x-axis provides an alternative representation.

A vector is drawn as an arrow in space. The projection of the length of the vector in each of the coordinate axes corresponds to the components of the vector along the three coordinates. Figure 2.3 illustrates a vector **A** (in this book, we follow the convention of denoting vectors by either boldface type, or by drawing an arrow over the variable name) drawn in two-dimensional space as an arrow, with its A_x and A_y components

[2]Boltzmann and Maxwell stated the ergodic hypothesis over one hundred years ago [70]. In the present context, it implies that the time average value of an observable variable—which is determined by the dynamics—is equivalent to an ensemble average, that is, an average at one time over a large number of replicas all of which may not have truly identical initial conditions.

showing. The magnitude A and the direction, the angle $\boldsymbol{\theta}$, are also shown. Here the usual coordinate geometry convention is adopted: the angle $\boldsymbol{\theta}$ is measured so as to be positive in the *counterclockwise* sense from the x-axis. The x and y components of the vector **A** are given by

$$A_x = A\,cos\,\theta, \tag{2.2}$$

$$A_y = A\,sin\,\theta, \tag{2.3}$$

Often a vector expressed in x and y components is written as (A_x, A_y). Knowing A_x

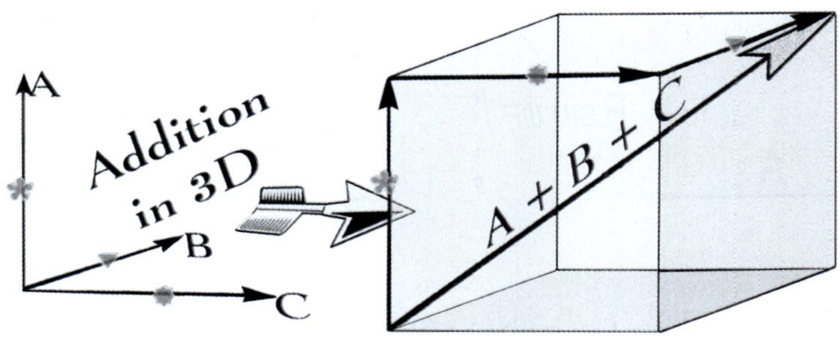

Figure 2.4: Combination of vectors that do not lie on the same plane.

and A_y, the magnitude A and direction $\boldsymbol{\theta}$ of the vector **A**, are obtained by applying the Pythagorean Theorem, and trigonometry.

$$A = (A_x^2 + A_y^2)^{1/2}, \tag{2.4}$$

$$\tan\theta = A_y/A_x. \tag{2.5}$$

2.2.1 Adding and subtracting vectors

We can add two or more vectors as follows. Let **A** and **B** be two vectors located at a point P. Their sum, indicated by **A+B**, is obtained as follows: We construct the parallelogram having the two vectors as its sides and let P′ be the vertex opposite from P. Then PP′ is the sum **A+B**. Subtracting vectors is just as easy. The negative of a vector is simply a vector of the same length, pointed in the opposite direction. To subtract a vector, we just add the negative value of the vector. In x and y coordinates, to make a vector negative, we just reverse the signs of both the x and y values. Vector addition in three dimensions simply involves not one but two applications of the parallelogram rule, in succession (Fig. 2.4).

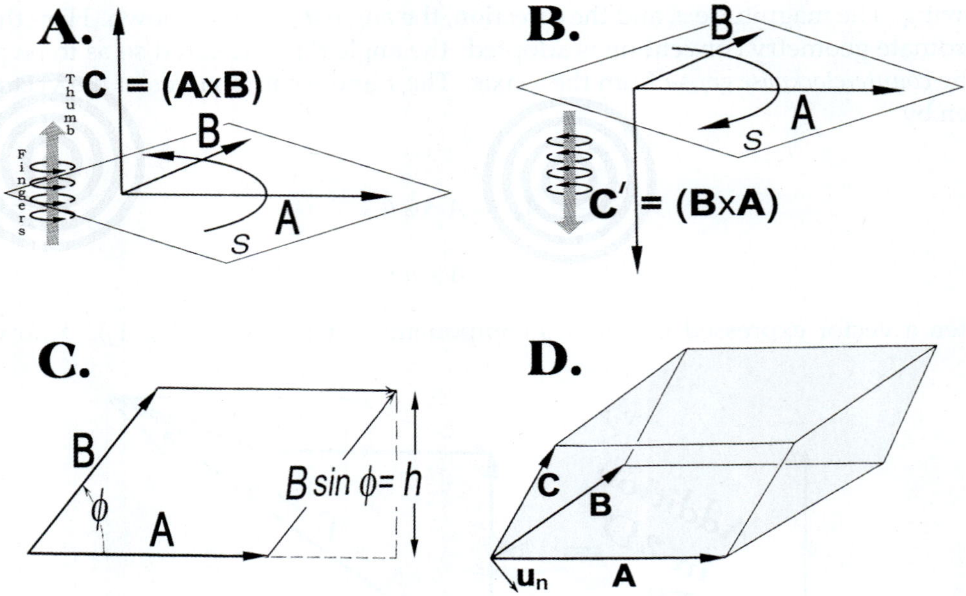

Figure 2.5: Panels A. and B. show that both $(\mathbf{A}\times\mathbf{B})$ and $(\mathbf{B}\times\mathbf{A})$ are perpendicular to the plane (S) of **A** and **B** but point in opposite directions. Panel C. shows that the area of a parallelogram is $(\mathbf{A}\times\mathbf{B})$. Panel D. shows that the volume of a parallepiped is given by the scalar triple product $\mathbf{A}\cdot\mathbf{B}\times\mathbf{C}$.

2.2.2 Dot product and cross product

Vectors can be multiplied in different ways, each of which has a slightly different interpretation. As vectors are quantities with direction, vector multiplication also depends on direction. The dot product represents multiplying one vector with the component of a second vector onto the first. Thus, the dot product of a vector with a unit vector is the projection of that vector in the direction given by the unit vector. The dot product of **A** and **B** is written as $\mathbf{A}\cdot\mathbf{B}$ and spoken as "A dot B"

$$\mathbf{A}\cdot\mathbf{B} = AB\cos\phi, \tag{2.6}$$

where, ϕ is the angle between the two vectors. An immediate consequence of this equation is that the dot product of a vector with itself gives the square of its length. The dot product is fundamentally a projection. If two vectors are parallel, the dot product is large and we get a large effect, but if they are perpendicular, it is zero. It follows immediately that two vectors are orthogonal if and only if their dot product vanishes.[3] If they are parallel, the dot product is just the product of the magnitudes. Note that the dot product produces a scalar result.

[3]The fact that two vectors are perpendicular if their dot product is zero may be used in more abstract settings, such as the theory of orthogonal functions and Fourier analysis—see Section 2.18, on pp. 82 ff.

The cross or "vector" product is used when the resulting quantity should also be a vector, and has a largest effect when the given vectors are perpendicular. The cross product of vector **A** with vector **B** is spoken as "A cross B." The product has a magnitude of

$$\mathbf{A}\times\mathbf{B} = AB\ sin\ \phi \tag{2.7}$$

and has a direction which is at right angles to both vectors and can be found using a "right hand rule": Start with the fingers of the right hand pointing in the direction of the first vector, **A**. The fingers are then rotated in the direction of the second vector, **B**, by closing the fist. The direction of your thumb gives the direction of the cross product vector, as is indicated in Figure 2.5. Physically, the magnitude of the cross product is the area of a parallelogram made from the two vectors (see Fig. 2.5).

2.2.3 The triple scalar product

This product is denoted by $\mathbf{A} \cdot (\mathbf{B} \times \mathbf{C})$ and arises when a cross product of two vectors, **B** and **C**, is combined with a third vector **A** by means of a scalar product. The triple scalar product has an important geometric property. If **A**, **B**, and **C** form the edges of a parallelepiped, the magnitude (absolute value) of their triple scalar product is the volume of that parallelepiped. As is indicated in Figure 2.5, the magnitude of the vector $\mathbf{B}\times\mathbf{C}$ is the magnitude of the area of the side; and the projection of **A** in the direction of $\mathbf{u}_n$, i.e., the direction of $\mathbf{B}\times\mathbf{C}$ is the altitude of the parallelepiped. We will utilize this important geometric tool in the computation of cardiac chamber volumes by the *"Prism Method,"* which does not invoke any geometric model assumptions and is described in Chapter 14.

2.3 Kinematics of circular motion and rotation

A concept basic to understanding rotational kinematics is that of the uniform circular motion, which is the motion of a particle along a circular arc, or a circle, with constant speed. This type of motion involves a continuous change in the *direction* of the velocity without any change in its magnitude, or *speed*. A change in the direction of the velocity vector, **v**, however, constitutes a change in velocity; this implies that a uniform circular motion is associated with an acceleration and, consequently, with a force, **F**. To keep the speed constant, the force, **F**, must always act *perpendicularly* to the direction of circumferential velocity. Since the latter direction is constantly changing, the direction of force—being perpendicular to it—should also be changing continuously, as is shown in the center panel of Figure 2.6. The direction of the velocity along the circular trajectory is *tangential*. Therefore, the direction perpendicular to the trajectory is the radial direction. This implies that force and acceleration in uniform circular motion point in the radial direction, as shown in panels a. and b. of Figure 2.6, and are *centripetal*, i.e., seeking the center or axis of rotation. As the centripetal force is passing through the axis of rotation,

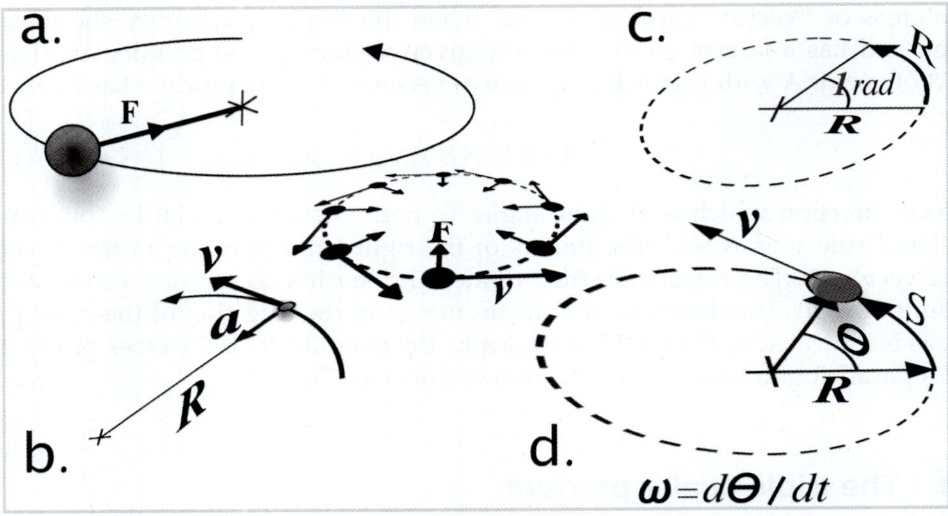

Figure 2.6: Pictorial representation of concepts basic to understanding uniform circular motion and rigid body rotational kinematics—explanation of symbols is found in the nearby text.

it does not give rise to a torque[4] and, thus, it does not cause acceleration in the tangential, or circumferential, direction.

Circular motion involves the following three quantities:

- **Angular displacement**: Circular motion brings on an angular displacement of the object. We define as angular displacement, $\boldsymbol{\theta}$, the angle that a line from the axis of the circular motion to a specified point on the object makes with respect to the positive x-axis; its magnitude, θ, is measured counterclockwise. As measure of the magnitude of the angle , we take the ratio of the length of the corresponding circular arc, S, to that of the radius of rotation, R: $\theta = S/R$; as a nondimensional unit of angular displacement we use the radian, *rad*, which is the angle swept out by an arc of length equal to the length, R, of the radius of the circle, as is shown in panel c. of Figure 2.6. In addition to magnitude, the angle, $\boldsymbol{\theta}$, has a direction parallel to the axis of rotation and the *right hand rule*, described in the preceding section, indicates the positive (counterclockwise) direction. Accordingly, in the formalism of physics, *angle* and *angular displacement* represent vector quantities.
- **Angular velocity**: The path described by a point P_R circling at distance R from the axis of rotation is R times as long as the arc S_r, which a point P_1 circling at the distance 1 *cm* from the axis describes during the same time interval. Consequently, P_R has R times the circumferential velocity of P_1. The velocity of P_1 is measured by the ratio of the length of the arc S_r, covered by it, to the time used. However, this

[4]A torque is force multiplied by the perpendicular distance of the line of action of the force from the axis of rotation.

arc is also the measure of the angle, θ, by which the object circled around the axis during the same time interval, t. Therefore, the ratio of the length of the circular arc, covered by a point at distance 1 *cm* from the axis, to the time taken is simultaneously a measure for the velocity by which the *entire* body describes this angle. It is called its *angular velocity*. As is shown in panel d. of Figure 2.6, the magnitude, ω, of the instantaneous angular velocity $\boldsymbol{\omega}$ is the rate at which the angular displacement *theta* changes with respect to time t: $\omega = d\theta/dt$. As for angular displacement, the line of direction of the angular velocity $\boldsymbol{\omega}$ is given by the axis of the circular motion, and the *right hand rule* indicates the positive direction. For uniform rotation, the magnitude ω of the angular velocity is constant.

- **Angular acceleration**: For nonuniform circular motion, the magnitude of the instantaneous angular acceleration **a** is the rate at which the magnitude of the angular velocity $\boldsymbol{\omega}$ changes with respect to time t: $a = d\omega/dt$; again, the *right hand rule* indicates the positive direction.

Generally, rotational motion involves turning, or *spinning*, of an object. At the beginning of a rotation, all its points start to move simultaneously along circles; at the end, they stop simultaneously. When the object has completed its rotation once, it regains the same position as it had at the start. The time interval, T, between the start and the end of a full rotation is the *period*. The greater the distance of a point from the axis, the longer is its circular trajectory during T, and it therefore has a larger circumferential (*viz.*, tangential) velocity than points closer to the axis. Assuming that the body is rigid, the paths and circumferential velocities of points at different distances from the axis are related. The object's rigidity forces all points that during rest lie on a straight line, to do so also during rotation. Although they may under steady-state conditions tend to approximate rigid-body rotation (see Fig. 2.19, on p. 62), rotating viscous fluid particles or volume elements do not commonly behave in such a simple fashion, but rotate in laminae that may exhibit relative motions relative to one another, shear strains and viscous (frictional) stresses, as well as complex secondary flow patterns, as we shall see in subsequent chapters.

2.4 Phasors and complex numbers

A phasor is a rotating vector with a constant magnitude and constant angular velocity. Angular velocity $\boldsymbol{\omega}$ is the angular distance $\boldsymbol{\theta}$ traveled per unit time, and angular acceleration is the rate of change of the angular velocity. Examples of phasor quantities are a voltage sinusoid or a sinusoidal harmonic of a compound arterial velocity waveform. The algebraic rules applicable to vectors can also be utilized for phasor operation. Thus, note the method of representing a sinusoid as a radius vector, or phasor, as shown in Figure 2.7. It is evident, therefore, that sinusoidal waveforms of the same frequency can be represented by fixed phasors with the angle between the radius vectors corresponding to the phase difference between the sinusoidal waveforms.

The conversion of the representation from the time domain into the phasor domain proceeds in the following manner. Let $s(t) = 100 \cdot sin\ \omega t$ represent a signal in the time domain. The value of the modulus is equal to 100; the phase angle is zero. Thus, the conversion from the time to the phasor domain is

$$\begin{array}{rcccl} & \text{Time domain} & \Longrightarrow & \text{Phasor domain} & \\ s(t) = & 100 \cdot \mathit{sin}\ \omega t & = & 100\angle 0^\circ. & \end{array} \tag{2.8}$$

After converting from the time to the phasor domain, we find that the techniques of vector or phasor algebra are now applicable. After any problem involving sinusoids has been solved in the phasor domain, the solution can be converted back into the time domain.

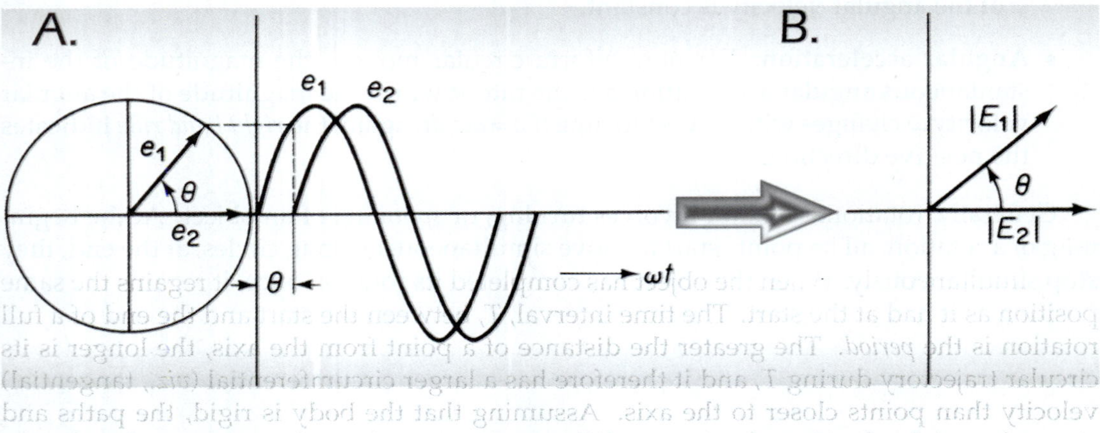

Figure 2.7: Panels A. and B. illustrate representation of two sinusoids as rotating vectors in the time domain and as phasors. For simplicity, the two sinusoidal signals depicted have the same angular frequency, ω and amplitude; e_1 leads e_2 by a phase angle θ.

2.4.1 Complex quantities

A complex number is a point that is represented by two orthogonal components, one along and the other at right angles to some arbitrary axis of reference. This point can also determine a radius drawn from the origin of the arbitrary axis to the point. The horizontal axis, or the abscissa, contains all real numbers, whereas the vertical axis, or the ordinate, is called the imaginary axis, since it contains so-called *imaginary* numbers.

In the complex plane shown in Figure 2.8, all real and imaginary numbers in the first quadrant are positive; the second quadrant contains negative real numbers and positive imaginary numbers. The third quadrant contains negative real and imaginary numbers, and in the fourth quadrant, the real numbers are positive and the imaginary numbers are negative. This type of plot on the complex plane is called an Argand diagram. Jean-Robert Argand (1768–1822) is famed for his geometrical interpretation of the complex numbers, where j is interpreted as a rotation through 90°, as we show next.

In conventional usage, the presence of either of the symbols j or i in front of a real number denotes a vertical element or imaginary number. Consider the complex plane

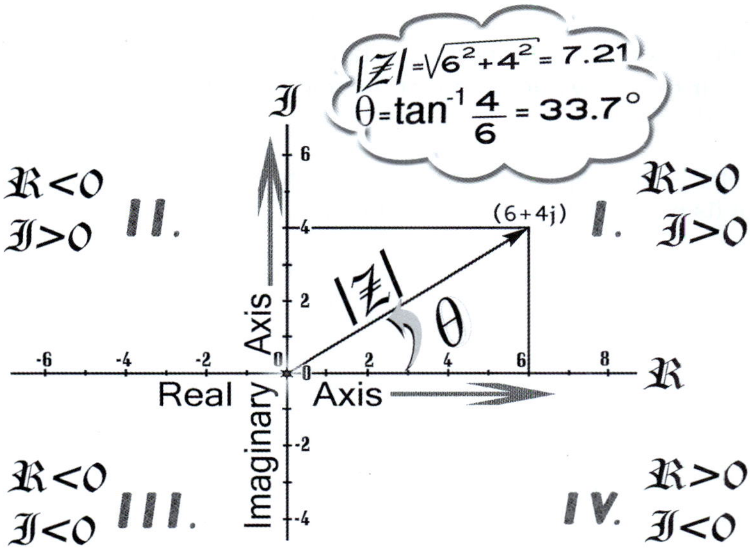

Figure 2.8: The Argand diagram gives us a way to picture complex numbers and it is not to be confused with the x–y plane. The area covered by the diagram is known as the complex plane where any complex number can be represented by a point—in this case, point $(6 + 4j)$.

shown in Figure 2.8. In this complex plane, a point is shown whose coordinates are six units in the horizontal (real axis) and four units in the vertical (imaginary axis) direction. This point represents a radius phasor equal to $6 + j4$. The definition of the operator j, and some integer powers of j that are derived directly from this definition are:

$$\begin{aligned} j &= \sqrt{-1} \\ j^2 &= -1 \\ j^3 &= -j = -\sqrt{-1} \\ j^4 &= +1. \end{aligned} \tag{2.9}$$

It is evident that when we multiply a given quantity by j, the quantity is rotated through an angle of $90°$ in a counterclockwise direction. The operation simply means a change of phase angle to lead by $90°$, or $\pi/2$ *rad*. On the other hand, division of a phasor by j causes it to be rotated through an angle of $90°$ in the clockwise direction. Division by j simply means a change of phase angle to lag by $90°$, or $\pi/2$ *rad* (cf. Fig. 2.9, on p. 49).

A complex quantity is a number consisting of a real part, $\Re(Z)$, and an imaginary part, or the j-component, represented by $\Im(Z)$. We may represent a complex number, Z, by any one of the following forms (see Figs. 2.8 and 2.9):

(i.) Rectangular.—The complex number, $Z = a + jb$, is said to be expressed in rectangular form. This form can be used, e.g., to describe a radius phasor in any one of the four quadrants of the complex plane, as shown in Figure 2.8, on p. 47. It is convenient to add or subtract complex numbers in rectangular form. When adding or subtracting in rectangular form, we add/subtract the real terms together, and add/subtract the j terms together.

(ii.) Trigonometric.—By inspection of Figure 2.8, the components of Z can be expressed in terms of its magnitude, symbolized by $\mid Z \mid$. Thus,

$$\Re(Z) = \mid Z \mid \; cos\,\theta, \qquad \Im(Z) = j \mid Z \mid \; sin\,\theta, \tag{2.10}$$

where,

$$Z = \sqrt{([\Re(Z)]^2 + [\Im(Z)]^2)} \quad \text{(modulus or magnitude)}, \qquad \theta = tan^{-1}\frac{\Im(Z)}{\Re(Z)} \quad \text{(direction or phase angle)}. \tag{2.11}$$

Therefore, $Z = \Re(Z) + j\;\Im(Z) = \mid Z \mid (cos\;\theta + j\;sin\;\theta)$. The position of the magnitude of Z is determined by the direction angle, θ. This form is called the trigonometric form and can be used to represent any given complex number or phasor (cf. Equation 2.8). If we plot the projections of a rotating phasor on the real and imaginary axes, against time, we shall have the plots of its oscillating real and imaginary components, respectively, in the time domain; allowing the angular frequency to be ω, we have

$$Z(t) = \mid Z \mid (cos(\omega \cdot t + \theta) + j\;sin\,(\omega \cdot t + \theta)). \tag{2.12}$$

When we consider separately the real or the imaginary part of the phasor representation of a complex variable, we must remember that what we really mean is the projection of the rotating phasor on the real or on the imaginary axis, respectively (see Fig. 2.9, on p. 49).

(iii.) Polar.—This is another convenient method of writing a radius phasor quantity. The polar form of a complex number is simply a vector at some angle to the reference positive real axis and is given as (see Fig. 2.8)

$$Z = \mid Z \mid \angle\theta^{\circ}. \tag{2.13}$$

This notation should be interpreted as the magnitude of Z making an angle of $\boldsymbol{\theta}$ degrees with the positive real axis, in the *counterclockwise* direction of rotation. It is convenient to multiply or divide complex numbers in polar form. When multiplying in polar form, we multiply the magnitudes ($|Z|$) together and add the angles. When dividing in polar form, we divide the magnitudes and subtract the angles. We also use the polar form when taking the reciprocal of a complex number, since the operation is conceptually a division; we take the reciprocal of the magnitude and change the sign of the angle.

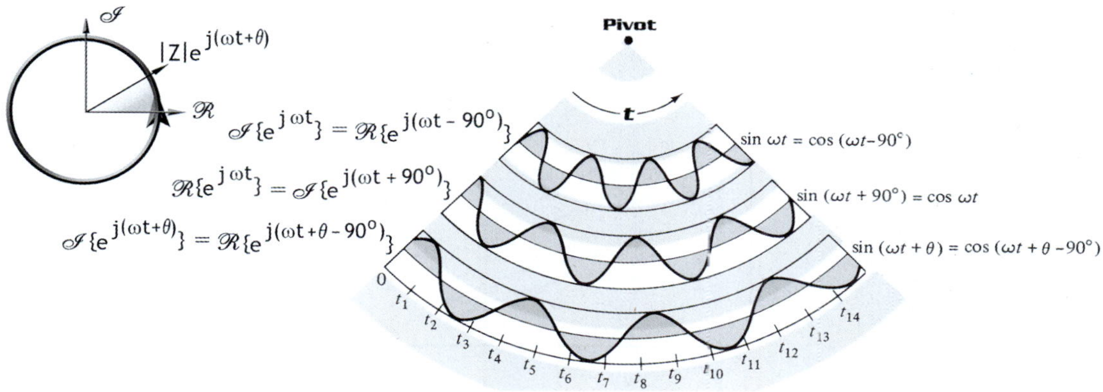

Figure 2.9: The correspondence between the complex exponential and the trigonometric formulations for phasor quantities. As time, t elapses, the complex exponential $\mid Z \mid e^{j\,(\omega\,\cdot\,t\,+\,\theta)}$ rotates counterclockwise, as shown in the inset. Its projections on the real, $\Re$, and imaginary, $\Im$, axes correspond to the oscillating cosine and sine functions, respectively.

(iv.) Exponential.—This relationship is derived by expanding the $cos\theta$ and $sin\theta$ functions into their infinite series representations. The next step is to expand e^{θ} into an infinite series and apply McLaurin's theorem of calculus. The final result is the exponential form for writing a complex quantity, namely

$$Z = \mid Z \mid e^{j \cdot \theta} \,. \tag{2.14}$$

Corresponding to the trigonometric form in Equation 2.12, for a rotating phasor we have (see Fig. 2.9)

$$Z(t) \;=\; \mid Z \mid e^{j(\omega\,\cdot\,t\,+\,\theta)} \,. \tag{2.15}$$

2.5 Fields and field lines

Many processes in mechanics and hemodynamics involve continuous media with their properties varying continuously in 3-D space and time. An example would be the velocity of blood within the beating heart chambers. Examples of continuous media are fluids, such as water and blood, gases, for example air, electromagnetic fields, etc. A field is a region of space for each point of which the values of one or several quantities of interest are defined [53, 90]. Alternatively, a field is a set of functions that describes one or several physical quantities at all points in a region of space. For a scalar quantity, the field is specified by a single magnitude at each point, such as the density, i.e., mass per unit volume, $\rho(x, y, z, t)$, measured in $kg \cdot m^{-3}$, or the pressure, $p(x, y, z, t)$, measured in $N \cdot m^{-2}$.

A field can be represented pictorially by sprinkling space with geometrical symbols of the corresponding quantity; for example, we picture a vector field as a "forest" of appropriately sized arrows covering space, the length and direction of each one corresponding

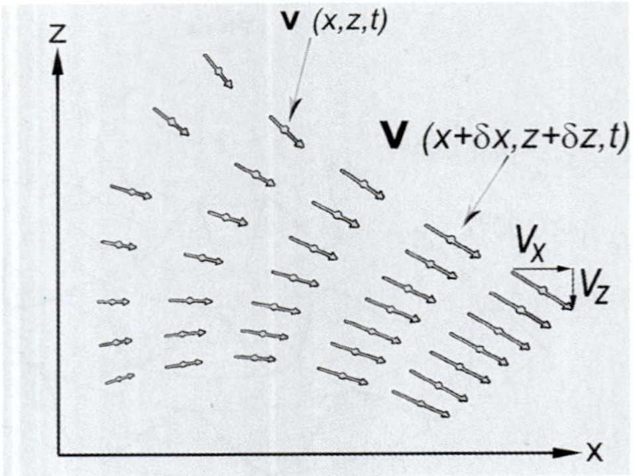

Figure 2.10: Velocity field with converging streamlines showing velocity vectors. Components V_x, and V_z, are shown for one velocity vector. At time t, a point with spatial coordinates (x, z) has one velocity, but another with coordinates $(x + \delta x, z + \delta z)$ has a higher velocity.

to the value of the vector field at that location. Therefore, for a flow-velocity field the physical quantity "velocity," $\mathbf{v}(x, y, z, t)$, is specified by a vector giving a direction as well as a magnitude.

A vector field line, such as an electric field line or a streamline (blood velocity field) is drawn such that the tangent to the vector field line at any point is in the direction of the vector variable, e.g., $\mathbf{v}(x, y, z, t)$, as exemplified in Figure 2.10. To draw a streamline, start out at any point in space and move a very short distance in the direction of the local velocity, drawing a line as you do so. After that short distance, stop, find the new direction of the local velocity at the point where you stopped, and begin moving again in that new direction. Continue this process indefinitely. Thereby you construct a line in space that is everywhere tangent to the local vector field. If you do this for many different starting points, you can draw a set of field lines that give a good representation of the properties of the velocity field. The field line separation gives an indication of the strength of the field. When the field lines are closer together, then the field is stronger and sketches of the field lines should reflect this—converging streamlines imply increasing velocity, i.e., acceleration, whereas diverging streamlines imply decreasing velocity, i.e., deceleration along the flow (cf. Fig. 2.10).

The concept of the *flow field* is fruitful because explanation of intracardiac blood flow phenomena depends upon the construction of models that go beneath the level of appearance, to the generative processes that describe the real *underlying* causes of phenomena. In classical mechanics the concept of a flow field embodies a domain of relational order, in which the state of one part of a fluid is connected by a precise[5] mathematical *relation* to the states of neighboring parts; accordingly, planetary dynamics involves the use of gravitational field theory to describe the motions of interacting bodies as an integrated whole.

[5]In physics, classical notions have to be abandoned or modified only when we go to realms, such as chaotic system dynamics or quantum mechanics, that are beyond our everyday experience, beyond the everyday physical environment.

Similarly, the intracardiac blood flow system consists of a single three-dimensional field, which unfolds in time according to particular laws.

2.5.1 Contour maps

Contour lines on contour maps bring to life the instantaneous spatial distribution of individual fluid dynamic variables in 2-D maps of a given flow field. The information contained in contour lines relates to intensity or magnitude, to rate of change or slope, and to overall pattern or shape of the distribution of the quantity plotted. Contour maps in three-dimensional space are obtained by fixing one of the independent spatial variables (z, for example) and then showing a plot for the two remaining dimensions, in which the curves represent lines of constant values of the function whose distribution in the field interests us. A series of such maps for various (fixed) values of z then will give a feel for the properties of the distribution. Color coding is common and makes detailed contour plots easier to read.

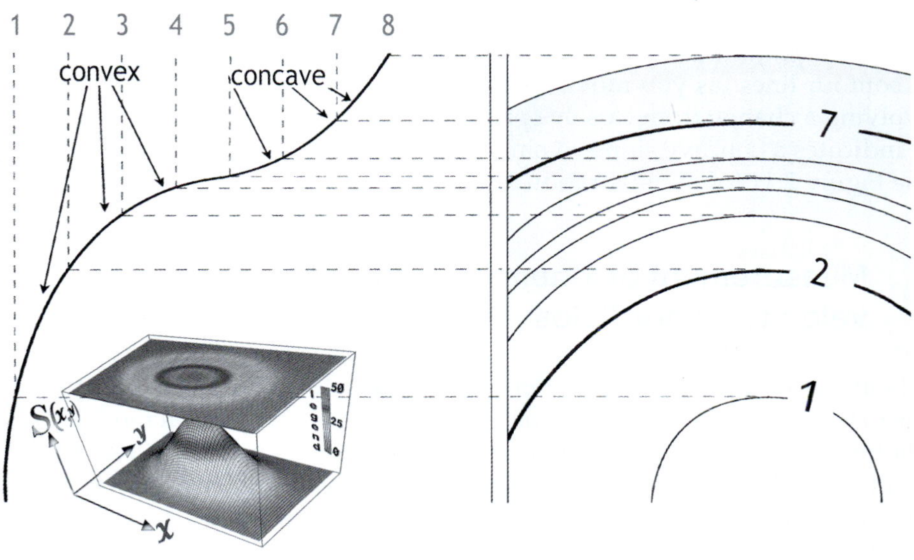

Figure 2.11: Widely spaced contour lines indicate low spatial rates of change or "slopes;" closely spaced contour lines indicate steep slopes. Slopes can be convex or concave. As is shown in the inset, a vivid way to portray a field is to fix one of the spatial dimensions, and then plot the value of the function as a height *vs.* the remaining spatial coordinates, i.e., as a *relief map*. The inset also depicts the geometry of 3-D–to–2-D orthogonal contour projection of a scalar quantity distribution in an $x-y$ plane (cf. Fig. 4.1 on p. 167).

Generally, if $f(x, y, z)$ is a function of three variables and c is a constant, then $f(x, y, z) = c$ is a surface in space, which is called a contour surface, or a level surface; e.g., if $f(x, y, z) = 4x_2+3y_2+z_2$, then the contour surfaces are ellipsoids. A contour line, or "level curve," traces a path of constant level of intensity or magnitude. Contour lines are also called *isovalue lines*, or *isolines*. The distance between adjacent contour lines, the "contour interval," will vary depending on local rates of change of magnitude of the quantity in different regions within the overall field. The contour interval will not vary on a single contour map, although some areas on a single map may have supplementary contour lines that fall between the regular contour lines. Contour intervals leave out any small-scale features that fall within their contour interval. Contour intervals are only representative of the general shape and slope of the distribution of the quantity that they depict, because they are limited by the resolution of the contour interval. To assess approximate magnitude values for points that do not lie on contour lines, we interpolate. With experience, a contour map user can learn to "read between the lines" and get more out of contour intervals than their literal intensity or magnitude content.

The overall pattern of the distribution of a flow-field quantity in cross-section is the most valuable information to read from a set of contour lines. Pattern is discerned by noting the curves and angles in the contour lines, both individually and in relationship to each other. Slope is directly related to spacing of contour lines. Widely spaced contour lines indicate gentle spatial rates of change or "slopes," and closely spaced contour lines indicate steep slopes (see Fig. 2.11). An important aspect of a slope is whether it is convex or concave. A pattern involving a change from widely spaced contour lines to closely spaced contour lines (as you move across) indicates a convex slope. On the other hand, one involving a change from closely spaced to widely spaced contour lines (as you move across) indicates a concave slope. A single slope can exhibit both characteristics; you can examine Figure 2.11 for an illustration of this situation.

2.5.2 Measurement of kinematic characteristics of velocity vector fields

Methods are available, generically denoted as particle image velocimetry (PIV), which allow us to visualize many flow kinematic characteristics in physical models of flow fields of cardiological interest—e.g., flow attributes of artificial heart valves. In these methods, small neutrally buoyant plastic polystyrene, polyamide, or hollow glass spheres in the range of 5–100 μm are dispersed homogeneously ("seeded") in the operating fluid (water). Any particle that follows the flow satisfactorily and scatters enough light to be captured by a digital camera can be used. The flow is lit with a series of pulses in a light plane so that only a sheet of the flow, the "plane of interrogation," becomes visible. The spheres move with the flow and show the path lines followed by fluid particles. In *single frame/single exposure* PIV, photographs are taken with an extended exposure time, such that each particle produces a streak the length of which is proportional to the local value of the velocity (cf. Marey's chronophotography method, depicted in Fig. 4.6, on p. 182). We may thus visualize the overall flow field in detail.

The use of a video recorder adds a further feature—the slow motion and looping effects permit us to scrutinize the flow in its development, and to repeat the observation as often as needed. Using these video recordings, we can quantify the flow field with methods of image processing. In *single frame/multiexposure* PIV and in *multiframe/*

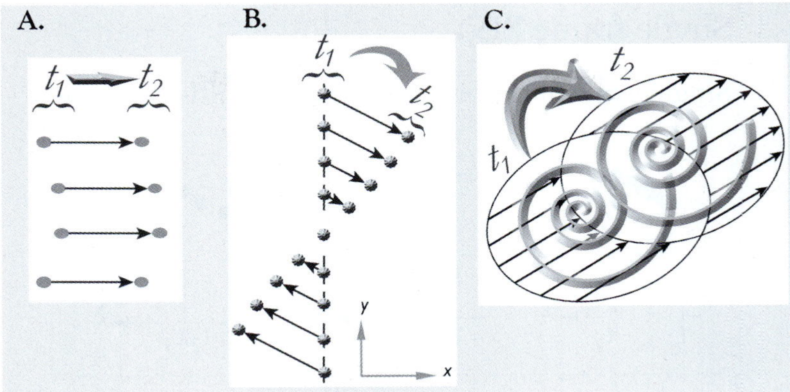

Figure 2.12: Velocity field kinematics. A. and B.: a point with spatial coordinates (x, y) at time t_1, has moved to another point with coordinates $(x+\delta x, y+\delta y)$ at time t_2. Velocity vector components, v_x, and v_y, are obtained by dividing the displacements by $(t_2 - t_1)$. C.: The evolution of coherent flow structures, e.g., eddies, can be visualized.

multiexposure PIV, we can calculate the velocity field from the displacement of the particles between different light pulse times, as shown in Figure 2.12. Such particle methods (Fig. 2.13) render an overview of characteristic patterns of motion within the flow field studied, and provide instantaneous velocity vector measurements in selected cross-sections of a flow field.

Two velocity components, e.g., v_x, and v_y are measured at all points with spatial coordinates (x, y) in each successive plane of interrogation in standard PIV systems; the third velocity component (v_z) is "invisible" due to the geometry of the imaging. This third velocity component can be derived by using two cameras in a stereoscopic arrangement. Use of such a stereoscopic approach permits recording of all three velocity components, resulting in instantaneous 3-D velocity vectors for the whole flow field.

2.6 The divergence

As we have just seen, a vector field is just a way of describing some quantity that is a vector [78]. For example, gravitational force is a vector. If, instead of a single point in a region of interest we want to refer to all points, we consider the gravitational field. Consider the gravitational force near a planet. It decreases in magnitude away from the planet's surface, but always has a direction toward the center of the planet. Vector fields that represent fluid flow velocity have an immediate physical interpretation: the vector at every point in space represents a direction of motion and speed of the corresponding fluid element. In such a vector field representation, we put arrows representing the field direction on a rectangular grid. The direction of the arrow at a given location represents the direction of the velocity at that point; we also make the length of the vector

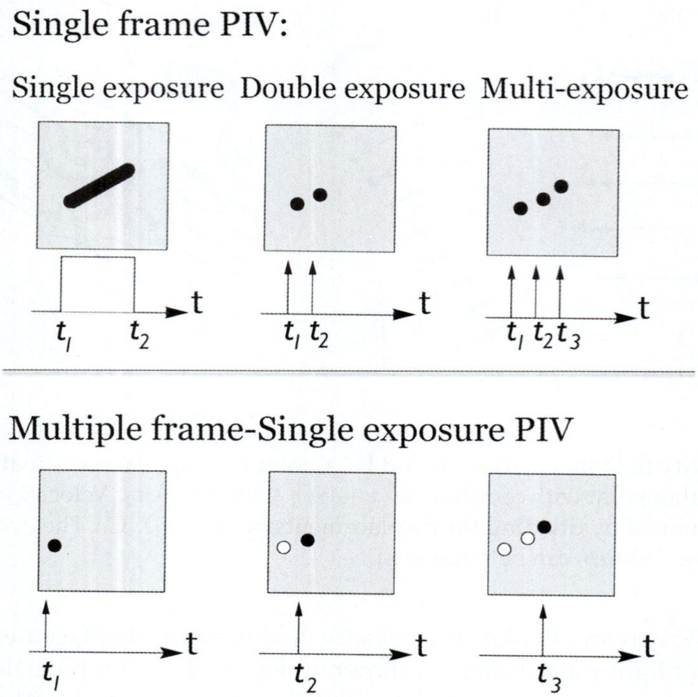

Figure 2.13: Representative techniques of Particle Image Velocimetry, PIV.

proportional to the magnitude of the velocity at that point. Sometimes we show only the direction, with all the vectors of the same length, and color-code the arrows according to the magnitude of the velocity.

The divergence ($\nabla\cdot$) quantifies the rate of change of a vector field and is a scalar field. It does not give any information about how that vector field changes with direction, it just gives a measure of how much a vector field $\mathbf{F}(x, y, z, t)$ is contracting or spreading apart at any given point. It is defined for three dimensions as

$$\nabla \cdot \mathbf{F}(x, y, z) = \frac{\partial F_x}{\partial x} + \frac{\partial F_y}{\partial y} + \frac{\partial F_z}{\partial z}. \tag{2.16}$$

The character used in the derivatives is a modified Greek delta (∂), and not a Roman d. This signifies that the derivatives are partial derivatives. A partial derivative of a function of more than one variable is a derivative that is taken with respect to one variable while holding the others fixed. For two dimensions, the partial with respect to z drops out.

In studying fluid flow, it is useful to think of a fluid parcel or particle, i.e., a notional bounded small volume of flowing fluid. Generally, an ideal fluid parcel can expand and contract along its path but cannot mix with the surrounding fluid. In other words, the volume of an ideal parcel is variable while its mass is constant. The divergence of the

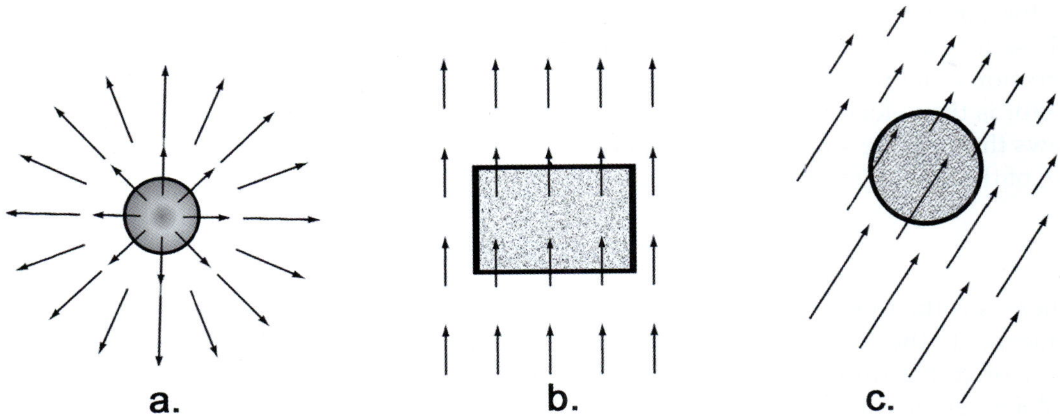

Figure 2.14: Velocity field regions with: **a.** positive, **b.** zero, and **c.** negative, divergences on the plane of the figure.

velocity field is a useful measure of compression (negative divergence) or expansion (positive divergence) undergone by the flowing fluid and of the corresponding compressive or distending stress on flowing fluid parcels or objects in the flow. In a diverging flow, fluid particles appear to magically materialize and "diverge" from a *source*; in the converse situation, fluid particles appear to "converge" toward a *sink* of particles, where they magically disappear. A fluid flow is incompressible if the divergence of the velocity is zero

$$\nabla \cdot \mathbf{v}(x, y, z) = \frac{\partial v_x}{\partial x} + \frac{\partial v_y}{\partial y} + \frac{\partial v_z}{\partial z}. \tag{2.17}$$

An incompressible flow that slows down along the flow axis must spread out in the other directions, and *vice versa*. If $\nabla\cdot\mathbf{v}(x, y, z) > 0$ in an incompressible flow region of a flow field, the flow is diverging (fluid is flowing out of a "source" in the flow field; cf. Fig. 2.14 a.). If $\nabla\cdot\mathbf{v}(x, y, z) < 0$ in an incompressible region of the flow field, the flow is converging (fluid is flowing into a "sink" in the flow field, for which the direction of the velocity vectors is reversed from that in Fig. 2.14 a.). A flow field's divergence at a given point describes the *strength* of the source, or sink, there. So, integrating the field's divergence over the interior of the region should equal the integral of the velocity field over the region's boundary. The divergence theorem of vector calculus, which is introduced in the next section says that this is true.

2.6.1 Flux and divergence of a vector

Consider a vector field that passes through a specified surface in space. For each element of this surface, the product of a surface element times the normal component of the field vector can be represented by the scalar product of the field vector with another vector whose length is equal to the area of the element and whose direction coincides with the direction of a line perpendicular to the element pointing outward (Fig. 2.15). If the field vector is the velocity of a fluid flow, **v**, then the product is the volume flux of liquid that flows through the surface element per unit time at the instant considered. Thus, the flux, dQ, of the velocity vector **v** through a surface element **ds** is defined as

$$dQ = \mathbf{v} \cdot \mathbf{ds} = \mathbf{v} \cdot \hat{\mathbf{s}}\, ds, \tag{2.18}$$

where, $\hat{\mathbf{s}}$ is the unit vector normal to the surface element of area size ds, so that $\mathbf{ds} = \hat{\mathbf{s}}\, ds$ is normal to the surface element as shown in Figure 2.15. If you find its representation as a vector counterintuitive, consider then that any surface element has both a magnitude and a given orientation. Hence,

$$dQ = \mathbf{v} \cdot \mathbf{ds} = \mathbf{v} \cdot \hat{\mathbf{s}}\, ds = v\, \cos\theta\, ds \tag{2.19}$$

and $v\ cos\ \theta$ is the component of **v** normal to the surface. Obviously, to obtain the flow through the surface, we only need to consider the component of **v** perpendicular to the surface; the flow along the surface is not relevant. Notice that the largest value of dQ occurs when $\theta = 0°$ (since $\cos 0° = 1$), and that $dQ = 0$ if $\theta = 90°$ (since $\cos\ 90° = 0$), so that in the latter case **v** does not cross the surface at all but is instead tangent to the surface. The integral of this product over the entire surface has a physical significance. It represents the volume of fluid crossing the surface per unit time at the instant considered.

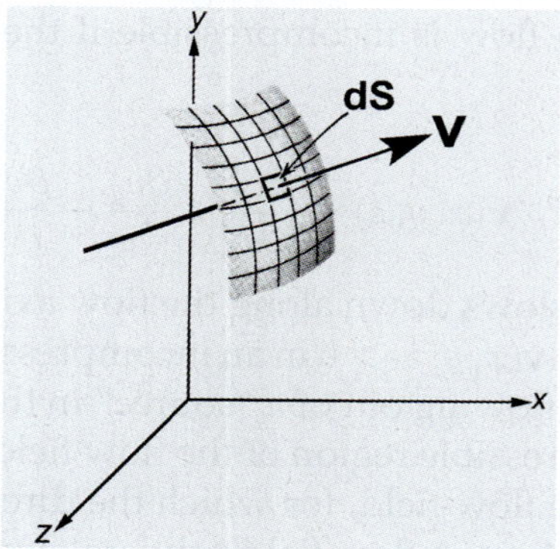

Figure 2.15: The flux, dQ, of the velocity vector **v** through a surface element **ds**, of a surface traversed by the fluid, is defined as $dQ = \mathbf{v} \cdot \mathbf{ds}$.

If the vector field is tangent to a surface, then the flux through the surface is obviously zero. The total flux of the velocity vector across the whole surface (rather than just a surface element) is

$$Q = \int_S \mathbf{v} \cdot \mathbf{ds}, \tag{2.20}$$

where the integral is evaluated over the entire surface, S. There are two types of surfaces, i.e., open surfaces and closed surfaces. A closed surface encloses a volume V, as is the case with a sphere. If the surface is closed so that it bounds a finite volume, then **ds** points outward from the volume. In this case the "Divergence Theorem" of Gauss gives

$$\int_S \mathbf{v} \cdot \mathbf{ds} = \int_V \nabla \cdot \mathbf{v} \, dV, \tag{2.21}$$

where the left integral is evaluated over the bounding surface, and the right over the enclosed volume. $\nabla \cdot \mathbf{v}$ is the divergence of the velocity. Hence, as is implied by this equation, it represents the net outgoing flux per unit volume and, in the general case of *compressible* flow, we have three important deductions (cf. Fig. 2.14, on p. 55):

1. If $\nabla \cdot \mathbf{v} = 0$, there is no net inflow into, or outflow out of, the region bounded by the given surface.
2. If $\nabla \cdot \mathbf{v} > 0$, the flow in the region is diverging, and (on balance) fluid flows out of the volume bounded by the given surface.
3. If $\nabla \cdot \mathbf{v} < 0$, the flow is converging, and fluid is flowing into the given volume.

The Divergence Theorem is a conservation law, since it states that the volumetric total of all sinks and sources, the volume integral of the divergence, is equal to the net flow across a flow region's boundary. With incompressible flow, the divergence is always zero, since no fluid mass is created or destroyed by the flow process itself. However, the illustrations in Figure 2.14 are still applicable *on the plane of the figure*; *compensatory* divergence components occur then, as needed, in the direction of the third coordinate axis, perpendicularly to the plane shown.

2.7 The gradient

Vector calculus deals with rates of change of functions in multiple spatial dimensions. For example, consider the elevation of a hill as a function of latitude and longitude. At a given point, you would like to know in what direction is the ground sloping, and how steeply. The function that would be used for this is called the gradient ($\vec{\nabla}$). While elevation is a scalar function, its slope has a direction as well as magnitude associated with it and is thus a vector. The gradient is a vector derivative of a scalar function and, letting f be the scalar function, it is defined in three dimensions as

$$\vec{\nabla} f(x,y,z) = \frac{\partial f}{\partial x}\boldsymbol{i} + \frac{\partial f}{\partial y}\boldsymbol{j} + \frac{\partial f}{\partial z}\boldsymbol{k}. \tag{2.22}$$

In other words, its component along each coordinate (or in any other desired direction) is equal to the partial derivative along that coordinate or direction; the arrow over ∇ is a reminder of the vectorial nature of the result of its operation on the scalar field $f(x,y,z)$.

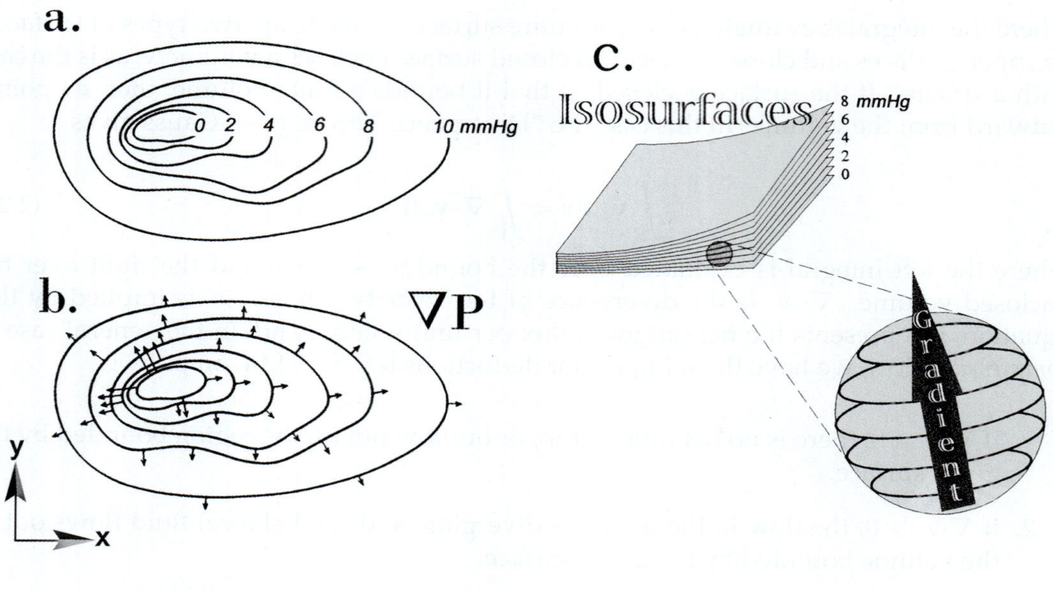

Figure 2.16: The gradient is just the generalization of slope to functions of more than one variable. **a.** Contour lines for 2-D pressure field (isobars). **b.** Vector field representing the corresponding pressure gradient: the gradient arrows are pointing in the direction of the maximum local rate of pressure *increase*, whereas the local pressure gradient force (not shown) would point in the opposite direction. **c.** 3-D representation in terms of *isosurfaces* and a local gradient vector.

The base vectors in 3-D Cartesian coordinates are the unit vector $\boldsymbol{i}$ in the positive direction of the x axis, the unit vector $\boldsymbol{j}$ in the y direction, and the unit vector $\boldsymbol{k}$ in the z direction. For two dimensions, the z-component drops off.

The gradient corresponds in length and in direction to the *maximal* rate of increase of the scalar function $f(x, y, z)$ from the point under consideration. Its direction is along that of the maximum rate of *increase* of $f(x, y, z)$; its magnitude equals the local value of the slope of $f(x, y, z)$. If we plot 2-D contours of constant pressure (p = constant), these "isocurves," or "level surfaces," are called "isobars" and $\vec{\nabla} p\,(x, y, z)$ crosses the isobars at right angles.

2.7.1 Pressure gradient force

Pressure is a scalar, but force is a vector; so we might expect on vector considerations alone that the two are related by the gradient. The force that tends to move a fluid as a bulk medium is due to a difference in pressure between two regions. Consider a cube of fluid where the pressure is lower on one of its sides than on the opposite one. The imbalance in pressure from one side of the cube to the other leads to a force in the direction of decreasing pressure. This "pressure gradient force" acts from areas of high pressure to areas of low pressure, and tends to drive flow from high-pressure areas to low-pressure areas. When expressed per unit volume of the fluid, it is equal in magnitude to the gradient of the pressure. However, the pressure gradient force or pressure difference force points in the direction *opposite* to the pressure gradient (see Fig. 2.16, on p. 58): physically the pressure gradient force pushes fluid away from regions of higher pressure to regions of lower pressure.

2.8 Circular motion

Imagine that a particle is subject to a force whose direction may change but whose magnitude remains constant. The particle's acceleration at any instant will be in the direction of the force at that instant. The change in the particle's velocity over a very short time will be a vector in the direction of the average acceleration. The new velocity at the end of this time interval will be the vector sum of the original velocity and the change in velocity. Now suppose that the changing direction of the force is such that the force is always perpendicular to the velocity. In this case, the force will bend the path of the particle into a circular line and the force vector and therefore the acceleration, **a**, will point toward the center of the circle (cf. Fig. 2.17). Under these conditions, the magnitude of the velocity

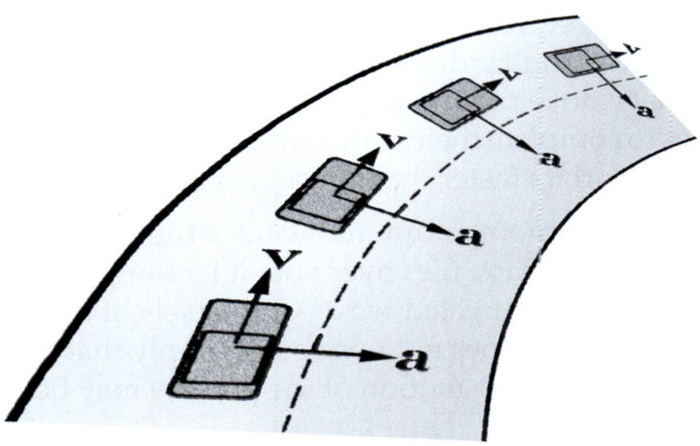

Figure 2.17: Any mass, such as a car, going around a bend at constant speed is nevertheless changing its velocity; it is accelerating. If the accelerating force is of constant magnitude (**A**) and acts always perpendicular to its velocity (v), then the car is deviating from its straight course at the same rate at every point of the bend, i.e., it goes around in a curve of constant curvature—a circle.

remains constant, and we have a uniform circular motion, meaning that the speed of the particle is constant. The magnitude of the acceleration, a, equals v^2/r, where v and r denote the magnitudes of velocity and radius, respectively. Any particle, or fluid parcel in a flow field, which moves in uniform circular motion, has an acceleration of magnitude v^2/r with a direction perpendicular to the velocity. Since the velocity is tangent to the circle, the acceleration vector is centripetal, i.e., it points toward the circle's center.

More generally, the path may be curved but not circular, and then the direction of the acceleration is along the *local* radius of curvature of the path. This centripetal acceleration contributes only to the change in direction of the particle, since it is perpendicular to the path and therefore cannot affect its speed along the path. If the total acceleration includes an additional component tangent to the path then the speed of the particle is affected as well.

By Newton' s Second Law of motion, the angular acceleration of a rotating object is directly proportional to the net force acting on it and inversely proportional to its inertial mass. Moment of inertia is the name given to rotational inertia, the rotational analog of mass for linear motion. It depends on mass and, most importantly, on how that mass is distributed with respect to the axis. For example, a large-diameter cylinder will have greater rotational inertia than one of equal mass but smaller diameter. The large-diameter cylinder will be harder to start rotating and harder to stop, because of the tendency to conserve angular momentum. When the mass is concentrated further away from the axis of rotation, the rotational inertia is greater.

For example, a skater doing a spin on ice rotates at a relatively slow speed with arms outstretched. But when they are brought close to the body and the axis of rotation, the spin becomes much faster, because the moment of inertia is reduced (cf. Fig. 14.25, on p. 792). Since the angular momentum remains constant, if the moment of inertia decreases, then the angular velocity must increase. This is the result of conservation of angular momentum. Celestial bodies also provide familiar demonstrations of the principle of conservation of angular momentum. Comets move rapidly when they come close to the sun, and then sometimes can take centuries to complete their path and return. Planets that are closer to the sun move around their elliptic orbits faster than those that are farther away.

A body can have angular momentum about the origin without any rotation being involved. When a northbound plane flies over you, it has angular momentum about you; its angular momentum vector is directed west. Conversely, if a fluid particle moves in a circular, or in any curved path, it does not necessarily imply that the particle itself rotates (see Fig. 2.18, on p. 61). The circular motion of the particle may be:

1. rotational—corresponds to the moon circling the earth while undergoing rotation, so as to keep the same "side" toward the earth.[6]

2. irrotational—corresponds to the irrotational mode of the hanging cars of a turning Ferris wheel.

2.9 Forced vortex motion

A flow with fluid particle rotation is that corresponding to a "forced vortex." Such a forced vortex is formed in a water containing cylindrical jar whose wall is suddenly set

[6]The moon is, in fact, *spiraling* centrifugally away from the earth, as a comparison of ancient and contemporary "growth rhythms" of the *Nautilus*, itself *spiral-shaped*, has confirmed [42].

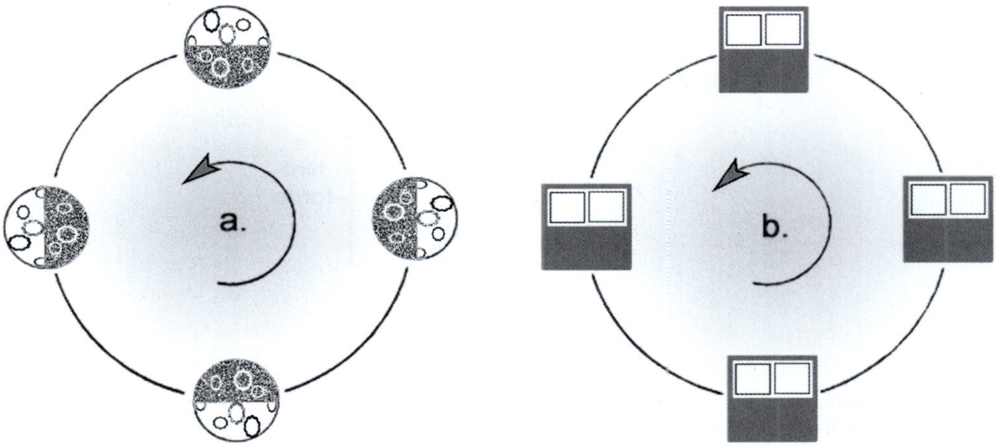

Figure 2.18: a. Circular motion *with* fluid particle rotation: Moon circling the earth always keeping the *same* side toward the center of orbit. This is also characteristic of rigid-body rotation. b. Circular motion *without* fluid particle rotation: turning Ferris wheel—a wheel rotating in the vertical plane at a constant angular speed carrying seated passengers (fluid particles).

into rotation at a constant angular velocity, about a vertical axis (see Fig. 2.19, on p. 62). We will have a propagation of momentum from one neighboring layer to the next by radial diffusion from the rotating curved walls. Convection due to hydrodynamic flows cannot, in fact, contribute to this propagation, because the water moves in a tangential direction, *perpendicular* to the radius. After a time, a steady state will be established[7] in which the vessel together with its contents will rotate as a single solid body, and all water particles will be rotating with uniform angular velocity, while the tangential velocity at any point will naturally be proportional to the radius. The water surface at any point must be normal to the total resultant force acting on a particle of water at that point. Because of the centrifugal force acting in addition to gravity, the total resultant force will have an inclination to the vertical, as shown in Figure 2.19. Consequently, the water surface, being normal to the *total resultant force,* is not horizontal—it forms part of a paraboloid of revolution. The surface curvature is crucial in neutralizing the centrifugal force.

The preceding description is rigorously true for an *infinitely* long cylinder. In a real situation, the bottom of the container creates an effect that eventually dominates the manner in which the velocity profile evolves at long times. The bottom layer of fluid in the jar is also set into rotational motion by viscous shear with the rotating *bottom wall,* i.e., independently of the effect of the curved container wall. A radial component of flow thus results, directed toward the axis of rotation. Near the bottom, momentum is no longer transferred toward the interior of the cylinder just by diffusion, but also by convection. This phenomenon is an example of *secondary flow,* a flow induced by, and superposed on, the principal flow field (see Section 9.5.5, on pp. 469 f., and Fig. 14.26, on p. 793).

[7] This will come about under the action of viscous shear forces (see Section 4.6, on pp. 190 f.), which will damp out all relative motion.

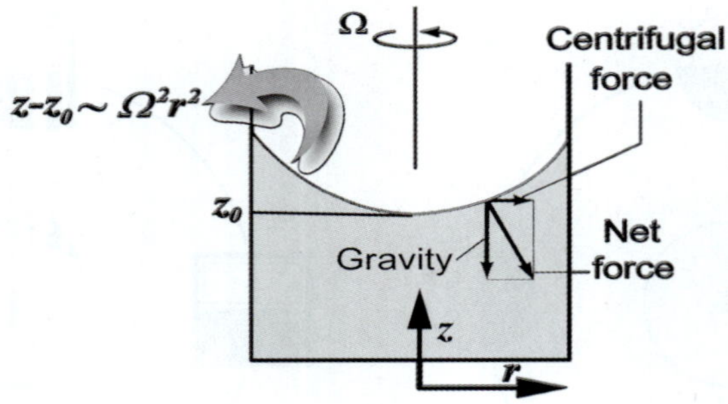

Figure 2.19: Elevation, z, of equilibrium surface of a rotating fluid in an open container, as function of radial coordinate, r. The surface slope is such that gravitational and local centrifugal forces combine into a net force everywhere aligned with the local normal to the surface—Ω is the angular velocity of the vessel and contents in "rigid-body" rotation.

2.10 The curl and vorticity

The curl, $\nabla\times$, tells us whether the flow field is twisting. Examples of this would be the bathtub vortex or a whirlpool in the sea. As you get closer to the whirlpool center, the spiraling velocity of the flow gets faster, and if you were to enter its region of influence in a canoe, the canoe would start to spin. This spinning motion of the water is a measure of the curl of the velocity. Conversely, the curl of the velocity quantifies the (local) intensity of rotation in the flow—it increases with the rotation rate.[8]

The curl of a velocity (or other vector) field is not a vector[9] although, like a vector, in three dimensions it is determined by three values as shown by

$$\nabla\times\mathbf{v}(x,y,z) = \left[\frac{\partial v_z}{\partial y} - \frac{\partial v_y}{\partial z}, \frac{\partial v_x}{\partial z} - \frac{\partial v_z}{\partial x}, \frac{\partial v_y}{\partial x} - \frac{\partial v_x}{\partial y}\right]. \tag{2.23}$$

However, it can be represented by a vector with length equal to the absolute value of the curl and direction normal to the plane of rotation. The curl of the velocity is given the special name, "vorticity," and it represents the amount of twisting or twirling in a flow. When the vorticity is zero, the flow is irrotational. Physically, a fluid particle in an irrotational flow keeps the same orientation (see Fig. 2.18).

2.11 The Laplacian

For functions of a single variable, a useful function is the second derivative. Thus, for motion in a straight line the second derivative of position is the acceleration. The corre-

[8] This accounts for why in European languages (e.g., Dutch, French, German, Italian) the notation *rot* **v** is used rather than *curl* **v**.

[9] It is sometimes called a pseudo-vector. It behaves like a vector otherwise, but, mathematically, it is a tensor.

sponding quantity for fields is the Laplacian ($\nabla^2 \equiv \nabla \cdot \nabla$), spoken as "del square," which is the divergence of the gradient of a scalar field. The Laplacian applies to a scalar function of position and is a scalar operator; if it is applied to a scalar field, it generates a scalar field.[10] The Laplacian is a measure of the difference between the value of a scalar function $f(x, y, z)$ at a point and its average value in an infinitesimal[11] neighborhood of this point.

Considering the elevation of a hill, if the gradient gave the steepness of the land, the Laplacian would give its curvature. The Laplacian of a scalar field $f(x, y, z)$ is given for three dimensions by

$$\nabla^2 f(x, y, z) = \frac{\partial^2 f}{\partial x^2} + \frac{\partial^2 f}{\partial y^2} + \frac{\partial^2 f}{\partial z^2} \,. \tag{2.24}$$

In two dimensions, only the x and y components apply. As an example of the use of the Laplacian, heat will diffuse through an otherwise uniform medium such that the Laplacian of the temperature becomes zero.

2.12 Average and instantaneous derivatives

Many quantities of interest in physiology and fluid dynamics deal with how a variable quantity, such as pressure or a fluid parcel's position, is changing in a flow field. For example, the velocity of a fluid parcel tells us how fast, and in what direction, its position is changing; accordingly, it is a vectorial quantity.

Setting aside directional aspects pertaining to the vectorial nature of velocity, the *speed* is defined as the rate of change, or the "derivative," of position with respect to time. To calculate the speed of an object, we observe how far an object went, and divide by the amount of time it took it to get there. However, the problem with this average derivative is that the answer will depend upon how much time you allow to pass when you make the calculation. The average speed over some finite time interval is defined in the way we think of the average rate of change, as the change in position divided by the change in elapsed time

$$v_{average} = \Delta x / \Delta t. \tag{2.25}$$

This definition of speed looks much like the definition of the slope, m, of a line

$$m = \Delta y / \Delta x. \tag{2.26}$$

The average speed, then, is just the slope of a line between two points on a plot of position *vs.* time.

In computational applications of fluid dynamics, we generally approximate derivatives by the "average" method over very small time intervals, but for some functions we can also specify the "instantaneous" value. The instantaneous velocity at a specific time is the velocity of the object of interest at that exact time. If we take the average rate of

[10] By convention, however, the Laplacian of a vector is meant to be a vector whose components are the Laplacians of the components of the original vector, in rectangular coordinates [59].

[11] Infinitesimal values are immeasurably small and capable of having values that approach zero as a limit.

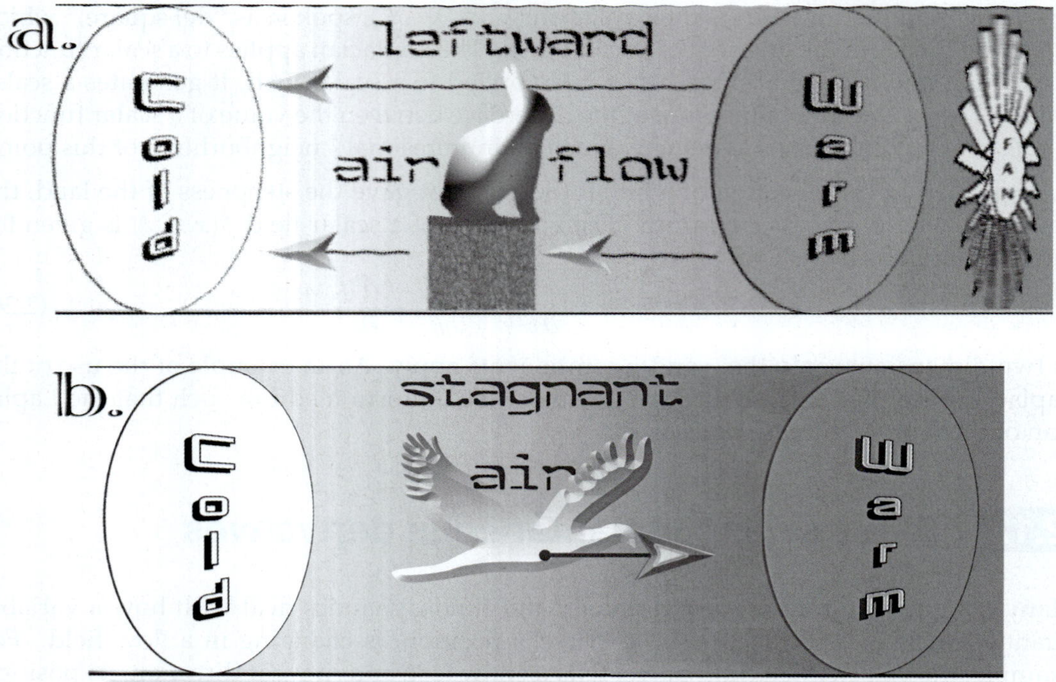

Figure 2.20: a. A stationary "observer," such as the sitting rabit, experiences an increase in temperature because the *local* temperature rises as a result of warm air flowing from right to left by the observer. b. A *moving* observer, such as the flying eagle, moves through a temperature field that is *constant* at each location. This "observer" detects an increase in temperature because he is *moving* through warmer-and-warmer regions.

change, and make the time interval over which we compute it smaller and smaller, we eventually arrive at a value that gets close to the instantaneous value of the derivative; e.g., the speed shown on the speedometer of a car is an instantaneous value.

Since the time interval over which we look at the change can never be *exactly* zero (if there is no change in time, how can there be change in position?) we have to consider what happens as the interval gets smaller and smaller. Technically, this means that the number we are trying to find for the instantaneous derivative, i.e., velocity, is the *limit*[12] that the value of $\Delta x/\Delta t$ approaches as Δt gets smaller and smaller. We write this as:

$$\frac{dx}{dt} = \lim_{\Delta t \to 0} \frac{\Delta x}{\Delta t}. \tag{2.27}$$

The limit as Δt approaches 0 of the function $\Delta x/\Delta t$ is said to be equal to the instantaneous derivative dx/dt, if the value of $\Delta x/\Delta t$ gets "closer and closer" to dx/dt as Δt gets "closer and closer" to 0. The instantaneous velocity is the slope of the tangent, a line drawn parallel to the curve of position as a function of time, at a specific time.

[12]The idea of a limit in the present sense goes back at least as far as Archimedes.

2.13 Total and partial time derivatives

We know from observation of various flows in nature—e.g., leaves, or debris, carried in a stream or a river—that the velocity of a fluid particle changes with time when the particle moves to a different location. This principle of a temporal change that is caused by a *motion* in the system is very general.

As an example, consider the situation in Figure 2.20, on p. 64, where an observer senses the temperature. In panel *a.*, warm air is transported leftward by the motion of the wind. The observer—the sitting rabbit—detects an increase of the temperature with time, so that $\partial T/\partial t > 0$. Note that in this expression the *partial* derivative symbol is used. In general, the temperature field is a function of both time and the space coordinates. For the stationary observer the space coordinates are fixed, which means that any change detected by him is due to the temporal change of the *local* temperature only. This is expressed by the partial derivative with respect to time, in which the time is varied but all other variables are kept unchanging. Let us now consider the situation in panel *b.* of Figure 2.20: here, an observer—the eagle—is flying along a temperature field that is constant with respect to time, so that $\partial T/\partial t = 0$. Now, the observer is moving from a cold region to a warmer region. This means that, just like the observer in panel *a.*, this second observer experiences an increase in the temperature. The total rate of change of the temperature is denoted by the *total* time derivative DT/Dt. This example demonstrates that DT/Dt can be larger than zero while $\partial T/\partial t = 0$.

Recapitulating, both observers in panels *a.* and *b.* detect a rise in temperature, but their description of this temperature change is completely different. The stationary rabbit feels an increase in temperature because the *local* temperature changes at his *fixed location*; this is described by the partial time derivative. The eagle detects an increase in temperature because he is *moving* to a warmer region in a *fixed temperature* field. This is described by the *convective* (pertaining to convection, or flow) time derivative. As a general rule, if the temperature field depends on all three space coordinates and on time, it may vary because of a combination of a change in the temperature at a fixed location and a movement of the observer; i.e., $T = T(x(t), y(t), z(t), t)$. In this notation it is shown explicitly that the space coordinates of any observation point depend on time as well. The total change in temperature is embodied in the *total* time derivative, DT/Dt, which is the instantaneous sum of the *local*, $\partial T/\partial t$, and the *convective*, $\mathbf{v} \cdot \nabla T$, components, where $\mathbf{v}$ denotes the velocity of the eagle and air behaves as an incompressible fluid, for our present intent.

The temperature field was used in this section only for illustrative purposes. The analysis applies to any function that depends on both time and the space coordinates. Also, in the analysis we brought into play "observers" to fix our minds. However, in general there are no observers and it is not imperative for anybody to be present to "observe" the change. The total time derivative is always related to the movement of a certain quantity. In the description of intracardiac blood flow, it concerns the motion of a parcel of blood that is being carried around by the flow. It should be noted that in the case of intracardiac flows there is an *additional* component of convective acceleration: it is contributed by the movement—contraction or expansion—of the walls of the cardiac chambers during pumping. To simplify understanding, consider, e.g., uniform radial collapse of the walls of a cylindical segment whose upstream end is closed and whose downstream end is open. By continuity considerations, to account for the flow contributed by the collapsing walls, the axial velocities will be higher as we move from the upstream end toward the downstream orifice. This implies a convective acceleration component attributable to the chamber wall movement. Its contribution to the axial velocity v_x is included in the expression $(\mathrm{v} \cdot \nabla)v_x$, which is the component in the x-direction of the vector $(\mathrm{v} \cdot \nabla)\mathrm{v}$.

2.14 Integration

To a mathematician, integration is about the accumulation [49] of change. It generally has three main applications, which are

1. The antiderivative (also referred to as indefinite integral): finding the family of functions that, if you take the derivative of any of them, you get the same desired result.

2. The integral (also referred to as definite integral): finding the area in between a curve, $y(x)$, on the x–y plane and the x-axis, between specified values of x.

3. Integration: the tracking of change undergone by a system over time, given some initial state of the system.

2.14.1 Antiderivatives

The first application listed above is the process of finding antiderivatives. The antiderivative of a function $f(x)$ is the function $g(x)$ whose derivative is equal to the original function, or $dg(x)/dx = f(x)$. However, since the derivative of a constant is zero, for any function there are more than one antiderivatives. The integral is not unique. For instance, consider the lines $g_1(x) = 5x + 6$ and $g_2(x) = 5x + 12$. Both have a slope of 5. Both of them could be considered the antiderivative of the function $f(x) = 5$. When we determine an antiderivative, we write it as

$$\int f(x)dx = g(x) + c, \tag{2.28}$$

where, the addition of the constant c reminds us that there are actually an infinite number of solutions to the problem.

Generally, we do not want infinite solutions; we want the *appropriate* solution. We can use the initial value of the state of the system, or "initial condition," to determine what value of the integration constant c to use when finding the appropriate antiderivative. Thus, the exact value of the antiderivative is not uniquely defined, unless we know the initial value of the solution, and the solution changes as the initial value changes.

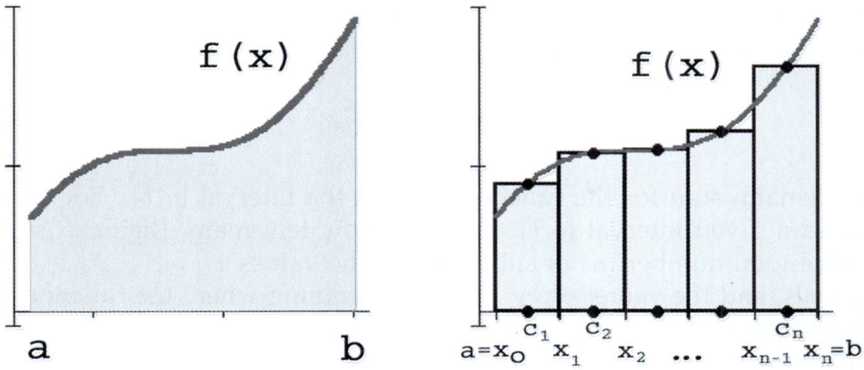

Figure 2.21: A continuous function $f(x)$ (left panel) and an approximation to this function that is constant within juxtaposed finite intervals (right panel). Rising out of the x-axis, Euclidean rectangles approximate the area underneath the curve $f(x)$. The area of the rectangles taken as a whole is the sum of their individual areas. The area beneath the curve is approximately the same as the area of the collection of those rectangles, amalgamated as the Riemann sum.

2.14.2 The area under a curve

The second application of integration entails finding the area under a curve. Consider the case of a car moving at constant velocity. Finding the distance, D, that the car covers is as simple as multiplying the time, t, over which the car drives by its velocity, $v : (D = v \times t)$. If we look at a graph of the constant velocity over time, the area between the line for velocity and the x-axis is given by v times t. The integral of velocity from the initial to the final time is just the area under the velocity *vs.* time curve. The same is true even if the velocity is not constant. The total amount of accumulated change in the position of the car moving at a variable velocity can generally be found by graphing the velocity of the car over time, and determining the area under the curve of the velocity from the initial to the final time—cf. the evaluation of the definite integral of $f(x)$ over x between the specific values a and b, in Figure 2.21.

Riemann Sum

To estimate the area between the x-axis and the graph of a function $f(x)$ on an interval $[a, b]$, we partition $[a, b]$ by choosing $(n - 1)$ points $x_1, x_2, \ldots, x_{n-1}$ in $[a, b]$, so that

$$a = x_0 < x_1 < \cdots < x_{n-1} < b = x_n.$$

On each subinterval $[x_{k-1}, x_k]$ we construct a rectangle of width $\Delta x_k = x_k - x_{k-1}$ and height $f(c_k)$ which reaches from the x-axis to the curve. If n is large enough, so that the width (x_k) of each strip is small, c_k can be any point between x_{k-1} and x_k, including the end points, without affecting appreciably the accuracy of the result.

By adding the areas of all the rectangular strips, we get an estimate for the area between the x-axis and $f(x)$. The sum

$$S = \sum_{k=1}^{n} \Delta x_k \cdot f(c_k) \tag{2.29}$$

is called a Riemann sum for the function $f(x)$ on the interval $[a, b]$. For a given function $f(x)$, and a given interval $[a, b]$, there are infinitely many Riemann sums, which depend on the total number (n) of subintervals, the values $x_1, x_2, \ldots, x_{n-1}$ determining the subintervals, and the values $c_1, c_2, \ldots, c_n$ determining where the function $f(x)$ is being sampled within each subinterval. To obtain a better approximation, a finer partition of $[a, b]$ (involving smaller subintervals) can be used. Of course, if the subintervals are narrower, there will be more of them. In the limit of $n \longrightarrow \infty$, which implies infinitely skinny rectangles, the area estimate of the Riemann sum will equal the true area under the curve, namely, the definite integral of $f(x)$ over x between a and b, which are the *limits* of integration.

Recapitulating, if the integral (the area under the curve) is taken between two specific values of *x*, the result is a single number, the area, and is called a *definite integral.* An *indefinite integral* is another function. To visualize it, we imagine that the first limit is x_0 and the second slides to the right from zero to infinity. As the right border moves, the two limits enclose more area, and the resulting area can be plotted against *x* and is considered a new function of *x*. The integral and the derivative are inverses of each other. That is, the derivative of the indefinite integral of *f(x)* is simply *f(x)* again, and *vice versa*, except for a possible additive constant.

2.14.3 Simpson's rule

The preceding simple linearization procedure depicted in Figure 2.21 provides a reasonable approximation to a definite integral, if we take a large number of steps. Clearly, the error in the approximation accrues from the fact that general graphs are curved and we are approximating them by straight linear segments. We can derive a formulation that takes into account the curvature of the graph; the result is a more efficient approximation referred to as *Simpson's rule.*[13] Simpson's rule is formed by approximating a general curve by a parabola. A parabola is the graph of a quadratic function $y = ax^2 + bx + c$; consequently, three pieces of information are needed to determine the coefficients a, b, and c. This implies that we must use three data points (x_0, y_0), (x_1, y_1), and (x_2, y_2), to specify the parabola.

Taking the width of each of the two intervals as $h = (b - a)/2$, it can be shown that:

$$\int_a^b f(x)dx \approx S_1 = \frac{h}{3}\left[y_0 + 4y_1 + y_2\right]. \tag{2.30}$$

[13] Simpson's rule, is named after Thomas Simpson (1710–1761), who developed it as a method for approximating the integrals of functions, assuming that they are nearly equal to the *quadratic arc* through three consecutive and equally spaced points.

This is Simpson's rule with one step. More generally, we can subdivide the interval into several slices and apply Simpson's rule on each subinterval. For instance, to use **n** steps, break the interval $[a, b]$ into $2n$ pieces, each of width $h = (b - a)/2n$. Call the **x** coordinates $x_0, x_1, \ldots, x_{2n-1}, x_{2n}$ and let $y_i = f(x_i)$. Then, we can obtain the general Simpson's rule equation:

$$\int_a^b f(x)dx \approx S_n = \left(\frac{h}{3}\right)[y_0 + 4y_1 + 2y_2 + 4y_3 + 2y_4 + \cdots + 4y_{2n-1} + y_{2n}]. \tag{2.31}$$

This is the same basic idea as the linearized sum depicted in Figure 2.21 on the preceding page, but here the algorithm is slightly different. Inside the sum, the end points are weighted once, while the odd values of y are weighted four times and the even values of y in the middle are weighted twice. This means that the coefficients for the "middle" terms alternate between 4 and 2, starting and ending with a 4 in the second and next-to-last term. Note that Simpson's rule must be used with an *even* number of subintervals (or "*strips*"), because each parabola is actually stretched across a *pair* of subintervals, not a single subinterval. The truncation error in Simpson's rule is proportional to h^4, i.e., it decreases with a decrease in strip width at the fourth power.

Simpson's rule is probably the most widely used approximation formula for numerical integration, and its extensive use is due to its simplicity, ease of application, and relatively high accuracy. In cardiac chamber imaging applications, where Simpson's rule is routinely employed, the data are less accurate than the formula, and consequently there is no need of considering the error due to the rule.

2.14.4 Accumulated change

Our understanding of physical processes commonly gives us direct knowledge of rates of change (or derivatives) of the quantities we are interested in, and not the quantities themselves. For example, Newton's law of gravity yields the acceleration (or the rate of change of velocity) of an object falling freely under the force of gravity. If we know the initial state, i.e., initial position and initial velocity of the object, we can accurately track the accumulated change in position of the object over time, and we can predict what the state of the system will be in the future.

The definition of velocity proceeded, in a previous Section, by taking the derivative of a variable, $\mathbf{P}(t)$, giving position as a function of time. One of the antiderivatives of velocity must be $\mathbf{P}(t)$. The vertical velocity function $v(t)$ of an object falling freely under the force of gravity is given by the integral of g, the constant acceleration due to gravity acting in the vertical direction, over the time of the free fall—note that the constraint "vertical" on velocity and gravitational acceleration causes these vectors to degenerate into scalar-like quantities

$$v(t) = \int g dt = g \cdot t + c_1. \tag{2.32}$$

The integral of the preceding vertical velocity function $v(t)$ over the time of the free fall

$$P(t) = \int v(t)dt = (1/2)g \cdot t^2 + c_1 \cdot t + c_2 \tag{2.33}$$

yields the vertical position $P(t)$.

In conclusion, note that to obtain $P(t)$ from acceleration, integration must be performed twice. Each integration yields a constant. The integration constants have a physical meaning. If no time of free fall has elapsed, $v(0) = c_1$ from the first integration equation. This observation reveals the physical meaning of c_1: it is the initial velocity of the falling object. Similarly, from the second integration equation

$$P(0) = c_2. \tag{2.34}$$

This observation in turn bestows c_2 its physical meaning: it is the initial vertical position, or height, of the falling object. Thus, if, e.g., the object is allowed to fall freely from a state of rest (zero initial velocity) at a height of 100 meters, after three seconds it will be at a height given by

$$P(3) = (1/2) \cdot (-9.81) \cdot 9 + 100 = 55.9\ m, \tag{2.35}$$

where, the acceleration force due to gravity amounts to $9.81\ m/s^2$ and is directed downward, i.e., in the negative z-axis direction (hence the minus sign).

2.15 Line and surface integrals

Vector functions, such as a velocity field and a force field, occur in physical applications involving fluid flow, and scalar products of these vector functions with another vector, such as distance or path length, appear with regularity. For instance, a line integral is used for the general definition of work in mechanics, as you may recall from a general physics course. When such a scalar product is summed over a path length where the magnitudes and directions change, that sum becomes an integral called a line integral. When the line integral is evaluated over a closed path, it is sometimes denoted as a cyclic integral, with a small circle superimposed on the integral sign; for instance, we define as circulation (see Section 9.3, on pp. 448 ff.) the line integral of the velocity, v, around any loop, or closed contour, L, within the flow field:

$$Circulation = \oint_L \mathbf{v} \cdot d\mathbf{l}.$$

An area integral of a vector function, such as velocity (**v**), can be defined as the integral on a surface, **A**, of the scalar product of **v** with the corresponding infinitesimal area element d**a**. The direction of the area element is defined to be perpendicular to the area at that point on the surface. The outward directed surface integral of the velocity over an entire closed surface, e.g., the net instantaneous volumetric outflow rate (Q) from a region, such as an ejecting ventricular chamber, enclosed by the surface **A** is denoted:

$$Q = \oiint_{\mathbf{A}} \mathbf{v} \cdot d\mathbf{a}.$$

2.16 The binary number system

Computers utilize the binary number system. In the binary system, information is extremely easy to store [17]. The binary system is based on only two numbers, zero and one, unlike our decimal system, which is based on numbers from zero through nine.[14] A system of ON and OFF switches is well suited to the binary system. Every 0 is marked by an OFF switch, and every 1 is marked by an ON switch. Binary digits are also very simple to work with mathematically; in fact, the computer can only do calculations on binary digits. Every time you calculate something on a computer using our standard decimal system, the computer converts it to binary, solves it, then converts it back to decimal and prints out the answer.

The binary system is the simplest number system, since it only has two numbers. One might think that the binary system is very complicated, but it is not. When you count in the decimal system, it goes like this: $0, 1, 2, 3, 4, 5, 6, 7, 8, 9$ and then you ran out of digits, so you make a two-digit number, 10. In the binary system, it is exactly analogous: $0, 1$, and you are out of digits. Now you make the binary number 10, which is equivalent to the decimal number 2. Then you go on: $10, 11, 100, 101$, and so on.

The binary numbering system works just like the decimal numbering system, with two exceptions: the binary only allows the digits 0 and 1 (rather than 0–9), and binary uses powers of two rather than of ten. Therefore, it is very easy to convert a binary number to decimal. For each "1" in the binary string, add in 2^n where "n" is the zero-based position of the binary digit. For example, the binary value 11001011 represents:

$$1 \cdot 2^7 + 1 \cdot 2^6 + 0 \cdot 2^5 + 0 \cdot 2^4 + 1 \cdot 2^3 + 0 \cdot 2^2 + 1 \cdot 2^1 + 1 \cdot 2^0 = 128 + 64 + 8 + 2 + 1 = 203. \quad (2.36)$$

To convert decimal to binary is conceptually the reverse, albeit slightly more cumbersome to implement, for most people.

2.16.1 Bits, bytes, and words

Bit is short for binary digit, the smallest unit of information on a machine. A single *bit* can hold only one of two values: 0, or 1. More information is accommodated by combining

[14]You can also think of the binary system as being based on powers of two, just as the decimal system is based on powers of 10. In the binary system you add another number place every time you reach another power of two ($2, 4, 8$, *etc.*) whereas in the decimal you add another place every time you reach a power of ten ($10, 100, 1000$, *etc.*).

consecutive bits into larger units. For example, a *byte* is composed of eight consecutive bits, numbered from zero to seven. *Bit* 0 is the low order *bit* or least significant *bit*, *bit* 7 is the high order *bit* or most significant *bit* of the byte. We refer to all other bits by their consecutive number. Since a byte contains eight bits, it can represent 2^8, or 256, different values. Generally, we use a byte to represent numeric values in the range $0, \ldots, 255$, and signed numbers in the range $-128, \ldots, +127$.

A computer *word* is a group of 16 bits. We number the bits in a word starting from zero on up to 15. Like the byte, *bit* 0 is the low order *bit* and *bit* 15 is the high order *bit*. When referencing the other bits in a word we use their *bit* position number. Observe that a word contains exactly two bytes. With 16 bits, you can represent 2^{16}, i.e., $65,536$ different values. These could be the values in the range $0, \ldots, 65,535$ or, as is usually the case, $-32,768, \ldots, +32,767$.

A *double word* is exactly what its name implies, a pair of words. Therefore, a double word quantity is 32 bits long, and encompasses four different bytes. Double words can represent 32-*bit* integer values; this allows encoding of unsigned numbers in the range $0, \ldots, 4,294,967,295$, and of signed ones in the range $-2,147,483,648, \ldots, 2,147,483,647$. 32-*bit* floating point values also fit into a double word. Analogous encoding considerations apply to 64-*bit* computer words, and so on.

2.17 Analog *vs.* digital signals and analog-to-digital conversion

A signal is a physical entity, such as a dc voltage or current, linearly proportional to pressure over a specified range. Signals are described by mathematical functions. In general, the particular function is only an approximation of the physical signal, especially when noise is considered. First, we need to distinguish between "continuous" *vs.* "discrete" and "analog" *vs.* "digital" signals [22,52,73,77].

i. Continuous-time signals are those signals that are defined at every instant of time over a continuous domain, such as an interval or a union of time intervals.

ii. Continuous-amplitude signals are those signals that can take any value coming from a continuous range; usually, this implies an uncountable number of possible values.

iii. Discrete-time signals are those signals that have a discrete domain—they take values only at a countable or (usually) finite set of points on the time line. Usually, these time instants are equally spaced.

iv. Discrete-amplitude signals are those signals that can take values only from a discrete range—a countable or (usually) finite set of values.

v. Analog signals are signals that are both continuous-time and continuous-amplitude.

vi. Digital signals are those signals that are both discrete-time and discrete-amplitude.

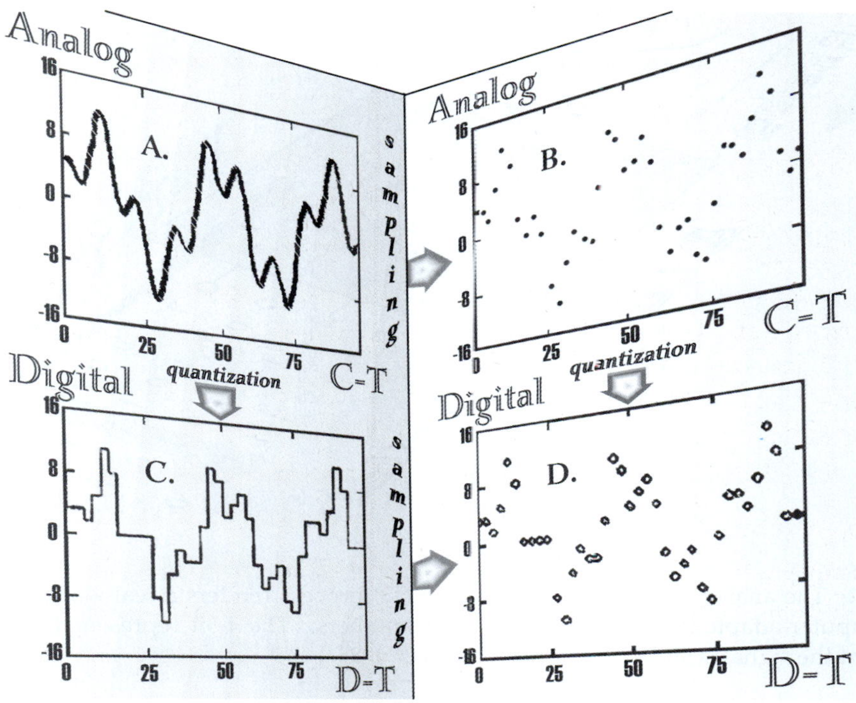

Figure 2.22: Digitization involves sampling and quantization. In the graphs, the horizontal axis is time and the vertical represents signal strength. Sampling and quantization are interacting sources of error; they arise in going, via panels B and C, from the analog signal of panel A to its digitized counterpart in panel D. D-T: discrete-time; C-T: continuous-time.

All signals stored as values in a computer (finite wordlength) are digital signals. Therefore, to be processed by computer, signals must obviously be presented in the appropriate digital format. The original analog signal, before processing, has to be converted into a digital one, it has to be *digitized*. The conversion of real-world analog signals into computer-understood digital signals involves sampling and quantization (see Fig. 2.22). Usually, digitizing and subsequent processing can be performed with good results by using available analog-to-digital converters (ADC) and standard digital signal processing (DSP) techniques, such as the discreet Fourier transform.

The process of converting a real-world analog signal into a computer-adapted digital form (bits) is called analog-to-digital conversion, or signal digitization[15] (see Fig. 2.23). Digitization involves sampling and quantization. Sampling is the conversion of continuous to discrete time; it entails taking "snapshots" of the amplitude or intensity of the

[15]Why use *digitize and digitization,* rather than *digitalize and digitalization*? When electronic engineers got to inventing digital techniques, the terms *digitalize* and *digitalization* had been appropriated by physicians, more than a century earlier, and pertain to administration of the cardiac glycoside *digitalis*, which is often used to treat congestive heart failure and certain cardiac arrhythmias.

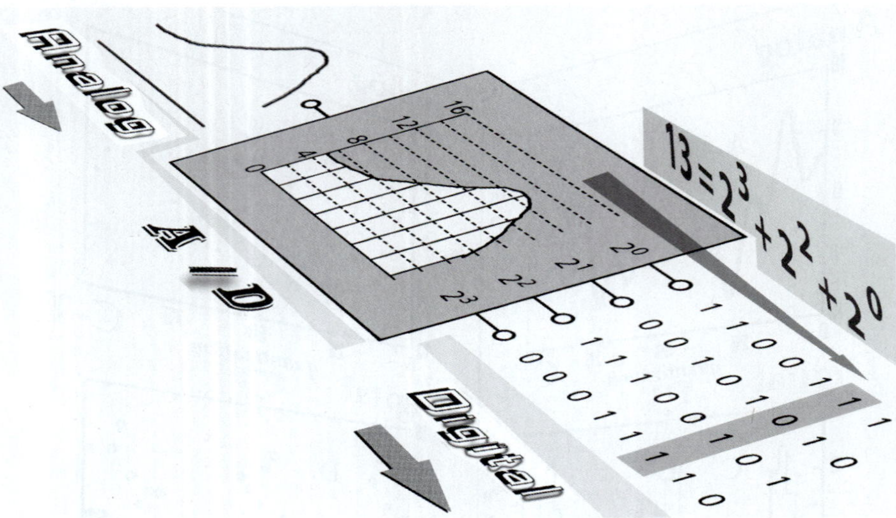

Figure 2.23: The analog-to-digital conversion (A/D) process renders a real-world analog signal into a computer-adapted stream of binary digit numbers. The 4-*bit* representation of the peak value, 13, of the signal is shown to correspond to $2^3 + 2^2 + 2^0$.

signal at discreet time intervals. Quantizing refers to the approximation of the signal value by a number, usually an integer, and almost always a number in the range of 0 to $2^N - 1$, where N is called the *bit depth* and typically varies from 8 to 16. *Bit depth* is the number of *bits* used to store information about the amplitude of the signal. Increasing the sampling rate (more samples acquired per unit time) and the *bit* depth (N), or the number of digital levels (2^N), allows a better representation of the input signal.

The quantization error occurs because we are approximating the continuous amplitude of the signal by a finite number of discrete *quantization intervals*, or *bins*. There is inherent uncertainty in digitizing any analog value, because values lying anywhere within a quantization interval are assigned the same nominal[16] amplitude value corresponding to that bin—see Figure 2.24, on p. 75, for a mental picture of this procedure. Thus, the original amplitude values cannot be recovered without error; the maximum possible error is equal to the quantization step size, which equals the range enclosing all amplitude values divided by the number of discrete steps, 2^N.

In practise, the D/A converter, the device that converts digitized to analog signals, assigns an amplitude equal to the value lying halfway in each quantization interval. Thus, the error introduced by converting a signal from analog to digital form and then back again to analog form becomes half the quantization interval for each amplitude value. Thus, the so-called "A/D error" equals half the width of a quantization interval (see Fig. 2.24). With larger N, there is a more accurate representation of the signal following its

[16]A nominal value is one that we assign to all measurements that fall within each of the series of successive approximating subranges or bins.

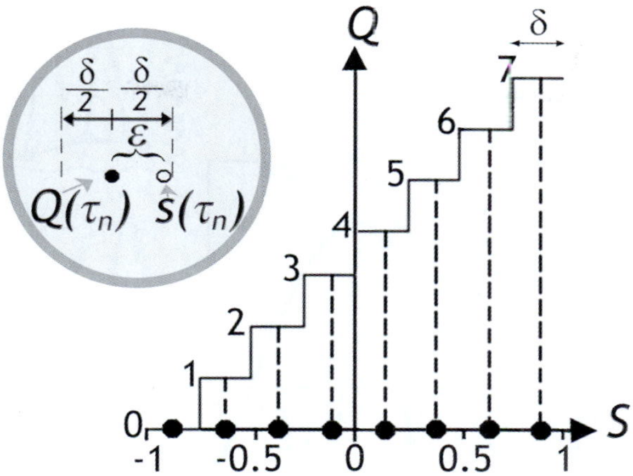

Figure 2.24: In analog-to-digital conversion, the analog signal can be rescaled to lie within a predefined range, $[-1, 1]$. A B-*bit* converter produces one of the integers $(0, 1, \ , 2B - 1)$ for each sampled input value. Thus, a three-*bit* converter assigns one of 8 integers between 0 and 7 to the voltage values in the range $[-1, 1]$; e.g., all values between 0.25 and 0.50 are assigned the integer value 5 and, upon conversion back to an analog signal value, they all become 0.375. As shown in the inset, the maximum error, ε, between the value, $S(\tau_n)$, sampled at time τ_n and its quantized representation, $Q(\tau_n)$, will be $\varepsilon \leq (\delta/2)$, where δ is the adjustable *quantization step*.

quantization—a higher fidelity. However, this calls for higher processing power, as well as more computer memory and storage.

Given the discrete-time samples of a signal, can we uniquely recover the original waveform? Generally, a reduction in the sampling interval—increase in the sampling frequency—increases the observable frequencies. Various sampling theorems address this issue more rigorously. Bear in mind that any periodic function can be reconstructed from a series of sine and/or cosine functions with appropriate amplitudes and frequencies. The Fourier transform of a periodic function is a mathematical transformation which finds the frequencies and relative amplitudes of the sine and cosine components of a periodic function. In the case of nonperiodic, or *aperiodic* signals, the Fourier series undergoes transition to the *Fourier integral.*

A *bandlimited* signal is a function of time whose Fourier transform is zero after a certain frequency. The Nyquist sampling theorem, a basic law of signal sampling theory, states that a bandlimited signal can be fully reconstructed from its samples, if the sampling frequency (f_s) is at least twice as high as the maximum frequency (W) in the bandlimited signal: $f_s > 2W$. This critical sampling frequency is also referred to as the *Nyquist* frequency, f_N. However, the sampled spectrum will have aliases at multiples of f_s (see Fig. 2.25 A.); frequencies larger than the Nyquist frequency are "folded back" and are spuriously added to frequencies smaller than f_N. An inordinately low sampling frequency can also miss the full amplitude of a pulsatile signal by sampling synchronously with its high, in-between, or low values (see Fig. 2.25 B.)

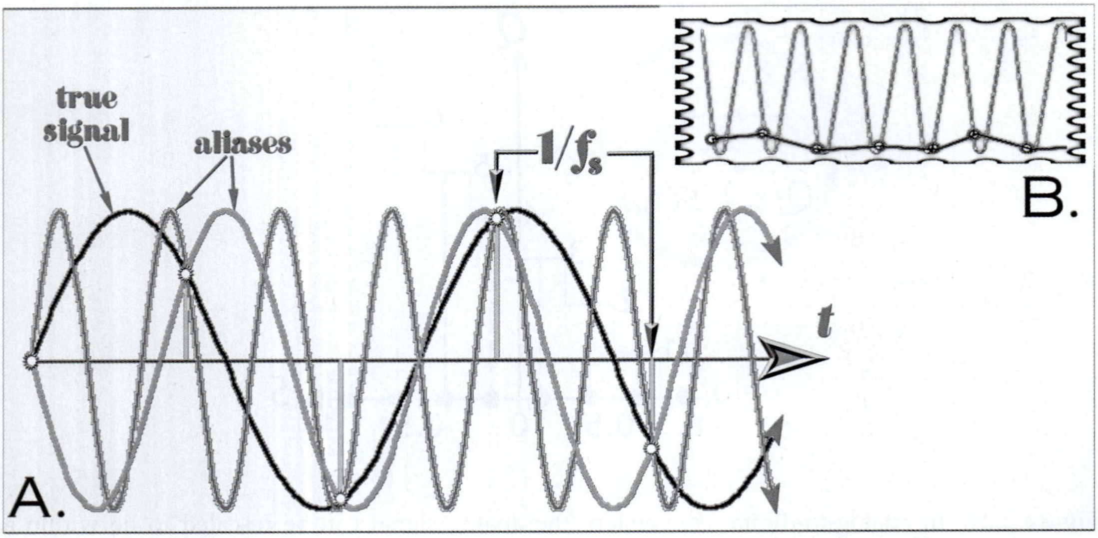

Figure 2.25: A. The true signal (sine function) is found to be fitting the sampled data. However, there are other sinusoids at higher frequencies, which can be drawn exactly through the same sample value points like the true signal. Such frequencies are aliases and the overlapping of them represents aliasing. B. Sampling synchronous with a pulsatile signal at its low values.

When $f_s > 2W$, an ideal "low-pass recovery filter" that passes fully the desired bandlimited signal whereas it attenuates infinitely all aliases generated by the sampler (see Fig. 2.26, panel a., top), can allow us to recover the signal exactly. We could then say that the output signal has a *flat* spectrum up to the *cut-off frequency*, above which its spectrum is *zero*. The Nyquist theorem does not take into account, however, the quantization error present in all digitizing systems. In effect, quantization is a noise source; it can be reduced, but it cannot be eliminated. In practice, we can enhance the signal-to-noise ratio (SNR) and improve the accuracy of digitization by using a narrow quantization step size and high-speed digitizing systems to sample at considerably higher rates, several times faster than the Nyquist criterion. A reasonable objective is to reduce quantization noise, so that it is smaller than other noise sources.

A related problem is the *clipping error*, which occurs when the analog signal exceeds the range of the quantizer. It is sometimes referred to as *saturation*. Clipping can be totally prevented by setting the range of the quantizer to the maximum input signal range. However, the quantization error is proportional to the overall range of the quantizer; thus, the increased range will result in a larger quantization error, a true *"Procrustean bed."* There is obviously a tradeoff between clipping and quantization. If the signal from the sensor is small relative to the input range of the A/D converter, then the step size is large relative to the signal and the resolution will be poor. If the input range is now reduced, the resolution will improve. However, if the input goes higher than the upper bound of the set input range of the converter, it will still give the upper bound number as its

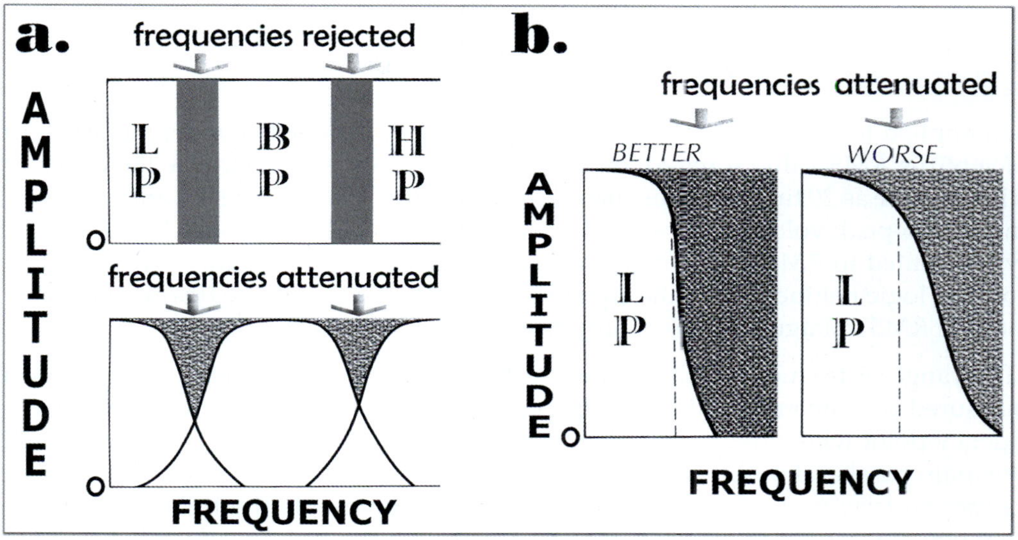

Figure 2.26: a. Low- and high-pass (LP, HP) filters permit the passage of low- and high-frequency components of signals, respectively; conversely, they ideally *reject* and, in reality, *attenuate* high- and low-frequency signal components. Band-pass (BP) filters permit passage of frequency components that lie between two limits. b. The cut-off frequency, indicated by the interrupted lines, is that frequency beyond which greatly reduced or no appreciable energy is transmitted; the sharper the demarcation between transmitted and filtered out frequencies, the better the filter quality.

output, *clipping* the signal. The conversion accuracy increases by matching the range of the quantizer to the amplitude of the signal as closely as possible, while avoiding clipping, and by increasing the number of resolution steps spanning the quantizer range.

2.17.1 The decibel scale and signal-conditioning filters

It is common to compare the intensity of two different signals, or of the same signal before and after performing a process—e.g., filtering—on it, by using ratios, V_{sig1}/V_{sig2}, and to represent such ratios in units of *decibels*. Actually, decibels (dB) are not really units, but are simply a logarithmic scaling of ratios. The decibel has several merits and is used in a wide variety of measurements in electronics. It provides a measurement of the effective power, or power ratio; the *log* operation compresses the range of values (e.g., a range of *1* to *1,000* becomes a range of *0* to *3* in *log* representation); when numbers or ratios are to be multiplied, they simply *add* if they are in *log* units; and the logarithmic characteristic is similar to human perception. The bel is inconveniently large for most applications, so it has been replaced by the decibel (*1/10* bel).

When applied to a power (*P*) measurement, the decibel is defined as *10* times the log of the power ratio:

$$P_{dB} = 10\, log\left(\frac{P_2}{P_1}\right), \text{ dB.} \tag{2.37}$$

When applied to a voltage ratio (or simply a voltage), the decibel is defined as *10* times the *log* of the *RMS* value squared, or the voltage ratio squared. Because the *log* is taken, this is the same as *20* times the unsquared ratio or value. If a ratio of sinusoids is involved, then peak-to-peak voltages (or whatever units the signal is in) can also be used, because they are related to *RMS* values by a constant (*0.707*), and the constants will cancel in the ratio. The logic behind taking the square of the *RMS* voltage value before taking the *log* is that the *RMS* voltage squared is proportional to signal power.

The range of frequencies that is passed by a low-pass, high-pass, or bandpass filter is measured by convention at the -*3* dB point [24, 86, 91]. This is, as we saw above, the frequency point where the amplitude response is attenuated by *3* dB relative to the level of the main passband output of the filter. For a bandpass filter two points are referenced: the *upper* and *lower* -*3* dB points. The -*3* dB point represents the frequency where the output power has been reduced by *one-half*. Decibel units are also useful when comparing ratios of signal and noise, the so-called signal-to-noise ratio (*SNR*). In spectrometry and medical imaging, the absorbance unit used to measure optical density is equivalent to -1 Bel, since just as the ear responds logarithmically to acoustic power, the eye responds logarithmically to brightness.

As is schematically summarized at the top of panel a., in Figure 2.26, ideal bandpass filters have no response below their lower -*3* dB cutoff, no response above their upper -*3* dB cutoff, and very steep response slopes approaching these -*3* dB points. Similarly, for low-pass filters, the bandwidth is from DC to the -*3* dB frequency; for high-pass filters, it is from the -*3* dB frequency to "infinity."[17] Although some real signals can be quite flat over selected frequency ranges, they are unlikely to show an abrupt cessation of energy beyond any given frequency. Figure 2.26, bottom of panel a., and panel b., shows more realistic spectral characteristics, where signal energy begins to decrease at a specific frequency but decreases *gradually* with frequency until there is no more energy in the signal. When the decrease in signal energy, referred to as the frequency *rolloff*, takes place gradually, then defining the bandwidth is problematic. If we are to define a single bandwidth for such a signal, we need to specify a cut-off frequency within the boundary between the region of substantial energy and the region of minimal energy. This boundary is somewhat arbitrarily defined as the frequency when the signal's *RMS* value has declined by *3* dB with respect to its average unattenuated value.

The -*3* dB boundary is not entirely arbitrary, however, because when the signal is attenuated by *3* dB, its *RMS* [18] amplitude is *0.707* of its unattenuated value and it has *one-half* the amplitude of its unattenuated power. Accordingly, this boundary point is also known as the *half-power point*. In medical instrumentation terminology, the terms *cut-off*

[17] For a high-pass *digital* filter the pass-band is limited to the maximum bandwidth, sampling rate, and word length that the filter order allows. After that, there is no pass-band!

[18] Root mean square (RMS) is the effective value or effective DC value that an AC signal represents. For a sinusoidal wave, the RMS value is 0.707 times the peak value, or 0.354 times the peak-to-peak value.

frequency, 3 dB point, and *half-power point* are synonymous. When a signal has both a low-frequency and a high-frequency rolloff end (see Fig. 2.26, middle signal in panel a.), the signal's frequency characteristic has two cut-off frequencies, one denoted as f_{low} and the other as f_{high}. In this case the bandwidth is specified as the range between the two cut-off frequencies (or 3 dB points), i.e., as $[f_{high} - f_{low}]$ Hz.

2.17.2 A/D conversion for images

Diagnostic image formation occurs when a specialized sensor registers radiation patterns following some kind of interaction of x-rays, ultrasound, radio frequency waves, or other detection means, with body tissues and organs. An image, therefore, represents an array of data samples representing some type of energy. A standard digital image is represented by samples in an equally spaced rectangular grid quantized at equal intervals of gray levels [9,14,26,39,41,76]. The spatial coordinate elements represent brightness and color and are referred to as *pixels, pels,* or *pict*ure *el*ements.[19] Therefore, image refers to a 2-D energy (mostly light intensity) function $IMAGE(x, y)$, where x and y denote the spatial coordinates and the value of the function $IMAGE$ at the point $[x, y]$ is proportional to the energy level of the image at that point.

Images should be acquired digitally or, if acquired in analog form, should be digitized to produce an array with a specified resolution of picture elements, with each element capable of representing a specified range of gray level intensities [12,89]. A/D conversion for images consists of sampling and quantization (see Fig. 2.27). The same principles apply to images as are described in the preceding section for analog signals in general. Instead of sampling in time, we sample in space (in both the x- and y-directions) using a hardware digitizer interfaced with the scanning apparatus. An image $IMAGE(x, y)$ can be thought of as a 2-D function of horizontal position x and vertical position y. The function usually represents signal intensity (e.g., proportional to the number of photons captured by the scanner), or color. You can think of digitizing an image as the *converse* of *painting-by-numbers*. In image processing, a high-pass filter provides image sharpening or edge enhancement when applied to the digital image array; a low-pass filter, commonly known as a *smoothing* filter, is generally used to remove image noise and speckle.

The rectangular area of a monitor screen used to display images is an "image raster." The raster is slightly smaller than the physical dimensions of the screen and varies for different resolutions.[20] For example, VGA resolution of 640×480 on a 19-inch monitor produces one raster, whereas SVGA resolution of $1{,}024 \times 768$ produces a slightly different raster. Using an A/D converter, each image raster is converted from a continuous voltage waveform into a sequence of voltage samples (see Fig. 2.27A).

A sampled, quantized image can be represented by a matrix of values—see Figure 2.27 for a mental picture of the process. Each matrix entry is an image sample, or a *pixel*. Each pixel gray level is quantized, i.e., assigned one of a finite set of numbers,

[19] *Pixel* is an abbreviation for *pict*-ure *el*-ement.

[20] The resolution is conceived here as the minimum significant image element (distance, area, or volume) that can be meaningfully interpreted from the displayed image.

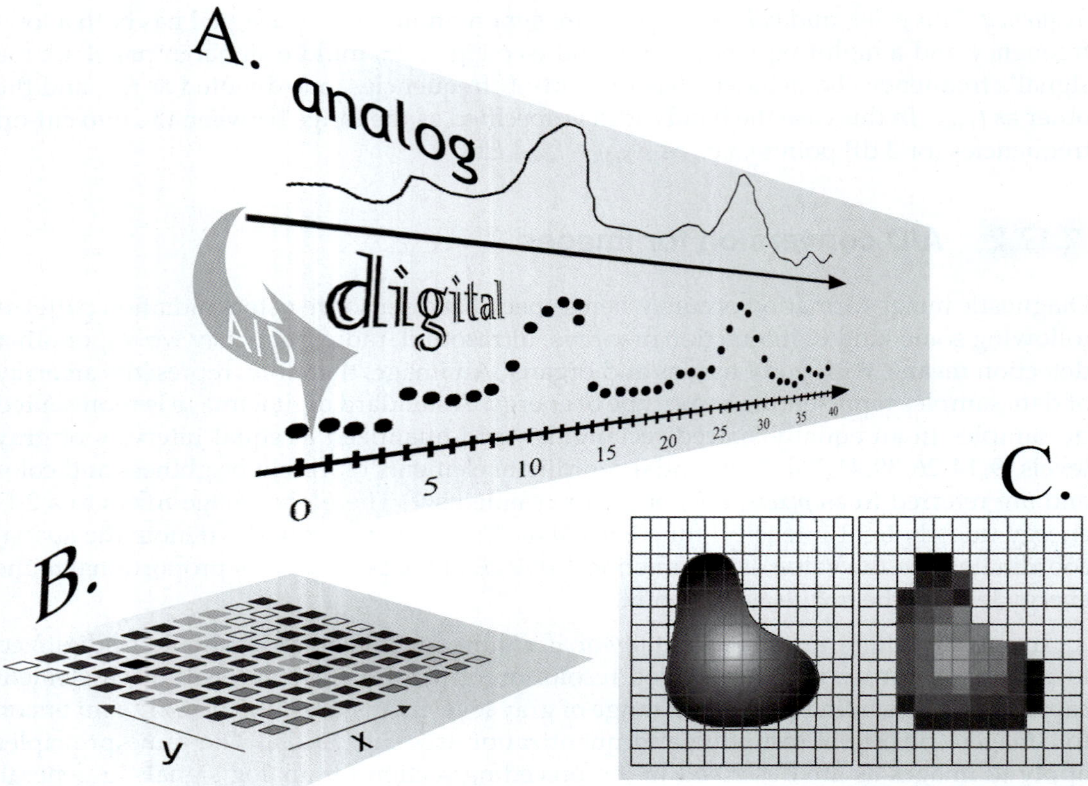

Figure 2.27: A. Continuous analog electrical signal from one scan line, and the corresponding sampled digital signal from one scan line, indexed by discrete (integer) numbers. B. Depiction of a 10×10 image array; each of the picture elements is called a pixel. C. Analog image projected onto a monitor screen (left), and result of its digitization comprising image sampling and quantization (right), which introduce spatial resolution and gray-scale depth errors.

generally integers, indexed from 0 to $(K-1)$. Typically, there are $K = 2^B$ possible gray levels. Each pixel is represented by B bits, where ordinarily $1 \leq B \leq 8$. The number of bits required depends upon the application. Video digitizers (*"frame grabbers"*) attached to medical imaging devices usually have a resolution of 8–12 bits ($256 - 4{,}096$ gray levels). Arguably, most humans cannot perceive more than 100 levels of gray scale, but the intensity perception by humans is nonlinear; therefore, the 10-*bit* or 12-*bit* linear scale is needed to accommodate the 6- or 7-*bit* human nonlinear scale [16]. For black-and-white images, 8 bits per pixel are adequate for display, but preferably 12–16 bits per pixel are needed for digital data analysis and for digitization of analog images. For color images, 24 bits per pixel is best. More bits reproduce finer-and-finer amplitude detail, an important consideration with medical and scientific imagery and visualization.[21] The number of quantization

[21] Thus, medical CT scans span a range of 4,096, or (2^{12}), gray-scale levels (see detailed discussion in

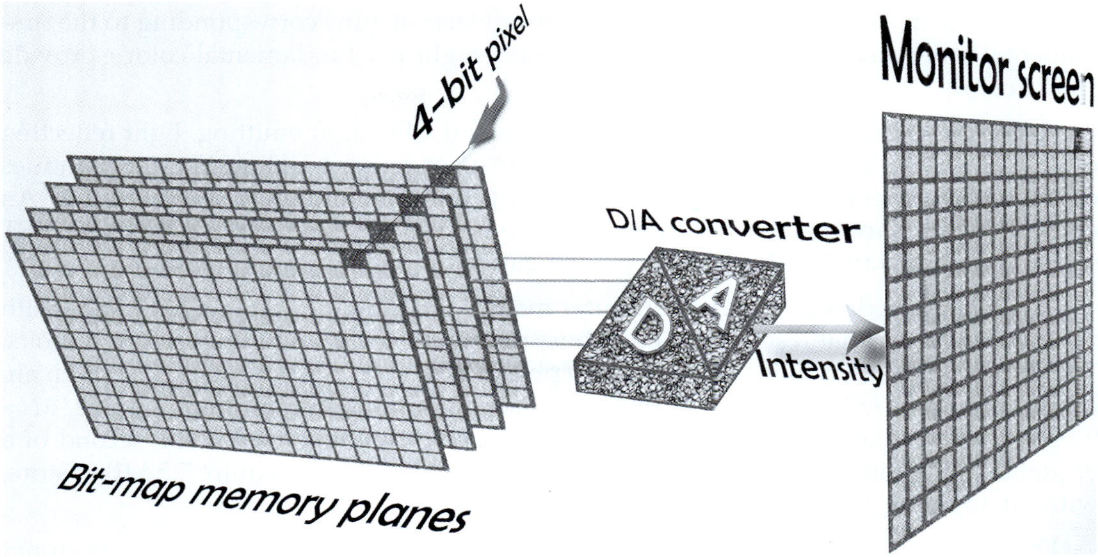

Figure 2.28: Black and white 4-*bit* screen (16 gray levels) with planar organization.

levels is properly determined by the signal-to-noise level achieved by the sensor used during the conversion of the specific intensity signal to an electric signal.

After quantization, some fine-grain information of the original image is liable to be lost, but the amount of information lost in this way can be negligible, provided that the "shade of gray" bin widths are small. Therefore, pixel intensities or gray levels must be quantized sufficiently densely, so that shades of gray useful in discerning morphologic or other mapped quantitative details are not lost.

A digital image is an array of numbers representing the sampled (row, column) image intensities, as indicated in Figure 2.27B. It is essential to sample the image sufficiently densely, i.e., with high spatial resolution; otherwise, the image quality will be severely degraded. This can be rigorously demonstrated mathematically in terms of the Nyquist sampling theorem, which was introduced in the preceding section, but the effects of the ensuing *pixelization* are very readily perceived visually.

Raster scan cathode ray tubes (CRTs) display images as a set of dots across each scan line. In principle, digital-to-analogue (D/A) converters are used in order to draw segments on the monitor screen by providing gray-scale levels to the individual pixels. In a simple planar organization, several *bit*-map plane memories connected in parallel encode the intensity of each raster pixel (see Fig. 2.28). Filled areas, colors as well as shading are possible, if special graphics solutions are used. The resolution depends on the number of scan lines and the modulation frequency. Color screens obviously need more

Section 10.1.3, on pp. 490 ff.). On the other hand inexpensive fax machines only need to detect the presence of ink and therefore can be 1-*bit* systems (ink/no ink).

bits. Shadow mask cathode ray tubes have three electron guns corresponding to the fundamental red–green–blue (RGB) colors. 24 bits—eight per fundamental color—provide 16,778 colors.

In flat plasma screens or liquid crystal displays (LCD), light emitting, light reflecting or light absorbing dots are formed at the intersection of orthogonal lines. Large quantities of electronic components are required for driving, selecting and scanning these dots. An embedded interface makes the screen look like an addressable memory, or like a CRT screen with horizontal and vertical synchronization pulses.

The total hard disk storage or computer memory required for one digital image with $2^M \times 2^M$ pixels spatial resolution and B bits/pixel gray-level resolution is $B \times 2^{2M}$ bits. The gray-level resolution is usually 1 byte/pixel, i.e., $B = 8$. An important exception are *binary* "black-and-white" images with $B = 1$. The spatial resolution is often 512×512 ($M = 9$). A standard-size image thus takes up one-quarter MB (megabyte). One second of a digital imaging video loop (TV rate = 30 images/sec) would thus require 7.5 MB to store, without applying digital image compression techniques.

Data transmission and storage are costly; in spite of this, most digital data are not stored in the most compact form, but in whatever way makes them easiest to use, e.g., individual samples from a data acquisition system, ASCII text from word processors, etc. Typically, these easy-to-use encoding methods require data files about twice as large as actually needed to represent accurately the information. Data compression is the general term for the various algorithms and programs developed to address the storage problem. A *compression program* is used to convert data from an easy-to-use format to one optimized for compactness; in contrast, an *uncompression program* returns the information to its original form.

2.18 Fourier transform and Fourier series

Digital signal and image processing [12, 48, 61, 89] have found many applications in cardiac imaging and flow studies, and can be extremely computer-intensive. Much effort has gone into the methods, but also into the development of fast algorithms and into computer architectures. Signal or image processing methods can be executed either directly in the time or spatial domain, respectively, or we can first transform the signals into another domain, such as the frequency (Fourier transform) domain, or another orthogonal function domain—cf. Figure 2.31, on p. 87, and the associated discussion. Then we can perform the processing in the appropriate transform domain, to be followed by the back-transformation (*inverse transform*) to the original time or spatial domain.

The Fourier transform,[22] named for Jean Baptiste Joseph Fourier (1768–1830),[23] is an

[22]The term "transform" means to change form or appearance. In terms of signal processing, a transform is normally a tool that is used to convert the signals from time domain or spatial domain to the frequency domain.

[23] Fourier was interested in heat transfer, and submitted a paper in 1807 to the Institut de France on the use of sinusoids to represent temperature distributions. The paper claimed that any continuous periodic

integral transform[24] that expresses a function in terms of sinusoidal basis functions, i.e., as a sum or integral of sinusoidal functions multiplied by some coefficients ("amplitudes"). A Fourier series is an expansion of a periodic function $f(x)$ in terms of an infinite sum of sine and cosine terms of different frequencies (see Fig. 2.29, on p. 84). Fourier analysis makes use of the concept that we can approximate real world signals and functions by a sum of sinusoids, each at a different frequency. In principle, there is very little distinction between the Fourier series and the Fourier transform (integral). One difference is that each applies to different classes of functions: the series to *periodic* functions and the integral to *aperiodic* functions.

Harmonic analysis represents the computation and study of Fourier series. It is extremely useful as a way to break up an arbitrary periodic function into a set of simple terms that we can substitute for it, solve individually, and then recombine to obtain the solution to the original problem, or an approximation to it to whatever accuracy is desired, or reasonable. The frequency of each sinusoid in the Fourier series is an integer multiple of the frequency of the signal that is being approximated. These sinusoid components are the harmonics of the original function. The more sinusoids included in the sum, the better the approximation. For a continuous-time, T-periodic function $g(t)$, the N-harmonic Fourier series approximation can be written as

$$g(t) \;=\; a_0 \;+\; a_1\, cos(\omega_0 t \;+\; \theta_1) \;+\cdots+\; a_N\, cos(N\omega_0 t \;+\; \theta_N), \tag{2.38}$$

where, the fundamental frequency ω_0 equals $2\pi/T$ rad/s, the coefficients $a_1, \ldots, a_N$ are nonnegative, and the phase angles fall between 0 and 2π radians ($0 \leq \theta_1, \ldots, \theta_N < 2\pi$). The complete Fourier representation includes both a magnitude spectrum (plot of a_n vs. ω_n) and a phase spectrum (plot of θ_n vs. ω_n).

In terms of signal processing, the Fourier transform takes a time series[25] representation of a function and maps it into a frequency spectrum. That is, it takes a function from the time domain into the frequency domain, and it decomposes the function into harmonics of different frequencies, as is summarized pictorially in Figures 2.29 and 2.30, on the next pages. The frequency domain contains exactly the same information as the time domain, just in a different form. If you know one domain, you can calculate the other.

---

signal could be represented as the sum of sinusoidal waves. Among the reviewers were two famous mathematicians, Joseph Louis Lagrange and Pierre Simon de Laplace. While Laplace and the other reviewers voted to publish the paper, Lagrange adamantly insisted that such an approach could not be used to represent signals with corners, i.e., discontinuous slopes, such as in square waves. The Institut de France bowed to Lagrange, and rejected Fourier's paper. It was only after Lagrange died that it was finally published, some 15 years later [82].

[24] For the mathematically inclined, an integral transform is a mathematical operator that produces a new function, $T_f(u)$, by integrating the product of the given function $f(t)$ and a so-called kernel function $g(t,u)$ between suitable limits, according to the following form: $T_f(u) = \int_\alpha^\beta f(t)\, g(t,u)\, dt$. T_f is a function of a parameter, denoted u in the defining equation. Thus, an integral transform maps one function into another which is a function of the parameter. There are several useful integral transforms [31,51,64]. Each of them corresponds to a different choice of the kernel function g. The original function and its transform comprise a *transform pair*.

[25] A *time series* is an experimental recording of a variable, or a set of discrete successive values extracted from such a recording, at equally spaced instants.

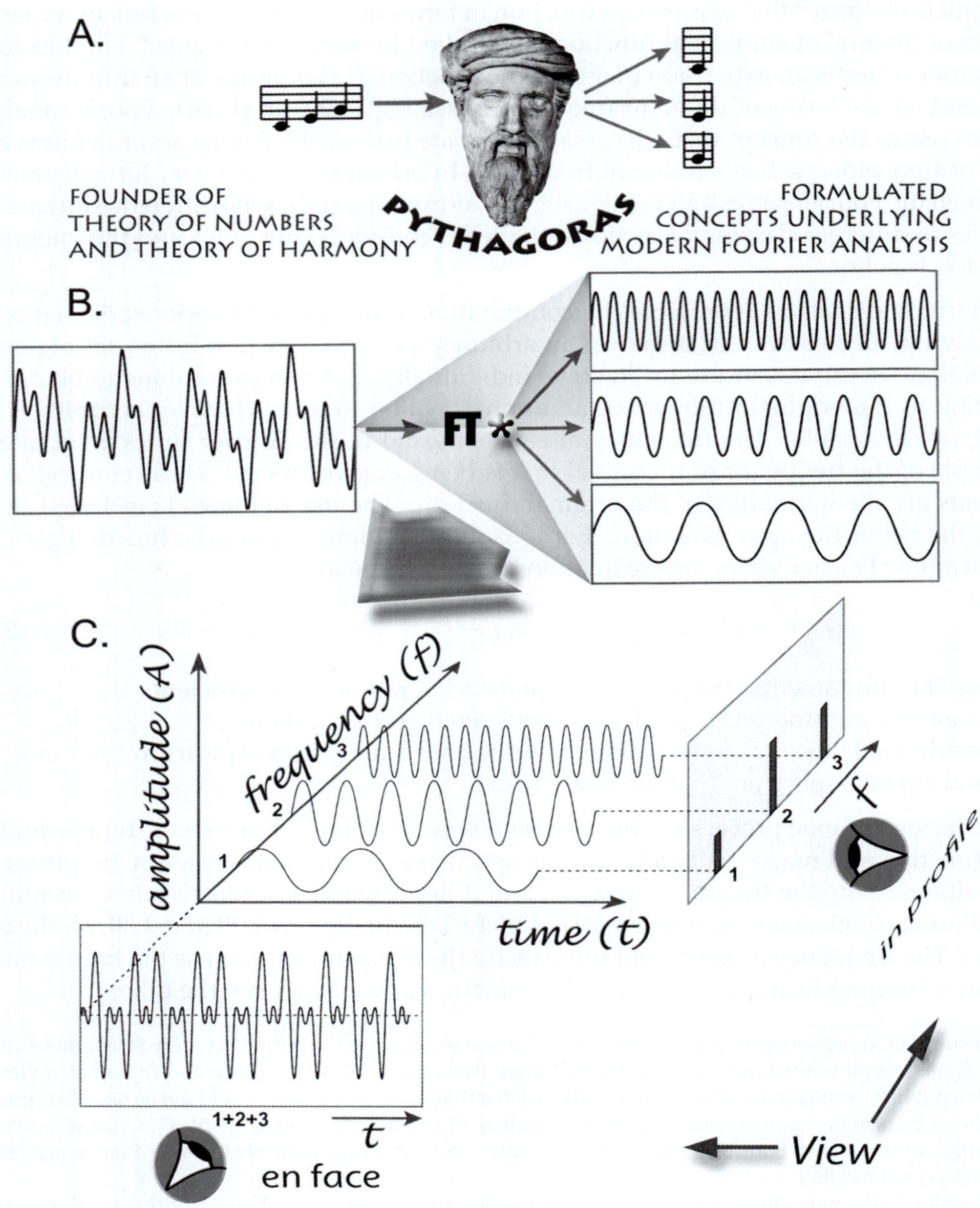

Figure 2.29: A. A chord *do-mi-sol* is heard by the ear, which recognizes by a Fourier transform (FT) the distinct notes (*do, mi* and *sol*) that make it up. B. Graphic representation of the Fourier transform of the composite signal into its three elementary frequencies. C. The Fourier transform allows transition from *amplitude vs. time* to *amplitude vs. frequency*: two distinct but *equivalent* viewpoints.

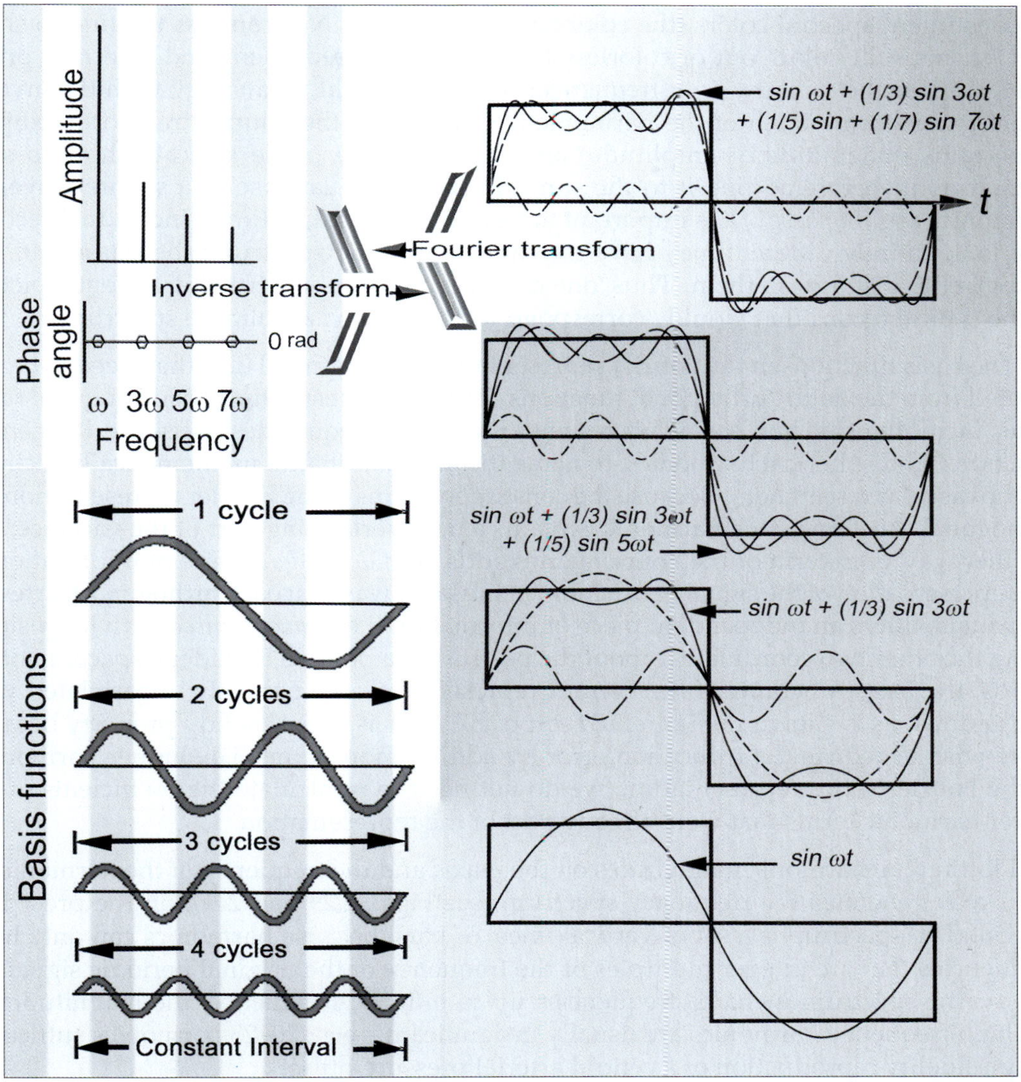

Figure 2.30: One-dimensional Fourier transform: the approximation of a *time*-domain square wave by a few sinusoidal components in the *frequency*-domain. The spectrum of the approximating wave is shown, plotted in terms of bar graphs of modulus and phase angle against angular frequency, ω_n—in this particular case, the phase angle happens to be identically *zero*-rad for all harmonics. The sense of the inverse Fourier transform is shown too. Because the Fourier representation comprises only orthogonal basis functions, each harmonic explains a nonoverlapping part of the variance. Thus, if we wish to reduce the truncation error by adding more harmonics, we do not need to recalculate the coefficients of the lower terms that were already part of the Fourier representation.

The Fourier transform acts like a prism, which breaks up white (colorless) light into its constituent spectral colors (the colors of the rainbow). Newton was the first to show that prisms split colors out of colorless light. He also used a lens and a second prism to recompose the rainbow light frequencies into white light, in analogy with the inverse Fourier transform. Each of the harmonic frequencies in the Fourier transform exhibits a modulus (magnitude or amplitude) and a phase. The phase indicates how to shift the harmonic before adding it to the sum. In the particular case of a square wave, all harmonics are *"in phase"*. It is important to bear in mind that, at times, individual records that look entirely different may have the same amplitude spectrum; the phase data are necessary to distinguish them. Thus, one must refrain from constructing a mental picture of the typical record that would "correspond to" a specified amplitude spectrum.

The basis functions in the Fourier representation are empirical (i.e., they need to be calculated from the data) "orthogonal functions." There is a near infinity of orthogonal functions, including sine and cosine waves with increasing frequencies, Bessel and Legendre functions, and spherical harmonics, to name the most familiar to mathematically inclined cardiovascular researchers. Because the constituent terms of the Fourier representation are orthogonal functions, each harmonic explains a nonoverlapping part of the variance; put another way, each term of the Fourier series adds an *independent* piece of information to the representation of the signal or function, in the same way that each orthogonal Cartesian coordinate offers an independent piece of information (i.e., *uncorrelated* with its position along the other two coordinates) about the position of a point in Euclidean space. In other words, the basis functions of the Fourier representation are perfectly uncorrelated with one another, as is shown in Figure 2.31, on p. 87. This is a very handy property because if we wish to reduce the truncation error by adding more terms, i.e., higher harmonics, to the Fourier series representation, we do not need to recalculate the coefficients of the lower harmonic terms that were already part of the representation.

Plotting the harmonic magnitudes on the y-axis and the frequency of the harmonic on the x-axis generates the frequency spectrum (see Figs. 2.29 and 2.30, on the preceding pages). The spectrum is a set of vertical lines, or bars, because harmonics can only have frequencies that are integer multiples of the frequency of the original periodic signal. In theory, the spectrum includes frequencies up to infinity; in practice, the magnitudes of the high frequency harmonics are usually insignificant—e.g., 20–25 harmonics suffice for a high-fidelity reproduction of a central arterial pressure pulse.

2.18.1 Fourier series for any interval

Although in common hemodynamic applications the Fourier representation is discussed in terms of a periodic function, its application is much more fundamental, because any section or interval of a well-behaved function may be chosen and expressed in terms of a Fourier series. This series will accurately represent the function *only* within the specified interval. If applied outside that interval it will not follow the function, but it will periodically repeat the value of the function within the specific interval. If we represent this interval by a Fourier cosine series, the repetition will be that of an even function;

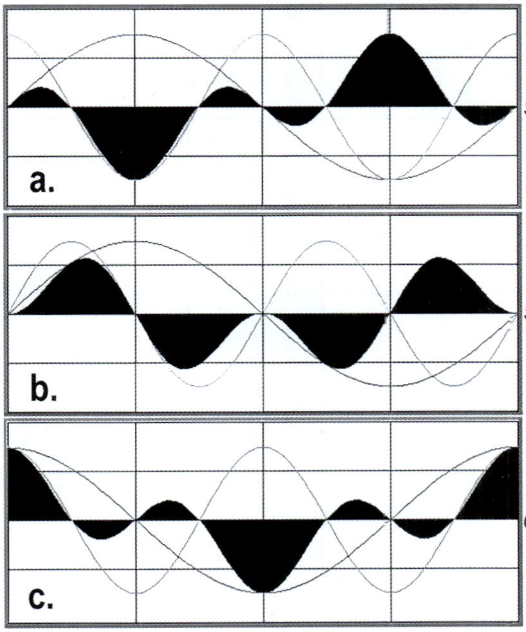

Figure 2.31: Sines and cosines are orthogonal functions. a. The product $\sin(nwt) \cdot \cos(mwt)$ for different n and m, i.e., *different harmonics*, always averages zero (black areas above and below the zero amplitude level cancel out) over a complete period of the lowest harmonic, or any integer multiple thereof. b and c. The products $\sin(nwt) \cdot \sin(mwt)$ and $cos(nwt) \cdot cos(mwt)$ each average $1/2$ when $n = m$ but again average zero for different n and m, i.e., different harmonics.

conversely, if the representation is a Fourier sine series, an odd function repetition will follow.

Suppose now that we are interested in the behavior of a function over only one-half of its full interval and have no interest in its representation outside this restricted region. In Figure 2.32, the function $f(x)$ is shown over its full space interval $-l/2$ to $+l/2$, but $f(x)$ can be represented completely in the interval 0 to $+l/2$ by either a *cosine* function, which will repeat itself each half-interval as an even function, or by a *sine* function, which will repeat itself each half-interval as an odd function. Neither representation will match $f(x)$ outside the region 0 to $+l/2$, but in the half-interval 0 to $+l/2$ we can write

$$f(x) = f_e(x) = f_0(x), \tag{2.39}$$

where, the subscripts e and o denote the even (cosine) or odd (sine) Fourier representations, respectively.

The arguments of sines and cosines must, naturally, be phase angles, and so far the variable x has been measured in radians. However, the interval l is specified as a distance and the variable becomes $2\pi x/l$, so that each time x changes by l the phase angle changes

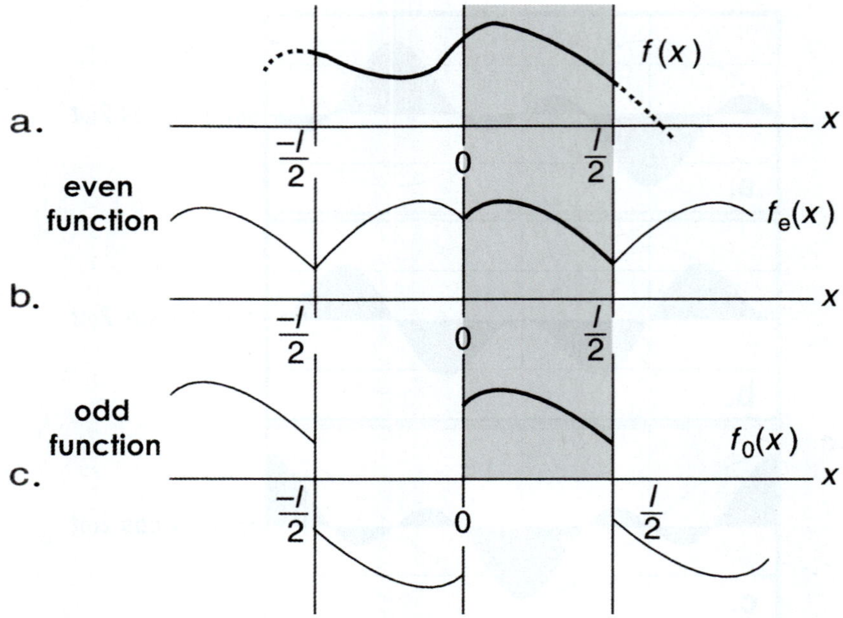

Figure 2.32: A Fourier series may represent a function over a selected half-interval. The function $f(x)$ depicted in panel a. is reproduced in the half-interval $0 < x < 1/2$ by $f_e(x)$, an even function cosine series in panel b., and by $f_o(x)$, an odd function sine series in panel c. These representations are valid only in the specified half-interval; their behavior outside it is purely repetitive and differs from the original function.

by 2π. If we follow the behavior of $f_e(x)$ and $f_o(x)$ outside the half-interval 0 to $+l/2$, we see that they no longer represent $f(x)$, as is shown in Figure 2.32.

2.19 Fourier analysis in image processing

It is important to realize that Fourier transforms are not limited to functions of time, and temporal frequencies. The discrete cosine transform (DCT), a form of Fourier analysis, is commonly used in image processing [9, 20, 71]. The procedure divides the image like a checkerboard into square patches of, e.g., 8×8 pixels. For each such patch there are 64 discrete Fourier components, which represent all possible spatial frequencies and phases along the x- and y-axes. Any eight-by-eight patch of the original image can be reconstructed by adding up various weighted combinations of these basic frequency elements, or *basis functions*. The zero-frequency component implies no spatial pattern modulation, i.e., just the average brightness of the whole image, and corresponds to the average brightness of the patch. If the patch has gradual variations in brightness over its entire width or height, then some of the lower frequency components will be strongly represented in the spectrum. Sharp edges and fine lines in the image require the high-frequency components to be properly represented.

Large amounts of cardiac imaging and intracardiac flow-field visualization data can create enormous problems in storage and transmission. The widespread, imaging and visualization use of information in the form of images has contributed to the development of data compression techniques. The design goal of image compression is to represent images with as few bits as possible, according to some fidelity criterion, to save storage and transmission channel capacity. All image compression techniques try to get rid of the inherent redundancy, which may be spatial (neighboring pixels), spectral (pixels in different spectral bands in a color-graphics visualization image), or temporal (correlated images in a sequence; e.g., video clips).

Fourier analysis is a useful method of image compression. It might seem at first that nothing is gained by converting to frequency space, since an 8×8 patch with 64 pixels also has 64 Fourier coefficients. However, not all the Fourier components are equally important; for instance, in a patch of nearly uniform color only the zero-frequency element has a significant weight, and the rest of the coefficients can be discarded. This situation is common enough to render Fourier compression worthwhile. Indeed, the discrete cosine transform is the main compression method in JPEG images.

We can also apply Fourier transforms in cardiac and intracardiac flow investigations, to analyze images and spatial frequencies [61,65]. As we have seen, the Fourier transform of an image generally encodes a whole series of sinusoids through a range of spatial frequencies, from zero up to the Nyquist frequency. The Nyquist frequency is the highest spatial frequency encoded in the digital image (cf. Section 2.20, on pp. 91 ff.) and depends on the resolution, or pixel size. The Fourier transform resolves all of the spatial frequencies present in an image simultaneously. A signal containing only a single spatial frequency is plotted as a single peak at point f along the spatial frequency axis, the height of that peak corresponding to the amplitude, or contrast of that sinusoidal component. The output of the transformation then represents the image in the frequency domain, while the input image is the spatial domain equivalent. In the Fourier domain image, each point represents a particular frequency contained in the spatial domain image.

High spatial "frequencies" are at larger distances to the optical axis than the low spatial "frequencies" that correspond to the larger structures or patterns in the imaged object. Imagine a fence consisting of vertical bars of constant distance. Its diffraction pattern would ideally be two dots at equal distance horizontally on both sides of the optical axis, as is shown in Figure 2.33. When changing the distance of the bars, these dots would move toward or off the optical axis in the horizontal direction, i.e., the closer the bars, the higher the spatial frequency and the larger the distance of the spots (see Fig. 2.33). The Fourier transform aims toward the reproduction of any given image as a summation of cosine-like component images. For that reason, images that are pure cosines have particularly simple transforms.

Figure 2.33A., on p. 90, shows two images with their transforms directly beneath them. The images are a pure horizontal cosine of 8 cycles and a pure vertical cosine of 32 cycles. Notice that the Fourier transform for each has just a single component, represented by two bright spots symmetrically placed on either side of the center, i.e., the origin of

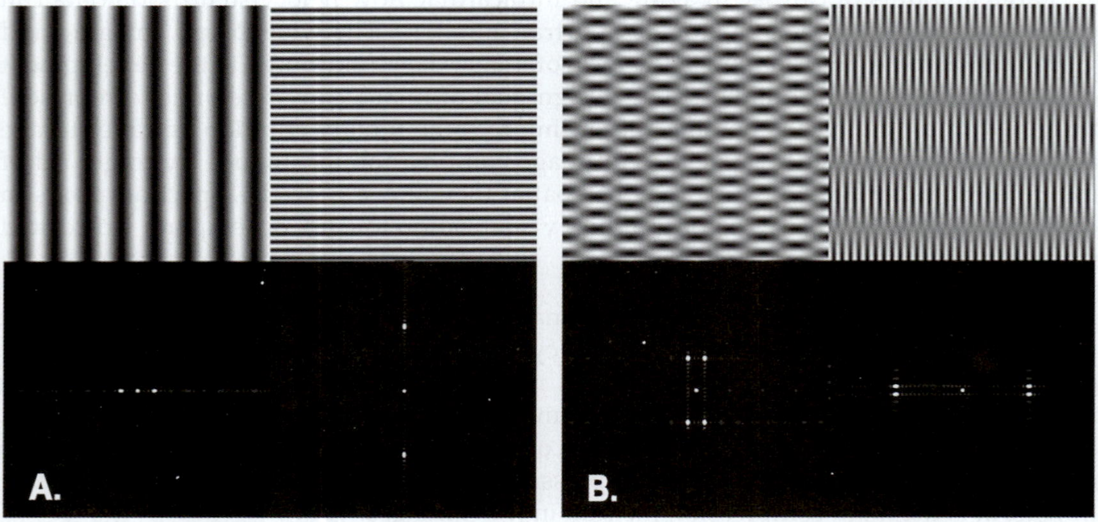

Figure 2.33: Simple cosine-like pattern images with their Fourier transforms directly beneath them; only the magnitude spectra are displayed—see explanatory details in the nearby text.

the frequency coordinate system.[26] A 2-D function in the x–y plane has a 2-D Fourier transform in the so-called u–v plane. Every pixel of the Fourier transform image is a spatial frequency value, and the magnitude of that value is encoded in the brightness of the pixel. The u-axis runs left to right through the center and represents the horizontal component of frequency; the v-axis runs bottom to top through the center and represents the vertical component of frequency. In both cases, there is a bright pixel at the very center that represents the (0, 0) frequency or "DC" term, which encodes the average brightness across the whole image. A zero DC term would imply an image with average brightness of zero, which would mean the sinusoid alternated between positive and negative values in the brightness image. But since there is no such thing as a negative brightness, all real images have a positive DC term, as shown here too. An extremely important property of the Fourier domain is that most of the image power is concentrated in the low frequency components near the center of the Fourier transform plot—this is analogous to the more familiar behavior of the Fourier transforms of hemodynamic signal waveforms, most of whose power is concentrated in the low frequency harmonic components, near the origin (*zero-frequency*).

Images usually have a large average value term and important low-frequency information; consequently, the transform images usually have some bright components near

[26] For mathematical reasons beyond the scope of this discussion, the Fourier transform also plots a mirror image of the spatial frequency plot reflected across the origin, with spatial frequency increasing in both directions from the origin. These two spots are always mirror-image reflections of each other, with identical peaks at f and $-f$, as shown in Figure 2.33.

the center. Notice that high frequencies in the vertical direction will cause bright dots away from the optical axis in the vertical direction, whereas high frequencies in the horizontal direction will cause bright dots away from the axis in the horizontal direction. The higher the contrast in the brightness image, the brighter the peaks in the Fourier transform image. Since there is only one Fourier component in these simple images, all other values in the Fourier transform images are zero, depicted as black.

Figure 2.33B. shows two images with somewhat more general Fourier components. They are images of 2-D cosines with both vertical and horizontal components. The panel on the left has 4 cycles horizontally and 16 vertically; the panel on the right has 32 cycles horizontally and two vertically. There is a gray band when the function goes through gray, which happens twice/cycle. Note that the Fourier images under consideration are just the *magnitude* spectra. The magnitude puts in view *how much* of a certain frequency component is present and the phase *where* the frequency component is in the image. In image processing, often only the magnitude of the Fourier Transform is displayed, because it contains most of the information of the geometric structure of the spatial domain image. However, if we want to retransform the Fourier image into the correct spatial domain after some processing in the frequency domain, we must make certain that both magnitude and phase of the Fourier image are preserved.

In principle, the Fourier image encodes exactly the same information as the brightness image, except expressed in terms of amplitude as a function of spatial frequency, rather than brightness as a function of spatial coordinate. An inverse Fourier transform of the Fourier image produces an exact pixel-for-pixel replica of the original brightness image. Fourier optics influence the diffraction pattern by, e.g., weakening or canceling certain spatial "frequencies." If, for instance, we want to enhance the edges in an image, then we have to attenuate the central regions in the diffraction pattern while passing the higher spatial frequencies (outer regions of the diffraction pattern) in their full intensity before imaging the diffraction pattern through a lens. Conversely, if we view an image using an overhead projector that is somewhat out of focus, the finest details will be blurred. We may think of such defocusing as amounting approximately to a linear filtering, which removes or attenuates high harmonics in the spatial Fourier decomposition of the image, above a cutoff frequency that depends on the defocusing.

2.20 Fourier analysis with computers

Several techniques are available that enable a computer to calculate the frequency spectrum of a signal. The first step in all cases is to convert the analog signal to a set of numbers for the computer to use. This requires the sampling of the signal at a regular interval, to give a stream of digital values. A fixed interval of time, the "sampling interval," separates each sampled value from the next. The number of samples obtained and the sampling interval combine to determine the length of time we look at the signal. The following definitions apply:

- f_s: sampling rate, in *Hz*; $dT = 1/f_s$: sampling interval; N: number of samples taken; $T = N \times dT$: total time period; $f_1 = 1/T$: frequency of the first harmonic, in *Hz*.

The traditional mathematical approach to Fourier analysis entailed the approximation of continuous waveforms. However, digital computer techniques can only deal with a set of discrete digital samples. The analog signal is continuous in time and it is necessary to convert this to a set of discrete values. This does not change the basic idea of harmonic analysis, but faithful reproduction of a continuous waveform is only possible if the sampling rate is higher than twice the highest frequency component present in the signal.[27] Keep in mind the following:

1. The spectra based on sampled waveforms can encompass at most only $N/2$ harmonics.

2. If the original signal contains more than $N/2$ harmonics, the higher frequency harmonics will cause errors in the magnitude spectrum. This type of error corresponds to "aliasing."

Digital or analog filtering of the input signal before performing the Fourier analysis, so that there are no frequency components above $N/2$, prevents undesirable aliasing.

2.20.1 Qualitative insight into the Fourier transform algorithm

What does the Fourier transform (FT) actually do? Starting with the time domain representation of an oscillating signal, it derives the individual frequencies of the sinusoidal components making up its compound waveform.[28] These frequencies are its *frequency content* in the frequency domain. Considering, for the sake of simplicity, only the *real parts* of oscillating signals, which are *cosine* waves (see Fig. 2.9, on p. 49), we can obtain an intuitive understanding of the FT, as follows.

We begin with the signal $s(t)$, whose frequency content we are investigating. We create a trial signal function $f_1(t)$, which oscillates at an initial guess of a frequency present in $s(t)$. We convert the two signals to digital form, and obtain their product digitally, i.e., on the computer. We then integrate over time. If the guess of the frequency was not good, the functions $s(t)$ and $f_1(t)$ do not match, and consequently their product, $s(t)f_1(t)$, has as many positive as negative excursions, so that the integral is close to zero. The low value of this integral corresponds to a low value of the spectral function $S(w)$ for $s(t)$ at the frequency (w_1) of $f_1(t)$. We repeat this process, scanning in succession for all frequencies that may be present in the signal $s(t)$. When the frequency w_j of the trial signal function $f_j(t)$ coincides with, or is close to, one contained in the signal $s(t)$, then

[27] This is, essentially, what is embodied in the Shannon–Nyquist sampling theorem—see H. Nyquist, Trans. AIEE, 47: 617–44, 1928; and C.E. Shannon, Proc. Inst. Radio Engin., 37: 10–21, 1949. The theorem also applies when reducing the sampling frequency of an existing digital signal.

[28] If the waveform is *aperiodic*, i.e., it does not repeat itself after a finite interval of time or distance, it has an infinite frequency content and its frequency spectrum is continuous.

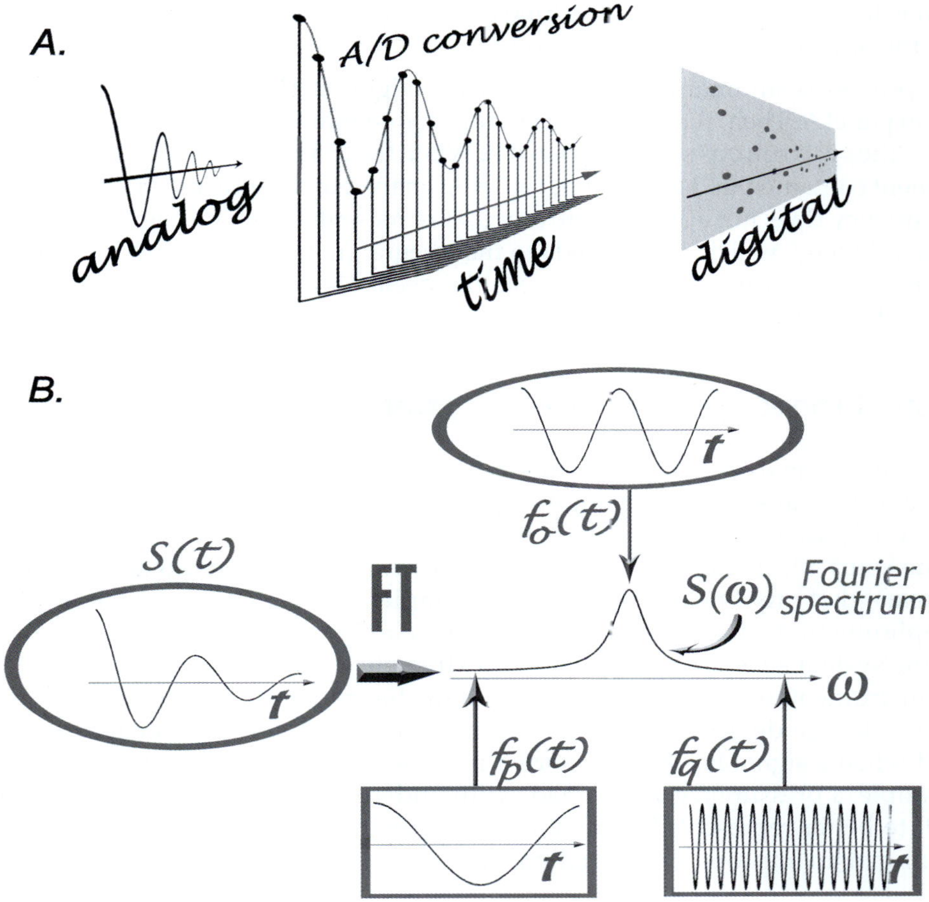

Figure 2.34: A. An analog signal in the time or spatial domain is converted to digital form by sampling its magnitude, or intensity, at a set of points separated from adjacent points by the *sampling interval*, and then storing the information as a set of discreet digital values. The total duration, or extent, of sampling is the aquisition interval. B. The Fourier transform (FT) detects and quantifies the intensities of the cosine wave components in the digitized representation of a time- or spatial-domain signal, e.g., $s(t)$, and then displays the "spectral function," $S(\omega)$, of the signal in the frequency (ω) domain.

positive and negative excursions will match in time and their product will be consistently positive. Accordingly, the value of the integral, *viz.*, the spectral function, will be high at that frequency. In other words, we are correlating the input signal with each basis function in its Fourier decomposition. The concept of correlation allows us to detect a known waveform contained in another signal, by multiplying the two signals and adding all the points in the resulting signal. The single number that results from this procedure is a measure of how similar the two signals are. Accordingly, each sample in the frequency domain is found by multiplying the time domain signal by the sine or cosine wave being looked for, and adding the resulting points.

The process is summarized schematically in Figure 2.34. The signals are digitized, as shown in panel A. Then, the FT algorithm steps sequentially through all possible frequency values in the spectrum, as shown in panel B. When the trial function frequency hits that of a component contained in the signal that is being analyzed, the integral shoots up. When the trial frequency does not approximate any that is present within the signal analyzed, then the spectral value, which corresponds to the integral, remains depressed. In this fashion, the Fourier transform detects *in principle* the oscillating components in a time-domain compound signal, and constructs the frequency spectrum for the signal. [29]

2.20.2 Frequency response of systems

Systems can be analyzed in the frequency domain by using the Fourier transform. Using the Fourier transform, every input signal can be represented as a group of sinusoidal waves, superposed on one another, each with a specified amplitude and phase shift. Likewise, the Fourier transform can be used to represent every output signal in a similar form. This means that any linear system can be completely characterized by how it changes the amplitude and phase of sinusoidal waves passing through it. This information is called the system's *frequency response*. It is extremely useful in assessing the fidelity with which instrumentation components, from transducers, through amplifiers, to recorders and mass storage devices, reproduce hemodynamic waveforms. Signal restoration can be used when a signal has been distorted in some way by instrumentation components. For example, a pressure recording made with underdamped equipment may be low-pass filtered, to better represent the pressure as it actually occurred. Another example is the deblurring of an improperly focused image.

2.20.3 Discrete (DFT) and Fast (FFT) Fourier transform

The discrete Fourier transform, DFT, is the sampled Fourier transform and therefore does not contain the set of all the frequencies forming a signal, but only a subset of them. This subset is just large enough to describe the time or spatial domain function with the desired fidelity—for inadequate resolution pitfalls, reexamine Figure 2.25, on p. 76. The Fourier transform is useful in a wide range of applications beyond hemodynamic signal analysis, such as 2-D and 3-D image analysis, image filtering, image reconstruction, and image compression. The usual purpose of applying a transform is to help make more obvious, or explicit, some desired information.

In the case of digital imaging, an important goal is to make explicit the spatial frequency composition of the image. The transformation is often followed by a thresholding

[29] In signal processing mathematical formalism, the method which basically underlies implementations of the Fourier transformation is *cross-correlation*: signals of varying frequency and phase are correlated with the input signal, and the degree of correlation in terms of frequency and phase represents the frequency and phase spectrums of the input signal (cf. Section 2.21, on pp. 95 ff.)

operation, which is intended to select the most prominent or relevant features. It may then be possible to apply an inverse transform, for reconstructing the geometry of the original image, but with the desired features (such as the endocardial boundaries, in cardiac segmentation applications) explicit or *enhanced*. The number of frequencies in the Fourier transform corresponds to the number of pixels in the spatial domain image, i.e., the images in the spatial and Fourier domains are of the same size. This can make for a daunting task when large images are transformed.[30] The most popular computer algorithm for generating a frequency spectrum is a special linear algebraic computation called the Fast Fourier Transform, or FFT.

As the name implies, the FFT is very efficient in terms of the number of operations required in its computation and this is a significant improvement, especially for large images. However, it does have one peculiarity that affects the way it is used. The FFT can only process a sampled waveform where N (the number of sampled data points) is a power of 2. Admissible values of N include $128, 256, 512, 1{,}024$, and $2{,}048$. If the number of data points does not meet the power of 2 requirement, one may interpolate the data set to satisfy this requirement. Alternatively, we can adjust the number of data points by resorting to the method of *zero padding*.

In fact, one of the fundamental principles of discrete signals is that zero padding in one domain (time, frequency) results in an increased sampling rate in the other domain (frequency, time). It can be shown that if a signal is extended by appending a string of zeros to the end of the signal at the same spacing as the available signal, then the Fourier transform of the resulting function will be the same as the Fourier transform of the original signal, except that the frequency resolution will be the reciprocal of the length of the *padded* signal. Thus, zero padding in the time domain also results in an increased sampling rate in the frequency domain and improves the attainable frequency resolution. This process is aptly referred to as "spectral interpolation" [81].

The FFT, like most computer algorithms, generates an exponential instead of a trigonometric Fourier series (see Fig. 2.9, on p. 49). The two series are identical except that the magnitudes generated by the exponential series are half the values of the trigonometric series. Most application software automatically compensates for this, and presents the magnitude spectrum as a trigonometric series.

2.21 Auto-correlation and cross-correlation

Cross-correlation is a standard method of estimating the degree to which two series are correlated. When the correlation is calculated between a series and a lagged version of

[30] To obtain the Fourier transform of a square (2-D) or cubical (3-D) image of size $N \times N$ or $N \times N \times N$, a double or triple sum, respectively, has to be calculated for each image pixel. However, because the Fourier transform is separable, it can be written in terms of a series of $2N$, or $3N$, 1-D transforms, and this decreases the number of required computations. Even with these computational savings, the ordinary 1-D DFT has N^2 complexity. This can be reduced to $N\ log_2 N$ if we employ the FFT to compute the 1-D DFTs. This is a sizeable improvement, in particular for large images.

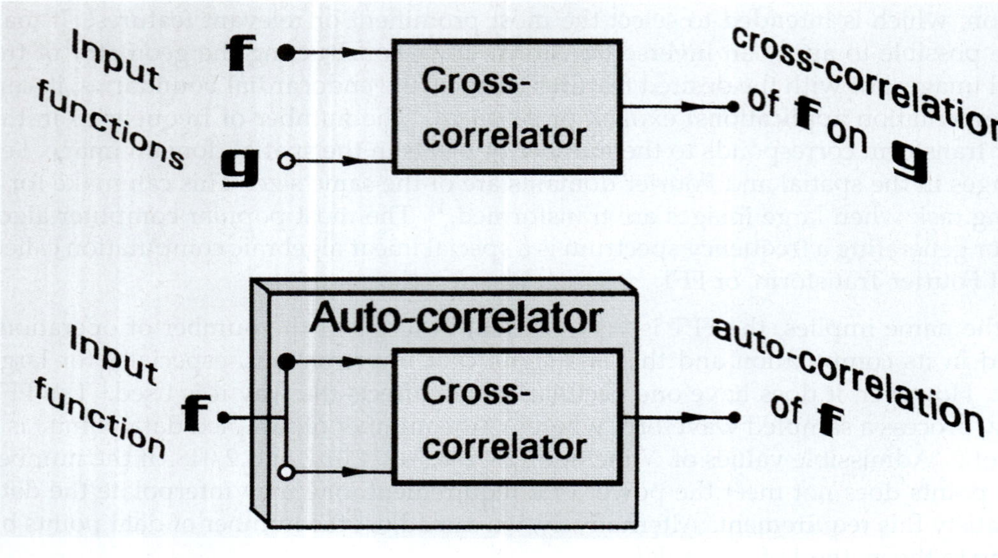

Figure 2.35: Diagrammatic views of cross-correlation and auto-correlation. A cross-correlator has different terminals for f and g; no output can emerge from an auto-correlator until the input is fully inserted.

itself it is called auto-correlation (see Fig. 2.35). Auto-correlation is a time-domain function that is a measure of how much a signal shape, or waveform, resembles a delayed version of itself. The auto-correlation is the simplest device to identify periodicities in a signal; its value can vary between *zero* and *one*. A periodic signal, such as a sine wave, has an auto-correlation which is equal to one at zero time delay, zero at a time delay of one-half the period of the wave, and one at a time delay of one period; in other words, it is a sinusoidal wave form itself. Random noise has an auto-correlation of one at zero delay, but is essentially zero at all other delays. Auto-correlation is sometimes used to extract periodic signals from noise. The continuous auto-correlation function reaches its peak at the *origin*, i.e., for zero time delay, τ, where it takes a real value representing the power contained in the signal. The same result holds in the discrete case. Moreover, the auto-correlation of a *white*, i.e., totally random, noise signal will have a strong peak at $\tau = 0$ and will be close to zero for all other τ. This shows that white noise has no periodicity.

Certain dual-channel FFT analyzers, having a variable delay setting facility between the channels, are able to measure auto-correlation. Generally, auto-correlation is used in signal processing for analyzing functions or time series of values, such as time domain hemodynamic signals. Any given hemodynamic signal $f(t)$ evolves with time, t, according to the frequencies present in its waveform. Auto-correlation is particularly valuable for finding repeating patterns in a signal, i.e., in determining the presence of periodic components in measured time series that commonly contain confounding noise. This determination can be accomplished by using the auto-correlation function, defined by the coefficients of linear correlation between the points corresponding to the common parts

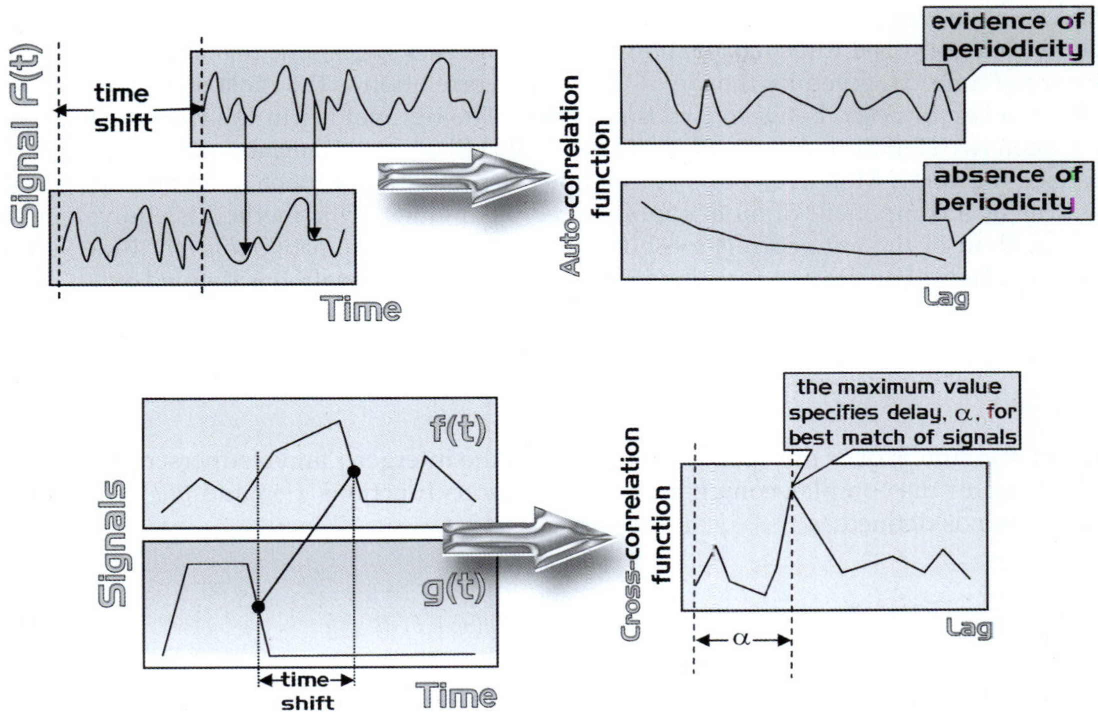

Figure 2.36: *Top*: The auto-correlation analysis. The correlation between the values of the time series $F(t)$ and $F(t+\tau)$ is calculated for various values of the lag τ. If the plot of the auto-correlation coefficient *vs.* the lag is of *oscillatory* form, it reveals the presence of periodicity in $F(t)$. *Bottom*: Cross-correlation of two time series $f(t)$ and $g(t)$. Each value of $f(t)$ is correlated with $g(t+\tau)$. The computed cross-correlation coefficients are then plotted *vs.* the lag τ. The *maximum* value in the plot indicates the time delay α, where maximum correlation is achieved.

of the original signal $f(t)$ and another signal—$f(t+\tau)$—for various values of τ; τ represents the variable *time shift*, or *delay*, parameter. The auto-correlation depends on f and τ, but is independent of t.

If the *correlogram*, i.e., the graph of the auto-correlation function *vs.* lag τ has at least a quasi-periodic form, it testifies to a periodicity in $f(t)$ (see Fig. 2.36). A cross-correlogram, is a graph of the cross-correlation coefficients for the values of the functions $f(t+\tau)$ and $g(t)$ for various values of the variable lag τ. A requirement for these computations is that $f(t)$ consists of equidistant data. If not, a new time series must be constructed using interpolation techniques.

The correlation between two signals (cross-correlation) is a standard method of estimating the degree to which two signals or time series of values, such as time domain hemodynamic signals, are correlated. Alternatively, it is the process of determining "how much" of one signal is in another. If the correlation is significantly nonzero, we may conclude that there is a direct correlation between the two series, but this effect is delayed by some time Δt, given by the lag τ. The cross-correlation is the most standard way to obtain a lag, or *delay*, between two time series. The optimal lag in the cross-correlation between two signals (input-output) will generally tell us something about the process that caused the delay. Moreover, cross-correlation is a standard approach to feature detection, as well as a component of more sophisticated techniques. This method is equivalent to the method of the auto-correlation but, in this case, data from two *different* time series are correlated. For discrete functions f_i and g_i, the cross correlation is defined as

$$(f \star g)_i \equiv \sum_j f_j^* \, g_{i+j}, \tag{2.40}$$

where the sum is over the appropriate values of the interger j and a superscripted asterisk indicates the complex conjugate. For continuous functions $f(x)$ and $g(x)$, the cross-correlation is defined as

$$(f \star g)(x) \equiv \int f^*(t) g(x+t) \, dt, \tag{2.41}$$

where, the integral is over the appropriate values of t.

In signal processing, cross-correlation, or sometimes simply *correlation*, is a measure of similarity of two signals, and is commonly used to find features in an unknown signal by comparing it to a known one. It is a function of the relative time shift, τ, between the signals, is sometimes called the sliding dot product, and has applications in pattern recognition. The cross-correlogram, is a graph of the cross-correlation coefficients for the values of the functions $f(t)$ and $g(t+\tau)$ for various values of the variable time lag, τ. The maximum value in the plot indicates the time delay α, where *maximum* correlation is achieved. A high correlation is likely to indicate a periodicity in the signal, with a period corresponding to the time delay. The cross-correlation at $\tau = 0$ will give only an indication of pattern similarity of the two sets of data without any time shifting. In fact, one approach to identifying a particular pattern within a larger image uses cross-correlation of the image with a suitable mask. Where the mask and the pattern being sought are similar, the cross-correlation will be high. The mask is itself an image data set that needs to have the same functional appearance as the pattern to be found.

An objective measure of the actual time shift between two similar patterns is the particular $\tau = \alpha$ value, at which the plot of the cross-correlation function *vs.* the time shift is maximized (see Fig. 2.36). This property is exploited in some Doppler methods for red blood cell velocity determinations, as is exemplified in Section 5.9.6, on pp. 289 ff. If a periodicity is documented, the next step may be to resolve the time series in a sum of periodic signals, and estimate their period and amplitude. This can be done using the Fourier transforms (mainly the DFT), which were considered in the immediately preceding Sections 2.18, 2.20, 2.20.1, and 2.20.3.

2.22 Differential equations

In order to represent the behavior of matter at the scale of human observations, classical mechanics has principles and laws, which are expressed by systems of governing equations. For a fluid, for example, general equations represent all its possible states, while its behavior necessarily obeys the principles and laws of physics. Differential equations are an excellent way to express many physical laws, which commonly involve change and rates of change of variables, in space and time. The ultimate objective is to find "the solution," a mathematical expression linking all states of a system that may be separated by long intervals of time and space. However, in general, this is too difficult to achieve by the straightforward application of the laws of mechanics. Accordingly, to start with we apply these laws to *neighboring* states of the system that differ infinitesimally[31] with respect to time and space.

We accomplish this by using differentials and forming from them a relation between derivatives and certain functions. Such a relation is a differential equation, in which time and space may enter as the independent variables [13,45,60,75,80]. In effect, a differential equation is an algebraic relation between variables that includes the rates of change of quantities of interest, as well as their instantaneous values.[32] The process by which we work out the general expression, relating states of the system separated by any desired intervals of time and space, from the differential equation is the "integration" of the equation. At times, change in "space" actually functions as a general concept, one standing in for change in some measurable independent variable other than space. The solutions, or integrals, generally involve arbitrary, and thus contingent, constants and functions; they correspond to the special so-called *boundary conditions* pertaining to the particular system. The boundary conditions are the mathematical statement of the *particular* constraints that pertain to the system, such as (for intracardiac flows) those imposed by the dynamic geometry of the moving cardiac chamber walls.

In any event, finding the solution, or "integrating" the differential equation, means finding an equivalent expression that does not involve derivatives. As a very simple illustration, a differential equation is $\frac{dy}{dx} = 2x$. A solution to this differential equation is $y = x^2 + 1$, because the derivative, dy/dx, is in fact $2x$. There are obviously other admissible solutions to this differential equation, and to other more difficult but much more valuable equations. This is the extensive mathematical field of differential equations. Numerical methods of solution are also available, which are very useful [3,18,21,28,36]. They can be applied to equations that we can express in analytical terms that contain infinite series expansions or special functions of mathematical physics [1,40,87] that are cumbersome to evaluate, but are essential when only numerical values are available to us, and no analytic expressions for the solution.

[31] The word *infinitesimally* is applied here to signify differences in amounts that are infinitely small, or less than any assignable quantity.

[32] It was Descartes (1596–1650) who clearly stated that an equation in two variables, geometrically represented by a curve, indicates a dependence between variable quantities. The idea of derivative came about as a way of finding the tangent to any point of this curve.

An *"ordinary"* differential equation is an equation that implicitly defines an unknown function, the dependent variable, and its derivatives with respect to a *single* independent variable. The order of a differential equation is the order of the highest derivative of the unknown function involved in the equation. Thus, Newton's second law of motion turns out to be a $2nd$-order differential equation, because the acceleration is the second derivative of the position with respect to time. A differential equation is said to be *linear* if each term in the equation has only one order of derivative, e.g., no term has both y and the derivative of y with respect to time. In addition, no derivative is raised to a power.

The boundary conditions on a differential equation are the constraining values of the function at some particular value of the independent variable. A problem in which time is the independent variable and where the values of the unknown function and its derivatives at some point are known is called an initial value problem. For example, if the equation involves the velocity, the boundary condition might be the initial velocity, the velocity at time $t = 0$. In order to have a complete solution, there must be a boundary condition for each order of the equation, namely two boundary conditions for a second order equation, only one for a first order differential equation. If a solution to a differential equation is found which satisfies all the boundary conditions, then it is the only solution to that equation; this is called the uniqueness theorem. If no boundary or initial conditions are given, we call the description of all solutions to the differential equation the general solution.

Generally, a *"partial"* differential equation is an equation that implicitly defines a function of *two or more* independent variables and involves partial derivatives of the dependent variables [2,5,6,23,25,29,33,35,56]. The fundamental governing laws of mechanics, such as Newton's equations of motion and the Navier–Stokes equations, are stated in terms of partial differential equations, i.e., these laws describe the spatiotemporal evolution of physical phenomena by relating time and space derivatives of physical variables. Accordingly, much of analytical and computational fluid dynamics is based on the study of partial differential equations. Derivatives arise in these equations because the derivatives represent natural quantities, such as velocity, acceleration (retardation is simply *negative* acceleration), force, friction, and flux. Hence, we have equations relating partial derivatives of some unknown quantity that we would like to find. For instance, if $\Theta(x, t)$ is the time-varying temperature of a long, thin metal bar at a distance x from the initial end of the bar, then under suitable conditions $\Theta(x, t)$ is a solution to the heat equation

$$\frac{\partial \Theta}{\partial t} = k \frac{\partial^2 \Theta}{\partial x^2}, \tag{2.42}$$

where, k is a constant. This is the diffusion equation. If time-varying velocity is substituted for the temperature, the same equation governs the evolution of the velocity profile over a suddenly accelerated plate. Its analysis can then provide good qualitative—and even semi-quantitative—insights into, e.g., the early development of the velocity profile in a central arterial trunk (ascending aorta, main pulmonary artery) during the upstroke of the ejection velocity waveform.

When a partial differential equation occurs in an application, our goal is usually that of solving the equation, where a given function is a solution of a partial differential equation if it is implicitly defined by that equation. That is, a solution is a function that satisfies the equation. Partial differential equations often occur in practice with boundary conditions, which are constraints on the solution and its derivatives at different points in space, and initial conditions, which are constraints on the solution and its derivatives at a fixed point in time.

2.22.1 Navier–Stokes equations

Fundamental physical principles describe the net variations of the flow-field variables. In general, and including the study of intracardiac flow, these principles are formulated by the Navier–Stokes equations. The Navier–Stokes equations embody one equation for conservation of mass and three equations for conservation of momentum, one along each coordinate in 3-D space; they are thus equal to the number of unknowns of the flow field, namely the pressure and the three components of velocity. The eponym commemorates the French engineer C. L. M. H. Navier, and Sir G. G. Stokes, who formulated them independently in 1822 and 1845, respectively [62,84].

As applied to intracardiac flows, the Navier–Stokes equations are a continuum expression of Newton's second law of motion for incompressible, viscous flow: the rate of change of momentum per unit volume of the flowing fluid equals the applied force per unit volume, which—as we saw in Section 2.7.1, on pp. 58 f.—is represented by the pressure gradient. They contain *first* order partial derivatives with respect to time and space, and *second*-order partial derivatives with respect to space [4].

To determine the rate of change of momentum at a point in the flow field, we must add, to the instantaneous rate of change of momentum with respect to time, any spatial difference in the rate at which momentum arrives at and leaves the neighborhood of the point. The influx and efflux of momentum involve *products* of velocity components and so we have a nonlinearity at the crux of fluid flow. As a result, there are very few exact solutions to the Navier–Stokes equations, mostly involving parallel incompressible flows (laminar flow in a cylindrical tube, between parallel plates, etc.), in which the influx and efflux of momentum at any point in the flow match exactly and the nonlinearity effect vanishes.

As indicated earlier in this section, the general solution to partial differential equations contains arbitrary functions and constants. In other words, although the Navier–Stokes equations govern the evolution of all intracardiac flows, for the complete solution and determination of a particular flow field, such as that of the right ventricle during diastolic filling, the particular circumstances of the flow must be taken into account. They correspond to contingent factors relative to the particular flow under study. To express them explicitly, we must specify the applying boundary and initial conditions (see also Chapters 12–14).

2.22.2 Solution of the Navier–Stokes equations

We note at this early juncture that, when applied to intracardiac flows, the Navier–Stokes equations must usually be solved numerically using computers [7,34,47,92], in

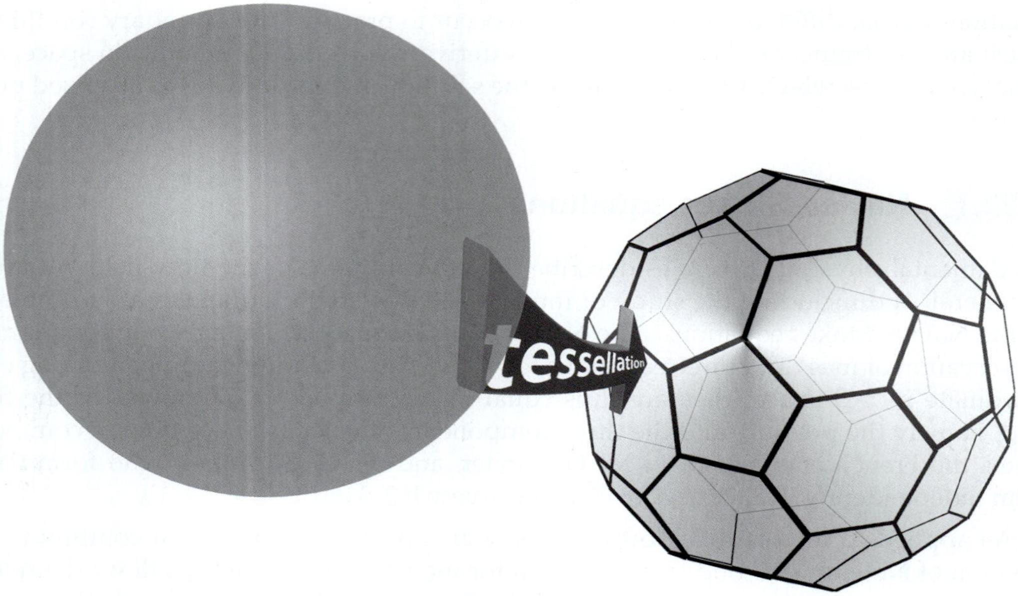

Figure 2.37: In tessellated surfaces the cells, or *faces*, are polygons; here, pentagons and hexagons. The 3-D region of interest, here a spherical chamber, is bounded by the faces and is demarcated by them.

a burgeoning field of modern research that is known as Computational Fluid Dynamics, or "CFD." Using sophisticated graphics methods developed in the ultramodern technological field of "scientific visualization," the results are then visualized on computer monitors to provide otherwise unattainable insights into the behavior of any complicated flow field, such as the intraventricular field during diastolic filling. Before embarking on any complex CFD simulation study, one should always consider the option of using a simplified analytical model [11,27,50]. While simulation offers a number of important advantages over analytical models, often these simpler models will suffice and will provide elegant insights into the dynamics of the processes that are being investigated.

Most of the impetus to the development of CFD and scientific visualization has come since the advent of powerful computers; their application to problems of increasing complexity in cardiovascular flows has taken place over the past 15 years, or so. Typical computers have finite-sized memories segmented into bytes and words of data (see Section 2.16.1, on pp. 71 f.) that correspond to floating-point numbers. This structure obliges us to represent the continuous intracardiac flow-field variables in the computational domain using a finite, albeit large, number of discrete real values (see Chapters 12–14). Consequently, the spatial domain is tessellated into computational *cells*, also called finite *elements*.

In discretized surfaces (see Fig. 2.37), the cells are triangles or, generally, polygons; these are small plane faces bounded by a closed path that is composed of a chain of straight line segments, called edges or sides, and the points where two edges meet are

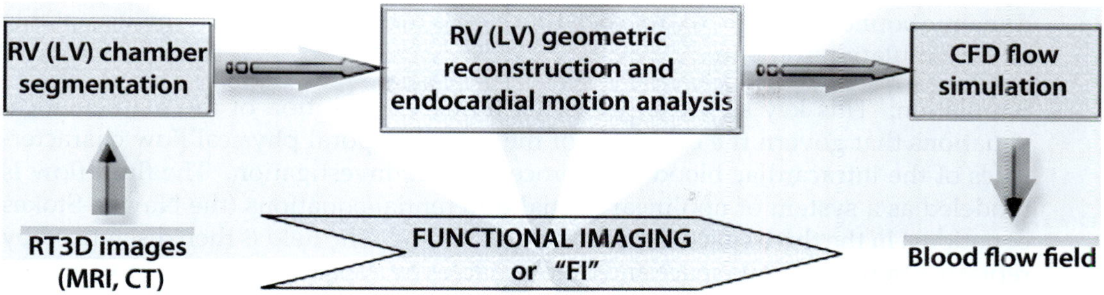

Figure 2.38: Flowchart of the Functional Imaging method. Input to the algorithm is a series of real-time, 3-D echocardiography (RT3D) images of the right ventricular (RV) chamber, and the output is the corresponding blood flow-velocity field in the right ventricle. CFD, computational fluid dynamics. (Reproduced from Pasipoularides et al. [69], with permission from the American Physiological Society.)

the polygon's vertices or corners. When discretized volumes are involved, the 3-D region is bounded by the faces, and is demarcated by them. The cells are then small control volumes that correspond to polyhedra, which are named according to their number of faces—the naming system is based on Greek, e.g., *tetra*hedron (4), *penta*hedron (5), *hexa*hedron (6), *octa*hedron (8), *dodeca*hedron (12), and so on. In any case, the 2- or 3-D region of interest is defined by a lattice of points, the *computational mesh*, or the *grid*. Usually, the values of the flow variables associated with these cells are evaluated at a specific time. Because the computer representation uses discrete numbers rather than continuous variables, the resolution in time is also broken up into discrete intervals. These intervals are denoted as *timesteps* and provide convenient increments over which to advance the numerical solution of the flow-field equations.

In brief, the entire modeling, simulation and visualization methodology entails the following distinct steps (cf. Fig. 2.38):

1. Image Acquisition: Various noninvasive 3-D imaging modalities provide a series of cross-sectional views of closely spaced "slices" of the heart, in which each type of tissue is recognizable by its unique "density" and shown in a distinct shade or color. This facilitates the automatic, or semi-automatic interactive, detection of the spatial boundaries (the endocardial surface) of the cardiac chambers.

2. Boundary Identification: For each timestep of the unsteady flow simulation, it is necessary to express the geometry of the walls of the cardiac chambers in terms of their Cartesian coordinates (with each imaging slice occupying a separate x–y plane, normal to the z-coordinate) and then to represent the boundary surface by a large set of contiguous triangles. This process is termed segmentation and it entails the application of various algorithms; a decimation algorithm can then reduce the number of triangles to a minimum by eliminating unnecessary triangles. The

dynamic boundary geometry for each timestep is then expressed in terms acceptable to the simulation software.

3. Simulation: This key step comprises the numerical solution of the mathematical equations that govern the evolution of the spatiotemporal physical flow characteristics of the intracardiac blood flow process under investigation. The fluid flow is modeled as a system of nonlinear partial differential equations (the Navier–Stokes equations) in the three space dimensions and in time. The field is then discretized by replacing the continuous space and time variables by a sequence of successive arrays, each composed of irregularly spaced points to form a finite element grid. It must be emphasized that, unlike analytical models, simulations do not provide a *closed-form*[33] solution to the problem under investigation. Instead, simulation provides answers to so-called *"what if"* questions, via a series of evaluation experiments; or, the results of complex simulation experiments can be analyzed using statistical techniques, such as analysis of variance, to determine the relationships between independent and dependent variables of interest. These approaches may disappoint some who expect models to provide closed-form answers to their question, and quickly.

4. Post-processing for Visualization: Suitable computational fluid dynamics (CFD) algorithms are then brought into play to provide the solution variables for all points in space at successive timesteps. In this way, pressure and blood velocities are calculated for all points in time and space throughout the flow field. In addition, the shear force at all points on the endocardial surfaces can be computed for each timestep. The computation is carried out over any phase of the cardiac cycle, and successive phases can be combined. It is fortunate that the time and skill level required for CFD simulation model-building is decreasing rapidly, as the power and flexibility of available marketed CFD software increases. Nevertheless, the time and effort required to formulate and implement a valid simulation model, and to conduct and properly interpret carefully designed experiments with the model, can still be considerable, even for the analysis of relatively simple cardiovascular flow systems.

5. Solution Data Base: The simulation software generates a flat file containing a vast amount of numerical data. These must be assembled in back-up memory to be accessible sufficiently rapidly for interactive displays of the solution and exploration of the evolving intracardiac flow phenomena. It is the purpose of the graphics hardware and flow visualization software to translate the myriad of numbers stored in memory into an easy-to-understand form.

We may someday soon be able to visualize the results of simulations of intracardiac blood flow in three dimensions using virtual reality techniques. The objective will be to enable clinicians and cardiac investigators to "take a walk" through the cardiac chambers

[33]In mathematics, an equation or system of equations is said to have a *closed-form solution* if, and only if, the solution can be expressed analytically in terms of a limited number of operations—e.g., the two roots of a quadratic equation can be expressed in closed form in terms of addition and subtraction, multiplication and division, and square root extraction. For many practical computer applications, it is reasonable to assume that other special functions of mathematical physics [1, 40, 87], such as the error function and the gamma function are "well-known," because computer software implementations are widely available.

and to observe how pressures and shear forces within the heart vary dynamically as it goes through its pumping cycle, in health and disease. This will provide better insights into multifaceted aspects of cardiac function and its aberrations, from molecular biology of endothelial adaptations and embryology, through comparative anatomy, physiology, and pathology, to diagnosis and medical and surgical management.

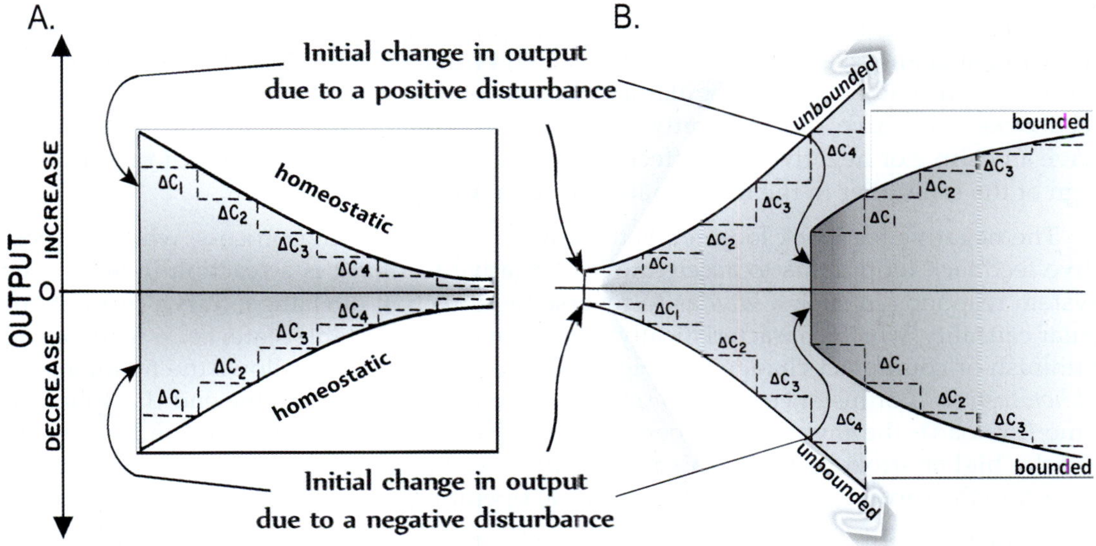

Figure 2.39: The output of a negative feedback control system might appear as shown in panel **A.** In this case, the ratios of successive to preceding values $\Delta C_2/\Delta C_1, \Delta C_3/\Delta C_2$, etc., of the controlled variable $C(t)$ are less than unity. Positive feedback may cause what is known as a vicious cycle, or it may not, depending upon the characteristics of the system, as is exemplified in panel **B.** In the case of the vicious cycle (*unbounded* response), the ratios $\Delta C_2/\Delta C_1, \Delta C_3/\Delta C_2$, etc., are greater than unity. When the response does not result in a vicious cycle (*bounded* response), the ratios $\Delta C_2/\Delta C_1, \Delta C_3/\Delta C_2$, etc., are less than unity.

2.23 Feedback mechanisms

Feedback is common in real-life events—e.g., it is sometimes observed when a microphone is in use, when some of the output signal is literally *fed back* into the system and causes the unpleasant screeching sounds. Feedback is a feature of any system in which the output, or result, affects the input of the system, thus modifying its operation. Feedback can, therefore, be useful; e.g., in the assembly of amplifiers where it is deliberately looped back into a system.

In physiologic systems, such as we encounter in the study of cardiac fluid dynamics [66, 67], most dynamic operating parameters, appropriate to a given physiologic state, must stay under control within a narrow range. Deviations from the optimal value of any controlled physiologic parameter can result from changes in the internal and external environments. In principle, a receptor system monitors the value of the parameter to maintain, and conveys it to a regulatory module via an afferent information pathway. Feedback is the message, from the sensor to the controller, of the difference between expectation and actual state.

There are two main kinds of feedback, by which a physiologic system may respond to incipient changes: positive and negative [32, 44, 55, 57, 74, 83, 88]. Hemodynamic systems contain many types of regulatory circuits, which comprise positive and negative feedbacks. "Positive" and "negative" do not imply that consequences of the feedback have a positive or negative final effect. They do not refer to desirability, but rather to the sign of the multiplier in the mathematical feedback equation.

The negative feedback loop tends to slow down an evolving process, while the positive feedback loop tends to accelerate it. Negative feedback is a reaction in which the system responds in such a way as to reverse the direction of change. It is a form of circular causality, which characteristically tends to maintain a stable state; i.e., a tendency to diminish or counteract change (see Fig. 2.39 A. on p. 105). This allows the maintenance of *homeostasis*. For instance, when a transient disturbance increases the end-diastolic volume (preload), the myocardial fibers increase their contraction strength and extent, to expel a higher stroke volume; this mobilization of the Frank–Starling mechanism tends to restore the cardiac volumes to their normal operating ranges, within a few beats.

In positive feedback, the response is to amplify the incipient change. Positive feedback is a form of circular causality, which acts as a growth-generating mechanism; i.e., the deviation of the system may grow continually larger (see Fig. 2.39 B., *unbounded* response) or it may tend asymptotically toward a new value (see Fig. 2.39 B., *bounded* response). Such responses typically have a destabilizing effect, so they do not result in homeostasis. They are seen in many a pathologic state, when they may sometimes progress on to a vicious circle (*unbounded* response). Although less common in normal physiologic systems than negative feedback, positive feedback loops do occur, usually resulting in so-called "virtuous circles" (*bounded* responses). For example, in an organism, most positive feedbacks provide for fast autoexcitation of elements of physiologic subsystems; for instance,

- in thrombosis, the presence of sticky platelets in a platelet plug, in turn stimulates other platelets to get sticky;
- in blood coagulation, the activation of at least one plasma factor in turn stimulates the transition to active of its own inactive form;
- in nerves, threshold electric potential triggers generation of the much larger action potential.

They play a key role in regulation of morphogenesis, growth, and development of organs, all of which are processes that represent in essence a rapid escape from some antecedent state.

Feedback and regulation are self-related. The negative feedback helps to maintain stability in a system in spite of external changes. It promotes homeostasis [8, 15], the summation of usually multifactorial regulatory processes by which viable internal conditions are maintained within the organism, independent of external variations. This homeostasis principle affirms that regulation and negative feedback control chains are essential ingredients in the maintenance of an organism's form and function. Positive feedback amplifies possibilities of divergences, i.e., changes in physiologic or pathophysiologic[34] states. It is a necessary condition for change, and gives the system the ability to access new points of equilibrium.

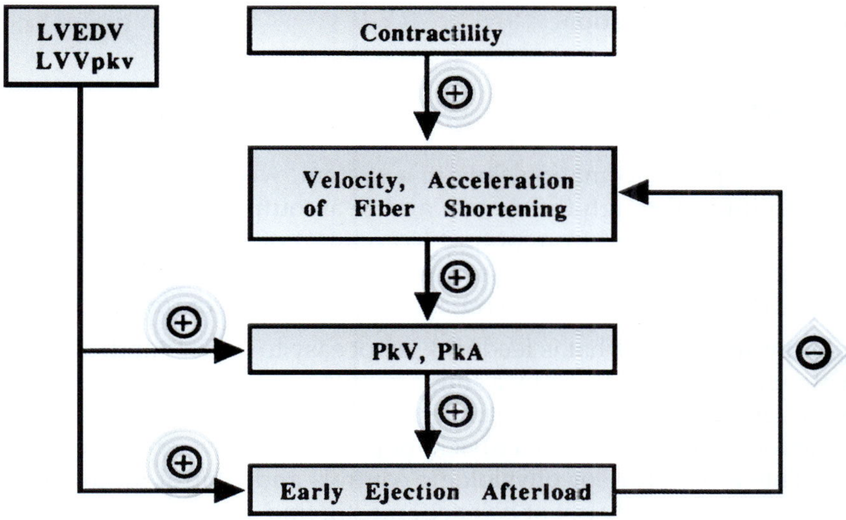

Figure 2.40: Diagrammatic representation of the interrelation between contractility, load on the ventricular myocardium and ejection variables. Note the negative feedback between the early ejection afterload and the peak velocity and acceleration of the ventricular myocardial fibers. LVEDV = left ventricular end-diastolic volume; LVVpkv = left ventricular volume at the time of peak velocity: PkA = peak outflow acceleration: PkV = peak ejection velocity. (Reprinted from Isaaz and Pasipoularides [38] by permission of the American College of Cardiology.)

Positive feedback, out of balance with negative feedback, leads to instability in a system. The heart is anatomically and functionally a "component" in a number of feedback control systems in the body, comprising hemodynamic, hormonal, and neuronal factors. Marked alterations in the dynamic function of diseased myocardium can alter the function of such feedback loops. The transition from a compensated ventricular function to a progressively decompensated one may result from conversion of a feedback control system that is stable, because of *negative* feedback, to a feedback control system that is unstable, because the feedback has become *positive*.[35]

[34]Pathophysiology is the study of the disturbance of normal mechanical, physical, and biochemical functions that characterize disease

[35]The system that previously responded to a perturbation by minimizing the effect of the perturbation,

In the example cited above, when a transient disturbance increases ventricular end-diastolic volume (preload), the myocardial fibers increase their contraction strength and extent, to expel a higher stroke volume; this tends to restore cardiac volumes to their normal operating ranges, within a few beats. Although effective and adequate in the acute situation, prolonged mobilization of the Frank–Starling mechanism carries potentially damaging side effects, when it persists over protracted periods. Increasing contractile strength by ventricular dilatation carries the risk of excessive myocardial oxygen demand because of the attendant increase in ventricular wall stresses at the larger chamber diameters—the law of Laplace [58]. In addition, there is risk of possible remodeling of the wall architecture to accommodate *persistently* larger chamber dimensions, which can be thought of as a positive feedback manifestation.

2.23.1 Feedback loop

In diagrams that depict information flow in a system, we usually draw arrowed lines, directed from an input through the system and to an output. We show the feedback by another arrowed line, directed from output to an input of the system, resulting in a loop on the diagram, which we recognize as a feedback loop (see Fig. 2.40). This notion is important; e.g., the feedback loop is a convenient place for a control mechanism.

In complex systems, just what is feedback is not easy to understand, and how to act on it is not always clear or determined by a single rule. A very complex system does not have a single controller. It has multiple controllers with multiple feedback loops on multiple levels of recursion. These various feedback loops learn, evolve and often compete with one another. This is a feature of physiologic controls and control redundancy. Systems built in this way can get wildly out of balance and still find a path back to stability. Indeed, going to the edge of nonstability is a strategy by which complex physiologic systems bring themselves to transformation and adaptation. As we noted above, such adaptations carry potentially damaging side effects when they persist over protracted periods. There is then qualitative transition from physiologic adaptation to disease.

2.24 Conclusion

We have reviewed mathematical tools and concepts that are very valuable in the study of intracardiac blood flows and support their better understanding. Clearly, the mathematical representation must and will be used cautiously and parsimoniously in what follows, to avoid overly reductive formulations which risk being abstruse, as well as artificial and irrelevant. There are indeed many occasions where ordinary language does provide satisfactory description of the evolution of intracardiac flow phenomena and allows valid prediction of some of their patterns. All the same, the mathematical modeling of the phenomena we are about to study can ensure a rational robustness for the analysis of their complex patterns and behavior.

---

subsequently responds to a perturbation by enhancing the effect of the perturbation—there is a qualitative change, recognized as transition to pathology.

References and further reading

Here are some useful references about mathematical methods. These references are cited in the text. They are available in every worthy bookshop and university library. It may help to read parts of some of them to find fuller accounts of concepts presented in this Chapter.

[1] Abramowitz, M., Stegun, I.A. Handbook of mathematical functions, with formulas, graphs, and mathematical tables. 1965, New York: Dover. xiv, 1046 p.

[2] Alger, P.L., Steinmetz, C.P. Mathematics for science and engineering. 2nd ed. 1969, New York: McGraw-Hill. x, 374 p.

[3] Antia, H.M. Numerical methods for scientists and engineers. 2002, Basel; Boston: Birkhäuser. xxii, 842 p.

[4] Aris, R. Vectors, tensors, and the basic equations of fluid mechanics. 1962, Englewood Cliffs, N.J.: Prentice-Hall. 286 p.

[5] Bajpai, A.C., Mustoe, L.R., Walker, D. Advanced engineering mathematics. 2nd ed. 1990, Chichester [England]; New York: Wiley. ix, 502 p.

[6] Bak, T.A., Lichtenberg, J. Mathematics for scientists. 1966, New York: W. A. Benjamin. xiv, 487 p.

[7] Bellomo, N., Preziosi, L. Modelling mathematical methods and scientific computation. 1995, Boca Raton, FL: CRC Press. xiv, 497 p.

[8] Bernard, C. Leçons sur les phénomènes de la vie communs aux animaux et aux végétaux. Avec une préface de Georges Canguilhem. 1967, Paris: Vrin. 14, xxxi, 404 p.

[9] Berry, E. A practical approach to medical image processing. 2008, New York: Taylor & Francis. xvi, 288 p.

[10] Bird, J.O. Engineering mathematics. 2007, Amsterdam; Boston: Newnes. x, 576 p.

[11] Bird, R.B., Stewart, W.E., Lightfoot, E.N. Transport phenomena. 2002, New York: J. Wiley. xii, 895 p.

[12] Bock, R.K., Krischer, W. The data analysis briefbook. 1998, Berlin; New York: Springer. v, 190 p.

[13] Boyce, W.E., DiPrima, R.C. Elementary differential equations and boundary value problems. 8th ed. 2005, Hoboken, NJ: Wiley. xviii, 790 p.

[14] Burger, W. Principles of digital image processing: fundamental techniques. 2009, New York: Springer.

[15] Cannon, W. B. The wisdom of the body. 1939, New York: W.W. Norton. xviii, 333 p.

[16] Carlbom, I., Chakravarty, I., Hsu, W.M. SIGGRAPH'91 Workshop Report Integrating Computer Graphics, Computer Vision, and Image Processing in Scientific Applications. SIGGRAPH Comput. Graph. 26: 8–17, 1992.

[17] Chaitin, G.J. Information, randomness & incompleteness: papers on algorithmic information theory. Series in computer science; v. 8. 1987, Singapore; Teaneck, NJ, USA: World Scientific. x, 272 p.

[18] Chapra, S.C. Applied numerical methods with MATLAB for engineers and scientists. 2008, Boston: McGraw-Hill Higher Education. xx, 588 p.

[19] Collins, R.E. Mathematical methods for physicists and engineers. 2nd corr. ed. 1999, Mineola, N.Y.: Dover. 385 p.

[20] Dahlhaus, R. Mathematical methods in signal processing and digital image analysis. 2008, Berlin: Springer. xiv, 292 p.

[21] Dahlquist, G., Björck, Å. Numerical methods. 1974, Englewood Cliffs, N.J.: Prentice-Hall. xviii, 573 p.

[22] Dallet, D., Silva, J.M.d. Dynamic characterisation of analogue-to-digital converters. 2005, Dordrecht: Springer. xx, 280 p.

[23] Davidson, R.C. Mathematical methods for introductory physics with calculus. 3rd ed. 1994, Fort Worth, TX: Saunders College Publishing. ix, 237 p.

[24] De Freitas, J.M. Digital filter design solutions. 2005, Boston: Artech House. xix, 463 p.

[25] Dixon, C. Applied mathematics of science & engineering. Introductory mathematics for scientists and engineers. 1971, London; New York: Wiley. xiii, 489 p.

[26] Dougherty, G. Digital image processing for medical applications. 2009, Cambridge, UK; New York: Cambridge University Press.

[27] Drazin, P.G., Riley, N. The Navier-Stokes equations: a classification of flows and exact solutions. 2006, Cambridge, UK; New York: Cambridge University Press. x, 196 p.

[28] Dunn, S.M., Constantinides, A., Moghe, P.V. Numerical methods in biomedical engineering. 2006, Amsterdam; Boston: Elsevier Academic Press. xviii, 615 p.

[29] Farlow, S.J. Partial differential equations for scientists and engineers. Dover books on advanced mathematics. 1993, New York: Dover. ix, 414 p.

[30] Feynman, R.P., Leighton R.B., Sands, M.L. The Feynman lectures on physics. 1963, Reading, Mass.: Addison–Wesley. 3 v.

[31] Franklin, P. An introduction to Fourier methods and the Laplace transformation. 1958, New York: Dover. 289 p.

[32] Hardie, A.M. The elements of feedback and control. 1964, London; New York: Oxford University Press. xi, 344 p.

[33] Harper, P.G., Weaire, D.L. Introduction to physical mathematics. 1985, Cambridge [Cambridgeshire]; New York: Cambridge University Press. xi, 260 p.

[34] Hoffmann, K.A., Chiang, S.T. Computational fluid dynamics for engineers. 4th ed. 2000, Wichita, Kan.: Engineering Education System. v2.

[35] Hopf, L., Nef, W. Introduction to the differential equations of physics. 1948, New York: Dover. v, 154 p.

[36] Hornbeck, R.W. Numerical methods. 1975, New York: Quantum. 310 p.

[37] Hull, M.H. The calculus of physics. 1969, New York: W. A. Benjamin. xiv, 132 p.

[38] Isaaz K, Pasipoularides A. Noninvasive assessment of intrinsic ventricular load dynamics in dilated cardiomyopathy. J. Am. Coll. Cardiol. 17: 112–21, 1991.

[39] Jähne, B. Digital image processing. 6th ed. 2005, Berlin; New York: Springer. xiii, 607 p.

[40] Jahnke, E., Emde, F. Tables of functions with formulae and curves [Funktionentafeln mit Formeln und Kurven]. 1945, New York: Dover. 8 p.l., 306, 76 p.

[41] Jan, J.r. Medical image processing, reconstruction, and restoration: concepts and methods. 2006, Boca Raton, FL: Taylor & Francis. xxiii, 730 p.

[42] Kahn, P.G.K., Pompea, S.M. Nautiloid growth rhythms and dynamical evolution of the Earth-Moon system. Nature 275: 606–11, 1978.

[43] Kant, I. Metaphysische Anfangsgründe der Naturwissenschaft (1786). In: Kants Werke. 1968, Berlin: Akademie–Textausgabe. vol. iv.

[44] Khoo, M.C.K. Physiological control systems: analysis, simulation, and estimation. 2000, New York: Wiley-IEEE Computer Society Press. xvii, 319 p.

[45] Knight, B., Adams, R. Complex numbers and differential equations. 1975, London: Allen & Unwin. 119 p.

[46] Kreyszig, E. Advanced engineering mathematics. 2006, Hoboken, N.J.: John Wiley. 1 v. (various pagings)

[47] Layton, W.J. Introduction to the numerical analysis of incompressible viscous flows. 2008, Philadelphia: Society for Industrial and Applied Mathematics. xix, 213 p.

[48] Leachtenauer, J.C. Electronic image display: equipment selection and operation. 2004, Bellingham, Wash.: SPIE Press. xix, 272 p.

[49] Leathem, J.G. Volume and surface integrals used in physics. 2nd ed. Cambridge tracts in mathematics and mathematical physics; no. 1. 1960, New York: Hafner. 73 p.

[50] Lightfoot, E.N. Transport phenomena and living systems; biomedical aspects of momentum and mass transport. 1973, New York: Wiley. x, 495 p.

[51] Lighthill, M.J. Introduction to Fourier analysis and generalised functions. 1958, Cambridge [England]: Cambridge University Press. viii, 79 p.

[52] Lyons, R.G. Understanding digital signal processing. 2004, Upper Saddle River, NJ: Prentice Hall PTR. xviii, 665 p.

[53] McQuistan, R.B. Scalar and vector fields: a physical interpretation. 1965, New York: Wiley. xiv, 314 p.

[54] Merritt, F.S. Applied mathematics in engineering practice. McGraw-Hill series in continuing education for engineers. 1970, New York: McGraw-Hill. xii, 289 p.

[55] Milhorn, H.T. The application of control theory to physiological systems. 1966, Philadelphia: Saunders. xiii, 386 p.

[56] Miller, K.S. Partial differential equations in engineering problems. 1953, New York: Prentice-Hall. vii, 254 p.

[57] Milsum, J.H. Biological control systems analysis. 1966, New York: McGraw-Hill. xiv, 466 p.

[58] Mirsky, I., Pasipoularides, A. Clinical assessment of diastolic function. Prog. Cardiovasc. Dis. 32: 291–318, 1990.

[59] Moon, P., Spencer, D.E. The meaning of the vector Laplacian. J. Franklin Inst. 256: 551–8, 1953.

[60] Murray, J.D. Mathematical biology. 3rd ed. 2002, New York: Springer. 2 v.

[61] Najim, M. [Ed.] Digital filters design for signal and image processing. 2006, Newport Beach, CA: ISTE Ltd. xv, 369 p.

[62] Navier, C.L.M.H. Mémoire sur les lois de mouvement des fluides. Mem. Acad. R. Sci., Paris, 6: 389–416, 1823.

[63] O'Neil, P.V. Advanced engineering mathematics. 2007, Toronto, Thomson. xix, 1204, 72, 14 p.

[64] Papoulis, A. The Fourier integral and its applications. 1962, New York: McGraw-Hill. 318 p.

[65] Parhi, K.K., Nishitani, T. [Eds.] Digital signal processing for multimedia systems. 1999, New York: M. Dekker. xxi, 855 p.

[66] Pasipoularides, A. Clinical assessment of ventricular ejection dynamics with and without outflow obstruction. J. Am. Coll. Cardiol. 15: 859–82, 1990.

[67] Pasipoularides, A. Cardiac mechanics: basic and clinical contemporary research. Ann. Biomed. Eng. 20: 3–17, 1992.

[68] Pasipoularides, A.D., Shu, M., Shah, A., Glower, D.D. Right ventricular diastolic relaxation in conscious dog models of pressure overload, volume overload, and ischemia. J. Thorac. Cardiovasc. Surg. 124: 964–72, 2002.

[69] Pasipoularides, A.D., Shu, M., Womack, M.S., Shah, A., von Ramm, O., Glower, D.D. RV functional imaging: 3-D echo-derived dynamic geometry and flow field simulations. Am. J. Physiol. Heart Circ. Physiol. 284: H56–65, 2003.

[70] Patrascioiu, A. The Ergodic hypothesis: a complicated problem of Mathematics and Physics. In: Cooper, N.G., Eckhardt, R., Shera, N. [Eds.] From cardinals to chaos: reflections on the life and legacy of Stanislaw Ulam. 1989, Cambridge; New York: Cambridge University Press. pp. 263–79.

[71] Pitas, I. Digital image processing algorithms and applications. 2000, New York: Wiley. 419 p.

[72] Poincaré, H., Maitland F. Science and method. 1914, London, New York [etc.]: T. Nelson and sons. 288 p.

[73] Proakis, J.G., Manolakis, D.G. Digital signal processing. 2007, Upper Saddle River, N.J.: Pearson Prentice Hall. xix, 1084 p.

[74] Riggs, D.S. Control theory and physiological feedback mechanisms. 1970, Baltimore: Williams & Wilkins. xv, 599 p.

[75] Scarborough, J.B. Differential equations and applications for students of mathematics, physics, and engineering. 1965, Baltimore: Waverly Press. xiv, 479 p.

[76] Semmlow, J.L. Biosignal and medical image processing. 2nd ed. 2009, Boca Raton, FL: CRC Press. xvii, 450 p.

[77] Sheingold, D.H. and Analog Devices Inc. Analog-digital conversion handbook. 1986, Englewood Cliffs, NJ: Prentice-Hall. xxi, 672, xxiii-xliii p.

[78] Shercliff, J.A. Vector fields: vector analysis developed through its application to engineering and physics. 1977, Cambridge; New York: Cambridge University Press. xi, 329 p.

[79] Shim, Y.T., Pasipoularides A., Straley C.A., Hampton T.G., Soto P.F., Owen C.H., Davis J.W., Glower D.D. Arterial Windkessel parameter-estimation: a new time-domain method. Ann. Biomed. Eng. 22: 66–77, 1994.

[80] Simon, W. Mathematical techniques for biology and medicine. 1977, Cambridge, MA: MIT Press. xii, 291 p.

[81] Smith, J.O. Mathematics of the Discrete Fourier Transform (DFT) with audio applications. 2007, Stanford, CA: W3K Publishing. 322 p.

[82] Smith, S.W. The scientist and engineer's guide to digital signal processing. 1997, San Diego, CA: California Technical Pub. xiv, 626 p.

[83] Society for Experimental Biology (Great Britain) and University of Cambridge. Zoological Laboratory., Homeostasis and feedback mechanisms. 1964, Cambridge [England]: Cambridge University Press. 460 p.

[84] Stokes, G.G. On the theories of the internal friction of fluids in motion, and of the equilibrium and motion of elastic solids. Trans. Camb. Phil. Soc. 8: 287–305, 1845.

[85] Sutton, O.G. Mathematics in action: applications in aerodynamics, statistics, weather prediction, and other sciences. 1984, New York: Dover. viii, 236 p.

[86] Thede, L. Practical analog and digital filter design. 2005, Boston: Artech House. xiii, 267 p.

[87] Tuma, J.J. Engineering mathematics handbook: definitions, theorems, formulas, tables. 3rd ed. 1987, New York: McGraw-Hill. xiii, 498 p.

[88] Tzafestas, S.G. Applied control: current trends and modern methodologies. Electrical engineering and electronics; 83. 1993, New York: Marcel Dekker. xxii, 1051 p.

[89] Watt, A.H. 3D computer graphics. 3rd ed. 2000, Harlow, England; Reading, Mass.: Addison-Wesley. xxii, 570 p.

[90] Williamson, R.E., Crowell, R.H., Trotter, H.F. Calculus of vector functions. 3rd ed. 1972, Englewood Cliffs, N.J.: Prentice-Hall. xii, 617 p.

[91] Winder, S. Analog and digital filter design. 2002, Amsterdam; Boston: Newnes. 450 p.

[92] Zienkiewicz, O.C., Taylor, R.L. The finite element method; v. 3. Fluid dynamics. 5th ed. 2000, Oxford; Boston: Butterworth-Heinemann. 3 v.

Chapter 3

Some Notable Pioneers

The search for truth is in one way hard and in another easy, for no one can master it fully nor miss it fully, but each adds a little to our knowledge of nature, and from all things assembled there arises a certain grandeur.

——Aristotle, quoted in Editorial in Circulation [123].

Thus you will see its shape and its function. [The heart] was created to dilate, to contract and to revolve the blood in its cells [= chambers], full of tortuous passages separated by rounded walls ... so that the motion of the blood ... will make an easier revolution in its swirling impetus.

——Leonardo da Vinci on the ventricles of the heart [89] .

If I have seen further it is by standing on the shoulders of giants.

——from a letter written by Newton to fellow scientist Robert Hooke, on 5 February, 1676.[1] [94]

Isaac Newton, and the pioneers recognized in this brief historical chapter serve as shining examples of dedicated workers on whose shoulders we are privileged to stand. There are many others in our blood-flow motivated fluid dynamic heritage. May we honor their memory and contributions.

[1]Robert Burton, an English clergyman who lived a generation before Newton, attributed a similar statement to the Roman poet Lucan: *"Pigmies placed on the shoulder of giants see more than the giants themselves."*

It is very hard to look forward—to imagine in any concrete way what developments in intracardiac flow-field visualization and analysis are going to affect clinical cardiology and basic science. Likewise, when we look backward, to the great advances of the past, it is almost impossible to comprehend the brilliance of achievement of the great medical and scientific pioneers, simply because we cannot free ourselves from our present insights. Before we start in on the main task of this book, it is good to remind ourselves of the difficulty of projecting ourselves outside our immediate intellectual and mental framework, either to look to the past, or to the future. Yet, if I had to characterize that part of scientific history which is important—indeed essential—for scientists and medical researchers, I would use the word *perspective*. By this, I mean the ability to see current work in relation to formative past events. How far back in time this perspective needs to extend depends on the particular topic. Interestingly, the father of Medicine, Hippocrates of Kos (ca. 460–370 B.C.), already knew that the heart is the origin of all the vessels; he was acquainted with the large vessels arising from the heart, the cardiac valves, the chordae tendineae, the auricles, and the closure of the semilunar valves. In the exploration of intracardiac blood flow, a very long historical perspective indeed is needed.... This brief, and admittedly spotty, survey of important historical people and their discoveries should facilitate a better appreciation of what is to follow in succeeding chapters.

3.1 Euclid, Ptolemy, and the origins of perspective and projective geometry

In our study of intracardiac blood flow phenomena, we will employ extensively scientific visualization methods. Though not strictly defined, the term *scientific visualization* refers to the visualization, usually on a monitor (2-D surface), of data that has a more or less inherent representation in 3-D space and time, like, e.g., discrete data defined on spatial, possibly time-dependent, computational grids. Perspective is the science which teaches how to represent 3-D objects on a 2-D surface, such as a monitor screen, so that the perspective image coincides with the one which is given by direct vision (see Fig. 11.2, on p. 587). Accordingly, in studying cardiac pumping function and intracardiac blood flow phenomena, we employ perspective in graphic reconstructions of dynamic 3-D datasets acquired by various medical imaging systems, as well as of multidimensional datasets derived from scientific computations and simulations of time-dependent intracardiac flows.

The theory of perspective can be developed from a single familiar fact: that the apparent size of an object decreases with increasing distance from the eye. Linear perspective has a history going back at least to Agatharchus, a scene painter for the great Greek tragedian Aeschylus in the 5th century B.C., who astonished his audience with his realistic depiction of depth through appropriate size reduction in the spatial layout of buildings. In fact, the first historical mentions of art, by Plato and contemporaries in the 5th century B.C., were provoked by the dramatic use of perspective in the scenery for the plays of Aeschylus and Sophocles. Agatharchus even wrote a commentary on his use of convergent perspective, whose effects inspired several contemporary and subsequent Greek geometers to analyze the projective transform mathematically.

In 300 B.C., Euclid wrote the first text on geometric optics, *Optica* [50], in which he defined the terms *visual ray* and *visual cone* and formulated mathematically the inverse relation of size to distance as a set of surveying propositions. Ptolemy's *Optica,* A.D. 140, was another text on geometric optics that included his theories of refraction. Later, in his *Geographia,* [53] Ptolemy (Claudios Ptolemaios) applied principles of geometric optics and projective geometry [2] to the projection of the spherical 3-D surface of the Earth onto a flat 2-D surface [11]; the first linear perspective construction is also ascribed to Ptolemy, in drawing his map of the world [45,46].

In more traditional metaphysical systems, such as Aristotle's, a distinction had been drawn between the realm of astronomy, which is subject to precise, intelligible mathematical laws, and the sublunar world of change and decay, which is only partially intelligible to mortals. The principal achievement of Ptolemy's *Geographia* turned on its demonstration of the possibility of using a regular mathematical grid system to map the entire known world. Ptolemy thereby showed how the Earth's surface could be comprehended in a uniform way in terms of a single mathematical system. Essential to this achievement was the idea that the grid not only must have the mathematical properties of an exhaustive tessellation, but also that it be transparent. Ptolemy's grid is not a part of any reconstruction of some abstract mathematical realm. It is designed, rather, to help us grasp this world as it really is. Ptolemy built upon other Greek geographers' discoveries, most notably those of Hipparchos, who conceived the revolutionary innovation of dividing the globe into 360° of longitude and latitude. Within this framework, Hipparchos decreed that every place on Earth could be fixed by the point at which the east-west circle of latitude and the north-south circle of longitude intersected, as measured by astronomical

[2]Projective geometry is the branch of geometry that deals with the relationships between geometric figures and the images that result from projecting them onto another surface. Familiar examples of projections are the shadows cast by opaque 3-D objects, radiographs, and videos or cine-loops displayed on a 2-D screen.

observation [19]. This Greek expertise was transmitted to the Roman Empire in, e.g., the accurate central vanishing points to be seen in the wall-paintings of Pompeii. Clearly, the Greek and Roman painters could evoke astonishing levels of three-dimensionality in their murals.

Not only in the Roman era, but subsequently in the 14th century, painters such as Cimabue, Giotto, and the Lorenzetti brothers made progress toward a more coherent approach to geometric perspective that sparked the eloquent visual representation that is the hallmark of Renaissance art. The "modern" origins of geometric perspective can be traced to the Masters of the Renaissance in Florence, Italy, in the early 1400s.[3] The artist and architect Brunelleschi demonstrated its principles, but another architect and writer, Leon Battista Alberti was first to write down rules of linear perspective for artists to follow. Leonardo da Vinci (see Section 3.3, on pp. 119 ff.), the first known proponent of scientific visualization, probably learned Alberti's system while serving as an apprentice to the artist Verrocchio in Florence. Leonardo was among the very first in "modern times" to take a scientific approach toward understanding how our world works and *how we see* it.

Nowadays mainly computers are employed for generating and displaying 3-D dataset representations; this connects the field of data visualization to computer science, in particular to computer graphics.

3.2 Aristotle

Aristotle (ca. 384–322B.C.) was born in Stagira, near Mount Athos at the northern end of the Aegean Sea. His father, Nicomachus, was the family physician of King Amyntas of the state of Macedonia in northern Greece. It is believed that Aristotle's ancestors had been the physicians of the Macedonian royal family for several generations. Having come from a long line of physicians, Aristotle received training and education that inclined his mind toward the study of natural phenomena. This education had long-lasting influences [48], and was probably the root cause of a less idealistic stand on philosophy, as opposed to Plato, in whose *Academy* Aristotle was a student until shortly after Plato's death [71].

Charles Darwin regarded Aristotle as the most important contributor to the subject of biology. On reading William Ogle's translation of Aristotle's *The Parts of Animals* [6], Darwin commented on Aristotle, the biologist: "I had not the most remote notion what a wonderful man he was. Linnaeus and Cuvier have been my two gods, though in very different ways, but they were mere schoolboys to old Aristotle." ((Letter to Ogle, Feb. 22, 1882) [64]).

[3]Note, in passing, that Christopher Columbus was motivated by the first printed Ptolemaic map of the world [45]. Ptolemy's *"Geographia,"* dating from around A.D. 140, was rediscovered and arrived in Florence in 1400 to great acclaim. The impact of Ptolemy's transparent grid system was so great that already by 1424 Florence had acquired the reputation of a center of cartographic and geographic study, and it is through commentaries on Florentine versions of *"Geographia,"* that its influence extended to Columbus.

Aristotle was a founder of scientific anatomy [126], and was perhaps the first to recognize that the blood vessels were a connected system arising from the heart and extending throughout the body. He was the first to apply the terms aorta and venae cavae. He discussed the structure of the heart in a few of his treatises, such as *Historia Animalium* and *De Partibus Animalium*, but his view was that the heart was the seat of the senses. He theorized that since the heart was "central, mobile, and hot, and well supplied with structures which served to communicate between it and the rest of the body, it was a singular and central organ, and so it was most suitable to being the seat of the soul." He did recognize correctly, however, that the heart was the source of motion of blood in the vessels and that blood was the distributor in the body of transformed food [122].

Aristotle's ideas basic to fluid mechanics are a lot closer to our contemporary knowledge [82,97,119]. All analytical fluid mechanics rests on the "continuum hypothesis" and the "continuity principle." Aristotle was the first to give their general formulation [3,4]: "The continuous may be defined as that which is divisible into parts that are in turn themselves divisible to infinity, as a body which is divisible in all ways. Magnitude divisible in one direction is a line, in three directions a body. Being divisible in three directions, a body is divisible in all directions. And magnitudes which are divisible in this fashion are continuous."

The observation of static and moving fluids and their effect on objects can be traced back to Aristotle, who conceived the notion that air has weight and observed that a body moving through a fluid encounters resistance. Another contribution of Aristotle to fluid motion was the principle of enforced motion, which was restated by Galileo, Huygens, and Newton: "It is impossible to say why a body that has been set in motion in vacuum should ever come to rest. Why, indeed, should it come to rest at one place rather than another? As a consequence, it will either necessarily stay at rest or, if in motion, will move indefinitely unless some obstacle comes into collision with it" [3]. Thus, Aristotle was the first, and Galileo and Newton only second and third, to formulate the concept of inertia [1,2,32,40].

In his *On the Heavens* [2–4], he developed the *distinction* between *natural* and *enforced* motion, which led him to conclude that "A body will necessarily either stay at rest or, if in motion, will move indefinitely unless some obstacle compels it to *change its state of motion*." He was also the first to perceive the action of frictional air resistance [3], stating that "When a body moves in the atmosphere, the surrounding air becomes hot and, in certain circumstances, it (the body) even melts." Aristotle was thus able to discern inertial and frictional effects, whose interplay underlies many fascinating fluid dynamic phenomena, including intra-cardiac flow vortices.

3.3 Leonardo da Vinci and Albrecht Dürer

Leonardo da Vinci (1425–1519) may be the first known proponent of scientific visualization; see Section 12.9.1 on pp. 668 ff. He developed techniques for observing the wind, by generating *smoke* in a tube and adding it to the wind at suitable points. Most remarkably,

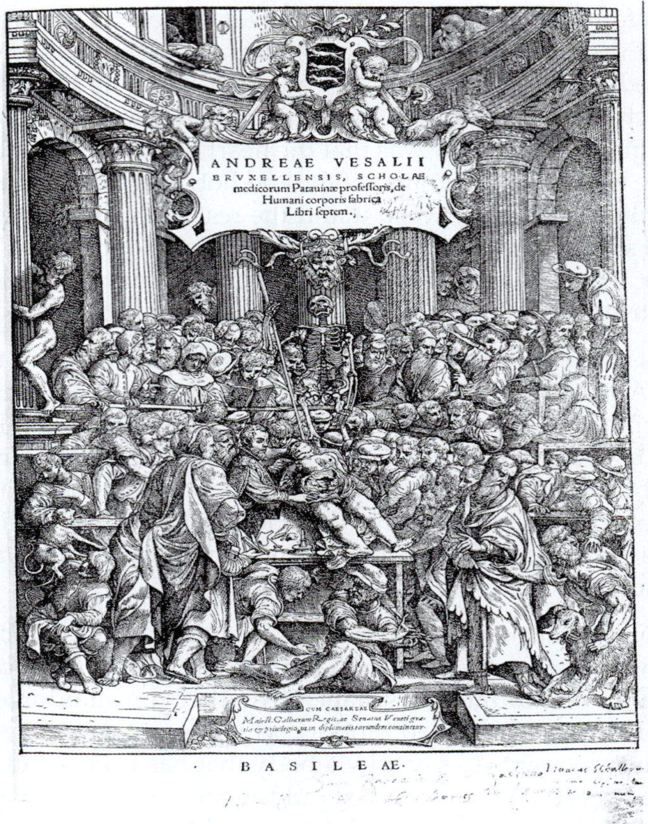

Figure 3.1: Andreas Vesalius, Title page of *De Humani Corporis Fabrica*. ©National Library of Medicine, Washington, DC.

he made actual experiments under controlled conditions. For this purpose, he used, among other things, a tank containing water mixed with fine millet,[4] through which he moved solids, observing the flow around and past them. Leonardo wrote: "The movement of water within water proceeds like that of air within air" [135]. His fascinating sketches provide an obvious early link between fluid dynamics and art.

One aspect of Leonardo's innovative technical contributions is his analysis of the components (the "organs") of machines, which he depicted in isolation from the other parts to which they were functionally connected. He was the first to regard machines as such an assemblage of distinct parts, rather than as an indivisible whole. In the thirty years from A.D. 1485 to 1515, Leonardo discovered that perspective was much more than a means for producing 3-D effects. Perspective was based on the assumption that every object has a fixed measured size; that size and shape within a given plane are constant, and that size varies only with distance.

[4]Millet is a fine, edible yellow grain, the seed of an annual grass; it is a common ingredient in bird seed.

Perspective enabled representation of complex organic forms, such as the human body, in methodical terms: from different viewpoints, as a whole, and in relation to its parts, with a result that its functions could be laid bare. It offered the same possibilities with respect to machines, which led to a catalog of different mechanical functions, including couplings, friction wheels, flywheels, brakes, pipes, and valves [117]. He applied the same method to the study of the human body whose organs, including the heart, he regarded as highly sophisticated *mechanical devices*. His vision of the anatomy of machines and man was enshrined in a progression of masterly drawings, which opened up the era of modern scientific illustration [10]. However, Leonardo's manuscripts are rarely tidy. Characteristically, each page stands autonomous and unrelated to the neighboring sheets, giving the impression of an apparently chaotic stratification of drawings and annotations, many with interspersed pedantic reminders for everyday tasks.

Leonardo focused his interest on visual elements and qualities. He added *tracers* to air and to water, in order to make visible flow patterns within. The shift to the visual that Leonardo spearheaded is an enhancement of vision over, above, and to the detriment of either full perceptual or nonvisual perceptions. For instance, descriptive anatomy at the time was often in tactile (hard, pliant, etc.) and olfactory (metallic, putrid, etc.) terms—bear in mind that in the Renaissance, refrigeration was not available! Da Vinci reduced this anatomy to a structural and analytical set of drawings based on his own human dissections. These drawings visually depicted muscles, veins, and heart valves in a way that was later emulated by the Belgian anatomist and physician Andries van Wesele, better known as Andreas Vesalius (1514–64), in his detailed account of human anatomy, *De Humani Corporis Fabrica*, which was first published in 1543 (see Fig. 3.1, on p. 120).[5]

The scientific revolution is often described as if it occurred primarily in the realm of astronomy. However, it owed as much to disciplines such as surveying and painting which, combined with perspective, established a vision of universal *measurability*. Remarkably, the origins of a truly modern kind of understanding of intracardiac flow patterns, albeit not of the circulation, can be traced readily back to Leonardo, who actually predated Harvey by one-and-a-half century. Leonardo's ideas were contrary to the prevailing teachings of authority. The authority in question, to whom Harvey refers repeatedly in his *de Motu Cordis* as the "Divine Galen," was Claudius Galenus [48, 116], the second-century (A.D. 129–210) Greek doctor *Galenos* ($\Gamma\alpha\lambda\eta\nu o\varsigma$), who was the attending physician to Marcus Aurelius Antoninus, the Roman Emperor, A.D. 161–180, and stoic philosopher, remembered for his moral precepts, written in Greek. Galen, called Gallien by Chaucer and other writers of the middle ages, proved that the nerves conducted a "force of contraction" from the brain to the muscles. He founded the sciences of neurophysiology and experimental anatomy. Galen correctly surmised [86] that the veins *communicate* with the arteries by *fine tubes*! His deductions concerning the function of the heart, however, were quite off the mark and somewhat quaint, when viewed from our modern perspective. Nevertheless, the Galenic view was coherent within itself and related neatly to a general medical theory that dealt with the body in terms of humors and spirits. Because of that coherence, it exerted a compelling grip on physicians' minds.

---

[5]It is of some interest that Vesalius' seven-volume masterpiece was created in collaboration with Johann Stephan von Kalkar, student of the great Renaissance Italian painter Ticiano (Tiziano Vecellio) [48].

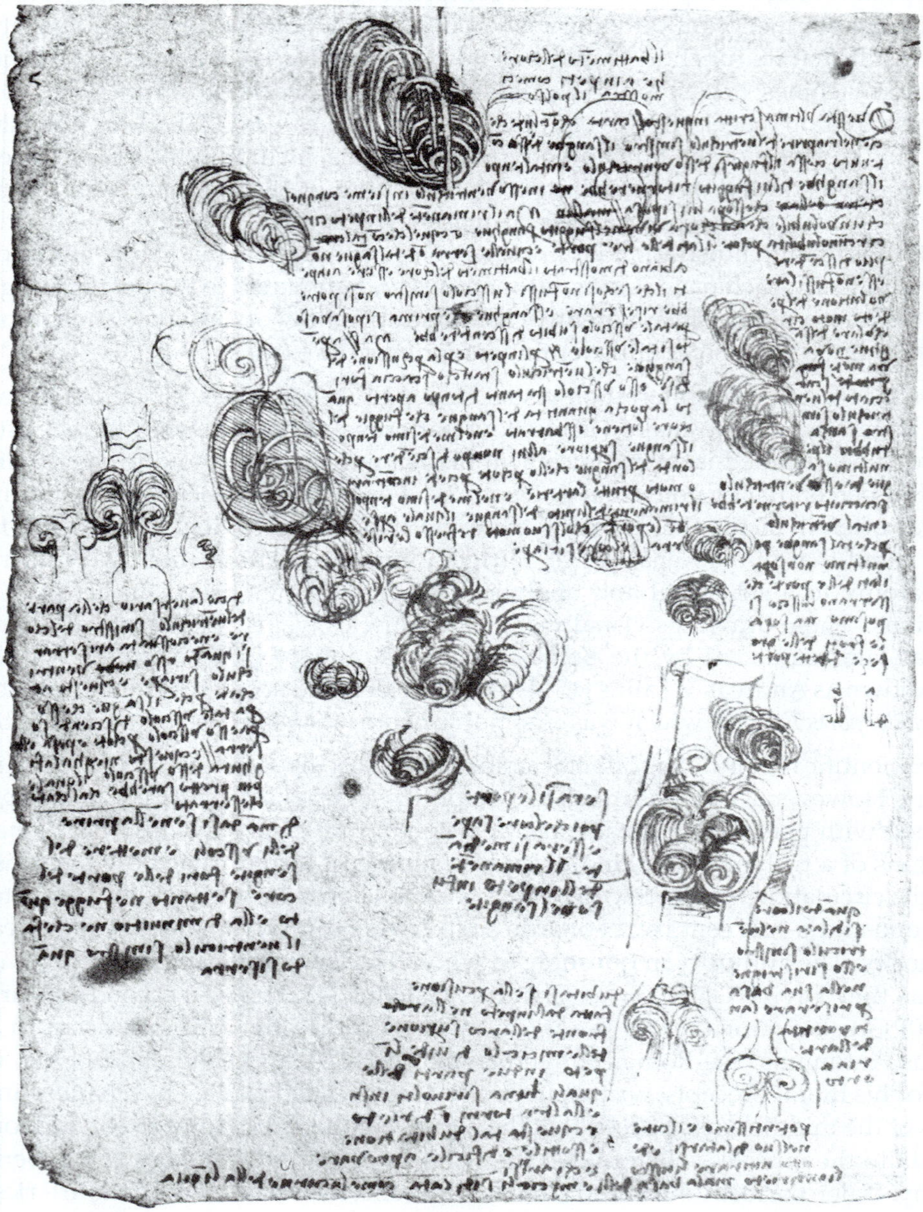

Figure 3.2: Hydraulics, called by Leonardo "the nature of water," was a subject of abiding interest for him, and he applied it to problems of hemodynamics. The representative figures and notes on this plate examine the question of the influence of blood vortices in the closure of the aortic valve. Drawings of the Heart, ca. 1513, Windsor Castle Royal Library I9083v. ©1994 Her Majesty The Queen of England.

Contrary to Galen, the properties that Leonardo typically associated with musculature he considered to be possessed by the heart tissue. Rather than assigning these qualities as being deceptive to the true function of the heart, as Galen decreed, Leonardo found the evidence suggestive of the function of the heart [83]. His own anatomic observations (he may have dissected as many as thirty human bodies) allowed him to come closer to a picture of the heart by today's standards. He suggested that the heart was actually the most powerful muscle in the body. The noble status of the heart that Galen arrived at via the distancing of the heart from mechanical, mindless movement, was entirely reversed by Leonardo. By taking the mechanical function of the heart and its muscular nature seriously, he was able to postulate as to how the muscle worked [83]. According to the theories inherited from Galen, the heart consisted of two ventricles separated by the interventricular septum, the atria being simply bulging appendixes of the veins. After much study, and unlike any of his predecessors, Leonardo came to consider the importance and independence of the chambers residing above the ventricles.

He realized that the upper chambers, which he denoted as auricles, were composed of substance that differentiated them from mere vasculature. Secondly, he realized that these auricles were made of material that allowed them to expand passively under stress and that contracted actively. Thus, rather than holding the inert role of draining conduits, the auricles were *active*. He also realized that the lower ventricles contract, and that their contraction occurs at a *distinct* time than in the auricles He argued logically that two opposite motions could not take place at the same time in the same subject. Therefore, if the right upper [auricle] and lower ventricles were the same, it would be necessary that the whole should cause one and the same effect at the same time, and not two effects subserving two diametrically opposite purposes.

Leonardo viewed the organs to be of perfect design [89]. However, unlike previous and contemporary authorities alike, he did not consider his observations tangential. Perfect design was reflected in contingent observations. Dividing membranes, valves, and opposing functions would not exist within the same chamber, if perfectly designed. By employing a visual, rational science, Leonardo was able to come to refreshing and insightful conclusions about the physical nature and function of the heart.

Characteristic of all Leonardo's work is the thorough integration of experimental and observational method and of reasoning with applications. We are now in a position to explore the dynamic discourse germinating in his mind between an evolving understanding of the body and its parts and his firmer understanding of the earth and its parts. The microcosm–macrocosm analogy, persistent since ancient times, was a world view that Leonardo elaborated throughout his own studies. Leonardo believed the earth and the body to be governed by universal mechanical laws. Thus, a beautiful reciprocal relationship emerged between an understanding of the heart and blood flow on one hand, and of the earth and its waters on the other, and fundamental principles were explored *by analogy* for their impact on both scales.

A first major analogy that Leonardo made was that the seas and blood were functionally the same in the living organisms of the earth and the human. Similarly, the water conduits and vasculature were of the same nature. In research about the heart's

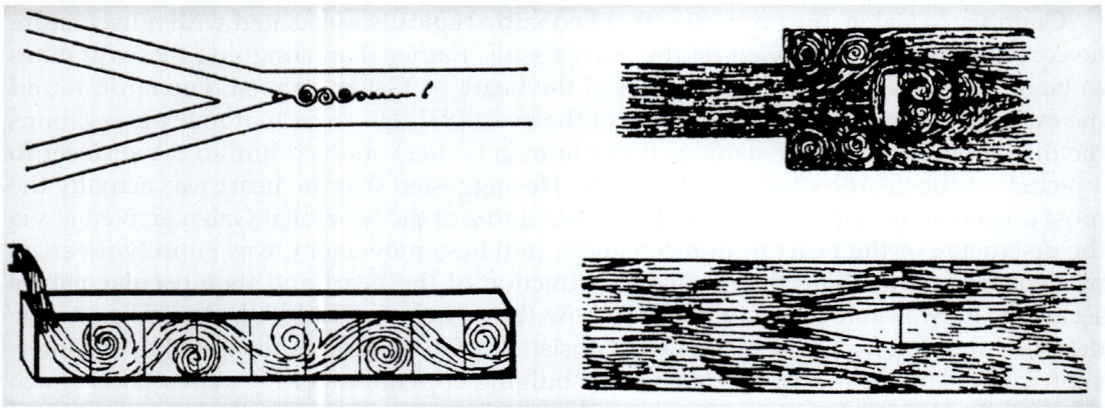

Figure 3.3: Sketches from Leonardo da Vinci visualizing flow patterns [93].

operation, Leonardo referred to experiments about water flow [31, 51, 83, 90, 93]. As to rivers—objects of vital interest in Renaissance times, because they offered the main means of communication—he said that one general law applies: where the flow carries a large quantity of water, the flow speed is great, and *vice versa*. Similarly, he stated that where a river becomes shallower, the water flows faster [98]. He enunciated and clearly understood the implications of the velocity–area law, namely, that the product of fluid mean velocity and cross-sectional area of a channel or duct is constant. This idea of *"continuity,"* or mass conservation, can be traced in all his drawings of air, water, and blood flows.

Having made canals, he observed the way undertows formed when the water flowed from a smaller conduit to a wider [115]. He applied this discovery to the blood's flow through the heart's valves (see Fig. 3.2, on p. 122), and was the first to draw and describe intracardiac vortical flows [83,91,92]. Having introduced quite a modern technique, flow visualization, in his experiments by means of floating particles in water (see Fig. 3.3), he even suggested further flow visualization studies by using glass models!

In fact, in McMurrich's delightful history of Leonardo da Vinci [105] we read: *"He pondered much over the nature of the eddies and whirlpools that must be formed within the cups of the semilunar valves, when these were brought together by the reflux of the blood on the completion of the contraction of the ventricle. There are several sketches representing theoretical possibilities for these eddies, but these did not satisfy; the eddies could not be actually observed in the heart and Leonardo proposed to make a glass model of the basal portion of the aorta in which the course of the blood could be seen."* His studies on a simple aortic root glass model to simulate flow dynamics was 400 years ahead of Osborn Reynolds' famous pipe flow visualization studies [63]. Da Vinci's drawings depict beautifully the formation of vortical structures in the sinuses of Valsalva, three cavities at the entrance region of the aorta. He visualized correctly the nature of vortex formation in confined cavities, and their role in the closure dynamics of the aortic valve.

Leonardo's observations on vortex motion were numerous [62] and most insightful. The modern concept of "rotation" or vorticity (i.e., the angular velocity of an infinitesimal fluid particle) was, of course, beyond the grasp of Leonardo. For him, vortices or eddies (*"retrosi"*) are simply curl-like, rotatory flow phenomena, which are directly visible, or can be made so by adding some millet to water, or by introducing smoke into the air. He made very numerous sketches of such vortices—cf. Figure 3.3, on p. 124. He not only observed the vortex-filled wake of obstacles, such as bridge supports, and the vortices at an abrupt expansion of a canal or at the discharge of a narrow jet into a much broader waterway, but he also observed, astutely, the less conspicuous vortices *upstream* of an abrupt contraction.

It seems that Leonardo clearly distinguished between all these curl-like vortices on one hand and, on the other, the helicoidal, circulatory swirls as observed in, e.g., a bathtub vortex away from its central core; today, such swirls are known to be essentially irrotational in that the fluid particles in them circulate but are free from "rotation." He made the following amazingly accurate quantitative observation:

"The helicoidal, circulatory motion[6] of any liquid is so much the faster, as it is nearer to its axis of revolution. This is a phenomenon worthy of admiration. It is known that the circular motion of a wheel is slower toward the middle than toward the periphery. However, this is not the case for the water. In each full revolution of the water, in the smaller circles as in the larger ones, the total amount of motion—taking into account both the velocity and the perimeter—is the same..." Thus, Leonardo anticipated one of the key concepts of modern hydrodynamics, that is, the notion of *circulation* (path times velocity), and aptly ascertained that in an irrotational flow this quantity is invariant with radial distance from the axis of the circulatory motion.

Interestingly, although it became a popular and very important fluid mechanics notion only in the twentieth century, the word "turbulence"[7] was apparently first introduced by Leonardo, who in approximately the year 1500 used it in the sense that is similar to its current meaning—see Section 4.14, on pp. 212 ff. He knew also that eddies of the most varied sizes are present in rivers and in the wind and the following passage is significant: "Of the things carried by the water, those will make the greatest revolution that are of least size. This happens because the great revolutions of eddies are infrequent in the currents of rivers, and the small eddies are almost numberless and large objects are only turned round by large eddies and not by small ones, whereas small objects revolve both in small eddies and large."

Albrecht Dürer, the German artist and mathematician (1471–1528), is arguably the greatest exponent of Northern European Renaissance art [110]. Dürer was a great admirer of his contemporary Leonardo da Vinci and was intrigued by the Italian master's studies of the human figure. After 1506, he adapted Leonardo's proportions to his own figures, as is noticeable in his drawings. Later in life, in the 1520s, he produced illustrated geometric treatises instructing artists in perspective and proportion [43]. Dürer's works

[6] See Neményi [108], p. 168.

[7] Derived from the Greek $\tau\upsilon\rho\beta\eta$, Latin *turba*, meaning *whirling confusion*, the term betrays at once the chaotic kinetic nature of the phenomenon and the rotational disposition of the eddies.

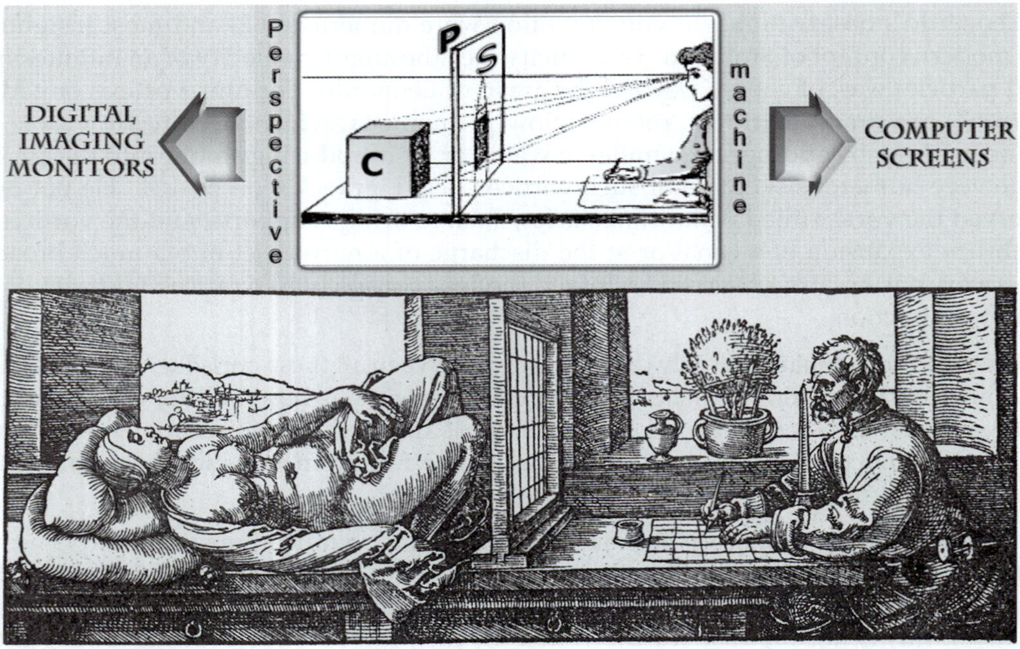

Figure 3.4: Bottom: *Zeichner des liegenden Weibes* (Artist drawing a recumbent woman), by Albrecht Dürer, in his *Underweysung der Messung* [43]. It depicts a *perspective machine*; note that the head of the artist is held immobile. It is only this rigid immobility that produces stable, measurable distances in the field of vision, allowing space to be measured or rendered as a construction. It is only thus that seeing can be subjected to the laws of Geometry. Inset: In this simplified sketch, P is the vertical transparent plane or picture, C is a cube placed on one side of it, and the painter is the spectator on the other side of it. The dotted lines drawn from the corners of the cube to the eye of the spectator are the visual rays, and the points on the transparent picture plane where these visual rays pass through it indicate the perspective position, S, of those points on the picture.

were related to scientific visualization issues in many ways, most obviously through their representation of nature. They include his pioneering and most successful efforts aimed at producing *realistic*, rather than idealized, images of natural objects. To this end, he pushed his skills as an engraver, drawer, and colorist, to the extremes. He also exploited geometry in his studies on the representation of the human body [133], and more generally for the translation of 3-D volumes into 2-D images. Indeed, he was a pioneer of Descriptive Geometry [125] and in imparting *depth* on flat images (cf. modern *computer graphics*).

Although it is true that he combined prints to create a sense of depth, his studies on *perspective* aimed at the *compression* of the 3-D visual experience onto a 2-D surface based on vanishing points and lines were of substantially higher novelty and significance. They were a real breakthrough toward the representation of depth and 3-D volumes, and have been universally used by artists and medical illustrators thereafter. Accordingly, he is credited with formalizing and refining linear perspective in Renaissance Art, having studied the principles of foreshortening and the creation of an illusion of depth by viewing a subject through a grid and then transposing the image onto a sheet of paper having an identical grid of lines on it [47], as is shown in Figure 3.4.

Perspective [132] represents figures and objects not as they are but *as we see them* in 3-D space, whereas Geometry represents figures not as we see them but *as they are*. When we have a front view of a figure such as a square, its perspective and geometrical appearance are the same, and we see it as it really is, i.e., with all its sides equal and all its angles right angles. The perspective only varies its size, according to the distance we are from it. However, if we place that square flat on the table and look at it sideways or at an angle, then we become conscious of certain changes in its form; the side farthest from us appears shorter than that nearest to us, and all the angles are different (cf. Fig. 11.2, on p. 587). Perspective gives the dimensions of objects in space as they appear to us, just as a perfect tracing of those objects on a vertical sheet of glass between us and them would do; indeed, the word is derived from *perspicere*, to "see through."

3.4 William Harvey, Marcellus Malpighi, and Giovanni Alphonso Borelli

The circulation of blood and the physiologic function of the heart as a pump were established by William Harvey (1578–657). He studied at Padua, which at the time was the most prestigious medical university in Europe. It was also one of the most Aristotelian. Paduan Aristotelianism differed from the brand taught elsewhere. At Padua, they taught Aristotle as a preliminary to medicine, not theology.

Although he is renowned as a scientific revolutionary, Harvey was a devoted Aristotelian who saw an underlying unity between various circular motions in the universe—the planets in the heavens, air and rain in the sky, blood inside bodies. As he put it, the heart "deserves to be styled the starting point of life and the sun of our microcosm just as much as the sun deserves to be styled the heart of the world [69]." In some ways, Harvey was not a radical reformer but a traditionalist who clung to many Aristotelian ideas. According to the gossipy diarist John Aubrey, Harvey "bid me goe to the fountain head and read Aristotle . . . and did call the neoteriques [upstart philosophers] shitt-breeches [8,59]."

Since the early fifteenth century, Padua had been ruled by Venice, which fostered freedom of thought. The latter attracted many of the ablest men of the time—among them Vesalius, Copernicus, Galileo, and William Harvey [22]. At Padua, Harvey was a pupil of Casserius and, most notably, of the great anatomist Hieronymus Fabricius of Aquapendente—that pretty little hill-town near Rome. It is perhaps more intriguing that Harvey was a contemporary of Descartes, who was an early modern proponent of the biomedical concept of *function*, which he connected intimately to the metaphor of living organisms as machines that are constructed from separate parts. For Descartes organisms were composed of parts, whose functions could be reduced to mechanical operations, in order to show that living organisms were simply *automata*. Descartes said: "I do not recognize any difference between machines made by craftsmen and the various bodies that nature alone composes" [25]. The great triumph of seventeenth-century physiology came when Harvey applied the mechanistic model of Descartes to the phenomenon of blood circulation and solved what had, since ancient times, been the most fundamental and difficult problem in physiology.

The anatomy theater in the University of Padua is much the same as in Harvey's day, and also the courtyard, or cloister, where the coat of arms of Harvey (his *stemma di famiglia*) is clearly to be seen, rather high up in the ceiling. Fabricius had already been Professor of Anatomy for thirty-five years when Harvey arrived in Padua, and had spent these years reviving the anatomical program of study of Aristotle. He had been studying the same kinds of things as Aristotle, such as the generation of animals, respiration, and the local motion of animals—and all not on man alone, but on animals or, in Aristotle's point of view, on "the animal." Others could not see in Aristotle's animal books an approach to anatomizing which to follow, but Fabricius could. It was this that Harvey appreciated, copied, and continued, perhaps as a result of his exposure in England—as an undergraduate at Cambridge University—to Aristotle's books on the soul, on analytic logic, on physics, on metaphysics, and so forth. This all came in very useful to his understanding of how to undertake research, especially in following Aristotle's approach to investigating animal anatomy.

In 1628, Harvey published his tract entitled *Exercitatio Anatomica de Motu Cordis et Sanguinis in Animalibus* [69]. Harvey (see Fig. 3.5, on p. 129) may be considered the father of modern quantitative experimental Physiology. Francis Bacon, sometimes viewed as the father of modern science, was at one time a patient of Harvey's. In his utopian masterpiece, the *New Atlantis* [81], Bacon probably had Harvey's anatomical dissections in mind when he described how the ideal scientists in the land of Bensalem kept "inclosures of all sorts of beasts and birds, which they use not only for view or rareness, but likewise for dissections and trials; *that thereby they may take light what may be wrought upon the body of man*."

In this context, we need to ask what led Harvey to see things completely differently than other researchers. It was not simply a matter of his using his eyes better, nor the fact that he used experiment, because his rivals did so too. Indeed, with respect to using one's eyes, the circulation of the blood is not something that is visible: it is the *deduction* of a quantitative argument about anatomical pathways, the capacity of the chambers of the heart, its rate of pulsation, and so on.

The circulation of the blood is certainly *not* something lying in front of one's eyes, just waiting to be found! In studying the circulation, Harvey started by measuring the quantity of blood in the body of an animal (he took an animal and cut a vein in order to extract all the blood) and saw that its quantity was limited. He went on to describe, in Chapter VIII of *de Motu*, which he titled "The circulation of the blood is proved by a prime consideration," how the blood that is put out by the heart in less than half an hour[8] would

[8] Despite the strong underestimate for the cardiac output, which Harvey himself recognized as a very conservative assumption, this quantitative argument supports *a fortiori* his wholly new concept of the *closed loop*.

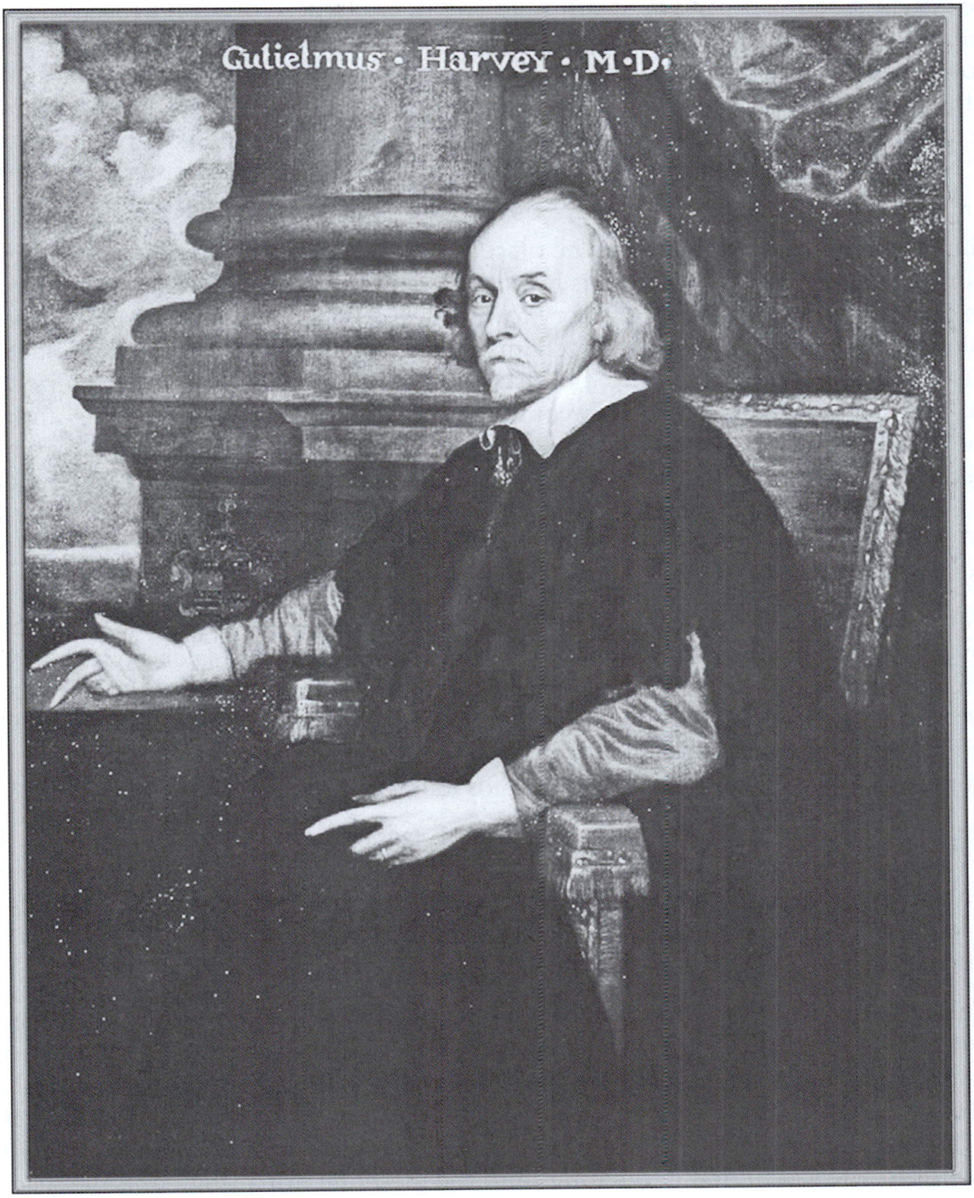

Figure 3.5: William Harvey, ca. 1655–1660. By unknown artist. Reproduced (oil color original), with permission from the Royal College of Physicians, London, England.

far exceed the weight of a man, and so he came to discuss the concept of a closed-loop circulation [66, 69]. This fact contrasted *dangerously* with the prevailing concept, according to which blood was produced continuously in the liver in order for it to be absorbed by the peripheral structures and tissues. The liver, Harvey reasoned, could not possibly manufacture that much blood. Rather, the heart must be the center of a system that *circulates* the blood; and the blood itself *passes* from the arterial into the venous system. This must stand as one of the most important early, and valid, inductions of modern science. How hard it is to really apprehend the prevalent intellectual constraints that seemed to bind the thought processes of the medical and scientific workers of Harvey's time!

Harvey demonstrated that when he placed a loop around a vein, it became turgid and then on closing another two segments he noticed that the blood did not go from the center to the periphery, but from the periphery toward the center. Therefore, he understood the function of venous valves and the mechanism of venous circulation, and postulated that the heart is a valved muscle pump that makes the blood circulate from the arteries to the veins. Without a microscope, Harvey could not see what connected the arteries and veins, but he perceived that a connection had to exist between the arteries and the veins and so predicted the discovery of "pores." However, he could not demonstrate them because he was not able to see the capillaries with the naked eye. Using the microscope [137], Malpighi and Spallanzani later discovered the capillaries in cold- and warm-blooded animals, respectively [116].

Harvey also introduced the concept of a "vis a tergo" (the *force from behind* carried out by the blood expelled from the left ventricle). Interestingly, Galen believed that the heart contained a distinctive muscle, that was capable of exerting a "vis a fronte" (the *force from the front* capable of spreading ventricular walls apart, after each systole [127]. The first idea about the heart as a "pressure–suction pump" has been attributed to the famous Greek physician, Erasistratus of Chios (304–250 B.C.).

Marcellus Malpighi (1628–1694) of Bologna was a student of Galileo Galilei. He is often called the father of microscopic anatomy, or "histology," because of his many important discoveries, including: the red corpuscles, to which he correctly attributed the color of blood, the layers in the epidermis, the renal glomerulus, the corpuscles of the spleen, and *fibra*, today's fibrin.

Malpighi's genius stemmed from being able to distinguish between what was false and what was true, since microscopes at that time produced truly illusory images [57]. Malpighi was the first to actually see the "missing link," represented by the capillaries, in 1660–61: a full thirty-two years after the publication of *de Motu Cordis*, and fifteen centuries after Galen surmised (see p. 121) that the veins communicate with the arteries by fine tubes. He saw it first in the lungs and the mesentery of a frog,[9] and the discovery was announced in the second of two letters, *"Epistola de Pulmonibus,"* addressed to his good friend the iatrophysicist[10] Borelli, and dated 1661. "I could clearly see that the

[9]Cold-blooded amphibians, including the frog, have capillaries and red corpuscles that are 3–4 times the size of those of warm-blooded animals.

[10]At the time, physicians and scientists who accepted the mechanical model of physiology were known as "iatrophysicists."

blood is divided and flows through tortuous vessels," wrote Malpighi, "and that it is not poured into spaces, but is always driven through tubules and distributed by the manifold headings of the vessels..." In extrapolating his findings to humans, Malpighi vindicated Harvey four years after Harvey's death.

Giovanni Alphonso Borelli (1608–1679) had been taught by one of Galileo's students and sought to understand animal physiology in terms of physical laws. Borelli investigated the circulation of blood during the lifetime of Harvey and recognized and described the *spiral arrangement* of muscle fibers in the cardiac ventricles in quite a remarkably modern-sounding way [20] (see Chapter 6). He pioneered in applying mathematical principles to the explanation of animal functions and is regarded as the founder of animal mechanics. In his *De Motu Animalium* (1680), he stated his theory of the circulation in eighty propositions and, in proposition *lxxiii.*, he formulated a supposed relation between the bulk and the strength of muscle fibers as found in the ventricles. In spite of his preoccupation with mechanical principles, Borelli introduced a chemico-physiological view of muscle innervation and muscular contraction. His ideas inspired investigators of muscle action to think in terms of chemical events behind muscular activity, and to create and utilize new techniques and instruments.

3.5 Leonhard Euler and Daniel Bernoulli

Other venerable researchers followed on Leonardo's footsteps, and the field of Hydraulics advanced greatly from the sixteenth century onward. When Newton published the "*Philosophiae Naturalis Principia Mathematica*" in 1687, the scientific community was still small, despite the pioneering work that had already been done in many areas of scientific inquiry. In the broader society, science was not yet held in especially high regard, and the notion that science might have a role in guiding everyday human affairs was barely a topic of conversation at the time, even among the natural philosophers ("natural" referring to what we think of as *science*). The "*Principia*" dramatically changed all that. It explained how nature worked on a universal scale, linking terrestrial and celestial physics under one set of laws with a precision that seemed almost magical. Over the next several decades, reason—meaning scientific reason as we know it today, in which mathematics, logic, and empirical evidence are joined—became the reigning intellectual paradigm. Reason's potential to allow humans to understand the workings of nature was seen as unlimited.

The magnificent advent of Hydrodynamics, which deals with fluid flow mathematically and theoretically, ensued in the eighteenth century. Among its early pioneers were Leonhard Euler (1707–83) and Daniel Bernoulli (1700–82), who were connected both by personal friendship and by common interests in the field of applied mathematics. In fact, Euler used his great analytic skills to put many of Bernoulli's physical insights into a rigorous mathematical form.

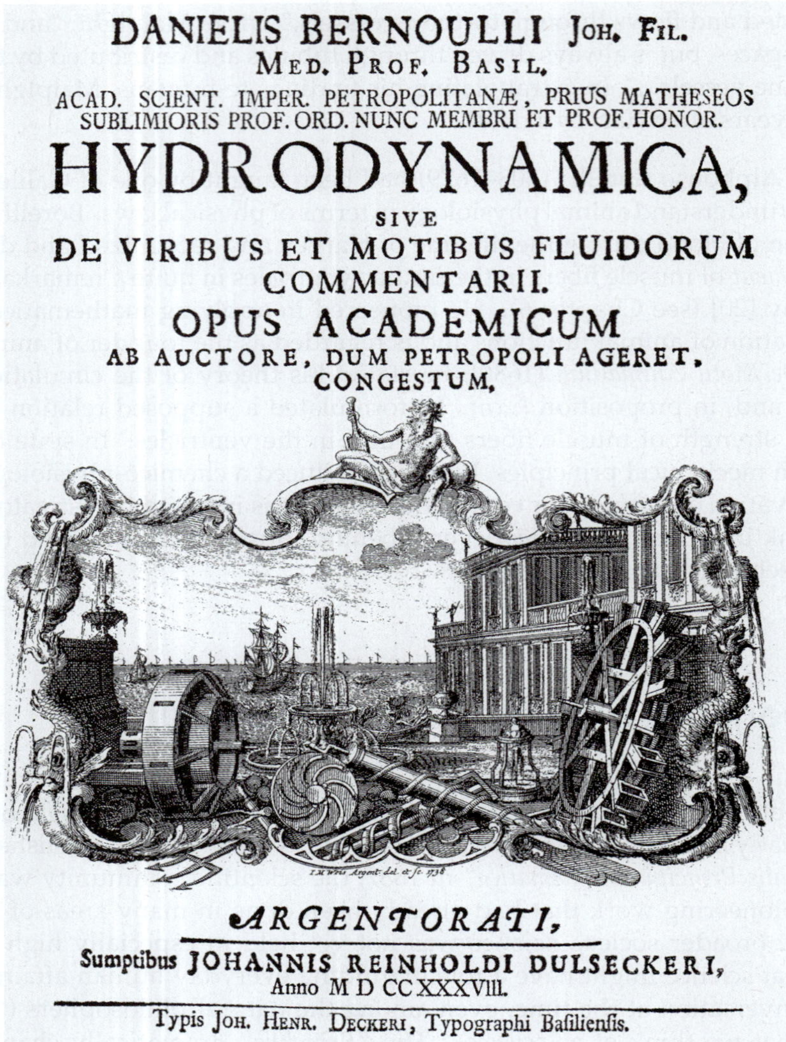

DANIELIS BERNOULLI JOH. FIL.
MED. PROF. BASIL.
ACAD. SCIENT. IMPER. PETROPOLITANÆ, PRIUS MATHESEOS
SUBLIMIORIS PROF. ORD. NUNC MEMBRI ET PROF. HONOR.

HYDRODYNAMICA,
SIVE
DE VIRIBUS ET MOTIBUS FLUIDORUM
COMMENTARII.
OPUS ACADEMICUM
AB AUCTORE, DUM PETROPOLI AGERET,
CONGESTUM.

ARGENTORATI,
Sumptibus JOHANNIS REINHOLDI DULSECKERI,
Anno M D CC XXXVIII.
Typis JOH. HENR. DECKERI, Typographi Basiliensis.

Figure 3.6: The frontispiece of Bernoulli's *Hydrodynamica* (1738), with the first *"modern"* use of the term—see discussion in text. (Reproduced, with permission, after minor retouching and manual despeckling, dust, noise, and scratch removal, from Dover [16].)

Euler's work in mathematics is vast [42]; he was the most prolific writer of mathematics of all time [38], and he developed the general hydrodynamic differential equations of motion for ideal (inviscid) flows. They are known as "Euler's equations," and will be developed in Chapter 4, along with their integral expressions in diverse applications that are recognized as variants of the so-called "Bernoulli equation."

Bernoulli, who was a physician [16], investigated the laws governing blood pressure as a professor of anatomy at the University of Basel, in Switzerland; in 1730 he formulated his "vis viva equation," with which most readers of this book may be acquainted, which relates pressure, density, and velocity. Bernoulli drew on the Greek word "Hydrodynamikè" for the field: he used it in the title (in Latin, as was customary at the time) of his treatise *Hydrodynamica, sive de viribus et motibus fluidorum commentarii*, which can be considered as the first textbook of the new discipline (see Fig. 3.6, on p. 132). Generalizing Evangelista Torricelli's (1608–1647) theorem concerning the velocity of a water jet leaving a well shaped orifice at the bottom of a tank [108], Bernoulli announced here the principle of "equality between actual descent and potential ascent" of a liquid mass, and, in connection with it, his energy theorem. With remarkably sound judgment, Bernoulli, while he emphasized and showed by example the "wonderful usefulness" of his theorem, at the same time warned against its inexactness. Less known is Bernoulli's work on medical subjects [65], including a manuscript on the physical performance of the heart, *De vita*, 1737, his most significant contribution to the subject.[11]

Interestingly, in a celebrated paper developing the wave equation and published by the Berlin Academy of Sciences in 1753 [17], Bernoulli elaborated his "superposition principle." His analysis of the motion of a vibrating string was that the displacement of every point on the string was the algebraic sum of the displacement produced by the fundamental and all its harmonics. This is the principal that found a more universal application in the hands of the French mathematician Baron Jean Baptiste Joseph Fourier (1768–1830) who used it in his "Analytical theory of heat," published in 1822, to express a mathematical function as an infinite series of sines and cosines (see Section 2.18, on pp. 82 ff.).

3.6 Hermann von Helmholtz

The theoretical equations for nonviscous fluid flow were deemed, however, to be of little or no practical use: calculation of the force exerted by a flowing fluid on a body, for instance, resulted in a very different outcome than that found by experiment. In 1868, a modern "Renaissance man," Hermann von Helmholtz (1821–94) published an important paper, which for the first time reconciled hydraulics and hydrodynamics (see Fig. 3.7, on p. 134). In it, he derived *theoretically* the contraction coefficient of a jet issuing from a 2-D orifice as 0.611. This agreed closely with the experimentally measured nominal[12] value of 0.60. Of considerable historical interest is the fact that Helmholtz was probably the first to link the Navier–Stokes equations to the Hagen–Poiseuille law [37]. Note that the simplified differential equation that Hagen and Poiseuille derived contains only *two* of the *30* terms of the complete Navier–Stokes equations for 3-D, incompressible, viscous flow.

Undoubtedly, Helmholtz is one of the greatest scientists of the post-Leonardo period.[13] Born in Potsdam, he was, on his mother's side, a descendent of William Penn,

[11] *De vita*, 1737; manuscript. In: Verh. Naturf. Gesell. Basel, 52 (1940–41): 219–234. St. 75. [Introd. and German trans. by O. Spiess and F. Verzár on pp. 189–218.]

[12] Nominal values are those that we can measure and control by ordinary means.

[13] Helmholtz lived in an era when science was identified with the *path to truth* and he did much to chart its course. He searched for principles that would unify the sciences, and he early recognized that knowledge of natural processes was the key to ascendancy over Nature. There was little room for doubt in this approach,

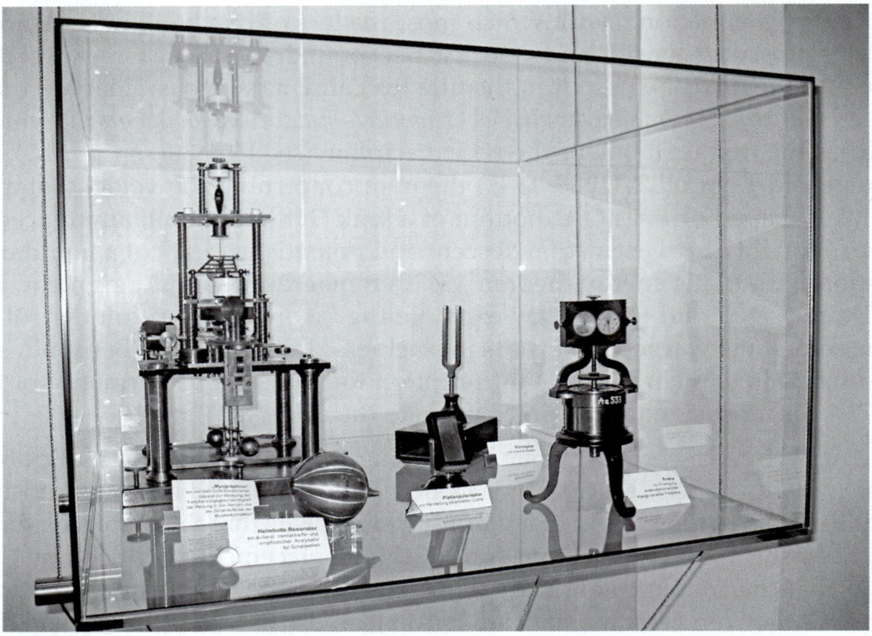

Figure 3.7: Helmholtz taught at several German universities; he had held the Chair of Physiology in Heidelberg, and that of Physics in Berlin. This photograph was taken by the author at the Old University Museum in Heidelberg, and shows several instruments developed and used by Helmholtz: on the left rear there is the *Myographion* and, in front of it, a *Helmholtz-resonator*.

the founder of Pennsylvania [70]. He stands for the whole diversity of scientific research (see Fig. 3.8, on p. 135) with an orientation toward technological and medical application [74]. He was one of the last true universal scholars [75]. Helmholtz reflected a natural science that spanned the fields of medicine and physiology, physics and mathematics, psychology and music, and chemistry and thermodynamics [24]. He devoted his life to seeking the great unifying principles underlying nature. His career began with one such principle, that of energy, and concluded with another, that of "least action."

Helmholtz's work was characterized by an undeviating reliance on mathematics and mechanism, and by the scope and depth of the mathematical and experimental expertise that he brought to science [76]. Research findings of lasting effect include, for example, his formulation of the law "On the conservation of energy." Studies on metabolism had led Helmholtz to this finding. He was the first to measure the wavelengths of ultraviolet light and to calculate the resolution capacity of the light microscope.

Helmholtz developed the "three-component theory of color vision," which took on a new significance with the coming of the age of color television and monitors (*RGB color*).

and the uncertainties of modern physics lay ahead. Ironically, it was one of Helmholtz's own students, Max Planck, who laid the foundations for this transformation.

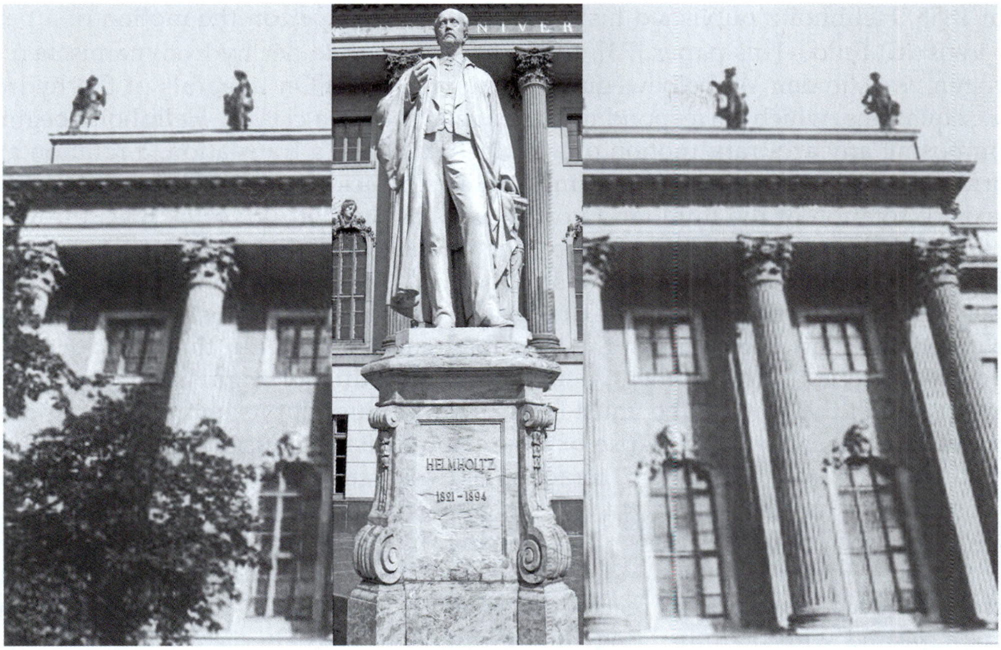

Figure 3.8: The Helmholtz monument in front of Humboldt University on the boulevard Unter den Linden, in Berlin. Helmholtz, who was known in Germany as the *Reichschancellor* of German physics, has the singular distinction of having been considered for, but refused, professorships at both Oxford (in 1865) and Cambridge (the Cavendish professorship, in 1871) [85].

While investigating the field of acoustics, he developed the theory of air speed in open tubes. His ophthalmoscope made the retina visible for the first time. He additionally developed the "ophthalmometer," for measuring corneal curvature. His philosophical writings examined the epistemological consequences of theoretical natural science.

His mathematical studies on vortex motion, air and water waves, and other flow-related phenomena also made Helmholtz one of the founders of modern fluid mechanics.[14] Like Jean Poiseuille and several other notables in the history of fluid dynamics who were also physicians, he undertook some of his studies of fluid flow in conjunction with the circulation of blood, but his discoveries proved to be of fundamental importance [77]. He became one of the greatest of fluid dynamicists and theoretical physicists, above all in the fields of conservation of energy and electrodynamics, who did not forget that he was a physician. "Medicine," he stated (see Chapter 17), "was once the intellectual home in which I grew up: and even the emigrant best understands and is best understood by his native land."

[14] Helmholtz was, in fact, the father of the *analogy* between *electrodynamics* and *hydrodynamics*. In his curl laws, he derived a formula for any arbitrary vector flux through a moving and simultaneously deformed area element, which was the basis for the so-called *Lorentz transformation equations* and Einstein's electrodynamics of moved bodies—dubbed the *"special relativity theory."*

In 1858, Helmholtz published his ground-breaking paper on the motion of a perfect (i.e., inviscid) fluid. This paper [73], titled "Über Integrale der hydrodynamischen Gleichungen, welche den Wirbelbewegungen entsprechen," [On integrals of the hydrodynamic equations, which correspond to vortex motions], is a classic. Helmholtz begins by decomposing any arbitrary motion of a perfect fluid into a translation, a rotation and a deformation; he then defines vortex lines as lines coinciding with the local direction of the axis of rotation of the fluid, and vortex tubes as bundles of vortex lines through an infinitesimal[15] element of area. He shows mathematically that the vortex tubes cannot begin or end in the fluid, i.e., they must "close up," (e.g., a smoke ring), and that in an inviscid fluid the particles in a vortex tube at any given instant must remain in the tube indefinitely, no matter how much the tube may get distorted. In the inviscid fluid the *strength of the vortex*, or its moment, defined as the product of angular velocity by cross-sectional area of the vortex tube, must be constant throughout its entire extent and must keep the same value with the lapse of time. Somewhat bemused, he summarized his theoretical conclusions regarding interaction of two circular vortex rings with a common axis of symmetry as follows: "If two vortex rings both have the same direction of rotation, they will proceed in the same sense. The ring in front will enlarge itself and move slower, while the second one will shrink and move faster. If the velocities of translation are not too different, the second will finally reach the first and pass through it. Then the same 'game' will be repeated with the other ring, so the rings will pass alternately one through the other." This game remains a favorite of many a computational fluid dynamics simulation and scientific visualization study to the very present.

In 1868 Helmholtz published a paper on what happens along the contact surface of two infinitely extended fluids if the one moves relative to the other [41]. In that publication, "Über dickontinuirliche Flüssigkeits-Bewegungen," [On discontinuous fluid motions], he pointed out that if a water jet issues from a sharp-edged orifice into a tank filled with water, a discontinuity in the velocity distribution is observed at the edge of the orifice. In his view, in a non-viscous fluid a whole surface of discontinuity separating the jet from the surrounding quiescent water can be assumed. Even though Helmholtz had doubts as to the stability of such a surface of discontinuity [108], he suggested that such a region of irrotational flow bordered by surfaces across which the velocity, but not the pressure, suffers a discontinuous change, should be investigated. The challenge was met by Lord Kelvin (see next paragraph). In spite of the tentative nature of this essay, it had a pivotal influence. Based on his concept of vortical motion, Helmholtz envisioned the infinitesimal boundary between the fluids as a plane of parallel vortex lines—a vortex sheet, akin to the one depicted in Figure 4.15, on p. 204. Because, according to his theory, the vortex lines stick to the fluid particles, the vortex sheet would move with half of the relative speed between both fluids, like a ball-bearing. In a real viscous fluid, the rotating motion of fluid particles would be communicated to neighboring particles; the slightest motion perpendicular to the boundary would (according to Bernoulli's law) cause pressure differences, which would further increase the deformation such that more and more fluid particles would be caught in a vortical motion, and the surface of discontinuity would become a vortex layer of a finite thickness.

[15]Infinitesimal means immeasurably small and capable of having values approaching zero as a limit.

Sir William Thomson, better known as Lord Kelvin (1824–1907), discussed Helmholtz's vortex sheet concept critically in a paper, "On the doctrine of discontinuity of fluid motion, in connection with the resistance against a solid moving through a fluid." The discussion focused on the problem of the stability of such vortex sheets. The analysis of the Helmholtz–Kelvin instability, as it came to be known (see Section 9.5.1, on p. 457 f.), became an active topic for research among theoretical fluid dynamicists over the following century [26,41].

It is striking that, prior to Helmholtz's papers, most of fluid mechanics had been concerned simply with what we call irrotational flow, where none of the individual little parcels of fluid have an intrinsic rotation or spin. That seminal paper was highly rigorous in its mathematical approach. It had a marked impact on future work on vortex motions by Helmholtz's friend, the Lord Kelvin. It is fundamental to our physical understanding of vortical flow phenomena in general, including those observed in intracardiac flows (see Section 7.13, on pp. 382 ff., in Chapter 7, and Chapter 14).

3.7 Étienne-Jules Marey

A contemporary of Helmholtz was Étienne-Jules Marey (1830–1904), the brilliant French physician and physiologist. He developed a vivifying, physiological approach to the study of the heart and other bodily organs and functions, which complemented the pathologic anatomic description of the eighteenth and early nineteenth century [128]. Marey set himself apart from other physicians of his time by choosing an area about which little was known. This choice, and the results of his research, placed him at the forefront of nineteenth-century medical research. In Marey's approach we witness, already remarkably perfected, the origins of sophisticated methods for the graphic encoding of living processes, and the early roots of the contemporary "Functional Imaging" approach [113] to the study of the heart and ventricular function.

His photographic techniques for the study of organ function and animal locomotion documented dynamic processes as they happen over time, involving time lapse techniques—which he developed—and overlapping frames. His experiments with what he called "chronophotography" led him to develop cameras with oscillating shutters controlled by clockwork-style gears, so that each exposure occurred at a precise interval from the one before it and the one after it. His photographic techniques directly influenced the invention of cinematography and special cinematic effects (see Fig. 8.5, on p. 420).

Marey took on the task of studying the movements of the organs, to learn more about their precise functions. His first study was in the circulation of blood. Since he disapproved of vivisection, he invented or modified apparatus, which would allow him to record movements without mutilating the animals that he was studying. He understood the enormous scientific value of using precision instruments to record complex phenomena, such as those pertaining to blood circulation. In 1859, he invented a "Sphygmographe," which allowed him to record the beating of the pulse. At the time, the Germans were at the forefront of research in this area, with such devices as Carl Ludwig's "Kymographion" *(Gk, wave-recorder).* In the Kymographion, which inspired Marey, the liquid metal mercury was the conducting medium that reacted on pressure. It took up the pressure of the arterial blood through a glass cannula inserted into an artery, as depicted in Figure 3.9; at the other end of the U-turn, the ups and downs of the meniscus of the metal were transmitted to a stylus that transformed them into inscriptions on paper mounted on a rotating cylinder. This was the first in a long line of recording instruments for studying the functions of the body, including the "Cardiographe," the "Pneumographe," the first "Polygraph," and so on.

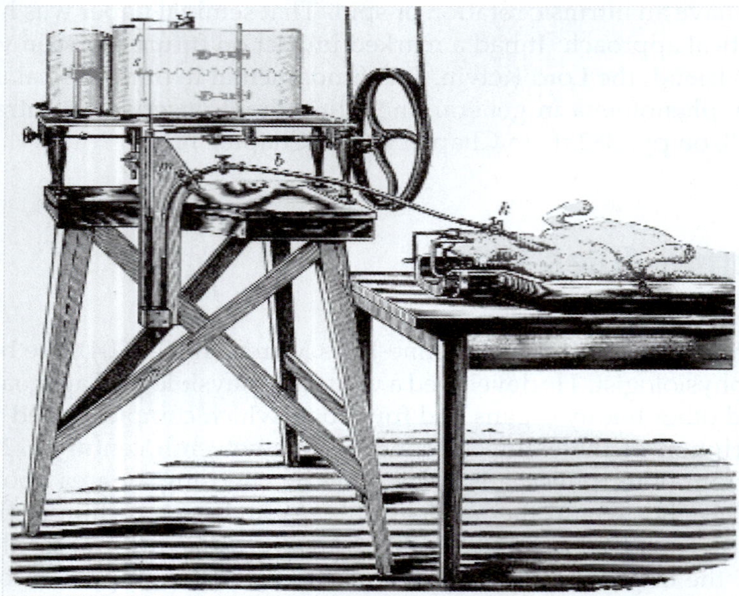

Figure 3.9: Kymographion employed in a blood pressure dog experiment. From Langendorff, O.: *Physiologische Graphik: Ein Leitfaden der in der Physiologie gebräuchlichen Registriermethoden* (Leipzig, Wien, 1891), p. 206, Figure 169.

Auguste Chauveau, a veterinary surgeon from Lyon, was to become Marey's collaborator in cardiac physiologic research. Chauveau invented his "Hémodromètre" in 1860 [27]. This was an instrument for recording the details of the velocity pulse by placing a tiny paddle in the axis of the stream within a cannula that was interposed in an artery. The movements of this paddle by an ingenious system of levers were transmitted to a tambour writing on a smoked drum. The recordings foreshadowed the details of quantitative records taken by means of modern electronic instruments.

In 1860, Marey invented an instrument for cardiac catheterization and the measurement of intracardiac pressures. With Chauveau, they inserted a double-lumen catheter version of the device through the jugular vein until the orifice of one tube lay in the right ventricle and that of the other in the right auricle, and a single-lumen catheter version

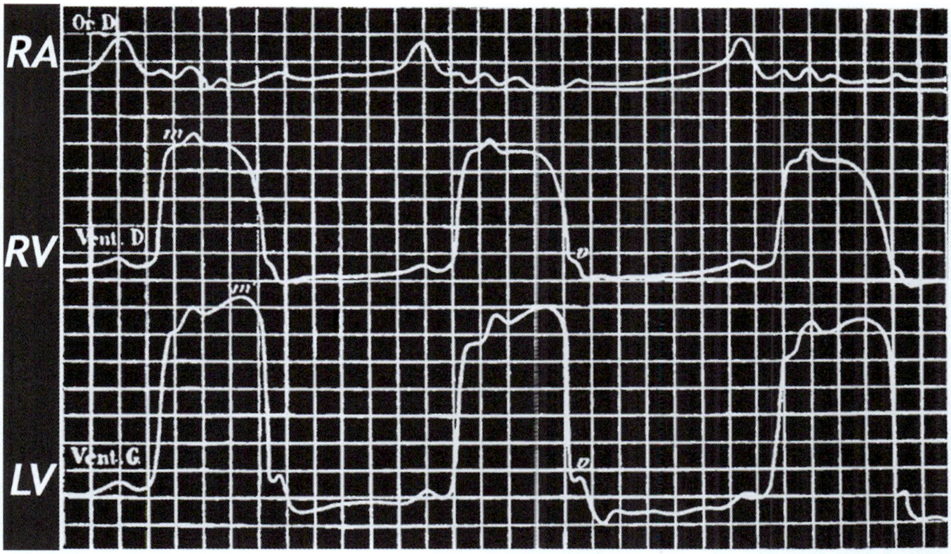

Figure 3.10: Tracings from the heart of a horse, by Chauveau and Marey at around 1861. The upper tracing (RA) is from the right auricle, the middle (RV) from the right ventricle, and the lowest (LV) from the left ventricle. The horizontal lines represent time, and the vertical amount of pressure. The breadth of one of the small squares represents one-tenth of a second. (From Marey, É-J, *La Méthode graphique*, Paris, 1878, p. 357 [103].)

from the carotid artery into the left ventricle of a conscious horse. The tubes were connected to small drums (*tambours*) with lever styluses that wrote on a steadily revolving recording cylinder covered with smoked paper (cf. Fig. 3.10, and Fig. 8.4, on p. 419). They recorded systolic pressure readings around 27 *mm Hg* in the right and 129 *mm Hg* in the left ventricle.[16] These measurements provided experimental support for the explanation advanced by Harvey for the difference between the wall thickness of the two ventricles: "[The] wall [of the right ventricle] is three times as thin as that of the left ventricle... The lungs are spongy, loose in texture and soft, and hence less force is required to extrude blood into them... the left ventricle needs greater strength and force to have extended its influence upon the blood throughout the whole of the body"—*De motu cordis*, Chapter 17 [69].

Marey and Chauveau's techniques of dynamic recording and analysis enhanced cardiac performance information with kymograph physiologic data regarding function, process, and movement of the working heart [28]. In their hands, the kymograph filled the cognitive vacuum produced by the failure of sensory observation and provided an encoded inscription of dynamic phenomena (e.g., cardiac pulsations, intracardiac pressure pulses) beyond the reach of sensory observation! Through it, physiology reorganized its

[16] Recherches sur le pouls au moyen d'un nouvel appareil enregistreur (sphygmographe), *Gazette médicale de Paris*, 14 avril 1860, no. 15, t. 15, 3e série, pp. 225–6 ; 21 avril 1860, no. 16, pp. 236–42 ; 12 mai 1860, no. 19, pp. 298–301.

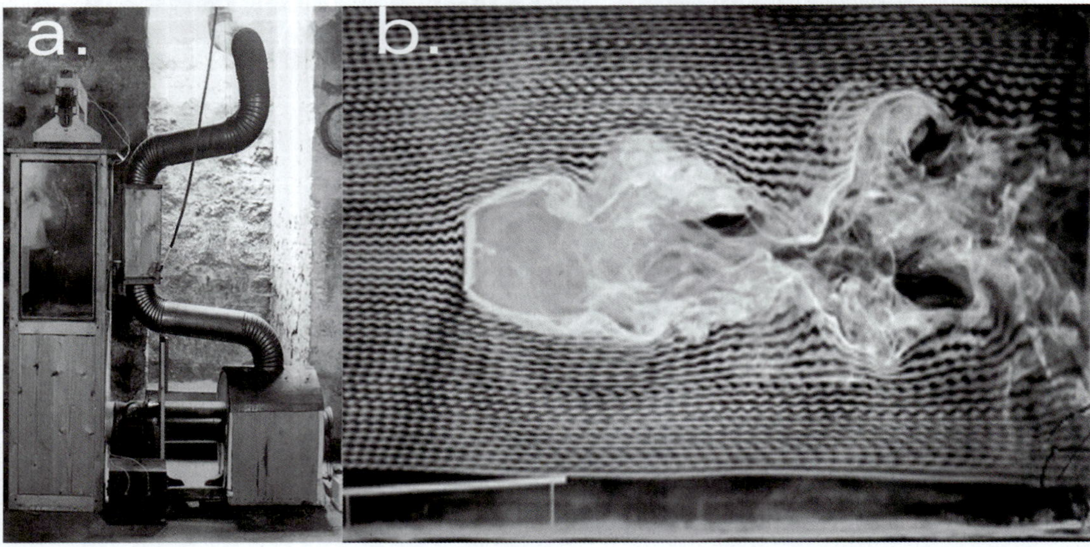

Figure 3.11: Marey was one of the first modern fluid dynamicists. He studied airflows by means of instant photography of smoke currents, which he produced in the "machine à fumée" (smoke machine) that he devised, one of the first modern aerodynamic wind tunnels (a). They revealed the diverse shapes of wisps of smoke according to the applying flow parameters and the geometry of the particular obstacles encountered in their trajectory (b). © Cinemathèque Française.

perception of the living heart, rendering it more *viewer-friendly*. Marey's emphasis on dynamic physiologic phenomena through technologies of inscription superseded Claude Bernard's (see below) "experiments of destruction." Even when Marey and Chauveau "invaded" the interior of the body, their purpose was not simply to open it up for observation. The magnitude of their achievement becomes clear when one recalls that autopsy was the chief investigatory technique of the nineteenth century. With a living animal body taking the place of the corpse, they obtained detailed physiological information regarding movement, hemodynamic processes and function of the heart during life.

An example of their inventiveness is to be found in the manner in which they established the detailed chronology of cardiac valve operation, including the reciprocal timing of atrioventricular *vs.* semilunar valve opening and closure. They did so by placing on their intracardiac catheter, at the level of the segment that traversed the valvular orifices an electrical contact-interrupter, such that it closed an electric circuit when the valvular leaflets abutted against it in the closed position and opened the circuit when they receded from it, upon valvular opening.

One can understand why Marey can be compared to Leonardo da Vinci. Their inventiveness and their visionary character made them scientists, technologists and artists. Marey's graphics have influenced some futuristic schools of modern art. Marey was exceptionally creative. He developed to the utmost man's ability to analyze visually and spatiotemporally. As he scrutinized what was real, he also saw what was possible, and understood how close the one was to the other: analyzing and developing what is real makes what is possible come true. Marey was a great visualizer and, just like Leonardo, he was also a great *visionary* who still inspires us today.

André Cournand, who shared the Nobel Prize for the introduction of cardiac catheterization in humans (see Section 3.10, on pp. 144 ff.), remarked on the great implications of the technique that Chauveau and Marey developed, using for the first time cardiac catheters to record phasic intracardiac pressures. According to Cournand, their 1863 monograph [29] represented "the first systematic description and interpretation of intracardiac pressure recordings" [35]. Their pressure recordings also revealed, for the first time, the duration of the phases of the cardiac cycle. Tracings that they published (see Fig. 3.10, on p. 139) showed that the time interval between the onset of atrial systole and that of ventricular systole was 0.2 seconds, that atrial systole lasted 0.1 seconds, and ventricular systole lasted 0.4 seconds. They also published simultaneous recordings of intraventricular and intra-aortic pressures, from which they speculated about the impact of some specific attributes of left ventricular systole on qualities of the aortic pressure pulse. Cournand concluded, "Their text goes into important detail regarding numerous other facets of cardiac pressure tracings in health and simulated disease . . . This work unquestionably is a milestone of the physiology of the heart" [35].

Marey's work and the images that he created are among the very sources of modernity [21]. Indeed, the origins of our Functional Imaging method [113] are to be found in his approach to cardiac physiology. Far from merely extending the senses, Functional Imaging's digitally encoded visualizations and plots of intracardiac flow variables actually fill the vacuum in direct sensory observation of intracardiac flow phenomena. Marey's theories were always supported by graphs, images, and direct impressions: he never lost this belief in the "trace" and the graphical record [100, 101, 103, 104].

For fluid dynamics, the climax of Marey's work came between 1899 and 1902, in his flow visualization studies. At a time when aerial exploits were occupying many researchers, there was a clear need to understand the behavior of the air around bodies of various shapes: balloons, airplanes, etc. Considering the flight of a bird, the nature of the wing movements had already been captured by Marey's chronophotography. However, for flight mechanisms to be understood, visualization of the behavior of the air which gives the wing its support was required. His last great work was the observation and photography of smoke trails (cf. Fig. 3.11, on p. 140), a fascinating spectacle that surely must have given him great visual pleasure. A huge number of glass plate photographs were taken in the course of those experiments [99, 102].

Marey presented his first photographic results to the Académie des Sciences in Paris on 16 July, 1900. Those photographs allowed a better understanding of the action of a bird's wing on the air. His design produced in a closed space with transparent walls a fan-generated current of air; and it introduced into this flow equidistant, parallel threads of smoke. In the path of these threads could be placed surfaces of different configuration, over which the smoke threads would deviate in different ways. The smoke trails were brightly illuminated in order to make instantaneous photographs of their changing appearance, as is shown in Figure 3.11. The speed of flow could be increased or decreased using a control attached to the fan. The room where Marey's ingenuous machine was set up, was darkened. As a magnesium flash exploded, a camera set up in front of the glass would capture the smoke trails in the capricious wanderings that they described, in the places where vortices formed.

3.8 Claude Bernard

History credits Marey's contemporary 19th-century French physiologist Claude Bernard (1813–78) with the "invention" of cardiac catheterization. In 1844, Bernard passed a catheter into both the right and left ventricles of a horse's heart retrogradely from the jugular vein and carotid artery. He was the first to perform a scientific study of cardiac physiology, and he set the stage for cardiac catheterization, as it is known today. Bernard's name is known to physiology students the world over for his idea of the internal environment, "le milieu intérieur."[17] He is one of the founders of experimental physiology and medicine. "His philosophy," wrote the 1977 Nobel laureate Rosalyn S. Yalow [15], "provides the basis for interdisciplinary research which has become increasingly important in modern science as the boundaries between the various disciplines appear to merge."

Bernard's masterpiece was his book "Introduction à l'étude de la médecine expérimentale," published in 1865 [12]. The thesis of the book fitted well with the times and brought him great recognition, notably election to the Académie Française. In essence, he argued that progress in medicine was only possible by the application of experimental physiology.

He emphasized the distinction between "observation," which consists in "noting everything normal and regular," and "experiment," which acknowledges the "variation or disturbance that an investigator brings into the conditions of natural phenomena." In particular, it is only through the stopping of a "normal" activity—its suppression or destruction—that the function of the subserving organ can be known. It is intriguing and a measure of his versatility and greatness that in one of his articles [13], which was aimed at a general audience, he expressed ideas regarding the heart as a seat of emotions that echo similar Aristotelian notions but with a psychosomatic medicine perspective.

Bernard's pioneering efforts in experimental cardiac catheterization evolved in parallel with much of the work of Marey and Chauveau, as well as other noted experimental physiologists of the period, such as Adolph Fick [80]. Interestingly, it was Bernard who coined the term "cardiac catheterization." Beginning in 1844, i.e., before the start of the younger Marey's studies, and continuing for almost 40 years, he developed and refined a technique for passing a catheter from the peripheral vasculature into the chambers of the heart [23]. His investigations, conducted on a variety of animal species, gave insight to questions concerning intracardiac temperatures and ventricular pressures, as well as providing a description of the anatomic and functional characteristics of aortic valve leaflets.

[17] He wrote: *La fixité du milieu intérieur est la condition de la vie libre* [14].

Thus, the catheter became an accepted tool in the understanding of cardiac hemodynamics and ventricular function.

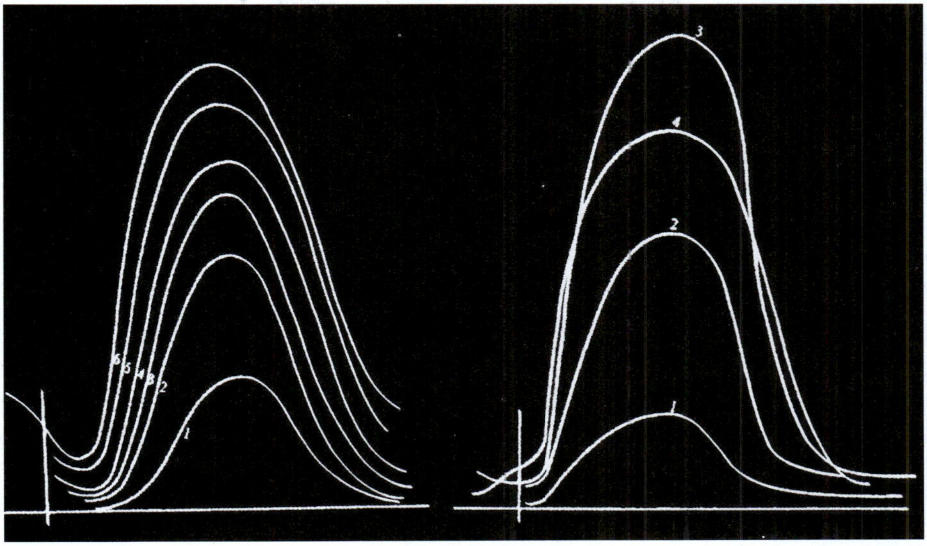

Figure 3.12: Otto Frank's demonstration of the effect of increasing filling or *preload* of the left ventricle of the frog heart on the isovolumetric pressure curve (end-diastolic filling pressure progressively augmented in successively higher-numbered curves). The peaks of the isovolumetric pressure curves generated by the ventricle rose with increasing end-diastolic filling (*left panel*). However, beyond a certain level of filling, the peak ventricular pressure declined (curve 4, in the *right panel*). Reprinted from *Zur Dynamik des Herzmuskels* [58].

3.9 Otto Frank, Ernest H. Starling, and Maurice B. Visscher

At the close of the nineteenth century, the prolific German cardiovascular physiologist and physician Otto Frank (1865–1944) examined the response to distension of the isolated frog heart, perfused with diluted ox blood. He found that the maximum systolic pressure generated during isovolumetric contraction was a function of end-diastolic ventricular pressure [58] (see Fig. 3.12). These seminal studies provided the first experimental demonstration of the importance of diastolic filling as a determinant of systolic ventricular myocardial function (see Section 15.6.1, on pp. 836 ff.).

In 1914, Ernest H. Starling (1866–1927), the brilliant "clinician's physiologist" [130] who originated the word "hormone" in his Croonian Lecture—the Royal Society's premier lecture in the biological sciences—of 1905, used an isolated heart-lung preparation and an apparatus to monitor the volume of the ventricles. William Harvey, whom Starling frequently referred to and in whose tradition he pictured himself, had demonstrated three hundred years earlier that the heart was not a "fount of fire" but a hydraulic apparatus. Starling proceeded by asking how this hydraulic apparatus worked, so that at one time it put out about four liters and at another time thirty-two liters per minute, and each time adjusted its output to the demands of the body. His heart-lung preparation enabled him to give the answer. From the beginning, there was the thrill of a new problem. He wrote [30] "To search out the intimate character of this power of adaptation is a problem almost as enthralling in interest as the demonstration of the circulation itself." He demonstrated that the ventricular stroke volume was a direct function of the end-diastolic volume. It is instructive to remember that Starling and his students obtained their results with recording instruments having distinct limitations. With the exception of the optical manometers used by Patterson, Piper and Starling [114], the available instruments were mercury and water manometers, a cardiometer and piston recorders [36].

In their 1926 publication, Starling and the eminent American physiologist Maurice B. Visscher (1901–1983) [18] wrote [131] "Experiments carried out in [our] laboratory have shown that in an isolated heart, beating with a constant rhythm and well supplied with blood, the larger the diastolic volume of the heart (within physiological limits) the greater is the energy of its contraction. It is this property which accounts for the marvelous adaptability of the heart, completely separated from the central nervous system, to varying load..."

Subsequent studies, published in 1954 [120], by Stanley J. Sarnoff (1917–1990), while he was Chief of the Laboratory of Cardiovascular Physiology at the National Heart Institute in Bethesda, revealed a modulation of the stroke work *vs.* preload relationship with stimulation of the heart by inotropic agents—a *homeometric* in contradistinction to the *heterometric* autoregulation of the heart by the Frank–Starling mechanism.

3.10 Werner Forssmann, André Cournand, and Dickinson Richards

The discovery of x-rays by Wilhelm Conrad Röntgen in 1895 [118] opened a new era in medicine. For the first time in history, it was possible to take a look *inside* the human body without the need for an incision. This *new kind of rays* created a revolution in diagnostic medicine and led to the development of radiology, as well as that of diagnostic cardiac catheterization and angiocardiography in humans. For over fifty years medical imaging

[18] During my medical studies at the University of Minnesota, I had the privilege to work for a while in the cardiac research laboratory of Dr. Visscher, who had collaborated with Starling at University College Medical School in London. From 1936 to 1968, Dr. Visscher headed the Department of Physiology at the University of Minnesota. Here, he conducted the combined weekly seminars (of which I have fond memories) between his Physiology Department and the celebrated Dr. Owen Wangensteen's Department of Surgery, sharing with all his expertise in physiology and other scientific disciplines. Visscher was a pioneer in this kind of strong interdisciplinary collaboration. Innovative heart surgeons Christiaan Barnard, C. Walton Lillehei, Norman Shumway, and many others had to spent part of their surgical residencies at the University of Minnesota as students in Visscher's physiology department.

was based entirely on x-ray images, and their popularity has continued to increase. Even today, x-ray images are the most requested diagnostic images.[19]

The subject of x-rays and human cardiac catheterization brings us to a 25-year-old surgical trainee named Werner Forssmann at the August Victoria Hospital in Eberswalde, near Berlin, Germany, in 1929. As a first-year medical student in the University of Berlin, where one of his professors was Rudolph Fick, Forssmann had learned of the experimental work of Bernard, Chauveau, and Marey. Because of the growing awareness about bacterial contamination, the cardiac catheterization procedure had not been performed in human subjects in the intervening years. Fascinated by those experiments revealed in Bernard's book, Leçons de Physiologie Opératoire [15], published in 1879, Forssmann wondered about applicability to humans. Nearly a century after the catheterization of the heart chambers in horses and dogs by Claude Bernard, under fluoroscopic guidance, Forssmann was the first to document human right heart catheterization, which he performed in heroic experiments on himself.[20]

Ignoring his departmental chief, and having tied his assistant to an operating table to prevent her interference, Forssmann used a narrow ureteral catheter that he advanced from an antecubital vein into his right atrium [56], and then climbed the stairs to the radiology department, to undergo a chest roentgenogram. He subsequently showed that the right-sided chambers could be visualized radiographically after injection of iodinated contrast media through a catheter into the right atrium, having again tried the method first on himself. Translated from the original German, he noted [55]: "I documented the position of the catheter with roentgenograms that I obtained by standing in front of the fluoroscope while observing the catheter in a mirror held by a nurse. In conclusion, I would like to point out the utility of this technique in providing new opportunities to research the metabolic activities and the actions of the heart." He thereby demonstrated that, in principle, the techniques well known from animal experiments could also be adapted safely for cardiac function studies in man [55].

This was naturally of paramount importance for a study of pathologic changes involving the heart, which could be reproduced with difficulty, or not at all at that time, in animal experiments. It also opened up better opportunities for röntgenologic angiocardiographic examinations of the right side of the heart and the pulmonary vessels, after injection of contrast medium directly into these organs. For this purpose as well, Forssmann made experiments on himself. It must have required firm conviction of the value of the method for him to undertake self-experimentation of this kind. His later disappointment must have been all the more bitter. It is true that the method was adopted in a few

[19] According to U.N. statistics [18, 136], in 2000 the annual diagnostic x-ray frequency per 1000 in the United States was estimated at 962, in Germany at 1254, and in Japan at 1477.

[20] Cases of self-experimentation were not very uncommon until the 1960s, but the trend gradually declined and is now extremely rare. The trend of self-experimentation has declined probably not because of a lack of dedication, but because of the growth of a more rational approach to medical research. In spite of the shortfalls of self-experimentation, researchers who endanger themselves at the altar of medical science should not be denounced as irrational. After all, why think of self-experimentation as foolhardy when we climb mountains, become test pilots, build bridges, and so on?

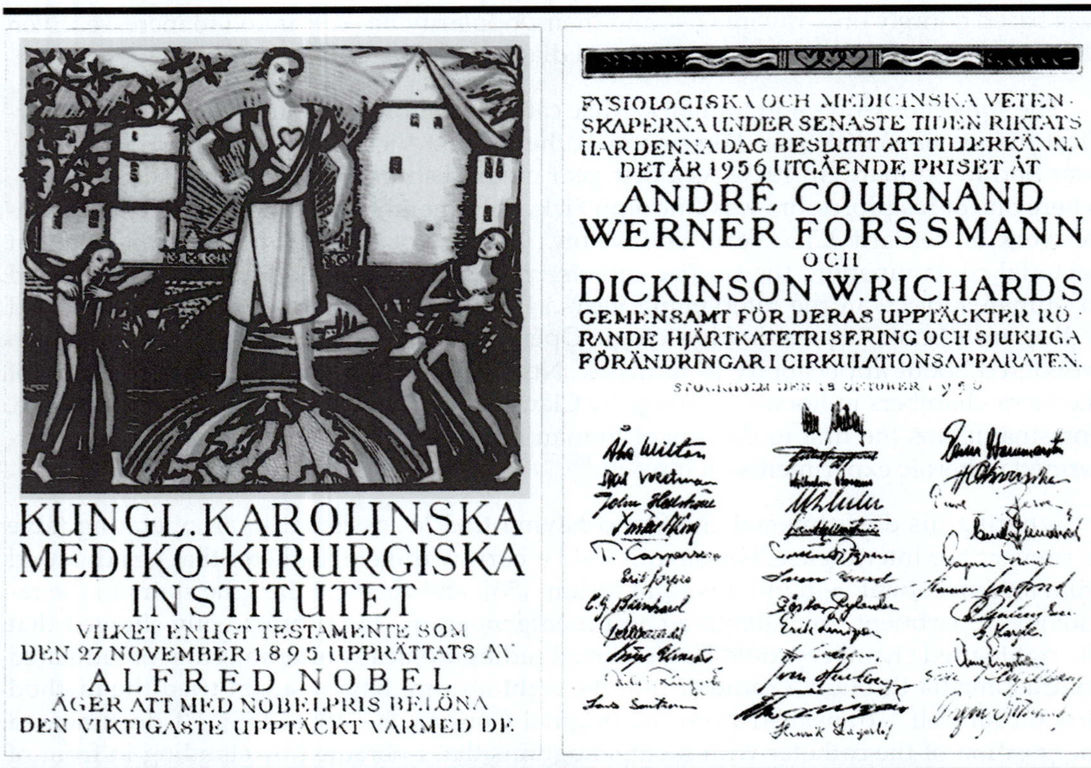

Figure 3.13: The Nobel Prize certificate presented to André Cournand, Werner Forssmann, and Dickinson Richards. (Gray-scale rendition of color reproduction appearing with the courtesy of Werner Forssmann's son, Prof. Dr. W. G. Forssmann, in [72], with the kind permission of the authors and Steinkopff Verlag.)

places—in Prague and in Lisbon—but, overall, Forssmann was subjected to criticism of such exaggerated severity that it robbed him of any inclination to continue.

In 1947, Lewis Dexter[21] expanded the clinical use of right heart catheterization with studies in patients with congenital heart disease and identified the pulmonary capillary wedge pressure as a useful clinical measurement. André Cournand and Dickinson Richards and their coworkers at the Cardiopulmonary Laboratory at Bellevue Hospital in New York subsequently proved the practical value of right and left heart catheterization and angiography definitively [34, 39]. Moreover, in 1941, Cournand and Richards employed the cardiac catheter as a physiologic diagnostic tool to measure cardiac output.

[21] I had the good fortune to see Dr. Dexter in action teaching when I was on the faculty at Harvard Medical School, where he continued to consult and attend teaching rounds of the Cardiovascular Division at the Peter Bent Brigham Hospital well into the late nineteen-eighties. One day in 1980, while making rounds at the Brigham, he suffered an acute myocardial infarction and underwent emergency coronary artery bypass grafting, performed by John J. Collins, Jr., MD. He survived this ordeal with no hypoxic brain injury and continued to teach for more than a decade.

Forssmann, Cournand, and Richards were awarded the 1956 Nobel Prize in Physiology or Medicine jointly for their discoveries concerning human cardiac catheterization and angiocardiography—a reproduction of their Nobel Prize certificate is given in Figure 3.13, on p. 146. In his acceptance speech, Cournand stated that "the cardiac catheter was...the key in the lock."

By this point, the value of hemodynamic measurements was being fully realized, and further developments came rapidly. In 1949, Hansen discussed in detail the measurement of pressures in the human organism [68]. While conducting an imaging procedure, Dr. Mason Sones—a pediatric cardiologist at the Cleveland Clinic—discovered that the catheter had accidentally entered the patient's right coronary artery and, before it could be withdrawn, 30 *mL* of contrast dye had been injected. He expected the heart to fibrillate, but it did not; thus, he discovered that the heart could tolerate intracoronary contrast dye injection. Using his specially designed catheters, Sones performed selective coronary arteriography in a series of more than 1,000 patients, and in 1962 he published a brief description of his technique [129]. This breakthrough would make possible accurate diagnosis of coronary disease and set the stage for future therapeutic interventions, such as coronary arterial bypass surgery and coronary angioplasty. The decade of the 1970s was characterized by substantial improvements in imaging systems and catheterization methods. Preformed catheters, introduced by Drs. Judkins and Amplatz, facilitated safe and expeditious catheterization from the femoral artery route and rapidly became more popular than the brachial artery approach pioneered by Dr. Mason Sones, which continued to be the preferred access for multisensor catheter (see Section 5.2, on pp. 243 ff.) studies.

3.11 Modern instrumentation

Cardiac imaging and evaluation of ventricular function have undergone a dramatic development during the past half century, following the introduction of catheter-tip micromanometers by Otto Gauer and his co-workers at the Mayo Clinic [49]. As regards modern hemodynamics instrumentation, I would attach primary importance to the application of multisensor micromanometric and velocimetric catheters for human right- and left-heart catheterization, by Huntly Millar and Joseph Murgo, with whom I worked over several years on their development and application to clinical cardiac fluid dynamics at Brooke Army Medical Center, where I was serving as the director of cardiology research [112].

In the 1980s, the clinical cardiac catheterization laboratories at Brooke Army Medical Center (BAMC) attained a peak of excellence unmatched anywhere else in the world. In collaboration with Mr. Millar's catheter development and manufacturing company, and with Honeywell and Siemens corporations, major developments occurred at BAMC in state-of-art transducer design, signal acquisition, and digital processing of multichannel physiologic signals obtained from human patients during clinical cardiac catheterization. Custom designed multisensor catheters provided a large number of simultaneous high-fidelity pressure and flow-velocity signals from the right and left heart in man, at rest and during a variety of physiologic and pharmacologic stresses. After processing by an analog system designed with special features for clinical hemodynamic and fluid dynamic measurements and simultaneous multiple imaging modalities, a dedicated computer entered these signals into a variety of programs designed for human clinical investigations. The overall capabilities of that system and the cardiologists and catheterization technicians working there were and remain unique in clinical cardiology, and represent a distinguished application of the principles of signal acquisition, processing, and analysis to biologic systems. In 2001, Huntly Millar was awarded the AAMI Foundation Laufman–Greatbatch Prize, for his contributions to the advancement of medical instrumentation.

A whole series of imaging modalities have been discovered and developed, thanks to scientific and technical advances accumulated in previous decades. Case in point, the evolution of ultrasonography dates back to 1880, when Pierre and Jacques Curie discovered piezoelectricity. The pioneers of echocardiography were Inge Edler and Hellmuth Hertz, who borrowed a sonar device from a local shipyard, improved it, and recorded cardiac echoes from Hertz's own heart. With their ultrasonic "reflectoscope," [7,44] the field of echocardiography emerged in Sweden. Doppler[22] echocardiography arrived in the 1960s, and the ink-jet printer (another invention by Hertz) supported the development of the color Doppler.

The activities in the field of ultrasound created a demand for some kind of printer suitable for the printing of color pictures. The first steps in ink jet printing were taken during the nineteen-sixties. The goal was that the ink-jet plotter would replace the conventional film for printout of medical images, such as x-rays, CT and ultrasound images, for patient records use in the future "digital" hospital. Hellmuth Hertz invented *ink jet* printing, a method for the electrical control of tiny colored ink droplets, which enabled him to put a dot of ink on a piece of paper in about one-millionth of a second. The pixel size was 0.1×0.1 mm, with continously variable color saturation in each pixel. The introduction in the 1960s of the Doppler principle to the medical use of ultrasound broadened the diagnostic spectrum of noninvasive techniques for measuring blood flow, flow-velocity and flow-velocity derived pressure gradients. With the development of Doppler echocardiography, the ink-jet printer proved useful in the development of the color Doppler technique [106].

In 1977, Edler and Hertz received the prestigious Lasker Prize. In Germany, Sven Effert and his colleagues identified atrial masses using cardiac ultrasound in 1959. At the University of Minnesota, John Reid and John Wild developed the first clinical ultrasound scanner. The American achievements in early clinical cardiac ultrasonography are credited to Harvey Feigenbaum [52], who led research in the new field and published the first book on echocardiography, in 1972.

Critical to the evolution of other powerful imaging methods in the last decades was the advent of high-speed computers that are necessary to handle the massive quantity and complexity of the computations involved in imaging. Among other notable achievements

[22]Christian Doppler (1803–1853) was an Austrian mathematician. Interestingly, his publications referred to changes in the wavelength of light as applied to astronomical events, and he never extrapolated his basic principle to sound waves. He drew an analogy of a ship moving toward, or retreating from, incoming waves. A ship moving out to sea would meet the waves with a higher frequency than a ship moving toward the shore.

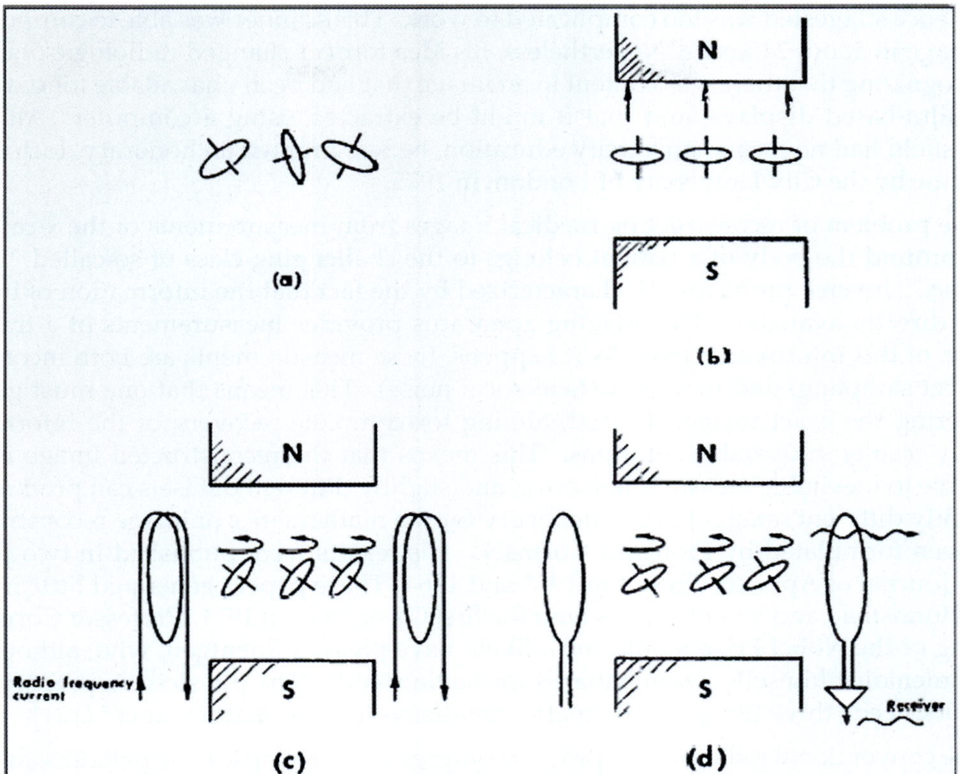

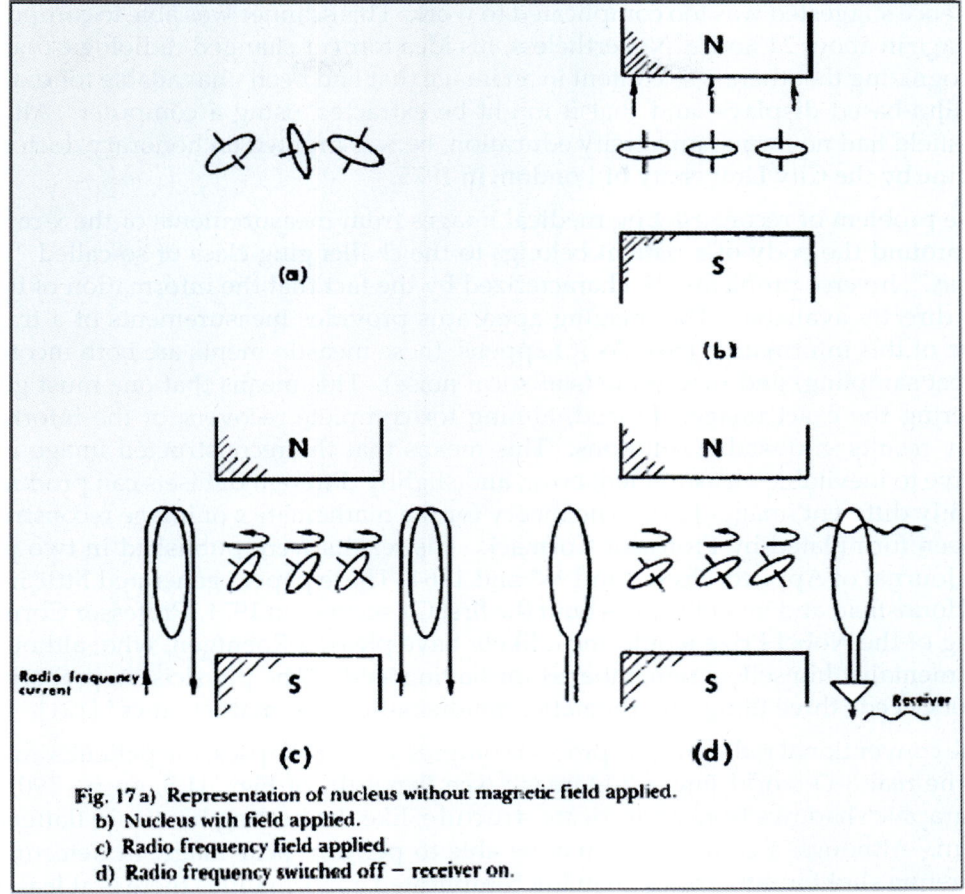

Fig. 17 a) Representation of nucleus without magnetic field applied.
b) Nucleus with field applied.
c) Radio frequency field applied.
d) Radio frequency switched off – receiver on.

Figure 3.14: Figure representing diagrammatically the usual *NMR procedure* for imaging by means of a strong magnetic field along the body to be studied. Reproduced, slightly retouched, from the published version [79] of the Nobel Lecture given on 8 December, 1979, by the co-inventor of *computed tomography (CT)*, Sir Godfrey Hounsfield. © The Nobel Foundation.

in recent decades, I would like to mention here the development of computer assisted tomography, digital angiography, real-time 3-D echocardiography, and magnetic resonance imaging.

3.11.1 Computer assisted tomography

Computer assisted tomography (CT, or CAT scans) was invented by the South African nuclear physicist Allan Cormack [33] and the British electronics engineer Sir Godfrey Hounsfield, who were recognized by the Nobel Prize in Medicine in 1979. Hounsfield was recognized for the engineering feat of designing a machine which theory and prior experience suggested was too complicated to work. This scanner was able to compute one CT image in about 24 hours. Nevertheless, his idea forever changed radiologic diagnosis by recognizing that there was content in an image that had been unavailable for diagnosis from film-based displays, and that it might be extracted using a computer. Although Hounsfield had no formal university education, he was granted an honorary doctorate in medicine by the City University of London, in 1975.

The problem of reconstructing medical images from measurements of the x-ray radiation around the body of a patient belongs to the challenging class of so-called *"inverse problems."* Inverse problems are characterized by the fact that the information of interest is not directly available. The imaging apparatus provides measurements of a transformation of this information [54]. As it happens, these measurements are both incomplete (discreet sampling) and inaccurate (statistical noise). This means that one must give up recovering the exact image. Indeed, aiming for complete recovery of the information usually results in unstable solutions. This means that the reconstructed image is very sensitive to inevitable measurement error, and slightly different datasets can produce significantly different images [134]. The theory for the mathematics of image reconstruction had been formulated by Professor Cormack. His results were published in two papers in the Journal of Applied Physics in 1963 and 1964. These papers generated little interest until Hounsfield and his colleagues built the first CT scanner in 1971. Professor Cormack's sharing of the Nobel Prize would most likely have pleased Roentgen, who, although an experimentalist himself, is remembered for having said: "The physicist in preparing for his work needs three things, mathematics, mathematics, and mathematics" [121].

The conventional radiographic process compresses, or collapses, the patient's anatomy from the real 3-D world into a 2-D image (see Panel III. of Fig. 11.5, on p. 590). The radiographic shadows from an intricate structure, like the beating heart, are flattened on the film. Although a cardiologist may be able to perform near magic in detecting and interpreting slight irregularities, in many complicated abnormalities there is at least some visual confusion. CT uses x-rays, an elaborate radiation detection system, and a computer that carries out millions of calculations to construct the image of a thin, bread-like slice of the patient's body. By eliminating the interfering patterns that come from over- and under-lying bones, organs, and tissues, CT provides ample contrast among blood and the various soft tissue interfaces, far better than standard radiography.

In 1971, Hounsfield presented a way to use CT clinically, and invented a machine to do so at EMI, then an English music record company [78,79]. It is really not surprising at all that CT was conceived by a *digital sound* recording engineer. It and MRI, which was soon to follow, entail *digital image* derivations, manipulations, and recording. It involved a *step* (not a big leap) from digitized sound element reproductions to digitized picture *(pixel)* and volume *(voxel)* visual element reconstructions of the body and its constituents. Hounsfield's instrument combined an x-ray machine and a computer to scan the body from many directions, and used algebraic reconstruction principles to manipulate the images in order to produce cutaway views of the interior. In x-ray CT, image density is measured in terms of *Hounsfield units*, abbreviated HU. The *Hounsfield scale* quantifies tissue types according to relative x-ray attenuation, ranging from air to bone; this digital scale, which represents numerically the image output of CT scanners, has become standardized in the years ensuing since its development by Hounsfield. Cormack had published essentially the same ideas in 1963. Using the so-called Radon reconstruction,[23] he developed the first technique for the inversion of the x-ray transform, the mathematical algorithm at the core of cross-sectional imaging. Indeed, the principles underlying CT are at the foundations of many other sophisticated imaging modalities in use today, most notably MRI (cf. Fig. 3.14, on p. 149).

In the mid-1970s, CT gave physicians a completely new way of seeing, and the resulting effect on patient care has been incalculable. More recently, CT has had to face stiff competition from MRI, which provides clinical information that is usually comparable, and at times far superior. CT scanning with cross-sectional or spiral data collection enabled a dynamic 3-D reconstruction and visualization of the beating heart, and a display of selected information in "measures and numbers."

3.11.2 Digital angiography

Digital angiography provides another path around the problem, alluded to above, of the collapse of bodily and organ anatomy from the 3-D world into a 2-D image, and it works well for blood vessels and cardiac chambers. In 1963 Ziedses des Plantes [138] described the principle of subtraction angiography, which allowed the removal of obscuring interfering structures from the image by adding the postcontrast image of a vessel to a negative of the pre-contrast radiograph. This technique received another enormous boost about 15 years later, thanks to an advance introduced by Mistretta, Ovitt, and their coworkers [107, 109], who demonstrated the automatic subtraction of the contrast and non-contrast images using *digital* means.

In digital subtraction angiography (DSA) the computer stores separate fluoroscopic images before and after injection of a contrast agent into the patient's bloodstream. It then subtracts, point by point, the first from the second image, and displays the result as a new image. This third, "difference" image highlights only those places where the two images differ, that is, where blood vessels hold contrast agent—all the confusing background patterns are cut out. This process, known as *mask mode subtraction*, increases the visual detectability of contrast-containing structures and their boundaries, enabling the development of applications such as intravenous ventriculography.

DSA was made commercially available initially by Philips Medical Systems, in 1980. The first rudimentary digital imaging equipment was introduced to the cardiac catheterization laboratory in 1981 and 1982. Most current digital angiography systems use some form of image enhancement (filtration) to improve image quality.

There is little doubt that some form of digital storage will soon replace entirely conventional cineangiography. The advantages of this conversion are numerous and reflect those of digital over analog processing methods, and digital archiving methods over cine film.

[23] In the context of tomography, the Radon transform data is often called a *sinogram*, because the Radon transform of a delta function is the characteristic function of the graph of a sine wave. Consequently, the Radon transform of a number of small objects appears graphically as a number of blurred sine waves with different amplitudes and phases.

Computer storage will enable duplication of digital studies, with each copy retaining quality identical to the original. Advanced local networking and communications technologies allow immediate viewing of angiograms from anywhere within a hospital or clinic, while rapid long-distance communications enable remote review and consultation.

3.11.3 Real-time 3-D echocardiography

Real-time 3-D echocardiography (RT3D) was developed by Olaf von Ramm, who made the early fully functional system available for my own work developing the Functional Imaging method [113] for visualization of intracardiac flow phenomena, at Duke University. Just like CT, this imaging method too is Sectional and can be used to "slice and dice" through the heart using the computer. It reveals internal organ structure in arbitrarily oriented directions *slice-by-slice*, in the way in which the thin slices of a loaf of bread—quite apart from their expediency—also reveal the internal structure of the loaf.

3.11.4 Magnetic resonance imaging

Magnetic Resonance Imaging (MRI), has origins that may be traced, if not to Thales of Miletus in Greek antiquity, at least to the seventeenth century. In 1600, William Gilbert, who studied medicine at Cambridge University and became physician to Queen Elizabeth I of England, published his widely celebrated *De Magnete*. Gilbert also *rediscovered* the extension of the attractive principle to amber (Gk. $\eta\lambda\epsilon\kappa\tau\rho o\nu$ = *ēlektron*, whence *electricity*), which was the first "modern era" essay into electricity;[24] this, in turn, ushered in scientific inquiry into electromagnetism, and led ultimately to MRI. On the way came the towering genii of Helmholtz, Michael Faraday, and James Clerk Maxwell. MRI's ultimate developers, Paul Lauterbur and Sir Peter Mansfield were awarded the Nobel Prize in Medicine in 2003 [61].

Lauterbur discovered the possibility of creating 2-D slice pictures of structures, by introducing gradients in the magnetic field used in MRI [84]. His discovery moved from the single dimension of NMR spectroscopy to the second dimension of spatial orientation ushering in MRI. He suggested a new way of forming an NMR image: as well as placing the sample in a uniform standing magnetic field to excite the hydrogen proton resonance, another magnetic field was applied in order to create a uniform gradient in magnetic field strength across the sample. In a seminal paper published in Nature in 1973 [87],[25]Lauterbur described his new imaging technique. He recognized that the *pictures* aquired by his method were a new kind of image, based on principles completely different from those behind other imaging methods. To emphasize this point, he coined the new word "zeugmatography" (Gk. $\zeta\epsilon\upsilon\gamma\mu\alpha$ = zeugma, meaning yoke or a joining together) as a description, "checking with a classical scholar for its fidelity to ancient roots

[24] In 1881, in a lecture delivered in London, Hermann von Helmholtz argued for the particulate nature of electricity, leading to the coining of the word *electron*.

[25] The paper was nearly not published, having been initially rejected by the editor as not of sufficiently wide significance for inclusion in Nature [88].

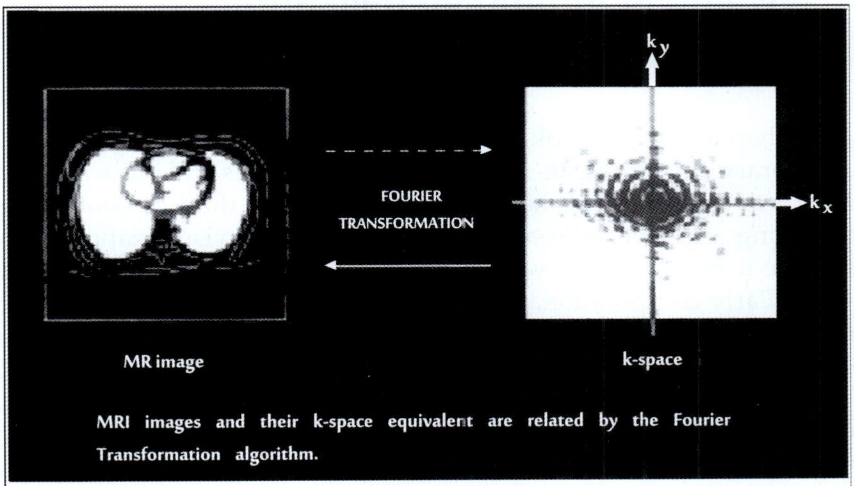

Figure 3. Diagram of a slice through the mediastinum showing the two lung fields and heart mass, also shown is the Fourier transform of this real-space image to the k-space map.

Figure 3.15: Illustration of the forward and inverse Fourier transforms, allowing a reversible transformation from real to so-called *k-space*. Reproduced (retouched) from the text of the Nobel Lecture, given on 8 December, 2003, by Sir Peter Mansfield [96]. © The Nobel Foundation.

and with a speaker of contemporary Greek to ensure that the meaning of "zeugma" had not shifted during later centuries" [88]. This term conjures up nicely the *joining together* of the weak gradient magnetic field with the stronger main magnetic field, allowing spatial localization. Because one side of the sampled object is in a higher standing magnetic field strength, the protons resonate at higher frequencies than those on the other side; and because it is a uniform gradient, position of the protons is coded linearly by frequency. The general idea is that inhomogeneous magnetic fields introduce locational coordinates into NMR signals. Also, because there is a stronger signal at the frequency of the position with a greater concentration of protons, it is possible to plot a frequency spectrum of proton concentration across the sample. By compounding several spectra, each one taken with the magnetic field gradient at a different angle across the sample, an image can be reconstructed by computed tomography [84].

Mansfield further developed the use of gradients in the magnetic field and showed how the signals could be analysed, to obtain a useful imaging technique [95] (see Fig. 3.15). He patented the method of selectively exciting and defining a slice in 1974. He later concentrated on so-called "echo-planar fast pulse sequences" and discovered how to achieve very fast imaging. Advances in high-speed computing and superconductive magnets have allowed rapid development of larger MRI machines with enormously improved sensitivity and resolution—a crucial step in making MRI a practical tool for use in cardiology and in the Functional Imaging method (see Sections 10.2 and 10.3, on pp. 505 ff. and 531 ff., respectively).

3.12 CFD and scientific visualization: merging numbers and images

In the ensuing chapters of this book, the reader will be introduced to the living history of major contemporary developments in cardiac fluid dynamics and intracardiac blood flow phenomena. These developments have been made possible through continuing advances in cardiac imaging and computer-assisted simulation and visualization of intracardiac flows, which are ushering in a new era in cardiac diagnostics and ventricular function investigations. Early computational fluid dynamics (CFD) analyses were performed in only two dimensions, to conserve memory space. Today, highly complex CFD problems may be solved relatively quickly and at a fraction of the cost of early analyses. Computer-mediated data-driven scientific visualization can be defined as the mapping of extensive datasets to a digital visual representation. In the context of intracardiac flow phenomena, this mapping is the transformation of numerical, instrument recording, or diagnostic imaging data into a visual mode that can be used to understand, document, synthesize, analyze, hypothesize, and communicate anatomic, physiologic, fluid dynamic, and clinical information.

The historical role and influence of visual models upon the process of conception, developing, and communicating scientific knowledge are well documented [9, 67]. Historically, visualization was defined as the process of creating and using images and visual models. Before the computer, hand drawings and diagrams served as conceptualizing, documenting, and didactic tools for early science. This process was employed by great scientists, and the Renaissance was the watershed regarding the use and intent of scientific and technological illustrations; text accompanied the most important and unforgettable illustrative visualizations (cf. Section 3.3, on pp. 119 ff.). The search for visual structure in science and nature continued to develop during the nineteenth century, as we saw earlier in this chapter. Visualization was brought to extraordinary pinnacles in the work of Leonardo da Vinci, of Albrecht Dürer, and, a few centuries later, of Étienne-Jules Marey (cf. Section 3.7, on pp. 137 ff.). They recognized fully the power of the scientific image and contributed to making our scientific culture a "visual" culture. Indeed, this chapter's synoptic overview from our rich scientific past to the current information revolution reinforces the idea that the process of visualization contributes to creativity and critical thinking.

The visual scientific culture is now coming of age in the digital revolution where images and numbers have merged—cf. Section A.1, on pp. 893 f., in the Appendix. Visualization is particularly valuable to the investigation of intracardiac fluid dynamics, where it plays a key role in providing researchers with insights into flow phenomena with basic scientific interdisciplinary correlations, and clinicians with faster decision-making capabilities.

Interactive and display technologies provide techniques to extract, view, integrate, and explore very large datasets that include instrumentation, imaging, and computational data. The overall process is inherently iterative, to explore different aspects of data and refine the visualization. Interactive real-time software applications provide iterative interrogation of datasets. Time evolution is a dimension of many datasets; accordingly, visualizations can also take the form of animated sequences of images.

Early CFD analyses were notorious for producing reams of numerical data output, readable only to the most dedicated scientists or engineers. The CFD codes of today include spectacular graphics, which display the output in a multitude of ways that even the most casual observers can understand. Indeed, a great strength of the contemporary CFD studies of intracardiac flows, which are emerging as a vital complement to animal experiment, is their clear and accessible output formats: color contours, vectors, and streamlines that can be easily appreciated by clinical cardiologists and surgeons, as well as by cardiovascular investigators and basic scientists—cf. Chapters 12–14, and 16. Scientific visualization is an indispensable tool helping to integrate diverse data and bring more insight into complex informational systems [60], such as those pertaining to CFD; it will play an increasingly important role in the continuing evolution of cardiology, cardiac imaging, and cardiac surgery.

References and further reading

[1] Aristotle, Apostle, H.G. Physics. 1969, Bloomington: Indiana University Press. xi, 386 p.

[2] Aristotle, Graham, D.W. Aristotle physics book VIII. Clarendon Aristotle series. 1999, Oxford; New York: Clarendon Press; Oxford University Press. xvii, 209 p.

[3] Aristotle, Guthrie, W.K.C. On the heavens. 1939, Cambridge, Mass.; London: Harvard University Press; W. Heinemann. xxxvi, 378, [1] p.

[4] Aristotle, Leggatt, S. Aristotle on the heavens, I and II. 1995, Warminster: Aris & Phillips. vii, 273 p.

[5] Aristotle, Ross, W.D. Aristotle's physics. A revised text with introduction and commentary by W.D. Ross. 1936, Oxford: Clarendon Press. xii, 750 p.

[6] Aristotle, Ogle, W. Aristotle on the parts of animals. Rev. ed. In: Aristotle's Works, 12 vols. 1968, Cambridge, MA.: Harvard University Press. x, 555 p.

[7] Åsberg, A.G. Ultrasonic cinematography of the living heart. Ultrasonics 5: 113–17, 1967.

[8] Aubrey, J., Dick, O.L. Aubrey's brief lives. 1999, Boston, MA: D.R. Godine. cxiv, 408 p.

[9] Baigrie, B.S. Picturing knowledge: historical and philosophical problems concerning the use of art in science. 1996, Toronto; Buffalo, NY: University of Toronto Press. xxiv, 389 p.

[10] Belt, E. Leonardo, the anatomist. Logan Clendening lectures on the history and philosophy of medicine; 4th ser. 1955, Lawrence: University of Kansas Press. 76 p.

[11] Berggren, J.L. Ptolemy's map of Earth and the heavens: a new interpretation. Arch. Hist. Exact Sci. 43: 133–44, 1991.

[12] Bernard, C. Introduction à l'étude de la médecine expérimentale. 1865, Paris: J.B. Bailliére.

[13] Bernard, C. Étude sur la physiologie du coeur. Revue des Deux Mondes, 1865 (1er mars): pp. 236–52.

[14] Bernard, C. Leçons sur les phénomènes de la vie communs aux animaux et aux végétaux. Avec une préface de Georges Canguilhem. 1967, Paris: Vrin. 14, xxxi, 404 p.

[15] Bernard, C. Leçons de Physiologie Opératoire. 1879, Paris: J.B. Bailliére.

[16] Bernoulli, D., Hydrodynamica, sive de viribus et motibus fluidorum commentarii. Opus Academicum ab Auctore, dum Petropoli ageret, congestum, Argentorati: Sumptibus Johannis Reinholdi Dulseckeri, Typis Joh. Henr. Deckeri, Typographi Basiliensis, 1738.— [English translation by T. Carmody and H.Kobus], 1968, New York: Dover. xv, 456 p.

[17] Bernoulli, D. Réflexions et éclaircissement sur les nouvelles vibrations des corde. Mémoires de l'Academie Royale des Sciences et Belles-Lettres, Berlin, 1753.

[18] Berrington de Gonzalez A, Darby S. Risk of cancer from diagnostic X-rays: estimates for the UK and 14 other countries. Lancet 363: 345–51, 2004.

[19] Berthon, S., Robinson, A. The shape of the world. 1991, Chicago: Rand McNally. 192 p.

[20] Borelli, G.A., Maquet, P. On the Movement of Animals (1680). 1989, New York: Springer-Verlag.

[21] Braun, M., Marey, E.-J. Picturing time: the work of Etienne-Jules Marey (1830–1904). 1992, Chicago: University of Chicago Press. xx, 450 p.

[22] Butterfield, H. The origins of modern science, 1300–1800. Rev. ed. 1957, New York: Macmillan. x, 242 p.

[23] Buzzi, A. Claude Bernard on cardiac catheterization. Am. J. Cardiol. 28: 405–9, 1959.

[24] Cahan, D. Hermann von Helmholtz and the foundations of nineteenth-century science. 1993, Berkeley: University of California Press. xxix, 666 p.

[25] Capra, F. The turning point. 1983, New York: Flamingo. 540 p.

[26] Chandrasekhar, S. Hydrodynamic and hydromagnetic stability [1961]. 1981, New York: Dover. 704 p.

[27] Chauveau, A., Bertolus G., Laroyenne L. Vitèsse de la circulation dans les artères du cheval d'après les indications d'un nouvel hémodromètre. J. Physiol. 3: 695, 1860.

[28] Chauveau A., Marey, É.-J. Appareils et expériences cardiographiques. Mémoires de l'Académie imperiale de Médicine. Tome XXVI, 268–319, 1863.

[29] Chauveau A., Marey É.-J. Appareils et expériences cardiographiques: Démonstration nouvelle du méchanisme des mouvements du coeur par l'emploi des instruments enregistreurs à indications continuées. Paris: J.-B. Baillière, 1863.

[30] Colp, R., Jr. Ernest H. Starling–his contribution to medicine. J. Hist. Med. Allied Sci. 7: 280–94, 1952.

[31] Cook, T.A. The curves of life: being an account of spiral formations and their application to growth in nature, to science and to art: with special reference to the manuscripts of Leonardo da Vinci. 1979, New York, London: Dover; Constable. xxx, 479 p.

[32] Cooper, L. Aristotle, Galileo, and the tower of Pisa. 1935, Ithaca, New York; London: Cornell University Press; H. Milford Oxford University Press. 102 p.

[33] Cormack, A.M., Representation of a function by its line integrals, with some radiological applications. J. Appl. Phys. 34: 2722–7, 1963.

[34] Cournand, A., Ranges, H.A. Catheterization of the right auricle in man. Proc. Soc. Exp. Biol. Med. 46: 462–6, 1941.

[35] Cournand, A. Cardiac catheterization: Development of the technique, its contributions to experimental medicine, and its initial applications in man. Acta Med. Scand. Suppl. 579, 1975.

[36] Daly, I.D.B. The second Bayliss-Starling memorial lecture. Some aspects of their separate and combined research interests. J. Physiol. 191: 1–23, 1967.

[37] Darrigol, O. Worlds of flow: a history of hydrodynamics from the Bernoullis to Prandtl. 2005, Oxford; New York: Oxford University Press. xiv, 356 p.

[38] Deutsche Akademie der Wissenschaften zu Berlin. and E. Winter, Die Registres der Berliner Akademie der Wissenschaften 1746–1766; Dokumente für das Wirken Leonhard Eulers in Berlin zum 250. Geburtstag. 1957, Berlin: Akademie-Verlag. xii, 393 p.

[39] Dickinson Chamberlin, M., Dickinson W. Richards, MD: through a grand-daughter's eyes. Coronary Artery Dis. 12: 79–82, 2001.

[40] Drake, S. History of free fall: Aristotle to Galileo; with an epilogue on "Pi" in the sky. 1989, Toronto: Wall & Thompson. 99 p.

[41] Drazin, P.G. Introduction to hydrodynamic stability. Cambridge texts in applied mathematics. 2002, Cambridge, UK; New York: Cambridge University Press. xvii, 258 p.

[42] Dunham, W. Euler: the master of us all. Dolciani mathematical expositions; no. 22. 1999, Washington, D.C.; Cambridge: Mathematical Association of America; Cambridge University Press. 185 p.

[43] Dürer, A. Underweysung der Messung mit dem Zirckel und Richtscheyt [1525] [Course in the art of measurement with compass and ruler]. 1972, Portland, Ore.: Collegium Graphicum. Alan Wofsy Fine Arts, distribution. 180 p. Illustrated. Facsimile reprint of the 1525 edition.

[44] Edler, I., Hertz, C.H. The use of ultrasonic reflectoscope for the continuous recording of the movements of heart walls. Kungl. Fysiografiska sällskapets i Lund förhandlingar 24: 1–19, 1954.

[45] Edgerton, S.Y. Jr. Florentine interest in Ptolemaic cartography as background for Renaissance Painting, Architecture, and the discovery of America. J. Soc. Architect. Histori. 33: 274–92, 1974.

[46] Edgerton, S.Y. Jr., The Renaissance rediscovery of linear perspective. 1975, New York: Basic Books, Harper and Row. xvii, 206 p.

[47] Edwards, B. Drawing on the right side of the brain: a course in enhancing creativity and artistic confidence. Los Angeles; New York: J.P. Tarcher; Distributed by St. Martin's Press. xiv, 254 p., [12] p. of plates.

[48] Eijk, P.J.v.d., Ancient histories of medicine: essays in medical doxography and historiography in classical antiquity. Studies in ancient medicine, v. 20. 1999, Leiden; Boston: Brill. viii, 537 p.

[49] Ellis, E.J., Gauer, O., Wood, E.H. Application of a manometric sound to the recording of intracardiac and intravascular pressures. Mayo Clin. Proc. 25: 49–51, 1950.

[50] Euclidis Optica et Catoptrica, 1557, Parisiis: ed. J. Pena. In: Francastel, P. Peinture et Société, 1951: Lyon, France.

[51] Fehrenbach, F., Leonardo. Licht und Wasser: zur Dynamik naturphilosophischer Leitbilder im Werk Leonardo da Vincis. 1997, Tübingen: E. Wasmuth. 378 p., [36] of plates.

[52] Feigenbaum, H. Evolution of echocardiography. Circulation 93: 1321–7, 1996.

[53] Fischer, J. [Ed.] Claudii Ptolemaei Geographiae Codex Urbinas Graecus 82, 2 vols. in 4, Codices e Vaticanis Selecti quam Simillime Expressi, vol. 19, 1932, Leiden: Brill; Leipzig: Harrassowitz.

[54] Fischer, B., Modersitzki, J. Ill-posed medicine—an introduction to image registration. Inverse Problems 24, 2008 034008 (16pp).

[55] Forssmann, W. Die Sondierung des rechten Herzens. Klin. Wschr. 8: 2085–7, 1929; [addendum, 1929; 8: 2287].

[56] Forssmann-Falck, R. Werner Forssmann: A Pioneer of Cardiology. Am. J. Cardiol 79: 651–60, 1997.

[57] Fournier, M. The fabric of life: microscopy in the seventeenth century. 1996, Baltimore, MD: Johns Hopkins University Press. 267 p.

[58] Frank, O. Zur Dynamik des Herzmuskels. Z. Biol. 32: 370–437, 1895.

[59] French, R.K. William Harvey's natural philosophy. 1994, Cambridge [England]; New York: Cambridge University Press. xii, 393 p.

[60] Friedhoff, R.M., Benzon, W. Visualization: the second computer revolution. 1991, New York: W.H. Freeman. 215 p.

[61] Geva, T. Magnetic resonance imaging: historical perspective. J. Cardiovasc. Magn. Reson. 8: 573–80, 2006.

[62] Gharib, M., Kremers, D., Koochesfahani, M.M., Kemp, M. Leonardo's vision of flow visualization. Exp. Fluids 33: 219 -223, 2002.

[63] Gibson, A.H. Osborne Reynolds and his work in hydraulics and hydrodynamics. 1946, London, New York: Pub. for the British Council by Longmans. 33 p.

[64] Gotthelf, A. Darwin on Aristotle. J. Hist. Biol. 32: 3–30, 1999.

[65] Grattan-Guinness, I. Daniel Bernoulli and the varieties of mechanics in the 18th century. Nieuw Archief voor Wiskunde (Mathematisch Instituut Universiteit Leiden) 1: 242–9, 2000.

[66] Graubard, M. Circulation and respiration: the evolution of an idea. Ideas in science. 1964, New York: Harcourt Brace & World. ix, 278.

[67] Hall, A.R. The scientific revolution, 1500-1800; the formation of the modern scientific attitude. 1962, London: Longmans. 394 p.

[68] Hansen, A.T. Pressure measurement in the human organism. Acta Physiol. Scand. 19, Suppl. 68: 1–230, 1949.

[69] Harvey, W. Exercitatio anatomica de motu cordis et sanguinis in animalibus (An anatomical disquisition on the motion of the heart and blood in animals). London, 1628. Translated by Robert Willis. Surrey, England: Barnes, 1847.

[70] Haas, L.F. Hermann von Helmholtz (1821–94). J. Neurol. Neurosurg. Psychiat., 64: 787, 1998.

[71] Hakim, J. The story of science. Aristotle leads the way. 2004, Washington, DC: Smithsonian Books. xiv, 282 p.

[72] Heintzen, P., Adam W.E. History of cardiovascular imaging procedures (as developed and/or applied in German cardiology). Z. Kardiol. 91: Suppl 4, IV/64–73, 2002.

[73] Helmholtz, H. v. Über Integrale der hydrodynamischen Gleichungen, welche den Wirbelbewegungen entsprechen. J. Angew. Math. 55: 25–55, 1858.

[74] Helmholtz, H. v. On thought in medicine (Das denken in der medizin). 1938, Baltimore: The Johns Hopkins Press. 27 p.

[75] Helmholtz, H. v., Atkinson, E. Popular lectures on scientific subjects. 1908, London; New York: Longmans Green. xiv, 348 p.

[76] Helmholtz, H. v., Kahl, R. Selected writings of Hermann von Helmholtz. 1st ed. 1971, Middletown, Conn.: Wesleyan University Press. xlv, 542 p.

[77] Helmholtz, H. v., Krigar-Menzel, O. Vorlesungen über die Dynamik continuirlich verbreiteter Massen. 2. ed. Vorlesungen über theoretische Physik; Bd. 2., ed. H.v. Helmholtz. 1925, Leipzig: J. A. Barth. viii, 247 p.

[78] Hounsfield, G.N., Computerized transverse axial scanning (tomography): part 1. Description of system. Br J Radiol 46: 1016–22, 1973.

[79] Hounsfield, G.N. Computed Medical Imaging–Nobel Lecture, December 8, 1979. Nobel Lectures, Physiology or Medicine 1971–1980, Editor: Jan Lindsten, World Scientific Publishing Co., Singapore, 1992.

[80] Hurst, J.W., Fye, W.B., Acierno, L.J. Adolph Fick: mathematician, physicist, physiologist. Clin. Cardiol. 23: 390–1, 2000.

[81] Jardine, L. Ingenious pursuits: building the scientific revolution. 1999, London: Little, Brown & Co. xx, 444 p.

[82] Judson, L. Aristotle's Physics: a collection of essays. 1991, Oxford [England] New York: Clarendon Press; Oxford University Press. 286 p.

[83] Keele, K.D., Leonardo. Leonardo da Vinci on movement of the heart and blood. 1952, Philadelphia: Lippincott. xviii, 142 p.

[84] Lai, C.-M., Lauterbur, P.C. True three-dimensional image reconstruction by nuclear magnetic resonance zeugmatography. Phys. Med. & Biol. 26: 851–6, 1981.

[85] Laidler, K.J. Energy and the unexpected. 2002, Oxford; New York: Oxford University Press. xiii, 146 p.

[86] Landois, L., Stirling, W. A text-book of human physiology including histology and microscopical anatomy, with special reference to the requirements of practical medicine. 4th ed. 1892, Philadelphia: P. Blakiston, son & co. xliv, 1156 p.

[87] Lauterbur, P.C. Image formation by induced local interactions: examples employing nuclear magnetic resonance. Nature 242: 190–1, 1973.

[88] Lauterbur, P.C. All science is interdisciplinary–from magnetic moments to molecules to men (Nobel Lecture). Angew. Chem. Int. Ed. 44: 1004–11, 2005.

[89] Leonardo, O'Malley, C.D., Saunders, J.B.d.C.M. Leonardo da Vinci on the human body: the anatomical, physiological, and embryological drawings of Leonardo da Vinci. 1952, New York: H. Schuman. 506 p.

[90] Leonardo, Schneider, M. Delle acque. 2001, Palermo Sellerio. 310 p.

[91] Leonardo, et al. Leonardo da Vinci: anatomical drawings from the Royal Library, Windsor Castle: 1983, New York: Metropolitan Museum of Art. 167 p.

[92] Leonardo, et al. Quaderni d'anatomia: tredici fogli della Royal Library di Windsor. Comunicazioni., ed. C. Universitetet i and i. Anatomiske. 1911, Christiania: Dybwad. 6 v.

[93] Leonardo da Vinci, Arconati L.M., Carusi E., Favaro A. Del moto e misura dell'acqua, libri nove ordinati da f. Luigi Maria Arconati. 1923, Bologna: Nicola Zanichelli. xxiii, 408 p., 3 l.

[94] Liggett, J.A. Fluid mechanics. 1994, New York: McGraw-Hill. xxviii, 495 p.

[95] Mansfield, P. Echo-planar imaging: multiplanar image formation using NMR. J. Phys. C. 10: L55–8, 1977.

[96] Mansfield, P. Snap-shot MRI–Nobel Lecture, December 8, 2003. *Les Prix Nobel*. The Nobel Prizes 2003, Editor: Tore Frängsmyr, [Nobel Foundation], Stockholm, 2004.

[97] Mansion, A. Introduction à la physique aristotélicienne. 2. éd., rev. et augm. ed. Aristote, traductions et études. 1946, Louvain: Institut supérieur de philosophie. xvi, 357 p.

[98] Marcolongo, R. Studi vinciani. Memorie sulla geometria e la meccanica di Leonardo da Vinci. 1937, Napoli: S. I. E. M.–Stabilimento industrie editoriali meridionali. xii, 364 p.

[99] Marey, É.-J. Animal mechanism: a treatise on terrestrial and aerial locomotion. 2nd ed. 1874, London: H.S. King. xvi, 283 p.

[100] Marey, É.-J. Développement de la méthode graphique par l'emploi de la photographie. 1885, Paris: G. Masson. vi, 52 p.

[101] Marey, É.-J. La circulation du sang à l'état physiologique et dans les maladies. 1881, Paris: G. Masson. iii, 745 p.

[102] Marey, É.-J. La machine animale: locomotion terrestre et aérienne. Bibliothèque scientifique internationale. 1873, Paris: Germer Baillière. x, 299 p.

[103] Marey, É.-J. La méthode graphique dans les sciences expérimentales et principalement en physiologie et en médecine. 1878, Paris: G. Masson. xix, 673 p.

[104] Marey, É.-J. Physiologie médicale de la circulation du sang, basée sur l'étude graphique des mouvements du coeur et du pouls artériel avec application aux maladies de l'appareil circulatoire. 1863, Paris: A. Delahaye. viii, 568 p.

[105] McMurrich, J.P. Leonardo da Vinci, the anatomist (1452-1519). 1930, Baltimore: Pub. for Carnegie Institution of Washington (Publication no. 411) by the Williams & Wilkins company. xx, 265 p., 2 l.

[106] Mehta, N.J., Khan, I.A. Cardiology's 10 greatest discoveries of the 20th century. Tex. Heart Inst. J. 29: 164–71, 2002.

[107] Mistretta, C.A., Crummy, A.B., Strother, C.M. Digital angiography: a perspective. Radiology, 139: 273–6, 1981.

[108] Neményi, P.F. The main concepts and ideas of fluid dynamics in their historical development. Arch. Hist. Exact Sci. 2: 52–86, 1962.

[109] Ovitt T.W., Christenson P.C., Fisher H.D. 3rd, Frost M.M., Nudelman S., Roehrig H., Seeley G. Intravenous angiography using digital video subtraction: x-ray imaging system. Am. J. Roentgenol. 135: 1141–4, 1980.

[110] Panofsky, E. The life and art of Albrecht Dürer. 1955, Princeton, N.J.: Princeton University Press. xxxii, 317 p., [148] p. of plates.

[111] Parvez, H., Parvez, S. [Eds.] Advances in experimental medicine: a centenary tribute to Claude Bernard. 1980, Amsterdam; New York: Elsevier/North-Holland Biomedical Press. xviii, 643 p.

[112] Pasipoularides, A. Clinical assessment of ventricular ejection dynamics with and without outflow obstruction. [Review]. J. Am. Coll. Cardiol. 15: 859–82, 1990.

[113] Pasipoularides, A.D., Womack, S.M., Shah, A., Von Ramm, O., Glower, D.D. RV functional imaging: 3-D echo-derived dynamic geometry and flow field simulations. Am. J. Physiol. Heart. Circ. Physiol. 284: H56–H65, 2003.

[114] Patterson, S.W., Piper, H., Starling, E.H. The regulation of the heart beat. J. Physiol. 48: 465–513, 1914.

[115] Pickover, C.A., Tewksbury, S.K. Frontiers of scientific visualization. 1994, New York: Wiley. vi, 284 p., [16] of plates.

[116] Porter, R. The greatest benefit to mankind: a medical history of humanity. 2003, New York: W W Norton & Co. xv, 831 p.

[117] Reti, L., Dibner, B. Leonardo da Vinci, technologist: three essays on some designs and projects of the Florentine master in adapting machinery and technology to the problems in art, industry, and war. 1969, Norwalk, Conn.: Burndy Library. 96 p.

[118] Röntgen, W.C. On a new kind of rays. Nature 53: 274–7, 1896.

[119] Sachs, J., Aristotle, and NetLibrary Inc. Aristotle's physics: a guided study. Masterworks of discovery. 1995, New Brunswick, N.J.: Rutgers University Press. xi, 260 p.

[120] Sarnoff, S. J., Berglund E. Ventricular function. I. Starling's law of the heart studied by means of simultaneous right and left ventricular function curves in the dog. Circulation 9: 706–18, 1954.

[121] Sarton, G. The discovery of X-rays. Isis 26: 349–69, 1937.

[122] Sarton, G. A history of science. 1952, Cambridge, MA: Harvard University Press. 2 v.

[123] Schaper, W., Buschmann, I. Collateral circulation and diabetes [Editorial]. Circulation. 99: 2224–6, 1999.

[124] Schneck, P. Geschichte der Medizin systematisch. 1. Auflage. 1997, Bremen und Lorch/Württemberg (Germany): UNI-MED Verlag AG, International Medical Publishers. 255 p.

[125] Schröder, E. Dürer–Kunst und geometrie. 1980, Basel: Birkhauser Verlag.

[126] Shaw, J.R. Models for cardiac structure and function in Aristotle. J. Hist. Biol. 5: 355–88, 1972.

[127] Siegel, R.E. Why Galen and Harvey did not compare the heart to a pump. Am. J. Cardiol. 20: 117–21, 1967.

[128] Snellen, H.A., Marey, E.-J. E.J. Marey and cardiology: physiologist and pioneer of technology, 1830–1904: selected writings in facsimile with comments and summaries, a brief history of life and work, and a bibliography. 1980, Rotterdam: Kooyker Scientific Publications. 264 p.

[129] Sones F.M. Jr, Shirey E.K. Cine coronary arteriography. Mod. Concepts Cardiovasc. Dis. 31: 735–8, 1962.

[130] Starling, E.H., Principles of human physiology. 1912, London: J.A. Churchill. xii, 1423 p. illus.

[131] Starling, E.H., Visscher, M.B. The regulation of the energy output of the heart. J. Physiol. 62: 243–61, 1926.

[132] Storey, G.A. The theory and practice of Perspective. 1910, Oxford: The Clarendon Press. xii, 272 p. illus.

[133] Strauss, W.L. [Ed.] Albrecht Dürer: The human figure. The complete Dresden sketchbook. 1972, New York: Dover Publications.

[134] Tenorio, L., Haber, E., Symes, W.W., Stark, P.B., Cox, D., Ghattas, O. Guest Editors' introduction to the special section on statistical and computational issues in inverse problems. Inverse Problems 24, 2008 034001 (5pp).

[135] Truesdell, C. Archive for history of exact sciences. 1960, Berlin; New York: Springer-Verlag. Vol.1, no.1/ [contributed and] edited by C. Truesdell, p. v.

[136] United Nations Scientific Committee on the Effects of Atomic Radiation. Sources and effects of ionizing radiation. 2000, New York: United Nations.

[137] Wilson, C. The invisible world: early modern philosophy and the invention of the microscope. Studies in intellectual history and the history of philosophy. 1995, Princeton, N.J.: Studies in intellectual history and the history of philosophy, Princeton University Press. x, 280 p.

[138] Ziedses des Plantes, B.G. Application of the Roentgenographic subtraction method in neuroradiography. Acad. Radiol. 1: 961–6, 1963.

Chapter 4

Fluid Dynamics of Unsteady Flow

Everybody reasons about Hydraulics, but there are few people who understand it...

——Count P. L. G. Du Buat, founder of the French hydraulics school, in his classic work *Principes d'Hydraulique*, 2nd edition, Paris, 1786. He was lamenting that the resistance to flow for most conditions was unknown; thus, channels and closed conduits could not be designed reliably.

Fluids in motion may behave in intricate ways, giving rise to a wide variety of complex flow phenomena [86]. In this chapter, we overview some of the varied phenomena that we will encounter in subsequent chapters, classified according to the kinds of forces that control them. We begin by noting that a fluid particle within a flow field responds to body and surface forces [68]. The gravitational force is the only body force considered here. The surface forces can be either normal or tangential (shear). It is an essential property of fluids that shear forces occur only if a fluid is flowing, and is thus being continually strained due to the relative motion of fluid particles. A fluid at rest, or one that is moving as a rigid body, is free of shear stresses. To a good approximation, the central cores of the proximal aortic and pulmonary arterial flows during the upstroke of the ejection waveform are totally dominated by inertial forces and move like a rigid body.

4.1 Inertial, viscous, and pressure gradient forces

Inertia allows a moving fluid to coast, after the removal of any driving force. Thus, we can stir creamer in our coffee, remove the spoon, and observe the motions that persist for a while. Viscosity resists the finite rates of fluid parcel deformation associated with such motions, and eventually brings the flow to rest. The resistance to finite rates of deformation produced by *viscosity* is also necessary for the motility of many microorganisms and the spermatozoa that operate at minuscule Reynolds numbers: it gives them something against which to push, to be able to swim. On the other hand, larger creatures, including humans, swim by pushing (leg "kick") or pulling (arms and hands action) against the *inertia* of the water.

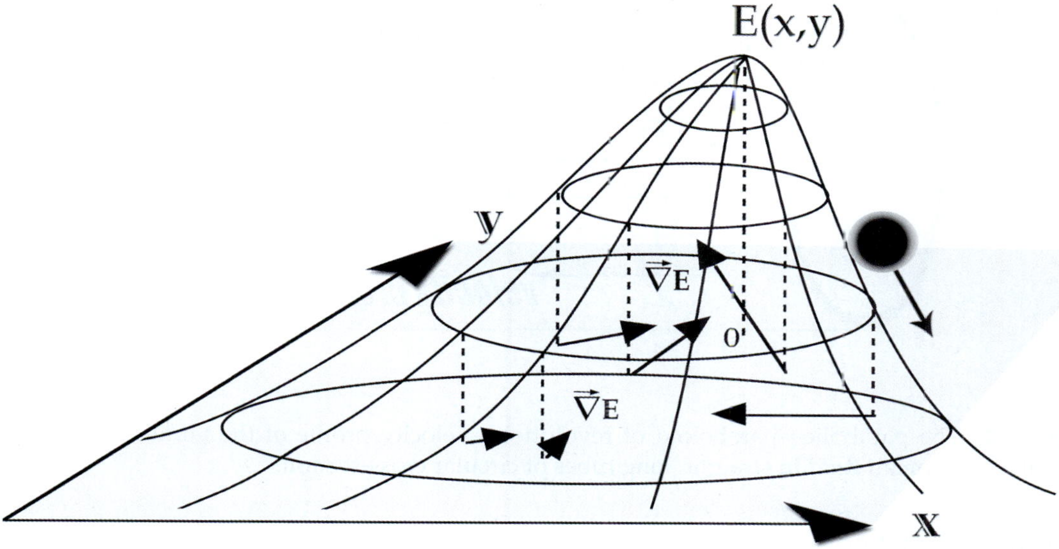

Figure 4.1: In two dimensions, we can visualize elevation as a contour map $E(x, y)$ for which E is the elevation of the land at the point (x, y). The vertical dashed lines indicate the elevation in the drawing. Representative contours of constant elevation are shown as ovals above, and one maximum (the summit) is present. The elevation gradient vector, $\vec{\nabla}E$, is 2-D in the $x-y$ plane; it is shown as an arrow for several representative points above. The direction of the vector $\vec{\nabla}E$ at each point is the direction of steepest *rise* and its magnitude indicates the steepness; note that $\vec{\nabla}E = 0$ at the summit—and at any maximum or minimum.

When analyzing the motion of fluids, it is convenient to hypothesize the presence of an inertial force density, equal to mass density times the total acceleration and acting in the direction of the acceleration. The problem of dynamics then reduces to one of a force balance, with the inertial force balancing out all other forces acting on a fluid element [30, 48, 89]. The simplest flows to analyze are those where the inertial forces are zero, i.e., where fluid acceleration terms are absent. One class of flows where inertial forces are absent encompasses the *fully developed* flows, like the familiar Poiseuille flow in long, straight tubes. Fully developed flows approach a certain invariant state in terms of appropriate variables, such as the velocity profile across a flow cross-section (see Fig. 4.2, on p. 168), or the axial pressure gradient. In these flows, the surface and body forces are in complete equilibrium. Neglecting the body force of gravity, the surface pressure forces exactly balance the surface viscous forces. Therefore, the viscous stresses at the walls determine the pressure drop in Poiseuille flow.

The expression for the inertial forces in fluids is a bit more complex than in solids, because in the study of fluid mechanics, the use of field description is preferred to the discrete particle or point-mass description. As shown in subsequent sections, the total

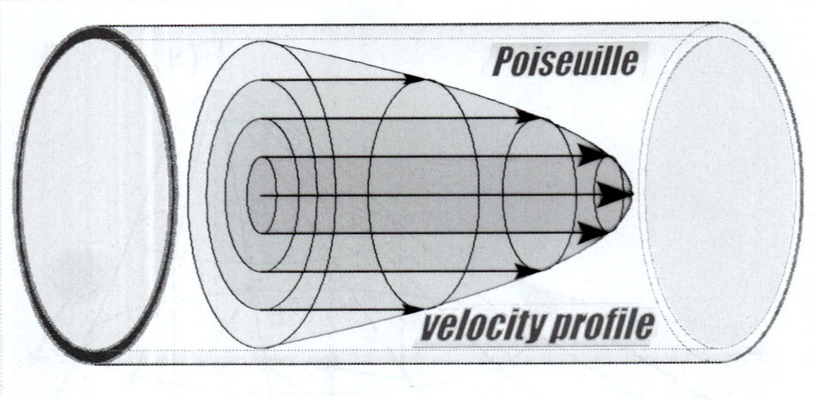

Figure 4.2: The parabolic—paraboloid of revolution—velocity profile of the familiar Poiseuille flow of a Newtonian fluid in straight, long tubes of circular cross-section.

acceleration of a fluid particle in the flow field is a combination of the local (i.e., unsteady) term and the convective term. Even when the flow is steady, i.e., the conditions at a fixed point in the flow field do not change with time—e.g., in a flow of an inviscid fluid about a cylinder (cf. Fig. 4.16, on p. 205)—fluid particles experience various accelerations as they move downstream. Thus, a particle in steady flow decelerates while approaching the cylinder, accelerates as it moves from the stagnation point up to the shoulder, decelerates on the downstream half up to the rear stagnation point, and then accelerates once again to the free-stream velocity far downstream.

Convective effects dominate most fluid motions of cardiovascular interest and are quite difficult to analyze, since the convective acceleration terms are nonlinear. Whenever the viscous forces are absent or negligible, the inertial force balances the pressure and the gravity forces, and the Euler equation governs the flow (Equation 4.10, on p. 181). Neglecting gravity, the net pressure force acting on a fluid particle is the *negative* of the pressure gradient. When the streamlines curve [62], the convective inertial force includes the centripetal force as well and, therefore, the pressure gradient then also has a component normal to the streamlines. Examples include the flow through a pipe bend or through a converging conduit. The equilibrium of pressure and inertial forces suggests that the pressure gradient is in the same direction as the (negative of) fluid acceleration (see Fig. 2.16, on p. 58).

Figure 4.1, on p. 167, provides a pictorial explanation for the need of the negative sign, in terms of a gravitational "rolling ball" analog: Just as the ball is rolling downhill—opposite to the direction of the maximum rate of *increase* of the elevation, so a pressure driven flow moves toward lower pressure—opposite to the direction of the maximum rate of increase of pressure, which is mathematically that of the pressure gradient vector, $\vec{\nabla} P$. Thus, in inviscid fluid motions, the pressure is higher where the velocity is smaller and *vice versa*, in the same way as the velocity of the ball in Figure 4.1 is lower at higher elevations and, *ceteris paribus*, highest at the bottom of the "hill." This fact is embodied in the Bernoulli equation.

The viscous stresses in a fluid depend on the severity of the rate of distortion produced, which depends on the velocity gradients [39, 77]. The Reynolds number, *Re*, measures the relative magnitude of inertial and viscous forces [30, 68, 86], and the viscous forces are significant only when *Re* is small. When $Re \ll 1$, we may neglect the inertial forces altogether and expect the pressure forces to be balanced by the viscous forces [48, 68, 86]. This is the Stokes flow regime of creeping flow. The other extreme, when $Re \gg 1$, is of greater interest for the analysis of intracardiac blood flow phenomena, since most of the cardiovascular flows outside the microcirculatory beds fall in this regime [53, 54].

Here, one expects the viscous effects to be negligible in the main stream outside a hydrodynamic *boundary layer*, suggesting that the flow patterns should be similar to those for inviscid flow except for the boundary layer and regions of separated flow. We will see in this chapter that the presence of viscosity, even if small, does give rise to a thin region next to the boundary surface where viscous shear effects are salient even when, at high Reynolds numbers, inertial effects are predominant over most of the flow. In this boundary layer, the viscous forces are of the same order as the inertial forces [67, 73].

The analytical solution of flow problems at high Reynolds numbers involves patching two solutions [13, 18, 29, 39, 53, 61, 74], one for the thin viscous boundary layer and the other for the remaining outer region where the flow is irrotational and is governed by the Euler and Bernoulli equations. Even though the boundary layer involves three types of forces, inertial, viscous and pressure, we know the pressure distribution *a priori*, from the irrotational outer flow, whose solution we obtain first. The dynamics of boundary layer flow underlie striking departures from ideal fluid flow behavior. If the pressure increases in the downstream direction, the boundary layer tends to separate from the wall, changing the entire flow pattern drastically. Consequently, the shear effects, which normally prevail in the narrow boundary layer region near the walls, letting the main flow to be approximately the same as predicted by inviscid flow theory, spread much farther into the flow field upon separation. The pressures at the rear of a bluff body (e.g., a circular cylinder) no longer follow the Bernoulli equation, and are lower than at its front. This *symmetry breaking* results in a net pressure drag, which, for bluff bodies, can be several orders of magnitude larger than the viscous shear drag.

Another paradigm of the complicated interplays of inertial (centrifugal) with viscous effects is the striking Taylor–Couette experiment, involving the movement of a fluid between two rotating cylinders (see Section 9.5.4, on pp. 463 ff.). This sets up a flow in which different parts of the liquid travel at different speeds, and recurring instabilities give rise to several fascinating flow patterns associated with breaking of successive flow symmetries. At very high rates of rotation, symmetry is, curiously, reestablished in the form of a highly turbulent flow regime with no discernible macroscopic coherent patterns.

I have outlined above only a few fluid-flow paradigms, which I chose to discuss in this chapter with an eye to the appreciation of complicated intracardiac flow phenomena and emerging advances in the field, which are the main subject of our interest. There is still a variety of phenomena, which we will not examine in this chapter, or will barely do so. Some of the books and papers listed in further readings at the end of this chapter dwell upon these in detail. However, the structure presented in this chapter should equip the reader to engage into a profitable study of intracardiac flows.

4.2 Fields

Envision a cubical region with a single mathematical point inside it. Place a second point somewhere else inside the cube, and allow the second point to approach the first until the spacing between the two is arbitrarily small. Do this repeatedly until the region is densely filled with points; i.e., so that there is no neighborhood inside the cube, regardless of how small, in which there is not at least one such point. We call this space of mathematical points a *continuum* (see also Section 1.6, on pp.16 f.). We will use this continuum of points to facilitate visualization of the *field* concept. First, we orient the cube in a Cartesian coordinate system. Then, to every point inside, we assign a color according to some specified rule. We call the color at any given point a "field variable," and the resultant whole a "color field." A field is a continuum of points with a physical quantity, in this case "color," assigned to every point according to some kind of rule. We will now consider two types of color field, each constructed according to a different rule.

Time-invariant continuous color field: Imagine a color field in which color changes progressively from left to right, perhaps starting with red at the left face of the cube and advancing smoothly through the rainbow to indigo at the right face. Let the colors remain non-varying with time. Such a field is classified as time-invariant or static. The first derivative in a given direction tells us how quickly the field variable (spectral frequency of the changing color) changes with distance as we move along this direction. The second derivative tells us how quickly the first derivative changes as we move along this direction. If the first and second derivatives are finite at every point inside the cube, they are said to exist everywhere within the field, and to be continuous functions of location. The field is then "well behaved."

Time-varying continuous field: In the preceding case, we assumed that the colors remained constant with time; i.e., that the field would appear the same regardless of when we look at it. Now, beginning with that color field, imagine that, at every point in the field, the color is continuously changing. Let us specify a rule for the change to help the conceptualization. First, imagine a line with the rainbow colors placed along it with red at the left and indigo at the right. Place a movable pointer on the line. Now pick a point in the field, and place the pointer at a corresponding color on the line. Let the pointer gradually move to the right until it reaches the end of the line. Then let the pointer move to the left, and so on, back and forth. Do this at every successive point along the left-to-right axis, letting the pointer move at the same rate each time. The overall effect is that at any individual point in the field, the full spectrum will be on display forwards and backwards, repeatedly. If we monitor a single point, the color at that point will change gradually through the rainbow. If we observe the field as a whole, waves of color will appear to be traveling back and forth.

This example is a time-varying, or dynamic, field. Since the overall color pattern repeats from time to time, the field is a periodic time-varying field, with the period equal to the time interval between any two successive snapshots in which the field appears the same. Points separated along the left-to-right axis will exhibit different colors in a snapshot at any given time, and this difference represents a phase-difference, or lag. Thus, a point near the left face might be going from red to orange at the same time that a point near the right face is going from green to blue. In general, time-varying, or unsteady, fields do not need to be periodic.

Unsteady blood flow fields: The properties of these time-varying fields depend on time because of dynamic changes in the driving pressure gradient, or in the size and shape of the containing walls. All intracardiac and great central vessel flows are highly unsteady [53, 54]. Of major interest in the study of intracardiac blood flow phenomena are *impulsive blood flows*. These are blood motions set up by the application of an impulse by the containing walls [27,35,53,54].

4.2.1 Impulse

Impulse is the application of concentrated or distributed forces of large magnitude for very short time periods. The impulse is the total momentum imparted, as when a hammer strikes a solid mass and sets it moving with high velocity. If the applied force is constant, the impulse, $\mathbf{I}$, is given by the product of the *constant* net force, $\mathbf{F}$, that is applied in order to change the velocity, and the time interval, Δt, of its application. It is equal to the induced net change in momentum, which is the product of the mass, m, multiplied by the net change in its velocity, $\Delta\mathbf{v}$:

$$\mathbf{I} = \mathbf{F}\,\Delta t = m\,\Delta\mathbf{v}. \tag{4.1}$$

The impulse of a *time-varying* force is calculated as the integral of the applied force with respect to time. Expressed in words, this means that to impart the greatest momentum to a mass, we must apply the greatest force possible and extend the time of its action as much as possible. However, even if the time of its action is short, a very large transient force can generate a large change in momentum. Ventricular ejection is a prime example of impulsive flow for which the inertial properties of blood, which relate to its mass, are pertinent while its viscous properties are typically quite irrelevant. In contrast, in the familiar steady Poiseuille flow, the viscous actions are pertinent and inertial effects are completely irrelevant.

4.2.2 The streamfunction

Consider a 2-D flow of an incompressible fluid on the $x-y$ plane. At some instant, t, we can draw a set of streamlines, which are lines tangent everywhere to the local instantaneous velocity vector [50,62,70,87]. Streamlines are drawn by joining a continuous line of points in the flow field by following the local instantaneous velocity vectors. Since the flow is 2-D, the streamlines will be identical in every plane that is parallel to the $x-y$ plane.

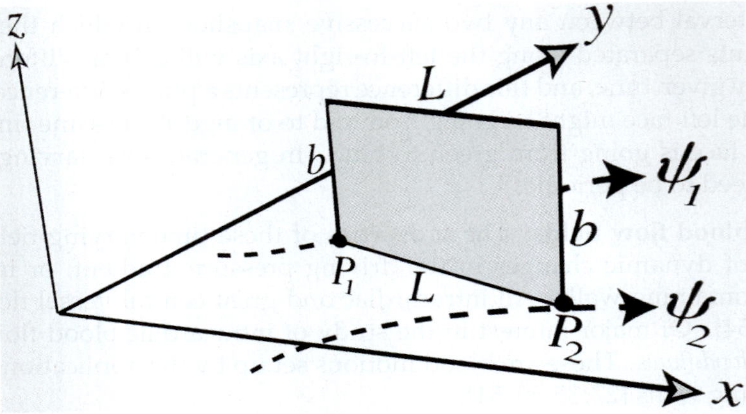

Figure 4.3: Schematic depicting a rectangular flow cross-section of area $b \cdot L$ perpendicular to the $x-y$ plane. One edge of this cross-section lies on the $x-y$ plane, and the end-points P_1 and P_2 of this edge lie on streamlines on which the streamfunction has the values ψ_1 and ψ_2, respectively. The difference in value of streamfunction between any two streamlines ψ_1 and ψ_2 a distance L apart equals the volumetric flow rate passing between the two streamlines *per unit width, b, normal to the plane of motion.*

If we draw a surface perpendicular to the $x-y$ plane and passing through a streamline, the instantaneous velocity vector will be tangent to it at every point and no fluid will cross this surface. Such a surface is designated a stream surface. Since no fluid can move across a stream surface, the groove bounded by any two stream surfaces can be regarded as a 2-D channel for fluid flow.[1]

If we take a pair of stream surfaces passing through streamlines S_1 and S_2 in the $x-y$ plane, and consider the region along the flow bounded by them, we may write the equation of volume continuity as

$$(vA)_1 = (vA)_2, \tag{4.2}$$

where, v_1 and v_2 are averaged velocities at cross-sections 1 and 2, and the inflow (A_1) and outflow (A_2) cross-sectional areas are selected perpendicular to the respective instantaneous velocity vectors. Equation 4.2 suggests that the spacing between streamlines increases where flow slows down and decreases where flow speeds up. The density of streamlines, thus, is a measure of the local fluid velocity. This is one reason why streamline patterns are used extensively as graphic descriptions of steady flow fields, or of instantaneous velocity patterns in unsteady fields [37,53,54].

In 2-D flow, a streamfunction (Ψ) can be defined as a measure of the volumetric flow rate of fluid between a pair of streamlines [27]. The streamfunction is specified only to within

[1] In a 3-D flow field, the streamlines that pass through a closed curve form a tubular stream surface. As for a 2-D flow, there is no flow across these stream surfaces, which can be visualized as conduits. They represent stream tubes and the instantaneous volumetric flow rate across any cross-section along their axis is constant, for incompressible flow.

a constant. As such, only *differences* in instantaneous (Ψ) values are physically relevant. Streamlines have a constant value of the streamfunction, since all the flow must be parallel to the streamlines—no flow crosses a streamline. For 2-D incompressible flow, continuity makes the local product of distance between streamlines and velocity a constant (cf. Fig. 4.3, on p. 172). Thus, the components, v_x and v_y, of the local instantaneous velocity vector in the flow field can also be found by differentiating the streamfunction with respect to the flow-field coordinates x and y:

$$\frac{\partial \Psi}{\partial y} = v_x \,, \qquad -\frac{\partial \Psi}{\partial x} = v_y . \tag{4.3}$$

4.3 Volume and surface forces: gravitational force and pressure gradient

A fluid particle or element is an idealization of the fluid, regarded to be small enough that the fluid motion does not disperse it. We never define the actual dimensions of a fluid particle: it is just assumed to be sufficiently small, regardless of whether this is close to the molecular limit or not. The approach is typical of "fluid thinking," where we attempt to understand difficult problems using simple arguments relating to basic length and time scales. It is possible to distinguish two kinds of forces, which act on a fluid element or particle [48, 68, 77, 86, 89]: 1) long-range forces like gravity, which decrease slowly with increase of distance; and, 2) short-range forces, which have a direct molecular origin.

Long-range forces: They act on all fluid particles. Gravity is the obvious and most important example. A consequence of the slow variation of long-range forces with position is that the force acts equally on all the matter within a fluid element and the total force is proportional to the size of any given fluid particle [48, 68]. Consequently, long-range forces are also designated as *volume* or *body forces*. For flow fields of cardiovascular interest, the relevant body force is gravity. The gravitational force per unit volume on a fluid particle is $\rho\,\mathbf{g}$, where $\mathbf{g}$ is the acceleration due to gravity, which points vertically downward.

Short-range forces: These are negligible unless there is direct mechanical contact between the interacting elements. Accordingly, the total of the short-range forces acting on the element is determined by the surface area of the element, while the volume of the element is not directly relevant. That is why they are also known as *surface forces* [77,86,89]. We consider the surface elements bounding any fluid particle of interest and specify the local short-range force as the total force exerted on the fluid on one side of the bounding surface by the fluid on the other side. The total force exerted across the volume element will be proportional to its area.

Pressure gradient: The assemblage of the unsteady pressure values on all of the points of a flow field is the instantaneous pressure field. The spatial distribution of the time-varying pressure values determines the instantaneous pressure force acting upon any fluid particle within an unsteady flow field [27, 35, 53]. This force, when expressed per unit volume of the fluid, is the pressure gradient, a vector quantity denoted as $\vec{\nabla}p$. Generally, the resultant of $\vec{\nabla}p$ in any direction is the rate of change of pressure in that direction—see Section 2.7 on pp. 57 f. By convention in cardiology, we use "pressure drop" and "gradient" interchangeably. Although gradient refers to the rate of change of pressure with distance, both expressions emphasize that, as far as flow is concerned, it is the differences in pressure that matter, not the pressure itself. The minus sign for the pressure gradient means that a blood particle has a positive acceleration when it moves from a region of higher to lower pressure, and *vice versa*.

In a flow field, different fluid particles are capable of different movements, and the distribution of the body and surface forces throughout the field is of the essence; moreover, the relative motion of the different fluid particles may affect both the body and surface forces. The way in which body forces (gravity) depend on the local properties (density) is evident, but the dependence of surface forces on the local properties and motion of the fluid generally requires fluid dynamics knowledge.

4.4 The flow-field equations

To describe the motion of a fluid, we must give its features at every point. For example, at different regions of a flow field, the fluid is moving with different velocities. To specify the character of the flow, therefore, we must give the three components of velocity at every point of the field and for any time. If we can find the equations that govern the velocity, then we will know how the liquid moves at all times. The velocity, however, is not the only variable that varies from point to point. In addition, there are other flow-field variables, such as pressure, which also varies from point to point, temperature, mass-density, and so on. In cardiac flow problems, the fluid mass-density (ρ) is constant—blood is essentially incompressible [53].

4.4.1 Introducing the conservation equations

When trying to understand a complex physical process, the best approach is to look for quantities which remain constant. Any such conserved quantity is often a signal that a conservation principle is at work, and that a more sophisticated analysis and understanding of the problem is possible. Fluid dynamic problems are solved using fundamental conservation laws, or equations derived from the conservation laws. A number of conservation principles have been identified in the study of flow phenomena; in general, three conservation laws can be used:

1. *Conservation of mass:* Matter is neither created nor destroyed. If a certain mass of fluid enters a volume, it must either exit the volume or increase the mass inside the volume. The conservation of fluid mass becomes the conservation of fluid volume if the density is constant. Equations derived from application of the conservation of mass principle are often referred to as *"continuity equations."*

2. *Conservation of momentum* (also called *Newton's second law of motion*): Momentum is defined as the product of mass and velocity. As such, it agrees with the intuitive definition of the term: objects with greater mass and velocity are harder to stop than smaller objects moving more slowly. In any closed system, such as a set of two colliding objects, the total momentum is conserved. The conservation of momentum includes the momentum flux and various forces on the boundaries of a flow region. Because forces are vectors and velocity carries with it direction as well, momentum does so too, and the momentum equation is vectorial. Hence in any given direction, the total momentum is conserved. The conservation of momentum and related equations are called *"equations of motion"* in the context of fluid flow.

3. *Conservation of energy:* The total energy in any fluid flow system remains constant. In considering conservation of the mechanical energy content of flowing blood, conservation of thermal energy is not taken into account explicitly, because relevant temperature-changes are small and hence there is no coupling between the energy and momentum equations in terms of blood density; in other words, heat generation and transfer effects do not affect directly intracardiac blood flow phenomena. Although it can be converted from one form to another, the total energy in a given system remains constant. Limiting attention to mechanical energy, the energy conservation principle is embodied in steady- and unsteady-flow formulations of the *Bernoulli equation*, modified—if need be—to allow for frictional losses.

All problems involving fluid flow are therefore solved by properly selected members of the same set of conservation equations. Conservation laws look different because we use different methods to measure, or "account for," each individual conserved property. For instance, conservation of mass uses mass: $d(mass)/dt = net\ rate\ of\ mass\ flow\ in$, because mass is something we can measure directly. On the other hand, conservation of energy or momentum cannot be dealt with easily in this form. This is because energy and momentum are not properties that we can measure directly.

Energy and momentum are abstract properties created to help us solve problems. We cannot measure them directly but must calculate their values and fluxes from quantities that we can measure. For example, we have to formulate the energy as the sum of the various components that we can measure or calculate: $d(potential - kinetic + flow)/dt = net\ rate\ of\ energy\ flow\ in$. This is really the same as if we wrote conservation of mass as: $d(solid + liquid + vapor)/dt = net\ rate\ of\ mass\ flow\ in$. Similarly, we recognize that although we cannot measure momentum directly, it is defined as the product of mass times velocity, and it flows into and out of any flow region of interest in several ways, including pressure gradient and shear forces acting on flowing particles. The equations become simpler as assumptions are made. Usually, the equation obtained with the conservation of momentum principle is simpler than the equation obtained with the conservation of energy principle. The customized forms of the equations specific to each problem differ by the applying flow geometry and other operating conditions, and by the simplifying assumptions made.

4.4.2 Equation of continuity

The equation of continuity expresses mathematically [24,30,48,66,68] the conservation of matter—if matter flows away from a point, there must be a decrease in the quantity remaining. If the fluid density is ρ and velocity is $\mathbf{v}$, then the mass that flows in a unit time across a unit area of surface is the component of $\rho\mathbf{v}$ normal to the surface. The rate of change of mass in a volume V equals the net rate of mass flow in or out of that volume; mathematically

$$\frac{d}{dt}\int_V \rho dV \quad = \quad -\int_S \rho\mathbf{v}\cdot\hat{\mathbf{s}}dS, \tag{4.4}$$

Rate of mass accumulation	=	Rate of mass inflow (outflow)
(depletion) in volume		across surface bounding volume

where, the volume (V) is fixed in space. The RHS of this equation is the instantaneous rate of mass discharge from V. The minus sign is necessary because when $\mathbf{v}$ and the unit outward normal vector $\hat{\mathbf{s}}$ to the surface element of area dS point in the same direction so that their dot product is positive, i.e., if $\mathbf{v}$ is outward and $\mathbf{v}\cdot\hat{\mathbf{s}} > 0$, the mass within V *decreases*.

From this equation, we can obtain mathematically [77,86,89] the differential form of the continuity equation for incompressible (ρ = const) flow:

$$\nabla\cdot\mathbf{v}(x,y,z) = 0\ . \tag{4.5}$$

The velocity field of an incompressible fluid has zero divergence. The divergence of the velocity is scalar, and it measures the net volumetric flux passing out through the surface of an infinitesimal[2] volume surrounding a point within the flow field. When multiplied by ρ, it expresses mathematically the rate at which fluid mass is appearing ("source") or disappearing ("sink") at the point. Thus, Equation 4.5 embodies the principle of conservation of mass for an incompressible (ρ = constant) fluid. The terms "source" and "sink" convey a clear physical meaning because they are directly related to a *source* of water as from a spout, and a *sink* as the sink in a tub. The streamlines diverge from the source while they converge toward the sink—cf. Figure 14.1, on p. 738. This justifies the term "divergence," because this quantity simply gauges to what extent streamlines originate (in the case of a source) or end (in the case of a sink). Equation 4.5 holds for steady and unsteady flows, although it does not contain a time-derivative term as the momentum equation does. In other words, for any time instant, the time-dependent velocity vector must obey the "stationary" continuity equation. The absence of the pressure variable in Equation 4.5 precludes linking between velocity and pressure, making the Navier–Stokes system incompletely coupled.

[2]Infinitesimal means immeasurably small; i.e., less than any assignable quantity.

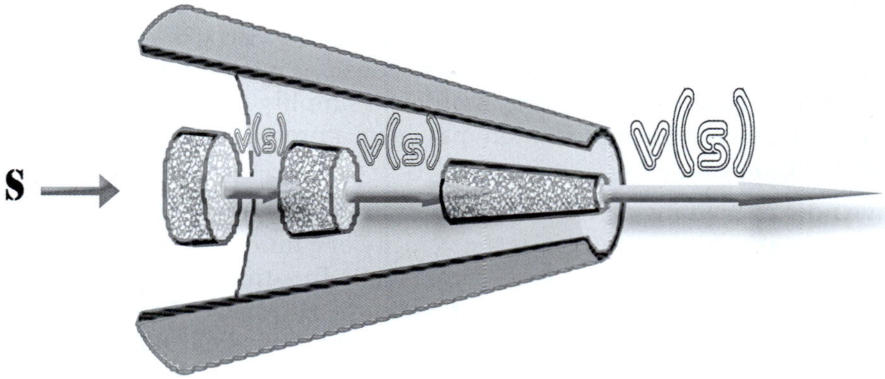

Figure 4.4: Convective change in streamwise velocity in a tapering flow field. A fluid particle accelerates as it moves successively through axial positions of narrower cross-section and higher velocity [$v(s)$]. This convective acceleration depends on the velocity gradient [$\partial v(s)/\partial s$] and on the velocity [$v(s)$], which determines how quickly the fluid moves through the spatial variations. (Modified from Bird, Murgo and Pasipoularides [6], with permission from the American Heart Association.)

4.4.3 Equation of motion

The equation of motion is, in its most fundamental form, a relation equating the rate of change of momentum of a selected fluid element and the sum of all forces acting on that fluid element. Newton's law [52] tells us how the velocity changes because of the applied forces. The mass of a fluid volume element times its acceleration, a, must be equal to the force on the element. Taking an element of unit volume, and writing the force per unit volume (force × density) as f, we have

$$\rho \cdot \mathbf{a} = \mathbf{f}. \tag{4.6}$$

The force density, f, is the sum of the following three terms, each having dimensions of force per unit volume:

i. The pressure gradient is a surface force acting normal (perpendicularly) to any surface element, and represents the pressure force per unit volume—as discussed in Section 2.7.1, on pp. 58 ff.

ii. The viscous force is a surface force per unit volume, and represents shearing (tangential) stresses.

iii. The body force is gravity, which acts with a force proportional to the fluid's mass density.

For now, we will ignore viscosity, making an approximation that describes an ideal fluid. An ideal fluid is one that is incompressible and has no viscosity. Ideal fluids do not actually exist, but it is at times advantageous to consider what would happen to an ideal fluid in a particular fluid flow problem, in order to simplify the analysis. It must be born in mind, however, that this simplification may have a profound impact, because it leaves out an essential fluid property.

We have now everything we need except for an expression for the acceleration. One might think, mistakenly, that if $\mathbf{v}(x,t)$ is the velocity of a fluid particle at some place in the fluid, the acceleration would be just $\partial\mathbf{v}/\partial t$; it is not. In a time-varying and nonuniform flow field, the velocity $\mathbf{v}(x,t)$ is a function of both time and space. The derivative $\partial\mathbf{v}/\partial t$ is the rate at which $\mathbf{v}(x,t)$ changes locally at a fixed point in the field. What we need is how the velocity changes for a flowing fluid particle because of changes in both time and its location within the field. We can express the total acceleration of the flowing fluid particle as [24,30,48,66,68,77,86,89]

$$\frac{D\mathbf{v}}{Dt} = \mathbf{a} = \frac{\partial\mathbf{v}}{\partial t} + \mathbf{v}\cdot\nabla\mathbf{v}, \tag{4.7}$$

$$\begin{aligned} Total\ acceleration &= Local + Convective\ acceleration, &(4.8)\\ (Lagrangian\ acceleration) &= (Eulerian\ acceleration). &(4.9)\end{aligned}$$

The differential operator $D/Dt = \partial/\partial t + \mathbf{v}\cdot\nabla$ is the *total*, or *material*, or *substantial* derivative—cf. Section 2.13 on pp. 65 f. The notation D/Dt emphasizes that the material time derivative includes both space and time partial derivatives, as is depicted in Figure 4.4, on p. 177. This follows from the Newton equation (Equation 4.6) in which the acceleration is the derivative of the velocity of a definite moving particle and not the derivative of the velocity at a fixed point. This change in velocity embodies two components:

a. there is the *local* change in velocity at the *instantaneous position* of the fluid particle, and

b. there is the change in velocity due to the *change in position* of the particle in the *nonuniform* flow field.

The material derivative is a scalar operator, so that the material derivative of a scalar variable, such as pressure, is a scalar quantity. The material derivative of a vector, such as velocity, is a vector.

Thus, there can be acceleration of fluid passing through a point even when the velocity at the given point is constant, i.e., even if the local (unsteady) acceleration, $\partial\mathbf{v}/\partial t$, is zero. It is possible then for the total acceleration, $D\mathbf{v}(x,t)/Dt$, not to be zero, because its second component, which represents the convective acceleration, is finite [53]. For steady flow, $[\partial\mathbf{v}/\partial t = 0]$, $\mathbf{v}$ is a static vector field and we can then speak of streamlines, which are the trajectories followed steadily by fluid particles. Streamlines connect velocity vectors in a flow field at a given instant, and are defined more precisely in Section 4.2.2 on pp. 171 ff. Trajectories are the actual paths taken by fluid particles.

If the flow is steady, i.e., the field of motion does not change in time, then fluid particles move along streamlines, and the streamlines coincide with particle trajectories. The streamlines can be found, in principle, by using the fact that the time derivative of the position of a fluid particle in a 2- or 3-D flow field is the velocity [27]. This approach leads to two or three, respectively, coupled differential equations for *x(t), y(t), and z(t),* [27, 62] which are difficult to solve. Fortunately, there are other, practical, ways of retrieving the streamlines. If the flow is unsteady, streamlines and flow particle trajectories may differ. Juxtaposed streamlines outline fluid layers, or laminae, in motion. When successive laminae are at distances of equal volumetric flux, the resulting picture gives information about regions of high and low velocities [27, 53, 62]. Closely spaced streamlines indicate relatively high linear velocities, and *vice versa*. Converging streamlines in a flow region imply convective acceleration [27, 53]; diverging streamlines, convective deceleration [58–60], as is illustrated in Figure 14.2, on p. 740.

4.4.4 Convective acceleration effects

It is most notable that the magnitude of the convective acceleration dictated by continuity considerations in 3-D flow situations is generally greatly enhanced relative to 2-D circumstances. Thus, for ideal flow in a cylindrical conduit, passage through a region along which there is a 50% reduction in diameter will not merely double but actually quadruple the velocity, since the latter is proportional to the volumetric flow rate and inversely proportional to the cross-sectional *area—viz.*, the *square* of the diameter. In the same context, if an ideal flow issues from an inlet into a typical expanding ventricular chamber, and is moving along streamlines that extend between the orifice and the inner surface area of the chamber, the convective deceleration will tend to be roughly proportional to the cube of the instantaneous radius of the chamber (cf. Fig. 4.5).

When we consider an outflow orifice, or sink, in the center of a chamber, we can readily visualize that the low pressure at the center "sucks" fluid toward it from the periphery. It is perhaps surprising that converting the sink into a central source, leaves the *convective* pressure field unchanged, with lower pressure at the center and rising toward the periphery (cf. Fig. 14.1, on p. 738). This is Bernoulli in action! To visualize this differently, concentrate attention on some fluid particles being driven outward, as shown in Figure 4.5. Since, by continuity, the outwardly directed speed decreases with streamwise distance from the central source, the particles slow down, and the acceleration that they experience is directed toward the center—*negative convective acceleration=convective deceleration*. A parallel argument shows that the acceleration of a particle on its way *toward* the sink from the periphery is again toward the center. Thus the convective acceleration is of the *same sense* in spite of the reversal of the velocity! This is an unexpected result, since intuitively one might have expected the acceleration to change sign too, when the sign of the velocity is changed.

The convective acceleration term represents the change of $\mathbf{v}(x, y, z, t)$ in the direction of the flow, and vanishes only when there is no variation of $\mathbf{v}$ along the stream. If all the fluid elements follow straight streamlines then this acceleration term is zero. Convective acceleration occurs where streamlines change direction. As an example, water

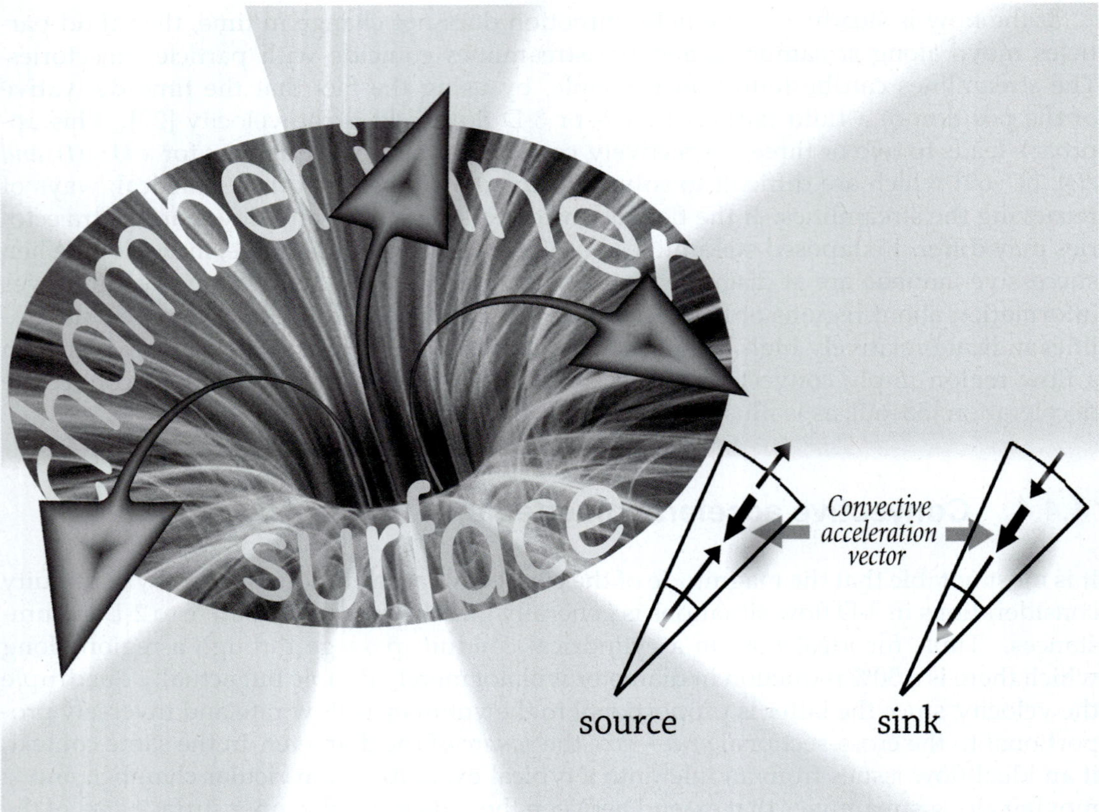

Figure 4.5: If an ideal flow issues from an orifice into an expanding spheroidal chamber, moving along streamlines extending between the orifice and the inner surface area of the chamber, the convective deceleration will tend to be proportional to the ratio of the instantaneous inner surface area of the chamber to that of the inlet. Lower right: the convective acceleration vector points in the *same sense* in spite of the reversal of the velocity of a particle on its way *toward* or *away* from the orifice.

flowing through a converging nozzle can be in steady state, so that at any location the velocity remains constant; however, the water accelerates convectively as the cross-section of the nozzle decreases and the streamlines converge. Of course, a fluid element can also accelerate by changing its speed along a straight streamline, if there is acting a local acceleration (cf. arterial pulse wave propagation). The concept of convective acceleration becomes clearer if we think of steady flow along circular streamlines, as we saw in Section 2.8, beginning on p. 59. Even though the rate of change of speed is then zero, there is a convective *centripetal* acceleration, which points toward the center of curvature of the streamline and is associated with the change in direction of the velocity of flow [59, 60].

Now we have all that we need for the equation of motion. Substituting the material acceleration from Equation 4.7 and expressing the force density as the sum of the pressure gradient and the gravitational force, we can make Equation 4.6 conform to the case of an inviscid and incompressible flow [27,30,53,68,77,89]:

$$\underbrace{\rho \times [\frac{\partial \mathbf{v}}{\partial t} + \mathbf{v} \cdot \nabla \mathbf{v}]}_{\substack{\text{Mass} \quad \text{Total} \\ \times \\ \text{density} \quad \text{acceleration}}} = \underbrace{-\nabla p + \rho\, \mathbf{g}}_{\substack{\text{Pressure} \quad \text{Gravitational} \\ + \\ \text{gradient} \quad \text{force density}}} . \tag{4.10}$$

This equation was derived by Leonhard Euler (see Section 3.5, on pp. 131 ff.) and is known as Euler's equation of hydrodynamics—one of a number of equations named after him in several areas of mathematics. The minus sign precedes the gradient, because mathematicians define the gradient function as pointing in the direction in which its argument (here, pressure) is *increasing*, whereas the net accelerating pressure force per unit volume points in the direction of *decreasing* pressure. Thus, the pressure gradient force is proportional and in opposite direction to the gradient of pressure, and at right angles to the isobaric pressure contours in the flow field (cf. Fig. 2.16, on p. 58).

We can similarly write the gravitational force per unit volume, which is acting *downward*, as minus a gradient as well, as $-\rho g \nabla \mathbf{h}$, where $\mathbf{h}$ represents *elevation* above a reference level, so that $\nabla \mathbf{h}$ is a vector of unit magnitude directed vertically upward, ρ is the constant mass density of the incompressible fluid, and g is the magnitude of the gravitational acceleration. We can then interpret $\rho g \mathbf{h}$ as potential energy per unit volume of the flowing medium.

Although the pressure acts as a normal stress at the surface bounding an element of fluid, it produces a resultant force on the element, which is the same as a body force per unit volume that is equal to $-\vec{\nabla} p$. This suggests that, under certain conditions, the pressure might play the part of a potential energy, as far as the total energy equation is concerned. In fact, for a static pressure field, the direct effect of the pressure on the energy of a fluid particle is the same as if the particle moved in a body-force field of potential energy p/ρ per unit mass. This representation of the effect of pressure embodies the work that can be done by it in accelerating a fluid particle, when there is conversion of pressure work into kinetic energy of flow.

4.4.5 Boundary conditions

The dynamic behavior of any flow, including intracardiac blood flows, is highly dependent on the environment where fluid motion takes place. The environment exerts its influence in terms of geometrical constraints to the fluid motion. Most flows of physiologic relevance "spend their life" in bounded domains, such as blood conduits and cardiac chambers, whose spatiotemporal geometry is quite complex and continuously changing. As with any physical system modeled in terms of partial differential equations (cf. Section 2.22 on pp. 99 ff.), the interaction between a physiologic flow and its bounding surfaces is mathematically prescribed by the type of boundary conditions that we apply on the flow-field governing equations, namely, the Euler or the soon to be considered Navier–Stokes equations. In principle, these boundary conditions pick-up specific solutions out of a whole class of possible ones, and ultimately dictate the large-scale features of the particular flow [24,30,48,66,68,77,86,89]. This forms the rationale behind the effort of trying to classify the types of flow patterns, which arise in connection with specific geometries, chosen in such a way as to obtain the best compromise between realism and simplification. The hope is, of course, that the flow regimes generated by more complex real-life geometries, can be sensibly analyzed, or understood, in terms of the "elementary" flow patterns associated with simpler but representative dynamic geometries.

4.4.6 Bernoulli's theorem for steady flow

We consider Euler's equation of motion in the limit of steady flow in which $\mathbf{v}(x, y, z)$ is a static vector field and the velocity picture remains unchanged in time. The fluid velocity is constant at all locations; the fluid is not static, but there is continuous fluid replacement along any trajectory by new fluid particles moving in exactly the same way. We can draw flow lines, or "streamlines," which are always tangent to the fluid velocity, as shown in Figure 4.6. For steady flow, they represent the paths of fluid elements. In unsteady flow, the streamline pattern changes in time and streamlines do not represent the path of a fluid particle at any instant.

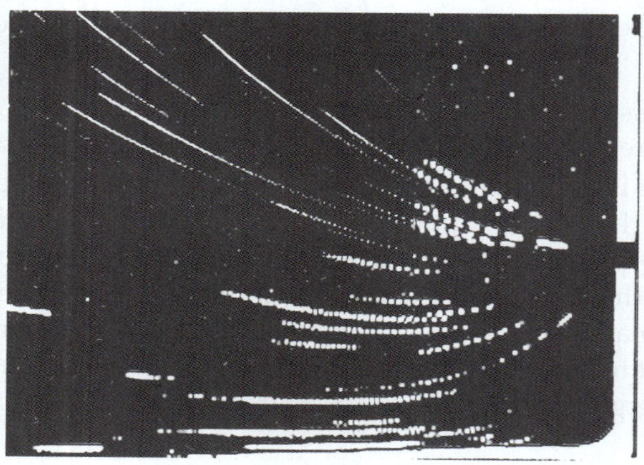

Figure 4.6: Chronophotography of streamlines upstream of an orifice, visualized by stroboscopic illumination of fine aluminum powder suspended in water. The method, introduced by Marey (1893) also allows estimation of magnitude and direction of local velocities. Convective acceleration occurs along the converging streamlines.

Taking the dot product with $\mathbf{v}$ of both sides of the Euler equation (Equation 4.10, on p. 181) for incompressible flow, and setting the time derivative (local acceleration) to zero for steady flow, we obtain [5,68,77,86,88]:

$$\mathbf{v} \cdot \nabla \left(p + \rho\, g\, h + \frac{\rho\, v^2}{2} \right) = constant. \tag{4.11}$$

For steady flow, when $\partial \mathbf{v}/\partial t = 0$, the material derivative D/Dt becomes $\mathbf{v} \cdot \nabla$, meaning that the quantity in parentheses does not change for a fluid particle for small successive displacements in the direction of its velocity, i.e., as it moves along a streamline. In other words, along a streamline the quantity in parentheses or "total head"—pressure plus the sum of the potential and kinetic energies per unit volume—maintains a constant value. This is *Bernoulli's theorem* for steady flow. For an irrotational and incompressible flow, Euler's equation of motion gives us directly the same result for the total head, namely

$$\left(p + \rho\, g\, h + \frac{\rho\, v^2}{2} \right) = constant \tag{4.12}$$

everywhere. Bernoulli's theorem is simply a statement of conservation of mechanical energy in the flow process. It shows that both gravitational potential energy and kinetic energy are interchangeable with pressure. Note that although Equations 4.11 and 4.12 have identical implications for the total head, the former equation applies along any particular streamline, irrespective of whether the flow is rotational or irrotational. The latter equation applies everywhere in the flow field but only for irrotational flow.

Moreover, the fluid's internal energy does not appear in either equation. This is because of the assumption of incompressibility. When ρ = constant, no $p\, dV$ (compression) work can be done on the fluid itself and, since inviscid flow is isentropic (no frictional dissipation of energy), the internal energy remains constant as well. Applied between two cross-sections of a streamtube in a steady flow field, the Bernoulli equation implies that the energy of the fluid contained between the two sections is constant. Any gains resulting from kinetic energy convected in at one cross-section and work done by pressure and gravity in accelerating a fluid particle are balanced exactly by complementary changes at the other.

When the pressure field is steady, the velocity field will usually be steady also, in which case the path of a fluid particle is a streamline. In terms of energy, we may say that, for steady motion of a frictionless fluid, the total energy per unit mass is constant for a fluid particle, provided this total includes not only the kinetic, but also the potential energies associated with the gravitational body-force field and the pressure field. In real life (as opposed to "ideal") flows, this total energy is not constant. Viscous stresses may act on the boundary of a fluid element and do work in accelerating it, so that its kinetic energy changes, and also in shearing it, so that its internal energy changes by internal friction. Moreover, the pressure field may be unsteady and the associated potential energy may change independently of changes in the other forms of energy of the element.

To see Bernoulli's formula in action, we will consider a few interesting situations to which it applies:

- **Blowing apart two sheets held close together:** If you hold two sheets of paper close together and try to blow them apart, they will, instead, come together! The

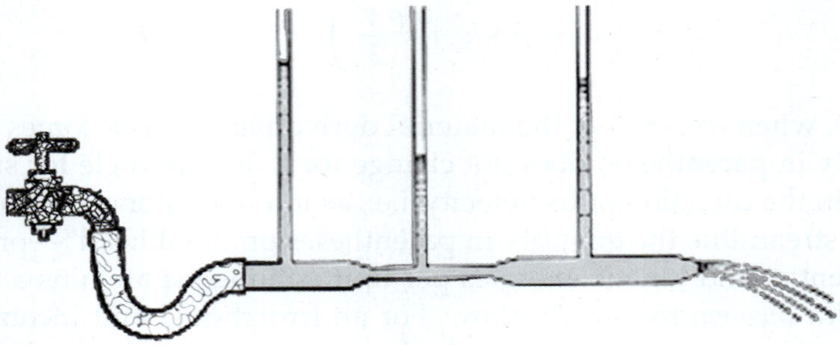

Figure 4.7: Flow through a horizontal pipe with small openings for manometric pressure measurement (pressure proportional to height of the water columns). The fluid in the manometric tubes is at rest and, consequently, the particles of the fluid in the openings are at rest too. Since pressure forces act equally in all directions, for the fluid particle in an opening to be at rest, the pressure produced by the water column in the corresponding manometer should equal the pressure p in the flowing fluid. If the diameter varies gradually, the pipe represents a stream tube in which the narrower the cross-section and greater the velocity, the smaller the pressure.

reason is that the air has a higher speed going through the constricted space between the sheets than it does outside. The pressure between the sheets is lower than the ambient (atmospheric) pressure and so they come together, rather than separating. The same mechanism underlies SAM, the systolic anterior motion of the mitral valve leaflets toward the interventricular septum, which is bulging into the left ventricular outflow tract, during ejection in hypertrophic obstructive cardiomyopathy [53].

- **Pipe with changing cross-section:** Consider now a horizontal pipe with changing cross-section, as shown in Figure 4.7, on p. 184, with water flowing in one end and out the other. Bernoulli's theorem says that the pressure is lower in the constricted area where the velocity is higher. We can demonstrate this effect by measuring pressure at the different cross-sections with small vertical columns of water attached to the pipe through holes small enough as not to disturb the flow. We measure pressure by the height of water in these columns. The pressure is lower at the constriction than on either side. If the area beyond the constriction comes back to the same value it had before the constriction, the pressure rises again. Bernoulli's formula anticipates that there should be complete *"pressure loss recovery"* and that pressure downstream of the constriction should be the same as it was upstream, but it actually is noticeably less. The reason that the prediction is wrong is the assumption of inviscid flow without any frictional effects. Despite the incomplete pressure loss recovery [53, 57], the pressure is definitely lower at the constriction (because of the increased speed) than on *either* side of it. To get the same amount of water through the narrower segment, the flow accelerates in going from the wide to the narrow part. The force that gives this acceleration comes from the drop in pressure in the *streamwise* direction.[3]

[3]In a Cartesian (x-, y-, z-) coordinate sense, x is defined as positive in the streamwise direction, i.e., downstream along the flow, y is defined as positive in the vertical direction, pointing upward, and z is taken

- **Flow up or down a pressure hill:** In a steady, incompressible flow, the average cross-sectional velocity can vary only if the flow cross-section changes. Flow in a hose is transformed to a swift jet by a *nozzle*. Bernoulli's equation shows that pressure must then be decreasing across the nozzle. Conversely, in a diffuser the flow cross-section *expands* and the flow is decelerated, in the streamwise direction. By Bernoulli's equation, the pressure must rise downstream, and this provides the force needed to *decelerate* the fluid. This interaction of geometry, velocity, and pressure is akin to the velocity of a bicycle increasing in rolling down a hill and decreasing in rolling up a hill. Effectively there is an analogous set of circumstances, as fluid flows up or down a *pressure hill*; down the pressure hill, the fluid speeds up and up the hill, it slows down. The pressure and velocity terms in Bernoulli's equation reflect that dynamic balance. An adverse pressure gradient can stop and even reverse the flow, causing flow separation from the wall, recirculation and eddying motions (see Section 4.9, on pp. 197 ff.). This is reminiscent of a roller coaster car that, having insufficient kinetic energy to overcome gravity and climb a hill, stops, *reverses* its motion and falls back instead.

- **Accessory external blood pump in fishes:** Consider now fish during fast swimming, a high-power activity. Operation of the Bernoulli mechanism should reduce the pressure at the widest part of their body, which contains the heart. Consequently, the faster a fish swims, the more the heart should expand, pulling in blood from both the front and the rear of the body, which are under higher external (ambient water) pressure. Fish and amphibians, contrary to mammals and birds, generally increase cardiac output by raising stroke volume rather than heart rate [71].

4.4.7 Vena contracta

At an abrupt contraction, the streamlines cannot follow the sudden change of geometry and hence they converge gradually from an upstream section of the wider conduit, as is indicated in Figure 4.8. However, immediately downstream of the junction of area contraction, the cross-sectional area of the stream tube attains its minimum, which is less than that of the narrower conduit. This section of the stream tube is known as vena contracta[4], and thereafter the stream widens again to fill the pipe. The flow of a fluid through an orifice similarly gives rise to a *vena contracta*. The fluid approaches the orifice with a relatively low velocity, passes through a zone of a convectively accelerated flow, and issues from the orifice as a contracted jet. If the orifice discharges liquid into the air, the orifice is said to have free discharge; if the orifice discharges under water, it is known as a submerged orifice. If the orifice is not too close to the bottom, sides, or water surface of the

in the cross-stream direction and is defined as positive increasing to the right when viewing downstream. Such a scheme is handy when considering flows that may change direction continuously along the stream. Thus, considering flow along a circular bend, the *streamwise* component is defined as positive following the flow along its circular path, as it changes direction.

[4] *L.*, literally, contracted vein.

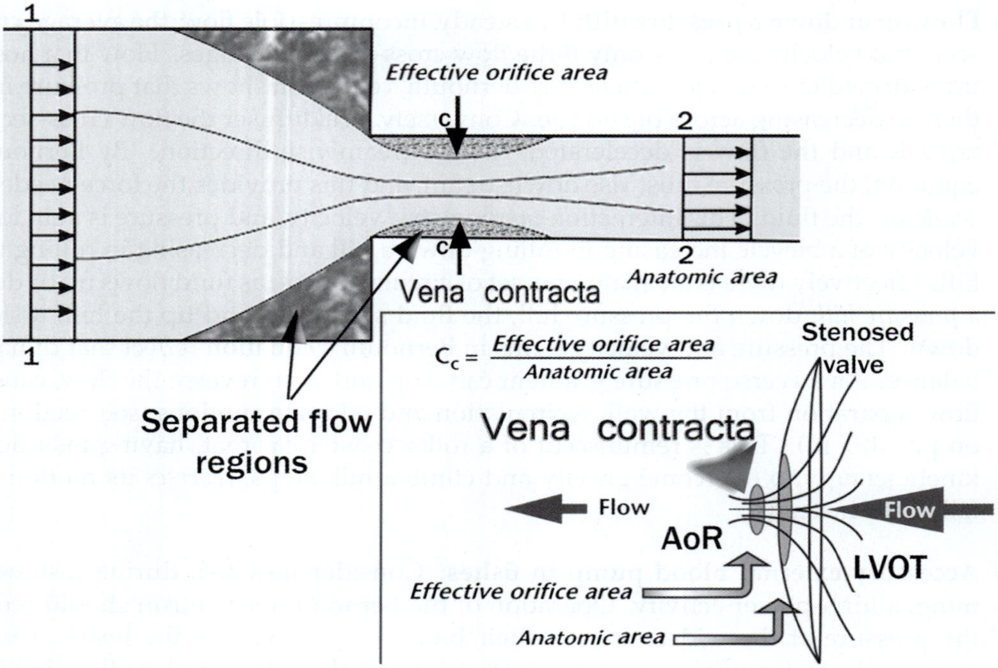

Figure 4.8: Looking at the streamlines across an abrupt contraction, you can see how they contract beyond it to a minimum streamtube when they all become parallel. This convergence is called the *vena contracta*; at this point, the velocity and pressure are uniform across the submerged jet. The ratio of the effective cross-sectional area of the *vena contracta* to the "anatomic" area of the conduit beyond the contraction is known as the contraction coefficient, C_c. AoR=aortic root; LVOT=left ventricular outflow tract.

container, the water particles approach the orifice along uniformly converging streamlines from all directions (see Fig. 4.6, on p. 182). Since these particles cannot abruptly change their direction of flow upon leaving the orifice, they cause the jet to contract. The station where contraction of the jet is maximal corresponds to the *vena contracta*. The velocity of flow in the converging portion of the stream tube, from station $1-1$ to station $c-c$ (*vena contracta*) in Figure 4.8, increases due to continuity and, accordingly, the pressure decreases in the streamwise direction, in compliance with Bernoulli's theorem (see Section 4.4.6, on pp. 182 ff.). In an accelerating flow, under a favorable pressure gradient, losses due to separation do not take place. But in a decelerating region of a flow field, e.g., from station $c-c$ to station $2-2$ in Figure 4.8, where the stream tube reexpands to fill the narrower conduit, flow separation ensues and minor losses take place, in a fashion similar to what occurs in case of a sudden geometrical enlargement. Hence, flow separation with recirculation ensues, and eddies are formed between the *vena contracta* $c-c$ and the downstream station $2-2$. Separation regions with recirculation and some flow energy losses are also observed just upstream of the contraction, where the streamlines diverge from the walls of the wider conduit, as is indicated in Figure 4.8.

4.5 A recapitulation: the unsteady Bernoulli equation

To recapitulate the preceding concepts on inertia-dominated flows, we consider now the dynamics of the intraventricular flow field during ejection [53,56,57]. This flow is governed by the Euler equation for the balance between the driving pressure force and the inertial forces associated with the acceleration of blood. Ejection velocity is a function of both time and position along a streamline. The total acceleration experienced by an intraventricular blood particle at any point in the ejection field is due to two effects:

1. the pulsatile acceleration applying *locally*, and
2. the interaction between the spatial gradient of the velocity in the ejecting chamber and the motion of the particle that is carrying it successively through regions of differing local velocities. This second effect gives rise to the *convective* acceleration component.

When spatial gradients in velocity exist (see Fig. 4.7, on p. 184), the local (unsteady) acceleration, $\partial \mathbf{v}/\partial t$, recorded by a stationary probe is in no sense a measure of the total acceleration, D/Dt, that a flowing blood particle experiences while moving past the probe.

Setting aside small hydrostatic effects, intraventricular ejection pressure (P) gradients must overcome only blood's inertia to its total acceleration, as shown in the hydrodynamic Euler equation (Equation 4.10, on p. 181). Its integration along the outflow axis, s, of the chamber yields the following form of the unsteady Bernoulli equation for the instantaneous pressure drop, in terms of the applying flow rate and its rate of change with time [53,56]:

$$\underbrace{\Delta P(s,t)}_{\substack{\text{Total}\\ \text{instantaneous}\\ \text{pressure drop}}} = \underbrace{A \cdot \frac{\partial Q_r}{\partial t} + B \cdot Q_r^2}_{\substack{\text{Local acceleration component} \; + \; \text{Convective acceleration component}}}. \tag{4.13}$$

Here, the subscript r signifies a reference position (for example, the aortic ring) for measurement of the volumetric flow rate, Q_r. The latter represents the flux (cf., Equation 2.20, on p. 57) of axial velocity through a flow cross-sectional area); its time derivative, $\partial Q_r/\partial t$ can be derived from the Q_r curve by time differentiation; A and B are integration coefficients depending both on the applying instantaneous ventricular chamber geometry and the density of blood.

We close this section with an application of an extension of the Bernoulli equation constant (see Equation 4.12, p. 183) to a uniform value along *any streamline* of an irrotational, laminar flow. We explore the flow with curved streamlines, as depicted in panel a. of Figure 4.9 on p. 188. We neglect hydrostatic pressure gradients and, to simplify the mathematical formalism, we consider *steady* irrotational flow, in which the pressure

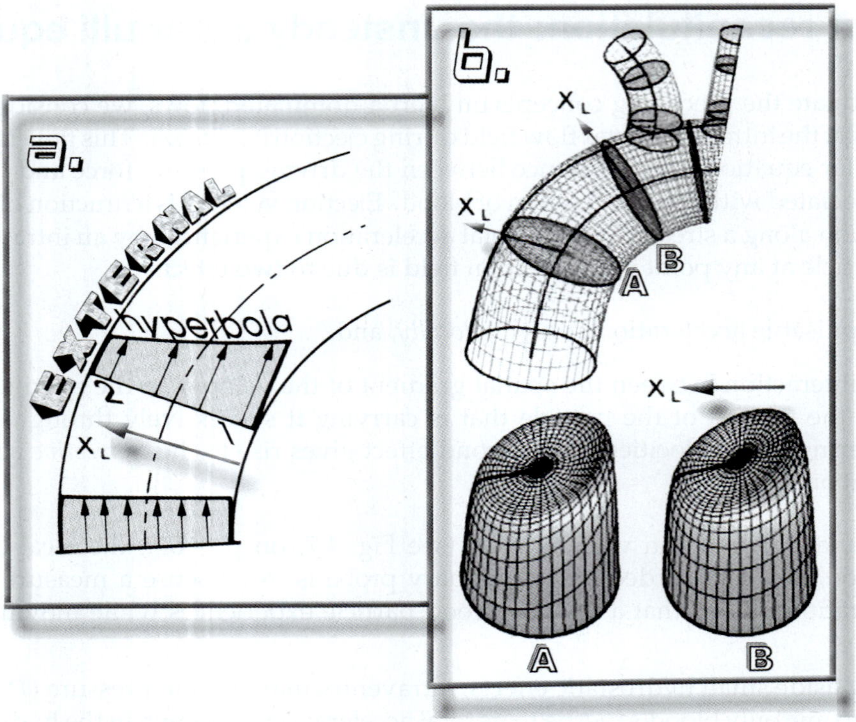

Figure 4.9: Panel a. Pictorial depiction of the modification of an initially uniform flat velocity profile as an irrotational, inertia dominated flow, negotiates the turn in a curved tube. Panel b. 3-D velocity profiles at maximum flow at two selected cross-sections in the ascending aorta, obtained in CFD simulations based on human geometric measurements using CAT scan imaging (this panel is based on data provided in [76]). The full time-dependent and 3-D Navier–Stokes equations were solved to obtain the flow field for an experimentally derived pulsatile flow waveform imposed at the aortic inlet to drive flow. Note the good agreement with the qualitative prediction for irrotational flow in panel a.—The direction of the local radius of curvature is indicated by arrows, X_L.

and velocity fields are independent of time, so that the *total* mechanical energy too can be taken to be independent of the time, t. If the velocity profile and pressure are uniformly distributed at the entrance to the region with curved streamlines, the sum of the (*instantaneous*, if the flow were *unsteady*) velocity and pressure heads will be a constant throughout the laminar flow field. This is a new statement, although its form may seem familiar from Section 4.4.6, on pp. 182 ff. There, for steady flows in general, the Bernoulli theorem (Equation 4.12, p. 183) stipulated that the sum of the velocity and pressure heads maintain a constant value along *any streamline*. For *irrotational* steady flows, however, it can be shown that the *same* constant value is taken on *all* streamlines.[5]

[5]This is a most important extension of the Bernoulli theorem; an extension which, itself, can be further extended to the case of *unsteady* irrotational flows.

As is developed later in Section 9.3, on p. 448 ff., the flow field under consideration here corresponds to a so-called *free vortex*. This implies that the distribution of the velocity across any specified diameter of the curved conduit and in the direction, X_L, of the local radii of curvature, conforms to a *hyperbola*—see panel a. of Figure 4.9. Let points 1 and 2 in Figure 4.9a. correspond to points 1 and 2 in the following Bernoulli equation:

$$p_1 + \frac{\rho v_1^2}{2} = p_2 + \frac{\rho v_2^2}{2} \, . \tag{4.14}$$

Allowing for the hyperbolic distribution of the velocities along the diameter under consideration, this equation can be rearranged to:

$$p_2 - p_1 = \frac{\rho C^2}{2}\left(\frac{1}{r_1^2} - \frac{1}{r_2^2}\right) , \tag{4.15}$$

where C is a constant, and r_1 and r_2 are the local radii of curvature for the two streamlines considered.

The above equation demonstrates that streamline curvature is the cause for the generation of pressure gradients and finite pressure differences *perpendicular* to the local flow direction. Pressure increases from the internal to the external border of the bend, while the local value of the axial velocity decreases. These *centripetal* gradients deflect the flow as needed, in order to negotiate the curve. This relation can be demonstrated in a familiar and striking way: if we make water rotate in a cup, the surface of the water rises toward the rim. The level of the surface is a *manometer*, indicating the pressure beneath. As the local radius of the curved flow path of the rotating water particles decreases, the required centripetal acceleration, and the local pressure gradient magnitude, increase strongly.

Apart from a nucleus surrounding the central axis of rotation (cf. Section 9.3, on pp. 448 ff.), the pressure is proportional to the reciprocal square of the local radius of curvature, generating a *hyperbolic* surface. This centrifugal pressure rise is also well-known for centrifuges.[6] Panel b. of Figure 4.9 shows that the aortic arch velocity profile at peak ejection flow conforms to a hyperbolic distribution, similar to the one just considered. These results, obtained in CFD simulations, have been corroborated by meticulous experimental measurements on dogs [19], and in human patients during open-heart surgery [75]. This hyperbolic profile, which characterizes irrotational flow in bends, is a consequence of the normally uniform distribution of the velocity at the aortic inlet, the irrotational character of the flow, and the curvature of the ascending aorta as it merges into the aortic arch.

[6] A centrifuge functions by swirling items in a liquid suspension around in circles and using their inertias to cause them to separate. The items have different densities (and other characteristics) that affect their trajectories as they revolve around the center of the centrifuge. Inertia tends to make them go straight, while the centripetal forces that are set-up in the centrifuge bend them inward. There is a tendency for the *denser* items to travel *straighter* than the less dense ones. Consequently, the denser items are found near the outside of the revolving container, where the centripetal force and the pressure are higher, while less dense items arrange themselves nearer the center of revolution. This distribution corresponds to a *manometric* indicator.

4.6 Viscosity

In the preceding sections, we discussed ideal fluid behavior, disregarding viscosity. We want to look at the behavior of real fluids, and therefore we have to include the effects of viscosity on the flow. To get some feel for the subject, we will describe qualitatively the actual flow behavior under various circumstances. The laws of motion of a fluid are contained in the Navier–Stokes equation for conservation of momentum in flow processes:

$$\underbrace{\rho \times [\frac{\partial \mathbf{v}}{\partial t} + \mathbf{v} \cdot \nabla \mathbf{v}]}_{\substack{\text{Mass density} \times \text{Total acceleration}}} = \underbrace{-\nabla p + \rho\,\mathbf{g} + \mathbf{f}_{\text{visc}}}_{\substack{\text{Pressure gradient} + \text{Gravitational force density} + \text{Viscous force per unit volume}}} . \tag{4.16}$$

In the Euler equation (Equation 4.10, on p. 181), we had neglected all viscous effects that correspond to the viscous force per unit volume, $\mathbf{f}_{visc}$. However, in ordinary fluids, it is almost never true that we can neglect the internal friction that we call viscosity. Most of the interesting things that happen come from it, in one way or another. For example, in Section 3.6 (pp. 133 ff.), we saw that the great physician-physicist Hermann von Helmholtz showed that in inviscid flow the circulation never changes. If there is none to start out with, there will never be any. Yet, circulation in ordinary fluids is an everyday occurrence.

We begin with an important experimental fact. In inviscid flows, there is no reason not to permit the fluid to have a velocity tangent to a solid boundary; only the normal component must be zero relative to the (impermeable) surface. There is no account of the possibility that there might be a shear force between the liquid and the solid. In fact, however, it turns out that in all circumstances checked experimentally [18,48,67,68,77,86, 88], the velocity of a fluid relative to the surface is exactly zero at the surface of a solid. Thus, the blade of a fan will collect a thin layer of dust that is still there after the fan has been churning up the air. Why doesn't the air blow off the dust? In spite of the fact that the fan blade is moving at high speed through the air, the speed of the air relative to the fan blade goes to zero right at its surface. So the very smallest dust particles are not disturbed. This is also the reason why you cannot blow fine pieces of dust from the surface of a table; only large pieces, which *stick up* into the breeze.

Navier and Stokes built upon the work of Cauchy to expand the scope of the Euler theory [24], in order to agree with the experimental fact that in all ordinary fluids, the molecules next to a solid surface have zero velocity relative to the surface. Characteristically, a liquid yields to any applied shearing stress, no matter how small [68,77,86,88]. In static situations, there are no shear stresses, but before reaching hydrostatic equilibrium, there must be shear forces present.

Tangential, "shear," forces reflect momentum transfer in a direction *perpendicular* to the motion of a fluid particle by diffusion of "faster" molecules into a region with "slower" molecules, and *vice versa*. Both these effects are characterized by the dynamic viscosity coefficient. Viscosity describes these shear forces which always exist in a moving fluid. Suppose that we have two parallel plane surfaces separated by a distance d in some viscous fluid like water, and keep the lower one stationary while the upper one moves parallel to it at some slow speed, u_0.

If you measure the magnitude of the force (F) keeping the upper plate moving, you will find that, at steady-state, F is proportional to the area (A) of the plates and to u_0/d. So the magnitude of the shear stress, F/A, is proportional to the velocity gradient, or rate of shear strain [68,77,86,88,89]:

$$\frac{F}{A} = \mu \cdot \frac{u_0}{d}. \quad (4.17)$$

The proportionality constant, μ, is the coefficient of dynamic viscosity, sometimes referred to as *molecular* viscosity [15].

Fluids for which the linear relation between shear stress and strain rate holds accurately are called *Newtonian*. Sir Isaac Newton (1642–1727) gave the definition of what we now call a Newtonian fluid with the following *Hypothesis:* "The resistance, arising from the want of lubricity in the parts of a fluid is, *ceteris paribus*, proportional to the velocity with which the parts of the fluid are separated from each other."[7] Particular forms of this equation applying in different instruments, e.g., the Brookfield viscometer, are used in viscosity determinations.

Viscous shear tends to remove any local anomalies in velocity, to give more uniform velocity gradients throughout the flow field. It is a diffusive process, in that the rate of momentum transfer by viscous shear is proportional to the momentum gradient, which for incompressible flow equals the velocity gradient, and to the momentum diffusivity, or dynamic viscosity. It is similar to solute diffusion and heat conduction. The energy needed for deforming a viscous fluid *completely* dissipates in the process; no energy for further deformation persists, and the deformation cannot be recovered. The presence of the viscous term, which involves second order derivatives, in the Navier–Stokes equations accounts for the irreversibility of real flows, including the intracardiac flow fields.

4.7 Viscous flow

Equation 4.17 can be generalized to show that the shear stress components are proportional to the spatial derivatives of the velocity components [24,30], and the proportionality coefficient, μ, is the ordinary dynamic viscosity, or coefficient of shear viscosity. Now we need an expression for the viscous force per unit volume, $\mathbf{f}_{visc}$, so that we may substitute it in Equation 4.16 in order to get the explicit equation of motion for a real, viscous, fluid. In the incompressible case [13,18,29,30,39,48,68],

$$\mathbf{f}_{visc} = \mu\nabla^2\mathbf{v}. \quad (4.18)$$

[7] In Book II of the *Principia*, Section IX [52].

This is the most frequently used approximation and we substitute it directly into Equation 4.16.

Viscous effects involve the momentum diffusivity, μ, and the Laplacian, ∇^2, of the velocity, v, in the Navier–Stokes equation. The Laplacian, which was introduced in Section 2.11, on pp. 62 f., measures the difference between the local and average values of a flow-field variable (in this instance, v) in an infinitesimal[8] neighborhood of a point within the field. In combination with the momentum diffusivity, it expresses the action of molecular agitation in resisting relative motion and smoothing away any velocity (momentum) gradients by the process of diffusion. The contribution of the viscous force per unit volume is non-negative, showing that a unidirectional transfer of energy to the internal energy of the fluid occurs in viscous flow, as is to be expected from the frictional character of viscous action. Generally, in pressure driven flows, the component in the streamwise direction of the Laplacian term in the Navier–Stokes equation represents the rate of mechanical energy loss per unit volume of flow along the flow path. In its effect on the fluid, this dissipation of flow-sustaining mechanical energy, by the action of viscosity, is equivalent to an irreversible addition of heat.

The mathematically inclined readers should note that first order derivatives appearing in the Euler equation (Equation 4.10 on p. 181), imply non-sheared, energy-conserving (hyperbolic) motion which is *reversible* because any initial condition can be recovered from an evolved one by merely inverting the sign of the speed. On the other hand, second order derivatives appearing in the Navier–Stokes equations (see Equations 4.16, on p. 190, and 4.18 above) imply energy and momentum dissipating diffusive (parabolic) motion in which the initial state can only be regained from an evolved one by inverting the sign of the diffusion coefficient, namely the dynamic viscosity. While negative speeds are perfectly acceptable in the physical world, negative momentum diffusion is not, because it must lead to gradient *intensification* rather than smoothing as is required by the second law of thermodynamics.

Notwithstanding the preceding general remark, it is worth mentioning that *negative* "effective" transport coefficients can show up during fluid motion under special conditions, as a result of local instabilities leading to self-organized spatiotemporal flow patterns [34, 47, 80].[9] The negative local entropy generation in a flow field is not in conflict with the second law of thermodynamics [91]. The law asserts that the entropy is always increasing in an isolated system, but a flow region is an open system that exchanges mass and energy with its neighboring regions. The given flow region may obtain a negative entropy flux from its neighbors, so that its entropy can be locally reduced while entropy in the neighboring regions increases. The total flow system should still have a positive entropy generation.

---

[8] *Infinitesimal* signifies immeasurably small and capable of having values approaching zero as a limit.

[9] In a more familiar context for readers with biomedical backgrounds, chemotaxis is used for intercellular signaling and is a spatiotemporal process involving cell aggregation, induced by a chemical substance that is denoted as a "chemoattractant." The chemoattractant diffuses in the cell-containing medium and attracts other cells by forcing them to move in the *uphill* direction of its gradient [1]. In the present context, by moving toward the site of increasing cell concentration, they are exhibiting a negative "effective" diffusion coefficient.

4.7.1 Brief remark on irreversibility

Ideal, inviscid flows are reversible, while real, viscous fluid flows are not. Consider the separated wake behind a cylinder (see Fig. 9.8, on p. 459) in a viscous fluid flow, at elevated Reynolds numbers; it will always appear *behind* the cylinder with respect to the oncoming flow direction. Thus, the viscous wake will change dramatically, "jumping" from one side of the cylinder to the other, as the flow direction changes. On the other hand, reversing the velocity at a "final" time and reversing the direction of time, will not change an ideal flow around the cylinder. We conclude that the possibility of a *reversible* zero drag ideal flow solution cannot be realized and that, instead, an irreversible turbulent wake solution with nonzero drag develops. In other words, the exact potential solution for "creeping-flow" with zero drag—*form drag*—at a vanishingly low Reynolds number is unstable; in its stead, at finite Reynolds numbers, turbulent wake solutions with nonzero drag develop.

Mathematically, the Euler momentum equation governs the evolution of *reversible* flow and involves only first order space derivatives. *Irreversible* viscous flow requires second order space derivatives, which are present in the Laplacian of the velocity that appears in the Navier–Stokes momentum equation. First order spatial derivatives imply convective motion, which is reversible because any initial condition can be recovered from an evolved one, by merely reversing the sign of the flow velocity. On the other hand, second order spatial derivatives imply diffusive motion in which the initial state might be regained from an evolved one only by inverting the sign of the diffusion coefficient, i.e., of the momentum diffusivity, $\nu\,(=\frac{\mu}{\rho})$,[10] in the momentum equation. Now, while negative speeds are perfectly acceptable in the physical world, negative momentum diffusion is not; as it was already noted above, it would lead to a spontaneous velocity gradient *enhancement*, rather than the smoothing required by an energy dissipative process.

4.8 Dimensions and units

In fluid dynamics—including intracardiac flows—observation and measurement are the basis of our insights. We are concerned with relationships of physical quantities, and these physical quantities have dimensions: length (L), mass (M), and time (T). These fundamental dimensions permit the expression of various other dimensions or physical quantities, such as area, volume, speed, and pressure. Whenever we write an equation that expresses a physical law, each term in the equation must have the same dimension or combination of dimensions. For example, the instantaneous intracardiac blood volume may be computed by

$$Total\ intracardiac\ blood\ volume = V_{RA} + V_{RV} + V_{LA} + V_{LV},$$

where, V_{RA}, V_{RV}, V_{LA}, and V_{LV} stand for the component volumes of the right atrium, the right ventricle, the left atrium, and the left ventricle, respectively. Each term has the

[10] Depending on the context, the term "momentum diffusivity" can be used for both the dynamic (μ) and the kinematic (ν) viscosities.

dimension of volume, L^3, and the equation is dimensionally homogeneous. Dimensional homogeneity is a general requirement in a single equation.

Similarly, neglecting gravitational effects, we may wish to write an equation for the mechanical forces per unit volume, acting on intraventricular blood during ejection. Such forces are inertial forces per unit volume (*INER*) that are associated with blood's mass density and oppose its acceleration, the pressure force per unit volume (*PG*) that is exerted by the contracting chamber's walls and corresponds to the accelerating pressure gradient, and the retarding viscous force per unit volume (*VIS*) that is associated with blood's dynamic viscosity.

$$INER = PG - VIS. \tag{4.19}$$

The dimensions of these forces must naturally be identical. Newton's second law states that force equals mass times acceleration, with the acceleration given as the rate at which speed changes over time. Since the dimension of speed is L/T, acceleration is characterized by L/T^2. In turn, the dimension of force is ML/T^2 or MLT^{-2}; therefore, the dimension of force per unit volume contains only mass, length, and time: $ML^{-2}T^{-2}$.

Returning to the summation of the forces resisting the forward motion of intraventricular blood, we must now make sure that all terms in the equation have the dimension of force per unit volume, $ML^{-2}T^{-2}$, to assure dimensional homogeneity. Also, note that these steps must be taken prior to deciding which system of units to use. The dimensional approach clarifies the physics of the problem in the selection of the relevant parameters. Most physical quantities that are needed in fluid dynamics can be derived from the three basic dimensions of mechanics given above. Once we have verified the dimensions of a given expression or equation, we can append units in order to provide numerical results. The choice of units is immaterial, but the same unit—e.g., the metric unit of force per unit volume, the newton per meter cubed (N/m^3)—must be used for each component of the equation.

Dimensional analysis, the basis of modeling physical phenomena, is a major contribution to both applied and basic science made by engineers. How do we go about dimensional analysis? For a given problem we attempt to identify the relevant physical parameters that govern the particular flow involved. We ask ourselves what conditions must be met to assure that different flows exhibit the same dynamic behavior. Obviously they must be geometrically similar, that is, they must look alike. Streamline patterns for them, marked by dye or smoke, must also look alike, with the only difference being a difference in scale. Such flows are called *similar*. We then search for a *similarity parameter*, i.e., a combination of variables expressing length, speed, and fluid properties that assures the dynamic similarity of the different flows. To ensure dynamic similarity, it is stipulated that the ratio of the forces acting on some fluid element in the different flow fields must be identical.

For the most part, important conceptions in science tend to be used metaphorically, as a basis for reasoning analogically. The result of such reasoning is the revelation of *patterns*. Geometry, similarity, and pattern are at the core of science. The geometric similarity of two figures when they differ from each other only in their scale of length (similar triangles, etc.) has been recognized since antiquity. More generally, mathematical similarity is defined for a category of systems represented by the same closed equations, with the same initial conditions and exterior forces acting upon each system, and with boundaries of the same form, i.e., geometrically similar.

With this in mind, the equations and conditions can be expressed in dimensionless terms, which are thus independent of the units of measurement. Lengths, times, and masses will then be related to the lengths, times, and reference masses characteristic of the phenomena under study. The flow-governing equations will then have the same terms without dimensions and with dimensionless coefficients, or similarity parameters, such as the Reynolds number, which take different numerical values for the different similar systems, according to their own properties. When the similarity parameters are equal, the equations of the systems are identical and their solutions are the same, when expressed in dimensionless terms. This condition is sufficient for these systems to be dynamically similar. There is, in such cases, an identity of relation that unites such homologous terms as forces and fluid particle trajectories. The solution, be it analytical or experimental, for *one* case is valid for *all* cases *similar* to it.

Similarity methods have proved useful in obtaining analytical solutions to flow problems that involve laminar boundary layers (see the next section), where the complexity of the flow processes precludes direct solution of the exact governing equations. The basic idea in the construction of these solutions is the observation that from one location x to another, the axial velocity, u, profile looks *similar* (hence, the term *similarity solutions*). Figure 4.10, on p. 196, shows that, although more and more fluid is held back near the wall as x increases, the longitudinal velocity is always $u = 0$ at the wall and $u = U_\infty$ sufficiently far from it. Imagine that two profiles $u_1(y)$ and $u_2(y)$ were drawn using the master profile depicted in Figure 4.10; like the elastic band of a swimsuit, this master profile can be stretched appropriately at x_1, and x_2, so as to fit the local velocity profiles. Mathematically, the stretching of a master profile amounts to writing

$$\frac{u}{U_\infty} = function(\eta), \tag{4.20}$$

where, the *similarity variable*, η, is proportional to y and the proportionality factor depends on x. The unknown function, which accounts for the shape of the master profile can be determined by solving the flow-governing equations cast in the language of the similarity transformation of Equation 4.20.

Similarity considerations permit predicting the behavior of phenomena belonging to a given category on the basis of the known behavior of another member of the same category. In such a case, it is sufficient to describe the phenomenon quantitatively as a function of similarity parameters. The dimensions of a physical quantity are associated with symbols, such as M, L, T, which represent mass, length and time, and each raised to rational powers. For instance, the dimension of the physical quantity, speed, is distance/time (L/T) and the dimension of a force is $mass \cdot distance/time^2$, or ML/T^2. Dimensional symbols, such as L, form a group: there is an identity, $L^0 = 1$; there is an inverse to L, which is $1/L$, and L raised to any rational power, p, is a member of the group, having an inverse of $1/L$ raised to the power p. The operation of the group is multiplication, with the usual

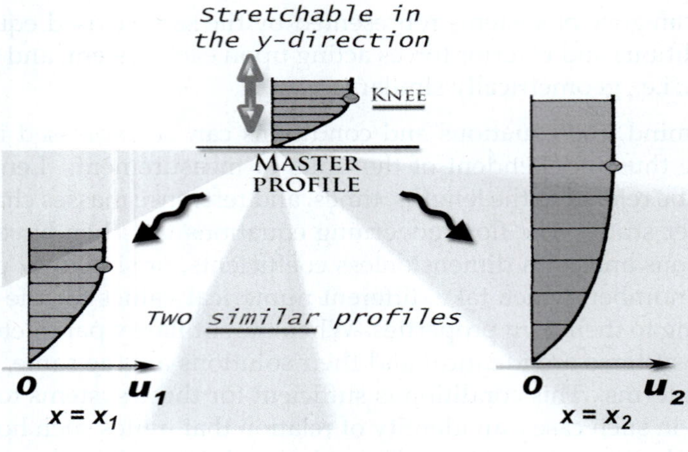

Figure 4.10: Construction of similar developing velocity profiles.

rules for handling exponents. In a very simple application, dimensional analysis may be used to check the correctness of physical equations: the two sides of any equation must be dimensionally homogeneous.[11]

Inertial forces in fluid flows depend on mass density—fluid mass per unit volume—and always act on a fluid particle. Viscous forces depend on viscosity, which gives rise to shear forces between neighboring fluid layers flowing at different velocities; usually, they counteract the inertial forces. Depending on the relative values of these two forces, fluid motion may be dominated by viscous or inertial effects. The inertial forces are given by Newton's second law of motion ($force = mass \times acceleration$). With a characteristic length, L, pertaining to the scale of the flow, and recalling the definition of density, ρ , we find ρL^3 for the mass of a fluid element taken as a cube. The acceleration, dU/dt, is given by the change of flow velocity U over the length of the element and takes place during the time interval L/U. Consequently, we find for the acceleration $U/(L/U) = U^2/L$. Finally, by this line of reasoning, we have for the inertial forces acting on an element of fluid: $\rho L^3 U^2/L \approx \rho L^2 U^2$, where the symbol "$\approx$," which represents a proportionality, may be used to connote "approximately." Next, we express the viscous force exerted by internal frictional shear, i.e., the shearing force per unit area linked to the dynamic viscosity, μ. For our fluid element, this area is accounted for by L^2 and, making use of Equation 4.17, on p. 191, we have for the viscous shear force: $L^2 \mu U/L \approx \mu LU$. Finally, from the two preceding expressions we establish the *ratio* of inertial, F_{in}, to viscous, F_{vis}, forces acting on the fluid element:

$$\frac{F_{in}}{F_{vis}} \approx \frac{\rho L^2 U^2}{\mu LU} = \frac{\rho LU}{\mu}. \tag{4.21}$$

[11]A corollary of this requirement is that scalar arguments to exponential, logarithmic and trigonometric functions must be dimensionless numbers. The logarithm of 3 *kg* is undefined, but the logarithm of 3 is approximately 0.477. This is attributable to the requirement for the Taylor expansion of these functions to be dimensionally homogeneous, which requires the square of the argument to be of the same dimension as the argument itself; for scalar arguments, this means that the argument must be dimensionless.

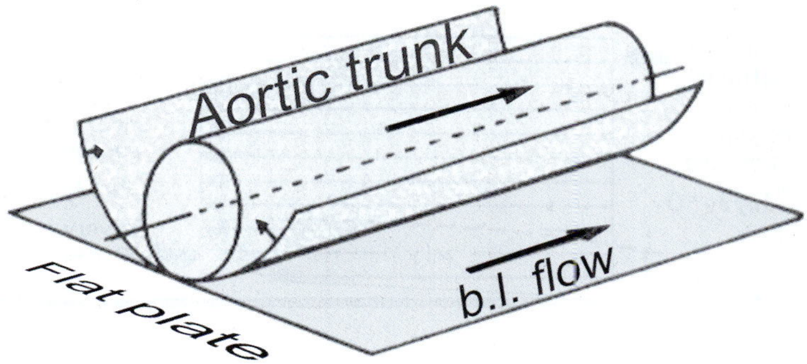

Figure 4.11: Rolling up a sheet into a tubular form shows why, provided the ratio of the boundary layer thickness to diameter (δ/D) is small, we may apply boundary layer analyses of flows over flat plates to physiologically important flow fields; b.l. = boundary layer.

The derived ratio of inertial to viscous forces is the Reynolds number [28], which will be discussed further in Section 4.11, on pp. 205 ff. Here, suffice it to note that high, or low, Reynolds numbers imply that the flow field is dominated by inertial, or viscous, effects, respectively. Intracardiac and large central vessel blood flows are generally characterized by high Reynolds numbers, implying that they are inertia-dominated.

Within a single category of flow systems—subject to the same forces, derived from similar initial conditions, and exhibiting the same geometric forms—it is not necessary to recast the governing equations in dimensionless form, in order to find the similarity parameters. They may be obtained by dimensional analysis and similarity theory, which provide empirical methods of finding universal relationships between variables that are made dimensionless by using appropriate scaling factors. In fact, all physical laws should be expressible in a form that is independent of the units of measurement employed.

Dimensional analysis is often applied in fluid dynamics as a conceptual tool, to understand physical situations involving a mix of different kinds of physical quantities. The method consists of choosing quantities that govern the category of the flow system under consideration and of determining their combinations that are dimensionless, i.e., that constitute similarity parameters. Experiments with models and on prototypes then permit predicting the behavior of all systems for which the given conditions of similarity are satisfied. Finally, empirical trials have to be performed.

4.9 Boundary layer and flow separation

The boundary layer is a layer near a wall in which we find concentrated cross-stream velocity gradients (see Fig. 4.12, on p. 198) and vorticity, i.e., rotation of fluid particles about their own axes as they flow. Boundary layers form because there can be no slippage between two adjacent fluid layers. Thus, there is a smooth variation in velocity from the boundary to the central core or mainstream, which can be moving at a relatively high

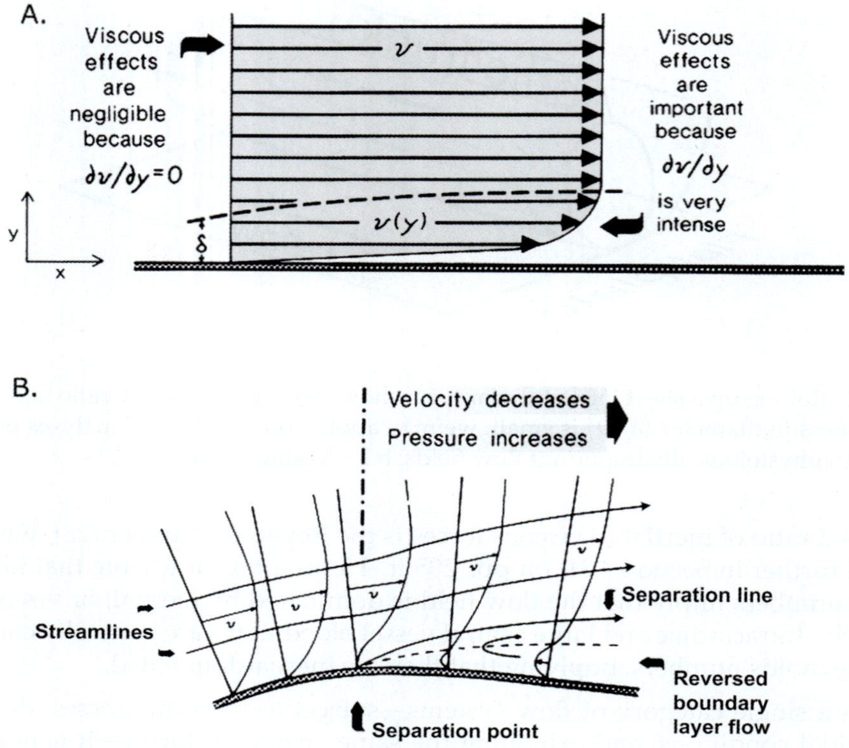

Figure 4.12: Pictorial sketches of a hydrodynamic boundary layer and flow separation. A. Across the thickness (δ) of the laminar boundary layer, the streamwise velocity (v) decreases from its mainstream value to zero relative to the wall to satisfy the "no slip" condition. Note how different the blunt core profile is from the parabolic profile of the familiar viscous Poiseuille flow. $\partial v/\partial y$ = cross-stream velocity gradient. B. A decrease in linear velocity along the flow is associated with an increase in pressure. The resulting adverse pressure gradient can arrest and even reverse the flow within the boundary layer, whereas its high streamwise momentum enables forward flow to persist in the quasi-inviscid main core. (Reproduced from Pasipoularides [53] by permission of the American College of Cardiology.)

speed past the wall surface. Outside the boundary layer, the flow moves with a blunt velocity profile and is effectively inviscid or "frictionless," because frictional forces require cross-stream velocity gradients to come into action (cf. Equation 4.17, on p. 191).

Of special interest for us is that intraventricular and central aortic ejection flows actually have *thin* boundary layers ("shear layers") and blunt, undeveloped velocity profiles.[12] It is this thinness of the ejection flow boundary layers, relative to the vascular

[12] Fully developed flows approach a certain invariant state in terms of appropriate variables, such as the velocity profile across a flow cross-section, or the axial pressure gradient. In sharp contrast to this behavior, unsteady, developing flows have continuously changing velocity profiles and other dynamic characteristics.

diameter, that allows us to apply engineering theory developed for boundary layer flow over flat plates to, e.g., ejection flow through the ventricular outflow tracts and adjacent great vessel trunks—this is explained visually in the topologic diagrams of Figure 4.11, on p. 197. There are many situations where pressure increases, rather than decreases, as one moves downstream in the flow. In most cases where this occurs the velocity, and hence the kinetic energy of the flow, are rapidly diminishing and, as predicted by Bernoulli's equation (Equation 4.12, on p. 183), kinetic energy is being converted to increasing pressure.

In Figure 4.12B., the cross-section available for the flow is increasing in the downstream direction. Since the total flow is unchanging, the average velocity in the larger cross-sections must be lower. Thus, the kinetic energy decreases and this brings about an increase in pressure (not all of the mechanical energy is recoverable since some is lost by viscous dissipation to heat, which is also occurring).

What is the consequence of this "adverse pressure gradient" on boundary layer behavior? This situation is illustrated in Figure 4.12B. Since both pressure force and wall shear force act in the direction opposite to the flow, the momentum of the flow diminishes. Moreover, the effect of the net force is greatest on the fluid near the wall, which has been slowing at a more rapid rate by the higher velocity gradient and consequent higher shear force. It then has less inertia and adjusts (changes its velocity) even more rapidly in response to the net force. Thus, the fluid near the wall eventually slows down to zero velocity and, since it experiences a net pressure force in the direction opposite to the flow, it actually begins to flow in that reverse direction. The result is the flow pattern shown on the right in Figure 4.12B.; the velocity is:

- zero at the wall,
- negative for some distance from the wall,
- then zero again and increasingly positive until it reaches the mainstream velocity.

In the cardiovascular system, separation can occur at any change in cross-sectional area or flow direction if the Reynolds number is high—e.g., cf. Figure 14.15, on p. 770. The point where the velocity gradient at the wall becomes zero is the "point of separation." Beyond that point, the locus of zero velocity points appears to be a pseudo-wall with its own boundary layer separated from the real wall by the newly created backflow region. Invariably, boundary layer separation comes with the formation of vortices.

In many situations, the conditions that bring about flow separation exist over only a short section of the flow path. Beyond that section, the boundary layer will reattach and boundary layer growth will continue in a normal manner. The region between the point of separation and the point of reattachment is the "separated flow" region. We have directed our attention at the components of velocity in the axial direction in this region, but it is evident that to conserve mass, fluid must flow into the back-flow zone of the separated region toward the downstream end and out of the back-flow zone near the upstream end. Thus, the overall motion is in a more or less elongated recirculating vortex pattern. For regions of flow separation, only numerical solutions can be obtained, by solving the incompressible Navier–Stokes equations using methods of computational fluid dynamics (CFD).

Separated flows may have open or closed recirculating streamlines. Unlike plain 2-D flows which have a single separation point with a downstream set of closed streamlines forming a recirculating "flow bubble," 3-D flows reveal more intricate recirculating patterns, with streamlines which do not form a closed recirculating bubble. With open streamlines, fresh upstream fluid enters and leaves the separation bubble simultaneously. Here, entering fluid particles leave the recirculating region sooner or later, depending on the applying flow rate and geometry. The velocities in such vortices are lower than the mainstream velocity owing to the viscous effects induced by the nearby wall, and any fluid captured in the vortex may recirculate for a long time.

Streamlining is useful for steady flows but it is unclear how a recirculation region should be defined in unsteady flows, since a region that appears to be recirculating (closed streamlines) at an instantaneous time-slice might actually be moving with the flow (open streamlines) at another instant of time. Examining streamlines to understand transient flows can be misleading, because any given streamline may change long before a particle could follow it. Streaklines need to be used.[13]

A useful concept in analyzing separation bubble flows is that of the so-called *residence time*. Essentially, one computes the amount of time that the fluid has been in or "resident" within the bubble. Residence time zero is defined as the time when the observation starts. On a closed streamline, the residence time is infinite. Open recirculating regions, on the other hand, mean that fresh upstream fluid continuously enters and leaves the separation bubble, simultaneously.

Most of the fluid within a separation region stays within that region for a considerable amount of time. Thus, a common feature of a separation region is that the residence time of the fluid within is much larger than that of the surrounding fluid. A residence time isosurface can consequently be used to distinguish this region. Therefore, residence time can easily produce the separation surface, for either steady-state or transient simulations in 2- or 3-D flows.

4.9.1 Unsteadiness and entrance length effects

All internal flows will have a certain *"entrance length."* Entrance, or entry, length is simply defined for steady flow as the length from the entrance of a conduit up to such a point that the flow is fully developed. In the case of unsteady flows, the dynamics are complicated by the fact that not only distance-related requirements pertain for the flow development, but available-time constraints, as well. A fully developed flow is one in which the boundary layer thickness is not changing, as it moves further downstream. In pulsatile, inertia-dominated flows in large central arteries, a fully developed Poiseuille flow profile does not come into being, because there is not enough time for such a profile

[13] Streaklines describe the motion of an injected massless material at a specific point in a flow field over a certain time interval. Therefore, any individual streakline is a family of such consecutive line segments.

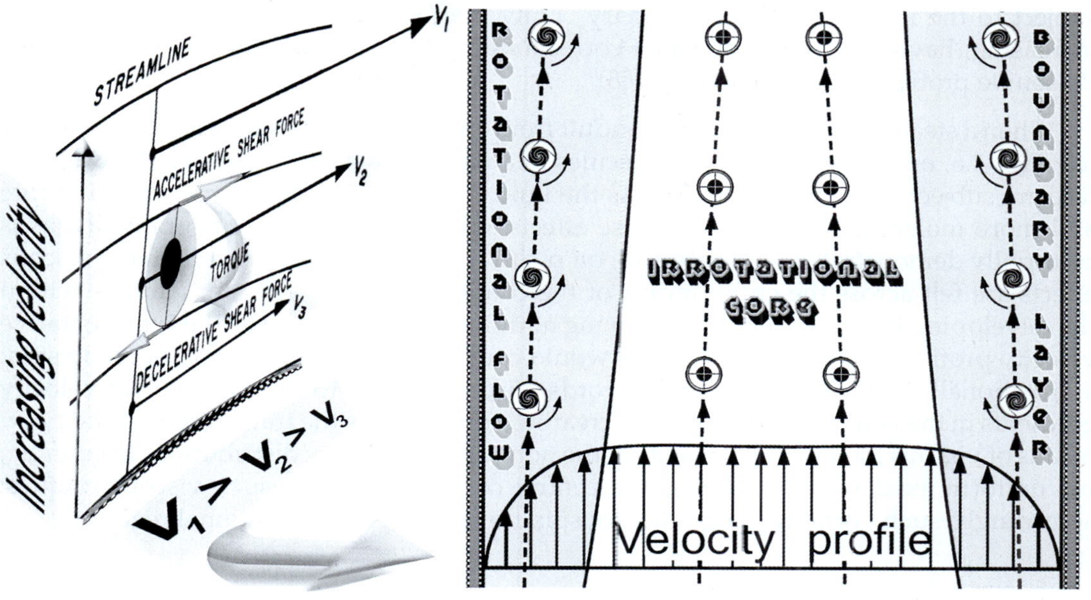

Figure 4.13: Because adjacent laminae within the developing boundary layer are moving at different velocities, viscous shear torques set the envisaged "vorticity gauges" spinning, as shown in the left sketch: this is rotational flow. The uniform axial velocities across the central core do not exert any net viscous torque; vorticity gauges are not spinning: this is the irrotational flow region.

to develop over any time interval within the cycle, before the pressure gradient reverses direction.

Assume that, at the onset of ejection, an accelerating—thus, *negative*—pressure gradient (-Π) is impressed along each proximal arterial outflow trunk, in the form of an abstracted step function in time, which is maintained until the velocity in each vessel reaches its observed maximum. Setting aside, temporarily, considerations of geometric "entrance effects," if such a negative pressure gradient (-Π) is steadily maintained long enough, the velocity tends to its corresponding maximum asymptotic value, which in a straight, cylindrical tube is the parabolic Poiseuille profile Purely from considerations relating to flow time-course, the developing velocity profiles are flat and akin to those applying in steady flow at the entrance region. In other words, at the very onset of ejection, due to the operation of -Π initially the blood in the corresponding proximal segment, virtually *in toto*, has forward acceleration Π/ρ. However, as the velocity is augmented, the restraining influence of the surrounding walls spreads further into the flowing blood, increasing the thickness of the boundary layer; *pari-passu* the central core, whose behavior is approximately ideal, and whose velocity is increasing with time (t) as $\Pi t/\rho$, where ρ is blood's density, is becoming narrower as t increases. It can be shown mathematically [55] that it would take a -Π application time of order $\rho R^2/\mu$, where μ is blood's dynamic viscosity and R the radius, for all or most of the parts of the flowing blood to become subject to the influence of the boundary. Only then will the velocity at the axis cease increasing, having attained the value corresponding to the "fully developed" parabolic Poiseuille profile (see Fig. 4.2, on p. 168).

When a steady flow first enters a conduit from an orifice on the side of a large container (cf. Fig. 4.6, on p. 182), only the molecules in a narrow "sleeve" closest to the wall surface are subjected to viscous effects. As the fluid moves further down the conduit, more and more molecules begin to feel these effects and the sleeve thickens gradually, as is pictorially demonstrated in Figure 4.13, on p. 201, until after one entry length the viscous effects are felt across the entire radius of the conduit. Because adjacent laminae within the developing boundary layer are moving at different velocities—see the representative velocity profile—viscous shear torques would cause spherical "vorticity gauges" to spin: a "rotational" flow regime. In other words, viscosity leads to the existence of velocity gradients in the neighborhood of walls, creating vorticity. It is the transport of vorticity, by means of viscous forces, which results in the nonuniform velocity distribution. In contrast, the uniform axial velocities across the central core do not exert such viscous torques; accordingly, such vorticity gauges do not spin there: this is the irrotational region.

4.10 Impulsive flows

Figure 4.14, on p. 203, demonstrates the impulsive mode of generation of intraventricular ejection pressure gradients and flows in humans, even under basal resting conditions in a supine posture at cardiac catheterization. Although transient, a forceful ejection pressure gradient can generate a high peak ejection velocity, because it delivers a strong impulse (see Equation 4.1, on p. 171) to intraventricular blood. The key phenomenon to be understood, in analyzing impulsively generated pulsatile ejection waveforms, is the global response of a fluid to a force field that is both impulsive and spatially localized. The fluid dynamic foundations are adaptations of classical arguments on fluid momentum and Kelvin's hydrodynamic impulse, which can be found in the incompressible flow theory part of the classic treatise of Lamb [40]. Depending on the nature (compressibility) of the fluid and its boundary conditions (e.g., depending on the presence of elastic or rigid boundaries) the response of the fluid will differ in detail, but it will always involve the propagation of pressure waves to large distances away from the forcing site and, therefore, it will involve the motion of fluid particles at large distances, as well. Methods for recording intracardiac hemodynamic events by solid-state multisensor (micromanometric and velocimetric) catheters have been developed [6,12,41,51,53,54,56,60,78,79].

The simultaneous pressure signals presented in Figure 4.14 were obtained [56] using a left heart catheter with two laterally mounted, solid-state micromanometers (Mikro-Tip™, Millar Instruments, Houston, Texas). The spacing between the two pressure sensors along the mildly curved catheter is 5 *cm* (see Fig. 5.7, on p. 244, and Section 5.2, on pp. 243 ff.); thus, the measured gradients represent pressure drops across a distance of approximately 5 *cm*, along the outflow-tract axis. The intravascular electromagnetic velocity probe was at the same location as the proximal (downstream) micromanometer.

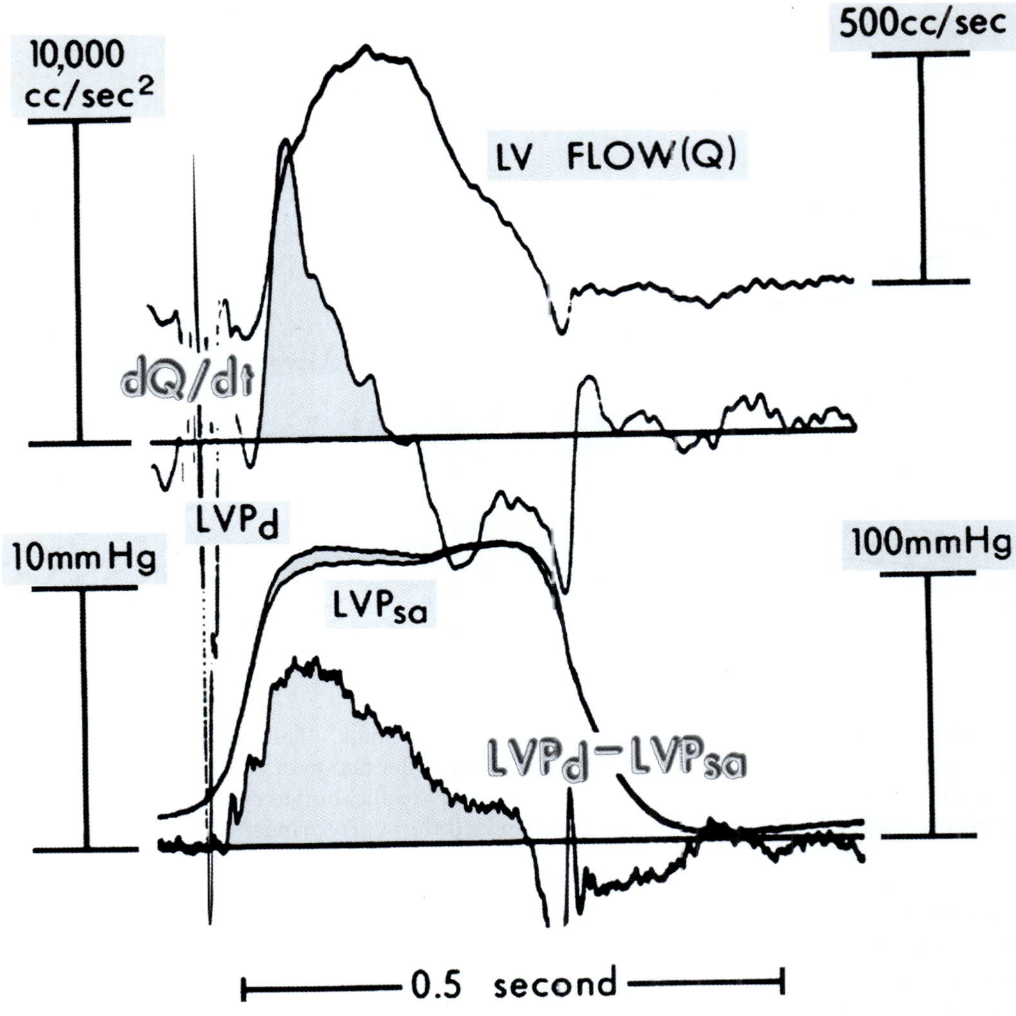

Figure 4.14: Left ventricular (LV) fluid dynamics in humans, obtained with a double pressure plus velocity microsensor catheter, during diagnostic cardiac catheterization. Deep (LVP_d) and subaortic (LVP_{sa}) left ventricular pressures are displayed at the bottom, with their instantaneous difference on an enlarged scale. The associated left ventricular outflow acceleration (dQ/dt) is shown in the middle and the volumetric outflow signal (Q) from the aortic ring, at the top. (Reproduced, slightly modified, from Pasipoularides et al. [56], with permission from the American Heart Association.)

The impulsive and transient nature of the flow implies that viscous frictional effects are negligible in the ventricular ejection field. They generally confine themselves only to very thin, unsteady and undeveloped, boundary layers [27, 53, 54, 56]. In effect, thin *vortex sheets* cover the endocardial surfaces in the outflow tract and the endothelial lining of the proximal large arterial outflow trunks. Across these sheets, the tangential velocity

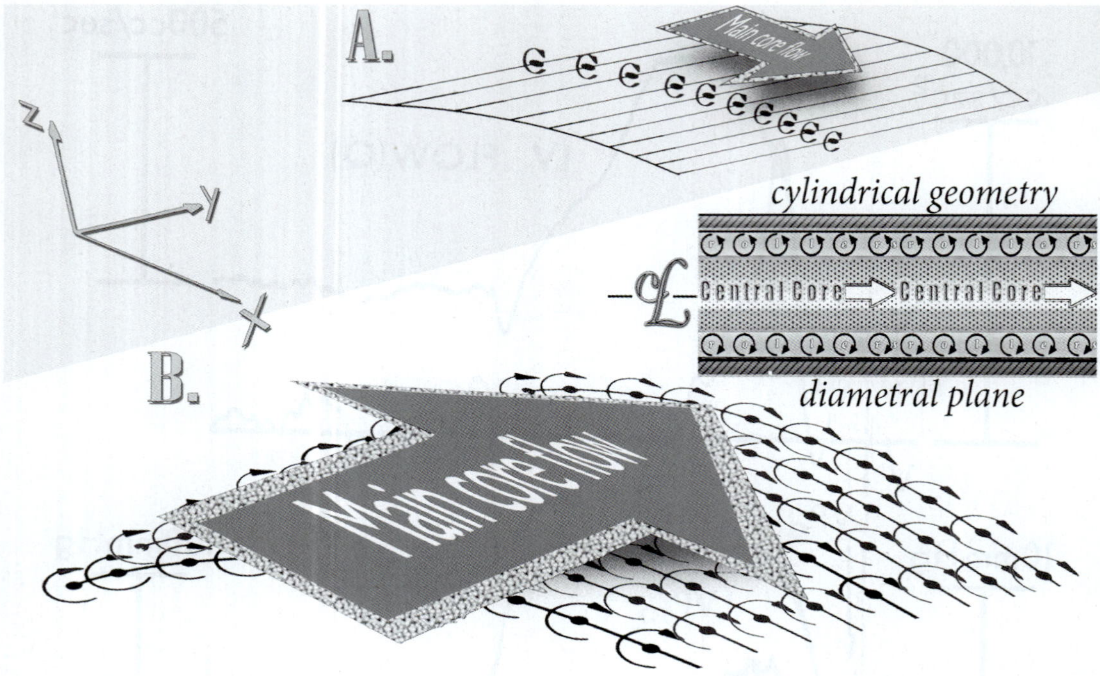

Figure 4.15: Side-by-side vortex filaments form a vortex sheet. The main flow is irrotational, "sliding" bodily by the bounding surface thanks to the roller action of the *vortex sheets* in the thin boundary layer. A.: global concept; B.: magnified. Inset: application to cylindrical geometry, with a central core sliding bodily over a series of juxtaposed thin vortex rings. c/L = centerline.

changes from zero to its instantaneous main core value. To visualize the concept of a vortex sheet, imagine an infinite number of straight infinitesimally thin vortices, or "vortex filaments," arranged side by side. These side-by-side vortex filaments form such a thin vortex sheet, as is shown schematically in Figure 4.15. The transverse vortices act as spinning fluid rollers that minimize friction at the fluid-solid interface.

Laminae of flowing blood within the boundary layer undergo intense shear, because viscous tangential stresses can be sufficient to yield the necessary retardation to zero at the wall only if the gradient of velocity is very steep (see Fig. 4.12, on p. 198) [53], due to the low viscosity of blood. The main core is irrotational, "slipping" bodily by the walls, as it were, thanks to the roller action of the vortex sheets in the thin boundary layer. Therefore, the dynamics of the main, or "core," flow outside the boundary layer conform closely to the inviscid fluid approximation. Without the action of viscosity to diffuse vorticity away from the wall, thus causing the boundary layer to thicken with the passage of time, the effect of the "no-slip" condition would not be discernible. The roller action of the vortex sheet would remain right at the wall and grow infinitely intense, while affecting the velocity in only an infinitely thin region. The flow would then be akin to a plug flow, having an unrestrained uniform stream velocity perpendicular to the boundary.

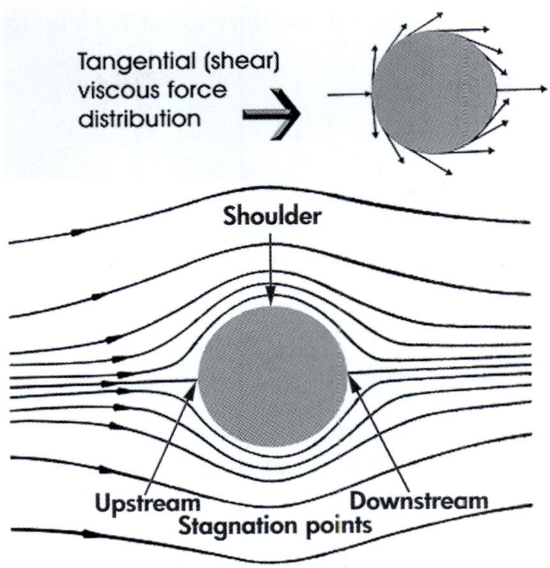

Figure 4.16: Streamline map constructed for 2-D flow across a long circular cylinder at a very low (<1) Reynolds number. Note the symmetries of the pattern: top-bottom, front-rear halves; only the top shoulder is pointed out. The viscous fluid exerts tangential viscous forces, whose distribution is depicted schematically in the inset.

4.11 Reynolds number

We will now examine interesting changes in the character of fluid flow that come about because of the viscosity term in the Navier–Stokes equations [48, 66, 68]. We will consider the flow of a fluid past a cylinder, as in Figure 4.16. The physical problem is this: we would like the solution for the flow of an incompressible, viscous fluid, past a long cylinder of diameter D. The flow should be given by the equations of motion and continuity, with the boundary conditions that the velocity at large distances is some constant velocity, say U (parallel to the x-axis), and at the surface of the cylinder it is zero. That specifies completely the mathematical problem, as we have already seen in Section 4.8, on pp. 193 ff. The specifically applying boundary conditions determine a unique solution of the general flow-governing (Navier–Stokes) equations, which is applicable to the particular flow at hand [86, 89]. In effect, knowing the velocity at the boundaries of the fluid allows determination of the appropriate velocity distribution for the specific flow geometry and fluid that has known constant mass density and dynamic viscosity.

In fact, if you look back at Equations 4.16 and 4.18, you see that there are two different parameters of the problem in the Navier–Stokes equations, μ and ρ, in addition to the two parameters in the boundary conditions, D and U. The viscosity and density appear only in ν $(=\mu/\rho)$, the kinematic viscosity or "momentum diffusivity." All these parameters which determine the appropriate flow-field dynamics condense into one factor, the

Reynolds number, Re [53,77,86,88], whose derivation is to be found in Section 4.8, on pp. 193 ff.:

$$Re = \frac{\rho\, U\, D}{\mu} = \frac{U\, D}{\nu}. \tag{4.22}$$

What this all means is that if, for example, we obtain the flow field for one velocity U_1 and a certain cylinder diameter D_1, and then ask about the flow for a different diameter D_2 and a different fluid, the flow will be the same for that velocity, U_2, which gives the *same* Reynolds number, that is, when

$$Re_1 = \frac{\rho_1\, U_1\, D_1}{\mu_1} = \frac{\rho_2\, U_2\, D_2}{\mu_2} = Re_2. \tag{4.23}$$

For any two situations that have the same geometry and Reynolds number, the flows will look the same, irrespective of the individual magnitudes of the particular parameters, which appear in the Reynolds number.

4.11.1 The role of the Reynolds criterion

A flow remains stably laminar until the Reynolds number exceeds a critical value Re_{cr}, and at $Re > Re_{\mathrm{cr}}$ it can become turbulent [48,66,68,77,86,88,89]. Re provides a criterion of the relative magnitudes of characteristic values of inertial forces and viscous forces. Inertial forces lead to the formation of marked inhomogeneities in the flow in response to any disturbance.[14] Viscous forces, on the other hand, level out any velocity differences in closely spaced points, i.e., they smooth out small inhomogeneities. It follows then that

- At small Re, when viscosity forces dominate over inertial forces, there can be no sharp inhomogeneities in the flow, i.e., hydrodynamic fields change smoothly, and the flow is laminar. Reynolds attributed to viscosity the role of the *discipline* of an army troop; conversely, the *larger* the troop (viz. L) and the more *rapid* the movement (viz. U), the higher the likelihood of disorder.
- At high Re, the smoothing action of viscosity forces proves to be weak, and random fluctuations—small-scale, sharp inhomogeneities—arise in the flow; i.e., the flow becomes more or less turbulent, depending on the applying Re.

These considerations explain the role and meaning of the Reynolds criterion. It should be noted that the character of the boundary layer changes as it develops along a bounding surface (see Fig. 4.17, on p. 207). Generally starting out as a laminar flow, the boundary layer thickens and undergoes transition to turbulent flow exhibiting a thoroughly disorganized appearance and fluctuating rapidly in space and time, with considerable fluid element inter-mixing; it then continues to develop along the surface, possibly separating from the surface under certain conditions, to form large eddies and regions of recirculating flow (see Section 4.12, on pp. 208 ff.)

[14] A disturbance is simply that which displaces, that which moves a flow field from one regime to another.

4.11.2 The limit of zero viscosity

The high Re flow regimes that we have considered in the previous sections are nothing like the corresponding inviscid flow solutions. This is, at first sight, surprising because Re is proportional to $1/\mu$, so $\mu \longrightarrow 0$, should be equivalent to $Re \longrightarrow \infty$. Yet, as we approach $Re \approx \infty$, the flow described by the (vectorial) Navier–Stokes equation (Equation 4.16, on p. 190) gives a completely different solution from the one corresponding to $\mu = 0$, as is illustrated in Figure 4.17. Note that the RHS of the Navier–Stokes equation is $1/Re$ times a

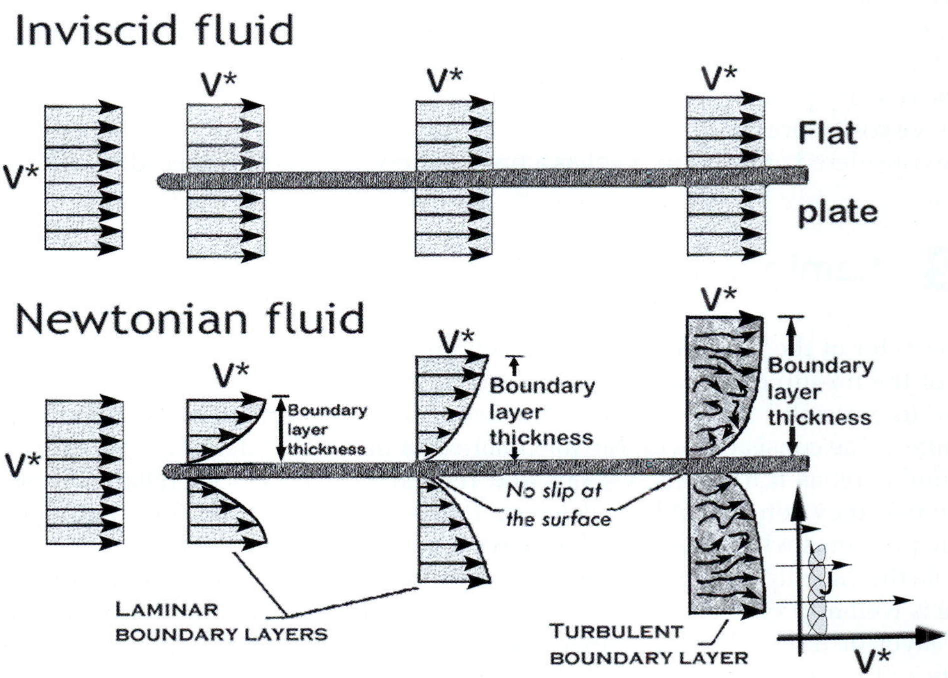

Figure 4.17: Inviscid flow along a flat plate compared to laminar and turbulent boundary layer flow with the same free-stream velocity. Velocity remains constant, at V*, in the free stream, and is zero at the surface, but the velocity gradient varies with downstream distance. In the turbulent boundary layer, the major mechanism of momentum transfer to the surface is through turbulent eddies, which is much more efficient than viscous molecular transfer. Accordingly, the turbulent boundary layer grows thicker at a faster rate than the laminar. Considering the competition between eddy motions and viscosity in the turbulent boundary layer, viscosity tries to return the mean flow to the parabolic laminar profile, while the eddying motions try to redistribute momentum uniformly across the boundary layer. The inset on the lower right depicts the direction of momentum (J) transport—perpendicular to V*—within the large-scale flow by the small-scale eddying motions (see discussion in text).

second derivative (Laplacian of the velocity; see discussion of Equation 4.18, on pp. 191 f.). This is the highest order derivative in the equation. What happens is that, although $1/Re$

may be very small, there are very steep variations of velocity and vorticity in the space near the flow boundaries [61, 67, 73, 74, 77]. These rapid variations compensate for the small coefficient, and the product does not go to zero with increasing Reynolds number.

The turbulent boundary layer flow can be considered as a state held in balance by the competing actions of eddies and viscosity. The eddying motions bring high-momentum fluid toward the wall, while viscosity tries to damp these motions, especially near the wall. The limiting cases resulting from these effects are sketched on Figure 4.17 and correspond to the flat-profile inviscid flow and the parabolic-profile laminar boundary layer solutions. If the viscous effects acted alone, we would revert to laminar flow with a *parabolic* velocity profile. If the eddying motions were allowed to act alone, unchecked by viscosity or walls, we would have a perfect redistribution of momentum, leaving a *uniform* velocity profile. The latter state can never practically be obtained, since there is always viscosity present, but it is *conceptually* useful. The state of turbulence can therefore be considered at a simple level as a balance between the two preceding effects.

4.12 Laminar and turbulent boundary layers

The character of the fluid flow near a solid boundary changes significantly by the imposition of the no-slip condition [82]. The no-slip condition makes the tangential velocity relative to any solid surface of flow contact go to zero, instead of allowing it to have any finite value consistent with the formulation of inviscid ("ideal," or "potential") flow. Real fluids are, as it happens, viscous and remain at zero velocity relative to any solid surface that they contact. What relevance, then, does the inviscid formulation have for realistic problems where the fluid does have a non-vanishing coefficient of viscosity? To reconcile the "no-slip" boundary condition with the fact that away from the boundary the regime is well-approximated by potential flow, Prandtl invented the "boundary layer"—a thin layer of fluid where the tangential velocity climbs rapidly from zero to the full velocity of the main stream [61, 67, 88]. Boundary layers typically thicken downstream [68, 73, 74, 77].

In presence of an adverse pressure gradient, as with increasing flow cross-section in the downstream direction, the low-velocity and low-inertia flow within the boundary layer may actually reverse its motion and form recirculating eddies, while the main central core flow may maintain its forward direction thanks to its higher forward velocity and inertia (see Fig. 14.1 on p. 738). It turns out that, except for the thin boundary layer and the recirculating eddy region, the flow may be very nearly given by the inviscid theory, i.e., by the equations of Euler (Equation 4.10, on p. 181) and Bernoulli (Equation 4.12, on p. 183). In the boundary layer, the inviscid approximation breaks down completely. In the case of flow around immersed obstacles, generation of vorticity can occur in the boundary layer and eddies can be swept back in the flow to become part of the wake behind the obstacle, a phenomenon that fascinated Leonardo da Vinci as we saw in Chapter 3.

The boundary layer does not have a constant fractional size, but thickens with increasing distance in the flow (or "streamwise") direction [61, 67, 73, 74, 77, 88]. We can relate the factors controlling this growth process in an approximate way by considering that the transverse diffusion length, δ, is of the order of $\sqrt{(\nu t)}$, where ν is the kinematic viscosity and t is the time of diffusion. Consider a flat plate parallel to an oncoming laminar stream of a viscous fluid of momentum diffusivity ν (see p. 205) and free-stream velocity V^*, as is illustrated in Figure 4.17. At a distance l from the leading edge, the time during which the viscous effects have diffused from the boundary is approximately $t \approx l/V^*$. Thus,

$$\delta/l \sim \sqrt{(\nu t)}\,/l = \sqrt{(\nu\,/\,lV^*)} = \sqrt{(1/Re)}. \tag{4.24}$$

This relationship is valid only at high Reynolds numbers, where $\delta/l \ll 1$. Because of this Re dependence, increasing the flow velocity decreases the boundary-layer thickness at any given station along the plate [67, 74]. The physical explanation for this is staightforward: with a higher mainstream velocity, at any position along the plate the boundary layer thickness gets smaller because it has had less time to grow.

4.12.1 Favorable and adverse gradient effects on the boundary layer

In most flow situations, there are regions of decreasing pressure and regions of increasing pressure in the flow direction [18, 29, 67, 74]. We first examine the effects of pressure decreasing downstream (a favorable gradient) [53]. The boundary layer upstream of the contracting portion of a flow may be thicker than the boundary layer emerging from it. How is this possible in view of the preceding paragraph? At each successive small increment in distance along the contracting portion of the flow, the pressure gradient causes a corresponding increase of the main flow velocity, by Bernoulli's equation. In the outer portions of the boundary layer, where changes in shear stress are small, the velocity increases by nearly the same amount. It is only very near the wall that the incremental increase in velocity is much lower than that of the free stream. The fluid velocity at the wall remains zero because of the no-slip condition. It is as if the edge of the boundary layer gets dynamically *squeezed toward the wall* along the contraction. The integrated effect is to further enhance the already high shear stress near the wall and decrease the lateral distance required for the velocity to attain, asymptotically, the mainstream value.

With a slightly diverging flow path, the free-stream static pressure increases in the flow direction, and this imposes on the boundary layer a positive (or unfavorable) pressure gradient. If the unfavorable gradient is small, then the increasing pressure in the free stream causes a corresponding decrease in the mainstream velocity, increases the boundary layer thickness, and decreases the wall shear stress, without causing flow separation. The positive pressure gradient decreases the velocity in the boundary layer and the mainstream by almost the same amount except very near the wall. Near the wall, the size of the decrement dwindles rapidly and must be zero at the wall. A major consequence of this process is to decrease the velocity gradient and shear stress at the wall. The deceleration of the flow imposed by a positive pressure gradient cannot be very large or sustained too long by the boundary layer fluid without the wall shear stress going to zero, followed downstream by local flow reversal [59, 60] (see also p. 208). For high Reynolds number, considerable shear develops in the boundary layer. The shear rate increases with increasing distance downstream, and if Re is large enough, a point may come where the boundary layer becomes unstable even without an adverse pressure gradient. A transition to turbulence can then take place, and a line of separation may then come between the smooth (laminar) and the irregular (turbulent) flow regions (cf. Fig. 4.17 on p. 207).

At high Reynolds numbers, we may treat viscosity as a small effect in a larger region of a flow field where potential flow applies. In the small region constituting the boundary layer, viscosity becomes important. Thus, except for special regions (boundary layers, separated flow areas, etc.), we may ordinarily ignore the effects of viscosity.

4.13 Mechanisms of mixing in fluid flow

The original experiments by Osborne Reynolds [63,64] on the onset of turbulent flow in a long pipe, rendering the motions of the flowing fluid visible by means of color bands, demonstrate the fundamental mechanisms of liquid mixing: In laminar flows, mixing may occur by streamline *convection* in the flow direction and by *diffusion* in directions normal to the flow streamlines. In turbulent flows, in addition, mixing is brought about by the *molar motions* of turbulent eddies. The erratic turbulent velocities convect fluid and solute in all possible directions.

The fundamentals of mixing [3,22] are extremely important in the study of cardiovascular flows. Mixing is a process or mechanism that promotes uniformity of concentration of any kind: solute, or dispersed particles. In static and flowing low-viscosity liquids and gases, diffusion is the primary cause of mixing. However, in high-viscosity liquids such as blood, convection is the dominant mechanism of mixing. Convection enhances mixing by increasing the interfacial area between regions of high and low concentration, which in turbulent flow is augmented by molar rearrangements of material produced by turbulent eddies (see next section). Once such regions are brought in immediate or close proximity by convection, diffusion takes over, *perfecting mixing at the molecular level*, where each solute molecule becomes *surrounded by solvent molecules*. In general, we recognize several interrelated mechanisms of mixing:

- **Diffusive mixing.** This is the only mechanism of mixing under *no flow* or *uniform flow* conditions, as is illustrated in Figure 4.18**a**. Due to molecular diffusion, the blotch of a dissolved colored species spreads out as it advances downstream, while its color weakens until complete mixing occurs, where almost every individual molecule of the solute is surrounded by solvent molecules.

- **Convective laminar mixing.** Consider laminar flow in a pipe. An islet of a colored species is injected at the inlet. Its particles are big enough, so that diffusion is negligible but are small enough that gravity is also negligible. The configuration of the island as it advances downstream is shown in Figure 4.18**b**. As can be seen from left to right, as the carrier liquid travels downstream, the colored islet is strained more and more, and to such a degree far downstream, that its *continuity breaks* and every solute particle is confined among solvent molecules. Observe that the mixing in

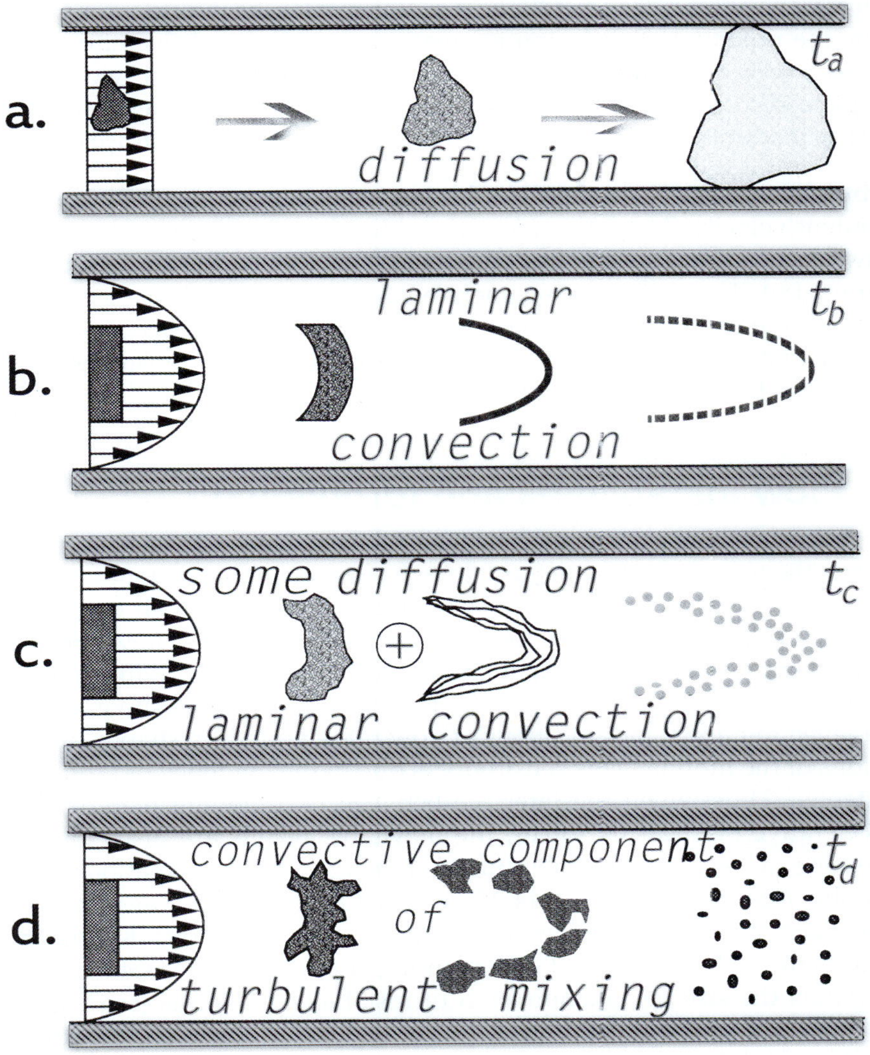

Figure 4.18: Schematic representation of the principal mixing mechanisms in flowing fluids. a. Diffusive mixing in uniform flow. b. Convective laminar mixing without diffusion. c. Convective laminar mixing with diffusion. d. Turbulent convective mixing without diffusion. t_i = time of last snapshot in each panel; typically, in intracardiac and large vessel flows, $t_a \gg t_b > t_c \gg t_d$.

Figure 4.18a is due entirely to the shear or elongational *deformation* of flowing material elements that is induced by the laminar flow.

- **Convective laminar and diffusive mixing.** When diffusion is not negligible, the situation of Figure 4.18 b. changes to that of Figure 4.18 c. Convective mixing due to deformation brings regions of low concentration in immediate or close contact with regions of high concentration—i.e., it increases the interface for mass exchange. Thus, the potential of diffusion is greatly intensified and this effect, when superimposed onto the convectively produced *macromixing* action, yields eventually a complete *micromixing*. The blotch of a dissolved colored species distorts and breaks apart as it adopts the velocity profile of the flow and it also diffuses.

- **Turbulent convective mixing.** In addition to the convective mixing of laminar flow, turbulent velocity fluctuations (erratic eddies) cause regions of high concentration to switch position continually with regions of low concentration, as is shown in Figure 4.18d. The bulk rearrangement of material by turbulence is called *distributive mixing*. Note that the stage of *ideal micromixing* occurs only as a result of diffusion, which is the only mechanism available to dissolve single molecules, and is consequently the last phase of any kind of mixing.

4.14 Flow instabilities and turbulence

For centuries, the complex nature of fluid flows has captivated our attention; as children, as adults, and as scientists and physicians. What attracts our attention is that flows in nature have a strong tendency to undergo flow regime changes. Indeed, it can be a thrilling, or a distressing, circumstance when small alterations in operating conditions produce large effects. This is true of fluid motions, which tend to be very sensitive and responsive, sometimes even to minute modifications of flow rates, boundary shapes, and of virtually all conditions of the motion. This sensitivity is due to the tendency of fluid motion states to be unstable. Thus, when the interface between two flowing materials experiences strong accelerative or shearing forces, the inevitable results are instability, turbulence, and the mixing of materials, momentum, and energy. Such a situation corresponds to the Helmholtz–Kelvin instability [4, 14, 16, 74] in which one fluid flows over another, e.g., wind over water, causing surface waves to grow. The Helmholtz–Kelvin instability is represented in the well known Van Gogh painting "La Nuit Etoilée" (Starry Night), where the artist paints the striking phenomenon of instability in clouds (see Fig. 4.19, on p. 213).[15] The general problem of transition from laminar to turbulent motion, with all of its ramifications, is a long-standing problem of fluid instability. The instability of a fluid motion can have positive or negative effects, depending on whether the result of the instability produces or destroys a desired property of the flow. Thus, for example, one may wish to avoid transition to turbulence in blood flow to reduce trauma to formed blood elements, or one may wish to promote it to enhance mixing.

Turbulence is the result of powerful flow instability and entails a random fluctuation in fluid motion superimposed on the ensemble-averaged (see Section 2.1, on pp. 37 ff.) time-course of a flow [8, 32, 46, 83]. Turbulence is important because it augments molecular transport and causes mixing within the fluid, a fact well known to anyone who has

[15] Some consider Starry Night to be Van Gogh's one greatest work of all. Starry Night was painted while he was in the asylum at Saint-Rémy, in Provence, and his behavior was very erratic at the time [7]. Unlike most of Van Gogh's works, Starry Night was painted from memory, and not outdoors [25].

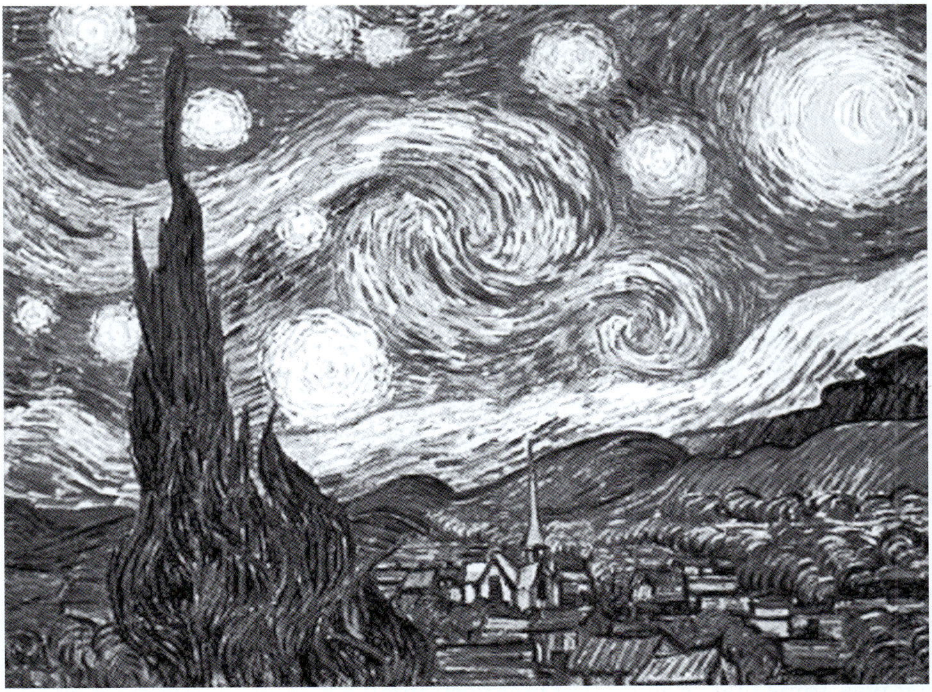

Figure 4.19: Detail of "La Nuit Etoilée," by Vincent Van Gogh. Reprinted by permission from The Museum of Modern Art, New York.

vigorously stirred sugar into a cup of tea. The effects of blood flow turbulence are of great clinical and basic science importance in both medical and surgical cardiology (cf. Chapters 7, 8, and 16). For example, several studies have focused on the role played by turbulence on cell and tissue behavior [38,42,72,90] .

4.14.1 Mechanisms of instability

Suppose that a given flow field is subjected to some disturbance. We would like to know if such a flow system can depart significantly from its original state, called "basic flow," or not [16]. If the disturbances are effective, large enough to extract sufficient energy from the basic flow and grow in the course of time, then the basic flow becomes unstable with respect to such disturbances. In effect, the mathematical solution, which governs the behavior of the basic flow system, will then he replaced by another, distinct, solution [84]. Such a transition is often evidenced by the emergence of a structure [9] that is periodic in space, or time. For instance, a small laminar stream of water from a faucet can give rise to regularly spaced *drops* due to an imbalance between gravity and surface tension.

More generally, the instability is associated with a loss of space-time symmetry by the initial flow considered. Hence, there will be transition from one basic flow to another due to the action of an instability. This can take place when a flow-regime controlling parameter, such as the Reynolds number (Re, see Section 4.11, on pp. 205 ff.) exceeds some critical value. Instability of the fluid flow can become established once the critical value of Re is exceeded.

Any sufficiently viscous fluid flow is hardly unstable, because an effect of viscosity is to dissipate the energy of any disturbance and thus high viscosity has the tendency to prevent flow destabilization. However, viscosity has a dual stabilizing–destabilizing effect, since it can also allow a disturbance to organize itself in such a manner that it can draw upon the energy available in the basic flow.[16] The momentum diffusion effect of viscosity can make some flows, such as parallel shear flows, unstable (see Section 9.5.1, on pp. 457 f.), while the same flows in the absence of viscosity remain stable. Thus, generally, flow boundaries tend to have an important effect in restricting the development of the types of the disturbances that are liable to come about [10]; usually the closer they are, the more stable the flow. However, boundaries sometimes give rise to strong shear in the adjacent layers, which is diffused outward by viscosity leading to instability.

Viscoelastic boundaries, such as cardiac and vascular walls, tend to confer flow stabilization compared to rigid-surface boundaries, a phenomenon discovered in studies of drag reduction by the skin of the dolphin [36,37]. Polymers in suspension similarly contribute to flow stabilization and drag reduction [11]. This effect is known as the Toms effect, because it was Toms that showed [85] that very small amounts of dissolved additives can suppress turbulent flow, or at least decrease turbulent flow energy losses to a considerable degree. The Toms effect leads to a decrease in the flow resistance, which can be as high as 75%, even though the amount of these polymer additives does not need to exceed 100 *ppm* [45].[17] Such small amounts of polymer additive are used to increase substantially the length of the water jet issuing from fire-pumps.

Acceleration, whether local or convective, of a laminar fluid flow has a stabilizing and deceleration a destabilizing effect. Intracardiac blood flows that are strongly time-dependent can have complicated stability characteristics [53,59,60]. The tendency for a fluid to move down a pressure gradient can amplify disturbances and lead to instability. When instability takes place in a fluid flow system, the effective disturbances responsible for the instability extract a sufficient amount of kinetic energy from the basic flow and pass it on to the growing disturbances. This upsets the equilibrium of the inertial, viscous, and pressure gradient forces that are operative on the basic flow. Depending on the particular laminar flow system, there may be several values of Re beyond which further flow regime changes occur, until laminar flow completely loses its laminar behavior. Streamlines and flow laminae get snarled and then completely confused; eddies and vortices form and spin, and they develop their own eddies in turn, and they dissolve without much obvious pattern.

[16] As an example, the flat-plate boundary layer—see Figure 4.17, on p. 207—has no inflection point in the flow and therefore should be inviscidly stable; nevertheless, it does become unstable due to the action of viscosity.

[17] ppm signifies "parts per million," i.e., the concentration of the additive does not need to exceed 0.01%.

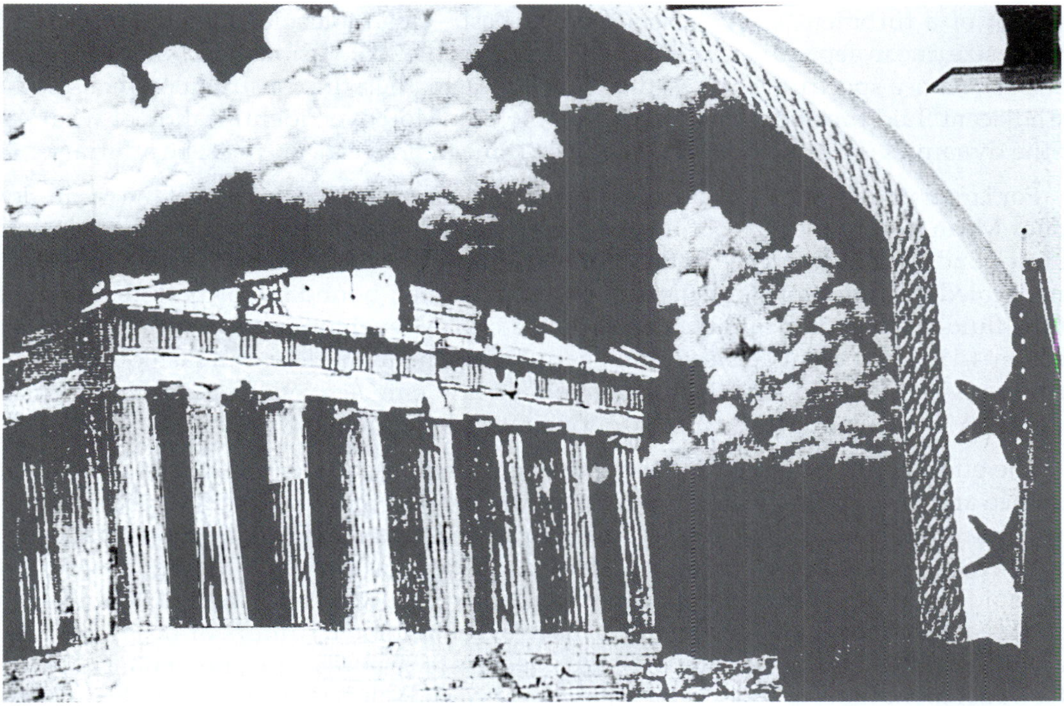

Figure 4.20: Portion from a mural of the Acropolis in a Greek restaurant in Fort Myers, FL (cf. Fig. 4.19, on p. 213).

An important feature of highly disturbed fluid flow systems are the erratic, fluctuating spatial structures of their motions which, in shear flow systems, correspond to eddies. We speak about the existence of turbulence in an intracardiac flow, if spatial and temporal changes in the flow field proceed much faster and have a character of random fluctuations in comparison with the changes in the pulsatile pressure and flow velocity, which are associated with the heart cycle [53, 57]. However, turbulent flows are not just fluids in a state of complete disorder and chaos. Rather, such flows are generally composed of the superposition of a number of organized motions that tend to persist in space and in time, the so-called vortical "coherent structures," possibly immersed in some unorganized background of random fluid disturbances. The search for coherent events in turbulent flows is [33] the embodiment of a human desire to find order in apparent disorder.

4.14.2 Turbulent eddies and mean flow

Turbulent eddies in a fluid superficially resemble individual molecules in a gas. They likewise bounce around in random fashion, carrying kinetic energy in their fluctuating velocities. Eddies also diffuse momentum (and any embedded materials), exerting pressure through momentum transport and bombardment against walls. However, the concept of a turbulent eddy is nebulous, at best. Gas molecules have an identifiable shape, size, mean separation, and mean free path between collisions. Turbulent eddies, in contrast, have a spectrum of sizes; they overlap each other; the constraint on their motion by adjacent fluid precludes any free path [8,46,83]. Moreover, identification of what part of the dynamics is turbulence and what part is mean flow can, at times, be arbitrary.

For larger eddies, the fluctuation scale may be an appreciable fraction of the mean-flow scale. Mean flow is that part of the dynamics that is directly associated with the macroscopic conditions; turbulence is the more erratic part of the flow that is associated with finer-scaled perturbations, arising from random initial, boundary, or bulk disturbances of the fluid, at Reynolds numbers exceeding a critical level for any specific geometry (cf. Section 4.11). Turbulent eddies drain energy from the main flow in a fashion similar to ordinary viscosity, and effectively act like a greatly enhanced viscosity or "momentum diffusivity." See Figure 4.17, on p. 207, for a mental picture of this behavior.

The effects of turbulence can be highly significant, increasing the fluid's effective resistance and enhancing the mixing of initially separated materials, such as the mixing of dust or sand into air [8,14,46,83]. It is easy to be deceived into thinking that turbulence is rare, because it often is not directly visible to the casual observer. Although water flowing rapidly through a transparent pipe may look completely smooth, touching the pipe can reveal vibrations, and auscultation may reveal audible murmurs or bruits beyond a valvular or arterial stenosis; similarly, the injection of dye through a tiny hole in the wall of a transparent tube, or of a radiopaque dye at cardiac catheterization, can demonstrate rapid downstream mixing. Both effects are a direct result of turbulent fluctuations.

Why is nature discontent with smooth fluid flow, especially at higher flow speeds? The answer may lie in the behavior of energy. Unlike momentum, energy has the peculiar ability to assume numerous and varied configurations. Momentum constraints, while restrictive, are helpless to prevent seemingly unpredictable energy rearrangements.

4.14.3 Turbulence energy: sources and sinks

Fluid flow implies the presence of energy, which can exist in any of various forms: kinetic, heat, turbulence. By kinetic energy we mean the motion energy carried by the main (mean) flow; heat energy refers to the kinetic energy of molecular fluctuations. Turbulence energy is at a scale between these first two: it is the kinetic energy of fluctuations large compared with the individual molecular scale but small compared with the mean-flow scale [8,14,23,46,83]. In contrast to mass and momentum, which are highly constrained by their conservation laws, energy behaves very capriciously. Although conserving the total energy, transitions among the many manifestations of energy occur continuously. It is, perhaps, a remarkable fact of nature that, because of such transitions, any system devoid of counteractive actions inevitably tends to move from order to disorder.[18]

Consider a fluid that has been set into smooth and uniform motion in a circular container. It has zero total (vector) momentum: as much is moving east, as is moving west at

[18] There are exceptions to this rule; they need not detain us here.

every instant. Tangential shearing drag on the walls slows the motion so that mean-flow kinetic energy is lost. Where does the energy go—to turbulence, or to heat? The competition is fierce, and heat always wins in the end, but fluids yield themselves to the inevitable only grudgingly. If possible, they transform at least part of their main flow kinetic energy to turbulence, as an intermediate step along the way.

The conversion of mean flow kinetic energy directly to heat is limited by the viscosity of the fluid and by the steepness of the main-flow velocity gradients. Main flow may be steady or unsteady (pulsatile) and is that part of the dynamics whose structure is comparable in size to the region of interest at a given level; finer dynamical scales of an erratic nature constitute the fluid's turbulence. However, the main flow for one observer may simply be the larger scales of a turbulence spectrum for an observer whose field of view is larger. Thus, the source of turbulence seen by one observer becomes the energy sink for the decay of turbulence at the larger scales of another observer. This principle and its generalizations have powerful consequences, leading to the concept of a "turbulence cascade," to which we next turn our attention.

4.14.4 Turbulence cascade

Visualization of turbulent flows shows various eddy structures—coalescing, dividing, stretching, and above all *spinning*. The total kinetic energy of turbulent eddies of an isolated fluid decreases with time due to viscous dissipation. Hence, a turbulent fluid can be in a steady state only if energy flows continuously into the system, so that the energy injection rate equals the rate of dissipation. The energy is transferred by instability processes toward the smaller turbulent eddy scales. If the energy is fed by stirring the fluid in such a fashion that the turbulence produced is homogeneous and isotropic, then Kolmogorov's theory—named after the great Russian mathematician who developed it in two papers published in 1941—can yield the energy spectrum of the eddies [14,23,46,83].

The turbulent velocity field is made of the multitude of eddies of *different* sizes. The Parthenon mural in Figure 4.20, on p. 215, is unconvincing exactly because it misses the vital *multiscale* characteristic of turbulence structures, which are admirably well exhibited in van Gogh's *Starry Night* painting in Figure 4.19, on p. 213. We somehow feed rotational kinetic energy into the system in a way able to produce large eddies. Eddies are describable as small whirlpools. That is, instead of flowing in distinct flow lines, the liquid rotates. These whirlpools are unstable and continue to break down into *successively smaller* whirlpools [59,60]. A mathematical analysis has shown [2] that van Gogh's *Starry Night* painting, created during a period of psychotic agitation of the artist, reflects the fingerprints of turbulence with such a realism that is even consistent with the Kolmogorov statistical scaling theory. Specifically, the probability distribution function (*PDF*) of luminance fluctuations (u) of pixels separated by a distance R in *Starry Night*, is the same as the *PDF* of the velocity differences (v) of pairs of points separated by a distance R in a turbulent flow, as predicted by Kolmogorov's theory.

In a pioneering work published in 1922, Lewis Fry Richardson formulated the concept that turbulence is organized as a hierarchy of eddies of various scales, each daughter-eddy

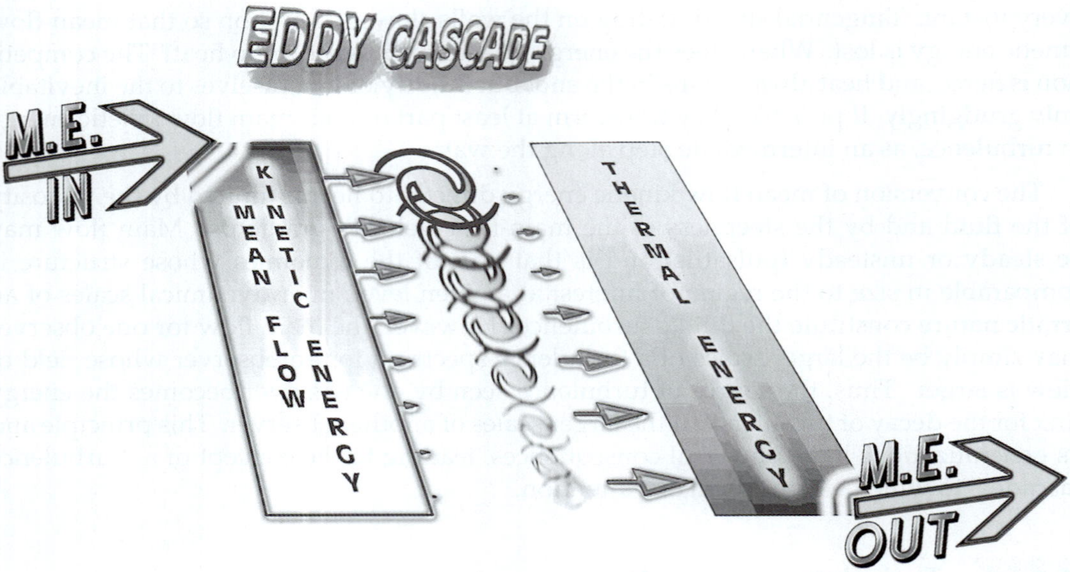

Figure 4.21: Mean flow kinetic energy transforms into turbulence energy and then to thermal energy. The relative amounts transported by each mechanism change as the size of turbulent eddies cascades down, as indicated by the arrow sizes. Most of the mean flow kinetic energy feeds into larger eddies, whereas substantial viscous dissipation into heat occurs only in the smallest eddy scales. Mechanical energy (M.E.) input is always higher that output from the flow system, because of these dissipative processes.

generation withdrawing energy from its immediately larger mother-eddy neighbor in a "cascading" process of eddy-breakdown. This picture was poetically immortalized in his book [65], which was inspired from observations of clouds and the verses of Jonathan Swift:

> "Big whorls have little whorls, Which feed on their velocity;
> And little whorls have lesser whorls, And so on to viscosity (in the molecular sense)"

This turbulence cascade is a familiar process. When we stir milk into coffee, uniformity of composition is arrived at as the result of a very complex pattern of motion, and the mixing process is much more effective than molecular diffusion. We recognize that when we wave the spoon about in the coffee we produce spoon- or cup-sized motions that quickly degenerate into much more complicated motions with smaller-size scales associated with them. The motions which spread tobacco smoke would be similar in kind: it is not long before the smoke smell can be detected in every corner of a room. Turbulent eddies diffuse the fluid itself, and with it any characteristic attached to it, such as color, chemical constitution, smell, and so on. Fluid parcels also possess heat, linear and angular momentum, and kinetic energy of rotation and of linear motion, relative to their surroundings.

These are features not attached permanently to the parcels: some may be diffused by turbulent transfer mechanisms, or by the action of pressure gradients, at a much greater rate than would occur through molecular diffusion.

At the critical Reynolds number, the kinetic energy of flow supports the growth of fluctuations (in space and time) and transition to turbulence is induced. The conversion of the energy of the main flow motion into the rotational kinetic energy of turbulent eddies in turbulent motion is *irreversible*. The *rotational* kinetic energy of turbulent eddies *cannot* be reconverted into kinetic energy of main flow motion. This is of primary importance in analyzing intracardiac flow fields (cf. Section 14.14, on pp. 789 ff.) both normally [59,60] and in the presence of turbulence [53,57], as occurs with heart valve pathology (cf. Section 16.2.2, on pp. 860 ff.).

We can now entertain the concept of redistribution of the energy of the main flow, which is not *directly* related to the conversion of the mechanical energy into thermal energy and, therefore, is independent of the fluid viscosity. In fact, the redistribution of the kinetic energy between the observed main flow motion and the fluctuating motion can also be considered in an ideal fluid. On the other hand, the conversion of the mechanical energy into thermal is impossible in an ideal incompressible fluid. Therefore, conversion of energy from the main flow motion into the turbulent motion of eddies can be determined, basically, only by the fluid inertia.

The eddy breakdown occurs in a random or "chaotic" fashion. Kolmogorov envisaged a self-similar cascade of energy from large length scales, set-up by the acting driving forces (e.g., stirring) to shorter length scales, where it is dissipated. *Self-similarity* implies that any subscale of the system is equivalent to the overall system.[19] Turbulent eddies, though, are only statistically self-similar—their magnified small scales do not superimpose on the entire system. Nevertheless, they do have the same general type of appearance.

Figure 4.21, on p. 218, gives a schematic pictorial depiction of the dynamics of the process. Large eddies can feed rotational kinetic energy to smaller eddies and these in turn feed still smaller eddies, resulting in the vigorous cascading of energy from the largest eddies to the smallest ones. Eddies can be as large as the smallest dimension of the turbulent stream and as small as about $0.1-1$ *mm* [26]. Energy does not build up at any scale; the intermediate eddies merely transmit this energy to the smaller. In this process, turbulence energy cascades to progressively smaller and smaller fluctuation scales, with the source of energy for each scale coming from the mean-flow velocity contortions of

[19] Two general geometric notions are to be distinguished. The first one relates to self-similarity, and the second to self-affinity. An object is self-similar if it is composed of smaller parts, each of which is an exact or approximate replica of the whole. Each small piece can be obtained from the original whole by a similarity transformation, or a contraction which reduces the original object by the same scale factor in all coordinates. A curve is said to be self-similar if, for every piece of the curve, there is a smaller piece that is similar to it. Many objects in the body, such as the bronchial or vascular trees, are statistically self-similar: parts of them show the same statistical properties at different scales. An affine transformation is one in which different coordinates are contracted by different factors. Objects with parts that are affine copies of the whole are labeled self-affine. Consider a trace of turbulent velocity measured as a function of time. Since velocity and time are independent of each other, the coordinate axes can be stretched (or contracted) independently. Such traces are not candidates for self-similarity, but for self-affinity. Both similarity and affinity are linear transformations.

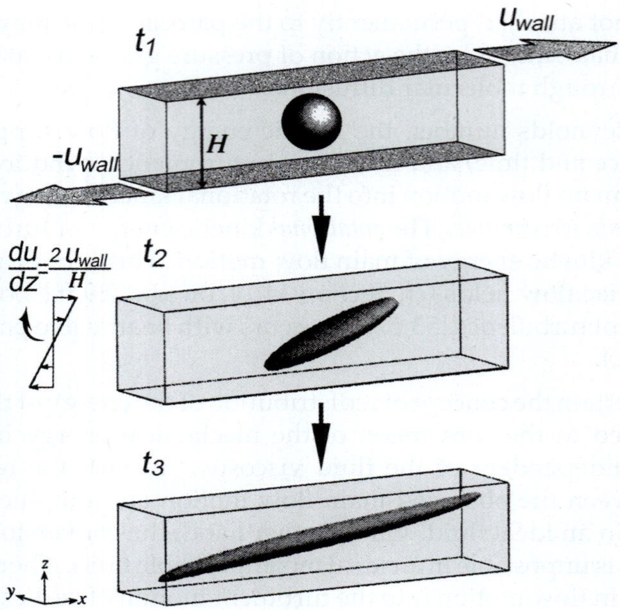

Figure 4.22: Schematic representation of shear-induced deformation of an initially (t_1) spherical region into progressively more elongated ellipsoidal forms at later times (t_2, t_3) in simple shear flow. A viscous fluid layer of thickness H along the z-axis is being sheared between two parallel plates moving in opposite directions along the x-axis with velocity u_{wall}, to establish a steady-state shear rate, or velocity gradient, of $2u_{wall}/H$.

the next larger scale [14, 23, 46, 83]. Phenomenologically, this cascade expresses itself in the development of a relatively disorderly flow from an initially relatively ordered flow, displaying large coherent vortex structures.[20]

Dynamically, we may visualize the fundamental turbulent mixing process as one of random eddy formation or "bursting" from the main stream, followed by decay of the highly energetic, highly nonuniform and highly convoluted eddying structures under the action of viscous shear and shear-induced deformations (see Fig. 4.22). This suggests that the turbulent energy cascade from larger to smaller scales is an overall randomly periodic creation and decay of the scales, rather than a pseudosteady state transfer between vortices of decreasing scale.

Possibly, the most distinctive feature of nonlinear dynamical systems in general, and of the turbulence energy cascade in particular, is that their physics is coupled at *all scales* of motion. This is in a blatant contrast with the much more comfortable behavior of linear

[20] In striking contrast to this phenomenon is the *self-organization principle* [31] of 2-D turbulence. The main difference between 3- and 2-D lies in the effect of vortex stretching. If a vortex is stretched, fluid is pulled toward its axis, and due to conservation of angular momentum it will rotate faster. In a 2-D flow, the mechanism of vortex stretching is absent, and this has important consequences for the dynamics: the kinetic energy of the flow actually shows a spectral flux *from small to large* length scales [21].

systems, in which each scale of motion evolves on its own, in a complete isolation with respect to other scales (cf. Fourier harmonics—Section 2.18, on pp. 82 ff.). At each stage of the turbulence energy cascade, there is competition for the rotational kinetic energy, part going into heat and part going into even smaller turbulent fluctuations. However, as the scale decreases, the characteristic eddy length decreases *pari-passu*, and the velocity gradients in the eddies become steeper and steeper. At the smallest of turbulence scales, energy goes directly to heat, as viscosity successfully "irons out" the fluctuations.

In an idealized steady state approximation of turbulence, exactly as much energy enters the fluctuation spectrum of motion at the largest scale as leaves it to become heat at the smallest scale. More accurately, there is some loss of energy to heat at every scale, but the loss at the smallest scale is dominant.

With each reduction in scale, turbulent motion of the larger scale becomes mean-flow motion of the smaller scale. Because each reduction in scale has approximately the same change in mean flow velocity occurring over a much smaller distance, velocity gradients become *steeper*, and a larger fraction of the turbulence energy goes directly into heat. It is the largest scales that contain most of the energy and thus exert the dominant effects on the main-flow dynamics. Main-flow kinetic energy feeds into large-scale turbulence, whereas thermal energy receives much of its energy from small-scale turbulence.

4.14.5 Pseudosound generation by turbulent flow

A striking manifestation of highly disturbed or turbulent blood flow in the heart and larger arteries is the generation of so-called "murmurs." Although they are considered as hydrodynamically generated sound, they are in fact better classified as *pseudosound*, a distintion that merits some attention.[21] We begin by noting that the ear detects pressure variations as small as 10^{-10} atm and can be damaged if subjected to variations in excess of 10^{-3} atm [20]. Generally, therefore, sound pressure variations are weak, as are their associated fluid motions, and the mechanics of sound can be understood within the context of linear theory. In linear theory, waves add without distortion; to wit, multiple concurrent conversations at a party do not interfere. In the case of pseudosound, unsteady pressures are nonlinearly related to fluid motion and are not organized like proper sound into propagating waves.

A laminar flow involving viscous shear at moderate Reynolds numbers may create a gentle hiss; a viscous turbulent flow at higher Reynolds numbers can create a roar. However the noise in both situations is confined and does not spread to the so-called *far acoustic field* [69]. Accordingly, it is termed *pseudosound*, because the noise is contained locally. It can affect a contiguous sensor, such as a catheter-tip micromanometer but decays as the inverse square of the distance. Similarly, the air stream about the unprotected ears of a motor cyclist can be painfully noisy to him, even though only a negligible fraction of the pressure variations within the turbulent eddies that bother him so much propagates away as true sound. These pressure variations can be made to propagate by the action of

[21] Pseudosound consists, in an elementary form, of the pressure disturbances generated by the rapid fluctuations of the local velocity, which characterize the velocity field of turbulent eddies [44].

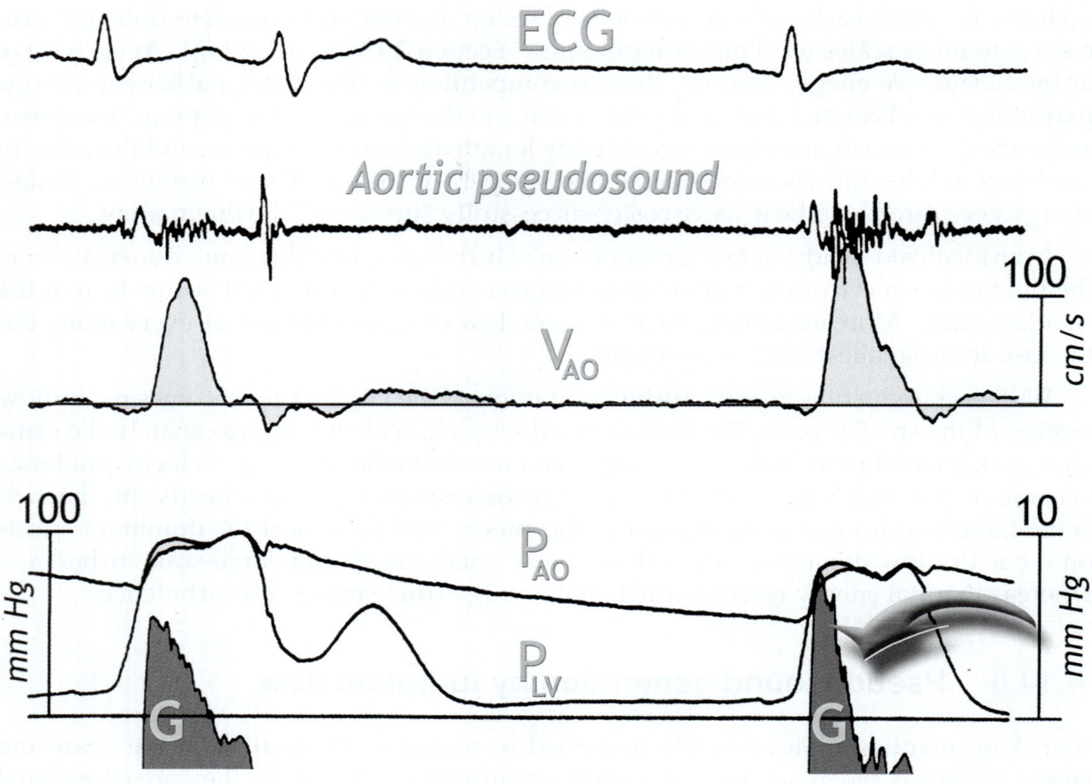

Figure 4.23: Simultaneous left ventricular (LV) and aortic root (AO) pressure (P) and velocity (V) signals obtained by Millar multisensor catheter. Also shown are electronically derived intraaortic pseudosound and instantaneous transaortic ejection pressure difference, or "gradient" (G), signals. Note the enhanced pseudosound, velocity, and peak accelerating gradient (abbreviated in duration) after the long compensatory pause.

a resonator [20], and that is the principle of the wind instruments. True sound, such as that created by a vibrating panel decays as the inverse of the distance.

An illustration of hydrodynamic pseudosound generation by disturbed flow in the heart is given in Figure 4.23, where pressure, ejection velocity and transaortic ejection pressure gradient signals are demonstrated in a normal sinus beat and a post-PVC[22] beat in a patient without any evidence of LV or aortic valve disease, at diagnostic catheterization to rule out cardiac causes of chest pain.

In Figure 4.23, a simultaneous intraaortic pseudosound signal that is derived from the aortic micromanometer[23] demonstrates acoustic range frequencies, which may not be

[22]PVC = premature ventricular contraction.

[23]It is of some interest that several of the micromanometric pressure transducers (piezoelectric, variable-capacitance, and strain-gauge types) originated, in fact, as microphones, namely devices used for acoustical measurements [81].

audible at the body surface without amplification. Their magnitude is seen to be strongly accentuated as the flow velocity increases in the post-PVC beat. This pseudosound signal is derived from the micromanometric aortic root sensor in a two-stage process that amplifies only the acoustic range frequencies: this selective isolation is accomplished by first passing the micromanometric signal through a high-pass filter (see Fig. 4.24, and also Fig. 2.26, on p. 77) and, in a second stage, through an amplifier that amplifies only the acoustic range frequencies. On the other hand, the transaortic ejection pressure gradient signal is obtained by electronically subtracting the aortic root from the LV chamber pressure signal, and then amplifying the difference signal nonselectively. Note that the instantaneous pressure gradient is displayed in Figure 4.23 at a scale with 10 times the sensitivity of the individual pressures scale.

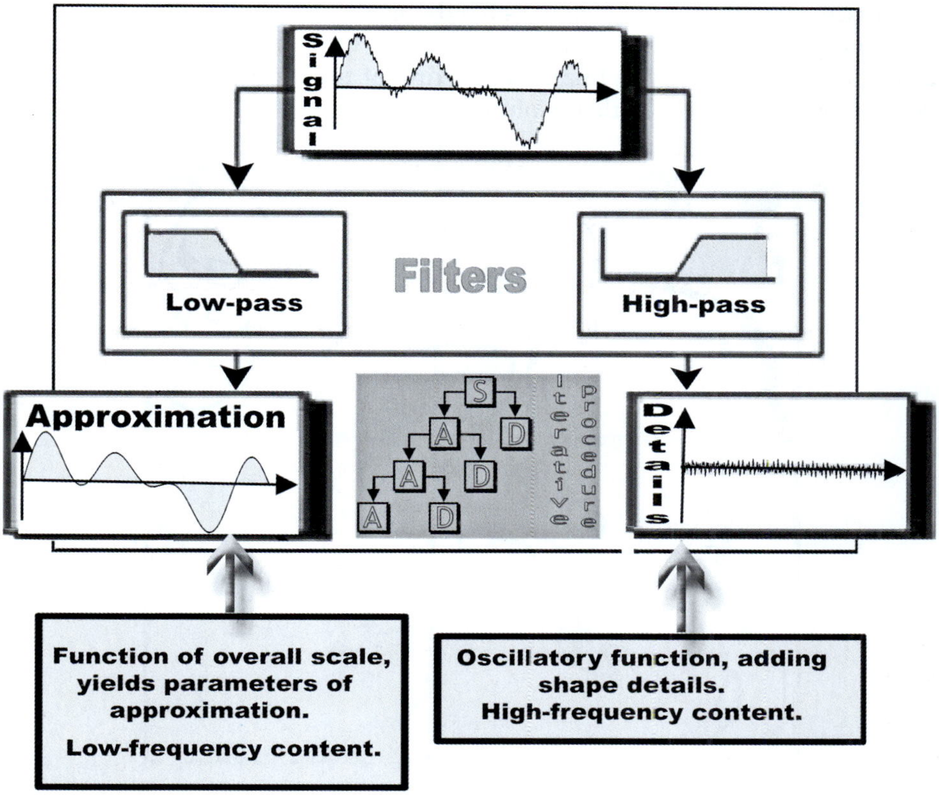

Figure 4.24: Schematic view of the stepwise decomposition of a pulsatile velocity or pressure signal (S) into low-frequency components, determining approximate overall shape (A), and high-frequency fluctuating components adding detail (D). The procedure can iteratively resolve a signal into multiple frequency bands by peeling off successively "remaining" higher frequencies (inset); alternatively, band-pass filters can be used (cf. Fig. 2.26, on p. 77).

4.14.6 Turbulent mixing

One of the consequences of inhomogeneity in a fluid system is that it gives rise to transport phenomena that lead to mixing. Mixing is a process, or mechanism, that promotes uniformity of concentration of any kind: solute, particles in suspension, heat. Even in laminar flow, in high-shear regions there are steep velocity gradients (strong inhomogeneity) transverse to the local direction of fluid motion (cf. Fig. 4.22).

In laminar flow fields, mixing may occur by streamline convection in the flow direction and by diffusion in directions normal to streamlines. Laminar mixing is due to shear or elongational deformations of fluid particles. Such shear motions allow fluid from one place to penetrate and convectively mix with other fluid because they can pull apart two initially close fluid elements. Thus, shear enhances species gradients and causes faster molecular mixing. Furthermore, convection enhances mixing by increasing the interfacial area between regions of low and high concentration. Once such regions make contact by convection, diffusion takes over, finalizing mixing at the molecular level, where solvent molecules surround each molecule of solute.

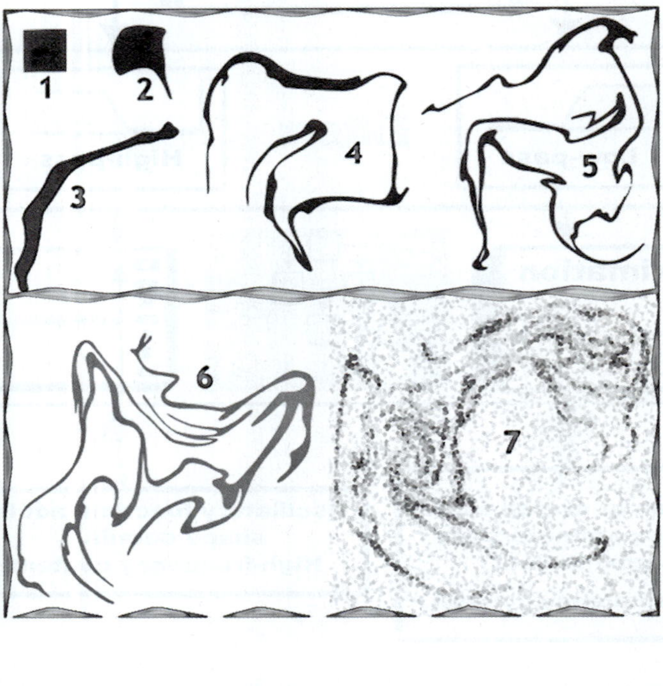

Figure 4.25: Turbulence enhanced mixing of a scalar quantity, e.g., the concentration of a compound. The eddying motions stretch and distort an initial (stage 1) blob of inhomogeneous fluid, giving rise to numerous interdigitating striations, until the ensuing (stage 6) increase in surface area and scalar property gradients enable molecular diffusion effects (stage 7) to proceed rapidly.

Since fluid elements carrying different physical quantities move around randomly under turbulence, we expect turbulence to augment the transport processes greatly [14, 23,

46, 83], compared to molecular diffusion mechanisms (see Fig. 4.25, on p. 224).[24] In turbulent flows, the turbulent molar motions intensify mixing due to bulk rearrangements of material [49], which bring about *distributive mixing*. These molar motions convect fluid and solute in all possible directions. Similar effects pertain to enhanced turbulent transport, as compared with molecular diffusion of heat. Thus, the warmth of a hot-water radiator is felt throughout an ordinary room in minutes rather than hours or days. This is caused by weak natural-convection turbulent currents, which are driven by air temperature and density gradients in the vicinity of the radiator.

Molar mixing similarly promotes dissemination of axial momentum in the normal direction and normal momentum in the axial direction, which together culminate in more *uniform* velocity distributions in turbulent as compared to laminar flows. Figure 4.25, on p. 224, shows the progression of mixing in a turbulent flow field. Velocity fluctuations cause regions of high concentration to spread out and switch position continually with regions of low concentrations. At successive stages, there is an increasing interfacial area of mass exchange between the black regions of high concentration and the white ones of negligible concentration, such that diffusion takes over and molecular mixing is carried out, denoted by a progressively spreading and weakening gray color. Eventually, complete mixing occurs, where solvent molecules will surround almost every single solute molecule. Complete mixing occurs only due to diffusion, which is the only mechanism available to accomplish the last stage of any kind of mixing.

Sir Geoffrey Taylor and Ludwig Prandtl, arguably the two giants of fluid mechanics of the twentieth century,[25] both formulated theories of turbulent diffusion. As the turbulent eddies move around the flow, they can transfer their momentum, substances in solution or suspension, and energy, between different regions of the flow much more effectively than molecular motions. A trailblazing idea, due to Prandtl, is that a turbulent flow can be equivalent to a "gas of eddies," the smallest eddies acting on the large ones in a diffusive manner. This picture, clearly inspired by the kinetic theory of gases, led him to the introduction of the concept of an *eddy viscosity*, which is much more effective for momentum transfer than the dynamic viscosity of the fluid.

You make use of the notion of turbulent diffusion when you stir coffee vigorously to mix sugar in it. If one puts sugar in the coffee and does not stir it, then the sugar mixes with the coffee only by molecular diffusion, which takes a very long time. On the other hand, if we stir the coffee, then we generate turbulence inside it and turbulent diffusion mixes up the sugar much more efficiently than molecular diffusion. Turbulent mixing is a natural consequence of large-scale rotation in flows, which brings widely separated fluid elements close together, where they can mix diffusively and can react chemically. In a similar context, we note that, in larger cardiovascular structures, the interaction of convection and diffusion effects gives rise to concentration boundary layers for substances that may be secreted or taken up by the walls. Such substances are transported convectively

[24] Molar motions, akin to but less intense than those prevailing in turbulent regimes, characterize so-called "secondary flows" (see Section 9.5.5, on pp. 469 f.) in laminar environments.

[25] Ludwig Prandtl founded the boundary layer theory that earned him the title of Father of Modern Fluid Mechanics—even G.I. Taylor addressed him as "our chief" [17]. Among his students were Blasius, Tollmien, Tietjens, Schlichting, Nikuradse, von Mises, von Kàrmàn, and many others [17, 43].

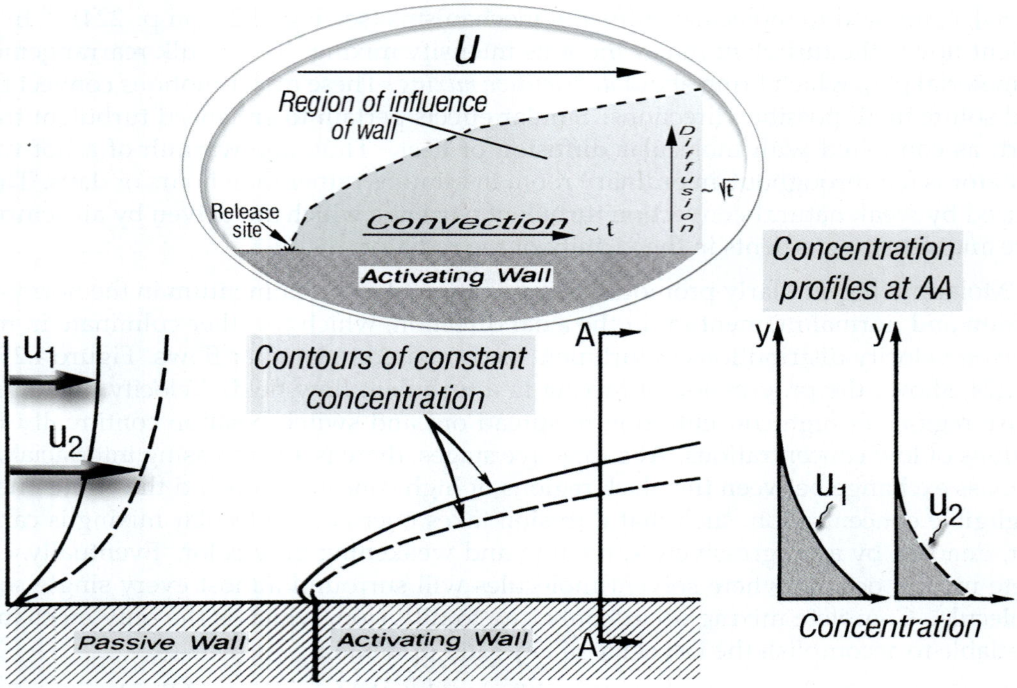

Figure 4.26: Development of concentration boundary layer on an activating wall area, under laminar flow conditions; u_1 and u_2 are different applying blood flow velocities; t is time. As is indicated in the inset, mass transfer within the laminar boundary layer in the axial direction (tangentially to the boundary) occurs as a result of convection with the flow, whereas in the radial direction (perpendicularly to the boundary), it occurs as a result of the generally much slower process of mass diffusion. Inception of turbulence can augment radial transport greatly, as is described in the text.

(distance $\sim t$) by the stream along the flow direction, but diffuse relatively slowly (distance $\sim \sqrt{t}$) perpendicularly to the wall in the radial direction (see Fig. 4.26). This produces a *concentration boundary layer*, across which the concentration changes from the value that applies at the wall to the value that applies in the main stream, similarly to the change in velocity across the hydrodynamic boundary layer.

The coupling of fluid motion with diffusion processes in blood and with biochemical processes needs to be emphasized. Movement of blood past a surface determines the rate at which constituents—including reactants—are brought into its vicinity. However, the residence time of individual constituents within a significant range of any specific point on the surface is reduced as the flow rate is increased. If there are activated or activating substances in the close vicinity of the surface, the effect of increasing blood-flow rate is to decrease the distance across the bloodstream (namely, perpendicular to the surface) to which the substance can penetrate before being swept downstream, out of the region of interest. Increase in blood flow rate does not mean that the concentration of a substance diffusing from the boundary surface is reduced all across the stream by dilution, but rather that the thickness of a *concentration boundary layer* of the substance in the bloodstream is reduced (see Fig. 4.26). Reactive constituents that are carried in the blood stream flow into the boundary layer; the thickness of this layer, the flux of reactive constituents, and their residence times all depend on the blood flow rate. Similar concepts govern the evolution of concentration boundary layers for transport in the reverse direction, namely, from endothelial lining to blood.

The inset in Figure 4.26, on p. 226 should aid understanding of the coupling of fluid motion with diffusion processes, which underlies the development of the concentration boundary layer. A highly schematic representative trajectory of a substance released at just a single site on the activating wall is shown. This trajectory embodies the effects of the two coupled processes on the spread of the substance: in the axial (streamwise) direction, the entrained substance covers a distance proportional to time, t; in the radial (cross-stream) direction, it covers a distance that is proportional to merely the square root of time, $\sqrt{t}$. Note the effect that accrues on the highly schematized, linearized trajectory, as the substance moves away from the wall and into higher axial velocity laminae: the slope of the linearized depiction of its trajectory becomes progressively smaller. The region of influence of the wall corresponds to the concentration boundary layer.

References and further reading

[1] Alberts, B., Johnson, A., Lewis, J., Raff, M., Roberts, K., Walter, P. Molecular biology of the cell. 4th edn. 2002, New York: Garland Science. xxxiv, 1463, [86] p.

[2] Aragón, J.L., Naumis, G. G., Bai, M., Torres, M., Maini, P.K. Kolmogorov scaling in impassioned van Gogh paintings. arXiv:physics/0606246 v1 28 Jun 2006.

[3] Aref, H. [Ed.] Chaos applied to fluid mixing. 1995, Oxford, UK; New York: Pergamon. vi, 380 p.

[4] Batchelor, G.K., An introduction to fluid dynamics. 2nd pbk. ed. 1999, Cambridge, UK; New York: Cambridge University Press. xviii, 615 p., 24 of plates.

[5] Bernoulli, D., Bernoulli, J. Hydrodynamics. 1968, New York: Dover Publications. xv, 456 p.

[6] Bird, J.J., Murgo, J.P., Pasipoularides, A. Fluid dynamics of aortic stenosis: Subvalvular gradients without subvalvular obstruction. Circulation 66: 835–40, 1982.

[7] Blumer, D. The Illness of Vincent van Gogh. Am. J. Psychiatry 159: 519–26, 2002.

[8] Bradshaw, P. An introduction to turbulence and its measurement. 1971, Oxford, New York: Pergamon Press. xviii, 218 p.

[9] Brunet, P. Pattern-forming instabilities: a phenomenological approach through simple examples. Eur. J. Phys. 28: 215–30, 2007.

[10] Bushnell, D.M., Hefner, J.M. [Eds.] Viscous drag reduction in boundary layers. (Progress in Astronautics and Aeronautics, Vol. 123) 1990, Washington, DC: American Institute of Aeronautics and Astronautics. xv, 517 p.

[11] Bushnell, D.M., Moore, K.J. Drag reduction in nature. Annu. Rev. Fluid Mech. 23: 65–79, 1991.

[12] Condos, W.R., Jr., Latham, R.D., Hoadley, S.D., Pasipoularides, A. Hemodynamics of the Mueller maneuver in man: right and left heart micromanometry and Doppler echocardiography. Circulation 76: 1020–8, 1987.

[13] Constantinescu, V.N. Laminar viscous flow. 1995, New York: Springer. xv, 488 p.

[14] Davidson, P.A. Turbulence: an introduction for scientists and engineers. 2004, Oxford, UK; New York: Oxford University Press. xix, 657 p.

[15] de Nevers, N. Fluid mechanics for chemical engineers. 3rd ed. 2005, New York: McGraw-Hill Chemical Engineering Series. xxiii, 632 p.

[16] Drazin, P.G. Introduction to hydrodynamic stability. Cambridge texts in applied mathematics. 2002, Cambridge, UK; New York: Cambridge University Press. xvii, 258 p.

[17] Eckert, M. The dawn of fluid dynamics: a discipline between science and technology. 2006, Weinheim, Germany; Chichester, UK: Wiley–VCH; John Wiley. x, 286 p.

[18] Evans, H.L. Laminar boundary-layer theory. 1968, Reading, Mass.: Addison–Wesley ix, 229 p.

[19] Farthing S., Peronneau P. Flow in the thoracic aorta. Cardiovasc. Res. 13: 607–20, 1979.

[20] Ffowcs Williams, J.E. Sound sources in aerodynamics—fact and fiction. AIAA J. 20: 307–15, 1982.

[21] Fornberg, B. A numerical study of two-dimensional turbulence. J. Comput. Phys. 25: 1–31, 1977.

[22] Fox, R.O. On the relationship between Lagrangian micromixing models and computational fluid dynamics. Chem. Eng. Proc. 37: 521–35, 1998.

[23] Frisch, U., Kolmogorov, A.N. Turbulence: the legacy of A.N. Kolmogorov. 1995, Cambridge, UK; New York: Cambridge University Press. xiii, 296 p.

[24] Galdi, G.P. An introduction to the mathematical theory of the Navier–Stokes equations. Springer tracts in natural philosophy; v. 38–39. 1994, New York: Springer–Verlag. v. <1–2 >.

[25] Gayford, M. The yellow house: Van Gogh, Gauguin, and nine turbulent weeks in Arles. 2006, Brighton, England: Fig Tree Press; Penguin. 368 p.

[26] Geankoplis, C.J. Transport processes and separation process principles: includes unit operations. 2003, Upper Saddle River, NJ: Prentice Hall Professional Technical Reference. xiii, 1026 p.

[27] Georgiadis, J.G., Wang, M., Pasipoularides, A. Computational fluid dynamics of left ventricular ejection. Ann. Biomed. Eng. 20: 81–97, 1992.

[28] Gibson, A.H. Osborne Reynolds and his work in hydraulics and hydrodynamics. 1946, London, New York: Pub. for the British Council by Longmans. 33 p.

[29] Goldstein, S., Aeronautical Research Council (Great Britain), Modern developments in fluid dynamics; an account of theory and experiment relating to boundary layers, turbulent motion and wakes. 1965, New York: Dover. 2 v. (xxviii, 702 p.).

[30] Granger, R.A. Fluid mechanics. 1985, New York: Holt Rinehart and Winston. xii, 884 p.

[31] Hasegawa A. Self-organization processes in continuous media. Adv. Phys. 34: 1–42, 1985.

[32] Hunt, J.C.R., Vassilicos, J.C. Turbulence structure and vortex dynamics. 2000, Cambridge, UK: Cambridge University Press. xiii, 306 p.

[33] Hussain, A.K.M.F. Coherent structures and turbulence, J. Fluid Mech. 173: 303–56, 1986.

[34] Indeikina, A., Chang, H.-C. Estimate of turbulent eddy diffusion by exact renormalization. SIAP (Society for Industrial and Applied Mathematics), 63: 1–41, 2002.

[35] Isaaz, K., Pasipoularides, A. Noninvasive assessment of intrinsic ventricular load dynamics in dilated cardiomyopathy. J. Am. Coll. Cardiol. 17: 112–21, 1991.

[36] Kramer, M.O. Boundary layer stabilization by distributed damping. J. Aeronaut. Sci. 24: 459–60, 1957.

[37] Kramer, M.O. The Dolphin's secret. J. Am. Soc. Nav. Eng. 73: 103–7, 1961.

[38] Ku, D.N. Blood Flow in Arteries. Annu. Rev. Fluid Mech. 29: 399–434, 1997.

[39] Lagerstrom, P.A., Moore, F.K. Laminar flow theory. 1996, Princeton, N.J.: Princeton University Press. 268 p.

[40] Lamb, H. Hydrodynamics. 6th ed. 1932, Cambridge [England]: Cambridge University Press. xv, 738 p.

[41] Latham, R.D., Westerhof, N., Sipkema, P., Rubal, B.J., Reuderink, P., Murgo, J.P. Regional wave travel and reflections along the human aorta: A study with six simultaneous micromanometric pressures. Circulation 72: 1257–69, 1985.

[42] Libby, P. Inflammation in atherosclerosis. Nature (Lond.) 420: 868–74, 2002.

[43] Liggett, J.A. Fluid mechanics. 1994, New York: McGraw-Hill. xxviii, 495 p.

[44] Lighthill, M.J. On Sound Generated Aerodynamically, I. General Theory. Proc. Royal Soc., A211: 564–87, 1952.

[45] Malkin, A.Ya., Isayev, A.I. Rheology: concepts, methods and applications. 2006, Toronto: ChemTec Pub. xii, 474 p.

[46] Mathieu, J., Scott, J. An introduction to turbulent flow. 2000, Cambridge, UK; New York: Cambridge University Press. ix, 374 p.

[47] McComb, W.D. The physics of fluid turbulence. Oxford Engineering Science Series, 25. Oxford Science Publications. 1991, New York: The Clarendon Press, Oxford University Press. xxiv, 572 p.

[48] McCormack, P.D., Crane, L. Physical fluid dynamics. 1973, New York: Academic Press. xxiii, 487 p.

[49] Meunier, P., Villermaux, E. How vortices mix. J. Fluid Mech. 476: 213–22, 2003.

[50] Merzkirch, W. Flow visualization. 2nd ed. 1987, Orlando: Academic Press. x, 260 p.

[51] Mirsky, I., Pasipoularides, A. Clinical assessment of diastolic function. Prog. Cardiovas. Diseases 32: 291–318, 1990.

[52] Newton, I., et al., Sir Isaac Newton's Mathematical principles of natural philosophy and his System of the world. 1934, Berkeley, CA: University of California press. xxxv, 680 p. incl. front. (port.) facsim.

[53] Pasipoularides, A. Clinical assessment of ventricular ejection dynamics with and without outflow obstruction. [Review]. J. Am. Coll. Cardiol. 15((4)): 859–82, 1990.

[54] Pasipoularides, A. Cardiac mechanics: basic and clinical contemporary research. Ann. Biomed. Eng. 20: 3–17, 1992.

[55] Pasipoularides, A. Contribution to the study of pulsatile flowsin large arterial branchings. PhD Thesis, University of Minnesota (Mpls). UMI (University Microfilms International)/Bell and Howell Information and Learning, 1972.

[56] Pasipoularides, A., Murgo, J.P., Miller, J.W., Craig, W.E. Nonobstructive left ventricular ejection pressure gradients in man. Circ. Res. 61: 220–7, 1987.

[57] Pasipoularides, A., Murgo, J.P., Bird, J.J., Craig, W.E. Fluid dynamics of aortic stenosis: Mechanisms for the presence of subvalvular pressure gradients. Am. J. Physiol. 246: H542–50, 1984.

[58] Pasipoularides, A.D., Shu, M., Womack, M.S., Shah, A., von Ramm, O., Glower, D.D. RV functional imaging: 3-D echo-derived dynamic geometry and flow field simulations. Am. J. Physiol. Heart Circ. Physiol. 284: H56–65, 2003.

[59] Pasipoularides, A., Shu, M., Shah, A., Womack, M.S., Glower, D.D. Diastolic right ventricular filling vortex in normal and volume overload states. Am. J. Physiol. Heart Circ. Physiol. 284: H1064–72, 2003.

[60] Pasipoularides, A., Shu, M., Shah, A., Tucconi, A., Glower, D.D. RV instantaneous intraventricular diastolic pressure and velocity distributions in normal and volume overload awake dog disease models. Am. J. Physiol. Heart Circ. Physiol. 285: H1956–65, 2003.

[61] Persen, L.N. Introduction to boundary layer theory. 1972, Trondheim: Tapir. 6 l., 210 p., l.

[62] Pozrikidis, C. Little book of streamlines. 1999, San Diego: Academic Press. xiii, 148 p.

[63] Reynolds, O. An experimental investigation of the circumstances which determine whether the motion of water in parallel channels shall be direct or sinuous and of the law of resistance in parallel channels. Philos. Trans. R. Soc. 174: 935–82, 1883.

[64] Reynolds, O. On the dynamical theory of incompressible viscous fluids and the determination of the criterion. Philos. Trans. R. Soc. 186:123–64, 1895.

[65] Richardson, L. F. Weather prediction by numerical process. 1922, Cambridge, England: Cambridge University Press, 236 p. [Reprinted by Dover Publications, 1965].

[66] Rogers, D.F. Laminar flow analysis. 1992, Cambridge, UK; New York: Cambridge University Press. xiv, 422 p.

[67] Rosenhead, L. Laminar boundary layers; an account of the development, structure, and stability of laminar boundary layers in incompressible fluids, together with a description of the associated experimental techniques. Fluid motion memoirs. 1963, Oxford, UK: Clarendon Press. 687 p.

[68] Rouse, H. Elementary mechanics of fluids. 1978, New York: Dover Publications. viii, 376 p.

[69] Russell, D.A. On the sound field radiated by a tuning fork. Am. J. Physics 68: 1139–45, 2000.

[70] Samimy, M., Breuer, K.S., Leal, L.G, Steen, P.H. A gallery of fluid motion. 2003, Cambridge New York: Cambridge University Press. x, 118 p.

[71] Satchell, G.H. Physiology and form of fish circulation. 1991, Cambridge; New York: Cambridge University Press. xvi, 235 p.

[72] Sato, M., Ohashi, T. Biorheological views of endothelial cell responses to mechanical stimuli. Biorheology 42: 421–41, 2005.

[73] Schetz, J.A. Foundations of boundary layer theory for momentum, heat, and mass transfer. 1984, Englewood Cliffs, NJ: Prentice-Hall. xxi, 309 p.

[74] Schlichting, H., Gersten, K. Boundary-layer theory. 8th rev. and enl. ed. 2000, Berlin, Germany; New York: Springer. xxiii, 799 p.

[75] Segadal, L., Matre, K. Blood velocity distribution in the human ascending aorta. Circulation 76: 90–100, 1987.

[76] Shahcheraghi, N., Dwyer, H.A., Cheer, A.Y., Barakat, A.I. and Rutaganira, T. Unsteady and three-dimensional simulation of blood flow in the human aortic arch. J. Biomech. Eng. 124: 378–87, 2002.

[77] Shapiro, A.H. Shape and flow; the fluid dynamics of drag. 1961, Garden City, N.Y.: Anchor Books. 186 p.

[78] Shim, Y., Hampton, T.G., Straley, C,A., Harrison, J.K., Spero, L.A., Bashore, T.M., Pasipoularides, A.D. Ejection load changes in aortic stenosis. Observations made after balloon aortic valvuloplasty. Circ. Res. 71: 1174–84, 1992.

[79] Shim, Y.T., Pasipoularides, A., Straley, C.A., Hampton, T.G., Soto, P.F., Owen, C.H., Davis, J.W., Glower, D.D. Arterial Windkessel parameter-estimation: a new time-domain method. Ann. Biomed. Engin., 22: 66–77, 1994.

[80] Starr, V.P. Physics of negative viscosity phenomena. 1968, New York: McGraw-Hill. xv, 256 p.

[81] Tavoularis, S. Measurement in fluid mechanics. 2005, Cambridge, UK; New York: Cambridge University Press. xiii, 354 p.

[82] Telionis, D.P. Unsteady viscous flows. 1981, New York: Springer-Verlag. xxiii, 408 p.

[83] Tennekes, H., Lumley, J.L. A first course in turbulence. 1972, Cambridge, Mass.: MIT Press. xii, 300 p.

[84] Thomas, M.D. On the nonlinear stability of flows over compliant walls. J. Fluid. Mech. 239: 657–70, 1992.

[85] Toms, B.A. Some observations on the flow of linear polymer solutions through straight tubes at large Reynolds numbers. Proc. Int. Cong. Rheol. 2: 135–41, 1949.

[86] Tritton, D.J. Physical fluid dynamics. 2nd ed. 1988, Oxford [England] New York: Clarendon Press; Oxford University Press. xvii, 519 p.

[87] Visualization Society of Japan. Fantasy of flow: the world of fluid flow captured in photographs. 1993, Amsterdam; Washington, DC: Ohmsha, Tokyo; IOS Press. 184 p.

[88] von Kàrmàn, T. Aerodynamics: selected topics in the light of their historical development. 2004, Mineola, NY: Dover. ix, 203 p.

[89] Whitaker, S. Introduction to fluid mechanics. Reprint 1981 w/corrections. 1981, Malabar, FL: Krieger. xiii, 457 p.

[90] Wootton, D.M., Ku, D.N. Fluid mechanics of vascular systems, diseases, and thrombosis. Ann. Rev. Biomed. Eng. 1: 299–329, 1999.

[91] Wu, J.Z., Ma, H.Y., Zhou, M.D. Vorticity and vortex dynamics. 2006, Berlin, Germany; New York: Springer. xiv, 776 p.

Chapter 5

Micromanometric, Velocimetric, Angio- and Echocardiographic Measurements

At the same time, I carried out my first experiments in angiocardiography. Here for the first time the living heart of a dog was successfully visualized radiologically with the aid of a contrast medium.—Werner Forssmann, Nobel Lecture, December 11, 1956.

——From *Nobel Lectures, Physiology or Medicine 1942–1962,* Elsevier Publishing Company, Amsterdam, 1964.

Science meets with two obstacles, the deficiency of our senses to discover the facts and the insufficiency of our language to describe them. The object of the graphic methods is to get around these two obstacles: to grasp the fine details, which would be otherwise unobserved; and to transcribe them with a clarity superior to that of our words.

——Étienne-Jules Marey, quoted by Aldo Luisada [25].

DYNAMIC GEOMETRIC, velocimetric and pressure field measurements on the heart are critical to understanding cardiac dynamics and intracardiac blood flow phenomena. An outcome of advances in computer technology and changing clinical perspectives has been, in recent decades, the rapid development of a wide range of techniques for imaging dynamic cardiac geometry, and for examinations of the unsteady (pulsatile) intracardiac pressure and velocity fields. Important in this regard are:

a. Cardiac catheterization and angiography, including digital subtraction angiography (DSA), and

b. echocardiography and Doppler velocimetry, various implementations of which we will study in both the present chapter and in Chapter 10.

c. Computed tomography (CT), and magnetic resonance imaging (MRI), which we will study in Chapter 10.

5.1 Hemodynamic data aquisition at catheterization

The cardiac catheterization procedure involves the acquisition of angiographic images and of hemodynamic and electrocardiographic waveforms, the calculation of cardiac output and intracardiac shunts, possible diagnostic provocations and operative interventions with post-interventional waveform acquisitions, and the evaluation of cardiac function based on those data [4–8,13,19,20,31,34,43,52,55]. At cardiac catheterization, the complete diagnostic picture of the heart, its valves, and the coronary and great vessels, is revealed by the integrated set of images, waveform measurements, and other collected recordings, frequently encompassing echocardiographic and Doppler datasets (see Fig. 5.1).

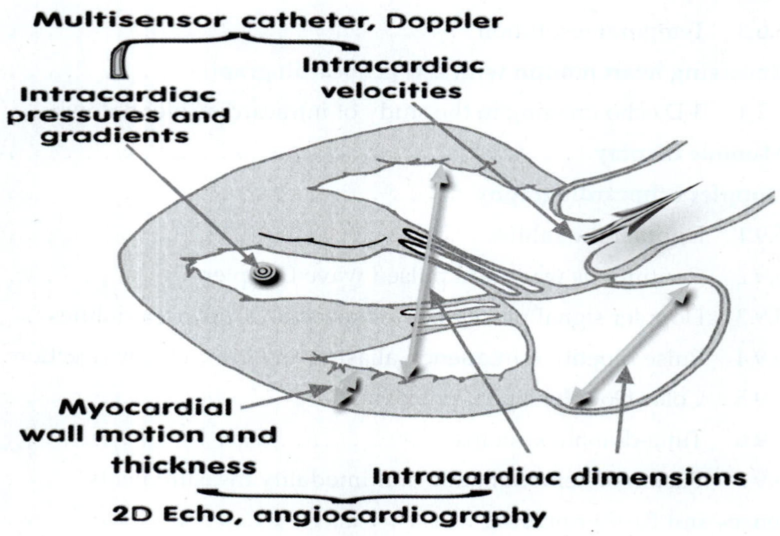

Figure 5.1: Dynamic geometric and hemodynamic measurements acquired at cardiac catheterization.

5.1.1 Hemodynamic data acquisition systems

Hemodynamic data acquisition systems interface between the world of physiological parameters, which are analog, and the world of digital representation and computation. The devices that perform the interfacing function between analog and digital worlds are the analog-to-digital (A/D) and digital-to-analog (D/A) converters. With current emphasis on digital imaging and storage systems, the interfacing function has become an important one; digital systems are used widely because they are accurate and relatively simple to implement. In addition, there is rapid growth in the use of workstations and personal computers to perform digital measurement, computer display and video signal processing functions.

Besides A/D and D/A converters, hemodynamic data acquisition systems contain transducers, "sample-and-hold" modules, gain amplifiers, filters, nonlinear analog functions, and analog multiplexers. The interconnection of these components is shown in the diagram of Figure 5.2, on p. 237; while the configuration depicted is a common acquisition system configuration, there are alternative ones. The inputs to the system are physiological

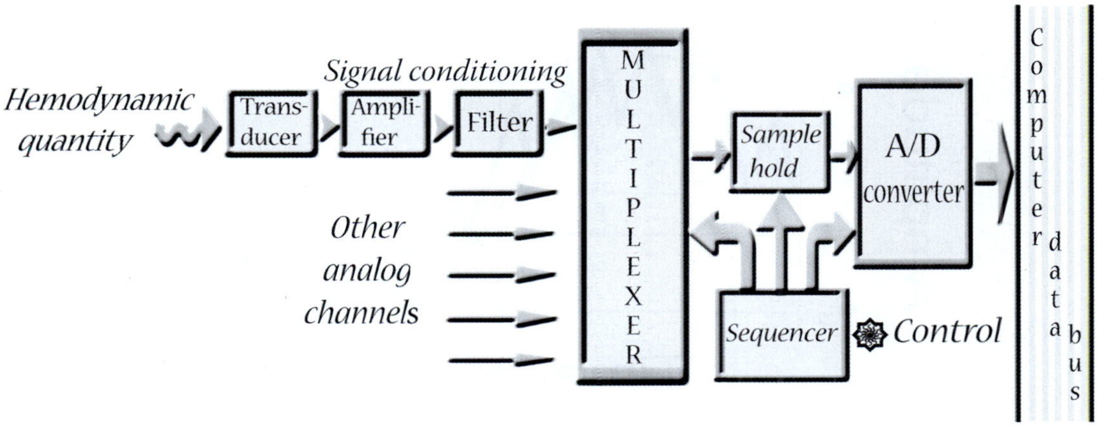

Figure 5.2: Catheterization hemodynamic data acquisition system.

parameters, such as pressure, flow, and acceleration, which are analog quantities. Each hemodynamic variable is first converted into an electrical signal by means of a transducer; once in electrical form, all further processing is done by electronic circuits.

Transducer outputs may be signals measured in millivolts or microvolts, too small for applying directly to low-gain, multiplexed data acquisition system input ports, so some amplification is necessary. Such signals are *first* amplified to an appropriate level before they can be further processed; otherwise, the amplifier noise, as well as interference voltages from various sources, would get amplified as well. For an improved signal-to-noise ratio (SNR), it is necessary to use dedicated, very low-noise *preamplifiers*.

Preamplifiers boost the transducer outputs to 1–10 V levels, and also condition the transducer signal (which may be a high-impedance signal, a differential signal with common-mode noise,[1] a current output, a signal superimposed on a high voltage, or a combination of these) for further processing. *Instrumentation amplifiers* are particularly suitable as preamplifiers, and have a committed response, e.g., the amplification of a voltage difference with a gain either fixed or selectable by means of a single resistor, or a jumper. Thus, differential amplifiers amplify differential-mode signals and reject common-mode signals. Instrumentation amplifiers typically have extremely low internal noise and drift and a moderate gain range.

An amplifier is expected to raise the level of input signals within its operating frequency range without any preference for any frequencies. This means that it must have a *flat* frequency response. Moreover, the performance of an amplifier should not have any

[1]Common-mode noise or interference is occasionally inherent in an instrument design, but most often it is inductively or capacitively coupled from an external source. A familiar example of common-mode noise is the 60-*Hz* signal induced on a pair of wires by nearby power lines. In this case, the noise signal is "common" to each of the two wires. Common-mode rejection quantifies the ability of a device to tolerate common-mode noise. For amplifiers, it is usually specified in dB (see Section 2.17.1, on pp. 77 f.), as the ratio of the differential mode gain to the common-mode gain.

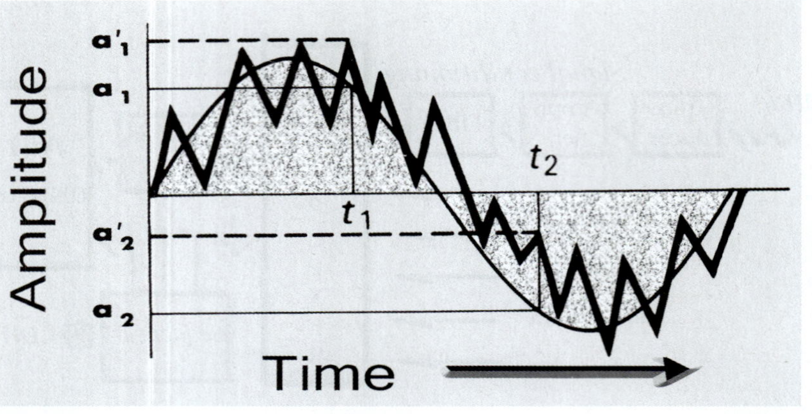

Figure 5.3: Effects of noise on analog signals. Noise on a signal can cause incorrect amplitude values to be read during analog-to-digital conversion. Sometimes the difference is small, as at time t_1, where the read amplitude ($a_1{'}$) is nearly the same as the true signal amplitude (a_1). In other cases, the difference may be considerable, as shown at time t_2, where the received amplitude ($a_2{'}$) is markedly different from the true signal amplitude (a_2).

deficiencies, imperfections or peculiarities that may lead to vitiating noise (see Fig. 5.3) and various forms of signal distortion (cf. Fig. 5.4, on p. 240).

The amplifier is commonly followed by a low-pass filter (see Fig. 2.26, on p. 77) that removes high-frequency signal components, electrical interference and electronic noise. It may also be followed by special nonlinear analog function circuits, called *function modules* [54], which can perform multiplication, division, squaring, and other mathematical operations on the signal, for cases in which it is preferable to condition and process signals by analogue rather than digital means.

The processed analog signals are next transmitted to a multiplexer, which can switch sequentially between the different channels. Each input is, in turn, connected by the multiplexer switch to the output of the multiplexer for a specified time interval. Because with multiplexing the samples from multiple channels are taken sequentially, they are not simultaneous: there is a delay between each successive signal, causing so-called *sampling skew* [60]. This introduces issues of relative timing between ostensibly simultaneous signal samples from the various recording channels, especially when instantaneous values of impulsively developed pressure gradients, or differences, are derived digitally from simultaneous measurements of rapidly varying intracardiac pressures. The multiplexer-induced delay can be predicted from the sampling rate used and the number of channels.

Sampling skew can be diminished by a more rapid sampling rate, but the amount of data thus recorded can become too great. Alternatively, the A/D converter can be set up to accept the samples from all the channels sequentially as quickly as it will run, then wait until the next sample batch is due. Suppose that eight channels are used and that the sampling rate is $100\ Hz$. The maximum sampling rate of the A/D converter may be much higher, say, 40 kHz. Then, using *burst mode* sampling, the A/D converter can be set up to record sequentially from all eight channels at this high rate, so that the incremental delay between successive signals is only 25 μs. When all eight channels have been sampled, the A/D converter waits the remaining 9.825 ms until the next burst mode sampling "point."

A method that effectively eliminates sampling skew altogether entails using a "sample-and-hold" circuit on each channel. The sample-hold circuit effectively acquires a *snapshot* of the value of the individual analog signal voltage when the A/D converter starts con verting and then holds it constant while the converter converts it into digital form. At each sampling "point," the signals on all channels are effectively frozen by the sample-hold circuit. Thus, the A/D converter can digitize each successive signal with no sampling skew. The resultant digital word (see Section 2.16.1, on pp. 71 f.) goes to the input of a digital circuit, or to the data bus of a catheterization lab computer, as is shown in Figure 5.2, on p. 237.

In sum, appropriate apparatus and software precondition analog hemodynamic signals and convert the preconditioned catheterization signals into their digital representations. The procedure includes preconditioning the analog signal, generating a quantity N of reference signals, comparing an amplitude of the preconditioned signal to an amplitude of the reference signals, to determine whether the preconditioned signal amplitude is greater than, less than or equal to reference signal amplitudes, and producing a timestamp at a time that the preconditioned signal and reference signal amplitudes are equal. The apparatus generally includes a preconditioner, a reference signal generator, and a quantity, N, of comparators [21]. The assembly of the N comparators receives the preconditioned signal from the preconditioner, separately receives a reference signal, and produces a digital signal (see Fig. 5.2, and Section 2.17, on pp. 72 ff.). The preconditioned analog signal, or the "original" analog signal, may be reconstructed from the digital representation.

5.1.2 Nyquist theorem and aliasing

Transforming a hemodynamic signal from the time domain to the frequency domain requires the application of the Nyquist sampling theorem: if a signal only contains frequencies less than a *cutoff, or Nyquist, frequency*, f_c or f_N, all the information in the signal can be captured by sampling it at a minimum frequency of $2 \cdot f_c$—see the detailed discussion in Section 2.17 of Chapter 2, on pp. 72 ff. However, experience suggests that while working in the frequency domain, the sampling rate must be set more than twice and preferably between five and ten times the signal's highest frequency component. Waveforms viewed in the time domain are usually sampled at 10 times the highest frequency (for most purposes, 30–40 Hz) required to faithfully reproduce the original signal and to retain accurate reproduction of the signal's highest frequency components.

If you fail to heed the sampling theorem, you not only lose the meaningful higher frequencies, but the frequencies above one-half the Nyquist frequency, f_N, actually fold back into the spectrum. Thus, when input signals are sampled at less than the Nyquist rate, spurious frequency components that are much lower in frequency than those actually

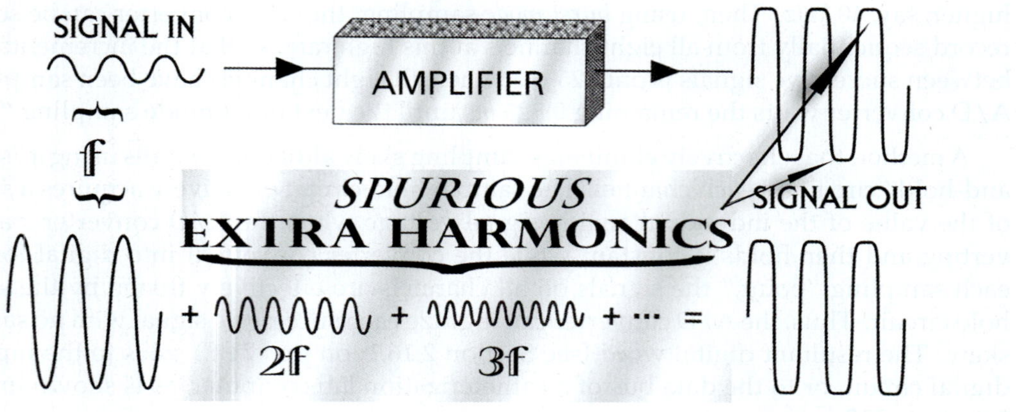

Figure 5.4: An amplifier may introduce *harmonic distortion* in the amplified signal. The amplitudes of the harmonic frequencies, which depend on the amplitude and the frequency of the applied input sine wave, are generally given as a *dB-ratio* with respect to the amplitude of the applied sine-wave input (see Section 2.17.1, on pp. 77 ff.). Their frequencies are usually expressed as a multiple of the frequency of the applied sinusoidal input signal.

composing the signal being sampled can appear in the time domain, a phenomenon that is referred to as *aliasing* (see Fig. 2.25 on p. 76). If, watching a western movie, you have ever seen the wheel of a fast-rolling wagon appear to be going backwards, you have witnessed aliasing. The camera's frame rate is not adequate to reproduce the rotational frequency of the wheel, and our eyes are deceived by the misinformation! Similarly, in recording music, with its many frequencies and harmonics, aliased components can mix with the real frequencies to yield dissonant distortions. The *disguising* of higher frequencies as lower frequencies is inherent in aliasing. To prevent aliases, an antialiasing, low-pass filter with a cutoff frequency greater than $(1/2) \cdot f_N$ may be applied judiciously,[2] in order to remove all of the contaminating high-frequencies.

5.1.3 Circular discontinuity and windowing

When pulsatile hemodynamic signals pass through a time-invariant, linear system, their amplitude and phase components can change but their frequencies remain intact. This process takes place when the continuous time domain signal passes through an A/D converter to the discrete-time domain. Sometimes, more useful information can be obtained from the hemodynamic waveforms by analyzing them in the discrete time domain with a Fourier series rather than reconstructing the original signal in the time domain. The sampled data pass through a Fourier transform function to cull out the fundamental and harmonic frequency information, as we discussed in conjunction with Figure 2.34 on

[2] Although the filter eliminates the aliases, it also prevents any other frequency components that are above the stop band of the filter from passing through.

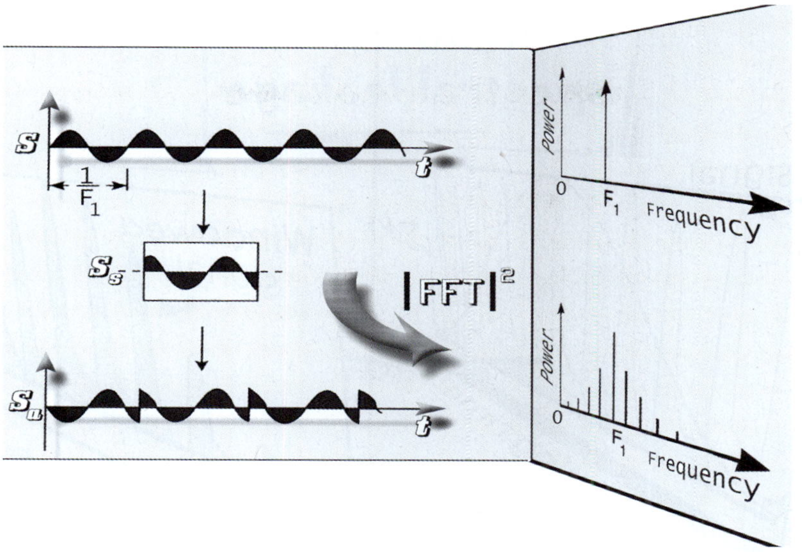

Figure 5.5: The power spectrum (shown in the graphs on the right) is the rms (*root mean square*) of the amplitude of each sine or cosine component of a waveform plotted at the frequency for that component. It graphs the "power," which is proportional to the *square* of the amplitude, versus the frequency for each sine wave in the reconstruction of the waveform. The FFT method finds negative as well as positive frequencies although, as is portrayed here, only the *positive* frequencies are needed to describe the periodic function. As is shown in the top panels, the true spectrum of a simple sinusoidal signal ($S(t)$) is a single line, or *impulse*. However, $S(t)$ is sampled through a finite time interval as $S_s(t)$, and the FFT assumes $S_s(t)$ to repeat indefinitely beyond the sampling time interval, as a new assumed periodic function $S_a(t)$. This leads to *spectral leakage*, depicted in the bottom right panel.

p. 93, in Section 2.18 in Chapter 2. The amplitude of the signal is displayed in the vertical axis, and the frequencies measured are plotted on the horizontal axis.

Real-time measurements are taken over finite time intervals. In contrast, Fourier transforms are defined over infinite time intervals, so limiting the transform to a discrete time interval yields sampled data that are only approximations. Consequently, the resolution of the Fourier transform is limited to approximately $1/T$, where T is the finite time interval over which the measurement was aquired. The Fourier transform resolution (higher-frequency content) can only be improved by sampling for a longer interval.

If we only measure the signal for a short time, the Fourier transform works as if the dataset were *periodic* for all time. If not quite an integral number of cycles fit into the total duration of the measurement, then when the Fourier Transform assumes that the signal repeats, the end of one signal segment does not connect smoothly with the beginning of the next. As a result of this, a finite time interval used for a Fourier transform can generate spurious oscillations, i.e., high *side lobes*, in the amplitude spectrum plot. This phenomenon is called *spectral leakage* (see Fig. 5.6). When the signal is periodic and

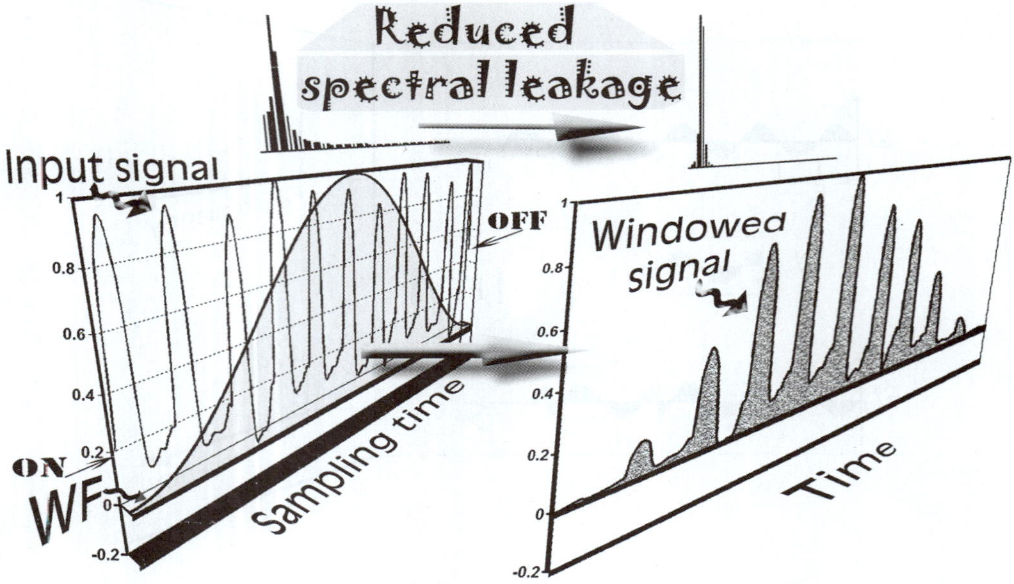

Figure 5.6: *Circular discontinuity* comes about by having the sampled signal effectively turn on (ON arrow) instantaneously at the beginning of the measurement and then turn off again instantaneously (OFF arrow) from a *different* arbitrary value at the end of the measurement. In this illustration, we employ a micromanometric right ventricular (RV) pressure pulse train from a dog with experimental RV pressure overload, normalized to the maximum value observed in the sample, to eliminate ordinate magnitudes disparity. Multiplying the sampled data, by a windowing function (WF) makes the ends of the windowed signal match by forcing them to be both *zero*.

an integer number of periods fill the acquisition time interval, or *aquisition buffer*, the Fourier transform turns out fine. When the number of periods in the acquisition is not an integer, the endpoints do not match and the result is spectral leakage.

From a geometric viewpoint, for the Nyquist theorem to work correctly, the data must have *circular continuity*. To understand what circular continuity is, draw a curve from end to end on a piece of paper and then form a tube with the curve on the outside by rolling the paper across the curve. Circular continuity exists if there is no "discontinuity" where the start of the curve meets the end of the curve. This means that the first point on the curve must be equal to the last point. In fact, the principle of circular continuity goes further: The slope of the curve at the start must equal the slope of the curve at the end. The slope of the slopes (the second derivative) must also be continuous. Discontinuities are by definition high-frequency changes in the data. If you do not have circular continuity and you reconstruct the curve from its Fourier representation, you will be violating the assumption that only frequencies of less than half of the sampling frequency are present in the data. If this occurs, there will be present in the reconstructed curve spurious oscillations that have high amplitudes at the endpoints of the curve. These oscillations become smaller the farther you get from the endpoints, but they become much more prominent if derivatives are calculated.

From a mathematical viewpoint, this is caused by the signal being effectively instantaneously turned on at the beginning of the measurement and then instantaneously turned off from a *different* arbitrary value at the end of the measurement. The result is a misinterpretation of the periodic signal by the Fourier transform procedure, as if there were a regular periodic discontinuity, causing spurious spectral components. These spurious oscillations can be eliminated by shaping the signal so that its ends match more smoothly. This is accomplished, as shown in Figure 5.6, on p. 242, by applying a function called *windowing*, that is, multiplying the sampled data by a weighting function that makes the ends of the sampled signal match by forcing them to be zero. In this way, their value is necessarily the same. Actually, we also want to make sure that the signal is going in the right direction at the ends, so as to match up smoothly. The easiest way to do this is to make sure neither end is going anywhere: that is, the slope of the signal at its ends should also be zero. Put mathematically, a *window function* has the property that its value and all its derivatives are zero at the ends. Any window function that rises and falls smoothly and gradually from zero decreases the spurious oscillations. There are different types of window functions available (Hamming window, Hann window, Bartlett window, and so forth), each with their own advantages and preferred applications [42].

5.2 Hemodynamic measurements

Basic hemodynamic measurements encompass simultaneous transvalvular and intracardiac pressure and flow velocity determinations using right- and left-heart high-fidelity multisensor catheters, as well as cardiac output (C.O.) assessments.[3] Endomyocardial biopsy and evaluation of intracardiac electrical activity can also be performed. Blood gas measurements allow localization of cardiac shunts accompanying congenital malformations, and are also needed for C.O. measurements by Fick's method.

The frequency response of the micromanometric pressure measuring system that is utilized can be determined by connecting to the chamber of a pressure generator (e.g., WGA-200,™ Millar Instruments, Houston, TX) and comparing the output pressure to a measured sinusoidal input pressure, by measuring the amplitude ratio and phase lag over a desired operating frequency range. Traditional fluid-filled catheter systems have a low resonant frequency (25–35 *Hz*) and therefore are prone to have a variety of inherent artifacts, with loss of signal integrity. Pressure damping due to air bubbles in the catheter lumen is common. Significant resonance and motion artifacts occur, which may interfere with accurate pressure and pressure gradient measurements. Because Millar micromanometric catheters measure pressure directly *at the source*, they minimize artifacts caused by the beating of the heart (catheter whip), patient movement, motion of the catheter inside the body, or inadvertent generation of pressure disturbances at any point along the length of the catheter. Other important advantages compared to a fluid-filled catheter are that there are no resonance artifacts, no dampening of pressure caused by

[3] C.O. is the volume of blood ejected by each ventricle per minute; various methods are used to calculate the C.O. The most commonly used are the Fick (most accurate, but cumbersome), indicator-dilution, and thermodilution (renders itself best to multiple, sequential determinations) techniques.

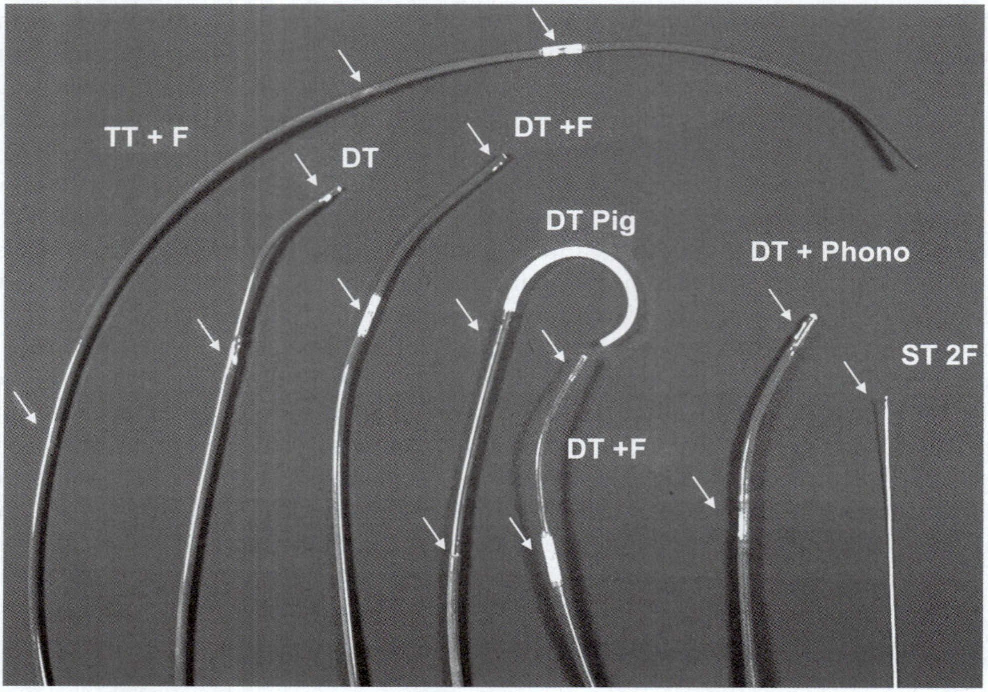

Figure 5.7: Representative Millar multisensor catheters—arrows indicate location of solid-state microsensors. DT = *double-tip* micromanometer catheter; ST = *single-tip* micromanometer; TT = *triple-tip* micromanometer; F = flowmeter velocimetric sensor; Pig = angiography (*"pigtail"*) catheter; Phono = phonocardiographic sensor; 2F = 2 French size.

the transduction of the pressure signal *after* transmission through a fluid column, and no frequency-dependent signal propagation time-delays.[4]

The Millar micromanometric catheters (Millar Instruments, Houston, TX) have a high bandwidth with a flat frequency response to 10 *kHz* [28,32], allowing for a true reproduction of fast transients in recorded pressure signals, which contain harmonics of varying frequencies, without loss of information [37–40]. They come with a variety of catheter-mounted micromanometric and velocimetric microsensors, and in a wide range of what is known as French sizes (see Fig. 5.7). "French size" is a scale used to identify the outer diameter of a catheter. French scale units are obtained by multiplying the outer diameter (O.D.) of the catheter, in *mm*, by 3. Consequently, multiplying the French size by 0.33 will give the outer diameter of the catheter in *mm*.[5]

[4] On the other hand, the proper use of these catheters, including retrograde crossing of the stenosed aortic valve, is difficult for those who do not use them regularly. Calibration requires the help of sophisticated laboratory staff who use these devices regularly.

[5] Another useful relationship is the multiplication of inches by 25.4 to convert to *mm*. It follows that, e.g., 6F = 1.98 *mm* O.D. = .078 in O.D.

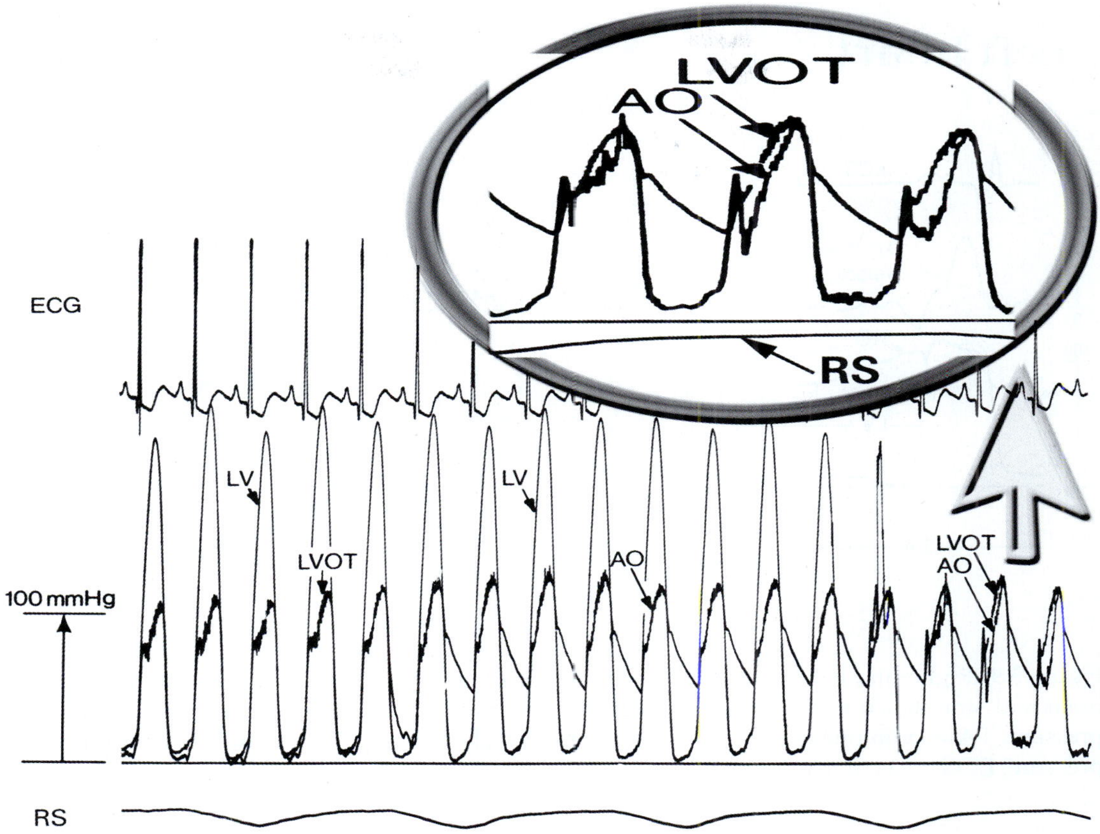

Figure 5.8: Catheterization hemodynamic data obtained from a patient evaluated for aortic stenosis by a left-heart Millar "double-tip" catheter—5 *cm* distance between the micromanometers. The catheter pullback reveals that the "transvalvular" pressure gradient is, nearly in its entirety, *intraventricular* in origin ("magnifying lense" inset). AO = aortic root pressure; LV = deep left ventricular pressure; LVOT = left ventricular outflow tract pressure; ECG = electrocardiogram; RS = respiration signal.

For measurement of left-heart transvalvular, or intraventricular pressure gradients, a left-heart catheter containing two equisensitive solid-state pressure sensors (Mikro-Tip,™ Millar Instruments) is used via a brachial (Sones technique) or a femoral (Judkins technique) arteriotomy approach. The catheter is directed into the left ventricle retrogradely through the aortic orifice, under fluoroscopic guidance. Figure 5.8 demonstrates micromanometric signals obtained at cardiac catheterization from a patient evaluated for aortic stenosis by a left-heart Millar dual pressure sensure ("double-tip") catheter. Catheter pullback shows that the "transvalvular" pressure gradient is, nearly in its entirety, *intraventricular* in origin. This important finding requires micromanometric measurement

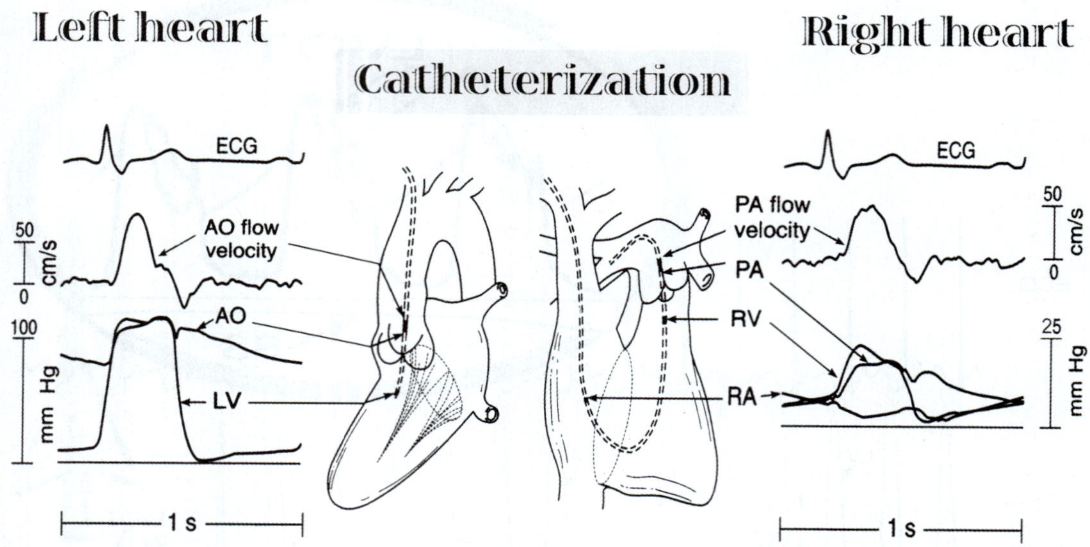

Figure 5.9: Right- and left-heart catheterization: representative Millar multisensor catheter placement and simultaneous hemodynamic signals. AO = aortic root pressure; LV = left ventricular pressure; PA = pulmonary arterial pressure; RV = right ventricular pressure; RA = right atrial pressure; ECG = electrocardiogram.

technology. A modification of this catheter for simultaneous velocity measurements contains an electromagnetic flow velocity probe adjacent to the downstream pressure sensor.

Patients undergoing cardiac catheterization are either unsedated or lightly premedicated and in a fasting state. After the hemodynamic studies—at rest and during supine submaximal bicycle ergometer exercise—are completed (cf. Fig. 5.9), the patient is allowed to return to a control state. The left-heart multisensor catheter is replaced with either an angiography catheter or a Millar injection catheter with a pressure sensor mounted just above the injection ports. Left ventricular biplane cineangiograms are then performed at 60–120 *frames/s* while injecting contrast medium with the patient in the 30° right anterior oblique (RAO) and 60° left anterior oblique (LAO) projections. Coronary arteriography using the Sones technique is also performed. For right-heart catheterization (see Fig. 5.9), the femoral, subclavian, internal jugular, or antecubital vein may be used for access. The right-heart multisensor catheter is passed into the right atrium; then, through the tricuspid valve, into the right ventricle; and, across the pulmonary valve, into the main pulmonary artery. Selective catheterization of the coronary sinus can also be performed.

Hemodynamic signals are displayed and calculations can be performed online. Specialized pressure control units and cables are necessary in order to interface pressure transducers on Millar (multisensor) catheters to physiological monitors and computer data acquisition systems. Such control units generally provide electronic calibration and transducer balance control, and some models have a built-in amplifier. Commercially available flexible displays allow the user to zoom in or out on different sections of the trace, while acquiring data. Recording channels can be calibrated into meaningful units, such as $mm\ Hg$, and chart data files can be exported to customized software for additional offline analysis. Mathematical operations, such as differentiation, integration, natural logarithm, division between two signals, Fourier transforms, and n-point time-series moving average filtering, which averages a rolling subset of elements of the digitized data, can be performed digitally on the acquired signals.

As was pointed out in Section 5.1.1, on pp. 236 ff., a factor that affects the relative timing of digitized hemodynamic waveforms from such multichannel measurements, and the accuracy of variables derived from them, is sampling skew arising because not all channels are sampled simultaneously. As was discussed in that Section, the time lag between sampling of each successive channel can be reduced or eliminated, by using burst mode sampling or sample-hold circuits, respectively.

5.3 Micromanometric and velocimetric calibrations

Before use, a hemodynamic sensor must first be connected to the data acquisition system. There are several signal conditioning considerations. Strain-based micromanometric sensors typically provide small signal levels. It is therefore important to have accurate instrumentation to amplify the signal before it gets digitized. Additionally, all bridge-based sensors require voltage excitation to return a voltage representing strain. This voltage source should be constant and at a level recommended by the manufacturer's manual. Excitation and amplification are necessary to accurately measure a sensor's electrical signal response. Once a measurable voltage signal has been obtained, that signal must be converted to actual units of pressure. Modern hemodynamic sensors generally produce a linear response across their range of operation, but some hardware or software is needed to convert the sensor's voltage output into a pressure measurement. The conversion formula depends on the type of sensor, and will be found in the user's manual provided by the sensor manufacturer. A typical conversion formula will be a function of the excitation voltage, the full scale capacity of the sensor, and a calibration factor.

A high resolution (e.g., 12-*bit*) analog-to-digital conversion of the calibration as well as of the hemodynamic signals can be carried out by a data acquisition card (e.g., the ATMIO16 plug-in card, by National Instrument, Inc., Austin, TX) in a workstation, or a personal computer. All the data can be continuously acquired and displayed on a monitor screen by a commercially available (e.g., the LabVIEW© software package, National Instrument Inc.) data acquisition system. To utilize maximum resolution of the analog-to-digital conversion, the magnitude of any of the input calibration and physiologic signals can be optimized before it reaches the A/D converter, by varying the software-controlled gain setting of the input amplifier. The data files are stored on hard disc; an external mass storage device may provide secondary backup for the recorded data.

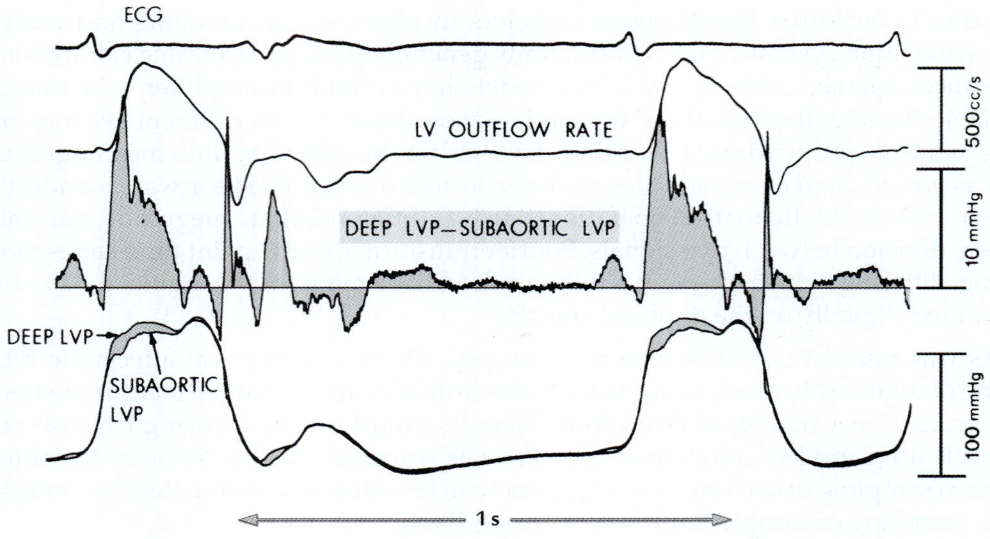

Figure 5.10: Oscillographic recording during supine bicycle exercise of a postectopic compensatory pause demonstrating the matching of the micromanometers to eliminate hydrostatic gradients and amplifier equisensitivity. ECG = electrocardiogram; LV = left ventricular; LVP = left ventricular pressure. (Reproduced from Pasipoularides [40] by permission of the American College of Cardiology.)

5.3.1 Micromanometric calibrations

To make measurements with maximum accuracy, micromanometric sensors should be calibrated prior to ("cal-in") and following ("cal-out") the hemodynamic data collections. This is best accomplished by mimicking the conditions to which they will be exposed *in-vivo*. This is done by placing the sensors under degassed sterile water or saline at body temperature, 37 °, and allowing them to temperature equilibrate prior to calibration or use. To minimize drift, micromanometric catheters should be presoaked in saline for at least 2 h before insertion. After catheter withdrawal at the completion of a study, the pressure with the micromanometric sensor barely submerged in saline at atmospheric pressure should be used as the zero reference.

The following procedures should be used as a guideline in establishing calibration technique. A tube communicating through a side-port with a mercury manometer should be connected to the airspace in an airtight container to be used to increase and decrease the pressure within, in measured steps. The sensor should be under the surface of sterile physiologic saline in the container. The volume of air in the chamber acts as a filter and dampens out rapid pressure transients and the effects of any undetected leaks. Calibration is accomplished by pressurizing the airtight container to several pressure levels and recording the output voltage values of the pressure amplifier for each level. The amplifier should be adjusted as described in the user's manual, to compensate for gauge offset and

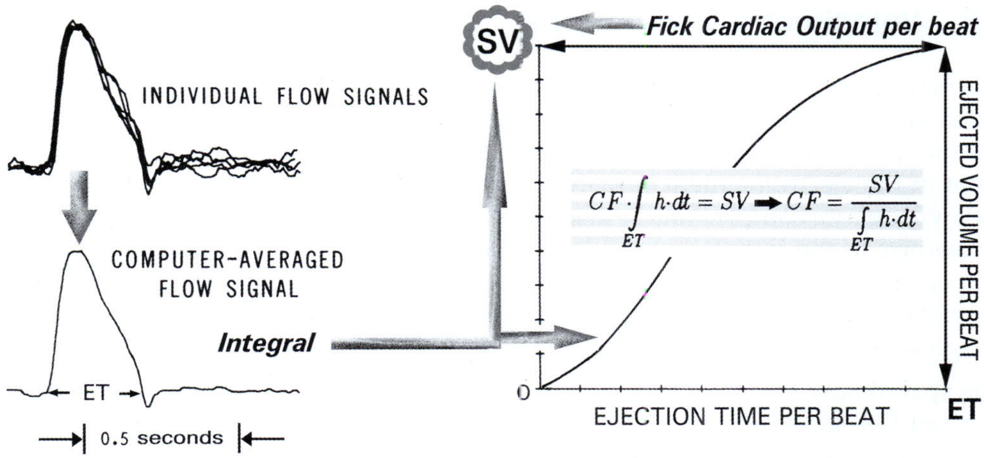

Figure 5.11: Volumetric flow scales for catheter-mounted intravascular flow probes are established by setting the summated systolic areas under the ensemble average of the steady-state flow velocity waveforms to be equal to the corresponding Fick-determined stroke volume—see discussion in text.

gain sensitivity. Typical output levels might be 0.00 *volts* at 0 *mm Hg*, and 2.50 *volts* at 150 *mm Hg*; the "zero" output represents a balanced bridge. Common calibration levels are 0, 25, 50, 75, 100, 125, 150, and 200 *mm Hg*.

Most micromanometric pressure gauges are sealed, and measure pressure relative to the internal pressure. As atmospheric pressure changes, the measured pressure will vary. It is good practice to measure and record atmospheric pressure while calibrating a pressure gauge and during any subsequent *in vivo* measurements. This will make it possible to normalize all measurements, which is particularly important when measuring small absolute intracardiac diastolic pressure levels; on the other hand, ambient atmospheric pressure fluctuations will cancel out when measuring pressure *differences*, or gradients.

These flow-associated gradients are generally superimposed on a simple hydrostatic pressure difference, usually not exceeding 1 to 2 *mm Hg* in the supine subject. That hydrostatic gradient needs no special fluid dynamic consideration, but must be suppressed in the recordings. This is done by *matching* the micromanometric signals, so that the superimposed pressure tracings appear to coincide during the extended no-flow diastasis periods, which are associated with the long compensatory pause following a postectopic beat (see Fig. 5.10, on p. 248). Offset nulling circuitry adds or removes resistance from one of the legs of the micromanometric strain gauge to achieve this "balanced" position. Offset nulling is critical to ensure the accuracy of the measurements. On digitized micromanometric data files, it can be readily accomplished digitally. When recorded (or adjusted *off-line*) in this fashion, the measured intraventricular and transvalvular pressure gradients embody only local acceleration, convective acceleration and dissipative components, which we will consider at length in subsequent chapters.

5.3.2 Velocimetric calibrations

The intraventicular or ascending aortic/pulmonary arterial root flow velocity signal is recorded simultaneously with the micromanometric pressure signals, the electrocardiogram, and a respiratory signal. A phase delay that increases linearly with frequency is inherent in the electromagnetic flowmeter circuitry. Such a linear phase shift versus frequency will delay a complex-shape time signal by a *fixed* amount of time without changing the waveform of the signal. Accordingly, it can be accounted for and corrected by a compensatory, small (few *ms*) forward time-shift of the velocity waveform. The exact amount of the shift is chosen so that, e.g., the onset of the sharp main upstroke of the ejection waveform signal comes to coincide with the crossover of the transvalvular pressure signals.

The spatial flow velocity profile in the ascending aortic or pulmonary root is assumed to be blunt [38–40, 49] and the flow velocity waveform representative of instantaneous *volumetric* flow rate. Each flow velocity signal is digitized at the desired rate (e.g., 200, 400, 500, 1000, or 2000 *Hz*) using a multichannel analog-to-digital converter coupled to the catheterization lab computer, and is stored to hard disc or other storage media. Data to be analyzed should span, at a minimum, two complete respiratory cycles.

Volumetric flow scales are established by setting the summated systolic areas under the flow velocity wave forms as equal to the Fick-determined cardiac output, scaled to the period of velocity signal integration. Letting the conversion factor be denoted as CF,

$$CF \int_{ET} h \cdot dt = SV \quad \Rightarrow \quad CF = \frac{SV}{\int_{ET} h \cdot dt},$$

where, ET is the ejection time, SV is the stroke volume, t is time, and h is the height (e.g., in *mm*) of the flow signal deflection from the baseline. The validity of using catheter-mounted electromagnetic flow velocity probes in studying ascending aortic/pulmonary arterial root flow in man has been established [10, 39, 40, 49]. A representative summary of this calibration method is shown in Figure 5.11. The calibration information is saved and applied to the acquired hemodynamic signals; it, along with the data files stored on hard disc, can be retrieved for off-line computer-aided data analysis.

5.4 Angiocardiography and digital subtraction angiography

Angiocardiography complements physiological studies, such as pressure recordings and measurements of oxygen saturation. It entails contrast medium injection for delineation of the dynamic geometry of the heart chambers, the coronary arteries, and the great vessels. It allows measurement of chamber volumes and assessments of anatomic and performance characteristics, including the function of the cardiac valves and the status of the coronary arteries. For coronary angiography special precurved coronary catheters (Judkins, Amplatz) for the right and left coronary arteries are used. Multiple projections are taken with hand injection of contrast material. Today, cineangiocardiography has been

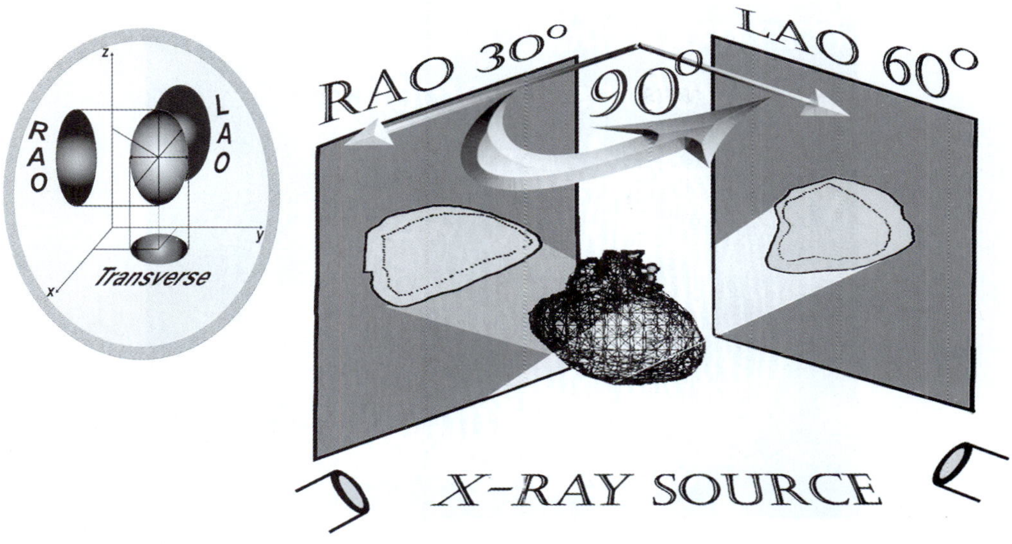

Figure 5.12: Although 2-D in principle, angiocardiography can provide orthogonal projections from two angles by using a *biplane* system; the transverse plane is omitted (inset). Selective enhancement of cardiac chambers (LV in the example sketched) can be accomplished by positioning a pigtail catheter through which contrast medium is injected.

mostly replaced by digital imaging modalities with *real-time* display on CRT, plasma, and LCD monitors. The images are also simultaneously transferred to online and archiving digital mass storage devices, such as hard disc and DVD.

Ventricular angiography is performed with a pigtail catheter.[6] In biplane left ventricular angiography, a 30° right anterior oblique (RAO–projection) and a 60° left anterior oblique (LAO–projection) view are simultaneously obtained. Biplane angiocardiography gives a 3-D perspective of the heart chambers and great vessels (see Fig. 5.12). Unlike static films, cinecardiograms can be monitored during the injection, and the sequence can be simultaneously recorded on videotape and replayed for analysis.

Calibration is performed on the basis of the dimensions of a radiopaque grid or a geometric solid (sphere, ellipsoid, etc.) of known dimensions. These objects are filmed after the ventriculographic procedure in the same position with respect to the x-ray system as the patient's, or experimental animal's, left ventricle during the examination. Volumes thus obtained are corrected for a systematic angiographic overestimation by an appropriate regression equation, specific to the particular laboratory. Standard quantitative angiographic calculations are performed from the RAO projection using the "area–length" method of Kasser and Kennedy [18], or by slice-summing methods, utilizing ventriculographic data.

[6]A pigtail catheter is an angiographic catheter ending in a tightly curled tip, which resembles a pig's tail and has several holes aimed at multiple directions; it minimizes recoil and the tendency of the catheter tip to jump out of the ventricle in response to the contrast-injection jet.

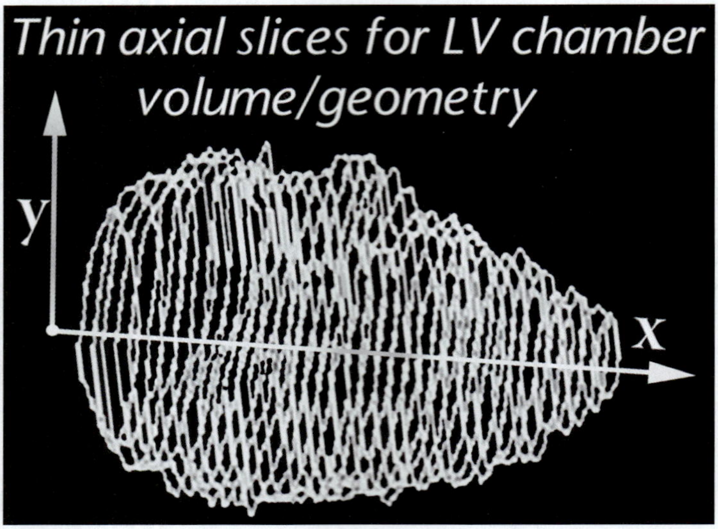

Figure 5.13: Assuming that the ventricular chamber is built by a stack of circular slices, its volume can be calculated using a Simpson integration algorithm (see Section 2.14.3, on pp. 68 f.).

For the area-length method, the ventricular area in the long axis view as well as the length from the ventricular apex to the level of the mitral valve are determined. The LV volume is estimated using these measurements in the equation $LV\ volume = (8/3) \cdot area^2/(\pi \cdot length)$. By assuming that the ventricular chamber is built by a stack of circular slices, the chamber volume is calculated using a Simpson integration algorithm (see Section 2.14.3, on pp. 68 f.). Contrast ventriculograms are traced interactively to delineate endocardial outlines, and the calculated axial chamber length L is subdivided into segments, ΔL_i, for which single or biplane short-axis diameters are determined. The chamber volume is then represented as the summed volumes of the juxtaposed graduated disks with thickness ΔL_i, as shown in Figure 5.13. The Riemann sum (see Section 2.14.2, on pp. 67 f.) of the disk volumes is then processed according to Simpson's rule, allowing for a smooth (*not stepped*) endocardial curvature.

Conventional angiocardiography uses ionizing radiation and has other disadvantages, including potential contrast-medium induced changes in circulatory dynamics and lack of soft tissue specific contrast. The radiological term *contrast* relates to the capacity of an x-ray beam detector, or transducer, to convert differences in photon fluence, i.e., the total number of photons reaching the detector per unit area,[7] across the x-ray beam into differences in optical density (radiographic film), image brightness (image intensifiers), electronic signal amplitude (electronic digital detectors), or some other type of representation in the imaging system.

[7] Photon fluence is related to photon flux, the number of photons reaching the detector per unit area per unit time.

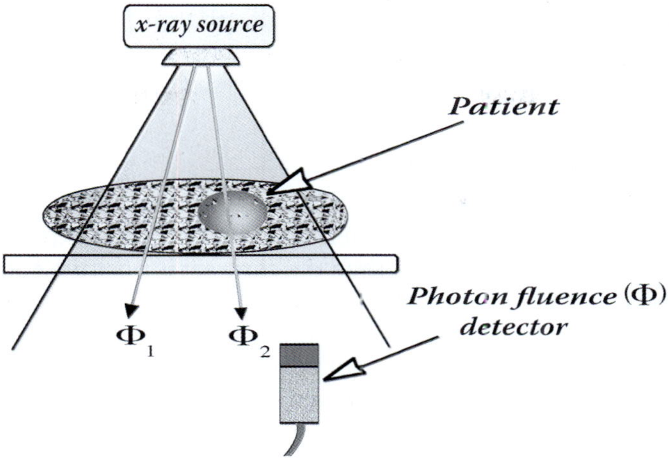

Figure 5.14: The radiographic contrast is defined to be the fractional difference in photon fluence, ϕ, between two adjacent scan areas.

In general the interaction of x-rays is with electrons, and thus an x-ray image is a map of the density of electrons from region to region within the body. Electrons are not heavy, but for each electron in a neutral atom there is one proton which is relatively heavy, plus one or two neutrons in most biological materials. Photons can be removed from a beam of x-rays by scattering, or by absorption. Accordingly, *attenuation* takes place by redirecting photons out of the beam (*Compton scattering* [16]), which takes energy away from the site of interaction, and by *absorption* in which energy is again removed from the beam but it is transferred locally to the tissues, as heat. The overall attenuation of x-rays is about proportional to mass of substance penetrated, and an x-ray image tends to be a map of the relative densities of matter within different parts of the region examined. Digital computed tomography is introduced below; it essentially assigns a numerical value of attenuation to each region in successive axial "body-slices," and it is the distribution of such numbers that is displayed (see Section 10.1, on pp. 484 ff.). For a given material, absorption is directly proportional to the number of grams per square centimeter of material placed in the path of the x-ray beam. The absorption coefficient of a given element varies with wavelength. It is sometimes handy with a group of wavelengths to speak of one average or *effective* value of the attenuation coefficient, which is like assuming a single wavelength. Similarly, it is often convenient to speak loosely of the output from an x-ray tube as if it were *effectively* all at one wavelength. Such an assumption is often inherent in the equations being solved, e.g., in computed tomography. As the wavelength is decreased by an increase in tube voltage, transmission through an absorber generally tends to increase.

Considering the x-ray beam photons on the detector-side of the patient, the radiographic contrast is defined to be the fractional difference in photon fluence between two adjacent areas. For example, if behind the patient, photon fluence of ϕ_1 is measured in one area while a photon fluence of ϕ_2 is measured in an adjacent area (see Fig. 5.14, on p. 253), then the radiographic contrast is defined to be

$$C(\phi) = \frac{\Delta\phi}{\phi_1} = \frac{\phi_2 - \phi_1}{\phi_1}. \tag{5.1}$$

For an opaque object, one where $\phi_2 = 0$ then $C = -1$, which is expressed by just saying that the contrast is 100%. When $\phi_1 < \phi_2$, then the contrast is positive and can exceed 100%. If $\phi_1 \approx \phi_2$, the object cannot be reliably differentiated from its background. X-rays can only discriminate between different tissues by the number of electrons capable of receiving the x-ray photon's energy. This number does not vary much in soft tissues (cf. Fig. 5.16, on p. 256), and contrast between different soft tissues—e.g., heart muscle and blood—can only be enhanced by the injection of a contrast medium.

The representation of a 3-D structure on a 2-D image[8] requires a collapse from three into two dimensions and is generally associated with foreshortening, as is depicted pictorially in panel Ia. of Figure 5.15, on p. 255. Certainly, the length of the observed rod does not change by rotating it in 3-D space, but the *projection* of this 3-D object onto the 2-D plane of vision (u, v) does. Physicists imprisoned in *Plato's cave* (see Section 11.1, on pp. 583 ff.) may be baffled initially by the fact that the lengths of *"shadow-objects"* are apparently not absolute. However, someone should eventually sense that the objects being observed behave as 2-D projections of a 3-D object that can be rotated in space. Mathematically, there is a quantity that is absolute and does not change under such rotations—namely, the length of the real rod. If this rod has a length L, while the length of the "shadow-rod" (i.e., the projection of L on the plane of vision) is l, then a cave mathematician, whom for the sake of argument we name Pythagoras, might suggest that there is a quantity, L, whose value does not change, and that is given by the relation $L^2 = l^2 + d^2$, where l is the projection of the rod on the plane of vision (u, v) and d is the projection of L perpendicular to this plane (see panel Ib. of Fig. 5.15).

As is illustrated further in panel II., a "cross-like" pattern on a plane may be distorted into an "x-like" pattern, when the plane is rotated by, e.g., $45°$ relative to the advantageous perpendicular line of vision, and into a simple 2-D "linear" pattern, when the plane is rotated by $90°$. This foreshortening is a consequence of the fact that, when any surface is viewed at such progressively larger angles, the image of the surface becomes "compressed" and occupies progressively smaller areas in the successive views.

Additionally, in radiography, information from *throughout a 3-D body part*, such as the thorax, is squeezed into 2-D and projected onto the film. In the process, subtle geometric structural information can become lost in the interplay of the image patterns created by all of the overlapped tissue structures, which may cause strong confounding variations in x-ray beam attenuation (see Fig. 5.16, on p. 256). 2-D x-ray images can hardly be used to delineate tissue topography at a particular depth without influence from tissue at other depths. Digital subtraction angiography (DSA) can circumvent this problem in studies of the cardiac chambers, and of arteries and veins [30].

[8]This vital topic is discussed at length in Chapter 11.

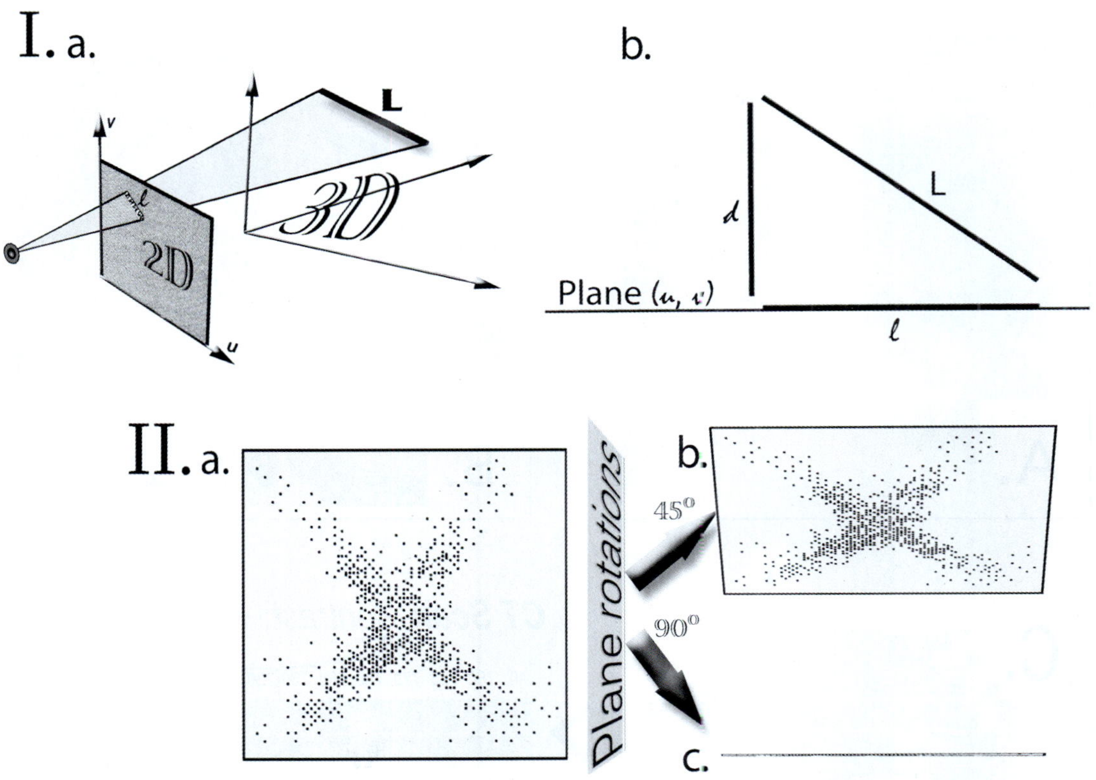

Figure 5.15: I. Viewing a 3-D structure in a 2-D image is generally associated with foreshortening. The rod of length L in (x, y, z)-space projects to a line of a generally shorter length, l, on the 2-D image plane. II. Apparent changes in the *shape* of a two-dimensional pattern or structure are also caused by changes in observational orientation relative to the imaging energy beam, which provide new "angles of sight," in going from a. to, say, b. or c.

Image subtraction is a simple, easy-to-understand and widely accepted method, and is applicable also to 3-D measurements obtained by CT angiography. In conventional DSA, a reference image is taken before contrast is injected, or reaches the region of interest. That reference image is then subtracted from subsequent images acquired after contrast injection. DSA uses these "before" (referred to as mask images, or "mask") and "after" (referred to as contrast images, or "contrast") radiographs to cancel out all tissues except the blood vessels that have just been filled with contrast agent opaque to x-rays (cf. Fig. 5.17, on p. 257). What remains is the "difference" x-ray image with the other, irrelevant (and unchanged) tissues rendered invisible, because nothing remains in the image, except for the contrast agent.[9] It may help with interpretation, however, to

[9]Before computers and digital x-ray image processing could be applied, radiographers or dark-room technicians used to spend considerable time manually exposing the subtraction mask film, matching the angiographic film and reproducing the image on the subtraction film to produce the subtraction angiogram.

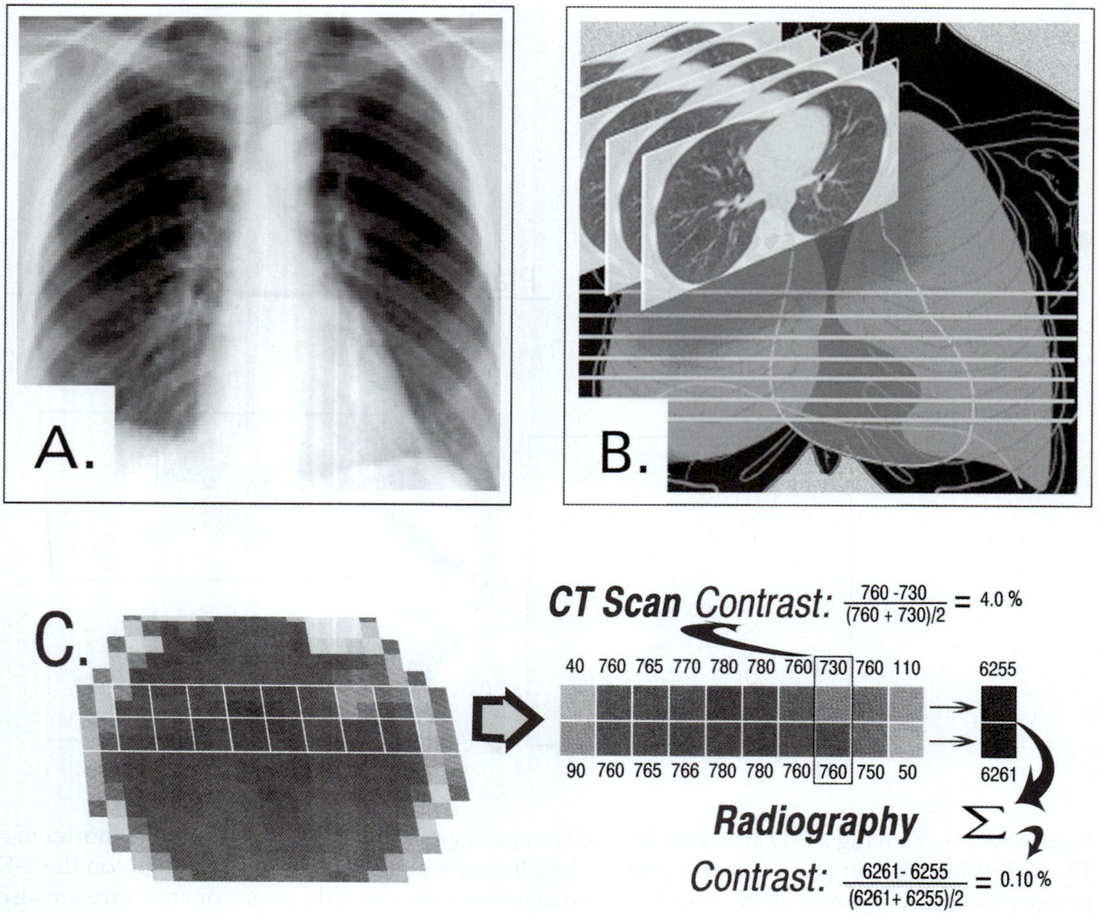

Figure 5.16: **A.** X-ray films are effectively "transilluminations" of the body. Various bodily structures are imaged overlapping each other and often need several views for visual understanding. **B.** Computed tomography images are thin x-ray generated slices through body structures. They present anatomy in a straightforward manner because they avoid confusion by multiple overlapping structures. **C.** In CT, contrast is determined by *local* tissue differences in x-ray attenuation, and is not confounded by tissue *overlap* and summation (Σ) effects.

reintroduce topographic context in the final "difference" image, via some faint background anatomy.

DSA assumes that tissues do not move between the scans. In fact, there are physiological motions (breath, heartbeat), which cause artifacts that appear as "blurring" in the reconstructed images. Some techniques model any such physiological motion as a periodic sequence and take images at a particular point in the motion cycle to achieve the

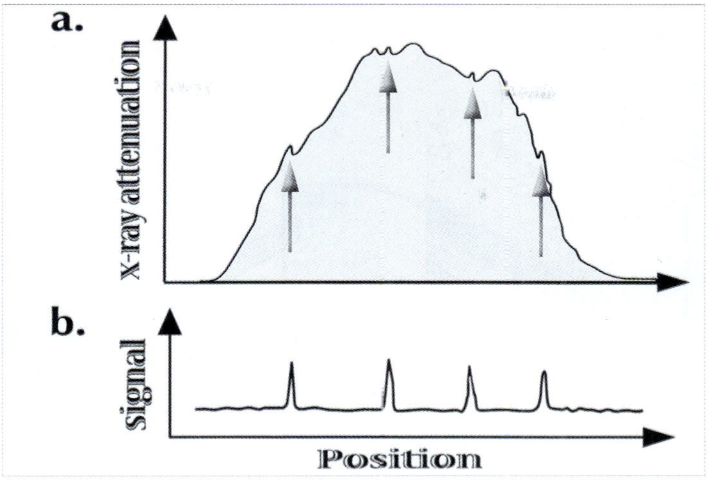

Figure 5.17: a. X-ray attenuation across a patient's body with contrast-enhanced blood vessels indicated by arrows. b. DSA-subtracted profile, with digitally amplified vessel signals on a homogeneous, featureless background.

effect of scanning a stationary object (similar to ECG triggering—see Section 10.2.9, on pp. 526 ff.). Various algorithms are available to correct more complex motions [26].

CT—*computed tomography* (the Gk. word $\tau o \mu \eta$ = tomé, conveys the meaning of a *cut*, or a *section*) uses a radically different strategy to achieve essentially the same end: the removal of extraneous but visually competing information. It does so in a way that makes possible the imaging of soft-tissue structural details (see Fig. 5.16, on p. 256), not just the cardiac cavities and blood vessel lumens. With new multidetector computed tomography (MDCT) it is possible to acquire high-resolution, 3-D images of the heart and great vessels. In MDCT, a two-dimensional detector element array replaces the linear array of elements that is used in typical conventional and helical CT scanners. The two-dimensional detector array permits the acquisition of multiple sections, or slices, simultaneously, and greatly boosts the speed of CT image acquisition.

The multiple tomographic images reconstructed in the axial plane are stacked to create a *"volume"* of imaging data from which a plane can be selected, as is depicted pictorially in Figure 5.18, so as to display optimally the image of interest. All the voxels in the acquired 3-D volume are stored in the computer, and it is convenient to think of the position of the storage of a number as corresponding to the position of a voxel in the cube. Any of the original planes can then be displayed by "calling up" the numbers representing the voxels in that plane and producing a proportional brightness on the monitor screen at the corresponding position. The gaps of missing data between the acquired tomographic images can be filled through interpolation of the values of adjacent, *nearest neighbor*, images, or other more sophisticated and more accurate interpolation methods (see Section 11.5.4, on pp. 601 ff.), which we will consider in some detail in Chapter 11. In this way, a solid cube of data is obtained.

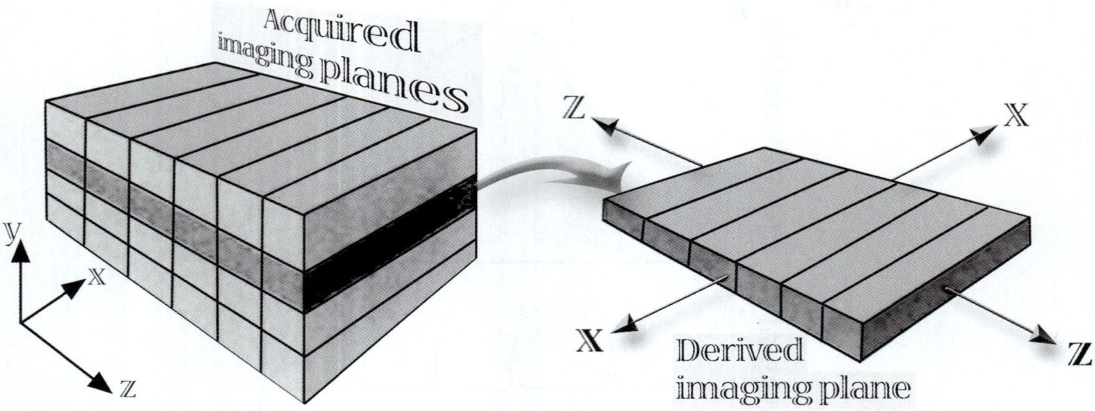

Figure 5.18: A large series of 2-D images along the body axis, acquired by multidetector computed tomography (CT), can be stacked to form a 3-D volume, from which any arbitrarily oriented imaging plane can then be derived to create a 2-D image, or "cut" through the data—a representative coronal plane is depicted. Unless isotropic 3-D resolution imaging is applied, the axial sections across a subject are more widely spaced than are the lines across the 2-D sections making the original projections; accordingly, the resolution in a tilted display will not be the same up and down as across the image.

It should be recognized that interpolation does not *create* information; rather, it increases the number of points with which the available information is represented; this is why interpolation tends to soften the image detail, unless the image size is reduced as well: then the smaller image appears to compress the detail and often results in an apparently sharper picture. After the volumetric dataset is obtained, any sequence of imaging data points can then be displayed from within the entire 3-D volume in order to show the appearance of planes other than the original ones through the subject. Such "slice and dice" planes of derived imaging data are 1 voxel thick, and their actualization generally entails the application of numerical interpolation routines. This process can be performed on an imaging console, or a computer workstation. Further examination of CT imaging and post-processing display techniques can be found in Chapters 10 and 11.

5.4.1 X-ray contrast media

X-ray contrast media are exogenous substances used to alter the contrast in x-ray imaging by affecting the attenuation of x-rays. The vast majority of x-ray contrast media are positive or radiopaque, i.e., they increase the attenuation of x-rays (see Fig. 5.17). In cardiovascular applications, iodine is the main component responsible for the increased attenuation. All water-soluble iodinated contrast media are derivatives of tri-iodinated benzoic acid. The derivatives are named monomeric when they contain only one benzene ring, and dimeric when they contain two benzene rings. Monomeric ionic contrast media are salts of derivatives of tri-iodinated benzoic acid.[10]

The ionic monomeric contrast media for intravascular use are so-called high-osmolar contrast media (HOCM), having an osmolality seven to eight times that of plasma in ordinary clinical use. This hyperosmolality is (partly) responsible for several adverse effects, including endothelial damage, bradycardia, a slight fall in systemic pressure, a rise in cardiac output, and increased pressure in the pulmonary circulation. The introduction of low-osmolar ("nonionic") contrast media (LOCM) has substantially reduced these side effects. The various water-soluble contrast media for angiography are all extracellular contrast media, and are excreted unmetabolized, by glomerular filtration. Undesirable hemodynamic side-effects and complications related to contrast media are significantly lower when using nonionic agents. With modern x-ray contrast media and adequate technique the risks of angiocardiography are very small.

5.5 Echocardiography

Echocardiography is a noninvasive technique and, along with Doppler velocimetry, it represents an important tool for evaluating the dynamic anatomy and the fluid mechanics of the heart. In real time, echocardiography provides considerable information on the motion of cardiac structures, including the endocardial boundary surface of the cardiac chambers. In clinical practice, it remains the method of choice because of its noninvasiveness, short examination times, and a relatively low cost and wide machine availability.

The basic components of all echocardiographic systems include a central processing unit (CPU), a transducer (or several different transducers, depending on the applications), a monitor, and a system to store the images. The CPU controls and processes the majority of the functions of the system. It is responsible for the input to the other components, such as the transducer and monitor. It also receives and analyzes electronic input from the transducer ultimately to assemble the image. The CPU also provides the interactive tools for analyzing and obtaining quantitative measurements from the images. All ultrasound systems have a CPU; however, only recent generation echocardiographic systems have the computing power and speed needed for high-resolution imaging at the high frame rates that are essential for intracardiac flow studies. These systems also have fully digital image processing capabilities and can be upgraded simply by updating software, as the technology advances.

The transducer generates the ultrasound waves and receives the reflected ones. Transducers contain piezoelectric crystals that vibrate when exposed to small electrical currents, thereby creating the ultrasound waves. The crystals also turn out small electrical currents when they are deformed by reflected sound waves. Sound waves produced by these

[10] The cations of the salts are mainly either sodium or meglumine, or a mixture of both. Sodium salts are generally more toxic to vascular endothelium and other tissues than meglumine. A mixture of sodium and meglumine has lower cardiotoxicity than either salts alone. Some manufacturers have partially replaced sodium with calcium and magnesium to reduce toxicity.

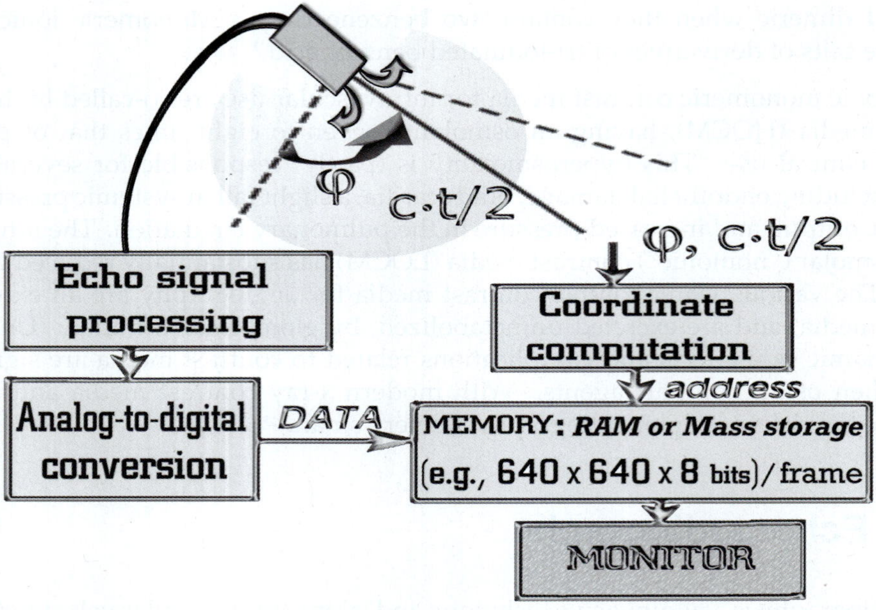

Figure 5.19: 2-D Imaging system diagram indicating how successive beam directions (φ) and ultrasound echo return times (t) to the transducer are linked to image display—c = effective sound propagation velocity.

crystals are focused into a beam and transmitted through the intervening soft tissues of the body to the beating heart. The transducer then halts briefly to receive the reflected sound waves. Each tissue through which the sound waves pass has slightly different acoustic impedance, which is proportional to the mass density of the tissue. At the interface of two different tissues, an acoustic impedance *mismatch* arises, and some sound waves are reflected. These reflected ultrasound waves interact with the piezoelectric crystals in the transducer to turn out a small current. These electrical signals are processed by the CPU using reconstruction software, and the images are put together and displayed on the monitor. Liquids, including blood, scatter almost nothing and appear black in the image. One of the prime advantages of an ultrasonic scanner is that it produces real-time images. Complete study image-sequences can also be saved as files on a mass-storage device, for off-line analysis.

Because of the freely maneuverable probe, ultrasonic imaging poses some problems. The spatial sampling of the produced data is commonly both inhomogeneous and unpredictable. Accordingly, mechanical arms can be fixed to the probe and its location and orientation can be measured, so as to track them reliably, for some research applications. State-of-the art echocardiographic systems can digitally accumulate in memory a limited number of frames; however, the image files must be stored on mass-storage media, such as DVD or CD, or on external or networked hard disk drives, to be transferred to another computer system, or a workstation, for research studies. Digital storage and archiving of images allows for easier retrieval and off-line analysis of data, and does not subject the

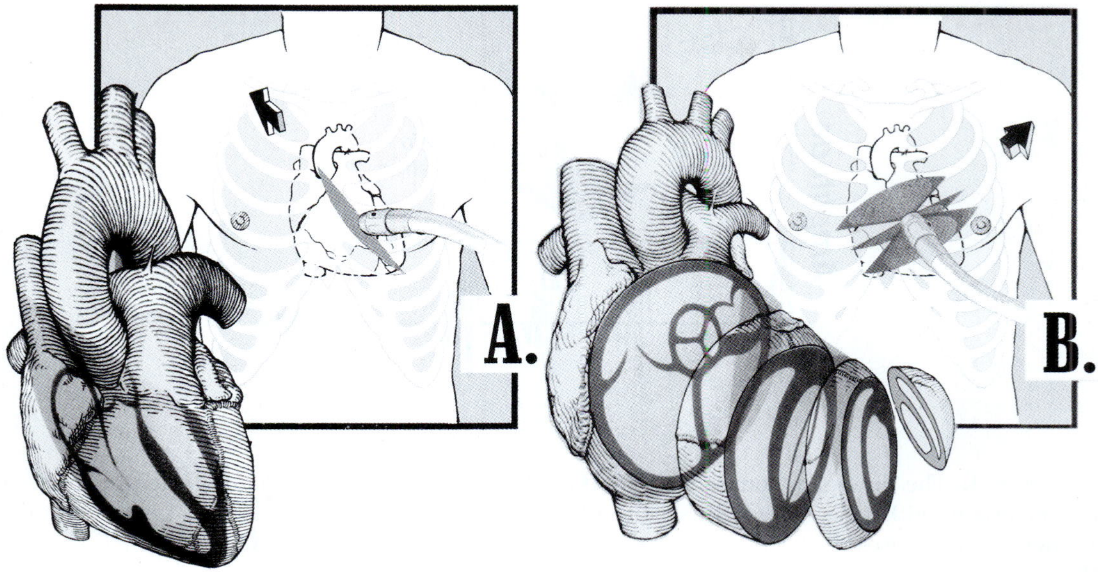

Figure 5.20: Standard 2-D echocardiographic images are described by the location of the transducer and the imaging plane used. Left panel: 2-D echocardiogram in a parasternal long-axis view is obtained with the imaging plane to the left of the sternum, parallel to the long axis of the heart. Right panel: parasternal short-axis views are obtained perpendicular to the long-axis view plane (aorta/left atrium, mitral, papillary muscle planes).

images to the loss of resolution that takes place when they are stored on analog videotape. With digital image storage, data analysis can be performed using the ultrasound system, or a compatible more powerful computer system.

5.5.1 2-D echocardiography

In real time, echocardiography provides detailed information on the motion of cardiac structures, including the endocardial surface boundary of the cardiac chambers [3,23,35, 36,41,45,46,50,53,59]. Echocardiographic imaging is based on detecting the reflections of an ultrasound wave by tissues. An ultrasound pulse is transmitted into the body with an overall average propagation speed of about $1{,}540\ m/s$ and, at the interfaces between tissues with different actual propagation speeds and mass-densities, partial reflections of the sound waves take place.

A B-mode image is a cross-sectional representation of tissue and organ topography, generated from the echoes arising by reflection of transmitted ultrasound waves at the underlying tissue boundaries and by their scattering from small irregularities within tissues. These reflections are detected when they return to the transducer and, by utilizing the angle of the ultrasound beam and the time of arrival of the reflections back to the

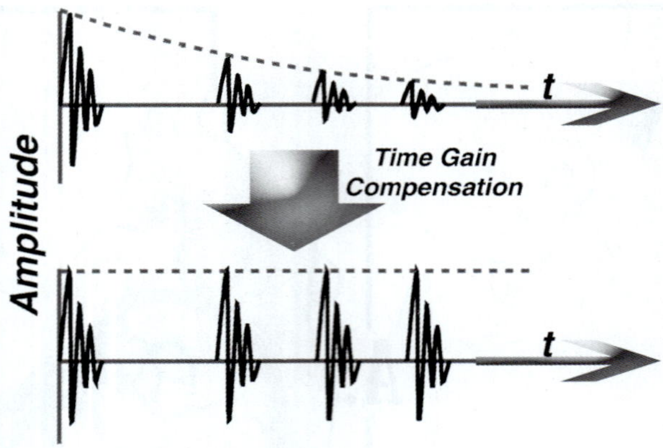

Figure 5.21: The time-gain-compensation (TGC) function increases the gain of the preamplifier exponentially with time, so as to offset the attenuation of the ultrasound as it passes through the tissues, which causes the echoes that originate from deeper in the body to be weaker. It reduces the dynamic range, i.e., the largest-to-smallest received signal amplitude ratio.

transducer, they are used to assemble an image of the organs and tissues that are being scanned, as is indicated in Figure 5.19, on p. 260. A digital echocardiographic image can be conceived as a matrix whose row and column indices identify a point in the image, and the corresponding matrix-element value identifies the gray level at that point. Each echo is put on view at a point in the image, which corresponds to the relative position of its origin within the body cross-section, resulting in a scaled map of echo-producing topographic features. The brightness of the image at each point is related to the strength of the echo, giving rise to the term B-mode, where B stands for *brightness*.

An illustration of some useful tomographic cardiac B-mode cuts is shown in Figure 5.20. The dynamic B-mode image bears a close resemblance to the sectional anatomy, which might be seen by eye, if the body part could be sliced through in the same plane. In approaching such tomographic "cuts" of the heart, irrespective of the imaging modality used, it is important to bear in mind that a 3-D object may have an infinite number of two-dimensional cuts and projections. Both the transmission of the ultrasound pulse through the body and the interaction between the pulse and the tissues of interest play essential roles in ultrasonic imaging. To obtain information on a specific part of the body, first, the ultrasound pulse must be aimed through an acoustic window and propagate from the scanner to the structure of interest; next, it must be partially reflected by successive tissue interfaces and travel back again to the receiving transducer. The real-time nature of the display means that motion of cardiac chamber walls can be observed, and their dynamic geometry quantitated.

Because of the attenuation of ultrasound passing through matter, the deeper within the body a reflection originates, the weaker will be the echo signal and the longer it will take to appear at the transducer. *Time-gain-compensation*, or *TGC*, uses the latter phenomenon to offset the former, by ramping-up the gain of the receiver throughout the

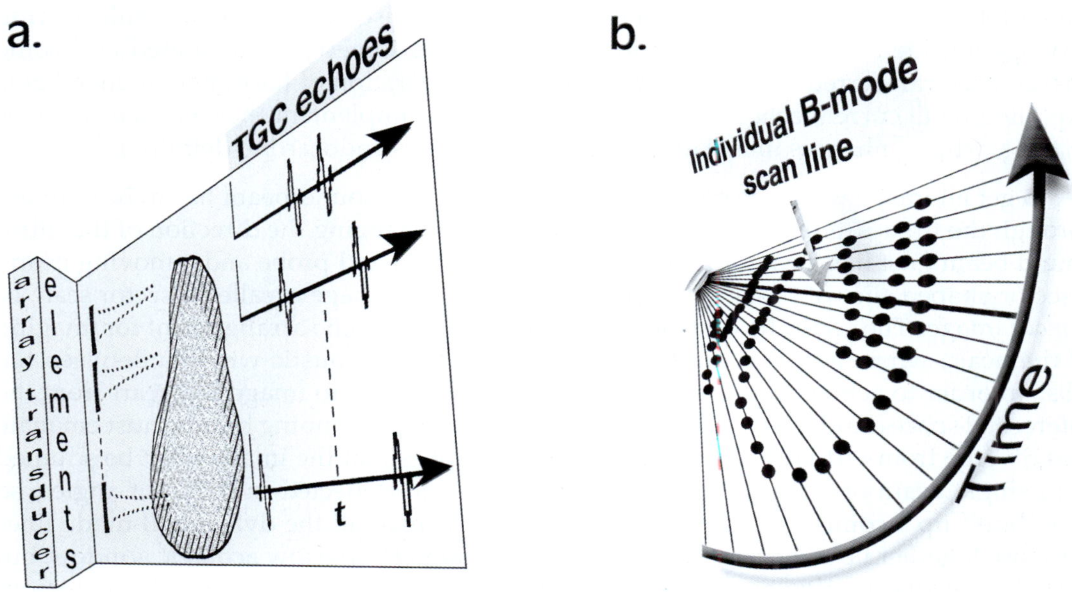

Figure 5.22: a. The focused array transducer elements insonify an organ's irregular boundaries from different positions. The received echoes from the front and back of the organ, with time-gain-compensation (TGC), are displayed *vs.* travel time (t). An image is formed as shown in b., based on the strength and arrival times of the received echoes. b. In *real-time* 2-D echocardiographic imaging, ultrasound data is spatially oriented against time and images are created at a fixed rate. A basic B-mode scan direction on the monitor is linked to the direction of an individual ultrasound beam. A 2-D echocardiographic image display can be built up from dynamic B-mode scans in many successive directions that are swept in time by the interrogating ultrasound beam. The beam sweeps over the field 30–90 times per second, which represents the frame rate.

time that a pulse travels into the body and its echoes are returning, so as to compensate for the attenuation of the signal with traversed distance. In effect, the deeper a reflecting tissue interface is found, the weaker its echo would be—but the *later* it will be detected and the *more* it will be amplified, as is shown in Figure 5.21. Note that the time-gain-compensation function increases the gain of the preamplifier exponentially with the *time* that the machine has been waiting for the return pulse, so as to offset the exponential attenuation of the ultrasound with *distance* traversed through the tissues; this time-distance equivalence has at its root the nearly *constant* ultrasound velocity through soft tissues and blood that relates these variables linearly.

Not only is the propagation of ultrasound through tissue subject to diffraction and a corresponding loss of power at increasing depth, it is also inherently *nonlinear*. Because of a pressure dependence of sound speed, the higher amplitudes travel at a higher speed, and the compressional portion of the wave is faster than the rarefactional, resulting in a change of the pulse waveform toward a triangular shape with a steepening wavefront. This process results in the generation of *harmonics* of the primary frequency in the original signal (cf. Fig. 5.24, on p. 267, and the associated discussion). As a result, during propagation the amplitude of the ultrasound pulse is somewhat attenuated and some energy gets transferred to higher harmonics. This generation of harmonic frequencies is exploited in all current echocardiographic machines to implement the so-called *harmonic imaging*, which enhances image quality [2] and improves endocardial definition.

To get an image with two spatial dimensions, the ultrasound beam has to be scanned through the tissues, either by moving the probe or by changing the direction of the ultrasound beam (just like a rotating radar antenna). With a fixed probe and a moving beam, a sector-shaped slice of tissue can be examined. Such an image is called a sector scan, or *S-mode* image. The sector field of view is the preferred scan-line arrangement for imaging of the heart, where access is normally through a narrow acoustic window between the ribs. In order to achieve a probe footprint sufficiently small to image the heart from the intercostal spaces, and with a sufficiently wide far field, the scanning beams must emanate and diverge from virtually the same point. This implies that the image must be scanned by a single beam originating from the same point and deflected in different angles, so as to build up a complete image. In such a sector format, all the dynamic B-mode lines are close together near the transducer and pass through the narrow acoustic window, but *diverge* after that to give a wide field of view at the depth of the heart. As is demonstrated pictorially in Figure 5.22, an ultrasound beam is sent out, and as all echoes along the beam are received, the B-mode line along the beam is retained, and a new beam is sent out in the neighboring region to build up the next B-mode line in the image. One full sweep of the sector by the beam will therefore build up a complete 2-D image.

This sweeping action can be achieved by a phased array sending a single beam that is stepwise rotated electronically. Each successive line in the image is formed after a slight angular rotation. Such a phased array with electronic focusing and steering can generate a beam sweeping through a pizza slice shaped sector. Beamforming by phased array also enables focusing of the ultrasound beam as is shown in Figure 5.23, on p. 265. Note that the beam is focused by delaying appropriately each of the channels, so that the return pulses from the focal point (or area) arrive at the processor at the same time.

Completion of each frame takes an interval equal to the time for transmitting and receiving the total number of pulses, which corresponds to the number of B-mode lines in the image. The temporal resolution is restricted by the sweep speed of the beam, which is limited by the speed of sound, since the echo from the deepest structure that is scanned has to return before the next pulse is sent out, at a somewhat different angle in the neighboring beam. The sweep speed can be increased by reducing the number of line scans in the sector, thus diminishing the lateral resolution, or by decreasing the overall sector angle, thus diminishing the extent of the scanned field. Contemporary 2-D echocardiographic systems can build up images with sufficient depth of scanning and resolution operating at about 30–90 FPS, which gives a fairly good temporal resolution for 2-D visualization of normal heart action, at least at normal or slow heart rates.

Intravascular ultrasound (IVUS) transducers use the *radial* format obtained by rotating the transducer at the tip of a catheter. The beam distribution is similar to that of beams of light from a lighthouse; B-mode lines all radiate out from the center of the field of view.

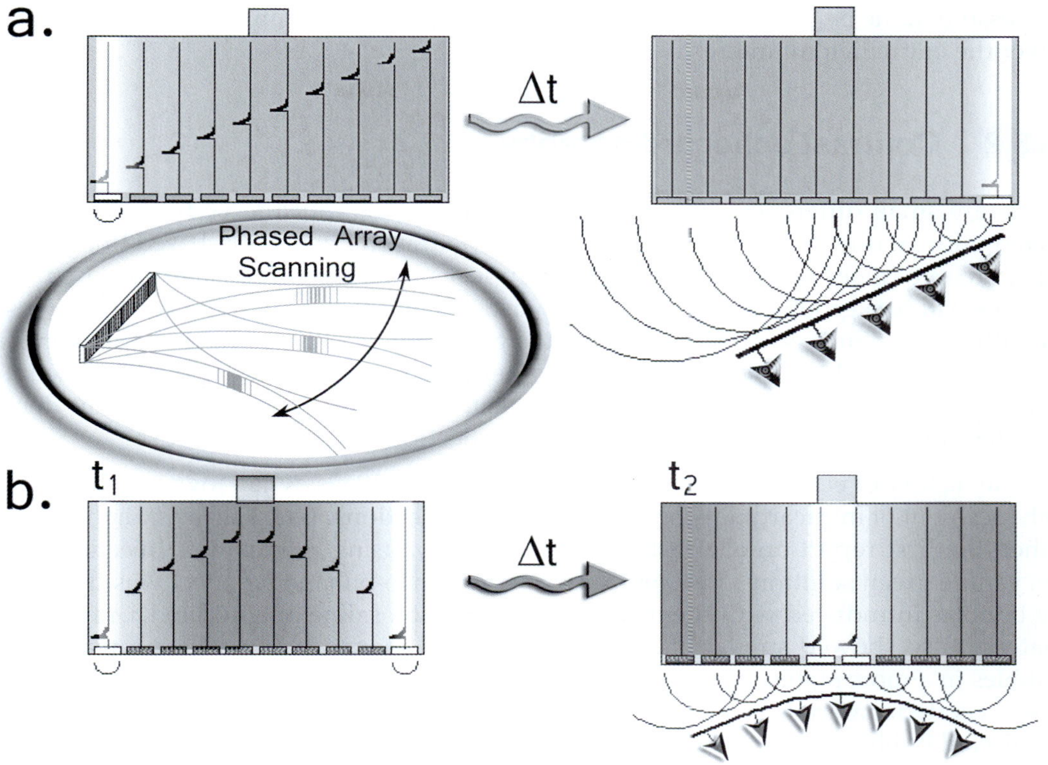

Figure 5.23: a. Electronic phasing used to steer a sound field: a linear time delay, or "phasing," pattern will cause an unfocused beam to be steered off the axis of the transducer, as is shown in the upper panels; steering is caused by the constructive interference of wavefronts emitted by the individual elements at different times. b. Electronic phasing used to generate a focused sound field: by phasing the individual elements appropriately, a cylindrically converging ultrasound wavefront can be formed, as is shown in the lower panels. These two patterns can be combined to steer and focus the sound field simultaneously, as is shown in the inset. In the diagrams, the activating voltage pulses are represented by the squiggles on the vertical time lines emanating from the array—with time (t) increasing vertically from the array surface; $t_1 - t_2 = \Delta t$.

Coronary IVUS provides quantitative information on lumen and vessel dimensions and atherosclerotic plaque severity, as well as qualitative information on plaque composition, in terms of hard and soft components, or calcification.

In cardiac applications, depending on the way the pulsing is performed and the reflections received, different information can be visualized and quantified. In 2-D echocardiography, B-mode imaging is applied to construct a cross-section of the heart, by assigning gray-scale values to the reflected ultrasound amplitudes in the individual pixels of a 2-D matrix, which makes up each image frame. Each image pixel is constructed in every successive frame by sending single ultrasound pulses through consecutive angles so as to cover the entire field of interest.

5.5.2 Contrast echocardiography

There are small differences in acoustic properties throughout the body that can be detected with an ultrasonic imaging system. Also, ultrasonic reflection-based imaging systems are extremely sensitive since echoes appear on nothing (i.e., superimposed upon only a small background of noise), rather than as a small change in some general intensity, as with x-rays. Since satisfactory contrast is generally present, extra contrast agents are less routinely used than with some of the other imaging modalities. However, the introduction of echo-enhancers with either different elastic properties or a different density (the determinants of acoustic impedance and reflection) intensifies contrast.

The history of echo-enhancers goes back to the mid-1960s, when Joyner first observed enhancement of intracardiac echoes during saline injections. Gramiak and Shah [14] published the first report on contrast echocardiography, using intracardiac injections of indocyanine green solutions, in 1968. The observed echo-enhancing effect was due to tiny air bubbles introduced with the injected fluid. Shaken saline or sonicated x-ray contrast material also showed similar effects. There ensued many attempts to encapsulate tiny bubbles in a more stable form. The field of contrast echocardiography depends upon the use of aerated materials being injected to outline the cardiovascular system. The progress of injected bubbles can be followed in ultrasonic images made in rapid succession.

Contrast agents for ultrasound interact with and form part of the imaging process. The technology universally adopted is that of *blood pool* agents, encapsulated bubbles of gas that are smaller than red blood cells and are therefore capable of circulating freely in the body. This imaging technique is based on the principle that microbubbles having a gas-liquid interface will backscatter the incident ultrasound. The bubbles scatter rather than reflect ultrasound because their diameter is much smaller than ultrasound wavelengths. The result of this behavior is the "opacification" of the medium containing the microbubbles, namely, blood. Moreover the bubbles exhibit an intravascular rheology similar to that of red blood cells [24] and are compressible. In recent years, better ultrasound contrast agents and imaging techniques have become available, with the aim to enhance the signal-to-noise ratio and allow detectable opacification of even small amounts of contrast agent. At present, the main targets of contrast-enhanced echocardiography in studies of ventricular function include the acquisition of images of improved quality, especially for endocardial border detection, and the assessment of myocardial perfusion.

An understanding of the basic principles of bubble composition and new available technologies is useful. For many years, the only available microbubbles were those obtained by hand agitation of saline solutions. Later on, sonication of 5% human albumin was used to obtain air bubbles of small size; afterwards, Albunex,™ a suspension of air-filled albumin microspheres in a 5% albumin solution, was developed. In this first-generation of contrast agents, the air used within the microbubbles reduced their overall durability and resulted in a short duration of effect before the bubbles were destroyed.

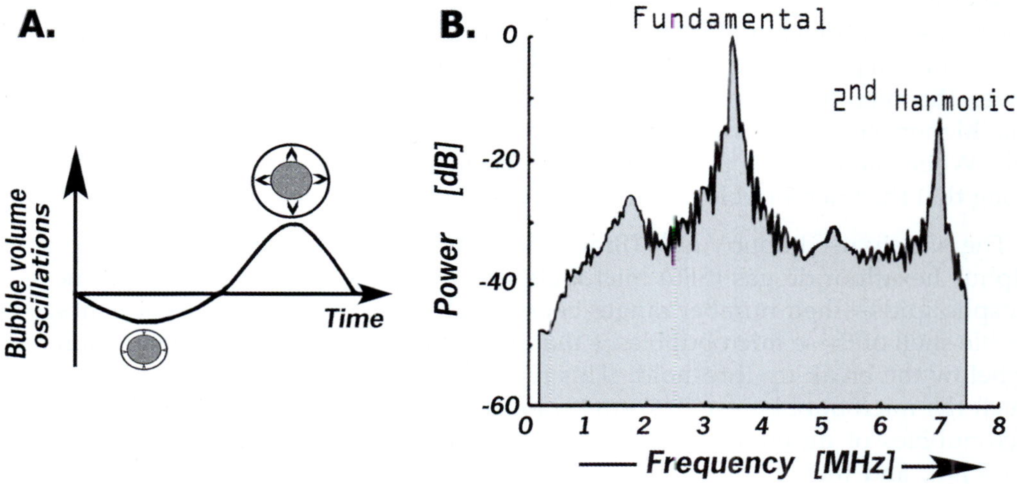

Figure 5.24: Bubbles in an acoustic field respond to the changes in pressure induced by the sound wave by changing in size. Their radius oscillates at the same rate as the incident ultrasound, radiating an echo. A. Nonlinearities in the microbubble-derived backscattered acoustic wave arise from the asymmetric bubble volume oscillations. B. Pictorial sketch of nonlinear frequency response characteristics of microbubbles exhibited in the backscattered acoustic power spectrum. There are distinct harmonic frequency peaks arising at multiples (at about 7 *MHz* in this example) of the actual insonation frequency (3.5 *MHz*), which are characteristic for the specific microbubble contrast agent.

Thus, although of small size, these microspheres were unable to cross the lung capillaries in sufficient concentration, so as to provide opacification of the left-heart chambers.

In recent years, more stable, second- and third-generation microbubbles have been developed. The major difference between the first- and later-generation contrast agents is the type of gas used within the bubble. The later-generation agents contain high molecular weight gases such as fluorocarbons, which are poorly soluble in blood. Another improvement is represented by changes in shell composition: some bubbles have no shell at all, while others, such as Definity™ and Optison,™ have shells constituted by lipids and protein surfactant. The surfactants lead to a decrease in surface tension and thus to a prolonged persistence in the bloodstream—once intravenously injected, bubbles larger than the capillary lumen remain trapped in lung capillaries. Most contrast agents contain microbubbles in the range of 2–10 μm but the range may extend to 25 μm [51]. Contrast agent may be administered as a bolus or by continuous infusion. Each mode of administration has advantages and disadvantages: bolus injection is the easiest way of introducing the contrast agent, but the contrast effect is relatively short lasting, with a peak opacification which may be too high. Continuous infusion requires improvised pumps, but can maintain a steady-state of microbubble concentration and less pronounced far field attenuation [58].

Microbubbles are unique contrast agents, in the sense that they are modified by the process used to image them [58]. The response of the microbubbles to the ultrasound field mainly depends on the power of the acoustic pressure wave. At very low insonation power, the microbubbles remain inert, simply backscattering the sound wave. At somewhat higher acoustic power, they start to *oscillate* at their resonant frequency, like a struck bell. When the acoustic power becomes too high, the resonant oscillations become so strong that the microbubble membranes burst and the bubbles break up.

The widely used SonoVue™ (Bracco SpA, Milan, Italy) is an aqueous suspension of sulphur hexafluoride gas (SF6) microbubbles surrounded by a thin and elastic shell of phospholipids—their number ranges between 2 and $5 \cdot 10^8$ per mL. The advantage of the flexible shell of these microbubbles is that the oscillation starts at low insonation powers, far below the break-up threshold. This results in a broad range of acoustic pressures in which the microbubbles oscillate continuously without bursting [15]. SonoVue contains microbubbles of different sizes, ranging between 10 *and* $1\ \mu m$, with a mean diameter of $2.5\ \mu m$, and their nominal resonance frequency (which depends mainly on the size of the microbubbles) is at $3.5\ MHz$ (see Fig. 5.24), ranging between 1 *and* $10\ MHz$, so that SonoVue covers the whole range of frequencies used for ultrasound imaging. Thus, strong contrast-specific signals can be obtained with all suitable ultrasound probes from low to high frequencies [15], and it is very effective for heart chamber opacification and delineation of the endocardial borders. This contrast agent can significantly improve ultrasound's ability to differentiate between normal and abnormal tissue. When used in combination with certain new, contrast-specific, imaging technologies, it creates a new imaging modality called "Contrast Enhanced Ultrasound," or CEUS [33].

5.6 Detection of endocardial borders

In 2-D echocardiography, the difference in reflected signal intensity between blood and myocardium allows identification of the endocardium, and the outlining of the cardiac chambers. Therefore, the endocardium, which acts as a specular reflector of the ultrasonic beam, provides an important contribution to the detection of cavity borders. It is well recognized that blood appears black on ultrasound imaging, not because it produces no echo but, rather, because the sound scattered by the blood cells at the low diagnostic frequencies is very weak, being 1,000–10,000 times weaker than that from solid tissues. Accordingly, it lies below the displayed dynamic range of the echocardiographic images.

Ultrasound imaging plays a crucial role in the identification of cardiac boundaries, especially those between the blood and the walls of the pumping chambers. Identification of the entire margin of the endocardium in views of the beating ventricles is an important component of any study of intracardiac flows during the cardiac cycle [22]. Although in some patients this boundary is seen clearly, in many the endocardial border is poorly defined, because of the presence of spurious echoes within the cavity that result in a reduction of useful contrast and a blurred haze between the wall and the cavity. By using contrast agents enhancing the signals from blood and opacifying the cardiac chambers of interest, the blood in the cardiac chambers can be rendered visible above the artifacts and a clear boundary can be seen, revealing the endocardial edges.

Technical developments over the past decade have focused on different microbubble constituents and effective methods of detection of their nonlinear signals. The ultrasound imaging apparatus extracts *nonlinear* signals to achieve the goal of separating microbubble from tissue signals with sufficient sensitivity to delineate boldly the endocardium-to-blood interface. Linear microbubble signals, due to simple backscatter, are too similar to the linear signals from the surrounding tissue. Blood signals are stronger with contrast agent, but the separation between tissue and microbubble is insufficiently crisp.

Luckily, strong nonlinear signals are created when an encapsulated gas is insonified, as the bubbles expand much more easily than they contract, as is shown in Figure 5.24, on p. 267. This is different from the behavior of tissue. Nonlinear fundamental signals originate from the same physical mechanism that generates the higher-order harmonics: asymmetrical expansion and contraction of the bubbles. Thus, a pulse with twice the compression pressure as another pulse will not generate exactly twice the returned signal, given that a microbubble resists progressively more strongly further compression, as it gets smaller.

5.6.1 Harmonic imaging

As microbubbles resonate in the ultrasound beam, they behave like a musical instrument and emit harmonic signals at multiples of the resonant frequency. Imaging microbubbles by selecting second harmonic signals is advantageous. A conventional phased array is used, with the receiver tuned to double the transmitting frequency, by means of a bandpass filter whose center frequency is at the second harmonic. The tissue and blood give an echo at the fundamental frequency, but the contrast agent undergoing nonlinear oscillation in the sound field emits the second harmonic, which is detected by the harmonic system. However, the higher frequency second harmonic bandwidth is subject to increased attenuation, limiting imaging depth. Moreover, echoes from solid tissues, as well as red blood cells, are suppressed. Real-time harmonic spectral Doppler and color Doppler modes (see Section 5.9, on pp. 280 ff.) have also been implemented on commercially available systems.

The pursuit of effective microbubble imaging ushered in unlooked for, but dramatic, enhancements in B-mode tissue image quality even without bubbles, because less haze is in evidence with second harmonic imaging. Studies have shown that contrast echocardiography improves image quality and completeness of wall segment visualization [61], especially in difficult-to-image patients and when harmonic imaging is used.

Moreover, it has been demonstrated that with contrast, harmonic imaging produces improvements over fundamental imaging in ventricular chamber opacification, endocardial delineation, and quantitative assessment of ventricular wall motion and systolic function [2]. Such improvements apply to rest as well as exercise echocardiography studies. As an ultrasonic wave propagates through tissue, energy at frequencies above the

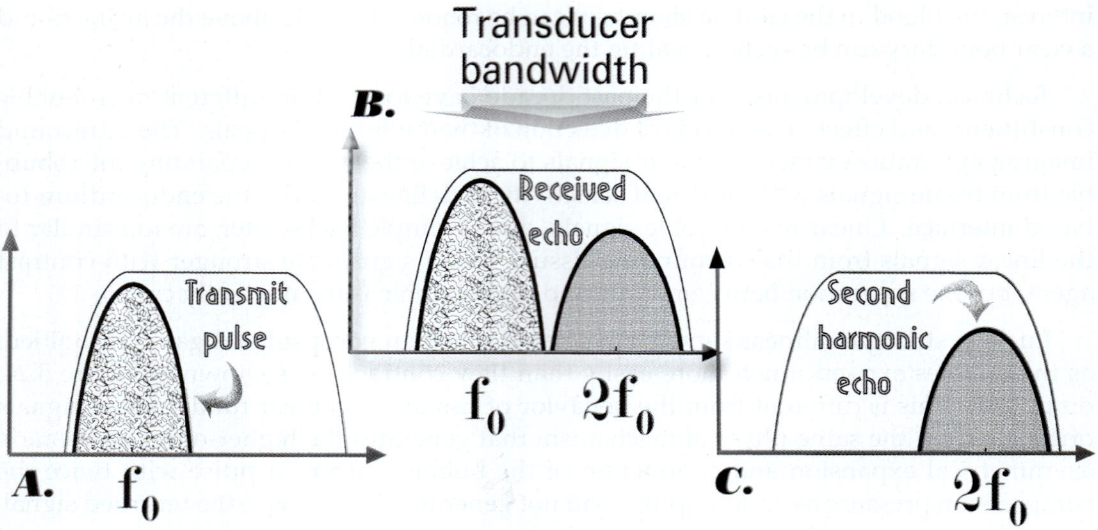

Figure 5.25: A. In second harmonic imaging, the pulse is transmitted at frequency f_0 using the lower half of the transducer bandwidth. B. The received echoes contain information at f_0 and $2 \cdot f_0$. C. The frequencies in the echoes around f_0 are filtered out and the image is formed from the $2 \cdot f_0$ part of the echo spectrum.

transmit-frequency range are gradually generated due to nonlinear propagation [9]. The importance of the effect increases as the applied acoustic pressure increases.

Tissue harmonic imaging has been found to improve ultrasonic imaging quality even without the use of ultrasound contrast agents [48]. Although the harmonic signal is weaker than the fundamental, it retains its "purity" better by only having to travel one way, from within the tissue (where it is generated) back to the receiver. Accordingly, the accumulation of noise and clutter is significantly reduced. Compared with standard mode, harmonic images typically show enhanced contrast and gray tone differentiation. Weak-echo, cluttering artifacts are particularly noticeable in liquid-filled areas, such as the cardiac chambers, and cloud the echocardiographic images making it difficult to identify with confidence anatomical features, including the blood-to-endocardium interface.

In harmonic imaging, the image is formed by using only the second-harmonic energy in the returned echoes, suppressing the weak cluttering echoes and enhancing those from the beam axis. This can result in a *clearer image*, improving the accuracy of diagnosis. Harmonic imaging can be achieved, as indicated in Figure 5.25, using a wide bandwidth transducer. To achieve good separation of the received second-harmonic frequencies from the fundamental frequencies, the frequency spectra of the pulse and the received echoes must be made narrower than for normal imaging. This results in an increase in the spatial pulse length, reducing the axial resolution of the system, as is explained in the next section.

5.6.2 Spatial resolution

Resolution, or the ability to distinguish two closely situated structures or events accurately, is an important concern for all imaging methodologies. If two echogenic features are not separated adequately in space, they produce overlapping ultrasound echoes that are not resolved on the display monitor. To be more precise, their echoes fuse together and they appear as one. If distinct echoes are not engendered initially by the reflectors in close proximity, the corresponding echogenic features will not be resolvable as discrete features. In echocardiographic imaging [47], spatial resolution has two facets: *axial* and *lateral*, which depend on different characteristics of the ultrasound pulses.

Axial resolution is the ability to distinguish two separate but closely positioned structures situated parallel to the propagation axis of the ultrasound beam. It is the minimum echogenic feature separation along the scan line that is necessary to produce separate echoes. Axial resolution (*mm*) is equal to one-half the spatial pulse length; its numeric value *decreases* as the ultrasound frequency increases. The smaller the axial resolution, the closer two reflectors can be along the ultrasound path and still be seen distinctly, and the finer the detail that can be resolved and the accuracy of echocardiographic dimensional measurements.

To enhance axial resolution the spatial pulse length must be decreased (see Fig. 5.26), by diminishing the ultrasound wavelength or the number of cycles in the pulse. Because the number of cycles per pulse is in general reduced to a minimum (one to three cycles) by transducer design, the way to improve axial resolution in practice is to increase frequency, so as to reduce wavelength. With the increase in frequency, however, comes a reduction in imaging depth because of a more intense attenuation of the ultrasound beam.

Lateral resolution refers to the ability to distinguish two adjacent but separate structures oriented perpendicularly to the axis of the sound-wave beam. It is the minimum echogenic feature separation across scan lines, which is necessary to produce distinct echoes when the beam is scanned across the echogenic features. Lateral resolution (*mm*) is equal to the beam width in the scan plane. As with axial resolution, a smaller lateral resolution value is better; it indicates finer imaging detail and accuracy of echocardiographic dimensional measurements. If the lateral separation between two echogenic features is greater than the beam diameter, two discrete echoes are created when the beam is swept across them.

The lateral resolution varies with distance from the transducer, along with the beam width. It is improved by reducing the beam diameter, namely, by *focusing*, with the best resolution attained at the focus (see Fig. 5.27A., on p. 273.). Focusing is accomplished through diverse means, incorporated in the transducer design. In most systems, it is achieved by curving the elements of the transducer or by electronically controlling them (cf. Figs. 10.39 and 10.43, on pp. 553 and 563, respectively). Lateral resolution is also influenced by the ultrasound wave frequency, with higher frequencies generally improving resolution [27].

Because both axial and lateral resolution improve with increasing frequency, higher frequency transducers would generally be preferred for accurate cardiac dynamic

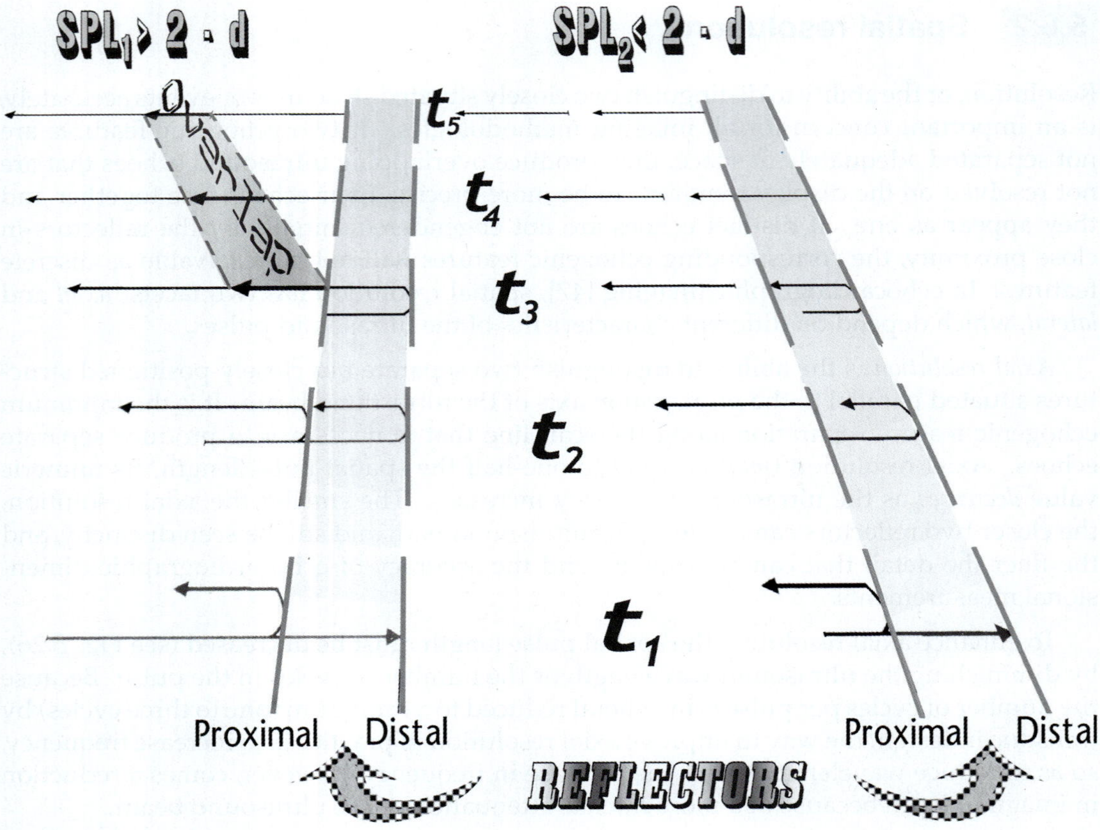

Figure 5.26: Axial resolution can be enhanced by increasing ultrasound frequency to yield a shorter spatial pulse length (SPL). On the left panel, the separation (d) of the reflectors is less than half the SPL and echo overlap occurs, so that the individual echoes cannot be resolved. On the right panel, reflector separation is again d, but resolution is achieved by shortening the SPL so that distinct echoes are obtained. Successive instants of time ($t_1, t_2, \ldots$) lapse from bottom to top in each panel.

geometric imaging. However, as the frequency increases, ultrasound wave penetration decreases. For example, a 5-*MHz* transducer will generally image to a depth of 12 to 15 *cm*, but a 10-*MHz* transducer may image to a depth of only 3–4 *cm*. Diagnostic ultrasound transducers generally have superior axial as compared to lateral resolution, even though the two may be similar in the *focal region* of strongly focused beams.

5.6.3 Temporal resolution

Temporal resolution, or the ability to distinguish two events in time, is an important consideration when imaging the beating heart. It is not as critical when imaging target organs

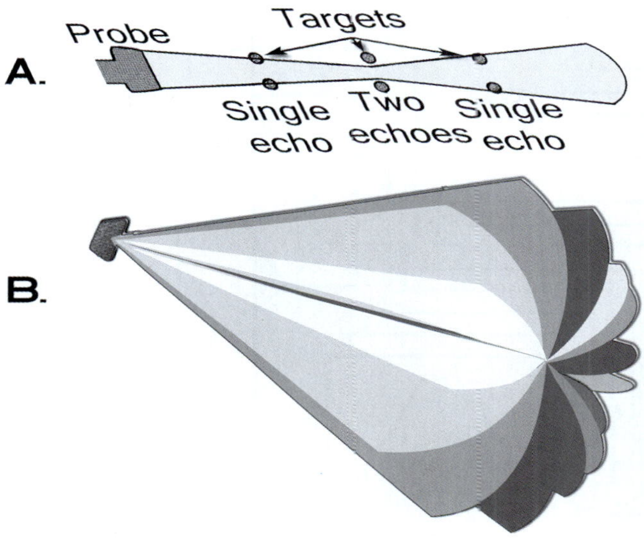

Figure 5.27: A. Two echogenic targets that are separated by the same distance can be seen as two in the focal zone but seen as one outside the focal zone, where the lateral resolution is lower. B. In rotational scanning the rotation of the imaging planes around a central axis results in oversampling nearer this axis of rotation and in undersampling farther from the axis.

that are relatively nonmoving, such as the kidney. Temporal resolution is determined by the number of complete image frames that can be acquired per second, generally expressed in Hertz. Depending on the applying frame rate, at which the ultrasound beam is scanned through the regional cross-sections, ultrasonographic instruments accumulate several frames per second in video memory. A rapid frame rate yields what appears to be a continuously changing echocardiographic image.

S-mode images (see description on p. 264) can be assembled in a movie. Such a movie is also called a *videoloop*, because it can be used to display repeatedly a number of cycles of a periodic phenomenon, such as a heart beat. While a 2-D echocardiographic videoloop is recorded, one will usually also record an ECG trace; the ECG has a number of distinctive peaks and valleys, which mark different events during the heartbeat and aid in the demarcation of successive phases of the electromechanical activity of the pumping heart.

The effective frame rate observed is limited by the *refresh rate* of the display monitor—i.e., the echocardiographic data may be entering the video memory at a frame rate of 100 *Hz*, but if the refresh rate of the monitor is 60 *Hz*, echo frames can be retrieved from memory and displayed at just 60 times per second. Nonetheless, there is an advantage to storing a frame rate that is a lot higher than the refresh rate of the display monitor, an important fact that is discussed in the following paragraphs.

When a frozen videoloop is put on view for interactive or manual quantitative geometric analysis, the individual successive frames retain the temporal resolution achieved

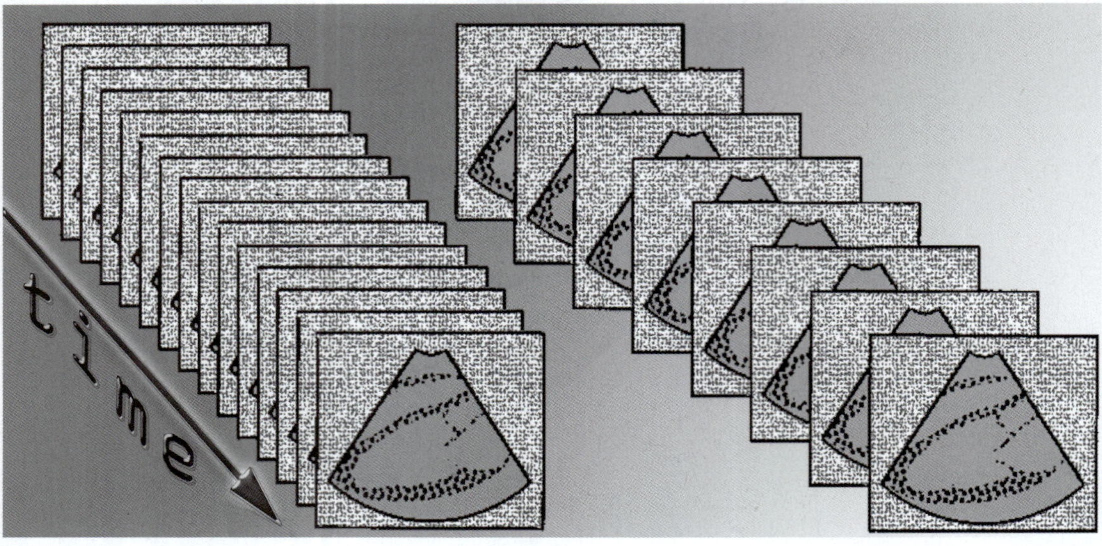

Figure 5.28: Interplay of frame rate and applying heart rate in determining effective temporal resolution. With a high frame rate, a specified interval of the cardiac cycle may be represented by 15–16 S-mode frames (left frame series); if the frame rate is cut down to half while the heart rate is maintained constant, the specified interval will be represented by only 8 frames (right S-mode frame series). The same effective reduction in the temporal resolution picture will result, in principle, if the frame rate (and the sampling interval between frames) is kept unchanged, but the heart rate is doubled in the right frame series compared to the left.

with the particular frame rate, e.g., 100 *Hz*. The importance of this becomes evident when the number of images acquired per cardiac cycle is evaluated. For example, at a heart rate of 90 *beats/min*, an acquisition frame rate of 30 *Hz* would result in only 20 images/cardiac cycle. Moreover, each image frame would be acquired over 5% of the cardiac cycle, making the accurate determination of continuously changing cardiac chamber dimensions unreliable. In contrast, imaging a heart beating at 60 *beats/min* with a frame rate of 120 *Hz* would acquire 120 frames over one cardiac cycle, greatly enhancing the temporal resolution. The interplay of frame rate and the applying heart rate in determining the effective temporal resolution is demonstrated in Figure 5.28.

When the freeze-frame mode is switched on, ultrasound beam scanning and/or fresh data entry into memory (during acquisition, or *off-line* analysis) are suspended, and the last frame entered is displayed continuously on the screen. Although the monitor continues to display what is in memory *at the refresh rate*, it is the *same* frame every time; accordingly, it appears as a static image. The introduction of freeze-frame technology on the ultrasound instruments permitted one to freeze, or effectively "stop," a single 2-D image and make cardiac geometric measurements. As a result of this development, echocardiographers and sonographers began making on-line measurements.

Freeze-frame, on-line measurements have become routine for not only 2-D echocardiography but for M-mode and Doppler, as well. A big advantage of freeze-frame technology is that one can create individual freeze frames, make the desired measurements, and have them immediately available during the examination. The measurements are usually made rapidly by an expert sonographer, and they are embedded into the video or digital recording. Upon review by the clinician, the measurements are available for interpretation. Even more crucial advantages of this method accrue for research studies.

Real-time echocardiographic imaging affords rapid and convenient acquisition of the desired images, with the display changing continuously as the scan plane traverses the region that is being examined. It allows quantitative imaging of the motion of moving structures (e.g., the endocardial borders), with the display at any individual scan plane changing constantly as the cardiac cycle unfolds. *Temporal resolution* is the ability of the echocardiographic display to distinguish closely spaced events in time and to present rapidly moving structures correctly. It is prescribed by the time (*ms*) from the beginning of one frame to that of the next. It therefore depends on the interval taken to acquire one complete frame, and improves as the acquisition frame rate increases.

The maximal frame rate, and thus the time resolution of the images, depends mostly on the time necessary for one pulse to propagate forward to the reflecting tissue interfaces of interest and back, and on the number of pulses used to construct the 2-D image. In current machines, where parallel beam forming is implemented, yielding several image lines with one ultrasound pulse, using an angle around 45°, a frame rate of about 150 *Hz* is attained. In the next section, we address issues pertaining to accurate resolution of heart motion with 2-D echocardiography.

5.7 Resolving heart motion with 2-D echocardiography

Beyond the straightforward information about heart position, size, and shape, we are particularly interested in following the dynamic geometric changes attendant to the motion of heart components, such as ventricular chamber walls and individual valve leaflets. The 2-D echocardiographic apparatus, however, does not sample the motion continuously. Instead, it samples the motion *intermittently*, at a frequency resolved by the mode of display and the depth of display.

The relationship between the sampling rate and the ability to depict accurately the motion that is being sampled is rather complex. A simple way of considering this problem is to recall the Nyquist theorem, which states (see Section 5.1.2, on pp. 239 f., and Fig. 2.25, on p. 76) that a sinusoidal component of frequency F must be sampled at least at twice its own frequency, or $2F$, to be followed. The sampling rate in an M-mode acquisition is the pulse repetition frequency and in a 2-D echocardiographic system, the *frame rate*. Thus, a pulse repetition frequency of 1000 *Hz* means that frequencies of 500 *Hz* and below would be encompassed in M-mode. At the same time, a 2-D echocardiographic system operating at 30 *frames/s* would *see* frequencies of 15 *Hz* and below, eliminating any possibility to detect high-frequency valve leaflet motions.

Very few cardiac structures vibrate at 500 *Hz*; therefore, a better question might be: how far do structures that need to be analyzed kinematically move between successive samples? Consider a valve leaflet moving at 100 *mm/s*, which is not uncommon for portions of a normal mitral valve. A sampling rate of 7.5 *Hz* then yields a distance of 13.3 *mm* between samples. At 15 *Hz*, the distance drops to 6.7 *mm*, and at 30 *Hz*, it is 3.3 *mm*. At 1,000 *Hz*, the displacement reduces to 0.1 *mm*. Clearly, the higher the sampling rate, the more faithful becomes the depiction of the kinematics of fast-moving heart components.

In the echo-ranging sonographic apparatus, the sampling rate is limited by the echo-ranging process, which requires echoes to return to the transducer, and the velocity of ultrasound through the tissues. An average soft tissue velocity of 1,540 *m/s* implies that it takes 13 μs ($13 \cdot 10^{-6}$ s) for an echo to arrive back to the ultrasound sensor for every cm of *round-trip* tissue travel. The maximum pulse repetition frequency, or PRF, possible in a sonograph is then determined, in part, by the depth of the most distant point that must be imaged. For instance, if the distance is 20 *cm*, then 20 $cm \times 13 \cdot 10^{-6}$ s$/cm = 260$ μs for echoes to arrive from that depth.[11] This represents a maximum nominal PRF of $1/(260\ \mu s)$, or 3,846 *Hz*. An M-mode sonograph operating at 1,000 *Hz* has no problems dealing with a 20 *cm* deep field of view, but a 2-D echocardiographic system clearly might.

A 2-D echocardiographic image is formed by displaying the echo-signals from many different ultrasound beam positions. Each pass of the ultrasound beam over its scanning limits defines one scanning frame. Each line within the scan used to make an image frame is called a *line-of-sight*. Typically, the lines/frame vary and can be as high as 256 or 512. In older systems, each line represented a single pulse-listen, echo-ranging cycle. Real-time scanning involves trade offs: higher resolution is achieved by increasing the number of lines (pulses) per degree of sweep angle; decreasing the depth of imaging increases the frame rate and the line density; by decreasing the size of the picture (scan angle), one can increase the density of lines per imaged field; and so forth.

Today, many phased-array and linear-array systems use a technique called *dynamic focusing*, where several pulse-listen cycles are used to make a *single* line on the 2-D image display. On every successive cycle, the beam focal zone axially changes position sequentially and only data acquired from each focal zone is used in the display. The number of pulse-listen cycles that are included in each image frame is a major determinant of the frame rate and the depth of imaging possible with any given 2-D echocardiographic system. This relationship is expressed in the equation:

$$FR = \frac{c}{D_{max} \times 2 \times N \times Z}, \tag{5.2}$$

where, FR is the frame rate (*Hz*), c is the effective speed of sound, D_{max} is the maximum imaging depth (2 accounts for the "round-trip" distance), N is the number of lines per frame, and Z is the number of focal zone positions if the system uses dynamic focusing. In a mechanical 2-D echocardiographic system or in a fixed focus phased-array scanner, Z

[11] To this time one should add the time required for the transducer to be switched from receiver to emitter mode—usually 10–20 μs.

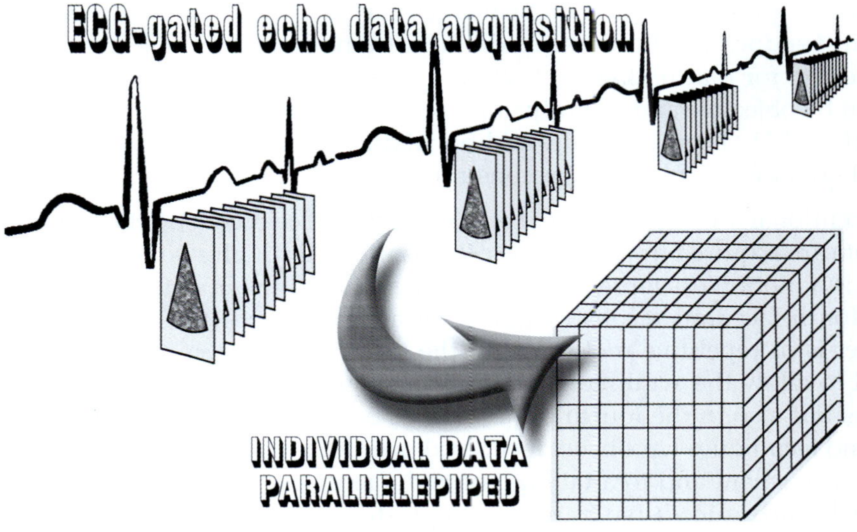

Figure 5.29: Multiple frames through the cardiac VOI, synchronized by ECG-gated 2-D echocardiography, are reformatted and transformed into a series of isotropic data cuboids, such as that depicted in the lower right, corresponding to instantaneous 3-D cardiac reconstructions. Such data cuboids serve as the basis for 3-D dynamic geometric analyses.

equals 1. The preceding equation shows that as either the depth of the scanned structures, or the number of lines per frame, or both are increased, the frame rate must be compensatorily reduced. Because of such limitations on frame rate, 2-D echocardiographic systems must trade off frame rate for lines-of-sight or depth of display.

5.7.1 3-D echo imaging in the study of intracardiac blood flows

The essential objective of any imaging technique for the investigation of the dynamic anatomy of the beating heart is an accurate 3-D display of cardiac morphology throughout a complete cardiac cycle. The reason for such an interest in the study of intracardiac blood flow dynamics is quite clear: 3-D imaging is necessary for the specification of the dynamic geometric boundary conditions of the flow field under normal or pathological conditions. The obvious requirement for reliable dynamic geometric measurements of the cardiac chambers is visibility of the entire endocardial border in cross-section. This can present difficulties, particularly on still frames used for interactive dimensional measurements, which entail manually tracing the endocardium and calculating instantaneous chamber shapes and volumes.

In routine clinical practice, spatial information is derived by mentally reassembling 2-D echocardiographic images obtained from different imaging planes. However, although endocardial borders may be visualized sufficiently well with moving images in video loops, signal dropouts and noise in the images may impair the accurate and reproducible delineation of endocardial borders in individual frame displays. Subjective procedures are subject to error; for that reason, 3-D echocardiography techniques have been developed to replace it by objective and reproducible computerized reconstructions, as is detailed in Chapters 10 and 11. There are many additional difficulties that can get in the way of fully automated quantification and 3-D reconstructions.

In conventional 3-D echocardiography, involving slice-reconstruction approaches, geometric data are acquired from multiple planes cutting through a volume of interest (VOI). If the VOI is a motionless target, only spatial tracking of the imaging plane movement is necessary for the accurate reconstruction of the acquired slices into 3-D images. However, if the target is in repetitive motion, as is the beating heart, temporal tracking must be performed to allow the acquired slices to be assembled correctly, not just in 3-D spatial dimensions but also in the fourth dimension of time in the cardiac cycle. Sophisticated methods and techniques have been developed in order to avoid image degradation caused by cardiac movement and to attain accurate dynamic geometric information. ECG gating, to synchronize successive frames through the cardiac VOI at corresponding points in the cardiac cycle, has successfully served this purpose (see Fig. 5.29).

To acquire a complete 3-D echocardiographic dataset, several hundred single images have to be collected and stored digitally. Prerequisite for a 3-D reconstruction of the instantaneous geometry of any cardiac chamber is a rectangular parallelepiped, or cuboid, an *isotropic* digital dataset comprising a multitude of cubic volume data elements, or *voxels* (see Fig. 5.29, on p. 277). Voxels are the mathematical basis for *any* 3-D reconstruction. (cf. Figs. 10.2, 10.3, and 10.4, on pp. 485, 486, and 488, respectively). The term "isotropic" signifies that the resolution is identical in all coordinate directions, and that the data density within the rectangle is homogeneous. In acquiring instantaneous 3-D images, the successive data cuboids are filled with 2-D echocardiographic information from transesophageal or transthoracic image acquisition methods. Gated image acquisition in preselected imaging planes can be accomplished by high-precision motion control modules using dedicated computer logic and encompassing a *stepper motor*.[12]

3-D reconstruction involves a succession of repeated steps of image processing. The first step is the elimination of problems arising simply because the imaging planes are recorded at different time points, and thus under varying conditions. Although several gating techniques are utilized for image acquisition, some variability is inevitable, and artifacts can be introduced by variations of the heart rate, global motions of the heart relative to the probe, and instability in the positioning of the transducer. Accordingly, various image processing algorithms have been developed for the identification, compensation, and suppression of such artifacts from the acquired 2-D frame sequences.

The next problem in 3-D dataset acquisition arises because the single imaging planes are recorded at different angles, resulting in non-homogeneous spatial data density. This is significant in rotational scanning since the rotation of the imaging planes around a central axis results in oversampling nearer this axis of rotation and in undersampling farther

[12] Stepper motors do as their name suggests: they "step" a little bit at a time, and have another characteristic, *holding torque*; this allows a stepper motor to hold its position firmly when not turning.

from the axis, in the deeper-lying structures (see Fig. 5.27B., on p. 273). After acquisition, image processing is needed to compensate for this: redundant data are eliminated and missing data are interpolated. Such adjustments can at times lead to heavy smoothing of geometric details, or to new artifacts.

After these preprocessing steps, the spatiotemporal geometric data matrices can be "sliced and diced" in any secondary direction in real-time, to display any desired "instantaneous" imaging plane on a dedicated viewing station, or to undertake computer studies of intracardiac flow. Brightness and contrast can be adjusted, and pseudocolors applied *(colorization)*, to obtain optimal image quality. Quantitative geometric analyses of the *dynamic* 3-D (effectively 4-D, time being the fourth dimension) datasets can be done using custom or commercially available dedicated software analysis systems (e.g., QLAB™ Advanced Quantification software, Philips Ultrasound, USA. and Tomtec 4D Cardio-view,™ Tomtec, Gmbh, Germany), for the measurement of intracardiac angles, distances, areas, volumes, and velocities.

Such software can readily provide numerical data and displays of 3-D renderings in gray scale or colorization, rapid generation of full 3-D wire-mesh instantaneous endocardial volumes, and global and simultaneous regional LV volume waveforms. The derived quantitative geometric data afford appropriate boundary conditions for patient-specific cardiac flow simulations and evaluations of intracardiac flows, as we will see in Chapters 10-14 and 16. Automatic multiplanar reconstruction (described in Section 11.5, on pp. 594 ff.), real-time 4-D display and volumetric, as well as area and distance measurements in 3-D, offer additional cardiodynamic geometric information, not available with any 2-D technology.

5.8 M-mode display

The M-mode display (motion mode) allows measurements of the rate and timing of the dynamic movements of the heart. As is discussed above (on p. 273) for the case of 2-D echocardiographic tracings, while an M-mode strip-chart tracing is recorded, one will usually also record an ECG trace. To acquire an M-mode display, the ultrasound beam is not steered as in B-mode but is aligned with the moving target under examination and held in position. Ultrasound pulses are transmitted along the beam and the echoes received in a normal pulse–echo sequence. As in B-mode scanning, the received echoes are used to control the brightness of the display line. However, in M-mode the beam remains fixed, while the display line is stepped across the display after each pulse–echo sequence.

Reflecting targets that are not moving with respect to the transducer show up as *straight lines* across the display. On the other hand, targets that are moving toward or away from the transducer show up as an *undulating line* pattern, as illustrated in Figures 7.14 and 7.15, on pp. 345 and 347, where the regular movements of the mitral and aortic valve leaflets can be followed. Dynamic geometric information relating to the movement of cardiac valves and of endocardial chamber boundaries can be obtained and measured.

5.9 Doppler echocardiography

Ultrasound can be used directly, by exploiting the familiar Doppler shift, to assess blood flow by measuring the change in frequency of the ultrasound scattered from the moving blood corpuscles [1,12,17]. This shift is the change in the observed frequency of the sound wave, compared to the sent frequency, which occurs due to relative motion between the observer and the source—e.g., changing pitch of an ambulance siren as it passes by. It enables ultrasound to be used to detect and measure the velocity of motion of blood and tissue. Most Doppler systems exhibit both spectral Doppler displays and color Doppler mappings of velocity; the magnitude of the Doppler shift frequency is proportional to the relative velocity between the source and the observer.

The detected Doppler shift frequency (f_{DS}) is the difference between the received frequency (f_S) and the sent frequency (f_R); it depends on the frequency of the transmitted ultrasound, the speed of the ultrasound through the tissue (c) and the velocity of the blood (v), as expressed by the Doppler equation:

$$f_{DS} = f_R - f_S = \frac{2 \cdot f_S \cdot v \cdot \cos\theta}{c}. \tag{5.3}$$

The ultrasound beam sent out by the transducer strikes the moving blood, so the frequency of ultrasound as experienced by the blood cells is dependent on their velocity relative to the transducer. The blood cells, in turn, scatter the ultrasound, some of which travels back to the transducer and is detected. The scattered ultrasound is Doppler frequency shifted again as a result of the motion of the blood cells, which now act as a moving source. Therefore, a Doppler shift occurs twice between the ultrasound beam being sent out and received back at the transducer; this accounts for the presence of the "2" in Equation 5.3.

The detected Doppler shift depends on the *cosine* of the angle θ, which is known as the angle of insonation, between the direction of the ultrasound beam and that of the blood velocity. This angle can change as a result of variations in the orientation of the probe or the direction of a time-dependent blood velocity. It is often desirable to adjust the angle of insonation to maximize the obtainable Doppler shift. The highest Doppler frequency shift from any specific blood velocity occurs when the velocity and the beam are aligned; that is when the angle of insonation is zero. This is so because the cosine function has a maximum value of ± 1.0 when the angle is $0°$ or $180°$, respectively, and a value of 0 when the angle is $90°$ or $270°$. Rearrangement of Equation 5.3 gives:

$$v = \frac{c \cdot f_{\text{DS}}}{2 \cdot f_S \cdot \cos\theta}. \tag{5.4}$$

Provided that the local, instantaneous, insonation angle θ is within about $18°$ from $0°$, good (within 5% of the *"true"* value) spectral velocity estimates can be obtained; similarly, for the opposite flow direction, when the angle θ is within about $18°$ from $180°$.

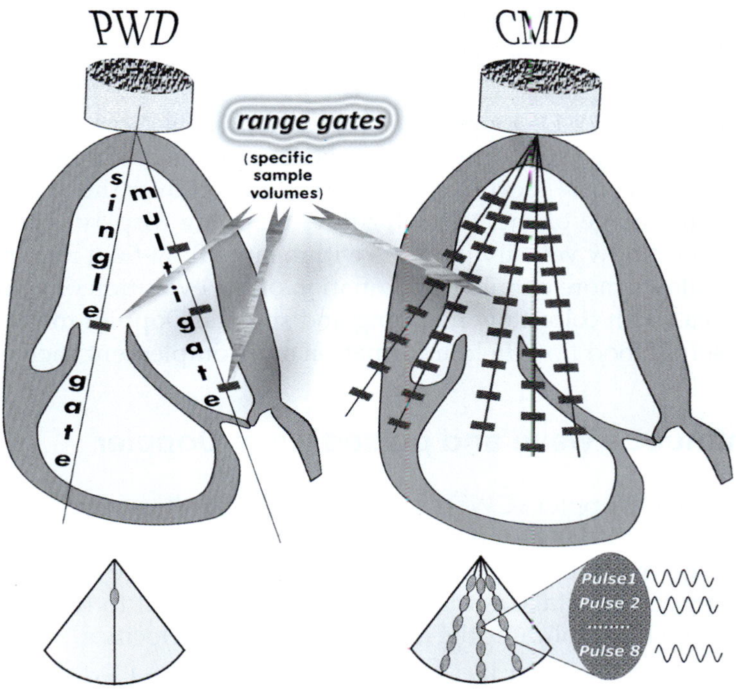

Figure 5.30: The main pulsed wave Doppler imaging modalities are pulsed wave *spectral* Doppler (PWD), which displays velocity information as frequency shift *vs.* time plots, as does continuous wave Doppler (CWD), and 2-D color flow mapping Doppler (CMD), which displays the velocity field information as a 2-D color image superimposed on an anatomic B-scan image. In CMD, color codes the magnitude and direction relative to the transducer of the instantaneous Doppler shift for each flow-field pixel, averaged over the pixel. In PWD, only one (or a few) range gate(s) are analyzed. In CMD, thousands of sample volumes distributed along many scan lines are examined by auto-correlation analysis (see Section 2.21, on pp. 95 ff.) using several (8 in this illustration) short, successive pulse trains, as is explained in Sections 5.9.5 and 5.9.6, on pp. 288 ff.

5.9.1 Doppler modalities

The main display modalities of Doppler ultrasound systems are [11]:

i. Spectral Doppler, which encompasses continuous wave (CWD) and pulsed wave Doppler (PWD). In CWD, ultrasound cycles repeat indefinitely, whereas in PWD, successive *pulses* each comprise a few (5–30) ultrasound cycles separated in time by gaps of no ultrasound.[13] Spectral Doppler presents all the velocity information in the format of frequency shift *vs.* time plots. In such plots, vertical distance from the baseline corresponds to Doppler shift, while the gray scale indicates the amplitude of the detected ultrasound

[13]This is to be contrasted with sonographic pulses, which are typically 2 or 3 cycles long; shorter pulses improve image quality.

with that particular frequency shift. The Doppler frequency shift is relatively easy to measure and to calibrate in the instrument, and a zero frequency shift corresponds always to zero velocity.

ii. Color flow mapping 2-D Doppler (see Fig. 5.30), which displays the Doppler information as a 2-D color image superimposed on the B-scan image (duplex scanning). Color represents the instantaneous, local Doppler shift averaged over the area of each pixel of the image. The advantage of the 2-D color flow mapping display is that it allows the visualization of blood flow velocity patterns within large flow-field regions. The spectral Doppler display allows more detailed examination of the evolution of velocity over time, within a small area. Both color flow mapping and spectral Doppler modalities provide a wide range of useful blood flow-field information and complement each other.

5.9.2 Continuous wave and pulsed wave Doppler

The continuous wave Doppler (CWD) systems send out ultrasound continuously. The pulsed wave Doppler (PWD) systems send out repeated short pulses of ultrasound. The foremost advantage of PWD is that the Doppler signals can be acquired from known depth(s); the main disadvantage is that there is an upper limit to the Doppler shift that can be detected, which complicates the estimation of high velocities.

In a CWD system there must be separate transmission and reception of ultrasound (see Fig. 5.31 a., on p. 283) using two elements, one which transmits continuously and one which receives continuously. Doppler signals are obtained from the region where there is overlap of the transmit and receive ultrasound beams. In a PWD system it is possible to use the same elements for both the transmit and receive functions. The region from which the Doppler signals are obtained is resolved by the *depth* and the *length* of the individual range gate(s) (see Fig. 5.31b. and c.), which can *both* be adjusted as needed. The output of the receiver is sampled at a rate corresponding to the time it takes for the transmitted pulses to leave the transmitting crystal and return from the depth of interest. The received signal is processed by the Doppler signal processor to extract the Doppler frequency shifts, which are then displayed in the form of spectral Doppler, or color-coded Doppler flow maps.

5.9.3 Doppler signal processing for spectral Doppler modalities

When ultrasound is sent out from the transducer, it will pass through regions of tissue and of blood. The blood will presumably be flowing, but tissues may also be moving; e.g., the heart moves in the course of the cardiac cycle and so do tissues in contact with it. The received ultrasound signal contains echoes from stationary and moving tissue, as well as echoes from flowing and, perhaps, from relatively stationary blood. The amplitude of the signal from blood is extremely small compared to tissue; typically 40 dB smaller (-40 dB is an amplitude ratio of 0.01, or 1%). On the other hand, maximal intracardiac and transvalvular blood flow velocities may amount to several m/s, whereas maximal velocities of mural myocardial tissue displacement may typically attain 10 cm/s, or so.

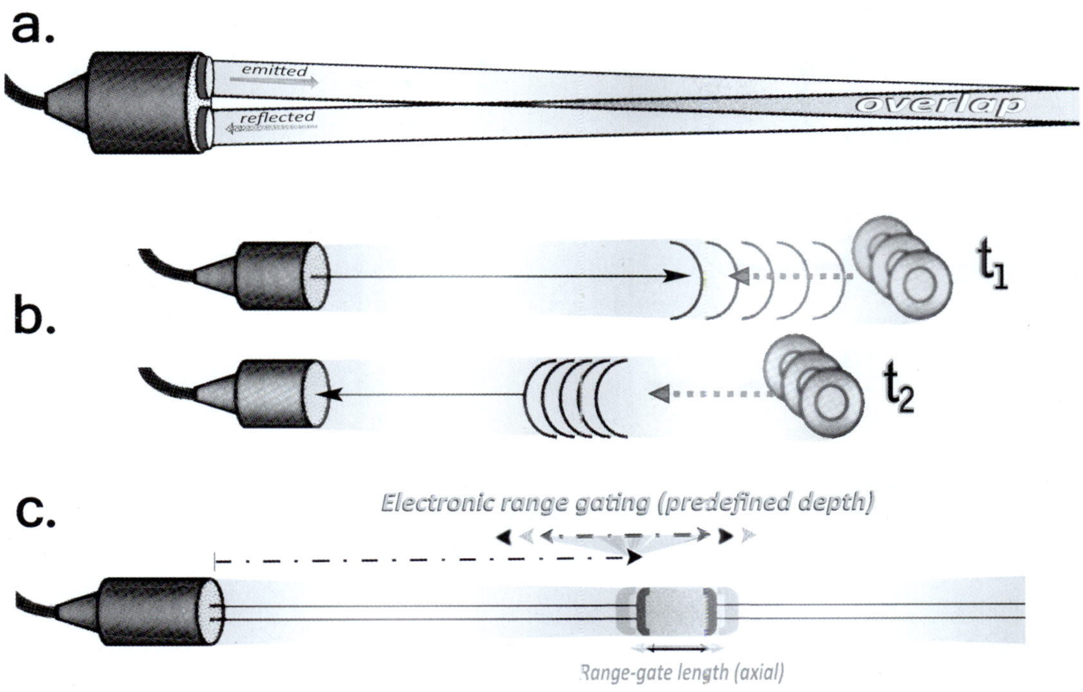

Figure 5.31: Spectral Doppler systems comprise continuous wave Doppler (CWD), which transmits ultrasound continuously, and pulsed wave Doppler (PWD), which transmits short ultrasound bursts, allowing Doppler signals to be acquired from one or multiple *known* depths. a. The CWD probe sends and receives continuously and simultaneously using two different piezoelectric crystals. The zone of overlap of the emitted and received beams is the measurement region, or "line of sight." b. The PWD transducer operates in a discontinuous fashion: at an instant t_1, it emits an ultrasound burst in the direction of the moving reflectors and then waits until it can receive the returning echo at a later time, t_2. c. The time-lag for the reception of the returning echo defines the depth of the range-gate. This depth and the axial length of the gate can be adjusted by the electronic controls of the Doppler system.

These different characteristics provide the means by which signals from actual blood flow can be separated from those produced by the surrounding walls. In fact, by implementing different filtering schemes, good advantage of these differences is taken in distinct applications based on the two sets of signals: applying a high-pass filter in Doppler flow, and a low-pass filter in Doppler tissue imaging (DTI). The heart valves, however, are solid structures which can move with the velocity of the passing blood, giving rise to high intensity signals (so-called "valve clicks" in the Doppler spectral recording [44], not to be confused with the auscultatory findings) attaining saturation of the Doppler spectrum, as is demonstrated in Figure 5.32, on p. 284.

Dedicated signal processing algorithms are applied to derive the Doppler signals from the received ultrasound echoes. They generally comprise *demodulation*, i.e., the separa-

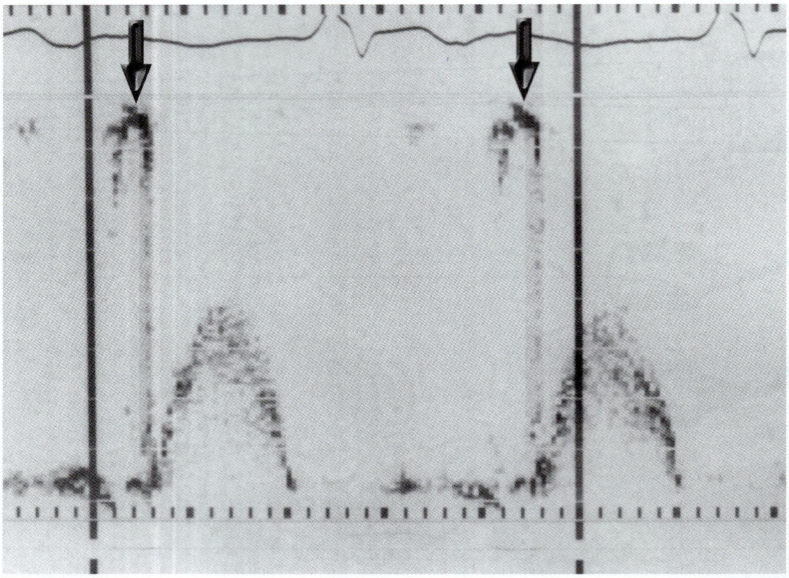

Figure 5.32: A typical ejection velocity curve from the right ventricular outflow tract showing the *valve clicks* (arrows) in the spectral recording. (Adapted, slightly modified, from Morera et al. [29], by permission of Elsevier Inc.)

tion of the Doppler frequency shift information from the underlying ultrasound signal received from tissue and blood, *high-pass filtering* for the removal of the tissue signal, and *frequency estimation* for the derivation of the Doppler shift frequencies and amplitudes. The Doppler frequency shifts created by flowing blood amount to a minute fraction of the transmitted ultrasound frequency. Equation 5.3 on p. 280 shows that, if the transmitted frequency is, e.g., 5 *MHz*, a flow velocity of 1 *m/s* will produce a Doppler shift of about 6.5 *kHz*, which is little over 0.1% of the transmitted frequency. Demodulation of the received signal removes the high transmit frequencies, but it leaves both the Doppler shift frequencies from blood flow and the *cluttering* large amplitude signal arising from the moving myocardial walls. At this stage it is actually not possible to distinguish the wall signal, known as "wall thump," from the actual blood flow velocity signal; this calls for another step, namely, high-pass filtering.

To correctly estimate the Doppler shift frequencies from blood, the Doppler signals from tissue are removed electronically by a special filter, the "wall thump" filter. It implements the simplest approach, adopted by many Doppler systems, which relies on a high-pass frequency filter. Wall filter performance is critical to the success not only of spectral Doppler systems, but of color flow-field mapping Doppler, too. A high-pass filter cut-off setting of 300 *Hz*, or more, is required since, e.g., valve leaflets are moving at relatively high speeds—$O(v) \simeq 10$ *cm/s*,[14] and the detection of high blood velocities

[14] An order of magnitude—$O(q)$, or $O \sim (q)$—estimate for a variable q is an approximation rounded to the nearest power of ten; e.g., an order of magnitude estimate for a quantity between about 5 and 20 is 10. The big-O, standing for "order of," is the capital letter O, and not the digit zero.

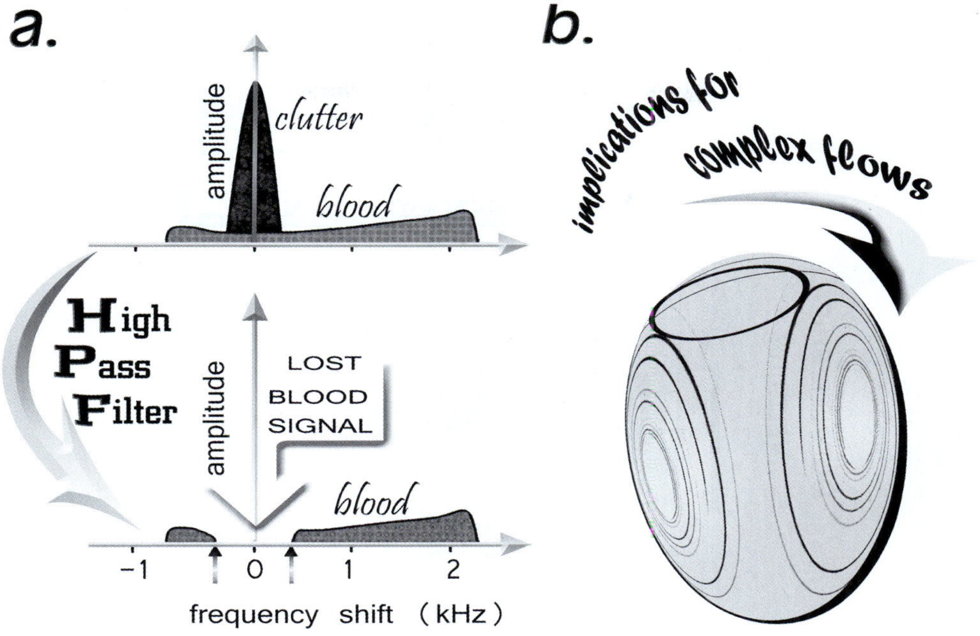

Figure 5.33: a. High-pass filtering is needed to remove the clutter signal from moving walls; a corollary of this is the concomitant loss of the lowest blood velocities. b. Moreover, at insonation angles close to 90°, the Doppler shift frequencies are low and are similarly removed by the clutter filter. These technical limitations have adverse repercussions for Doppler measurements of the kinematics of complex intraventricular blood flow fields, which are characterized by velocities in many directions and in close proximity to moving walls—see diastolic filling vortex, Chapter 14.

is of interest. Removal of frequencies below a certain threshold removes the Doppler-shift components derived from the walls. An unfortunate consequence of this process, however, is that the very low intraventricular blood velocities in the vicinity of the chamber walls are also removed, since this filter of the ultrasound receiver also removes the signal from slowly moving blood, as is shown in Figure 5.33a. This fact compromises the detection, demonstration and measurement of slow blood flow velocities in, e.g., the vicinity of the expanding walls during early diastolic filling. That the detected Doppler frequency shift is proportional to the cosine of the angle of insonation, between the direction of the ultrasound beam and that of the local blood velocity, is critical too. This angle may shift as a result of variations in the direction of blood velocities in time-dependent flow fields. It is often impossible to adjust the angle of insonation to maximize the obtainable Doppler shifts for complex unsteady fields with multidirectional instantaneous velocities.

The Doppler frequency shift from any specific blood velocity actually vanishes when the velocity and the beam are completely unaligned and the angle of insonation is $\pm 90°$.

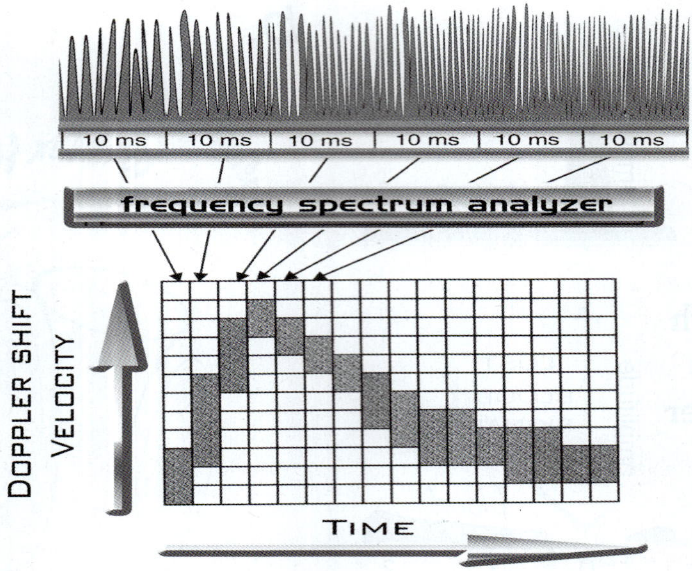

Figure 5.34: Schematic display of some aspects involved in the construction of a sonogram from the received pulsed Doppler signal. In this illustrative example, a complete spectrum is produced every 10 *ms* by frequency spectrum analysis, and each of these spectra is used to produce the next vertically swept "line" (or *window*) in the Doppler shift or velocity *vs.* time waveform.

This is so because the cosine function, which has a maximum absolute value of 1.0 when the angle is 0° or 180°, becomes 0 when the angle is ±90°. These technical limitations of the most prevalent method for clinical velocity measurements have had adverse repercussions in the appreciation of the kinematics and dynamics of intraventricular blood flow fields, and the recognition of related intraventricular blood flow phenomena, as is indicated pictorially in Figure 5.33**b.** We will address this important, albeit poorly appreciated, topic and will develop it at considerable length in Chapter 14.

After filtering, the Doppler shift frequency dataset is passed on to the process of frequency estimation. CWD systems display the time velocity waveform, either in the form of spectral Doppler, or in the form of a single trace that might, for instance, correspond to the maximal velocity at each successive time. A *spectrum analyzer* calculates the amplitude of all of the frequencies present within the Doppler signal, typically using the fast Fourier transform, or FFT,[15] which produces a complete spectrum every 5–10 *ms* (see Fig. 5.34). The computed Doppler shift can be displayed in frequency shift units (*kHz*), but most instruments solve the Doppler equation internally and output their display as linear velocity (in *cm/s* or *m/s*). The brightness in the spectral display reflects the power, or amplitude, of the Doppler signal component at that particular frequency shift or velocity.

[15]The FFT is discussed in Section 2.20.3, on pp. 94 ff.

Intracardiac blood velocities and the corresponding Doppler spectra are, generally, dynamic and nonstationary. The FFT works best on long samples with stationary spectra, and frequency resolution improves with longer samples but at the expense of temporal resolution of the unsteady velocities under examination (see Section 5.1.3, on pp. 240 ff.). To render the technique practicable for Doppler signal quantitation, special adjustments are made, which include the following:

- Short (1–10 *ms*) samples are taken and a stationary condition is assumed over each successive short interval—clearly, this condition is violated, especially during strong accelerations.

- Windowing is applied to the samples, which effectively yields a kind of *quasiperiodicity*, as is described in Section 5.1.3 on pp. 240 ff.

Despite its limitations, the FFT remains the archetype for Doppler signal analysis.

5.9.4 Pulse repetition frequency, aliasing and low velocity rejection

In PWD systems the basic steps of demodulation, high-pass filtering and frequency estimation are basically the same as for CWD. There is, however, an essential difference between CWD and PWD systems: in PWD a received ultrasound signal is *not* available continuously, as it is for CWD, and the location of the selected Doppler gate(s) (see Fig. 5.30, on p. 281) defines the range of depths from which each Doppler signal originates. The returned echoes received by the Doppler probe are amplified and demodulated. The demodulated signal is then sampled by a *sample-and-hold* (see Section 5.1.1, on pp. 236 ff.) circuit that is triggered by time-delay pulses. The time delay allows the selection of the location(s) at which the Doppler shift frequency is monitored. A low-pass filter removes frequencies above the Nyquist limit, which is represented by 1/2 PRF, and a high-pass wall filter removes unwanted high-amplitude, low-frequency signals, such as those from cardiac walls. The demodulated, filtered signal is digitized following *windowing* (see Section 5.1.3 on pp. 240 ff.), to minimize spectral leakage and distortion (cf. Figs. 5.5, on p. 241, and 5.6, on p. 242). The ensuing Fourier analysis yields the desired spectrogram or velocity displays.

Each PWD signal is thus contained within a series of multiple—depending on the applying pulse repetition frequency—consecutive, received short-segment samples of the demodulated Doppler signal that pass the individual receiver gate(s) once per pulse repetition period. These are fed to the sample-and-hold unit, where the demodulated Doppler signal is "recreated" from the small samples, and is revealed by the ensuing signal processing. The processed signal from any given gate has the same overall shape as the output from the CWD following demodulation, so that the velocity *vs.* time signals displayed from CWD and PWD appear similar.

A shortcoming of the pulsed Doppler is the limit of the highest Doppler frequency, or maximal velocity, that it can measure. This is determined by the PRF, which has to be at least twice as high as the maximal Doppler frequency, in order to avoid *aliasing*—see discussion in Section 5.1.2, on pp. 239 ff. This may pose a problem when measuring high velocities, e.g., in the ventricular outflow tracts during peak ejection. Because the round-trip pulse transit times from *deeper*-depth ranges are *longer*, a conflict exists invariably between range and maximum measurable velocity, and an increase in range means a decrease in the maximum velocity measurable by PWD. Accordingly, most modern ultrasonic imaging apparatuses are equipped with both CWD and PWD capabilities.

As we saw earlier, the maximum Doppler frequency that can be measured unambiguously is half the pulse repetition frequency. If the blood velocity being measured and the Doppler angle combine to give a Doppler frequency value greater than half of the PRF, aliasing and ambiguity in the Doppler signal ensue. The PRF is itself constrained by the range of the sample volume. The time interval between sampling pulses must be adequate for a pulse to make the return journey from the transducer to the reflector and back. If a second pulse is sent before the preceding one is received, the receiver cannot tell the reflected signals from the two pulses apart, and ambiguity in the range of the sample volume ensues. As the depth of investigation increases, the round-trip time of pulses to and from the scatterers increases, reducing the PRF for unambiguous ranging. The result is that the maximum measurable Doppler frequency decreases with depth.

Low pulse repetition frequencies are needed to examine low blood velocities, because the longer interval between pulses allows the scanner a better chance of discerning slow flow regions. Aliasing will occur if low pulse repetition frequencies or velocity scales are used and high velocities are present in the interrogated flow field. Conversely, if a high PRF is used to examine high velocities, such as those applying during the upstrokes of the E- and A-waves of diastolic filling near the inflow valve orifices of the ventricular chambers, low velocities that apply concurrently near the expanding walls are inadvertently missed. As noted at the outset of this section, the high-pass wall filter removes low-frequency (low velocity) signals, compounding this instrumentation-dependent systemic removal of low concurrent velocities (see also Section 14.4, on p. 742).

5.9.5 Color Doppler signal processing

The basic concept of the color Doppler is similar to that of the pulsed Doppler devices, which extract the mean Doppler shift frequency from a sample volume that is defined by the beam width and the individual range gate length. The only exception is that the color Doppler instruments are capable of estimating the mean Doppler shifts of hundreds of sample volumes along a scan line in a very short period of time, on the order of 30–50 *ms*. To be able to do so, they exploit fast algorithms, which use auto-correlation (see Section 2.21, on pp. 95 ff.) rather than the slower fast Fourier transform procedure.[16] Once the auto-correlation function is known, simple arithmetic operations remain, which are computationally more efficient (and hence faster) than the FFT, for computation of the mean frequency and the variance at each sample volume and corresponding pixel.

Range resolution in pulsed Doppler is achieved by transmitting a short burst of ultrasound. Following the burst, the received signal is cross-correlated with a delayed version

[16] One such algorithm is based on the Wiener–Khinchine theorem, which specifies that the auto-correlation function $H(\tau)$ of a function $f(t)$ is the Fourier transform of the power spectrum $P(\omega)$ of $f(t)$.

of the transmitted burst as a reference signal. The transit time of the transmitted pulse to the region of interest and back again is equal to this delay. Thus, the sampling volume can be moved to different positions along the beam by changing this delay. The implications of this are clear: flow at different depths, or at different points within the flow field can be selectively monitored.

Color Doppler flow imaging systems are *duplex scanners*, capable of displaying both B-mode and Doppler blood flow data simultaneously in real time. Color flow imaging uses fewer, shorter pulse trains along each color scan line of the image to give a mean frequency shift and a variance at each small area of measurement. This frequency shift is displayed as a color pixel. The scanner then repeats this for hundreds of scan lines to build up the color image, which is superimposed onto the B-mode image. The transducer elements are switched rapidly between B-mode and color flow imaging modalities, to give an impression of a combined (*"fused"*) simultaneous image. The pulses used for color flow imaging are typically three to four times longer than those for the B-mode image, with a corresponding loss of axial resolution.

In the flow images, each pixel indicates the Doppler shift. The frequency of the reflected ultrasound is Doppler shifted according to the speed of the blood in the direction away from or toward the probe. The false-color Doppler flow image is superimposed on a gray-scale B-mode tissue image. Although in principle any arbitrary color mapping scale might be used for the velocity, most systems employ a red-based scale for blood flowing in one direction (*toward* the transducer), and a blue-based scale for blood velocities in the opposite direction (*away from* the transducer). Eight or more shades of color are used in most systems to depict gradations in the magnitude of the velocity. Typically, the lighter the color, the higher is the corresponding velocity; speeds higher than 1 m/s are color-coded yellow and white *irrespective* of flow direction. Since the basic idea of Doppler flow mapping is similar to that of pulsed Doppler, the maximal Doppler frequency that can be detected without *aliasing* is at best one-half of the PRF (cf. preceding paragraph).

5.9.6 Time-domain systems

Another method for calculation of blood velocity is to divide the distance traveled by ultrasound-scattering blood cells by the time taken. This principle is used in time-domain Doppler systems, which use the pulsed wave approach [57]. Figure 5.35, on p. 290, shows the position of moving scatterers, which are red blood cells in the blood, and the corresponding echo train F(s) for two consecutive ultrasound pulses. For the second pulse the scatterer target and the site of origin of its echo are located further away from the transducer along the flow path s. The estimation of the blood velocity is performed as follows:

- Calculation of the depth from which echoes are received is carried out automatically by the machine from the time between transmission and reception of the echo, assuming the average soft tissue speed of sound, c, to be 1,540 m/s. The distance,

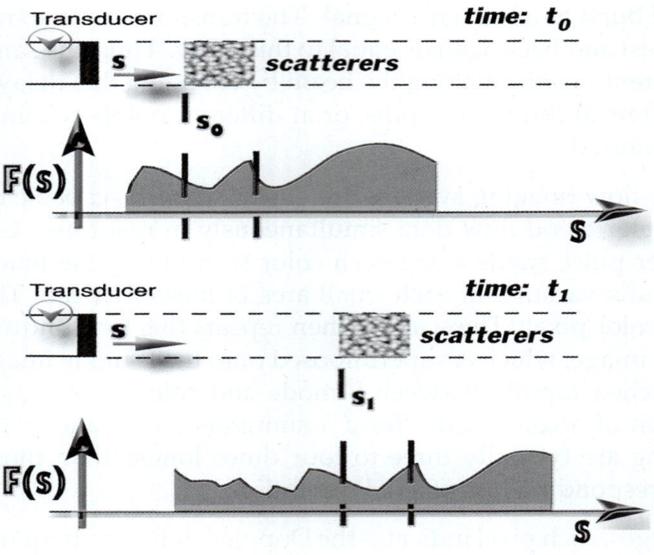

Figure 5.35: Pictorial representation of cross-correlation for time-domain velocity estimation. A volume of scatterers is shown moving along the flow path s with velocity v, from s_0 at time = t_0 to s_1 at time = t_1. F(s) signifies the received echo waveform.

$(s_1 - s_0)$ traversed between the two consecutive pulses is estimated from the difference between the corresponding depths:

$$(s_1 - s_0) = \frac{c(t_1 - t_0)}{2}. \tag{5.5}$$

The factor of 2 in the preceding equation allows for the total *"round-trip"* distance traveled by the ultrasound, which is two times the depth of the moving target from which the echoes originate. The time-domain system estimates the difference in the time the echo is received between consecutive echoes by performing a temporal cross-correlating of the echo trains or waveforms, $F(s) = F(ct/2)$, that are collected at different times, t_o and t_1.

- The cross-correlation function can be used to determine the delay of one signal with respect to another (see Section 2.21, on pp. 95 ff.). The cross-correlation function of the two continuous time echo waveforms is defined by:

$$r_{t_0,t_1}(\tau) = \int_{-\infty}^{\infty} F_{t_0}(t) F_{t_1}(t - \tau) dt, \tag{5.6}$$

where, $r_{t_0,t_1}(\tau)$ is the cross-correlation function, and $F_{t_0}(t)$ and $F_{t_1}(t)$ are echo waveforms obtained at t_o and t_1. A cross-correlation time lapse between the received signals $F_{t_0}(t)$ and $F_{t_1}(t)$ can be estimated by computing their cross-correlation function as the *time shift*, or *delay* τ, is varied; it is effectively given by the value of τ

for which r_{t_0,t_1} is maximized. In practice, when processing digital signals, the windowed cross-correlation $F_0 \star F_1$ of the digitally sampled received ultrasound signals $F_0(n)$ and $F_1(n)$ is given as:

$$F_0 \star F_1 = \sum_{n=N_1}^{N_2} F_0(n)F_1(n-d), \tag{5.7}$$

where, N_1 and N_2 define a window in time to which the correlation is applied. The value of the *dummy time* variable, d, which maximizes $F_0 * F_1$ is chosen as the *time delay* between the two echo waveforms.

- Considering the equations in the preceding paragraph, what is happening is the second waveform or time series is *"being slid past the first"* and, at each shift, the sum of the product of the newly lined up terms in the series is computed. This sum will be large when the shift (delay) is such that similar structure in the two samples lines up. Once the cross-correlation time delay is ascertained, it can be substituted for $(t_1 - t_0)$, the time difference between consecutive echoes, in Equation 5.5 and the distance traversed, $(s_1 - s_0)$, can be computed. The velocity, v, of the red blood cell scatterers moving in the direction of the ultrasound beam can then be calculated from the following equation, if $(t_1 - t_0)$ is set equal to T, the pulse repetition period of the transmitted pulses:

$$v = \frac{s_1 - s_0}{T}. \tag{5.8}$$

5.9.7 Fusion of hemodynamic multimodality measurements

Ultrasound imaging captures dynamic, real-time images that can be analyzed to obtain quantitative structural and functional information on the beating heart. This real-time format gives ultrasound imaging particular advantage in imaging moving targets, such as the heart and blood. Its various imaging modes and formats add to its versatility as well as its capability and adaptability. Other than magnetic resonance imaging, no other imaging modality can provide the same structural and functional information that can be obtained by ultrasound techniques. Modeling of moving anatomic structures is complicated by the complexity of motion intrinsic and extrinsic to the structures. However when motion is cyclical, such as in the heart, effective dynamic modeling can be approached using modern fast imaging techniques; they provide 2-D structural data from which 3-D volume images throughout the cardiac cycle may be reconstructed, yielding dynamic 4-D views of cardiac chamber pulsations (see Section 10.4, on pp. 547 ff.). Motion information can then be extracted by examining and tracking the 2- to 4-D image data.

The integrative study of intracardiac flow dynamics requires analysis of *multidimensional* spatial and temporal variables and complex hemodynamic measurements, such as those that are surveyed in this chapter. Visualization of the cardiac chambers and intracardiac flows in 3-D is now possible. Multimodality, multidimensional data obtained from diverse hemodynamic measurement systems, including multisensor catheters, angiography, and ultrasound, provide largely complementary hemodynamic data. Therefore, it is important to "fuse" or combine such complementary data into a composite form, which can provide synergistic information about cardiac fluid dynamic function.

Interestingly, the feasibility of multimodality registration of 2- and 3-D cardiac ultrasound images with cardiac SPECT images, with the aim to simultaneously present the complementary anatomical and perfusion information gleaned from the two unconnected modalities, has already been demonstrated in a clinical context [56]. Similarly, the fusion of cardiac anatomical and fluid dynamic CFD simulation data has the potential to improve on the sensitivity and specificity of the individual approaches for diagnosing subtle but important intracardiac flow and ventricular function changes, as is developed in Chapters 12-14 and 16. Moreover, the availability of a variety of interactive display tools for quantitative hemodynamic and imaging information can significantly enhance the analysis of structure-to-function relationships and of morphomechanical correlations in health and disease, as has already been emphasized in Section 3.12, on pp. 154 ff.

References and further reading

[1] Allan, P.L.P. [Ed.] Clinical Doppler ultrasound. 2nd ed. 2006, Philadelphia, PA: Churchill Livingstone Elsevier. viii, 373 p.

[2] Al-Mansour, H.A., Mulvagh, S.L., Pumper, G.M., Klarich, K.W., Foley, D.A. Usefulness of harmonic imaging for left ventricular opacification and endocardial border delineation by optison. Am. J. Cardiol. 85: 795–9, 2000.

[3] Anderson, B. Echocardiography: the normal examination and echocardiographic measurements. 2nd ed. 2007, Manly, Qld., Australia: MGA Graphics. 337 p.

[4] Aviles, R.J., Messerli, A.W., Askari, A.T., Penn, M.S., Topol, E.J. [Eds.] Introductory guide to cardiac catheterization. 2004, Philadelphia, PA: Lippincott Williams & Wilkins. xiii, 155 p.

[5] Baim, D.S., Grossman, W. [Eds.] Grossman's cardiac catheterization, angiography, and intervention. 7th ed. 2006, Philadelphia, PA: Lippincott, Williams & Wilkins. xvii, 807 p.

[6] Bashore, T.M. [Ed.] Invasive cardiology: principles and techniques. 1990, Toronto; Philadelphia: Decker; Saint Louis, MO: Sales and distribution, United States and Puerto Rico, C.V. Mosby Co. x, 318 p.

[7] Butler, R., Gunning, M., Nolan, J. Essential cardiac catheterization. 2007, London; New York: Hodder Arnold. 317 p.

[8] Carabello, B.A., Narula, J., Young, J.B. [Eds.] Valvular disease. 2007, Philadelphia, PA: Saunders. vii, 487 p.

[9] Carstensen, E.L., Bacon, D.R. Biomedical applications. Ch. 15, pp. 421–43, In: Nonlinear Acoustics, M.F. Hamilton, D.T. Blackstock [Eds.] Chestnut Hill, MA: Academic Press, 1998. xviii, 455 p.

[10] Condos, W.R., Latham, R.D., Hoadley, S.D., Pasipoularides, A. Hemodynamic effects of the Mueller maneuver by simultaneous right and left heart micromanometry, Circulation 76: 1020–28, 1987.

[11] DeGroff, C.G. Doppler Echocardiography. Ped. Cardiol. 23: 307–33, 2002.

[12] Evans, D.H., McDicken, W.N. Doppler ultrasound: physics, instrumentation and signal processing. 2nd ed. 2000, Chichester, UK; New York, Wiley. xxviii, 427 p.

[13] Fogel, M.A. [Ed.] Ventricular function and blood flow in congenital heart disease. 2005, Malden, MA: Blackwell Futura. xii, 380 p.

[14] Gramiak, R., Shah, P.M. Echocardiography of the aortic root. Invest. Radiol. 3: 356–63, 1968.

[15] Greis, C. Technology overview: SonoVue (Bracco, Milan). Eur. Radiol. 14 Suppl. 8: P11–5, 2004.

[16] Hubbell, J.H. Review and history of photon cross section calculations. Phys. Med. Biol. 51: R245–62, 2006.

[17] Jawad, I.A. A practical guide to echocardiography and cardiac Doppler ultrasound. 2nd ed. 1996, Boston, MA: Little, Brown. x, 405 p.

[18] Kasser, I.S., Kennedy, J.W. Measurement of left ventricular volumes in man by single-plane cineangiography. Invest. Radiol. 4: 83–90, 1969.

[19] Kern, M.J. The cardiac catheterization handbook. 4th ed. 2003, Philadelphia, PA, Mosby. xx, 650 p.

[20] Kern, M.J., Lim, M.J. [Eds.] Hemodynamic rounds: interpretation of cardiac pathophysiology from pressure waveform analysis. 3rd ed. 2008, Hoboken, NJ: J. Wiley.

[21] Kester, W., NetLibrary Inc., Analog Devices Inc. Engineering staff. Data conversion handbook. 2005, Amsterdam; Boston: Elsevier/Newnes. xxi, 953 p.

[22] Lang, R.M., Bierig, M., Devereux, R.B., Flachskampf, F.A., Foster, E., Pellikka, P.A., Picard, M.H., Roman, M.J., Seward, J., Shanewise, J.S., Solomon, S.D., Spencer, K.T., Sutton, M.S., Stewart, W.J. Recommendations for chamber quantification: A report from the American Society of Echocardiography's guidelines and standards committee and the chamber quantification writing group, developed in conjunction with the European Association of Echocardiography, a branch of the European Society of Cardiology. J. Am. Soc. Echocardiogr. 18: 1440-63, 2005.

[23] Leeson, P., Mitchell, A.R.J., Becher, H. [Eds.] Echocardiography. 2007, Oxford, UK; New York: Oxford University Press. xxv, 549 p.

[24] Lepper, W., Belcik, T., Wei K., Lindner, J.R., Sklenar, J., Kaul, S. Myocardial contrast echocardiography. Circulation 109: 3132–5, 2004.

[25] Luisada, A.A. The heart beat: graphic methods in the study of the cardiac patient. 1953, New York: Hoeber. xii, 527 p.

[26] Meijering, E.H.W., Niessen, W.J., Viergever, M.A. Retrospective motion correction in digital subtraction angiography: A review. IEEE Trans. Med. Imag. 18: 2–21, 1999.

[27] Merritt, C.R. Physics of ultrasound. In: Rumack, C.M., Wilson, S.R., Charboneau, J.W. [Eds.] Diagnostic Ultrasound. 1998, St. Louis, MO: Mosby. p 3–35.

[28] Millar, H.D., Baker, L.E. A stable ultraminiature catheter-tip pressure transducer. Med. Biol. Eng. 11: 86–89, 1973.

[29] Morera, J., Hoadley, S.D., Roland, J.M., Pasipoularides, A., Darragh, R., Gaitan, G., Pieroni, D.R. Estimation of the ratio of pulmonary to systemic pressures by pulsed-wave Doppler echocardiography for assessment of pulmonary arterial pressures. Am. J. Cardiol. 63: 862–6, 1989.

[30] Moodie, D.S., Yiannikas, J. Digital subtraction angiography of the heart and lungs. 1986, Orlando, FL: Grune & Stratton. xi, 191 p.

[31] Mullins, C.E. Cardiac catheterization in congenital heart disease: pediatric and adult. 2006, Malden, Mass.: Blackwell Futura. x, 932 p.

[32] Murgo, J.P., Giolma, J.P., Altobelli, S.A. Signal acquisition and processing for human hemodynamic research. Proc. IEEE 65: 696–702, 1977.

[33] Nelson TR, Fowlkes JB. Contrast-enhanced ultrasound: an idea whose time has come. J. Ultrasound Med. 26: 703–4, 2007.

[34] Otto, C.M., Bonow, R.O. [Eds.] Valvular heart disease: a companion to Braunwald's heart disease. 2009, Philadelphia, PA: Saunders/Elsevier.

[35] Otto, C.M. Textbook of clinical echocardiography. 4th ed. 2009, Philadelphia, PA: Saunders/Elsevier.

[36] Otto, C.M. [Ed.] The practice of clinical echocardiography. 3rd ed. 2007, Philadelphia, PA: Saunders/Elsevier. xx, 1153 p.

[37] Pasipoularides, A., Murgo, J.P., Bird, J.J., Craig, W.E. Fluid dynamics of aortic stenosis: Mechanisms for the presence of subvalvular pressure gradients. Am. J. Physiol. 246: H542–50, 1984.

[38] Pasipoularides, A., Miller, J., Rubal, B.J., Murgo, J.P. Left ventricular ejection dynamics in normal man, in Melbin, J., Noordergraaf, A. [Eds.] Proceedings of the VIth International Conference and Workshop of the Cardiovascular System Dynamics Society. Philadelphia, PA: University of Pennsylvania, pp. 45–8, 1984.

[39] Pasipoularides, A., Murgo, J.P., Miller, J.W., Craig, W.E. Nonobstructive left ventricular ejection pressure gradients in man. Circ. Res. 61: 220–27, 1987.

[40] Pasipoularides, A. Clinical assessment of ventricular ejection dynamics with and without outflow obstruction. J. Am. Coll. Cardiol. 15: 859–82, 1990.

[41] Poelaert, J., Skarvan, K. [Eds.] Transoesophageal echocardiography in anaesthesia and intensive care medicine. 2nd ed. 2004, London: BMJ Books. x, 350 p.

[42] Press, W.H., Teukolsky, S.A., Vetterling, W.T., Flannery, B.P. Numerical recipes in C++: The art of scientific computing. 2nd ed. 2002, Cambridge, UK: Cambridge University Press. xxvi, 1002 p.

[43] Ragosta, M. Textbook of clinical hemodynamics. 2008, Philadelphia, PA: Saunders/Elsevier. xi, 249 p.

[44] Reddy, A.K., Jones, A.D., Martono, C., Caro, W.A., Madala, S., Hartley, C.J. Pulsed Doppler signal processing for use in mice: design and evaluation. IEEE Trans. Biomed. Eng. 52: 1764–70, 2005.

[45] Roelandt, J., Pandian, N.G. [Eds.] Multiplane transesophageal echocardiography. 1996, New York: Churchill Livingstone. xiii, 257 p.

[46] Ryding, A. Essential echocardiography. 2008, Edinburgh; New York: Churchill Livingstone. xii, 251 p.

[47] Schiller, N.B., Shah, P.M., Crawford, M., DeMaria, A., Devereux, R., Feigenbaum, H., Gutgesell, H., Reichek, N., Sahn, D., Schnittger, I. Recommendations for quantitation of the left ventricle by two-dimensional echocardiography. American Society of Echocardiography Committee on Standards, Subcommittee on Quantitation of Two-Dimensional Echocardiograms. J. Am. Soc. Echocardiogr. 2: 358–67, 1989.

[48] Shapiro, R.S., Wagreich, J., Parsons, R.B., Stancato-Pasik, A., Yeh, H.C., Lao, R. Tissue harmonic imaging sonography: Evaluation of image quality compared with conventional sonography. Amer. J. Roentgenol. 171: 1203–6, 1998.

[49] Shim, Y., Hampton, T.G., Straley, C.A., Harrison, J.K., Spero, L.A., Bashore, T.M., Pasipoularides, A.D. Ejection load changes in aortic stenosis: observations made following balloon aortic valvuloplasty. Circ. Res. 71: 1174–84, 1992.

[50] Silvestry, F.E., Wiegers, S.E. [Eds.] Intracardiac echocardiography. 2006, London; New York: Taylor & Francis. viii, 124 p.

[51] Skyba, D.M., Kaul, S. Advances in microbubble technology. Coron. Artery Dis. 11: 211–9, 2000.

[52] Stouffer, G.A. [Ed.] Cardiovascular hemodynamics for the clinician. 2008, Malden, MA: Blackwell Futura. ix, 302 p.

[53] Sutton, M.St.J., Oldershaw, P., Kotler, M.N. [Eds.] Textbook of echocardiography and Doppler in adults and children. 2nd ed. 1996, Cambridge, MA: Blackwell Science. xiv, 983 p.

[54] Tavoularis, S. Measurement in fluid mechanics. 2005, Cambridge, UK; New York: Cambridge University Press. xiii, 354 p.

[55] Vetrovec, G.W., Carabello, B.A. Invasive cardiology: current diagnostic and therapeutic issues. 1996, Armonk, NY.: Futura, Inc. xiii, 618 p.

[56] Walimbe, V., Zagrodsky, V., Raja, S., Jaber, W.A., DiFilippo, F.P., Garcia, M.J., Brunken, R.C., Thomas, J.D., Shekhar, R. Mutual information-based multimodality registration of cardiac ultrasound and SPECT images: a preliminary investigation. Int. J. Cardiovasc. Imaging 19: 483–94, 2003.

[57] Walker, W.F. The significance of correlation in ultrasound signal processing. In: Insana MF, Shung KK [Eds.] Medical imaging 2001: Ultrasonic imaging and signal processing. San Diego, CA: SPIE2001; 4325: pp. 159–71.

[58] Wei, K., Skyba, D.M., Firschke, C., Jayaweera, A.R., Lindner, J.R., Kaul, S. Interactions between microbubbles and ultrasound: in vitro and in vivo observations, J. Am. Coll. Cardiol. 29: 1081–8, 1997.

[59] Wiegers, S.E., Plappert, T., St. John Sutton, M. [Eds.] Echocardiography in practice: a case-oriented approach. 2001, London: Martin Dunitz. viii, 536 p.

[60] Young, S.S. Computerized data acquisition and analysis for the life sciences: A hands-on guide. 2001, Cambridge, UK; New York: Cambridge University Press. x, 237 p.

[61] Yu, E.H., Skyba, D.M., Sloggett, C.E., Jamorski, M., Iwanochko, R.M., Dias, B.F., Rakowski, H., Siu, S.C. Determination of left ventricular ejection fraction using intravenous contrast and a semiautomated border detection algorithm. J. Am. Soc. Echocardiogr. 16: 22–8, 2003.

Chapter 6

Cardiac Morphology and Flow Patterns: Structural–Functional Correlations

The fibers of the heart are not straight and parallel to each other but curved and coiled. They are amazingly intricate. Their texture is not similar to that of a wicker-basket, as Vesalius believed, but they are arranged in a more complicated way. Immediately underneath the pericardium, from the basis of the heart and from the circular tendinous orifices of the vena cava and pulmonary auricle, and from the origins of the aorta and pulmonary arteries, a layer of fleshy fibers spreads. These fibers are parallel to each other and they are orientated from the basis straight to the apex of the heart where they are diversely curved and intertwined, reflecting toward the cavities of the ventricles. This layer is followed by other layers of fibers, oblique and descending in spirals. They are more and more inclined and orientated also toward the apex of the heart. Before reaching the apex, they intersect and cover each other and other ordinary fibers. Hence they are deviated to the inside and partly reflected in oblique and transverse spirals like scythes (sickles), towards the base of the heart. Part of them seem to compose internal columns to which the strings of the tricuspid and mitral valves are attached and others are intertwined transversally and form the cavity of the right ventricle.

——Giovanni Alfonso Borelli: *De Motu Animalium* [On the Movement of Animals] (1680). Translated by P. Maquet [9] (slightly modified).

THE HUMAN HEART HAS A COMPLEX ANATOMIC STRUCTURE and is a dynamic organ in constant motion. The myocardium is a complex fibrous continuum which contains not only the muscle cells but also an extensive network of connective tissue. It is reasonable to suppose that this tissue can contribute to the expansion of the ventricles during diastole [66]. The heart walls consist mainly of myocardial fibers (a series of longitudinally and laterally connected cardiomyocytes), which are joined in bands that *"present an exceedingly intricate interlacement"* [25]. What may, at first, appear to be more or less distinct layers of longitudinal, diagonal, and horizontal musculature are in reality connected band segments encompassing complex spiraling fibers, which are clearly visible after preparatory treatment, such as boiling. The organization of cardiac ventricular muscle fibers has long been recognized as of great importance in our understanding of cardiac function and the determination of the direction of the fibers has been the subject of investigation and speculation for many centuries. As I note in Section 7.8, on pp. 367 ff., a simple geometrical analysis shows that during the diminution of the luminal area of a circular ring that retains the same ring area, the inner (endocardial) circle must shorten *much more* than the outer (epicardial) one. The *thicker* the wall, the *more pronounced* becomes this effect. Nevertheless, a pure ring muscle cannot cause the near disappearance (very low end-systolic chamber volumes) of the lumen without inner paddings.[1]

On the whole, the inner changes of the heart muscle are much more striking than the outer ones (cf. Fig. 6.1, on p. 300), so that when observing an active heart from the outside the changes seem much smaller than they are in reality. In the left ventricle, the inner longitudinal fibers, the trabeculations and the papillary muscles also work through their thickening as they form pads of muscle that block off the lumen like bolsters (see Fig. 6.1, and also Fig. 7.26, on p. 368) greatly confining the lumen, something which would not be possible through the effect of the ring muscles alone. This is a reason why the chamber wall cannot consist exclusively of ring fibers. Another reason is that, with the lack of an elastic longitudinal reinforcement, the wall would suffer a *longitudinal rupture* due to the inner pressure developed during systole. Such functional considerations suggest that complex myofiber distributions across the cardiac chamber walls are to be expected—see also Section 7.6, on pp. 358 ff. Despite considerable advances in correlating myocardial structure and function, there is still lack of consensus and heated controversy [1,2,10,12,18,32,33,36,37,39,58,59] concerning the 3-D arrangement and workings of the myocardial fibers within the ventricular muscle masses.

6.1 The heart is a helix

Geometrically, the heart is a tightly wound helix that contains an apex. Grant [24] briefly and succinctly summarized earlier work on the muscular histoarchitectonics of the left

[1]During the embryonic stage, the pads of the endocardium (*endocardial cushions*—see Chapter 15) at the sites of subsequent development of the outflow and inflow valves, serve the same purpose, namely, shutting off luminal continuity.

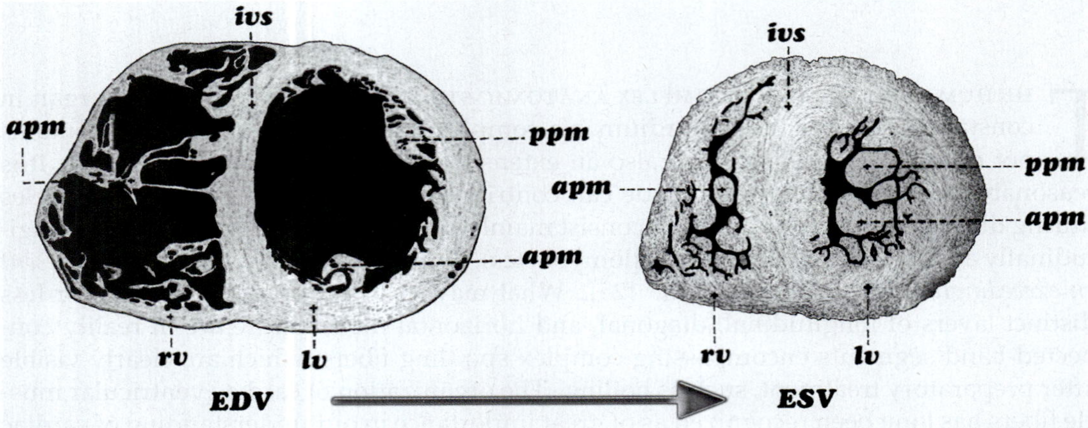

Figure 6.1: The papillary muscles and the *trabeculae carneae* work through their systolic thickening to form pads of muscle that block off the ventricular lumen like bolsters, thus allowing more complete emptying and the attainment of low end-systolic blood volumes; apm = anterior and ppm = posterior papillary muscle; ivs = interventricular septum; lv = left and rv = right ventricle; EDV = end-diastolic and ESV = end-systolic volume. (Adapted, modified, from Sklavounos [51].)

ventricle. He described the pioneering work of Lower [21] and Mall [40] and pointed out that Lower drew attention to the twisting of the myofibers. Grant compared this twisting to a *twisted large rope, or hawser*.[2] But he adroitly noted that there is an important difference between the generations of twist in a hawser, which can be isolated from one another, and those in a section of myocardium, where there is a smooth *syncytial continuity* from the smallest to the grossest "generation." Grant also discussed the possible role of embryonic development in myocardial morphology.

The cardiac helix form was described in the 1660s by Lower [21] as having an *apical vortex*, at which the muscle fibers go from outside in, in a *clockwise* way, and from inside out, in a *counterclockwise* direction; he made the point explicitly that the thin apex of the left ventricle was devoid of myocardium, the endocardial and epicardial layers being continuous at this site [21] (see Fig. 6.2, *inset A.*). This weak place in the heart wall is functionally reinforced by the fact that contraction begins here. In his *"Triebwerk,"* Krehl [34] described in 1891 the continuity of the subepicardial and subendocardial fibers at the level of the mitral orifice, and at the apex of the left ventricle, where they invaginate.

The nineteenth-century Scottish anatomist J. Bell Pettigrew investigated the spiraling course of the muscle fibers that form the walls of the ventricles of the heart. He discovered that the layers of muscle fibers were interconnected [43,44]; i.e., they are not like nested layers of onion skin, but are *continuous* sheets of helical fibers (see Fig. 6.2, on p. 302). He [43] and Keith [32] enunciated, about a century ago, the fact that the heart walls are formed

[2]A hawser consists of several ropes twisted helically around each other; each of them, in turn, consists of smaller ropes twisted helically about each other, etc., down to the individual strands of hemp, which are also twisted about each other.

on the basis of a *modified blood vessel wall*, rather than a collection of discrete muscle entities resembling the skeletal musculature. Pettigrew's communication presented to the Royal Society of London, in November 1859, which formed the subject of the Croonian Lecture for 1860 [44], summarizes an absolutely monumental work, which has influenced—directly, or indirectly—every one of his epigones in this area of research. It should be studied by everyone interested in myocardial morphology, and its dynamic mechanical correlations and implications.

The combination of clockwise and counterclockwise vortices is common in nature. Such a natural *reciprocal spiral* structure is exemplified in the sea shell. If one draws the tip of a coiled top shell outward, the collapsed spiral configuration elongates into a helix, very similar topologically to the arrangement of the heart muscle fibers [11]. Counterclockwise and clockwise spirals exist within our fingertips (fingerprint patterns) and this harmonic pattern of clockwise and counterclockwise spirals is clear-cut and readily evident at the apex of the heart, as we saw in a preceding paragraph.

According to the eminent German anatomist Benninghof, the outer muscle fibers begin at the base of the heart and sweep down in the aforementioned *counterclockwise* curves to the apex. There they loop around and form the so-called *vortex cordis* (heart vortex), as is displayed schematically in Figure 6.2, *inset* A. The fibers that begin at the front of the heart enter the *vortex cordis* at the back of the heart, while those that begin at the back sweep around to the front. These outer fibers loop around each other, to delineate the apical vortex [2], and then insert themselves into the inside of the muscular wall and spiral back upward, as inner layers. Some of them radiate into the papillary muscles that anchor the atrioventricular valve leaflets to the walls. Fibers that lie deeper at the base of the ventricles spiral down in a *clockwise* pattern. They coil in more tightly and form nearly horizontal *ring-like* loops around the body of mainly the left ventricle before they sweep upward again to the base of the ventricles.

The internal and external spiral loops were previously called the *bulbospiral* and *sinospiral* muscles, which go from without to within in a *clockwise* and from within to without in a *counterclockwise* spiral, respectively.

6.2 Ventricular myoarchitecture is intertwined with intraventricular blood flow

Since a muscle like the heart retains its form, we think of it as being a solid that nevertheless can change its shape drastically during the cardiac cycle, but when we recognize that muscle consists of about 75% water, we begin to think of it in more fluid terms. The spiraling and looping pattern of the myocardial fibers, including the *vortex cordis*, is a reflection of intracardiac blood movements. In the heart, form and movement unite in a rhythmical process in space and time; the organ, a form in space, is simultaneously a movement in time. As is developed at length in Chapters 14 and 15, the blood streaming through the filling ventricles in the course of most of diastole also creates loops and vortices. Like the mural fibers of the heart, this movement is very complex and intricate. The myofibers of

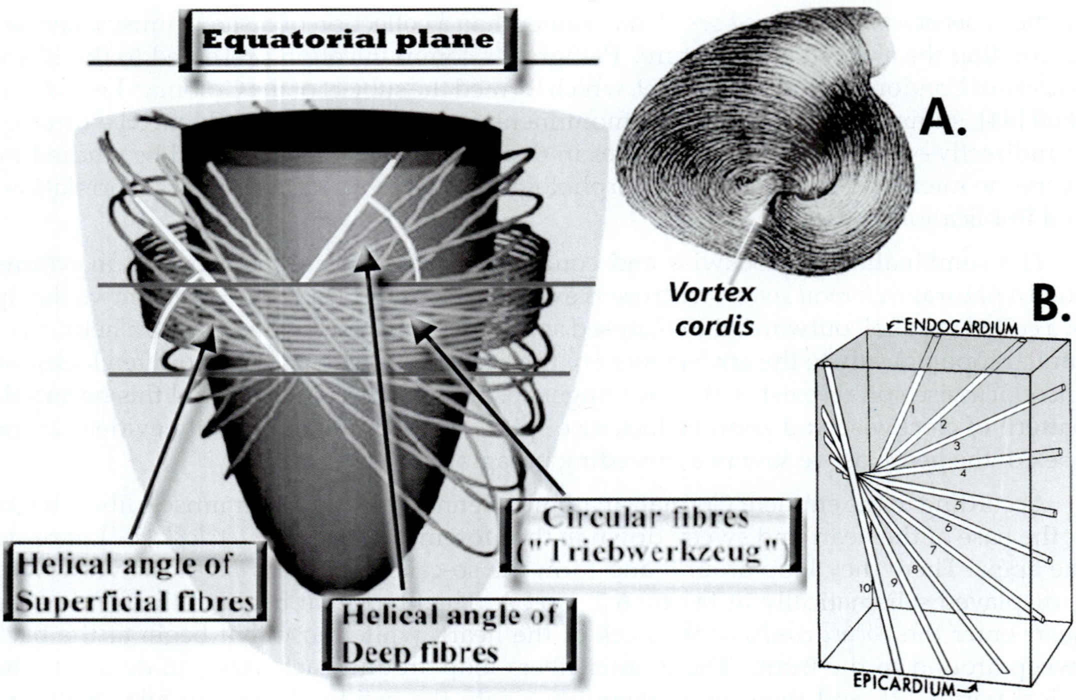

Figure 6.2: Diagrammatic representation of the variation in the angle of the long axis of the myofiber aggregates, when assessed relative to the ventricular equator; this is the so-called helical, or *"helix"* angle. Note the different helical angles subtended by subepicardial and subendocardial layers of the left ventricular walls. The helical angle was shown by Streeter and colleagues [53–55] to vary at different depths within the left ventricular wall; it varies by up to 180° transmurally. The circular fibers of the middle layer, the *"Triebwerkzeug,"* or actuating fibers, first described by Krehl [34], are parallel to the left ventricular equator. (Adapted, slightly modified, from Anderson et al. [3], with permission of Wiley-Liss, Inc.) Inset A. illustrates the *vortex cordis* and Inset B. an LV wall segment showing progressive shift in mean fiber orientation. (Insets A. and B. are slightly modified from Buckberg [11] and Spotnitz [52], respectively, with permission of The American Association for Thoracic Surgery and Mosby-Year Book, Inc.)

the cardiac walls are a physical replication of the creative fluid flow movements which they enclose.

In a way, what the blood does as a fluid has fashioned the muscular histoarchitectonics of the cardiac ventricles, as they are depicted in Figure 6.2. In spiraling paths, myofibers sway down to the heart's apex and then rise again to its base. They make the same movements and emphasize the revolving vortical streaming of the filling vortex within the ventricles. Therefore, intraventricular blood flow and the pattern of the muscular histoarchitectonics of the heart are mutually intertwined.[3] This mutuality is put on view already during the embryonic development of the heart.

[3]See also Section 16.7, with all its subsections, on pp. 876 ff.

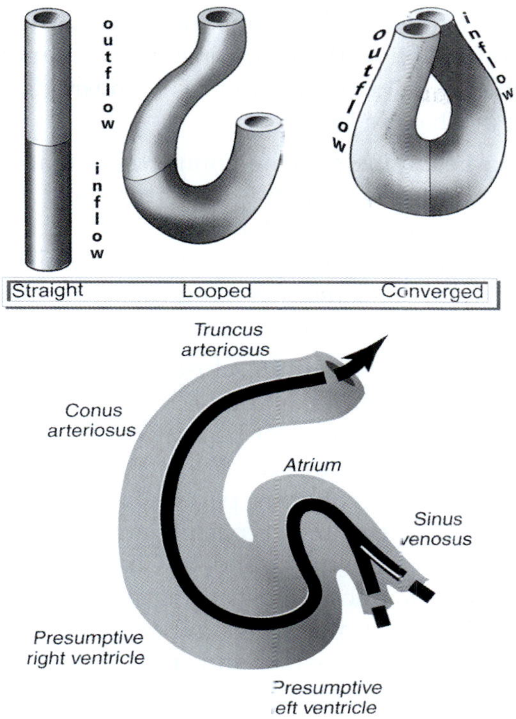

Figure 6.3: Cardiac muscle cells converge along the ventral midline of the embryo to form a beating *linear heart tube* composed of distinct myocardial and endocardial layers separated by an acellular matrix, the cardiac jelly. The linear heart tube undergoes *rightward* looping, which is essential for proper orientation of the right and left ventricles, and for alignment of the heart chambers with the vasculature. The molecular mechanisms governing cardiac looping remain unknown. Each cardiac chamber will balloon out from the outer curvature of the looped heart tube in a segmental fashion.

Early in its development in a *confined* space, the elongating linear heart tube begins to form loops that redirect blood flow, as is shown in Figure 6.3. The embryonic circulatory fluid, or *hemolymph*, is squeezed peristaltically from the caudally located venous pole toward the cranially located arterial pole. Meanwhile, the heart tube is looping three-dimensionally, while keeping the arterial and venous poles close together. It is evident that flow patterns and wall geometry are intricately linked. The complex loop results in a tight inner curve and a wider outer curve with predictable differences in flow and shear patterns; ensuing local expansion of the outer curve results in chamber formation [46]. But even before the heart has developed septa separating its four chambers from each other [29], the blood already flows in two separate streams through the heart. The blood streams flowing through the right and left sides of the developing heart do not mix, but stream and loop by each other, just as two distinct currents in a body of water. In the boundary zone between the two currents, the septa dividing the right and left sides take their origins. Therefore, the movement of the oxygenated and deoxygenated blood streams somehow provides delimiting signals governing the inner differentiation of the heart, just as the looping heart tube redirects the flow of intraluminal blood. Blood movement and heart differentiation are inexorably linked, as is discussed in Chapter 15.

The coiling, looping heart fibers create contractions that, in ways that remain to be established in future studies (see Section 16.7, on pp. 876 ff.), mirror and facilitate the dynamic trajectories of the intraventricular blood, both in diastole and in systole. The heart muscle does not work, as we often envisage it, opening and closing as a fist, first forming a tight fist in systole and then relaxing the fist in diastole. Rather, the cardiac cycle includes a much more complex array of myofiber movements.

Consider that every fluid flow in a finite, closed space must inexorably lead to rotation with vortex formation (see Section 9.6, on pp. 473 f.). This follows from the conservation law of matter, namely, that matter cannot be destroyed, as it also cannot be generated, within the framework of classical physics. Every movement of a material particle in a continuum must influence its neighboring particle, either by displacing it or by attracting it to follow. Contemplate the archetypal phenomenon of vortex formation, as we examine it in Section 1.5, on pp. 10 ff., and in Chapter 9. As we saw in Section 1.5, wherever any qualitative differences in a flowing medium come together, vortical formations occur. Such differences may be: slow and fast; solid and liquid; warm and cold; heavy and light (for instance, saline and fresh water)... At the surfaces of contact there is always a tendency for one layer to roll in upon the other (see Fig. 9.7, illustrating this "Helmholtz–Kelvin instability," on p. 458). If the difference in speed between neighboring layers reaches a certain degree, vortex formations occur; these always originate in the surfaces of contact involved in the movement. Similarly, vortices come into existence when, e.g., a stream gets stalled against its boundaries. The stalled stream breaks up and rolls over on itself, as occurs in the course of diastolic ventricular filling (see Fig. 7.37, on p. 389, and Chapter 14).

Right at the endocardial boundary, the flow of the stream has zero velocity relative to the endocardial border itself—in principle, this is why you cannot blow fine pieces of dust from the surface of a table (see Sections 4.9, on pp. 197 ff., 4.10, on pp. 202 ff., and 4.12, on pp. 208 ff.). At increasing distances from the boundary, the flow moves with higher velocities and the difference in rates of flow causes the stream to *"trip over itself,"* as it were, to curl around on itself just as a wave curls when rushing up the beach. Upper layers of water overshoot the more slowly moving lower layers and the water is drawn into the hollows in a circular motion. Some idea of the development of inner surfaces, as these layers flow past each other, can be gained if one imagines how the pages of an unbound stack slide over one another when they are bent or squeezed back and forth. This presents us with an intriguing formative principle: the fluid laminae folding over and finally curling under to form a circling vortex.

In wrapping around on itself, the vortex appears to be a prototypical model of spatial enclosure and exists by *"bleeding energy"* from the mainstream. The statement, earlier on this page, that rotation follows from the conservation law of matter for a finite enclosure is purely kinematic.[4] In contrast to inviscid vortex rings, which do not decay, real vortex

[4]The restriction "kinematic" means that the forces that cause the motion, or maintain it, are of *no concern*.

rings lose energy and speed. They decelerate not only through loss of energy due to friction but also through entrainment and incorporation of new fluid. This fluid must be set into rotation and increases the size and moment of inertia (see Section 2.3, on pp. 43 f.) of the vortex ring.

Just like the inflow into the developing and developed cardiac chambers, the myofibers of the heart are also reflecting the fact that they grow over "confined" geometric wall structures. Moreover, they must embody in their vortical paths creative morphomechanical interactions with the intraluminal flow movements which they encircle. In spiraling paths they swing down to its apex and then rise again to its base. They make the same movements and emphasize the revolving diastolic vortical streaming of the blood within the left and right ventricles (see Figs. 7.37, on p. 389, and 16.4, on p. 877), as well as the atrial chambers [22].

6.3 Ventricular myoarchitecture engenders compound motion patterns

Myocardial contraction patterns combine with the LV myofiber architecture to cause the heart to contract downward, oscillate somewhat to the sides, and also to generate torsion, *"wringing"*[5] the ventricle in systole and storing energy that could conceivably be abruptly released in diastole, so as to contribute to early vigorous LV filling, efficiently and with low intracardiac pressures. If it occurred, such a release would be most advantageous under conditions of tachycardia with high adrenergic drive and inotropy. Studies using myocardial markers have shown that LV torsion is proportional to contractility. Then, during isovolumic relaxation the musculature untwists and, subsequently, in early diastole the base of the ventricles moves upward. Only the interwoven, helicoidal, ventricular muscle fibers can bring into being such a compound pattern of motion. Circumstances under which stored strain energy is, in fact, released in diastole, so as to contribute to LV filling, remain to be actually identified in animals or humans.

Systolic torsion varies regionally and is greatest in the apical and inferior walls. Torsional deformation occurring during systole (twist) unwinds (untwist) during isovolumic relaxation [16]. Detailed investigation of the phenomenon has established that the untwisting process and filling of the left ventricle are quite *distinct*; Rademakers et al. [48] showed that more than 50% of the untwisting occurs *before* the mitral valve opening, whereas circumferential lengthening occurs *after* the opening of the mitral valve. The length and torsion angle of both epicardial and endocardial myofiber segments are *not* changing simultaneously during diastole, since the torsion decreases most sharply *before* mitral opening, whereas length increases sharply *after* mitral valve opening. The right ventricle exhibits a similar systolic torsional shift, supporting the hypothesis that the heart acts as a double bellows with both free walls approaching the septum during contraction [16].

[5] It appears that the analogy originated with Borelli, who proposed that left ventricular ejection involved torsional deformation in a manner analogous to wringing out a wet towel [9,65].

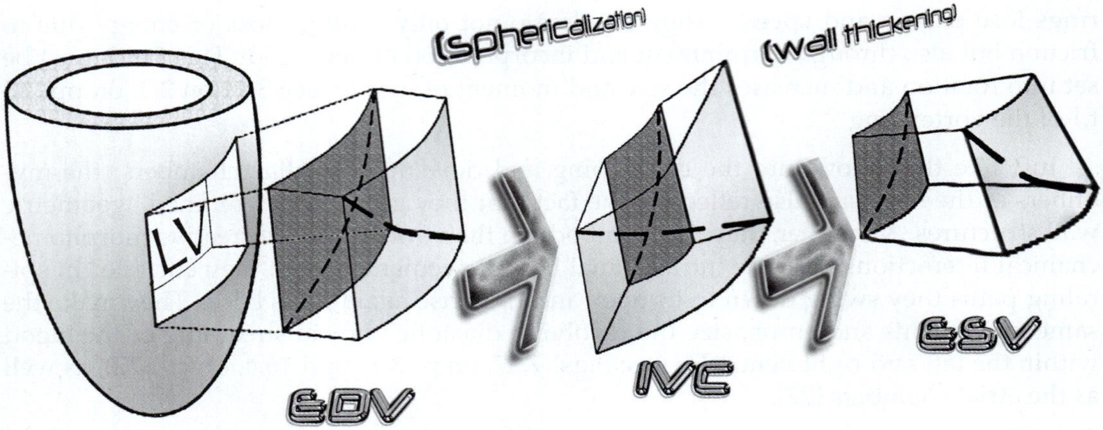

Figure 6.4: During the isovolumic contraction phase (IVC), the shortening of the *inner*, right-handed helix, myocardial fibers is accompanied with stretching of the subepicardial *(outer)*, left-handed helix, fibers; the chamber maintains the end-diastolic volume (EDV), but becomes more spherical *(sphericalization)*. This dynamic deformation process satisfies isovolumic wall mechanics, as does the ensuing ejection phase, during which there is substantial mural thickening, as all myocardial fiber-layers shorten and thicken, especially the inner layers.

There is no *a priori* reason to assume that the global organization of the myofibers in the cardiac walls can be inferred with confidence from any study restricted to the local organization at one or a few mural sites in the developing or adult heart. In recent years, several key parameters of LV function, previously measurable only on experimental animals by invasive instrumentation, have become available by noninvasive means, including LV torsion and recoil. Magnetic resonance imaging can be used to track globally and locally magnetically tagged myocardium, demonstrating distinct effects of preload, afterload, contractility and relaxation on LV torsion and untwisting. As is illustrated in Figure 6.2, on p. 302, the fibers of the human left ventricle are arranged in a complex fashion, with epicardial myofibers directed in a counterclockwise and endocardial in a clockwise spiral from apex to base. Therefore, there is transition in the orientation of fibers through the wall of the left ventricle (see Fig. 6.2, *inset B.*, on p. 302), with epicardial fibers oriented obliquely, midwall fibers oriented horizontally (the *"Triebwerkzeug,"* i.e., actuating fibers, of Krehl [34], or *ventricular constrictor layer* of Rushmer [50]), and endocardial fibers oriented obliquely but in the opposite direction from the epicardial fibers [26].

The helical myocardial fibers within the ventricular walls are arranged in syncytial fashion and assemble into transmural branching laminar sheets, or myolaminae [15]; recent results indicate that the myolaminae are highly discontinuous and thus begin and end many times between the inner wall and the outer wall [28]. Analysis of canine dynamic myocardial geometry [47, 63] has shown that at the epicardium shortening is predominantly aligned in the direction of the myofibers. However, at the endocardium, maximal shortening occurs at 90° from the myofiber direction [47, 64]. This *"cross-fiber shortening"* is most likely accomplished by the physical rearrangement of myofibers or fiber bundles [63], induced by contraction of inner layers with differing fiber orientations. This rearrangement occurs along cleavage planes that separate sheets of myocytes in which the myofibers are arranged in branching patterns 4 to 6 cells thick, and it is associated with transverse shearing deformation [35]. These myoarchitectonic shifts allow the endocardium to shorten in two orthogonal directions, producing extensive thickening in the third (radial) direction to conserve volume (see Fig. 6.4). Physiologists have long understood that changes in the macrostructure of the wall (cellular rearrangement) must account for the difference between wall thickening, which on the inner wall may exceed values of 40% measured by a variety of techniques, and the much lower estimates of myocyte thickening, such as the 8% diameter increase estimated by simple conservation of volume in an individual myocyte shortening by 15%. Recent work [13, 17] has clearly illustrated the importance of the regional structure of the ventricular wall in amplifying fiber shortening to produce wall thickening. This myocardial rearrangement mechanism clarifies, in part (see also Section 7.8, on pp. 367 ff.), the marked systolic endocardial thickening that accompanies normal ejection [47,62].

Marked differences in the extent of myofiber shortening have been observed among human and between human and canine experimental studies. The extent of fiber and cross-fiber shortening in the left ventricle of normal and abnormal human hearts is unclear, in large measure because it is influenced by many dynamic (contractile state, systolic loading, see Sections 2.23 and 7.9, on pp. 105 ff. and 369 ff., respectively), geometric, and histoarchitectonic factors. Using radiopaque beads [64] and MR tagging [47] in anesthetized dogs, fiber shortening was shown to be 8%. Using echocardiography, adjusted with geometric models, fiber shortening was calculated at 21% in normal human subjects and 18% in subjects with LV hypertrophy and normal global function [6].

MR tagging, a noninvasive method of marking specific segments of myocardial tissue [7,27,61], is a promising technique with which regional strains, including fiber shortening and cross-fiber shortening, can be studied noninvasively in humans. In MR tagging, a pattern of temporarily changed magnetization is created in the tissue. The pattern is imaged, as it moves with the tissue and undergoes deformation during the cardiac cycle. From the acquired image sequence, which gives detailed information on the spatial and temporal distribution of myocardial deformations, tracings of mural regional myocardial strains can be determined. Using MR tagging, fiber shortening was found to be 30% in normal subjects and 21% in patients with LV hypertrophy [42].

In stable patients with idiopathic dilated cardiomyopathy, fiber axial shortening was found, by magnetic resonance tissue tagging, to be markedly reduced from values around 15%, similar in the normal human epicardium and endocardium [38]. Cross-fiber shortening is the dominant strain in the normal human endocardium and exceeds 25%. Also, the transmural transition in anatomic fiber orientations is not significantly altered in these patients, and consequently, although cross-fiber shortening is reduced, it is still the dominant endocardial strain. Significant interactions between layers of the human left ventricle occur during systole in both normal subjects and patients with idiopathic dilated cardiomyopathy.

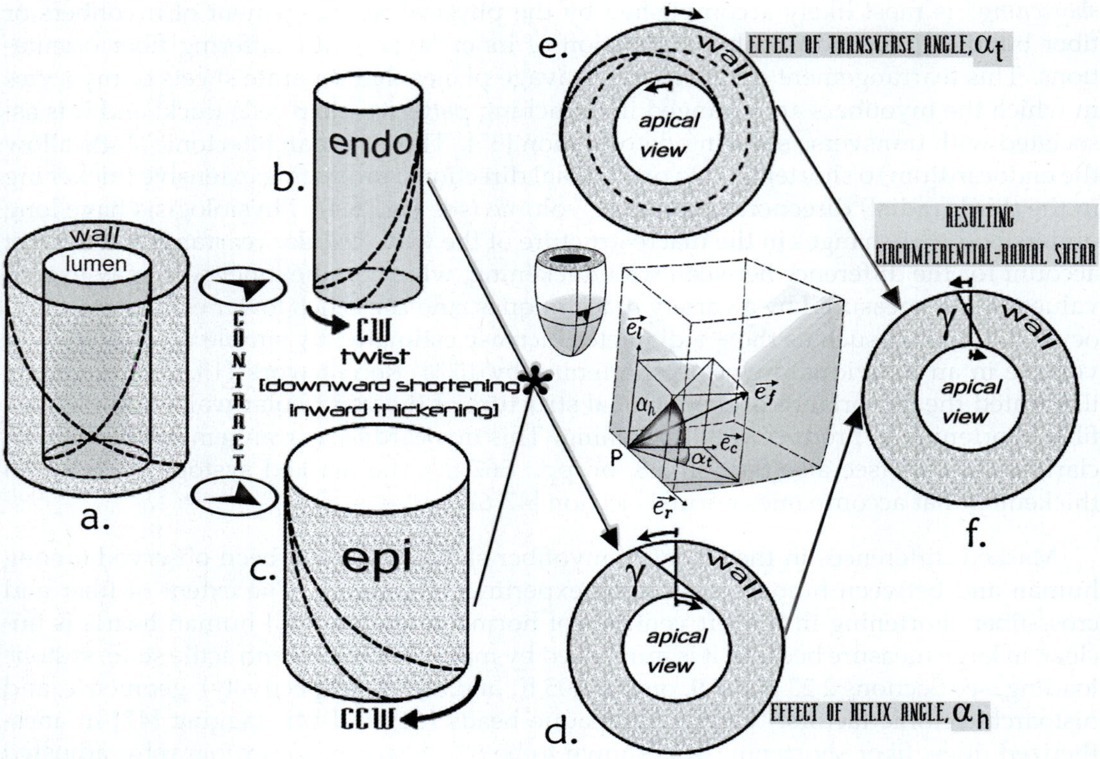

Figure 6.5: Influence of helix angle, a_h, and transverse angle, a_t, on transmural shear strain in a cylindrical model of the left ventricle. In the absence of a transverse angle (drawing a.), shortening of the myofibers (- - - - -) brings about a clockwise (cw) apical rotation of the subendocardium (viewed in apex-to-base direction) (drawing b.), and a counterclockwise (ccw) rotation of the subepicardium (drawing c.). In the apex-to-base view of short-axis images, this yields a positive circumferential-radial shear strain (drawing d.), as indicated by the shear angle γ. This shear strain is counteracted by a negative circumferential-radial shear strain component, resulting from the negative transverse angle, a_t, in the apical part of the ventricle (drawing e.). The total accruing shear strain (drawing f.) depends on the dynamic balance between the two effects. Inset: ellipsoidal model of LV geometry showing helix, a_h, and transverse, a_t, fiber angles. The fiber angles at any mural point P are defined from projection of the fiber direction, $\vec{e_f}$ on planes spanned by the local transmural, $\vec{e_r}$, longitudinal, $\vec{e_l}$, and circumferential, $\vec{e_c}$, directions. (Adapted, strongly modified, from Ubbink et al. [61], with kind permission of Elsevier.)

6.4 Ventricular myoarchitecture and shear strain minimization

Since LV rotation and twist originate from the dynamic interaction between oppositely wound epicardial and endocardial myocardial fiber helices [4], models based on uniform myocardial fiber structure cannot explain dynamic wall movement in normal subjects, and are likely to have significant limitations if used to investigate left ventricular function in disease [26]. Quite intricate structural-functional interplays are at play, at times in quite unsuspected ways. Considering, for instance, the simple cylindrical LV model of Figure 6.5, on p. 308, when myofibers are activated, the endocardial and epicardial layers tend to shorten in the axial direction, thereby increasing the circumferential strain, E_{cc}. On the other hand, when the circumferentially arranged midwall fibers are activated, the opposite happens, as the circumference shortens. Consequently mechanical equilibrium between layers with axial or circumferential fibers may be expected to govern the ratio of circumferential and axial shortening of the LV walls through the cycle. The time course of the circumferential-radial shear strain, E_{cr}, is predominantly related to the subendocardial and subepicardial layers, with their oblique fibers, since these layers exert a torque across the wall thickness. As is shown in Figure 6.5, contraction of subendocardial myofibers would cause a clockwise apical rotation, when viewing the apex in *apex-to-base* direction; shortening of subepicardial myofibers would cause the opposite effect. Accordingly, the contraction of the subendocardial and subepicardial layers generates a transmural shear load within, e.g., a short-axis slice.[6] This shear load must be compensated by a shear deformation of the tissue in the *endo-to-epi* interposed layers.

In the absence of an *endo-to-epi* component of fiber orientation, i.e., with zero transverse angle ($a_t = 0$, in Fig. 6.5), this shear load would only be counteracted by the passive myocardial tissue, which has a low stiffness; for this reason, mechanical equilibrium would be reached at large shear strains E_{cr}. If, on the other hand, myofibers cross over between inner and outer layers of the wall, as expressed by a nonzero transverse angle a_t, then these active and therefore stiff myofibers participate in sustaining the shear load, and the resulting shear deformation is reduced (see Fig. 6.5). Effectively, therefore, the intricate mural myoarchitectonics allow, *inter alia*, the avoidance of excessive shear strains and deformations of intramural structures, including relatively fragile components of the microvasculature.

6.5 The intraventricular blood as a myocardial *"hemoskeleton"*

The intraventricular blood does not only sustain passively pressure forces generated by the myocardium that surrounds it, but also provides a support (a fulcrum) to the myocardium to generate its contractile stresses. Considering the intraventricular blood as the myocardial *"hemoskeleton"* is appropriate, in order to emphasize this specific function. And it is well established, both physiologically and clinically, that different preload levels (*viz.*, dynamic changes of the *hemoskeleton*) can have an enormous influence on ventricular performance. From a physics viewpoint, applying the principles of a lever of the

[6] Because of their larger effective radii and mass the subepicardial fibers dominate and account for the normal rotation gradient in the LV *apex-to-base* direction, entailing a counter-clockwise rotation of the apex and a clockwise rotation of the base.

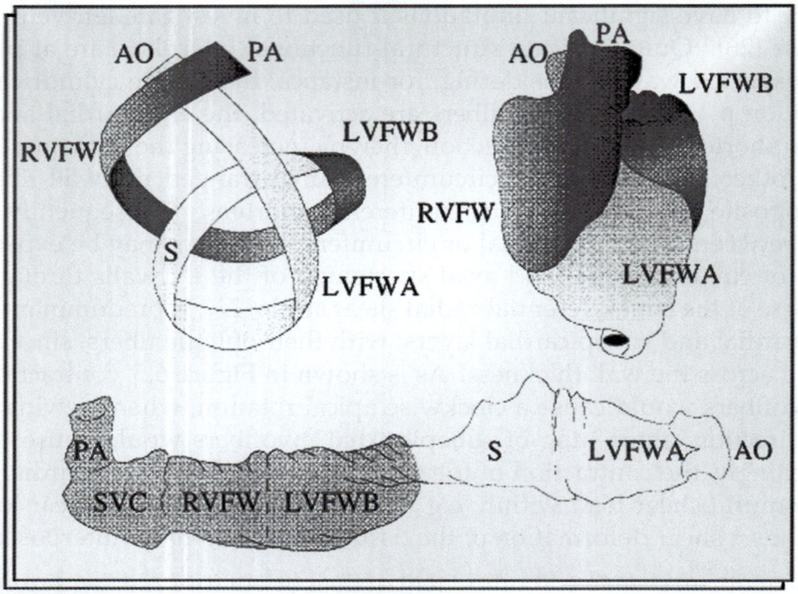

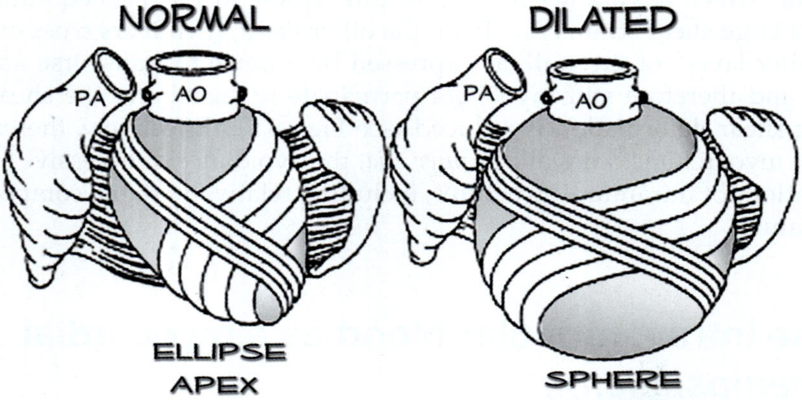

Figure 6.6: Top panel, the *Torrent-Guasp model* of the unique ventricular muscle band. Bottom panel, geometric change in size and shape during ventricular dilatation in congestive heart failure: the elliptical heart with a helical fiber orientation becomes spherical and develops a more transverse myofiber orientation, as the apex is lost in conjunction with the dilatation. AO, aorta; LVFWA, left ventricular free wall apical; LVFWB, left ventricular free wall basal; PA, pulmonary artery; RVFW, right ventricular free wall; S, septum; SVC, supraventricular crest. (Top panel, modified from Jouk et al. [30], with permission from Springer; bottom, modified from Buckberg [10], with permission from Elsevier.)

"first-kind," the dynamic hemoskeleton could modify the mechanical efficiency of contracting myocardial fibers by altering, as it were, the relative lengths of the curvilinear lever arms. The term *"dynamic"* used here to qualify the hemoskeleton, suggests that the support that it provides to the enfolding myocardium varies according to consecutive alterations of intraventricular blood volume (*viz.*, shifting fulcrum location) all through the cardiac cycle.

6.6 Torrent-Guasp's *"flattened rope"* or muscle band

The Spanish cardiac morphologist Torrent-Guasp envisioned the heart muscle as looking like a *"flattened rope"*, or like a helical ventricular myocardial band, with three parts: a beginning and an end at the aorta and pulmonary artery; a wraparound wide loop that he called a *basal loop*; and a smaller helix that he called the *apical loop* [57] (see Figs. 6.6, and 6.8). He based this unique flattened rope model, which is *topologically different* than the classic Benninghof myocardial fiber model [8], on phylogenetic development considerations. Indeed, it has been proposed and disputed [39] that the spatial orientation of Torrent-Guasp's ventricular myocardial band model (basal and apical loops) might be the mature morphological correlate of twists and torsions of the embryonic heart loop.

At 20 days of life, the circulatory system of a human embryo looks like that of worms *(helminthes)*, 1 billion years ago; a gastro-vascular tube with hemolymph, irregular tubular peristaltic activity and absence of a pumping organ, or "heart." At 25 days of life, a clear-cut venous system and an arterial system with a single pump develop, mirroring the circulation of fishes *(pisces)*, more than 400 million years ago. At 30 days, the embryologic heart contains a patent ventricular septal defect and an atrial septal defect (mixed blood, because of the ASD and VSD), so that it is similar to the amphibian and reptile hearts of 200 million years ago. At last, at 50 days of life, there is an intact atrial and ventricular septum, typical of birds *(aves)* and mammals, with separate pulmonary and systemic circulations, so that, within 50 days of embryonic development, our cardiac *ontogeny* recapitulates 1 billion years of *phylogeny*.[7]

In fact, blunt dissection along the natural muscle cleavage planes allows the heart to become completely unscrolled, a single muscle band extending between the aorta at its termination and the pulmonary artery at its beginning. In other words, a unique muscular band or *("flattened rope")* can be obtained by *unfolding* an intact heart, as is displayed in the top panel of Figure 6.6, on p. 310! This ventricular muscle band describes two spirals in space, as it extends from the pulmonary artery to the aorta, defining a helicoidal structure which enfolds and delimits the right and left ventricular chambers [11,57,60].

In view of their topography, the first spiral is designated as the basal loop (BL) and the second as the apical loop (AL). In each of these loops, it is practical to recognize two

[7]According to the biogenetic principle of Ernest Haeckel, *ontogeny*, i.e., the stages of development, especially of the embryo, is the abridged and accelerated recapitulation of *phylogeny*, i.e., the evolutionary history of the species. However, this idea is now largely discredited because evolution does not conserve phenotype but genotype, and phylogenetic memory does not necessarily produce morphological equivalents during ontogenesis, but rather appears in a form of "fast running" genetics programs [59].

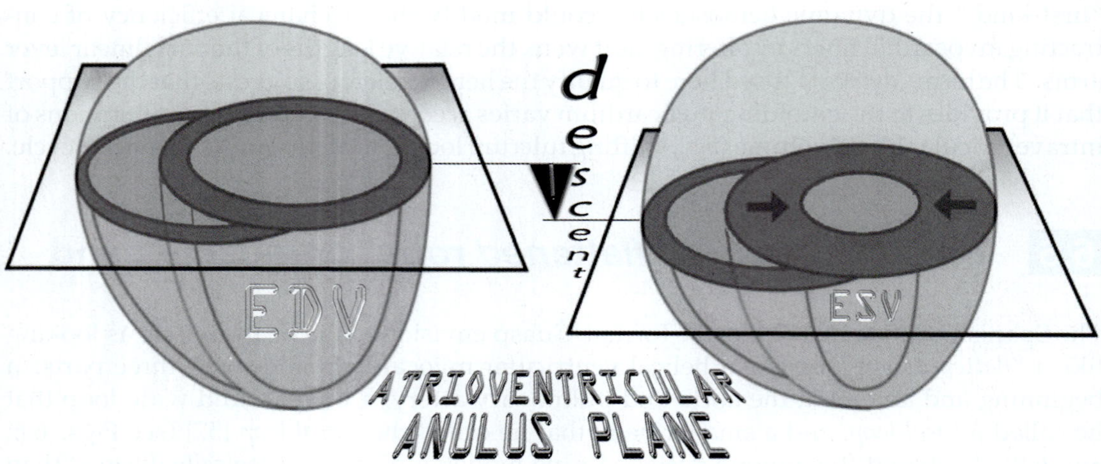

Figure 6.7: The forces that are developed during systolic contraction by helically arranged heart muscle fibers have components directed along the longitudinal axis of the heart. During systolic ventricular ejection, they bring about a shortening of the longitudinal ventricular axis and a *descent* of the atrioventricular anulus plane, and thus the atrium is simultaneously deepened. This process is called a *"shift of the valve plane."* The total external cardiac volume remains relatively invariant, as the atria become enlarged in the process—cf. Figure 7.22, on p. 359.

constitutive segments: in the BL, the right segment, which corresponds to the RV free wall, and the left segment, which partakes in structuring the LV free wall; in the AL, we recognize the *descending segment*, with fibers coming down from the ventricular base to the apex, and the *ascending segment*, with fibers rising from the apical to the basal regions (see Fig. 6.8, on p. 314).

The specialized spatial arrangement of the descending and ascending segment fibers and the presence of the dynamic hemoskeleton *(vide supra)* lead to complex interplays during the cardiac cycle. Verticality, obliqueness, and conical configuration, although not exemplified in an even way, may be regarded as common attributes for both the ascending and the descending segment fibers. Predominant verticality in descending-segment and obliquity in ascending-segment fibers, along with their X-crossing (see Fig. 6.8) within the apical loop, underlie the opposite effects that are, as is detailed below, produced by their respective contractions.

For the Torrent-Guasp model, sequential systolic contraction along the myocardial band is pivotal, starting in the right ventricle and then proceeding along the underlying muscular folds in the rope-like model. There is first contraction of the right segment of the basal loop; it proceeds around the loop toward its left segment to surround the left ventricle. The next step is contractile motion of the basal loop and subsequently there is sequential activation to contraction of both descending and ascending segments of the apical loop. Finally, the heart relaxes in diastole. This sequence of motion defines the rapid sequence of contraction along the band. As a result of contraction of the basal loop, there is a squeezing action on the left ventricle, as the outer ring develops a stiff outer *"shell"* that constricts or compresses the apical loop. The next motion is a downward twisting, akin to the *wringing of a rag*, of the muscle fibers that shorten and thicken, thereby making the heart eject. Next ensues the progression of contraction into the ascending segment, which brings about twisting and thickening in the opposite direction, as is depicted in Figure 6.8, on p. 314. This sequence is followed by relaxation to allow the ventricle to fill during the remainder of diastole.

Functionally, the basal loop, with myofibers running in a transverse direction perpendicularly to the long axes of the ventricles, behaves like a circular muscle embracing the entire apical loop. Conversely, the descending and ascending segment fibers of the AL, run in predominantly vertical directions, almost parallel to the ventricular long axes, but with opposed obliqueness so that they cross each other at about 90° (see "X-crossing" in Fig. 6.8). At the beginning of systole (i.e., isovolumetric phase), the successive contractions of the right segment and the left segment, respectively, of the basal loop of the ventricular myocardial band result in a tight embrace of the AL, an initial change in size and shape of the atrioventricular valve orifices, and an increase of the chamber pressure.

The ensuing contraction of the *descending segment* then produces three simultaneous actions: shortening of the ventricular longitudinal axis, counterclockwise (viewed from the apex) rotation of the ventricular base, and a further change in size and shape of the atrioventricular orifices. The preceding three actions reflect the distinctive spatial arrangement of the myofibers of the descending segment of the apical loop at the start of their contraction. Due to their predominantly vertical course, the ventricular base is forced to descend toward the relatively motionless apex[8] (see Fig. 6.7 and Section 7.6, on pp. 358 ff.), thus producing a longitudinal shortening of the conical compound ventricular mass. The slight obliquity of the descending segment fibers underlies the counter-clockwise (viewed from the apex) rotation of the ventricular base, which implies a torsion of the ventricular cone akin to the *wringing* of a wet mop (see footnote on p. 305, and Fig. 6.8, on p. 314). Finally their conical configuration, reflecting that of the compound ventricular mass, causes a continuous reduction in the dimensions of the ventricular base, as it descends toward the narrower, apical part of the cone.

The last distinct part of the ventricular muscle band to contract during systole, according to the Torrent-Guasp model, is the *ascending segment* of the apical loop, whose length is greater than that of the descending segment [11, 58–60], and whose fiber inclination, or obliqueness, exceeds that of the descending, even in a relaxed state. Prior to its own contraction, the ascending segment sustains a progressive elongation by the contraction of the descending segment (see Fig. 6.8, right). As was mentioned above, the predominant longitudinality of the descending segment fibers results in an abrupt downward displacement of the ventricular base; *pari-passu*, the initially small but (as ejection progresses) increasing obliquity of the descending segment fibers, gives rise to the aforementioned counterclockwise (viewed from the apex) rotation of the ventricular base. Apart from its "wringing" effect, this movement increases the curvilinear extension of

[8]The apex should he considered as relatively stationary, because it cannot change its position in the pericardium without leaving a vacuum in its place; it cannot take the pericardium with it because this is attached to the diaphragm.

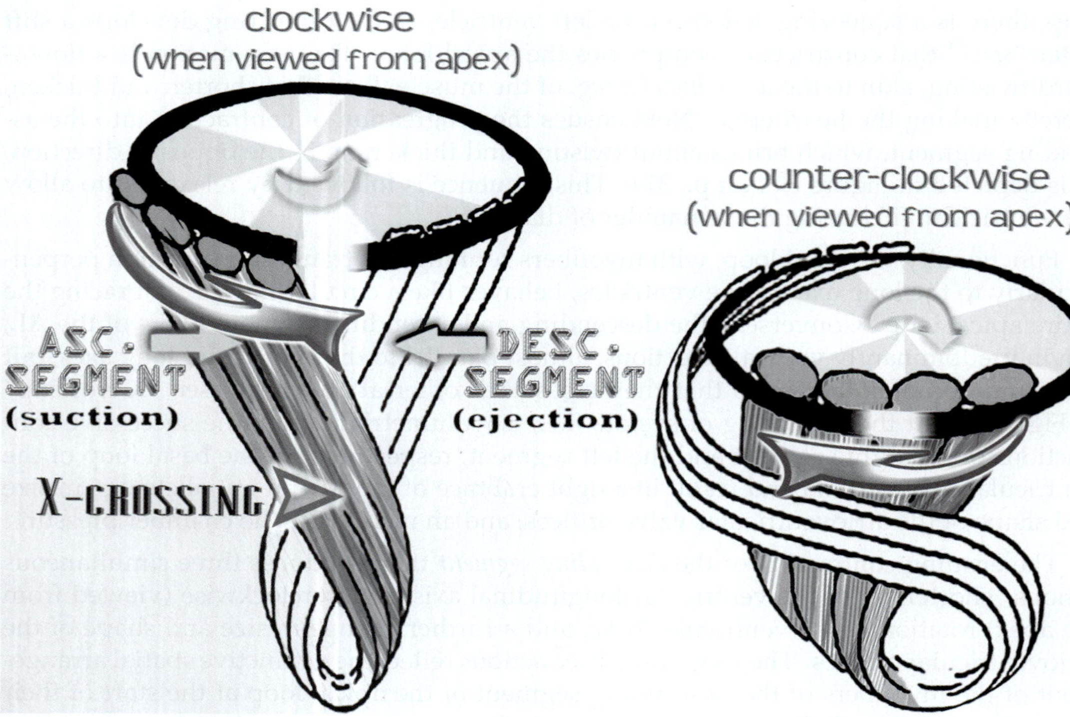

Figure 6.8: Schematic representation of the action of the two segments of the apical loop of the *Torrent-Guasp model*. Right panel: contraction of the descending segment (thickened, dark-striped fibers) compels the base to perform a descent, a counterclockwise rotation, and a diameter reduction. Left panel: subsequently persisting contraction of the ascending segment (thickened, dark-striped fibers) obliges the ventricular base to perform an ascent, a clockwise rotation, and a diameter enlargement. See Section 6.7, for Buckberg's modifications to the model.

the ascending segment to a maximal extent, at which the hemoskeleton is represented by the residual blood volume inside the ventricular cavity. According to Torrent-Guasp, the ascending segment *commences* its own contraction from this configuration.

At this juncture, it is crucial to recognize two essential considerations of the Torrent-Guasp model: first, that the obliquity of the relaxed ascending segment has been augmented as a result of the contraction of the descending segment; secondly, that the impending contraction of the curvilinearly extended ascending segment employs as a fulcrum the smallest possible (residual volume) hemoskeleton, and thus derives a maximal leverage for the straightening out action to be described next. Therefore, the contraction of the ascending segment brings about a simultaneous shortening and a pronounced straightening out of its fibers (see Fig. 6.8, left). This dynamic process underlies the *prima facie* paradoxical fact, which is a crucial attribute of the Torrent-Guasp model: ventricular chamber *elongation*, subserved by muscular *contraction*. In sum, the contraction of the ascending segment engenders three simultaneous actions: an abrupt lengthening of the ventricular longitudinal axis, a *clockwise* (viewed from the apex) rotation of the ventricular base, and an increase in size and change in shape of the atrioventricular valve orifices.

6.7 Implications of the Torrent-Guasp model

In sum, the main features of the Torrent-Guasp model are as follows:

According to Torrent-Guasp, the generally accepted concepts of the mechanics of ventricular pumping are questioned. The apical loop of the ventricular myocardial band is the principal force generator of the heart. There are no global movements of systolic chamber contraction and diastolic dilatation but, rather, of active ventricular muscle shortening and elongation with twisting (similar to the wringing of a wet towel) and untwisting, to allow for both the ejection of blood and for a contraction-induced (ascending segment of the apical loop) suction for ventricular chamber filling. The torsional deformation is built up during ejection (main systolic wringing motion, counterclockwise when viewed from the apex), imparted by contraction of the descending-segment fibers. The contraction of the ascending segment of the apical loop occurs during the last part of classical systole and the first part of diastole, which is, therefore, not a passive but rather an *active* phase.

Subsequent animal studies by Buckberg's group used sonomicrometric crystals, placed into the left and right segments of the basal loop of Torrent-Guasp's model, and into the descending and ascending components of the helical apical loop, as well as the wrap around posterior LV wall. These allowed them to correlate the *sequence* of regional contraction with pressure and dimension tracings, and to determine sequential contraction characteristics with the display of LV pressure [10]. Their data supported the anatomic concept of the helical heart surrounded by an external buttress, but demonstrated that the *timing mechanisms* differ from those that Torrent-Guasp deduced from his autopsy observations of the basal and helical loop configuration. The sequential contraction of the basal loop was confirmed.

The compression phase (or LV chamber narrowing) was found to be due to both segments of the basal loop, and the descending segment, a finding that goes against Torrent-Guasp's deduction. The sequence of shortening went from the descending segment to the posterior segment (0.10 *ms* later) and then to the ascending segment, 80 *ms* later. Importantly, the onset of ejection correlated with the positive *dp/dt* and corresponded to the onset of contraction of the ascending segment, implying a *"co-contraction"* of the *descending* and *ascending* segments. Such a *"co-contraction"* explains the *transmural* twisting during ejection, a phenomenon that is demonstrated by MRI tagging.

The early ascending segment contraction contributes to this *"co-contraction"* [10], contradicting Torrent-Guasp's notion that the descending segment causes ejection and the ascending segment begins contracting at a later time to generate suction, as it continues to shorten after shortening ceases in the descending segment. Thus, the two segments' reciprocal oblique fiber orientation can allow longitudinal lengthening during the ascending segment's continuing contraction. Buckberg emphasized that such ongoing motion during the hiatus after the descending segment stops is a critical finding, as it introduces the concept that (some) problems in diastolic dysfunction (could) have a muscular origin, and could become managed by altering calcium pathways related to muscular *contraction*.

The modified Torrent-Guasp model can explain nicely the observed longitudinal LV shortening and increased *sphericity* early in contraction, and the subsequent longitudinal lengthening (with possible development of LV suction) very late in systole and early in diastole, during what conventionally corresponds to isovolumic relaxation. However, meticulous MRI observations have established that there exists a *dissociation* between left ventricular untwisting and its diastolic filling, which is actually accentuated by catecholamines.[9] The longitudinal lengthening may contribute to LV pressure decay.

The Torrent-Guasp theory is very intriguing, but it is still awaiting scientific proof of its validity, and delineation of the particular circumstances under which it is more likely to be applicable. If it were shown to be valid, it would obviously offer radically new insights into systolic and diastolic ventricular function, insufficiency, and failure. Moreover, it would open up new fields of investigation and guide development of innovative corrective surgical procedures, pertaining to the pathology of the ventricular myocardial band and its segments. Thus, congenital cardiac abnormalities, such as a univentricular heart, would represent structural defects arising as a result of incomplete or incorrect scrolling of the ventricular myocardial band; in tetralogy of Fallot, the corrective operation would be to place a misplaced or lacking infundibular septum in its proper location.

Moreover, in the failing, dilated, spherical left ventricle there is no pointed apex (see Fig. 6.6, on p. 310). The apical muscle loop assumes a more transverse orientation, losing the mostly vertical normal configuration. Accordingly, the arrangement of the outwardly displaced papillary muscles of the left ventricle becomes more horizontal, allowing mitral regurgitation. The geometry of the heart is changed from that resembling the ellipsoidal American football to one similar to a round basketball (see Fig. 6.6). In partial ventriculectomy, resection typically takes place at the obtuse margin, which becomes ballooned in dilated cardiomyopathy and, therefore, according to the law of Laplace is the site of major mural stress overload.

The apex is typically widely resected because it is rounded in the dilated heart, as is shown schematically in the bottom panel of Figure 6.6, and, hence, overloaded. By measuring focal tension within the myocardial fiber mesh [49], it has been concluded that the shape and topography of resection have a major impact on the resulting redistribution of wall stress. New surgical ventricular restorative procedures for the failing dilated spherical left ventricle [14,45] would aim at restoring the elliptical shape in the remodeled spherical ventricle; i.e., at reestablishing the American football shape through a partial left ventriculectomy (aneurysmectomy, Batista, Dor, and other cardioreduction procedures [5,19,20,56]),[10] while rebuilding (*"pacopexy,"* [11]) the apical region.

[9]Any suction effect would obviously be most beneficial under conditions of tachycardia and high adrenergic drive, as they apply, e.g., in the "fight-or-flight" reaction.

[10]The salutary effects of such interventions that decrease the diastolic convective deceleration load (CDL) by diminishing diastolic ventriculoannular disproportion, as well as by promoting stronger diastolic intraventricular vortical motions, are discussed at length in Chapter 14.

At present, some supporting evidence for the unique ventricular muscle band may be found in Gorodkov et al.'s [23] corrosion casts documenting the spiral trabeculae of descending loop markings on cavity blood, in Jung et al.'s [31] MRI evidence of spiral velocity and strain development, and in the review by Buckberg [10] of data showing co-contraction of the descending and ascending loops during ejection along with *ongoing contraction* [12] of the ascending loop during "isovolumetric relaxation." Nevertheless, other researchers [18] inspecting the sonomicrometric data presented in Dr. Buckberg's review have claimed that it is their reading of the presented data that ascending segment contraction is overwhelmingly associated with ejection, isovolumic relaxation slightly, and early filling hardly at all; most ($\approx$80%) of the shortening of the ascending segment occurs during ejection, and the remaining ($\approx$20%) of shortening likely occurs before deep LV pressure falls below left atrial pressure. If the heart has not yet started filling at the end of the ascending segment contraction, how can Torrent–Guasp's idea of systolic filling (via anterior segment contraction) be fully supported by these sonomicrometric data?

Conclusive validation of the ventricular muscle band model remains to be developed in the future. All the same, Torrent-Guasp's insightful unraveling of cardiac structure and his morphomechanical correlations have opened pathways toward a revolution that will allow others to grow from his achievements. His unscrolling of the transverse basal loop and oblique apical loop to create a cardiac helix surrounded by an outer buttress has true elegance and profound implications for understanding cardiac normality and disease.

References and further reading

[1] Anderson, R.H., Sanchez-Quintana, D., Niederer, P., Lunkenheimer, P.P. Structural-functional correlates of the 3-dimensional arrangement of the myocytes making up the ventricular walls. J. Thorac. Cardiovasc. Surg. 136: 10–8, 2008.

[2] Anderson, R.H., Ho, S.Y., Redmann, K., Sanchez-Quintana, D., Lunkenheimer, P.P. The anatomical arrangement of the myocardial cells making up the ventricular mass. Eur. J. Cardiothorac. Surg. 28: 517–25, 2005.

[3] Anderson, R.H., Ho, S.Y., Sanchez-Quintana, D., Redmann, K., Lunkenheimer, P.P. Heuristic problems in defining the three-dimensional arrangement of the ventricular myocytes. Anat. Rec. Part A, 288A: 579–86, 2006.

[4] Ashikaga, H., Criscione, J.C., Omens, J.H., Covell, J.W., and Ingels, N.B., Jr. Transmural left ventricular mechanics underlying torsional recoil during relaxation. Am. J. Physiol. Heart Circ. Physiol. 286: H640–7, 2004.

[5] Athanasuleas, C.L., Buckberg, G.D., Stanley, A.W., et al. Surgical ventricular restoration in the treatment of congestive heart failure due to post-infarction ventricular dilation J. Am. Coll. Cardiol. 44: 1439–45, 2004.

[6] Aurigemma, G.P., Silver, K.H., Priest, M.A., Gaasch, W.H. Geometric changes allow normal ejection fraction despite depressed myocardial shortening in hypertensive left ventricular hypertrophy. J. Am. Coll. Cardiol. 26: 195–202, 1995.

[7] Axel, L. Biomechanical dynamics of the heart with MRI. Annu. Rev. Biomed. Eng. 4: 321–47, 2002.

[8] Benninghoff, A. Die Architektur des Herzmuskels. Eine vergleichend anatomische und vergleichend funktionelle Betrachtung. Morph. Jahrb. 67: 262–317, 1931.

[9] Borelli, G.A., Maquet, P. On the Movement of Animals (1680). 1989, New York: Springer-Verlag.

[10] Buckberg, G.D. Architecture must document functional evidence to explain the living rhythm. Eur. J. Cardiothorac. Surg. 27: 202–9, 2005.

[11] Buckberg, G.D. Basic science review: the helix and the heart. J. Thorac. Cardiovasc. Surg. 124: 863–83, 2002.

[12] Buckberg, G.D. Letter to the Editor. Reply to Criscione et al. Nature is simple, but scientists are complicated. Eur. J. Cardiothorac. Surg. 28: 364–365, 2005.

[13] Cheng, A., Nguyen, T.C., Malinowski, M., Daughters, G.T., Miller, D.C., Ingels, N.B. Jr. Heterogeneity of left ventricular wall thickening mechanisms. Circulation 118: 713–21, 2008.

[14] Cohn, J.N. Structural basis for heart failure: ventricular remodeling and its pharmacological inhibition. Circulation 91: 2504–7, 1995.

[15] Costa, K.D., Takayama, Y., McCulloch, A.D., Covell, J.W. Laminar fiber architecture and three-dimensional systolic mechanics in canine ventricular myocardium. Am. J. Physiol. Heart Circ. Physiol. 276: H595–607, 1999.

[16] Covell, J.W., Ross, J. Systolic and diastolic function (mechanics) of the intact heart. Chapter 10. In: Page, E., Fozzard, H.A., Solaro, J.R. [Eds.] Handbook of Physiology, Section 2, Volume I: The Heart. 2002, New York: Oxford University Press. pp. 741–75.

[17] Covell, J.W. Tissue structure and ventricular wall mechanics. Circulation 118: 699–701, 2008.

[18] Criscione, J.C., Rodriguez, F., Miller, D.C. Letter to the Editor. The myocardial band: simplicity can be a weakness. Eur. J. Cardiothorac. Surg. 28: 363–4, 2005.

[19] Dor, V. Surgery for left ventricular aneurysm. Curr. Opin. Cardiol. 1990;5:773–80.

[20] Eisen, H. J. Surgical ventricular reconstruction for heart failure [Editorial]. N. Engl. J. Med. 360: 1781–4, 2009.

[21] Franklin, K., Lower, R. Tractus de Corde, London, 1669. 1932, Oxford: Oxford University Press.

[22] Fyrenius, A., Wigström, L., Ebbers, T., Karlsson, M., Engvall, J., Bolger, A.F. Three dimensional flow in the human left atrium. Heart 86: 448–55, 2001.

[23] Gorodkov, A., Dobrova, N.B., Dubernaud, J., Kiknadze, G., Gatchetchiladze, I., Oleinikov, V., Kuzmina, N., Barat, J., Bacuey, C. Anatomic structures determining blood flow in the heart left ventricle. J. Mater. Sci.: Mater. Med. 7: 153–60, 1996.

[24] Grant, R.P. Notes on the muscular architecture of the left ventricle. Circulation 32: 301–8, 1965.

[25] Gray, H. Anatomy, Descriptive, and Surgical ("Gray's Anatomy," 1901). 1977, New York: Bounty Books.

[26] Greenbaum, R.A., Ho, S.Y., Gibson, D.G., Becker, A.E., Anderson, R.H. Left ventricular fibre architecture in man. Br. Heart J. 45: 248–63, 1981.

[27] Guttman, M.A., Zerhouni, E.A., McVeigh, E.R. Analysis of cardiac function from MR Images. IEEE Comput. Graph. Appl. 17: 30–8, 1997.

[28] Harrington, K.B., Rodriguez, F., Cheng, A., Langer, F., Ashikaga, H., Daughters, G.T., Criscione, J.C., Ingels, N.B., Miller, D.C. Direct measurement of transmural laminar architecture in the anterolateral wall of the ovine left ventricle: new implications for wall thickening mechanics. Am. J. Physiol. Heart Circ. Physiol. 288: H1324–30, 2005.

[29] Icardo, J.M. Development biology of the vertebrate heart. J. Exp. Zool. 275: 144–61, 1996.

[30] Jouk, P.-S., Usson, Y., Michalowicz, G., Grossi, L. Three-dimensional cartography of the pattern of the myofibers in the second trimester fetal human heart. Anat. Embryol. 202: 103–18, 2000.

[31] Jung, B., Schneider, B., Markl, M., Saurbier, B., Geibel, A., Hennig, J. Measurement of left ventricular velocities: phase contrast MRI velocity mapping versus tissue-doppler-ultrasound in healthy volunteers. J. Cardiovasc. Magn. Reson. 6: 777–83, 2004.

[32] Keith, A. The functional anatomy of the heart. Br. Med. J. 1918: 361–3.

[33] Kocica, M.J., Corno, A.F., Carreras-Costa, F., Ballester-Rodes, M., Moghbel, M.C., Cueva, C.N.C., Lackovic, V., Kanjuh, V.I., Torrent-Guasp, F. The helical ventricular myocardial band: global, three-dimensional, functional architecture of the ventricular myocardium. Eur. J. Cardiothorac. Surg. 29(Suppl 1): S21–40, 2006.

[34] Krehl, L. von. Beiträge zur Kenntniss der Füllung und Entleerung des Herzens. Abh. Math-Phys. Kl. Sächs. Akad. Wiss. 17: 340–83, 1891.

[35] LeGrice, I.J., Takayama, Y., Covell, J.W. Transverse shear along myocardial cleavage planes provides a mechanism for normal systolic wall thickening. Circ. Res. 77: 182–93, 1995.

[36] Lunkenheimer, P.P., Redmann, K., Anderson, R.H. The architecture of the ventricular mass and its functional implications for organ-preserving surgery. Eur. J. Cardiothorac. Surg. 27: 183–90, 2005.

[37] Lunkenheimer, P.P., Redmann, K., Westermann, P., Rothaus, K., Cryer, C.W., Niederer, P., Anderson, R.H. The myocardium and its fibrous matrix working in concert as a spatially netted mesh: a critical review of the purported tertiary structure of the ventricular mass. Eur. J. Cardiothorac. Surg. 29(Suppl 1): S41–9, 2006.

[38] MacGowan, G.Y., Shapiro, E.P., Azhari, H., Siu, C.O., Hees, P.S., Hutchins, G.M., Weiss, J.L., Rademakers, F.E. Noninvasive measurement of shortening in the fiber and cross-fiber directions in the normal human left ventricle and in idiopathic dilated cardiomyopathy. Circulation 96: 535–41, 1997.

[39] Männer, J. Ontogenetic development of the helical heart: concepts and facts. Eur. J. Cardiothorac. Surg. 29(Suppl 1): S69–74, 2006.

[40] Mall, F.P. On the muscular architecture and growth of the ventricles in the human heart. Am. J. Anat. 2: 417, 1911.

[41] Olson, R.E. Physiology of cardiac muscle. Chapter 10. In: Hamilton, W.F., Dow, P. [Eds.] Handbook of Physiology, Section 2, Volume I.: Circulation. 1962, Washington, D.C.: American Physiological Society. pp. 199–237.

[42] Palmon, L.C., Reichek, N., Yeon, S.B., Clark, N.R., Brownson, D., Hoffman, E., Axel, L. Intramural myocardial shortening in hypertensive left ventricular hypertrophy with normal pump function. Circulation 89: 122–31, 1994.

[43] Pettigrew, J.B. Design in nature, illustrated by spiral and other arrangements in the inorganic and organic kingdoms as exemplified in matter, force, life, growth, rhythms, etc., especially in crystals, plants, and animals. With examples selected from the reproductive, alimentary, respiratory, circulatory, nervous, muscular, osseous, locomotory, and other systems of animals. 1908, London, New York: Longmans, Green, and Co. 3 v.; vol. 2, pp. 506–18.

[44] Pettigrew, J.B. On the arrangement of the muscular fibres of the ventricular portion of the heart of the mammal. Proc. Roy. Soc. Lond. 10: 433–40, 1860.

[45] Pfeffer, M.A., Braunwald, E. Ventricular remodeling after myocardial infarction: experimental observations and clinical implications. Circulation. 81: 1161–72, 1990.

[46] Poelmann, R.E., Gittenberger-de Groot, A.C., Hierck, B.P. The development of the heart and microcirculation: role of shear stress. Med. Biol. Eng. Comput. 46: 479–84, 2008.

[47] Rademakers, F.E., Rogers, W.J., Guier, W.J., Hutchins, G.M., Siu, C.O., Weisfeldt, M.L., Weiss, J.L., Shapiro, E.P. Relationship of regional cross-fiber shortening to wall thickening in the intact heart. Three-dimensional strain analysis by NMR tagging. Circulation 89: 1174–82, 1994.

[48] Rademakers, F.E., Buchalter, M.B., Rogers, W.J., Zerhouni, E.A., Weisfeldt, M.L., Weiss, J.L., Shapiro, E.P. Dissociation between left ventricular untwisting and filling. Accentuation by catecholamines. Circulation 85: 1572–81, 1992.

[49] Redmann, K., Lunkenheimer, P.P., Dietl, K.H., Cryer, C.W., Batista, R.J.V., Anderson, R.H. Immediate effects of partial left ventriculectomy on left ventricular function. J. Card. Surg. 13: 453–62, 1999.

[50] Rushmer, R.F., Crystal, D.K., Wagner, C. The functional anatomy of ventricular contraction. Circ. Res. 1: 162–70, 1953.

[51] Sklavounos, G.L. Human Anatomy [*Ανατομικη του Ανθρωπου*]. 3rd ed. 1934–38, Athens: S.T. Tarousopoulos Press. 3 v.

[52] Spotnitz, H.M. Macro design, structure, and mechanics of the left ventricle. J. Thorac. Cardiovasc. Surg. 119: 1053–77, 2000.

[53] Streeter, Jr. D.D., Sponitz, H.M., Patel, D.J., Ross, Jr. J., Sonnenblick, E.H. Fiber orientation in the canine left ventricle during diastole and systole. Circ. Res. 24: 339–47, 1969.

[54] Streeter, Jr. D.D., Hanna, W.T. Engineering mechanics for successive states in canine left ventricular myocardium. I. Cavity and wall geometry. Circ. Res. 33: 639–55, 1973.

[55] Streeter, Jr. D.D., Hanna, W.T. Engineering mechanics for successive states in canine left ventricular myocardium. II. Fiber angle and sarcomere length. Circ. Res. 33: 656–64, 1973.

[56] Sutton, M.G., Sharpe, N. Left ventricular remodeling after myocardial infarction: pathophysiology and therapy. Circulation 101: 2981–8, 2000.

[57] Torrent-Guasp, F., Buckberg, G.D., Clemente, C., Cox, J.L., Coghlan, H.C., Gharib, M. The Structure and Function of the helical heart and its buttress wrapping. I. The normal macroscopic structure of the heart. Semin. Thorac. Cardiovasc. Surg. 13: 301–19, 2001.

[58] Torrent-Guasp, F., Kocica, M.J., Corno, A., Komeda, M., Cox, J., Flotats, A., Ballester-Rodes, M., Carreras-Costa, F. Systolic ventricular filling. Eur. J. Cardiothorac. Surg. 25: 376–86, 2004.

[59] Torrent-Guasp, F., Kocica, M.J., Corno, A., Komeda, M., Carreras-Costa, F., Flotats, A., Cosin-Aguillar, J., Wen, H. Towards new understanding of the heart structure and function. Eur. J. Cardiothorac. Surg. 27: 191–201, 2005.

[60] Torrent-Guasp, F., Ballester, M., Buckberg, G.D., Carreras, F., Flotats, A., Carrió, I., Ferreira, A., Samuels, L.E., Narula, J. Spatial orientation of the ventricular muscle band: physiologic contribution and surgical implications. J. Thorac. Cardiovasc. Surg. 122: 389–92, 2001.

[61] Ubbink, S.W.J., Bovendeerd, P.H.M., Delhaas, T., Arts, T., van de Vosse, F.N. Towards model-based analysis of cardiac MR tagging data: relation between left ventricular shear strain and myofiber orientation. Med. Im. Anal. 10: 632–41, 2006.

[62] van Dalen, B.M., Soliman, O.I., Vletter, W.B., Ten Cate, F.J., Geleijnse, M.L. Age-related changes in the biomechanics of left ventricular twist measured by speckle tracking echocardiography. Am. J. Physiol. Heart Circ. Physiol. 295: H1705–11, 2008.

[63] Waldman, L.K, Fung, Y.C., Covell, J.W. Transmural myocardial deformation in the canine left ventricle: normal in vivo three-dimensional finite strains. Circ. Res. 57: 152–63, 1985.

[64] Waldman, L.K, Nosan, D., Villarreal, F., Covell, J.W. Relation between transmural deformation and local myofiber direction in canine left ventricle. Circ. Res. 63: 550–62, 1988.

[65] Yacoub, M.H. Two hearts that beat as one. Circulation 92: 156–7, 1995.

[66] Yellin, E.L., Meisner, J.S. Physiology of diastolic function and transmitral pressure-flow relations. Cardiol. Clin. 18: 411–33, 2000.

Chapter 7

Cardiac Cycle and Central Pressure, Flow, and Volume Pulses

As a basis for initiating analysis, five lines are drawn [perpendicularly to the timeline of simultaneous recordings of hemodynamic variables from the cardiac chambers and great vessel roots] to indicate the customary subdivisions that have been used by others and myself in analyzing the cardiac cycle. Lines 1–2 demarcate the interval usually designated as the isometric contraction phase; 2–3 limit the ejection phase; 3–4 comprise the early diastolic relaxation phase; 4–5 include the rapid inflow phase and the balance of the cycle comprises the phase of diastasis terminating in auricular systole. In considering the time limits of these phases, the desirability of further subdivision will be discussed.

——Carl J. Wiggers, 1921.—Excerpt from his elegant description [156] of the phases of the cardiac cycle, which is often referred to as the "Wiggers' Diagram," a graphic summary correlating hemodynamic, volumetric, acoustic, and electrocardiographic events during the normal cardiac cycle.

The heart is a hollow organ weighing well under a pound and only a little larger than the fist, in absence of abnormal enlargement and hypertrophy. Its tough, muscular walls (myocardium) are surrounded by a fibrous bag (pericardium) and are lined by a thin membrane (endocardium). A wall (septum) divides the heart cavity down the middle into a "right heart" and a "left heart." Each side is divided again into an upper chamber (atrium or auricle) and a lower chamber (ventricle). Atrioventricular valves (the "mitral," on the left, and "tricuspid," on the right) regulate the flow of blood through the heart, and semilunar valves (pulmonic and aortic) to the root of the pulmonary artery and the aorta. A detailed survey of cardiac functional morphology is offered in Chapter 6.

The function of the two ventricles, operating as positive displacement pumps, is to deliver with every beat a stroke volume of blood into the roots of their outflow trunks. The cardiac output (C.O.) equals the product of the effective stroke volume (S.V.), of the right or left ventricle, by the heart rate (H.R.).

7.1 Low- *vs.* high-pressure operation: the disparate needs of diastole and systole

The pumping left ventricle forms the central link between the low-pressure and the high-pressure systems of the circulatory ensemble, which are depicted diagrammatically in Figure 7.1. The low-pressure system begins with the postarteriolar microcirculatory beds and comprises systemic vascular, right cardiac, pulmonary vascular, and left atrial components [20, 25, 26, 72, 85]. Their hemodynamic coupling to the left ventricle in diastole enters in the determination of its diastolic filling and loading *(preload)* [26, 76]. The extracardiac high-pressure system is represented by the systemic arterial ensemble from the aortic root through the arteriolar resistance vessels. Its input impedance [65, 66, 78, 82, 102] enters in the determination not only of left ventricular systolic loading *(afterload)*, but of *coronary perfusion* patterns as well [126, 152]. Representative intraluminal pressure levels in the low-pressure system are of the order of 10 *mm Hg*; in the high-pressure system, they are higher by one order of magnitude. The left ventricle in diastole

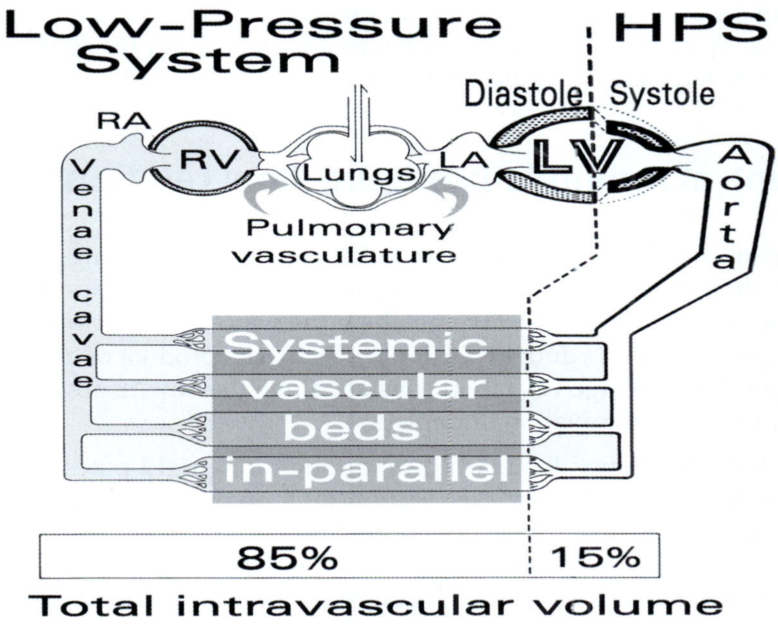

Figure 7.1: Partition of the circulatory ensemble into a *low-* and a *high-pressure system* (HPS). R = right; L = left; A = atrium; V = ventricle.

is functionally a part of the low-pressure system. Its filling patterns reflect the interplay of atrioventricular fluid (including valvular) and wall dynamics [38, 76, 83, 98, 144, 162]. In some degree, filling patterns are affected also by contiguous pericardial and right ventricular pressures [26, 38, 76, 77, 79, 98]. The left ventricle in systole becomes part of the high-pressure system and its contraction and ejection patterns reflect again the intimate interactions of ventricular wall and fluid dynamics [31, 54, 88, 130]. Accordingly, the left ventricle must be adapted to the widely disparate functional-structural requirements of both systole and diastole, states in which both the thickness and curvature of its walls drastically change within each beat [36, 86].

Moreover, almost all forms of heart disease alter ventricular topography; the changes in ventricular configuration may in themselves set the stage for cardiac dysfunction. For instance, excessive wall hypertrophy in response to systolic pressure overloading is associated with diminished ventricular distensibility and, not uncommonly, with increased muscle stiffness, both of which may then be responsible for impaired diastolic function [75, 76, 98]. Clearly, a good conceptual grasp and a quantitative understanding of the dynamics of the interaction of the ventricle with its diastolic and systolic loading patterns in health and disease are desirable. Such understanding is necessary in delineating, and hopefully forestalling, the transition from gradually accumulating quantitative adaptive changes of the chronically overloaded ventricle to the qualitatively new reactions, which transform normal adaptation into pathology with impaired performance.

The following sections provide a concise but comprehensive picture of current knowledge of diastolic and systolic ventricular and myocardial mechanics,[1] as they relate to the cardiac cycle. It should set the stage for a better appreciation of the chapters that follow, in which we will delve into the fluid dynamics of ventricular ejection and filling.

7.2 Central pulsatile pressure-flow relations

A flowing stream may change its velocity either because the driving pressure gradient changes with time (flow pulsations), or because the flow boundaries (and, for laminar flow, the streamlines) converge or diverge along the way: by the *continuity principle* (see Sections 4.2.2, on pp. 171 ff., and 4.4.2, on pp. 176 f.), the product of cross-sectional area by the corresponding average velocity is constant along the flow, in absence of interposed region(s) of transient accumulation or depletion.

In steady, fully developed laminar flows, through long rigid pipes of uniform cross-section—beyond the "entry length" (see Section 4.9.1, on pp. 200 ff.) needed for development of the Poiseuille profile under the action of liquid viscosity—flow is maintained by the steady pressure drop (gradient) along the axis, according to Poiseuille's law. There is no acceleration of fluid particles in fully developed Poiseuille flow, and thus inertial effects do not enter in the flow behavior. In Poiseuille flow, the force that the steady pressure gradient exerts on the liquid is completely balanced only by the viscous resistance to flow.

Central[2] pulsatile flows, on the other hand, are characterized by pressure gradients varying in time. The pressure gradient has to overcome the inertia of intracardiac blood masses and adjoining intraluminal blood columns, in order to accelerate or decelerate the

[1] The term "ventricular" pertains to attributes of the ventricle as a hollow organ; "myocardial" denotes properties of the tissue as a structural material.

[2] The term "central flows" denotes inertia-dominated flows in the cardiac chambers and the contiguous intrathoracic trunks of the great vessels, namely, aorta, pulmonary artery, venae cavae, and pulmonary veins.

flow. In fact, inertial effects are normally much more prominent in determining the basic behavior of central flows than frictional effects attributable to blood viscosity. Afterall, according to Newton's First Law every material body (including liquid masses) would continue in its state of rest, or preexisting motion, unless it is compelled by an external force to change that state. And, from Newton's Second Law of Motion, it follows that large instantaneous values of pressure gradient (that is, force per unit volume of moving blood) are necessary, in order to overcome blood's inertia to both local and convective acceleration components during ejection. Blood's inertia is of course associated with its finite mass per unit volume, or mass density, and is totally independent of its viscous behavior.

Consider central pulsatile (phasic) pressure gradients at instants when they may be reversing; for example, when a previously accelerating gradient becomes adverse or decelerating in action: at the instant of reversal, the pressure gradient passes through zero on its way to becoming adverse. However, at the instant when the gradient becomes zero the flow velocity is not zero, because the central blood mass or column still has the velocity that it gained under the action of the pressure gradient over the previous *accelerating* time interval. The central flow does not come to rest until the combined actions of primarily the now adverse (decelerating) pressure gradient and, only secondarily, of blood viscosity have overcome its momentum and tendency to maintain its preexisting state of motion; this is a process requiring a finite, albeit small, time interval.

A case in point from daily life may be instructive. Perhaps it will help those who have traditionally thought in terms of resistive pressure–flow relationships to understand how blood may continue to flow forward across the cardiac valves, even after the transvalvular pressure gradient has reversed. Once a car is accelerated to a certain velocity, turning its engine off does not stop it instantaneously. The vehicle's momentum allows for continued forward motion despite the fact that the only forces acting on the automobile are wind and road resistance—forces opposing its onward motion. Generally, pulsatile pressure gradients (gradients varying in time) acting on blood masses must first accelerate them and then decelerate them, when the gradients become adverse. Consequently, in absence of abnormal stenosis of the flow passages, central blood flow *velocities*, resulting from phasic accelerations and decelerations, must *lag* behind the swiftly changing *pressure gradients* and measured instantaneous *pressure differences* that are responsible for them.

In addition, inertial effects are primarily responsible for the fact that the cardiac pumping chambers must develop greater forces to eject a given stroke volume at higher than at lower heart rates. This rate dependency is again readily ascertained by trying to accelerate a car from 0 to 60 *mph* in 10, as compared to 60, *seconds*. The inertial forces required by the former task are much greater than by the latter.

7.2.1 Central velocity profiles

The action of liquid viscosity is manifested in viscous forces that tend to eliminate differences of velocity between adjacent laminae in a stream. Such viscous effects and the requirement that liquid at the wall must have zero velocity relative to the wall surface, by

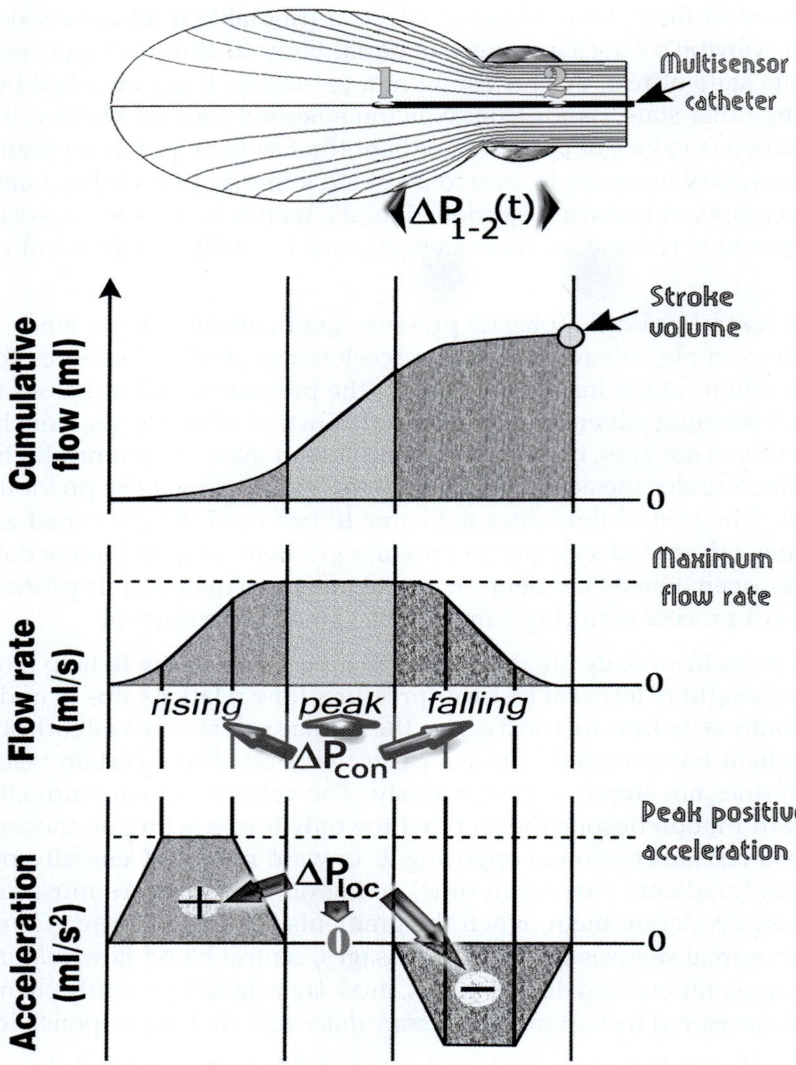

Figure 7.2: *Schematic development of pulsatile flow.* In early ejection, outflow accelerates to a peak rate. The ejection flow rate does not revert to zero until a *(decelerating)* pressure gradient has overcome blood's momentum; this requires an interval of negative acceleration, or *deceleration*. The time integral of outflow rate over the ejection period is the *stroke volume*. There is strong convective acceleration in the outflow tract, as shown by the confluent streamlines in the top panel. The total *transvalvular* instantaneous pressure drop normally embodies convective and local acceleration components—$\Delta P_{1-2} = \Delta P_{con} + \Delta P_{loc}$. At peak flow, $\Delta P_{loc} = 0$ while ΔP_{con} is at its peak level; during the flow *upstroke*, both components are present and acting in the *same* sense; during the *downstroke*, both components are present but are acting in *opposite* senses.

the "no slip" condition (see Sections 4.9, on pp. 197 ff., 4.10, on pp. 202 ff., and 4.12, on pp. 208 ff.), result in the parabolic velocity profile of fully developed Poiseuille flow in a long pipe under a given steady pressure gradient.

Central pulsatile blood flows are, in contrast to the more familiar Poiseuille flow, dominated by inertial effects and almost all the driving phasic pressure gradient goes into acceleration or deceleration, i.e., into overcoming blood *inertia* as is shown in Figure 7.2, on p. 328, rather than viscous forces. Viscous effects are generally predominant over inertial effects only in the immediate vicinity of the flow boundaries. The velocity profile-shaping action of blood viscosity does not have enough time to penetrate deep into the main core of the flow. Thus, central pulsatile profiles are far from fully developed: they are essentially flat (cf. Section 4.10, and Fig. 4.15 on p. 204).

7.3 Notable factors affecting central pulse magnitudes and waveforms

Several physical factors influence pressure pulse magnitudes and waveforms in the cardiac chambers and the trunks of the great vessels, under normal and pathological operating conditions. The following are most notable.

a. *Pressures in contiguous vascular segments or chambers, and in surrounding spaces.*

Transmural pressure (and intraluminal lateral pressure) pulses in a given short vascular segment or chamber depend on the flow conditions at its inflow and outflow sites. Central pulsatile flows have essentially flat velocity profiles. Frictional pressure drops across short central vascular segments are normally negligible, and are associated with the *viscoelasticity* of the pulsating vessel *walls*, rather than with blood viscosity effects.

Neglecting gravitational actions, the instantaneous value of the *total* or *stagnation* pressure (P_T) at any point of a central flow field is

$$P_T(t) = P_L + \frac{\rho v^2}{2}, \tag{7.1}$$

where, ρ is blood density, v is the velocity of the effectively inviscid core, $\frac{\rho v^2}{2}$ is the instantaneous "kinetic pressure," and P_L is the corresponding "lateral pressure." You can visualize the action of the kinetic pressure readily: if you blow down through a straw on a water surface, you can make a dimple in the surface, suggesting that where the air is brought to rest, just below the tube, the pressure is greater than at the sides, where the air is moving outwards (cf. Fig. 7.3, on p. 330). Since central flows are markedly pulsatile, P_T as well as $\frac{\rho v^2}{2}$ and P_L are functions of time.

Because central flows have essentially flat velocity profiles, total pressure as well as its lateral and kinetic pressure components are virtually uniformly distributed across most of the vascular cross-section. It is the lateral pressure, P_L, pulse, rather than P_T, that tends to distend the wall of the segment (or chamber). Accordingly, the rate of change

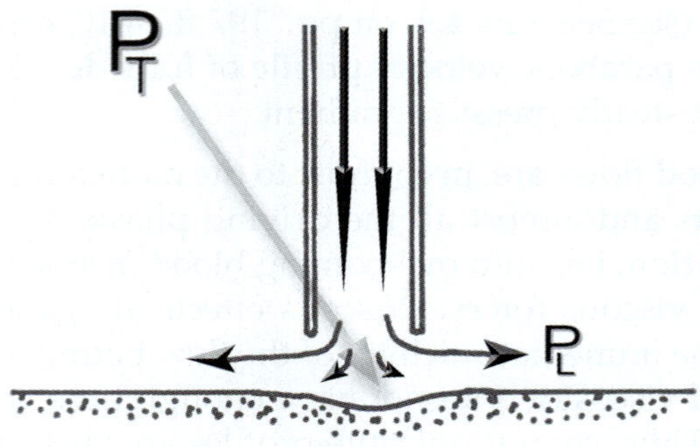

Figure 7.3: The pressure is lower where the air moves, P_L, than where it is brought to rest, P_T.

in volume depends on the rate of change in P_L. Thus, the lateral pressure pulse and the volume pulse depend not only on $P_T(t)$, but also on its instantaneously applying *apportionment* into lateral *vs.* kinetic pressure components.

When the pressure is independently raised only at the outflow site of a given segment, an augmented impediment to the outflow ensues and it decelerates. Blood accumulation (positive rate of change of volume, V, with respect to time—dV/dt) occurs in the segment as its transmural pressure rises. This rise in transmural pressure is in fact produced by flow deceleration in the segment, which reduces $\frac{\rho v^2}{2}$ to the advantage of P_L. A greater proportion of the $P_T(t)$ that is available at the segment's inflow site becomes transformed into $P_L(t)$ as $\frac{\rho v^2}{2}$ decreases, and thus the distending transmural pressure rises.

Because the relation between pressure and volume in cardiovascular organs is generally nonlinear, the transmural pressure pulse amplitude for a given volume change usually rises considerably with advancing vascular distension. The greater the time averaged value of transmural pressure and P_L in the segment, the greater is usually the superposed pressure amplitude for a given phasic volume change.

Perivascular pressures can generally influence cardiac chamber and vascular geometry. During each respiratory cycle, the changing intrathoracic and intrapleural pressures affect all cardiac chambers and intrathoracic vessels, except those that are apposed to alveoli. For the alveolar capillaries, the transmural pressure, which is the pressure that determines their caliber, is given as the difference between intracapillary and alveolar pressures. The transmural pressure of all cardiac chambers and other intrathoracic vessels is determined, in principle, as the difference between the intraluminal and the intrapleural or, more generally, the intrathoracic pressures (see Fig. 7.4). There are practical difficulties in estimating perivascular from intrathoracic pressures; pericapillary pressures approximate under quasi-static conditions the ambient atmospheric pressure, but the prospect exists for tissue forces, such as alveolar surface tension, to decrease pericapillary pressure to somewhat *subatmospheric* levels.

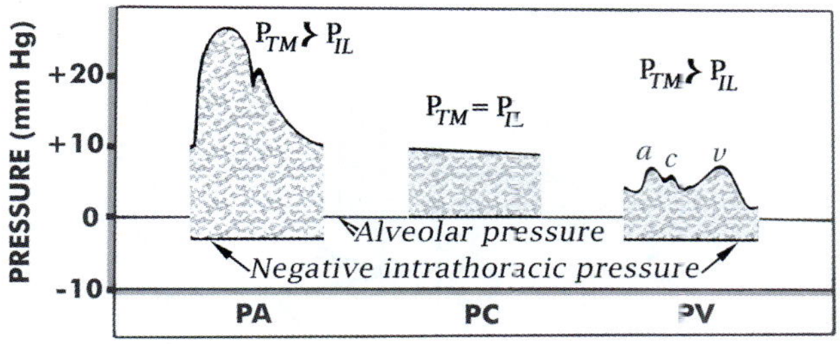

Figure 7.4: Difference between the intraluminal (P_{IL}), which are referred to atmospheric pressure, and the transmural (P_{TM})pressures, which are referred to perivascular pressure, in the case of the pulmonary vasculature. The patterned area represents the transmural pressure. In the pulmonary capillaries (PC), which are exposed to alveolar pressure, the intraluminal and transmural pressures are virtually identical in magnitude. Conversely, in the pulmonary artery (PA) and veins (PV), the transmural pressure exceeds the intraluminal pressure by the magnitude of the applying negative intrapleural pressure.

Figure 7.5, on p. 332, exemplifies the effects on intracardiac and large intrathoracic vessel pressures and flows of the fall in intrathoracic pressure to strongly intensified subatmospheric levels, induced by a sustained Mueller maneuver, i.e., a forced inspiratory effort against a closed glottis. Intracardiac pressures and pressure pulse waveforms are also affected by transient disturbances from surrounding spaces. For instance, a transient increase in external pressure (by a cough) produces a sharp rise in cardiac intraluminal lateral pressures, P_L.

The transmural pressures of the cardiac chambers, given by the differences between the intraluminal and the external effective pressures, determine their degree of filling and diastolic, as well as systolic, loading conditions and function [26,53,76,105]. Ordinarily, the negative pressure of the intrathoracic cavity and, more specifically, of the pericardial space surrounds the heart, and this negativity contributes greatly to the effective filling pressures. However, at times the negative pressure becomes weakened or completely lost; e.g., opening the chest immediately shifts the heart and the intrathoracic, extra-alveolar, vessels from negative pressure surroundings to atmospheric pressure. A more drastic change is induced by accumulations of pericardial or intrapleural fluid, pericardial constriction, pneumothorax, or mediastinal compression, all of which can cause intensive positive pressure on the outside of heart and impair its function even more than the open-chest state [26,53,105], as is depicted in Figure 8.17, on p. 433.

b. *The venturi effect.* By continuity considerations, a moderate luminal constriction along a central flow field results in flow acceleration and increased velocity at the constricted site. In the immediate vicinity of the constriction the kinetic pressure component rises and the lateral pressure component falls. As long as the constriction is not too great, frictional losses are negligible and the total pressure remains constant. A catheter tip with a micromanometric sensor (or pressure hole leading via a fluid-filled lumen to an external strain gauge) facing the oncoming flow measures the instantaneously applying *total* pressure, or *stagnation* pressure. In contrast, if the microsensor (or hole) faces laterally, then it will register the instantaneous *lateral* pressure. When frictional losses

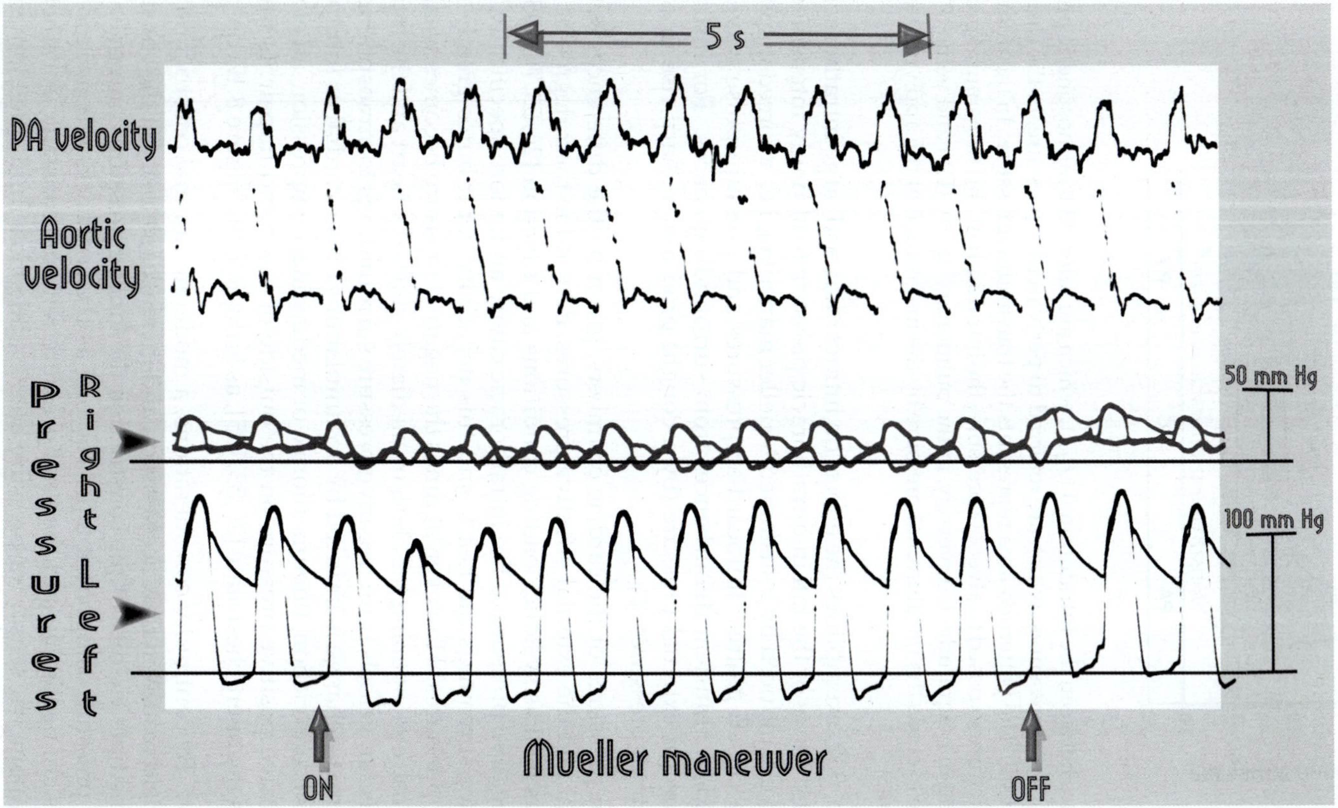

Figure 7.5: Hemodynamics during the Mueller maneuver, in a subject studied during elective cardiac catheterization with right and left-heart multisensor micromanometry. Simultaneous right and left-heart pressures and pulmonary arterial and aortic flow velocities and pressures are shown. (Redrawn, slightly modified, from Condos et al. [26], with kind permission of the Am. Heart Assoc.)

are negligible, *total* pressure is not affected by convergence or divergence of the flow streamlines. *Lateral* pressure falls where the streamlines converge, and rises again where they diverge, as is pictorially shown in Figure 7.6 on p. 334. *Kinetic* pressure undergoes changes complementary to those of the lateral pressure, in line with the requirement that total pressure is not affected by the flow geometry. These inter-relations of kinetic and lateral components associated with convective (geometric) flow-field acceleration or deceleration along the flow in the absence of significant frictional losses are known as the *venturi effect*. One must keep in mind the venturi effect not only because of its importance in explaining some features of central (lateral) pressure and volume pulses, but also because it may introduce considerable errors and uncertainties in hemodynamic mensurations, depending on the unsteady orientation of micromanometric sensors or catheter holes relative to the oncoming blood stream.

Measured pressure waveforms may be distorted not only by venturi effects but also by artefacts, including so-called catheter tip "entrapment" by a valve leaflet, endocardium, or vascular intima during part of the cycle, catheter obstruction by clotted blood, etc. Central hemodynamic waveforms may also be distorted by inadequate operational characteristics of measuring instruments, e.g., inappropriately damped liquid-filled catheter-external manometer systems with inadequate frequency response characteristics.

c. *Chamber volume and effective volume modulus.*

We may define an incremental volume modulus as $E_v = (\frac{dP_L}{dV})V_o$. V_o is an applying "original" volume, increasing with advancing distension $\frac{dP_L}{dV}$, itself depending on the applying V_o as well as on the particular segment and its physiologic state, is an index of effective "elastic wall stiffness." Since

$$dP_L = E_v \cdot \frac{dV}{V_o}, \tag{7.2}$$

a given change in volume (dV) will be associated with a greater change in lateral (transmural) pressure when the applying V_o is small than when V_o is large. This effect is moderated however, because E_v rises faster than V_o, since the elastic stiffness $\frac{dP_L}{dV}$ itself generally rises with increasing distension. If the effective successive volume strains $(\frac{dV}{V_o}'s)$ for a given volume increment, dV, did not become smaller as the applying V_o increases with advancing distension, the corresponding $dP_L's$ would be even higher than they are at larger volumes $(V_o's)$.

d. *Blood inflow vs. outflow rates.*

Lateral (P_L), and thus transmural, pressures generally change when net accumulation or loss of blood occurs at a given vascular segment. Then, the instantaneous time rate of change of intraluminal volume (V) is

$$\frac{dV}{dt} = Q_i - Q_o, \tag{7.3}$$

where Q_i and Q_o denote the simultaneous rates of flow into and out of the segment, respectively. If Q_i exceeds Q_o, $\frac{dV}{dt}$ is positive and there is net accumulation; if $\frac{dV}{dt}$ is negative, there is net blood loss from the segment.

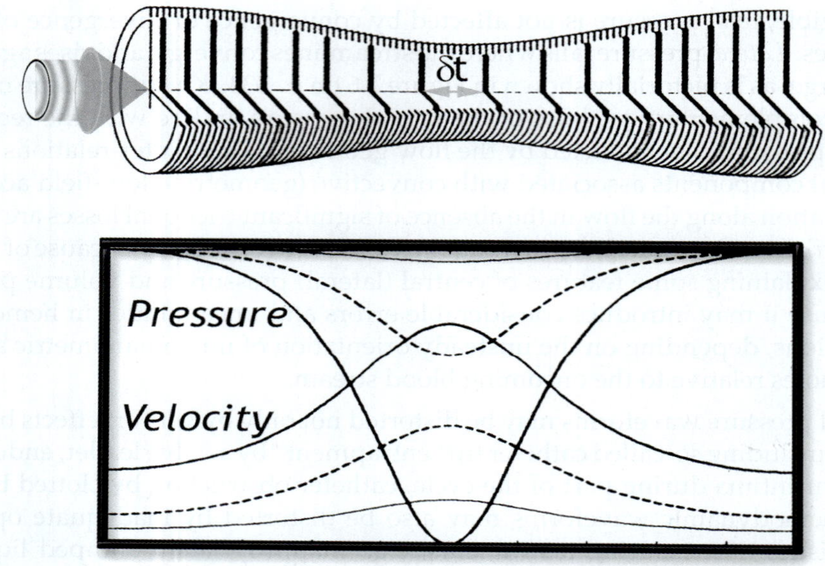

Figure 7.6: One-dimensional flow in a symmetric venturi tube. The *time lines* of the flow in the tube, every adjacent pair of which is separated by the same time interval, δt, are shown in the top panel. The distance between adjacent lines is proportional to the locally applying axial flow speeds. Pressure and velocity distributions along the axis of the venturi tube are shown in the bottom panel. The relation between velocity and pressure distribution along the tube depends strongly on the value of the inlet velocity of the tube, as illustrated, because pressure change is a quadratic function of the axial velocity change.

Generally, when $\frac{dV}{dt}$ is positive, pressure tends to rise, and *vice versa*. The simultaneous time rate of change of pressure, $\frac{dP_L}{dt}$, corresponding to an instantaneous value of $\frac{dV}{dt}$, may be estimated, if pressure *vs.* volume plots are available for the given segment under comparable operating conditions. In principle,

$$\frac{dP_L}{dt} = \frac{dV}{dt} \cdot \frac{dP_L}{dV} = (Q_i - Q_o) \cdot \frac{dP_L}{dV} \,. \tag{7.4}$$

Note that the instantaneous value of $\frac{dP_L}{dV}$ varies not only with the level of distension, but also with the physiologic state (*vide infra*) and the operating P_L and V levels.

e. *Active stress development by cardiovascular organ walls.*

Phasic cardiac action (pressure, volume and flow pulsations), and varying myocardial "contractility" exert strong shaping influences on central (intracardiac and large vessel) pressures. Under various circulatory states, active stress development by vascular smooth muscle tends to modify both mean central pressures and pulse pressure amplitudes.

7.4 Factors affecting heart filling

There are a number of factors whose intricate interplay influences venous return and blood flow into the heart.

Right atrial filling is dependent upon many interacting factors, which include:

- The **skeletal muscle pump**, which squeezes deep-vein blood orthogradely through the venous valves toward the heart, as a *vis-a-tergo*, or force from behind (see Fig. 7.7, on p. 336).
- **Respiratory pump movements**, which decrease intrathoracic and augment intraabdominal pressure, as the diaphragm descends with inspiration, helping to aspirate venous blood into the thorax. However, during a *sustained* Müller maneuver (see discussion of Fig. 7.5, on p. 332, in Section 7.3), there is an increased impedance to venous return to the right heart, which results from a *collapse* of the great systemic venous trunks at the thoracic inlets [26], confirmed by 2-D echocardiographic measurements in normal subjects. This collapse is responsible for the great augmentation of the hydrodynamic driving pressure for flow from the extrathoracic large veins to the right atrium. Viewed differently, the effort to increase the driving pressure for venous flow toward the right heart by greatly reducing the downstream (right atrial) pressure is ineffectual. Although the intensely negative intrathoracic pressure keeps the *intrathoracic* venous channels patent by maintaining a positive transmural pressure, it cannot buttress in a similar way the extrathoracic venous channels that collapse at the thoracic *inlets* [26]. The fluid dynamic difficulty in increasing flow by "suction" during the sustained Müller maneuver is akin to that experienced in attempting to suck water through a collapsible wet straw.
- **Venous tone** (state of smooth muscle contraction), which modulates venous capacitance.
- **Posture** (supine, standing upright), which brings into play intricate interactions between gravity and integrative cardiovascular reflexes.
- The **intravascular blood volume**, which interacts with the effective vascular compliance to determine the mean intravascular systemic pressure, which drives systemic venous return back to the right atrium.
- The **downward swing of the atrioventricular valve plane** toward the cardiac apex during ventricular contraction; this tends to enlarge the atria reducing intraatrial blood pressure, pulling blood from the venae cavae as a *vis-a-fronte* or force from the front (see Fig. 7.7)—the heart is a combined pressure and suction [140] pump.

Ventricular filling, in turn, is dependent upon:

- **Atrial contraction**, the atrium acting as a *booster pump* for the corresponding ventricle; passive blood flow under the action of the resulting driving pressure gradient

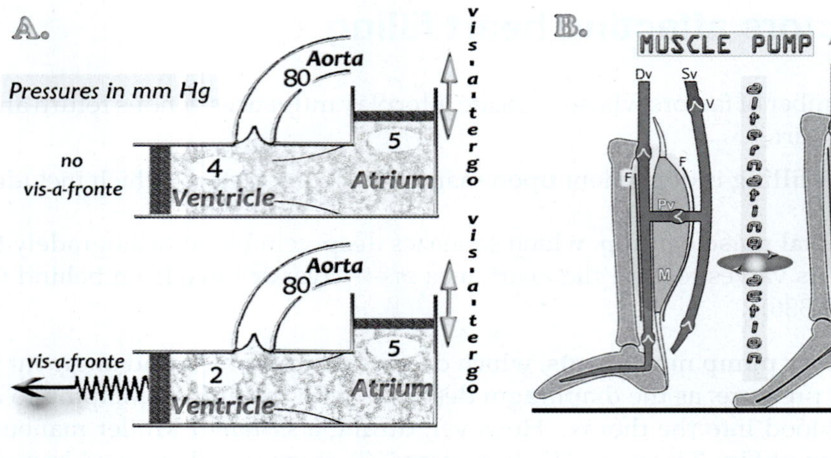

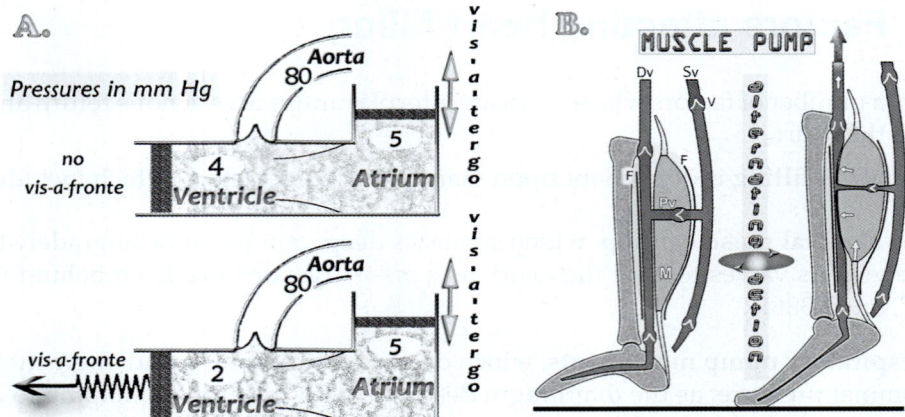

Figure 7.7: A. Physical analog illustrating the increase of the atrioventricular pressure difference by a *vis-a-fronte*, or force from the front, while maintaining a positive ventricular diastolic transmural pressure. The action of the *vis-a-tergo*, or force from behind, is straightforward. B. Action of a representative skeletal muscle pump, the calf muscle pump. The valves in small and medium-sized veins ensure that blood flow occurs in the orthograde direction only. The contractions of skeletal muscles near a vein, especially deep veins (Dv) within muscle fascial (F) compartments but to a lesser extent superficial veins (Sv) too, compress blood, helping push it toward the heart, as a *vis-a-tergo*. Blood then rushes, during relaxation, from the superficial into the deep veins via the perforating veins (Pv)—this is a *vis-a-fronte* action for blood in the superficial veins. During normal standing and walking, the *alternating cycles* of contraction and relaxation that accompany normal movements assist venous return.

and inertial venous return forces complements active ventricular relaxation, which acts to "suck" blood into the ventricles, as a *vis-a-fronte* (see Fig. 7.7).

- **Upward movement of the atrioventricular valve plane**, which assists in the translocation of blood volume from the atria into the ventricles.
- The nonlinear passive **ventricular chamber compliance**.
- The **pericardial constraint**, which acts to impede any overdistension of the cardiac chambers. The pericardium, a fibrous connective tissue sac, limits ventricular filling, as does also the high level of passive wall tension developed at high end-diastolic ventricular volumes.

The volume of the whole heart remains relatively constant throughout the cardiac cycle (see Section 7.6, on pp. 358 ff.); as the ventricles contract, eject blood into the great vessels and decrease in volume, blood is pulled into the atria increasing their volume—a *push-pull* arrangement. During ventricular relaxation the atrioventricular valve plane recoils upward, facilitating blood inflow into the ventricles from the atria, as a *vis-a-fronte* (see Fig. 7.7). Conditions which diminish ventricular compliance (concentric ventricular wall hypertrophy, myocardial infarction, cardiomyopathy, pericardial tamponade, etc.), limit ventricular filling.

7.5 Hemodynamic events of the normal cardiac cycle

The ability to examine the sequence of events responsible for cardiac pumping was enhanced by the development of the electrocardiogram to follow the electrical activity of the heart and of pressure transducers to monitor its mechanical activity. In the early 1920s, Carl Wiggers (see opening quotation to this chapter), who had spent several months in 1912 as an apprentice to Otto Frank in Munich, provided his classic rigorous descriptions of the simultaneous electrical and mechanical events of the cardiac cycle [156, 157]. Over the last three-to-four decades, advances in instrumentation, including recordings of phasic atrioventricular and semilunar transvalvular pressures and flows by multisensor catheterization, digital subtraction angiography and noninvasive cardiac imaging, have afforded us a superior understanding of the hemodynamic events of the cardiac cycle. Six or seven phases of cardiac mechanical activity may be delineated, depending on heart rate and, thus, on the total diastolic time available for ventricular filling.

The fluid dynamics of left and right ventricular filling have been studied extensively, and by diverse multidisciplinary research approaches [18, 27, 38, 53, 75–77, 85, 96, 98, 103, 105, 106, 108, 109, 145, 162]. Stimulated by such research, noninvasive imaging and Doppler echocardiography are becoming established as useful methods for assessing diastolic function [3, 30, 45, 76, 145, 162]. Information on diastolic ventricular function is based on Doppler and MRI flow velocity measurements in the ventricular inflow tract The derived parameters are very sensitive, but not at all specific. The reason is that many diverse factors, intrinsic and extrinsic to the left and right ventricles, enter in the determination of their inflow volumetric rates and velocity patterns (cf. Fig. 7.13, on p. 344).

The interplay between all these factors in determining ventricular filling is complex and quite protean,[3] reflecting constant adaptation to shifts in the operating environment. Various integrative simulation models are available and offer powerful means for interpreting this interplay and for visualizing its expression in the polymorphic Doppler patterns of mitral and tricuspid inflow [145]. Such models show how the early transmitral inflow velocity time course, in particular, may be affected by changes in ventricular compliance and relaxation properties, atrial pressure and compliance, and valvular morphology. They have provided considerable new insights on the complex interplay of these variables in shaping the diastolic filling patterns [89].

7.5.1 Semilunar valve closure and phase of isovolumic relaxation

Carl Wiggers coined the term "*proto*diastole" (Gk. *proto-*, first, hence, a combining form meaning *first in time*) to denote the earliest stage of diastole, which comes on the heels of the ejection phase, and is depicted as interval I in Figure 7.8, on p. 338. During protodiastole, the outflow valves of the cardiac ventricles get sealed completely by a transient backsurge of some reversed flow in the root of the outflow trunks, and against the almost fully apposed semilunar cusps.

[3]*Protean* is derived from Proteus, an ancient Greek god who had the ability to change his shape at will—think also of the constantly shifting form of the ameba proteus, under the microscope.

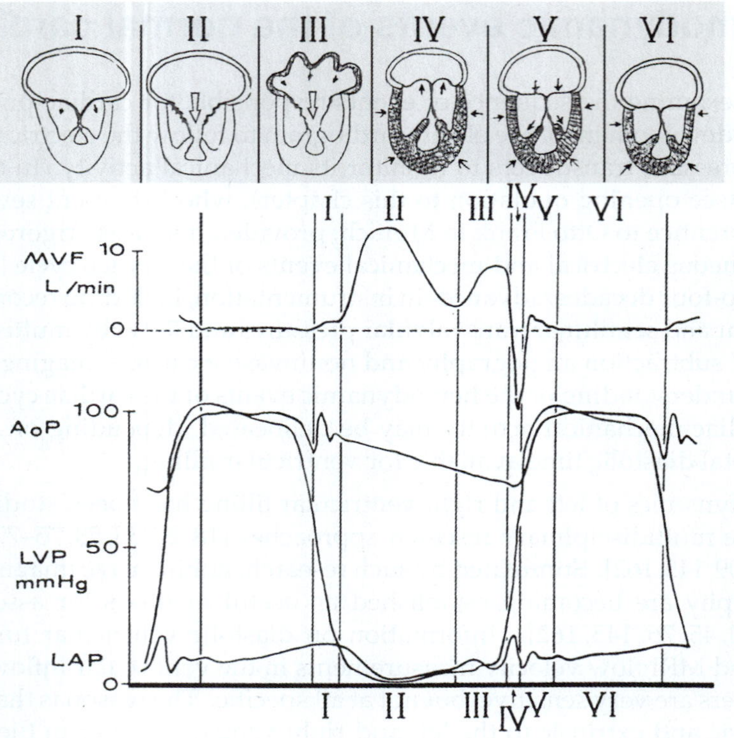

Figure 7.8: Graphic presentation of the six phases of normal mitral valve flow (MVF) in the course of the cardiac cycle, and their relationship to the left atrial (LAP), left ventricular (LVP), and aortic (AoP) pressures. (Redrawn, slightly modified, from Nolan et al. [85], with kind permission of the authors and the American Heart Journal.)

The almost fully apposed dynamic placement of the cusps by the end of the ejection phase prevents any significant leakage and a loss in pumping efficiency. Leakage loss, which would otherwise accompany valve closure by reversed flow, is normally held to less than 5% of the stroke volume (maybe less than 2–4 *mL* of blood). Part of the negative spike in flow recordings from the roots of the outflow trunks is associated with the recoil of the cusps, transiently billowing toward the ventricles, and, in the case of the aorta, to blood surging into the coronaries proximal to the flow probe.

Following semilunar valve closure, ventricular pressure falls sharply during the isovolumic relaxation phase. This phase is concluded when atrial exceeds ventricular pressure and the atrioventricular valves open. During isovolumic relaxation, as the ventricular pressure falls, the cusps of the atrioventricular, or "A–V," valve—mitral on the left, and tricuspid on the right—start to recoil toward the ventricle, and there is an apparent small flow (blood displacement) toward the ventricle. During this interval, ventricular shape changes take place. According to the elegant, sonomicrometric, conscious dog studies of Rankin et al. [119], during the initial isovolumic phase of diastole there ensues a change

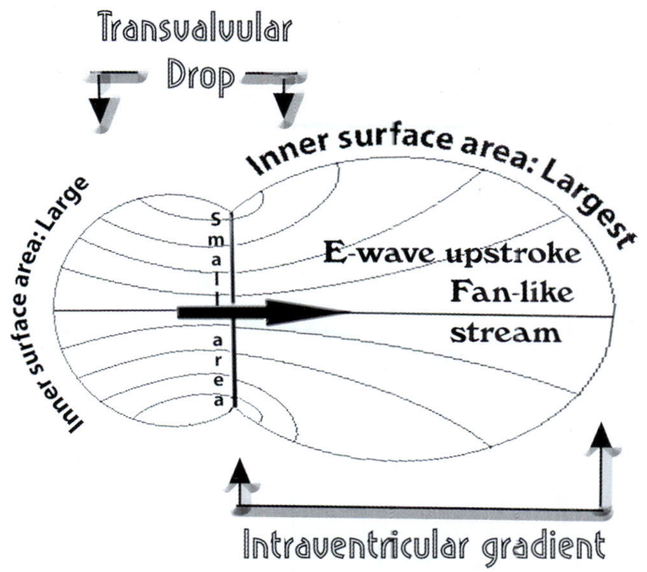

Figure 7.9: During the E-wave upstroke, flow is *confluent* between atrial endocardium and tricuspid orifice and *diffluent* between the latter and the ventricular walls. There is convective acceleration up to the orifice and convective deceleration beyond it. Therefore, atrioventricular transvalvular pressure drops embody a convective acceleration, whereas intraventricular diastolic filling gradients (which are examined in Chapter 14) embody a convective deceleration during the E-wave upstroke. (Reproduced, slightly modified, from Pasipoularides et al. [109], by kind permission of the American Physiological Society.)

in LV chamber geometry to a more spherical shape, a *sphericalization*. This shape change is opposite in direction to that observed during isovolumic contraction and has recently been confirmed by high-resolution, multiple-segment, sonomicrometric studies in sheep [41].

7.5.2 Atrioventricular valve opening and rapid ventricular filling phase

Inflow valve opening in the physical sense and the onset of rapid ventricular filling coincide well with the instant of reversal of the atrioventricular pressure difference across the atrioventricular valve cusps: blood rushes into each ventricle, which is at its end systolic volume (ESV). Early diastolic filling is rapid because of continued ventricular relaxation. During the rapid filling phase, which is depicted as interval II in Figure 7.8, on p. 338, most of the atrial blood content, which had been accumulating during the preceding four phases, is discharged passively into the ventricle. The so-called y-descent of the atrial pressure is a reflection of brisk atrial decompression with the initial outpouring of atrial blood into the ventricle (see Fig. 7.10, on p. 340).

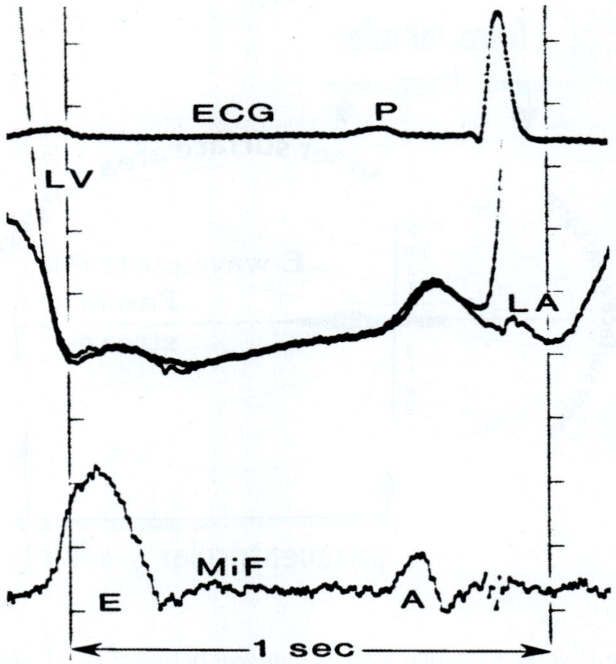

Figure 7.10: Transmitral pressure–flow relationships throughout diastolic filling in a human subject, obtained using multisensor catheters during diagnostic cardiac catheterization. Mitral inflow acceleration is associated with a positive atrioventricular pressure gradient and deceleration with an adverse gradient. E and A, early filling and atrial waves on mitral inflow velocity signal, MiF; LV and LA, left ventricular and atrial pressures. (Reproduced from Mirsky and Pasipoularides [76], by kind permission of the W.B. Saunders Company, a division of Elsevier.)

It is seen, on careful examination of the pressure tracings in Figure 7.8, on p. 338, that the measured A–V pressure difference does not reverse until well into the downstroke of the rapid filling phase wave ("*E*-wave") of the mitral inflow rate recording. This is attributable, primarily, to the *exact placement* of the pressure measurement sites within the atrioventricular flow field (cf. Fig. 7.9); secondarily, to technical problems related to the presence of the circular mitral electromagnetic flow transducer, which causes a mild degree of "mitral stenosis," and to the external strain-gauge manometer methodology that was available to Nolan and his collaborators at the time of these pioneering measurements.

Figure 7.10 exhibits normal dynamic measurement patterns; it was obtained at cardiac catheterization for the evaluation of chest pain on a patient who was found to have normal ventricular function, using a left-heart multisensor Millar catheter. Figure 7.10 demonstrates that at around the time of the peak of the *E*-wave in the rapid filling phase, there occurs the *reversal* of the measured A–V pressure gradient. The now *adverse* transmitral pressure gradient is responsible for the ensuing deceleration of the early filling *E*-wave. The important topic of the relationship between A–V *transvalvular* and *intraventricular* pressure gradients is examined in detail in Chapter 14.

During the 1970s, studies of diastolic mechanics assessed *passive* mechanical properties of the fully relaxed left ventricle (i.e., chamber volume, wall mass and composition), physical *constraints* extrinsic to it (i.e., the *pericardium* and the other cardiac chambers within it), and the dynamics of isovolumetric ventricular *relaxation*, an active myocardial process [39,74]. It had been well known, since the classic studies of Carl Wiggers[4] on the cardiac cycle in the 1920s, that during the early rapid filling phase (i.e., from atrioventricular valve opening to minimum diastolic pressure) ventricular chamber dimensions are *increasing* while the transmural distending pressure is *declining* [158]. Thus, the processes going on during this early period are neither purely passive nor purely active. This led me by 1980 [97] to postulate that total measured left ventricular diastolic pressure (P_M) is determined by two overlapping processes, namely,

a. the *myocardial relaxation*-induced decay of actively developed pressure, (P_R); and,

b. the concurrent *buildup* of passive filling pressure (P^*), as shown in Figure 7.11,

and to develop a comprehensive mathematical model for diastolic dynamics [98]. Further application of this model has allowed detailed evaluations of the role of active and passive dynamic factors in diastolic ventricular mechanics in health and disease [36,76,87,96,98, 105,106,110].

At normal or abnormally low heart rates, the rapid ventricular filling phase evolves into the slow filling phase; at high normal or abnormally fast rates, it *merges* with the active filling that is caused by atrial systole (see Fig. 7.12, on p. 343).

7.5.3 Phase of slow ventricular filling

The rapid filling phase may be followed by a slower phase, which is denoted as "diastasis." During the period of diastasis, atrial and ventricular pressures remain essentially equal while no or little inflow is taking place. This is the least stable event in the cycle, as is represented pictorially in Figure 7.12, on p. 343. It is present at extraordinarily low normal or abnormally slow heart rates; cf. the top two panels in Figure 7.12. The use of the term *diastasis* to denote a marked reduction in ventricular inflow rate may need some reappraisal in view of this Figure's vituline data, since at rates higher than 80/*min*, slow filling is phased out completely—at 80/*min*, the volumetric inflow rate does not fall below, say, 7,000 *mL/min* at any time during "slow" filling. At 50 *beats/min*, it may fall below 2,000 *mL/min*, which might correspond to linear velocities of around 5 *cm/s*, or less.

[4]As noted on p. 337, Wiggers who studied under Otto Frank is credited with formulating the details of the cardiac cycle; Frank had perfected optical manometers and capsules for precise measurement of intracardiac pressures and volumes.

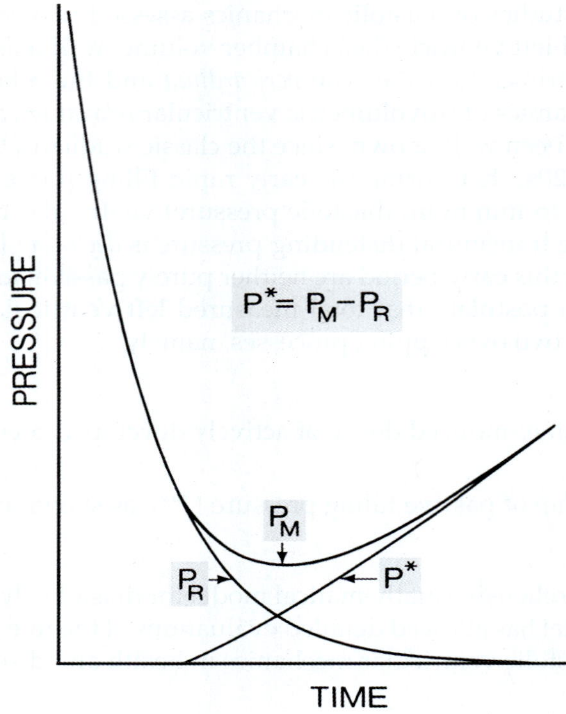

Figure 7.11: Schematic representation of the instantaneous diastolic left ventricular measured pressure (P_M) as the sum of the decaying relaxation pressure (P_R) and the increasing passive filling pressure (P^*), after Pasipoularides. (Reproduced, slightly modified, from Pasipoularides et al. [98], by kind permission of the American Heart Association.)

7.5.4 Phase of atrial systole

Toward the end of the filling phase, atrial contraction creates anew an accelerating transmitral pressure gradient, and is responsible for suddenly *reaccelerating* atrial blood onward, augmenting atrioventricular valve flow and producing the late-filling atrial wave (A-wave) in diastolic inflow recordings (Figs. 7.8 and 7.10). At higher heart rates, when no period of diastasis is observed, the E and A waves may merge to a greater or lesser extent [85]. This atrial action, which is depicted as interval IV in Figure 7.8, "tops-off" the end-diastolic intraventricular volume (EDV) and pressure (EDP) by the so-called "atrial kick." Since there are no competent valves at the atrial inflow sites, the transient rise in atrial pressure causes flow deceleration or even a transient flow *reversal* in the central veins. The latter effects are manifested with variable intensity, depending primarily on:

i. the magnitude of central vein flow and, thus, on its momentum and the applying inertial forces;

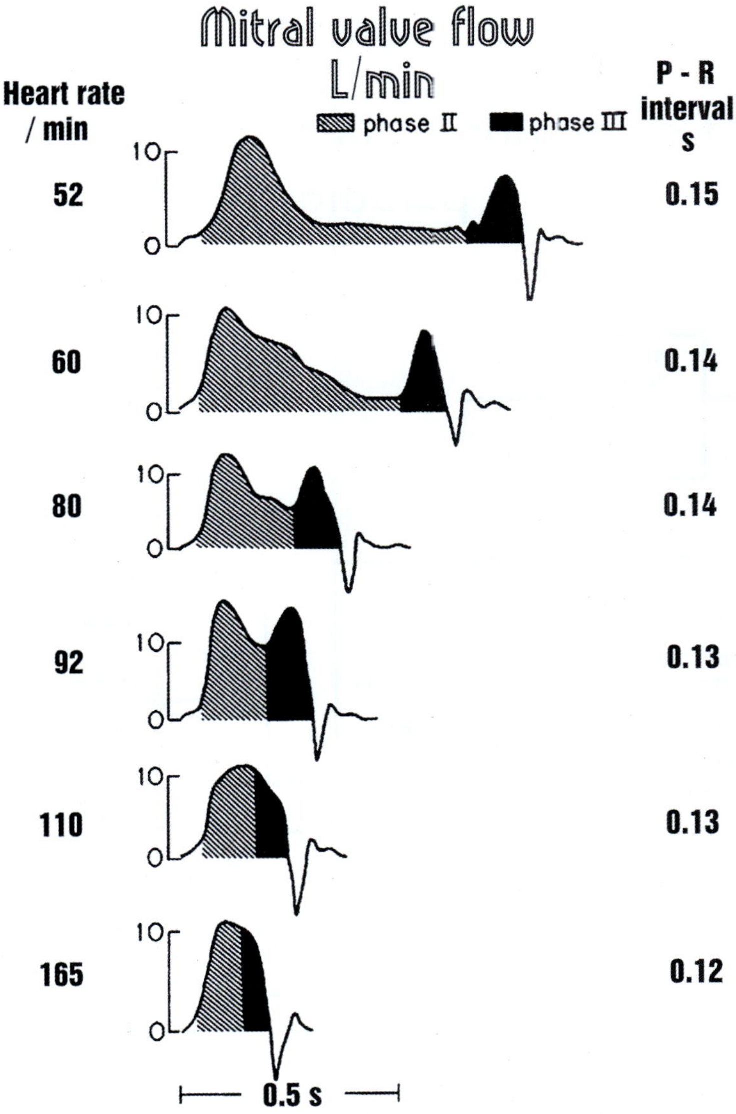

Figure 7.12: Effect of heart rate on mitral valve flow. Representative experimental transmitral flow signals throughout diastolic filling are shown in an anesthetized, open-chest calf, obtained via a nonobstructing electromagnetic flow transducer sutured to the atrial wall at the mitral anulus. Mitral valve flow is shown at six different heart rates from 52 to 165 *beats/min*. The P–R intervals are normal for each heart rate. The area enclosed by Phase II flow is crosshatched, while the area under Phase III flow is solid—cf. Fig. 7.8. At heart rates exceeding 92 *beats/min* there is no secondary reacceleration of flow into a distinct atrial *A*-wave during Phase III. (Slightly modified from Nolan et al. [85], by kind permission of Mosby Company, a division of Elsevier.)

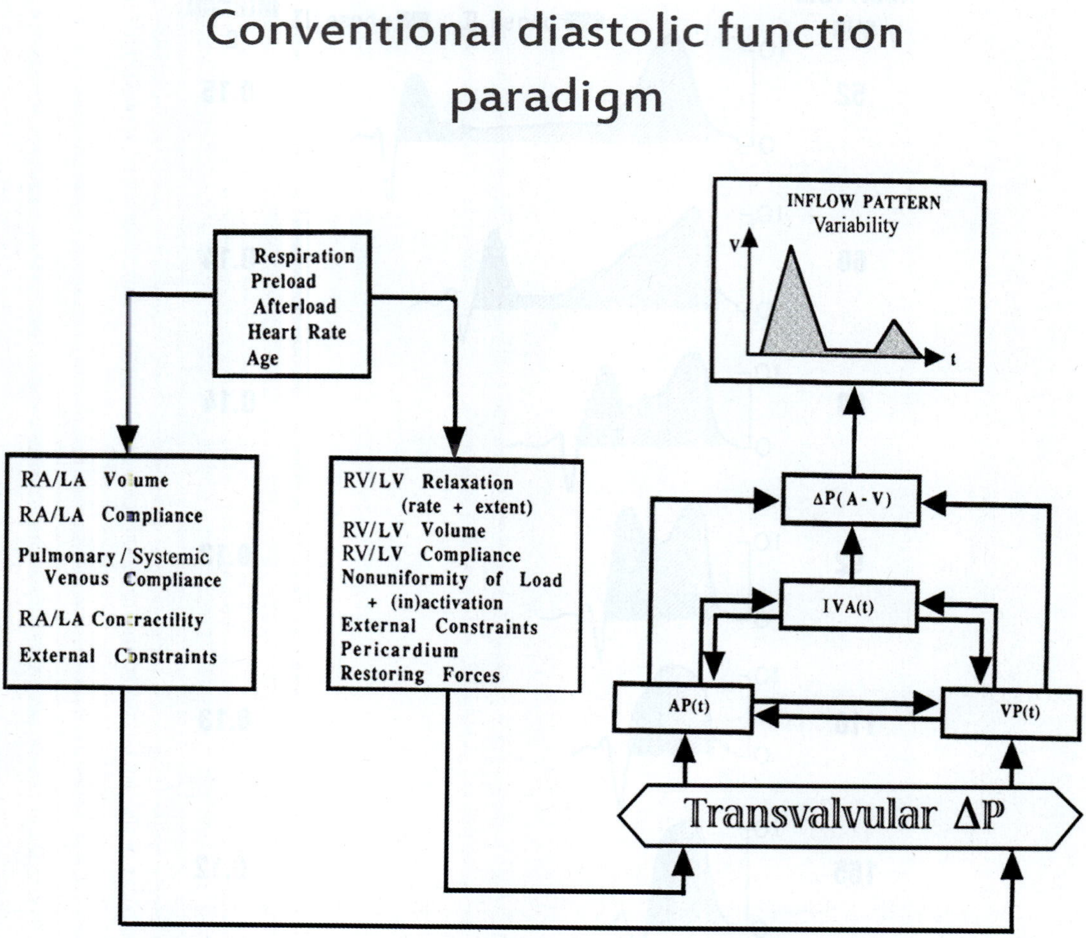

Figure 7.13: The determinants of ventricular inflow patterns and diastolic filling include factors intrinsic and extrinsic to the ventricle. A = atrial; V = ventricular; IVA = inflow valve area; P = pressure; ΔP = pressure difference, or "gradient"; t = time. (Redrawn, slightly modified, from Pasipoularides [89], by kind permission of the Biomedical Engineering Society and Springer.) The new diastolic function paradigm, which is depicted in Figure 14.27, on p. 796, complements and acts in parallel with the traditional one, which is shown here.

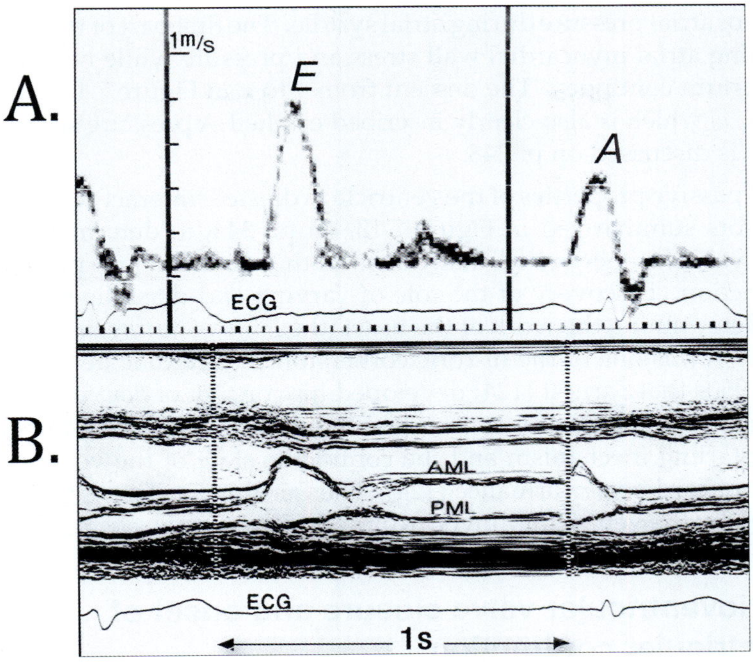

Figure 7.14: Pulsed-wave Doppler recording (A.) and M-mode echocardiogram (B.) from a normal human subject. The recordings have an identical cycle length and are synchronized by the ECG signals. They demonstrate normal relationships of transmitral flow velocity and mitral valve motion; the tracings were not adjusted for an expected 10–20 ms electronic circuitry delay in the Doppler display. Early transmitral flow rapidly accelerates to a peak (E) at 0.8 m/s, which exceeds the velocity peak of atrial contraction (A). Echocardiographic anterior (AML) and posterior (PML) mitral leaflet motion mirrors changes in mitral inflow, with minimal leaflet motion during diastasis when mitral inflow is low. The rapid deceleration of early mitral flow, brisk E–F slope of valve motion, and large Doppler E/A wave ratio reflect normal LV filling. Vertical lines are separated by one second. (Reproduced from Mirsky and Pasipoularides [76], by kind permission of the W.B. Saunders Company, a division of Elsevier.)

ii. the effective compliance of venous segments in the immediate proximity of the right and the left atrium and, thus, on the ability of such venous segments to transiently accommodate blood regurgitating from the atria; and,

iii. on body posture, and the applying gravitational effects.

Normal atrial pressure curves exhibit two primary positive humps, a- and v-waves, and two interposed troughs, the negative x- and y-waves (see Fig. 7.18, on p. 352). As atrioventricular flow gets decelerated following the peak of the E-wave, atrial pressure rebounds and rises toward the foot of the a-wave with continuing (pulmonary, or systemic) venous return. The transition to the more prominent ascent to the peak of the a-wave is due to active stress developed by the atrial myocardium and the resulting augmentation of atrial pressure during atrial systole. The first part of the ensuing x-descent reflects declining atrial myocardial wall stress and pressure while net loss of blood from the relaxing atrium continues. The descent from a to x in Figure 7.18 is interrupted by a transient peak, c, which is also clearly inscribed on the LA pressure signal in Figure 7.10, on p. 340, and is discussed on p. 348.

Active and passive properties of the ventricle in diastole interact with its venous return, and other factors summarized in Figure 7.13, on p. 344, to determine its end-diastolic pressure and volume, the *preload* that distends the chamber just prior to the onset of systolic contraction. Discovery of the role of varying end-diastolic volume, *heterometric regulation*, in determining the work of the heart (the *Frank–Starling mechanism* or *Starling's law of the heart* [12]) is one of the historic cornerstones of cardiac hemodynamics. It was not until the 1950s that Sarnoff [124] developed his concept of *homeometric regulation* and a "family of Starling curves," over the same range of EDV, which integrated the roles of the Frank–Starling mechanism and the contractile state of the ventricle as two major determinants[5] of cardiac performance [124]. The third major determinant is the *afterload*, the load driven by the ventricular myocardium during systolic ejection.

7.5.5 Atrioventricular valve closure and onset of ventricular contraction

Closure of the atrioventricular valves defines the onset of the "true" isovolumic contraction time (ICT) and opening of the semilunar valves its termination. In normal hearts, the *A–V* valves attain most of their closure before the onset of ventricular contraction; this is the result of two actions:

i. the *thrust* of the intraventricular diastolic vortex,[6] swirling between them and the chamber walls, on the mural side of the valve leaflets; and

ii. the sharp ventricular inflow deceleration following the peak of the atrial A-wave, with the associated *pressure gradient reversal* along the inflow tract.

The inertia of the inflowing stream causes persistence of forward flow for several *ms* after the reversal of the micromanometrically recorded high-fidelity pressure gradient between the atrium and the ventricle. Shortly after the initiation of the electric depolarization of the ventricular myocardium, identified by the Q-wave of the electrocardiogram, the ventricular walls begin to contract, actively increasing the intraventricular pressure and closing the inlet valves. Because of the two preceding reasons, there is normally no loss of pumping efficiency, as the case would be if A–V valve closure depended solely on actual inflow *reversal* effected by the ensuing ventricular myocardial contraction.

[5]Indeed, according to current concepts, length-dependent force changes (Frank–Starling) and inotropic alterations (Sarnoff homeometric autoregulation) of contractile performance may have the same or related underlying mechanisms. In both cases, the increase in contractile force may be due to an increased extent of calcium activation of the contractile elements. It is important to appreciate, in this context, that the contractile force of the ventricle can be modulated not only by altering the free calcium ion concentration in the myoplasm, but also by altering the *responsiveness* of the myofilaments to calcium [71].

[6]The formation and possible functions of the intraventricular diastolic vortex are considered at length in Chapter 14.

7.5.6 Phase of isovolumic contraction and semilunar valve opening

With the onset of ventricular contraction the adverse transmitral gradient decelerates the A-wave to zero. Zero flow is virtually synchronous with atrioventricular valve closure (see Fig. 7.14, on p. 345). Isovolumic contraction normally proceeds without change in the actual intraventricular blood volume since both inflow and outflow routes are cut off; this isovolumic phase is depicted as interval IV in Figure 7.8, on p. 338. The isovolumic process does not preclude changes in the *shape* of the ventricular cavities and their boundaries—the inflow and outflow valve leaflets, and the ventricular walls. Actually, physiologic asynchronous contraction while activation is still spreading during the isovolumic contraction time (ICT), with different LV regions acting as either contractile or *in-series* elastic elements, leads to interesting flow and pressure transients [115, 127, 139, 159].

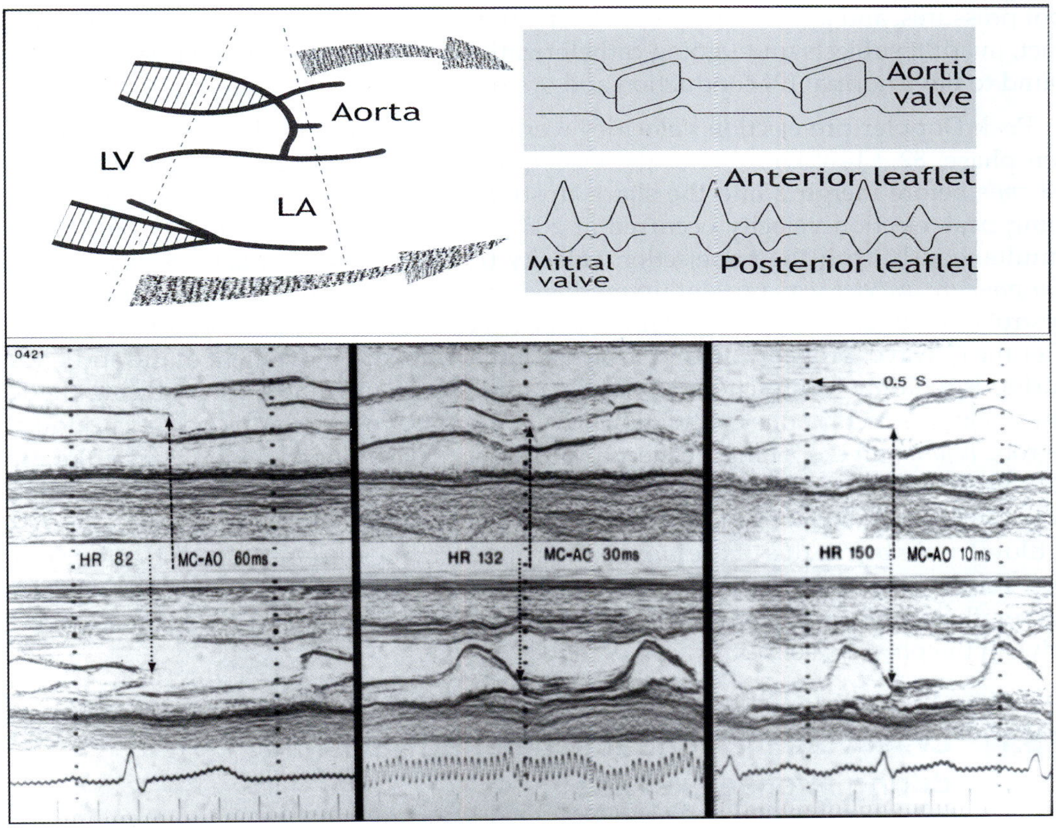

Figure 7.15: Parasternal long axis view with dual M-Mode simultaneously visualizing the movement of the mitral and aortic valve leaflets, as diagramed in the top panel; particular attention was given to imaging *mitral closure* (MC) and *aortic opening* (AO), identified by dotted line arrows in the lower panels. The duration of the *true* LV isovolumic contraction time is gradually curtailed during progressively stronger exercise, gauged by heart rate (HR). (From Pasipoularides et al. [99].)

As pressure builds up in the ventricle, the closed mitral leaflets are displaced toward the atrium and this may be recorded by the flowmeter as a backflow *spike.* This apparent flow reversal (toward the atrium) (see Fig. 7.8, on p. 338) is attributable to the billowing of the apposed valve cusps into the atrium. The bulging of the A–V valve cusps into the atrium as ventricular pressure rises during isovolumic contraction is also responsible for the transient interruption of the x-descent by the sharp c-peak in the atrial pressure signal (see Figs. 7.8, 7.10, and 7.18, on pp. 338, 340, and 352, respectively); since the atrially displaced blood is trapped beneath the A–V valve cusps, this is not a true regurgitation.

Blood displacement into the roots of the outflow trunks starts with the semilunar valve cusp edges still more or less apposed (see Fig. 7.33, on p. 384). A polymorphic "isovolumic contraction wavelet" marks the ICT on the micromanometric aortic root pre-ejection pressure signal, as is demonstrated in Figure 7.18, on p. 352. We investigated these ICT phenomena [99] by analyzing simultaneous ECG, micromanometric LV and aortic root pressures, and pulsed-Doppler velocity measurements obtained from the LV outflow tract, in adult subjects undergoing catheterization for evaluation of chest pain, who were found to have normal LV conduction and systolic function.

Peak Doppler pre-ejection velocities were found to occur in the isovolumic contraction phase, 82 $\pm$14 (SD) *ms* after the ECG Q-wave; they attained maximal values of 31 $\pm$8 *cm/s* before merging into the sharp upstroke of the main ejection velocity. The ensuing peak ejection velocity occurred at 203 $\pm$22 *ms* and reached 89 $\pm$ 19 *cm/s*. Nearly simultaneously with the pre-ejection velocity (r: -0.90), the distinct *isovolumic contraction pressure wavelet* was present, immediately preceding the onset of the aortic pressure upstroke, in all cases in the micromanometric aortic root signal. It occurred 80 $\pm$13 *ms* after the Q-wave, probably arising from the initial outward movement of the aortic valve during isovolumic contraction, just before aortic valve opening. Thus, during the ICT, physiologic asynchronous contraction accelerates intraventricular blood toward the aortic root *before* valve opening in the physical sense. This phenomenon assists the rapid outflow acceleration of early ejection. Intraventricular pressure, rising rapidly during isovolumic contraction, must exceed slightly the end-diastolic pressure in the roots of the outflow trunks before this phase is over. This upstream pressure *excess* provides the driving force for the acceleration of the effective arterial blood columns,[7] which initially displaces the semilunar cusps forward and then effects their separation and the "opening" of the valve in the physical sense.

7.5.7 LV isovolumic contraction period vanishes during intense exercise

As early as 1912, Henderson and Johnson used physical models to examine the dynamics of mitral valve closure and deduced that "if the flow of fluid through a model valve ceases rather abruptly, the inertia of the moving fluid carries it onward, leaving a wake of

[7] The effective length of the intraluminal blood columns that need to be accelerated and displaced distally along the outflow arterial trunk axis depends on the time-dependent interplay of arterial trunk inductance (longitudinal impedance) and capacitance (transverse impedance) functions [128, 129].

negative pressure which could close the valve with no regurgitation whatever" [46]. Support for this conclusion in animal experiments was provided by Nolan et al. [85], who pioneered the use of the electromagnetic flowmeter to the *in vivo* measurement of transmitral flow. These early investigators concluded that, following the atrial contraction, the momentum of transmitral flow required a reversed pressure gradient for deceleration. Studies from Yellin's laboratory on open-chest dogs gave similar results [63, 162]. They showed that mitral closure in instrumented, anesthetized, open-chest dogs is not simultaneous with the crossover of LV–LA pressures at the onset of LV contraction but actually follows it by approximately 50 *ms*. This delay is generally accepted to be the result of the inertia of blood traversing the mitral valve in late diastole.

These studies were concerned with closure of the mitral valve following atrial systole and deceleration of left ventricular inflow. They do, however, raise some interesting questions regarding the conventional subdivisions of the cardiac cycle, at least under conditions of vigorous physical activity or exercise. In particular, could the left ventricular isovolumic contraction period vanish altogether during intense exercise? We examined this question in the late 1980s [99]. As the intensity of exercise increases, several things progressively occur:

- the heart rate rises, causing a shortening of the diastolic filling time,
- the stroke volume rises slightly, and
- left ventricular contractility rises.

The first two of these changes should combine to yield an increase in the momentum of blood flowing into the left ventricle in late diastole, with a resultant increase in the delay between the timing of the atrioventricular pressure crossover and the actual mitral closure. Moreover, the *preejection period*, the time from the ORS complex of the ECG to aortic valve opening, is known to decrease during exercise, as a consequence of the augmented adrenergic activation and myocardial contractility. During exercise, these two effects should act in concert to *squeeze* the isovolumic contraction period.

This idea suggested to us that the *true isovolumic contraction time* ("true ICT," the time from *mitral valve closure* to *aortic valve opening*) [8] should shorten considerably during exercise. In severe exercise, the cumulative force (or *impulse*, see Section 4.2.1, on p. 171) required to close the mitral valve might become so great that the left ventricular pressure could exceed aortic root diastolic pressure prior to mitral valve closure. This would result in aortic valve opening prior to mitral valve closure, thus eliminating the true isovolumic contraction period.

We studied nine normal volunteer subjects (8 male, 1 female; ages 16–35), who were subjected to basal measurements followed by progressive semi-recumbent bicycle ergometer exercise to maximum exertion [99]. During exercise dual simultaneous M-mode echocardiography was performed of the mitral and aortic valves, directed by 2-D echocardiography in the parasternal long axis. M-mode signals were recorded on a strip chart

[8] This "true ICT" interval is to be distinguished from the conventional definition of ICT, which extends from the crossover of A–V *pressures* to the crossover of the LV and aortic *pressures*.

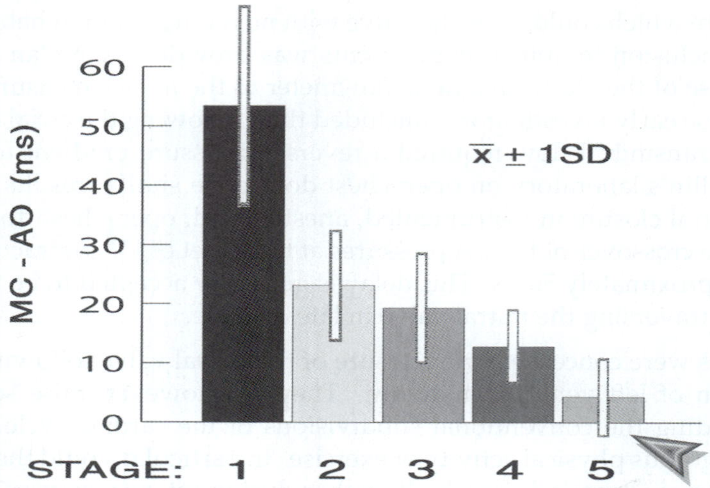

Figure 7.16: The *true* LV isovolumic contraction time is curtailed with progressively more vigorous exercise, and vanishes at heart rates around 175 *beats/min*. Stage 1 corresponds to rest (R–R interval: 0.867 ±0.137 *s*), Stage 5 to strenuous exercise (R–R interval: 0.365 ±0.026 *s*). In some cases at high exercise heart rates, negative MC–AO intervals ensue—highlighted by the arrowhead (see an example in Fig. 7.17, on p. 351). (From Pasipoularides et al. [99].)

recorder at 100 *mm/s* paper speed during progressive levels of exercise, at workloads designed to produce heart rates of 100, 125, 150, and 175 *beats/min*. Particular attention was given to imaging mitral closure and aortic opening (see Fig. 7.15, on p. 347). Imaging of Doppler LV inflow from the apical four-chamber view was also performed at each stage. The records were analyzed manually and beats were selected on the basis of having both mitral valve closure and aortic valve opening clearly identifiable, as in Figure 7.15. A minimum of 50 interpretable *beats* was obtained on each subject at each stage.

The top panel of Figure 7.15 illustrates the dual simultaneous M-mode echocardiography imaging method that we used, and the bottom shows representative strip chart tracings. These tracings demonstrate an example of the rapid curtailment of the true ICT, which comes about with progressively more strenuous exercise. Figure 7.16 summarizes the results obtained in our nine normal volunteers. An illustrative example of a total elimination of the true ICT with opening of the aortic valve occurring about 20 *ms* prior to mitral valve closure is provided in Figure 7.17, on p. 351.

7.5.8 Phase of ventricular ejection

With the onset of ventricular ejection, a sharp increase in pressure is produced in the great vessels (aorta and pulmonary artery). Accordingly, this phase, which extends over intervals V and VI in Figure 7.8, on p. 338, may be taken to start with the onset of the major systolic upstroke *(anacrotic swing)* of the pressure pulse from the root of the ventricular

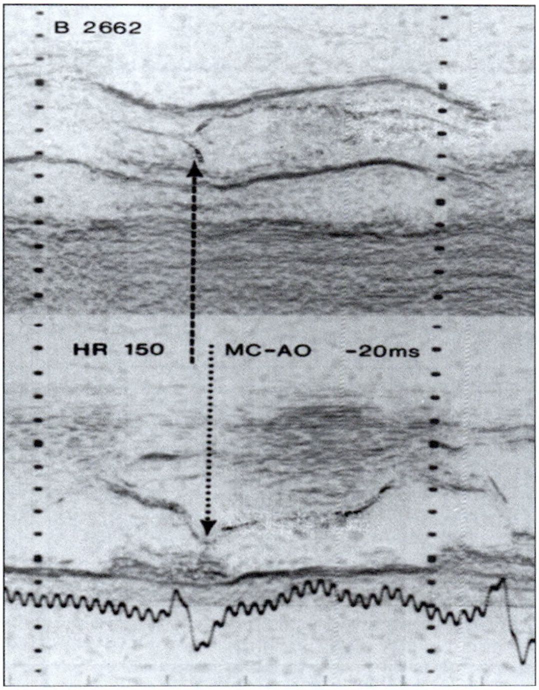

Figure 7.17: Parasternal long axis view with dual M-Mode simultaneously visualizing the movement of the mitral and aortic leaflets (cf. Fig. 7.15); particular attention was given to imaging *mitral closure* and *aortic opening*. In severe exercise, the cumulative force, or *impulse* required to close the mitral valve, is so great that the LV pressure can exceed aortic root end diastolic pressure prior to mitral valve closure. This results in the aortic valve opening ahead of mitral closure, eliminating the true ICT, as is demonstrated here. (From Pasipoularides et al. [99].)

outflow trunks. During the initial part of ejection there is a small apparent forward flow at the atrioventricular valve; it is associated with papillary muscle shortening, which pulls the shut atrioventricular valve cusps toward the ventricle.

The ongoing x-descent in the left atrial pressure tracing (see Fig. 7.18, and Fig. 7.22, on p. 359) continues for as long as blood accumulation into the atrial chamber cannot counteract the tendency of pressure to fall, because papillary muscle shortening is now pulling the mitral valve cusps and the anulus plane downward into the ventricle, effectively reducing the passive stress on the relaxed atrial walls. Continuing blood accumulation into the atrium accounts for most of the ensuing ascent toward the peak of the so-called v-wave in the atrial pressure tracings (see Fig. 7.18). The culmination of the v-wave in left atrial pressure is associated not only with maintained blood inflow, but also with the rebound of the mitral valve cusps and the reascension of the A–V valve-anulus plane during the ensuing isovolumic ventricular relaxation.

Peak systolic pressures may be reached in the latter part of the ejection phase, because of pulse wave reflections that get superimposed on the primary pressure wave generated

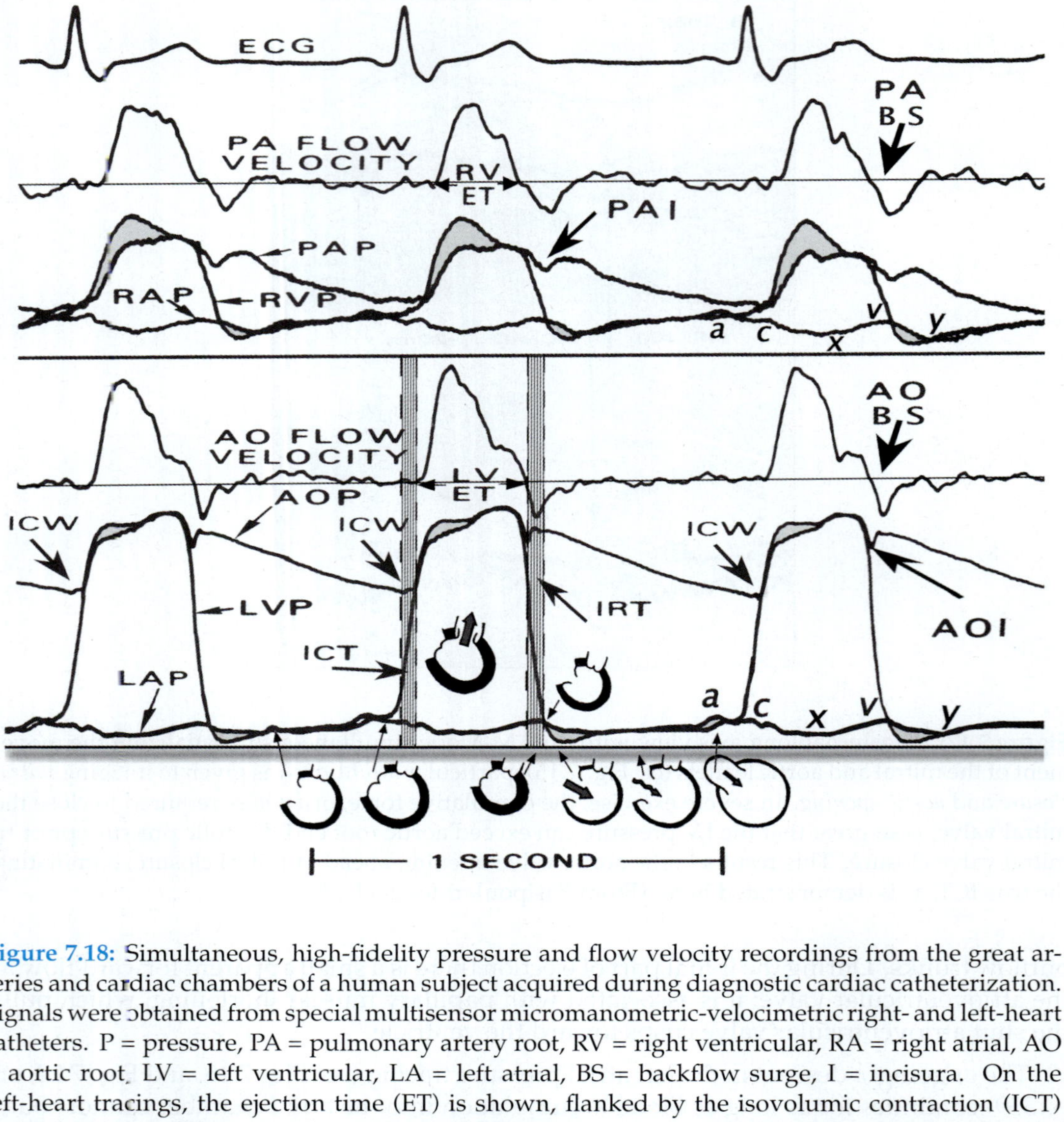

Figure 7.18: Simultaneous, high-fidelity pressure and flow velocity recordings from the great arteries and cardiac chambers of a human subject acquired during diagnostic cardiac catheterization. Signals were obtained from special multisensor micromanometric-velocimetric right- and left-heart catheters. P = pressure, PA = pulmonary artery root, RV = right ventricular, RA = right atrial, AO = aortic root, LV = left ventricular, LA = left atrial, BS = backflow surge, I = incisura. On the left-heart tracings, the ejection time (ET) is shown, flanked by the isovolumic contraction (ICT) and relaxation (IRT) times. The polymorphic "isovolumic contraction wavelet" (ICW) marks the ICT on the micromanometric AOP signal. The *a*, *c*, *x*, *v*, and *y* waves on the RAP and LAP signals are discussed in the text.

at the root of the aorta [126, 128].[9] In late ejection, ventricular pressure falls below that in the outflow trunk, outflow stops a short time thereafter, and the semilunar valves close.

[9] The pressure waveform that is recorded at any site of an arterial tree, and in the corresponding ventricular chamber during ejection, is the sum of a forward traveling waveform, which is the waveform generated by ventricular ejection, and a backward traveling waveform, which is the "echo" of the incident pressure wave reflected at multiple, more or less remote, peripheral sites.

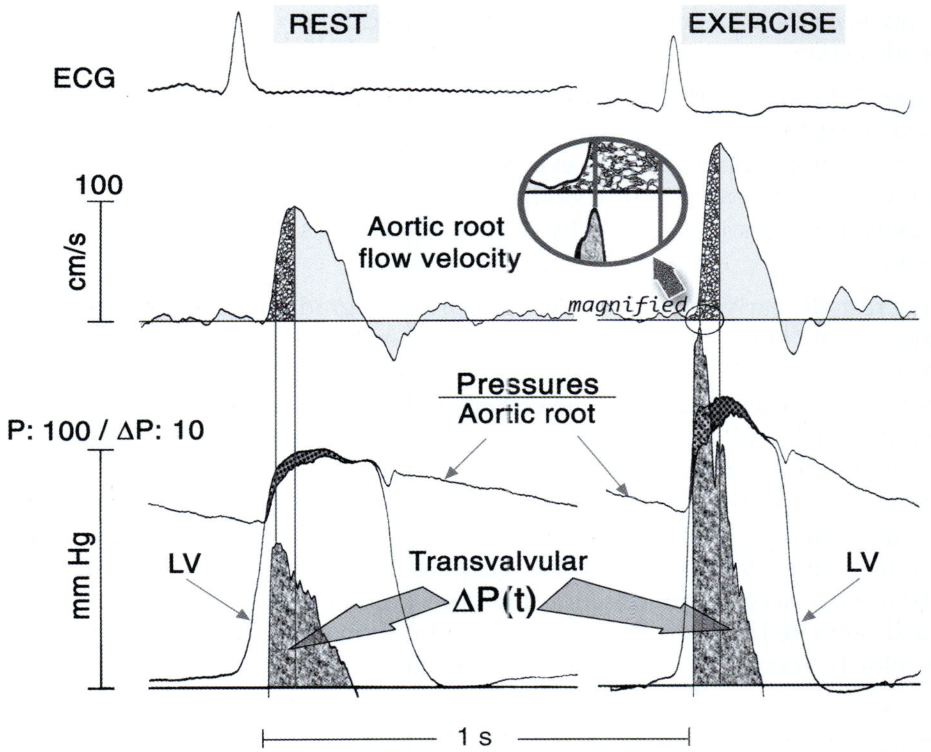

Figure 7.19: Representative left ventricular (LV) fluid dynamics at rest and during supine bicycle exercise in man via double pressure/velocity microsensor catheter: LV and aortic root pressures are displayed at the bottom, with their electronically derived instantaneous difference (ΔP) during the early systolic time interval that LV exceeds aortic root pressure on a blown-up scale. The associated LV outflow linear velocity signal from just beyond the aortic ring is shown in the middle panel and the electrocardiogram (ECG) at the top. Note the impulsive early systolic development of the driving pressure gradient and outflow velocity, which are strongly augmented during exercise, when the peak gradient is attained very near the foot of the velocity signal ("magnifying lense" inset).

As was discussed in Section 7.5.1, on pp. 337 ff., during protodiastole the outflow valves of the cardiac ventricles get sealed completely by a transient backsurge of some reversed flow in the root of the outflow trunks, and against the almost fully apposed semilunar leaflets; this is demonstrated in Figure 7.18, on p. 352. The end of the ejection phase is signaled by the zero-flow (baseline) crossing by the flow signals recorded at the roots of the outflow trunks. In absence of such flow signals, it is taken by convention to coincide with the *incisura* in the pressure tracings from the roots of the great vessels (see Figs. 7.18 and 7.19). This practise invariably overestimates the true ejection time, which can nevertheless be correctly measured noninvasively using velocity signals from the ventricular outflow tracts or the roots of the outflow trunks, as can nowadays be readily done using Doppler ultrasound.

In Figure 7.19, simultaneous left-sided pressure and outflow velocity signals, obtained with a left-heart Millar *Mikro-tip*® multisensor catheter, are demonstrated at rest and during submaximal supine bicycle exercise.[10] Peak early systolic accelerating pressure gradients occur very early in left ventricular systole. Aortic root flow velocity peaks shortly thereafter; this is followed by a more declivitous decline of the velocity to the zero baseline.

During rest, the early systolic accelerating pressure gradient normally remains positive for approximately 80% of the true left ventricular ejection time—i.e., the duration of the positive outflow velocity signal. Flow velocity returns to its zero baseline *after* the reversal of the pressure gradient but *before* the dicrotic notch in the aortic root pressure, which is the conventional delimiter of "end-ejection." With submaximal exercise, however, normal subjects must deliver approximately the same, or a slightly increased stroke volume, in a shorter systolic ejection time. Thus, the applying outflow acceleration (slope of the velocity–time curve) levels are higher and the return to the zero-flow baseline occurs relatively later in systole, as compared with the resting state. In addition, the peak of the transvalvular accelerating ejection pressure gradient is strikingly increased and its duration abbreviated in exercise, whereas the duration of the forward-flow phase of the ejection velocity waveform at the aortic root is lengthened.

These physical characteristics of the transvalvular ejection flow are best analyzed by considering the equation of motion (see Section 4.4.3, on pp. 177 ff., and Section 4.5, on pp. 187 ff.). It governs the pressure–flow relations across the tapering flow region, encompassing the outflow tract and valve, interposed between the main ventricular chamber and the root of the outflow trunk. By the unsteady Bernoulli equation for the instantaneous pressure gradient (cf. Equation 4.13, on p. 187), the instantaneous transvalvular ejection pressure differences comprise two inertial components, which are associated with local and convective acceleration forces. These pressure differences, or "gradients," measured during ejection go into overcoming blood's inertia to *local* and *convective* accelerations, imparted on it in the course of ejection. Viscous losses make only a nominal contribution to pressure gradients within the ejecting chamber and in the aortic root beyond a normal valve, in contrast to what happens beyond a stenotic valve, where viscous dissipation effects become important. In the normal heart, viscous influences are confined to a very thin boundary layer close to the wall of the outflow tract and trunk; the main stream within the collapsing chamber is effectively inviscid, as is the ascending aortic flow [88].

The convective and local acceleration components, when combined, give the total acceleration imparted on blood moving in the unsteady, nonuniform, velocity field between the micromanometric sensors. In a pulsatile velocity field local inertial effects are always present, irrespective of whether field taper also introduces convective acceleration components (for convective effects associated with *collapsing walls* in absence of taper, see discussion on pp. 65 f., of Section 2.13). The presence of the local inertial effects, which

[10] These signals were obtained during diagnostic catheterization for evaluation of atypical chest pain in an informed human subject, who was found to have no cardiovascular abnormality.

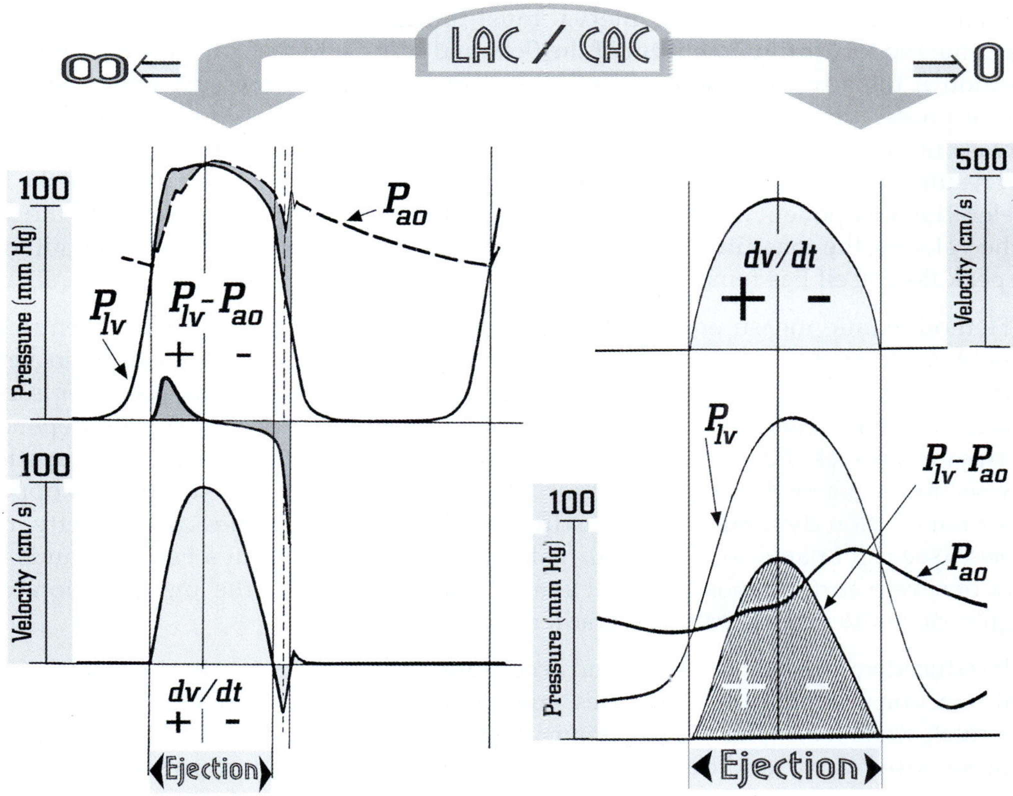

Figure 7.20: The paradigmatic relationships between the instantaneous transvalvular pressures, the corresponding pressure differences (the so-called "gradients"), and the ejection velocity waveforms under conditions of an exteme predominence of either the *local* acceleration component ("LAC," left panels) or the *convective* acceleration component ("CAC," right panels) of the total measured transvalvular pressure drop.

depend on the applying instantaneous time-rate of change—$\partial v / \partial t$—of the velocity, rather than on the magnitude itself of the applying instantaneous velocity (v), not only contributes to the instantaneous pressure gradient magnitude but also introduces a phase lag between pressure gradient and pulsatile velocity. Such a lag will be *more or less evident*, depending on the relative magnitudes of the local and convective inertial effects.

As a consequence of being related to the rate of change of flow, the pressure gradient component developed in response to the time varying velocity is related, at any instant of time, to the *slope* of the velocity curve. Thus, when the rate of change of velocity is greatest, the local acceleration component of the total pressure gradient will be greatest; when the rate of change of flow is zero, then the local acceleration component of the gradient will be zero (see lower left-hand panel of Fig. 7.20). Not only can flow be maximum when the pressure gradient is zero, but positive flow can occur during periods of adverse gradients, because a finite time interval must transpire before an adverse gradient can overcome the forward momentum of the flow and bring it to rest, on its way to reversing direction if the adverse gradient persists [88, 89, 101]. Thus, pressure and velocity are "out of phase," in an inertial system in which local acceleration effects are present. An increase in the rate of change of flow without changing the absolute magnitude of peak flow results in an increase in the slope of the upstroke of the velocity curve. Since the local acceleration component of the total pressure gradient is directly proportional to the slope of the velocity, the magnitude of ΔP will increase despite the fact that the magnitude of the peak flow itself has remained constant.[11]

Hemodynamic measurements demonstrate that transvalvular and intraventricular, particularly subvalvular, pressure drops and gradients are very pronounced in ventricles with stenotic outflow valves. The influence of an enhanced streamwise taper is much stronger on convective than on local acceleration gradients, since the former depend on the square whereas the latter on the square root of the ratio of downstream to upstream flow-section areas of the tapering region [88, 100]. Thus, in aortic stenosis, as opposed to normal ejection dynamics, pressure drops and pulsatile velocities can be pretty much *in-phase* (see right panels of Fig. 7.20). This is equally as important a hemodynamic hallmark of severe aortic stenosis (see Section 8.2, on pp. 410 ff.) as the augmentation of the magnitude of the driving pressure gradients [37, 88, 100, 101].

If reduced volumetric velocities and accelerations did not prevail in aortic stenosis, the cavity ejection pressures in severe cases would have to rise to levels unattainable even with very thick walls [88]. This would occur irrespective of turbulent jet losses downstream of the stenosed valve, and despite normal or subnormal aortic root pressure levels. It is referable to the fact that the convective acceleration component, in particular, increases in proportion to the square of the velocity [37, 88, 100, 101]. Contrary to conventional thinking, it is not "turbulent valve losses" that account for the great augmentation of ventricular load in aortic stenosis. Viscous dissipation in the separated flow beyond the stenosed valve simply accounts for the incomplete recovery of static pulsatile pressures as stream cross-section reexpands distal to the stenosis. Such turbulent dissipation of kinetic energy downstream of the stenosed valve *spares* the systemic arterial tree from the ravages that would be associated with the substantial recovery of abnormal ventricular systolic pressures in excess of 200 *mm Hg*, which are needed to rapidly force ejection through the strongly confluent subvalvular flow field [88, 100].

At peak flow, when the local acceleration is zero, practically the entire pressure gradient is due to the convective acceleration effect, since viscous losses are normally negligible. Thus, the closer the peak flow to the peak of the pressure gradient, the greater the convective acceleration component; the closer the peak flow to the return of the pressure gradient to zero (on its way to negative, flow-decelerating values), the lesser the convective acceleration component—in both cases, relative to the local acceleration forces. Figure 7.19 reveals that peak ejection flow occurs closer to the peak gradient, indicating a predominance of the convective effect, under both rest and exercise conditions. This

[11] For further understanding of the fluid dynamics, see Chapter 4, on the Fluid Dynamics of Unsteady Flow, particularly its Sections 4.4.3 and 4.5, on pp. 177 ff. and 187 ff., respectively.

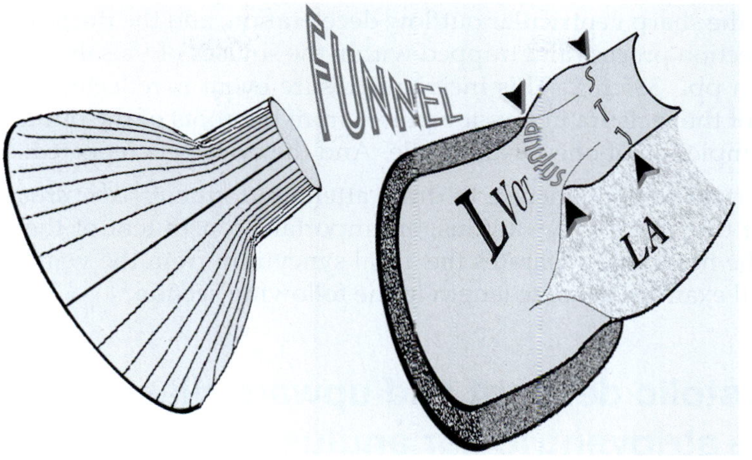

Figure 7.21: The exact positioning of the upstream sensor, deep within the *wide* LV chamber or in the *tapering* outflow tract (LVOT), affects the magnitude of the convective effect contribution to the transvalvular pressure gradient, measured by a double-tip micromanometric catheter. STJ: sinotubular junction.

is strongly corroborated by the ensuing outflow deceleration in the presence of a positive pressure "gradient" ($\Delta P(t)$), an effect which becomes less pronounced during exercise. Thus, the local acceleration forces undergo more of a strengthening during exercise compared to the convective acceleration component. Such relative comparisons may be influenced considerably by the *exact placement* of the upstream and downstream pressure measurement sites within the LV–aortic root flow field (cf. Fig. 7.9, on p. 339). LV outflow traverses first a subvalvar region, the left ventricular outflow tract, and then the aortic root, which extends from the level of the crown-shaped anulus to the level of the sinotubular junction.[12] The ventricular outflow tract acts as a funnel to increase blood flow velocity. Therefore, when the upstream sensor is in the *narrower* LV outflow tract, convective effects will seem artificially slighter than when the upstream sensor is in the *wider* deep LV chamber (cf. Fig. 7.21).

The ejection phase has been divided into a rapid ejection period and a reduced ejection period. Direct flow recordings from the roots of the outflow trunks have demonstrated the variability of the outflow waveforms under various normal or abnormal cardiovascular states. Although the classic time estimates as to the duration of the two conventional subdivisions of the ejection phase appear to lack general validity, it may be stated that during the first two-thirds of ejection about three-quarters of the stroke volume is expelled. What is more important however, is that during the final 15%, or so, of the ejection time flow drops off rapidly, and only a few milliliters of blood are expelled.

By the time that the phase of ventricular ejection ends, the outflow valve cusps are already in the almost fully-apposed state under the action of pressure gradient reversal

[12]The sinotubular junction is the boundary between the downstream edge of the sinuses of Valsalva and the tubular aorta.

connected to the sharp ventricular outflow deceleration, and the thrust of vortices formed during the ejection process and trapped within the sinuses of Valsalva (see Sections 7.13.2 and 7.13.3, on pp. 385 ff.). This incipient closure event is reflected in the sharp initial downstroke of the incisura in *pressure* pulses from the roots of the outflow trunks, which marks the completion of one cardiac cycle. And the cycle gets repeated...

It is important at this juncture to draw attention to the *variable area piston*-like cyclic excursions of the mitral valve anulus, an important constituent of the fibrocollagenous skeleton of the heart that separates the atrial syncytium from the ventricular syncytium, which we will examine at some length in the following section.

7.6 Systolic descent and upward diastolic recoil of the atrioventricular anulus plane

Ejection is effected by a systolic reduction of the ventricular chamber volumes, a process which can be conceptualized in two ways:

i. Each ventricle is able to reduce its volume by a lateral contraction alone. In this case, its length would remain the same, if the shortening and thickening of the heart muscle only causes a diminution of the inner volume and no increase in the length of the chamber.

ii. It can contract longitudinally, which would produce a shortening of its length accompanied by a reduction in effective short-axis dimensions, because of the lateral thickening that occurs as the muscle shortens.

The muscular layers surrounding the ventricular pumping chambers are depicted in Figure 7.22 schematically, so as to reveal some important functional consequences of their geometry.[13] The myocardial fibers in these helical superimposed layers are oriented roughly in three general directions: the obliquely arranged internal (deep) and external (superficial) layers of spiral muscles enclose the circumferentially arranged *medial constrictor* layer, which is especially prominent in the left ventricle.[14] The internal and external investments of both chambers are composed of the same muscle bundles, which are strongly twisted at the apex forming the *anatomic vortex* of the heart, and then spiral in opposite directions from the apex toward the base. The direction of force development by the contraction of the inner and outer layers of spiral muscles is indicated by the arrows in

[13]Chapter 6 provides a detailed overview of the functional morphology of ventricular myocardium.

[14] The functioning of hollow muscular pumping organs with optimal efficiency, at the myofiber and sarcomere levels, imposes a histoarchitectonic constraint: it requires the presence of spiral (supplying longitudinal action) as well as circumferential muscle layers in the wall. By mass conservation considerations, during the diminution of the lumen of a circular ring, which retains a constant annular (transverse) area, the inner circumference must shrink down to a much shorter length than the outer one. Another reason for such a histoarchitectonic requirement is that with the lack of an adaptable longitudinal reinforcement, the wall would be liable to suffer a longitudinal rupture, due to the inner pressure developed during systole by the powerful circumferential fibers (see also introduction to Chapter 6, on p. 299, and Section 7.8, on pp. 367 ff.).

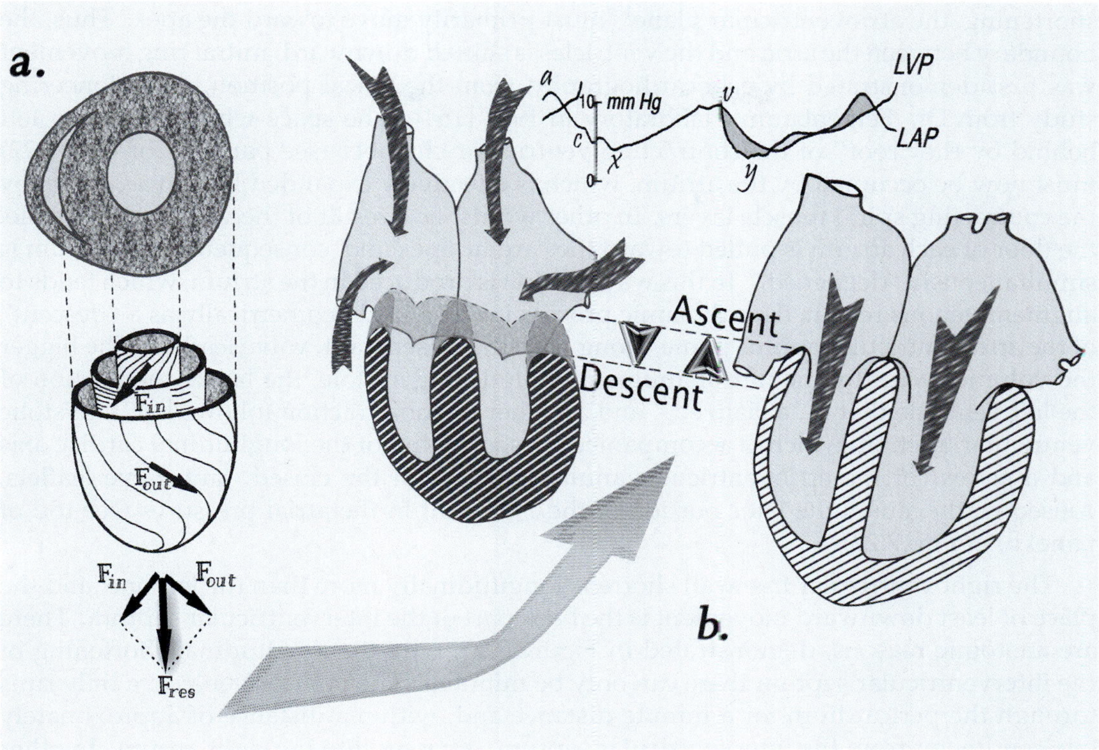

Figure 7.22: Panel a. The geometric resultant, F_{res}, of the forces F_{in} and F_{out} that are developed during systolic contraction by the inner and outer spiral heart muscle layers, respectively, is directed along the longitudinal axis of the heart. Panel b. Systolic ventricular ejection is consequently accompanied, as pointed out by the large arrow, by a shortening of the longitudinal cardiac axis and a *descent* of the atrioventricular anulus plane, along with the closed, taut, valve leaflets, which causes the x-descent exemplified in the left atrial pressure signal, LAP; LVP denotes left ventricular pressure. The A–V valve leaflets are prevented from being everted into the atria by the restraining chordae tendineae that anchor them onto the papillary muscles (not shown). During muscle relaxation and lengthening in early diastole, the reverse process occurs, encompassing an *ascent* of the atrioventricular anulus plane into previously "atrial space," while the apposed valve leaflets are being pushed "head-on" by atrial blood and forced to rapidly swing open into the ventricular chambers. (See text for details.)

panel a. of Figure 7.22. As is shown by the vector addition inset at the bottom of this panel, the resultant force is directed along the axis of each chamber, tending to produce a longitudinal shortening of the ventricles.

During this longitudinal shortening of the ventricles the tip of the heart should he considered as relatively stationary, since it cannot change its position in the pericardium without leaving a vacuum in its place; it cannot take the pericardium with it because the pericardium is attached to the diaphragm. Hence, during this ventricular longitudinal shortening, the atrioventricular plane[15] must primarily move toward the apex. Thus, the boundary between the atria and the ventricles is shifted downward; mitral ring movement was first demonstrated by echocardiography, from the apical position, in a pioneering study from Dr. Feigenbaum's laboratory in 1967 [164]. The space which is thereby left behind by the "roof" of the contracting ventricular chamber (see panel b. of Fig. 7.22) must now be occupied by the atrium, which is effectively expanded like an *accordeon* by the contracting spiral muscle layers. In other words: as a result of the ventricular systole, the floor of each atrium is pulled toward the cardiac apex and, consequently, the atrium is simultaneously "deepened." In this way, suction is produced in the atrium, which tends to augment venous return. This dynamic process is visualized geometrically as a "descent" of the atrioventricular anulus plane, along with the closed, taut, valve leaflets. The bigger the volume swept by the mitral anulus motion during systole, the larger the portion of the left ventricle that is "atrialized," and a higher ejection fraction follows [149]. Systolic ventricular ejection, which is accompanied by shortening of the longitudinal cardiac axis and a *descent* of the atrioventricular anulus plane with the closed, taut valve leaflets, consequently causes the later portion of the x-descent in the atrial pressures (see top of panel b. of Fig. 7.22).

The right ventricular free wall shortens longitudinally more than the left one, and the place of least downward movement is the back part of the interventricular septum. There are anatomic reasons, demonstrated in Figure 7.23, why the longitudinal shortening of the interventricular septum there can only be minimal. The inferior vena cava only runs through the pericardium for a minute distance and, within a distance of approximately one centimeter from the interventricular septum, it passes into the right atrium. In other words, its penetration into the diaphragm is followed immediately by entrance into the atrium. If the ventricular border of the atrium were now to move in systole strongly downward, the short segment of the atrial wall between it and the vena cava would have to be very considerably stretched, and the coronary sinus might also be distorted. Furthermore, with each systole the inferior vena cava would be drawn over the edge of the diaphragm, at its foramen. It is also noteworthy, in this context, that in the right ventricle those chordae tendineae that start at the septum and go to the middle part of the valve leaflets have absolutely no or only very short papillary muscles: when the septum shortens only slightly, there is clearly no need for large papillary muscles which in systole would shorten and pull the leaflets downward.

It is the normally more developed left ventricular musculature that contributes most of the pull on the fibromuscular atrioventricular anulus plane that forms the roof of both the ventricles. Accordingly, changes in the contractile state of the *left* ventricle are reflected to a variable extent on *right*-heart venous return dynamics, and in corresponding pressure and flow measurements and diagnostic signs classically looked for by past generations of clinicians, during the physical examination of heart failure patients [67, 68]. Various types of cardiac hypertrophy and dilatation can modify the proportion, and relative strength of the circumferential and the deep and superficial spiral muscle layers. This may alter dynamic ventricular function patterns. To wit, should any hemodynamic disturbance arise from diseases such as ventricular septal defect, pulmonary stenosis, pulmonary

[15] To my knowledge, the important valve plane (*German*: Ventilebene) concept was put forward by von Spee, who coined the term in 1909 [131].

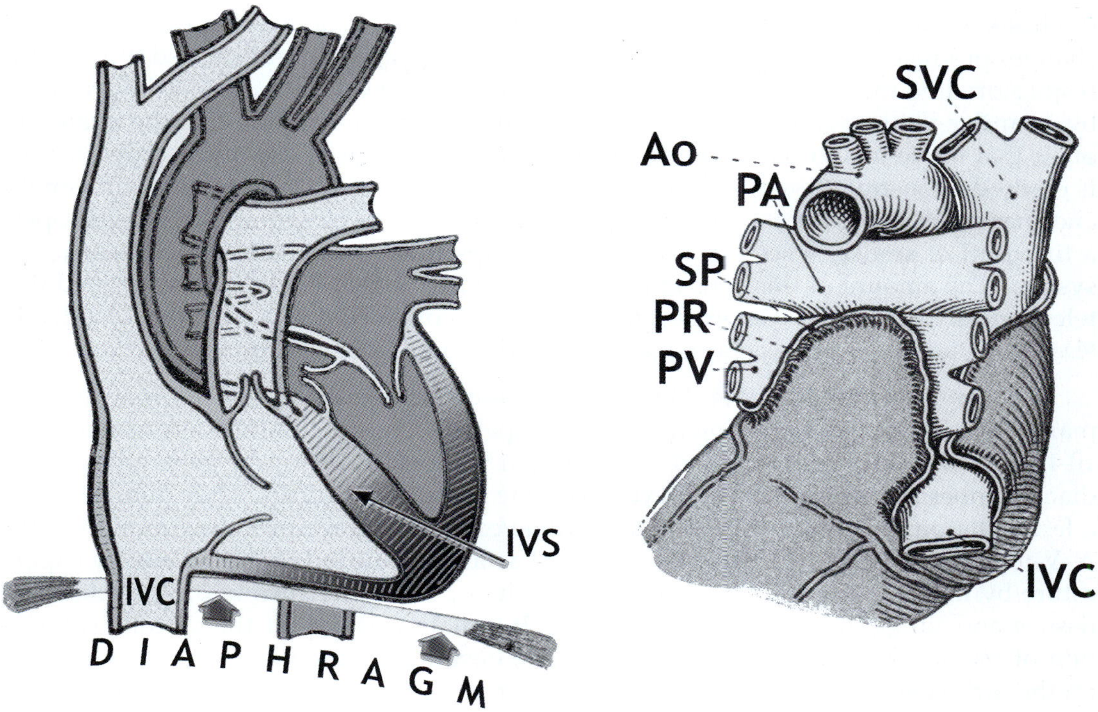

Figure 7.23: The inferior vena cava (IVC) only runs through the pericardium for a minute distance and, within a distance of approximately 1 *cm* from the interventricular septum, it passes into the right atrium. If the ventricular border of the atrium were to move in systole strongly downward, with each systole, the inferior vena cava would be drawn over the edge of the diaphragm, at its foramen. IVS = interventricular septum; PR = pericardium, SP = serous pericardium; PV = pulmonary veins; PA = pulmonary artery; Ao = aorta; SVC = superior vena cava.

hypertension, or hypertrophic cardiomyopathy involving the right heart, the systolic descent of the tricuspid floor becomes impeded; this, in turn, blunts the systolic accentuation of the central systemic venous return flow pattern. For this abnormal *systolic phase* behavior of an otherwise anatomically normal tricuspid valve, Kalmanson and his associates proposed the term "tricuspid dysfunction" [55].

The possibility of such an accordeon-like mechanism contributing to stroke volume was actually recognized very early—a systolic shortening of the heart was emphasized by William Harvey. More recently, in 1932, Hamilton and Rompf [42] deduced from experimental studies that cardiac pumping entails the movement of the atrioventricular plane toward the apex in systole and away from apex in diastole, while the apex remains fairly fixed and the outer cardiac contour relatively constant. The heart works as a reciprocating pump, alternately expanding the atria and the ventricles, without displacing significantly the surrounding tissue. The view that the heart remains relatively constant in volume in diastole as in systole (see Fig. 6.7, on p. 312) was actually formulated by Hamilton on the basis of an analysis of the cardiopneumogram. He maintained that cardiac volume changes produce pressure changes within the lungs which, when transmitted through the respiratory tree and corrected for the elastic "give" of the chest walls, seem to be produced by a cardiac volume change of 1 or 2 *mL*. He noted that his assertion that the quantities of air that move in and out of the chest during the cardiac cycle are of the order of 1 *mL* is easily demonstrated by a simple experiment [42]: "If one fills the mouth with smoke and maintains respiratory standstill with the internal nares closed and the glottis open, a tiny puff of smoke is seen to issue from the lips toward the end of each ventricular systole. The amount of this is usually not more than 0.5 *mL*." These authors argued that teleologically one might well expect that the heart is organized so as to move blood, and *blood alone*, and does not waste energy moving the contiguous tissues about.

The Hamilton and Rompf [42] hypothesis was confirmed in 1985 by Hoffman and Ritman, in studies on dogs utilizing the dynamic spatial reconstructor (DSR) system (cf. Fig. 10.4, on p. 488, and the associated discussion in Section 10.1.1) for the generation of cardiac chamber reconstructions and cyclic volume computations [50]. They demonstrated a fairly stationary apex, constant outer cardiac contour and reciprocating motion of the A–V-plane, and emphasized that this mode of action minimized pumping energy expenditure by moving blood *into* the heart rather than pulling the surrounding mediastinal tissues and lungs inward during systole.[16] It is noteworthy that the systolic contraction of the atrial myocardium just prior to the ensuing ventricular contraction will tug on the atrioventricular plane, pulling it away from apex. As a result of this action, the atrial contraction contributes to the *total stroke length* of the piston-like descent of the atrioventricular plane. During tachycardia, when diastole is disproportionately abbreviated, this atrial contribution to stroke volume and cardiac output can become substantial.

Representative pressure curves from both atrial chambers show, in general, a marked drop in pressure (the x-descent in the RAP and LAP traces in Fig. 7.18, on p. 352) coinciding with ventricular systole, an expression of the suction in the atrium caused by the descent of the atrioventricular valve anulus plane. It is not important whether by this means the pressure drops to "negative" (to be precise, *subatmospheric*) values. If the blood flows fast enough into the expanding atrium, the atrial pressure will not become negative.

During ejection, as blood is pushed into the ascending aorta toward the head, Newton's Third Law requires that the ejecting heart move in the opposite direction, toward the feet.[17] Since the diaphragm opposes such a bodily downward movement of the heart during ejection, what occurs is mostly a descent of the base that contains the aortic anulus. This mechanism acts to supplement the direct effect of the myocardial contraction, which is depicted in Figure 7.22, on p. 359. The subsequent rapid reascension of the atrioventricular anulus plane contributes to the early diastolic intraventricular volume replenishment, in addition to the early E-wave inflow that is directed toward the inner chamber surface.

[16] Clinically, palpation of the apex beat suggests that the cardiac apex moves *toward* the chest wall during systole, not *away* as it would by an inward apical squeeze; the distance traversed by this movement is negligible, i.e., the apex is fairly stationary.

[17] This explains the bouncing of the needle seen when one stands quietly on a sensitive spring-loaded scale, and provided the rationale for *ballistocardiography*, once used to estimate stroke volume [56].

The mitral anulus recoil motion relative to the ventricular apex is a function of the systolically deformed ventricular chamber shape and myocardial fiber histoarchitectonics along with myocardial viscoelastic and active relaxation characteristics. It is promoted by the early transmitral flow momentum influx (acting again in accordance to Newton's Third Law but in opposite direction to the momentum outflux through the aortic anulus during ejection), and is influenced by the *mitral apparatus* [9, 117] characteristics, including papillary muscle-chordal restraint and fluid-structure interaction between blood and mitral leaflets. Several studies [34, 44, 61, 155] have suggested that the mitral anulus recoil velocity and displacement in early diastole can be used as indicators of diastolic performance; e.g., the peak recoil velocity of the mitral anulus away from the LV apex in early diastole is reduced in patients with impaired diastolic relaxation [44]. As the atrioventricular ring plane moves back upward with the valve open, it allows the ventricular space to "slide over," as it were, and engulf some atrial blood. Working before the advent of MRI and second harmonic 2-D echocardiography, and on the basis of meticulous, elegant human studies using gated myocardial scintigraphy, echocardiography, and coronary angiography, Lundbäck [70] stressed the importance of such a "gripping" action.

During the cardiac cycle the changes in the area of the mitral anulus and its alternating descent-ascent excursions encompass a volume that is part of the total LV volume alteration during both emptying and filling. Interestingly, the upward diastolic recoil of the mitral anulus increases the net velocity of mitral inflow by as much as 20% [57,149]. Moreover, the myocardial tissue volume is regarded as nearly incompressible and, aside from slight cyclic changes in intramural vessel filling, the total volume of the heart is fairly constant during the entire heart cycle—see also Section 7.8, on pp. 367 ff. Accordingly, the displacement of myocardial wall tissues toward the apex during systolic long axis shortening must bring about a radial (lateral) expansion of the shortening walls and a volume reduction by encroaching on the chamber's short-axis diameters, in addition to the volume reduction directly produced by the anulus descent.

Contraction of the mitral anulus was detected by many old surgeons who performed closed commissurotomies for relief of mitral stenosis in the 1950s. The excursion of the mitral anulus accounts for an important portion of the total LV filling and emptying in humans. Recent work [23] on humans, using transesophageal echocardiography (TEE) and extending the pioneering investigations of Tsakiris and his coworkers first at the Mayo Clinic and then in Canada [150, 151], has shown that mitral anulus *up-and-down* excursions, along with shape and area changes contribute significantly to the total cyclic LV volume change. The mitral anulus excursion volume was found to represent about 20% of the total LV stroke volume and to correlate strongly with it. Peak mitral anulus area occurred during middiastole, and over 90% of the reduction in anulus area from peak to minimum took place *before* the onset of LV systolic contraction. These recent findings suggest an *atriogenic* influence on mitral anulus physiology and also a *sphincter*-like action of the mitral anulus that may facilitate ventricular filling and aid competent valve closure. These subtle but important effects complement the more familiar and straightforward *reservoir*, *conduit*, and *booster-pump* atrial functions.

The pulmonary arterial and ascending aortic roots are affixed to the anterior part of the atrioventricular plane, and are also attached to mediastinal structures adjacent to the

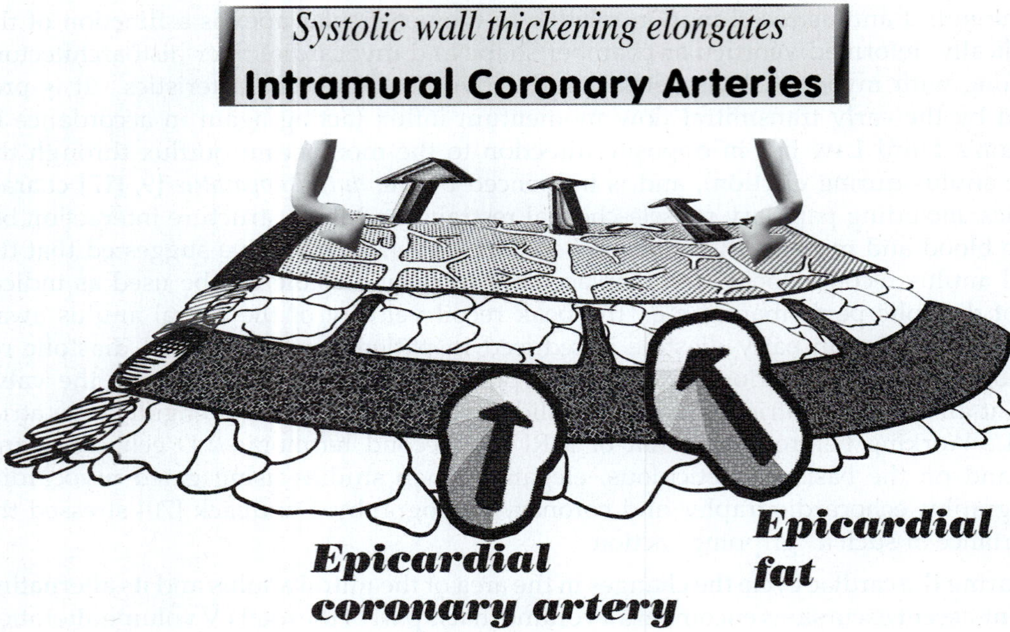

Figure 7.24: An elongation with a complementary reduction of diameter of the intramural perforating coronary arteries must accompany systolic ventricular wall thickening during ejection, in view of their disposition and manner of branching off the large subepicardial coronary arteries.

heart. Therefore, when during systole the atrioventricular plane moves in the direction of the apex, its posterior segment will move more freely than the anterior. This brings about a swinging *rotary motion*, causing the cardiac apex to beat against the chest wall, and giving rise to the palpable cardiac impulse.

7.6.1 Atrial stiffness and ventricular systolic load

The descent of the atrioventricular anulus plane that occurs normally during ejection has an interesting implication: conditions, such as atrial fibrillation, which increase atrial wall stiffness opposing atrial elongation in response to the pull exerted by the ventricular myocardium, would effectively augment the ventricular myocardial systolic load. Indeed, fast-multislice computerized tomography was used, by Drs. Hoffman and Ritman at Mayo Medical School [50], to study the atrioventricular anulus plane motion in dogs in sinus rhythm and atrial fibrillation. Heart rate was maintained constant between the two conditions by pacing, using a bipolar coronary sinus pacing catheter. Lines were drawn in space at the level of the A–V valve plane at end-diastole and end-systole. Meticulous measurements revealed that in atrial fibrillation there was a 60 % reduction in the extent of A–V valve plane descent. This valve plane motion reduction was a consistent finding in all dogs with atrial fibrillation, suggesting that *atrial stiffness* may play a significant role in ventricular afterload, by resisting the systolic RV and LV contraction-based long axis shortening. This may yield a significant relative increase in the work load, particularly of the right heart. Moreover, by thus influencing atrial wall strain, the strength of ventricular contraction may modulate the release of cardiac hormones, such as atrial natriuretic peptides [32].

Further investigations [51] applied the method of Suga et al. [137, 138], which uses the P–V relationship along with an estimate of ventricular volume at zero pressure to calculate the total ventricular work, along with a contrast dilution technique to measure myocardial blood flow. Using the pressure–volume loops in atrial fibrillation as compared with sinus rhythm for both left and right ventricles, total work was consistently less, on the order of 20%, in atrial fibrillation as compared with paced sinus rhythm. On the other hand, as total work was found to be less in atrial fibrillation, myocardial blood flow in the LV free wall was found to be greater in atrial fibrillation as compared to paced sinus rhythm by an average of 16%. This suggests a dissociation between calculated total work and myocardial blood flow, and highlights the importance of atrial–ventricular interactions, which enter into the total ventricular systolic load (cf. Fig. 7.27, on p. 370). Atrial stiffness may, therefore, impede ventricular emptying and contribute to the total ventricular myocardial work of contraction. Such an effect might also be introduced by hardening of the ascending aorta.

7.7 Coronary vessel effects restoring diastolic heart shape

It can be observed experimentally that an expansion of a freshly excised animal heart suspended in a physiological solution occurs when the coronary arteries are injected from the aorta under pressure of 120 *cm* of water, in effect an "erectile" response to vascular engorgement. One can also see clearly an unfolding of the right atrioventricular anulus. Considering that in the intact, closed-chest state this movement can further be supported by the elastic forces of the lung and chest wall which maintain subatmospheric intrapericardial pressures, these observations suggest a potential role for the coronary vascular tree in aiding the diastolic change of form of the ventricles. The influence of the coronary vascular tree on cardiac extension in diastole can come about in two distinct ways:

a. **Through the elasticity of blood vessels that undergo distortions during systole.** In the left ventricular chamber wall, there is a large number of perforating intramural arteries, running radially across the wall thickness. On the basis of their disposition and their manner of branching off the main subepicardial coronary arteries, an elongation of these intramural arteries must occur as a result of the systolic wall thickening, as is indicated in Figure 7.24, on p. 364. In the ensuing diastole, these arteries would tend to retract, thus "thinning" the systolically thickened chamber walls. Moreover, the *refilling* blood vessels interposed between inner myocardial muscle fiber surfaces that had been squeezed together by the contraction of enveloping outer muscle, especially

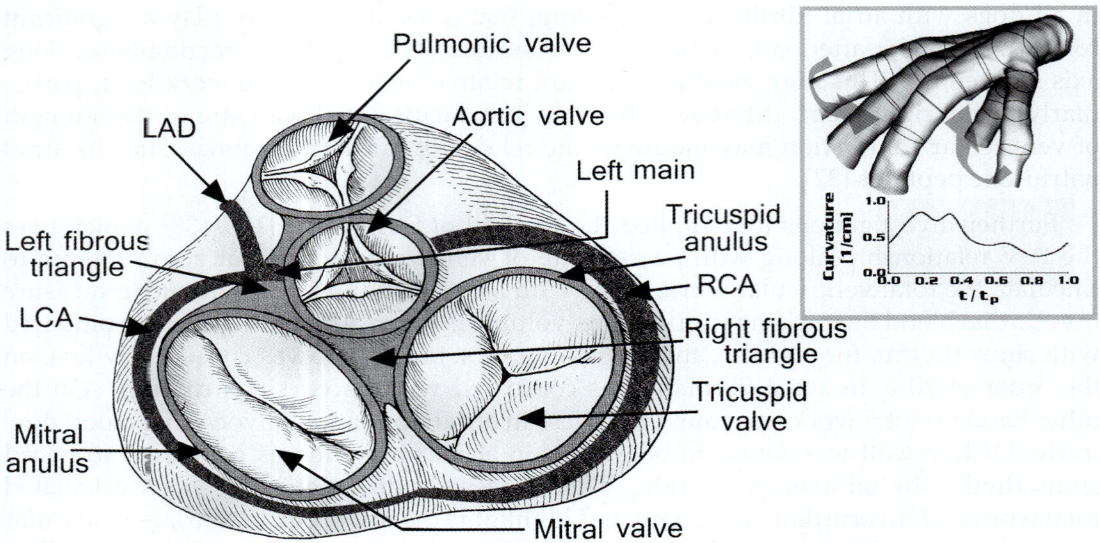

Figure 7.25: Diagrammatic view of the base of the heart, after excision of the auricles and the trunks of the great arteries. The anuli of the inflow and outflow ventricular valves along with the left and right fibrous triangles make up the fibrous skeleton of the heart. The right (RCA) and the left main coronary artery with its continuation, the circumflex coronary artery (LCA), encircle the atrioventricular anuli. The branches of the coronary arteries encircling the atrioventricular anuli take off predominantly in a single direction, toward the heart's apex; only the left anterior descending (LAD) branch is shown. The inset has been redrawn modified from Prosi et al. [116], and shows alternating variations of the local coronary artery curvature during a cardiac period of length t_P, measured on a subject undergoing diagnostic catheterization.

the veins and sinusoidal channels (cf. Fig. 7.26, on p. 368), could push the muscle fibers apart from each other, thus helping expand the heart wall.

b. **Through a variety of fluid dynamic mechanisms.** Flow dynamic influences are manifested in terms of intravascular pressure and velocity of flow. The right and left main coronary arteries display a strong curvature (see Fig. 7.25) around the auriculoventricular sulci.[18] The arteries are kept in place by adipose and connective tissue (cf. Fig. 7.24, on p. 364), which is in turn connected to the fibrous skeleton of the heart. The left main and its continuation, the circumflex coronary artery lie in the left auriculoventricular sulcus, and the right coronary artery lies in the right auriculoventricular sulcus. Their circular disposition in the sulcus between the auricles and ventricles reminded the ancient anatomists of Greece of a wreath encircling the head; accordingly, they were named *stefaniaiae arteriae*, wreath-like arteries; hence, the Latin form, *arteriae coronariae.* In a conduit curved in such a fashion, the outer area is greater than the inner one. Accordingly, the surface which sustains pressure must be greater outward than inward.

[18]Sulci, *pl.* of sulcus [L.], a groove.

This unequal distribution of pressure force causes a hydraulic tendency for the curved vessel to stretch outward and straighten, much like a *Bourdon tube*[19] pressure gauge.

Another mechanism that must be considered involves the inertia of blood flowing in a curved tube, which tends to make it flow straight in the direction of the tangent. Thereby, it bounces against the outer wall and causes a straightening and stretching of the curved tube there. The same mechanism applies to winding blood vessels and likewise causes a stretching. Thus, forces result which, in diastole, could expand the atrioventricular anuli that had been *squeezed down* in size (circumference and cross-sectional area) in systole.

A pushing upward and outward of the atrioventricular anuli and valve plane, by the main coronary blood vessels lying in the auriculoventricular sulci encircling them, would also be conceivable as a third fluid dynamic effect, as follows: The branches of the coronary arteries encircling the plane of the atrioventricular anuli *(vide supra)* take off predominantly in a single direction, namely, toward the heart's apex. This causes gaps on the apical side of the wall of the arteries encircling the atrioventricular anuli and valve plane. The opposite wall lying toward the atrium has a larger surface, and consequently receives a larger total pressure force, which yields a net force pointing upward and outward. Moreover, blood flowing into the apically directed branches of the left main, circumflex and right coronary arteries should exert on the parent vessel walls opposite their orifices a thrust that is directed upward and outward—by Newton's Third Law, or a "water-pistol," or "squid-propulsion" effect. This effect could be one additional factor that causes a return of the atrioventricular anuli to diastolic size, and the ascent of the valve plane, which during systole had descended toward the apex.

7.8 Systolic wall thickening and mural cyclic volume shifts

When considering the geometry of ejection, on the short-axis cross-section of the LV chamber, we are faced with a muscular anulus whose lumen must become narrower during systolic ejection. For conservation of mass, its surface area must not be reduced; on the contrary, it is expected to increase somewhat in size because the longitudinal axis of the chamber shortens. The mathematical conditions of the diminution of such a ring underlie the functioning of hollow muscular organs, including muscular arteries and arterioles.

Geometrical analysis shows that during the diminution of the luminal area of a circular ring that retains the same ring area, the inner (endocardial) circle must shorten *much more* than the outer (epicardial) one. The *thicker* the wall, the *more pronounced* becomes this effect. This is also a reason why the chamber wall cannot consist exclusively of ring fibers. Another reason is that, with the lack of an elastic longitudinal reinforcement, the

[19]The Bourdon tube is a curved metallic tube with an oval cross-section that tends to become circular as the distending pressure rises, while the tube straightens causing a measurable displacement.

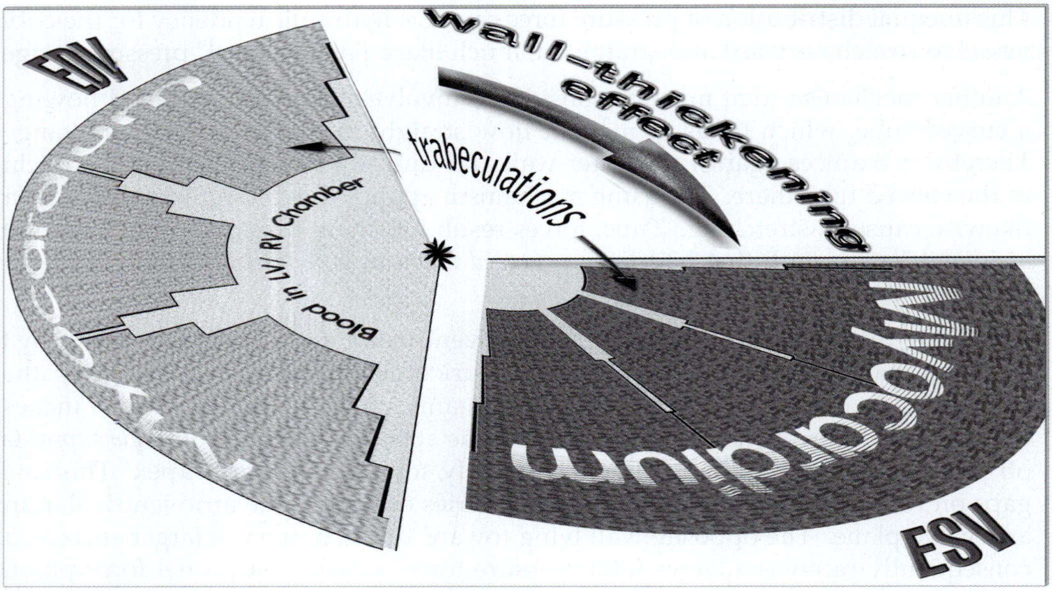

Figure 7.26: Schematic depiction of *squeezable* blood-filled spaces that connect to the ventricular chamber and are interposed between the *trabeculae carneae*. During diastole, there is a net shift of blood from the lumen into these mural spaces. There are more capacious spaces in the inner wall, which are filled with blood and have direct connection to the ventricular chamber. During systole, there is a net flow out of the *squeezable blood-filled spaces* and into the contiguous chamber lumen (cf. Fig. 6.1, on p. 300). This makes the mural spaces smaller and allows accommodation of the *trabeculae carneae* within a smaller enveloping circumference. The associated cyclic mural volume changes are much larger than could be accounted for by the intravascular volume changes of the intramural coronary vasculature, which pertain to the *coronary erectile effect*. EDV, ESV: end-diastolic and end-systolic ventricular chamber volume, respectively.

wall would suffer a *longitudinal rupture* due to the inner pressure developed during systole. Furthermore, the distance between the midwall and the inner circle increases more markedly in the course of the contraction than that between the midwall and outer circle. With reference to the left ventricle, this means that the inner (subendocardial) parts of the muscular system are inevitably pushed *further* toward the lumen during systole. During this process, they are rearranged in folds whose walls offer a larger receptive area to the postsystolic in-rushing blood flow of the rapid upstroke of the E-wave to expand the ventricular walls.

Experimental measurements [4] show that, as the wall thickens during ejection and chamber collapse, there are actual *systolic decreases* in volume in all layers of the ventricular myocardium. This suggests that the source of the *diastolic* volume increases would either be the epicardial coronary vessels or the ventricular lumen. Because previous studies have not shown a large negative venous blood flow [24], which would contribute the mural volume increase during diastole, the volume source appears to be the ventricular lumen. There are blood-filled spaces within the ventricular walls that communicate with the ventricular lumen. In fact, there are three cardiac mural structures that make up blood-filled spaces within the myocardium, which may contribute to the myocardial volume change during the cardiac cycle, which is much larger [4] than might have been expected from coronary intravascular volume shifts.

The first potential structure is anatomical communication between coronary vessels and ventricular lumens [2,153], including the Thebesian veins. The second potential structure that would provide for cyclic volume change within the ventricular myocardium is represented by cleavage spaces between myolaminar sheets [4], which undergo dynamic change during the cardiac cycle, contributing to the wall volume decrease during contraction. The third potential structure is sinusoidal blood-filled spaces interposed between ventricular trabecular tissues; these spaces shrink in size in the transition from end-diastolic to end-systolic volume configuration, as is represented pictorially in Figure 7.26, on p. 368.[20] Novel observations of this function of the ventricular trabeculae carneae and associated luminal sinusoids have been made lately by advanced cardiac imaging systems [112,113]. An exaggerated form of trabeculation is present in a congenital condition denoted as *noncompaction* of the ventricular myocardium, or *hypertrabeculation* [8].

Recent studies have established that the trabecular tissue extends as much as 50% from the endocardial border into the LV wall in human hearts, and a condition similar to the noncompaction state but less pronounced is observed in 91% of normal subjects [112,113]. The trabecular tissue is most regularly prominent in the apical regions near the papillary muscles, which do not attach directly to the compact mural myocardium but to the trabecular tissue [5]. It is important to recognize that the systolic reduction of mural volume by this mechanism allows more complete chamber emptying and attainment of small end-systolic volumes, which necessitate substantial ventricular wall thickening, especially in relatively thick-walled ventricles. Another possible function of the trabeculations is discussed in Section 16.7.4, on pp. 879 f.

7.9 Complementarity and competitiveness of intrinsic and extrinsic ejection load components

The ventricular systolic ejection load represents pressure against which the walls contract and is to be distinguished from *myocardial systolic load*, or wall stress, to which it is related by complex cardiomorphometric and histoarchitectonic factors. The total ventricular systolic load, or afterload, determines the manner by which the mechanical energy generated by the actin–myosin interactions in the ventricular walls is converted to the

[20] Discrepancies between routine *angiographic* and *echocardiographic* ventricular areas and volumes can be explained by considering that, whereas echocardiography detects the *inner* contour of the chamber cuts, excluding the papillary muscles and trabeculae, angiography delineates the *outer* silhouette of the chambers, including the papillary muscles and the trabeculae. For volume calculations, this overestimation of the angiographically derived areas is generally taken into account by using a correction factor that results from comparison with *true volumes* (by water displacement) of ventricular casts.

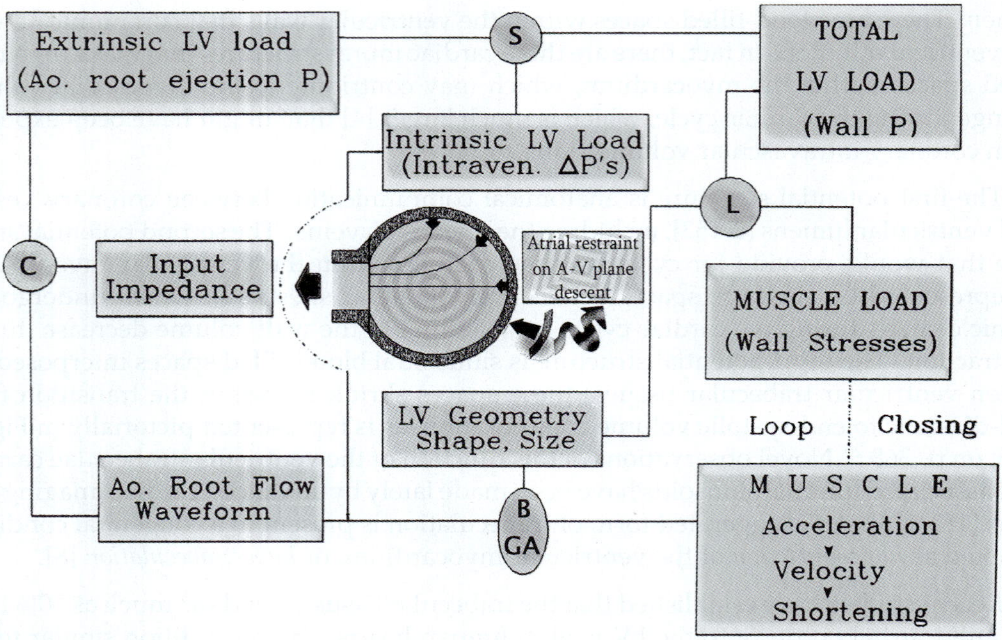

Figure 7.27: Framework for the study of systolic loading in the *in situ* heart and *complementarity* and *competitiveness* in the dynamic interactions between the intrinsic and extrinsic left ventricular (LV) load components. AO = aortic; Intraven = intraventricular; P = pressure. C denotes the mathematical operation of convolution, S denotes summation, L denotes operation of the Laplace law, B and GA denote Bernoulli effects and geometric actions, respectively. (Redrawn from Pasipoularides [88] by kind permission of the American College of Cardiology.)

work that pumps blood through the circulation. Under any given contractile state, increased afterload reduces ejection rate and stroke volume. Conversely, when afterload decreases, a larger volume is ejected at higher ejection velocities [14, 54, 75, 88]. This reflects the inverse force–velocity relation of working muscle [35,54,88].

In the 1980s, my clinical coworkers and I undertook intensive analytical and fluid dynamic studies of ejection (see Chapter 8), combining multisensor micromanometric and velocimetric catheterization, angiocardiography, and imaging and Doppler echocardiography, in patients evaluated for all kinds of heart disease, and others found to have normal ventricular function [88]. These studies demonstrated intraventricular ejection gradients of substantial magnitude in the human left ventricle in the absence of any organic or dynamic outflow obstruction [88,94,95,101] and delineated characteristics distinguishing them from obstructive gradients and transvalvular pressure drops [88,104,128]. Larger gradients can occur in the presence of what I have termed [88] *systolic ventriculoannular disproportion*, when blood is ejected rapidly from an enlarged chamber through a normal-sized aortic anulus [49, 54, 88], as may occur in aortic regurgitation. Large gradients may reach 30 *mm Hg* or more in the special case of cavity obliteration without

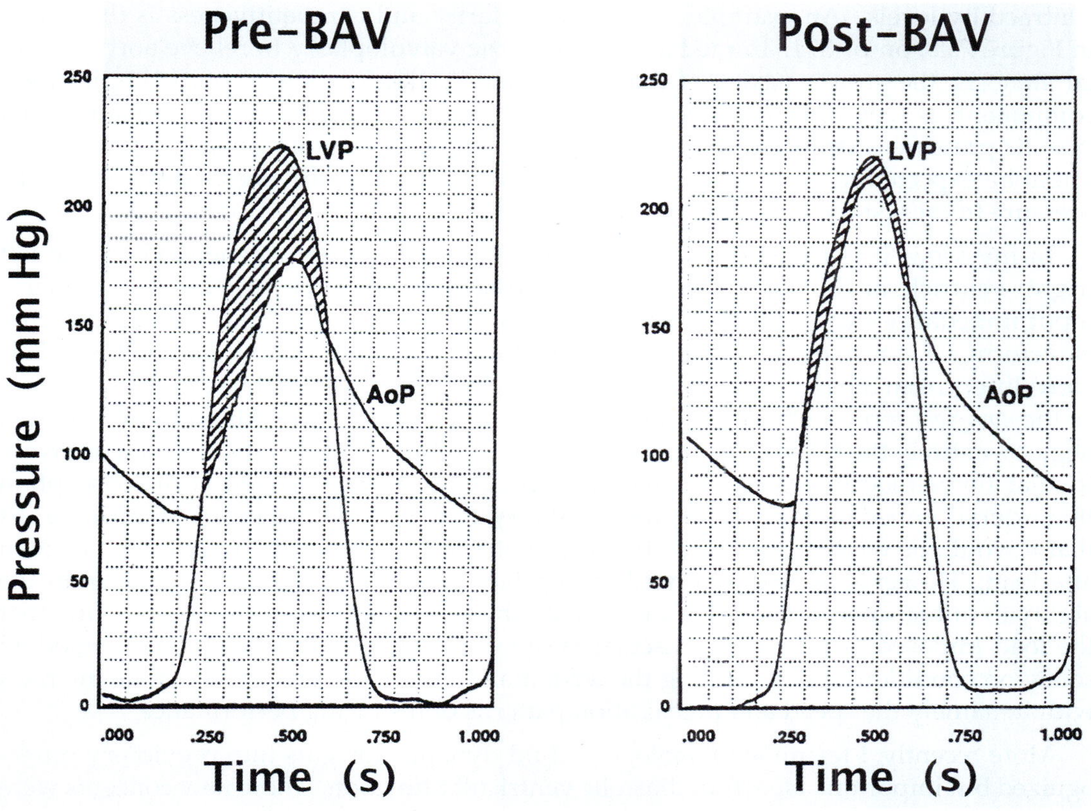

Figure 7.28: *Complementarity* and *competitiveness* between the intrinsic and extrinsic components of the total left ventricular systolic load. Immediately after balloon aortic valvuloplasty (BAV) to relieve stenosis, the great reduction of the ventricular ejection gradient (*competing* intrinsic component, hatched area) is counterbalanced by a *complementary* increase of the aortic root systolic pressure (extrinsic component). LV systolic pressure (total systolic load) remains unchanged—does not decrease acutely. AoP: aortic pressure; LVP: left ventricular pressure. (Redrawn from [128] by kind permission of the American Heart Association).

obstruction, in hypertrophic cardiomyopathy [88,95]. Ejection gradients of this magnitude are not uncommon in the presence of left ventricular (or, long standing right ventricular) outflow tract obstruction, including aortic (pulmonic) valvular stenosis [14,88,100].

Through this work, I developed the view that total ventricular systolic load comprises both *extrinsic* (the aortic root ejection pressure waveform) and *intrinsic* (flow-associated *intraventricular* pressure gradients) fluid dynamic components [54, 88, 94, 101]. Figure 7.27, on p. 370, provides a framework for the study of systolic loading dynamics in the *in situ* heart. I subsequently introduced the concept of *complementarity* and *competitiveness* [88], in the dynamic interaction between the extrinsic and intrinsic components of the total ventricular and myocardial systolic loads, under any given set of preload and contractility levels. An example of complementarity and competitiveness is illustrated in Figure 7.28, on p. 371. Immediately after aortic valvuloplasty to relieve aortic valvular stenosis, the *great reduction* of the ventricular ejection gradient (competing intrinsic component) is seen to be counterbalanced by a *complementary increase* of the aortic root systolic pressure (extrinsic component). Consequently, instead of decreasing acutely—as might be expected in absence of complementarity and competitiveness—the LV systolic pressure (total systolic load) remains unchanged [128] acutely.

In my view, it is the interaction of the ejection flow patterns generated by the left (right) ventricle at the aortic (pulmonary arterial) root with the systemic (pulmonary) input impedance that gives rise [92, 93, 126, 128, 129] to the aortic root systolic pressure waveform, i.e., the extrinsic component of the total ventricular systolic load [88, 89]. This view differs from the widely quoted formulation, by Milnor [73], of the arterial impedance as the *complete* representation of the ventricular afterload. Firstly, Milnor's formulation neglects entirely the intrinsic component of systolic ventricular loading (i.e., the intraventricular flow-associated pressure gradient). Secondly, Milnor arrived at his conception that arterial impedance, *per se*, represents the systolic load on the heart, because he felt that it would be wrong to conclude that the ventricle plays a part in determining its own afterload. However, invoking a need to deprive the intact pumping ventricle from the ability to influence its afterload is somewhat arbitrary. It is tantamount to accepting that the load imposed on, e.g., the muscular system of a cross-country runner is embodied solely on conditions characterizing the terrain and not on the way in which he interacts with it, namely the speed and acceleration patterns of his racing performance.

More recently, I formulated analogous fluid dynamic insights into previously unrecognized but important aspects of diastolic ventricular function. These new concepts were derived using our Functional Imaging method [91, 107], and are developed at length in Chapter 14. The method encompasses real-time 3-D echocardiography, sonomicrometry, and computational fluid dynamics, and has shown chamber dilatation in volume overload to underlie formerly unappreciated alterations in the intracardiac diastolic flow field, with major physiological and clinical implications [90, 91, 107–109]. A new mechanism, the *convective deceleration load* [108, 109], was revealed to be an important determinant of diastolic inflow during the upstroke of the $E-$wave. Its magnitude affects strongly peak E-wave velocities. The larger the chamber, the larger becomes the convective deceleration load. This underlies our concept of a *diastolic ventriculoannular disproportion* [107–109].

These innovative concepts on the dynamic interaction between the extrinsic and intrinsic components of the total ventricular systolic load, manifested in their complementarity and competitivenes under any given set of preload and contractility levels, have important clinical implications [88–90]. As one example, they could explain why changes in aortic valve area after balloon aortic valvuloplasty have not correlated with short-term clinical outcome. Moreover, they have been born out by findings of a recent serial study by Nemes et al. [81] of patients with aortic stenosis who underwent aortic valve replacement (AVR) and were investigated prospectively. As expected, stenosis severity and left ventricular mass decreased significantly after AVR. However, proximal aortic luminal diameter pulsatile changes (systolic minus diastolic dimensions) increased only progressively, and aortic stiffness decreased only at one-year to levels comparable to age-, gender-, and risk factor-matched controls. Some might find it counterintuitive that the pulse pressure in uncorrected severe AS tended to be greater than at 12 months after AVR.

However, within the scope of the integrative framework for ventricular loading, we can interpret the findings of the study by Nemes and his coworkers as follows [90]: Before AVR, aortic stiffness was greatly elevated from control in severe AS. The authors suggest that endothelial dysfunction, ischemia, and other factors [7] might bring about the increased stiffness. In any case, this stiffening augments the aortic input impedance, so that not only the intrinsic but also the extrinsic component of the total systolic LV load are elevated. Although measurements are not available immediately post-AVR, Figure 7.28, on p. 371, and findings post-balloon valvuloplasty [90, 128] suggest that the great reduction of the systolic ejection gradient (intrinsic component) can be transitorily counterbalanced by a complementary increase of the aortic root systolic pressure (the extrinsic component). The measurements 3 weeks, 6 and 12 months after AVR show the ensuing gradual decrease in aortic stiffness and in the extrinsic component of the systolic LV load. This decrease abets the immediate sharp drops in the peak and the mean transaortic pressure gradients, which reflect the intrinsic component of the systolic load. *Pari passu* with these changes in systolic LV load, LV mass and geometry tend to revert to normal.

Clearly, the pulse pressure before AVR is greater than at 12 months post-AVR because of the gradually ensuing substantial decrease in aortic stiffness, which was demonstrated for the first time by that seminal study! Its remarkable findings underscore the need for serial studies to detail mechanisms underlying the evolution of the interplay between the intrinsic and extrinsic components of LV load in the setting of interventions aimed at relief of aortic stenosis [90].

A related intriguing phenomenon in AS is "pressure loss recovery" [88, 89], in which some of the intrinsic LV load going into convective acceleration of the flow upstream of the stenosed orifice [100] is *regained* as the flow re-expands in the aortic root. Aortic stiffness may be an unrecognized determinant of this recovery [90]. Pressure loss recovery is considered at length in Section 16.2.2, on pp. 860 ff.

7.10 Asynchronism between right- and left-sided events

Quantitative, rather than qualitative, differences characterize the hemodynamics of the two sides of the heart (see Fig. 7.29, on p. 374). Corresponding hemodynamic events exhibit a distinct, albeit small, asynchronism even under normal conditions. This asynchronism arises from the pattern of cardiac excitation, and from the dissimilar hemodynamic operating conditions, most notably the dissimilar operating pressure levels. The effects of contrasting operating conditions are moderated by the morphomechanical adaptations of the two ventricles to their unequal arterial input impedances and pressure levels. As is shown in Figure 7.29, the phases of:

- isovolumic ventricular contraction, and
- isovolumic ventricular relaxation

are normally slightly longer for the left than for the right ventricle. The phases of:

- ventricular ejection, and
- ventricular filling

are slightly longer for the right than for the left ventricle.

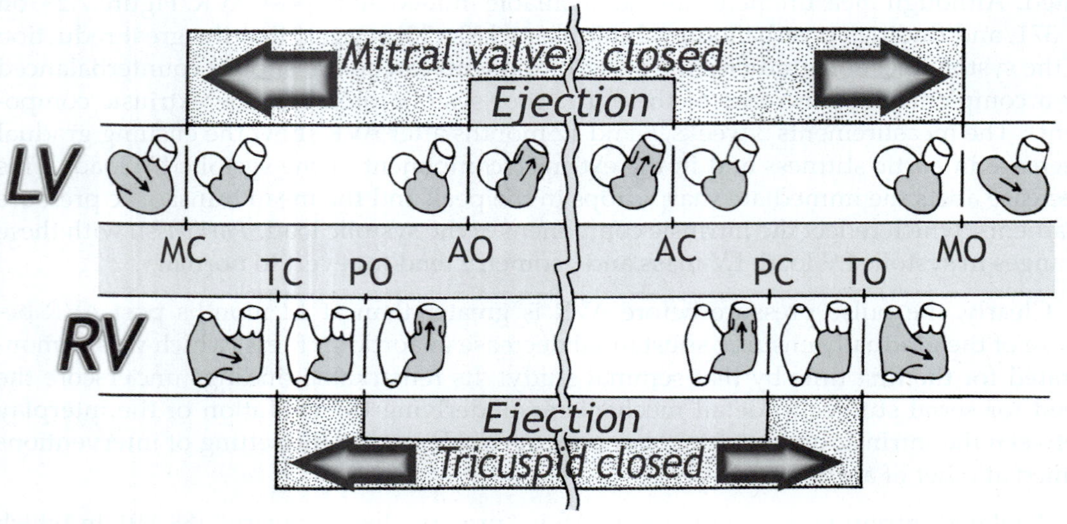

Figure 7.29: Asynchronism of cardiac cycle dynamic events between the left (LV) and right (RV) sides. A = aortic valve; M = mitral valve; P = pulmonic valve; T = tricuspid valve; C = closure; O = opening.

The ability of the relatively thin-walled, weak right ventricle to eject in a time comparable with that taken by the thick-walled left ventricle an essentially equal stroke volume is remarkable. It is attributable to the low input impedance of the pulmonary vasculature [62], which is, in turn, ascribed to the low elastic resistance of pulmonary arterial walls, and the low pulmonary arteriolar flow resistance.

Transient imbalances in ejected blood volume between the two ventricles are buffered by complementary changes in cardiac and pulmonary vascular volumes. It is nevertheless striking to think how effectively the asynchronism between the two sides is minimized under varying normal and even abnormal circulatory conditions, while preserving a relatively balanced state with only small discrepancies in stroke volume between the two sides. *Heterometric* and *homeometric* regulation and vascular reflex adjustments, may all have to play their homeostatic roles in maintaining such a safe and versatile coupled pumping operation!

7.11 Indices of myocardial contractility from central pressure and flow tracings

Because of obvious clinical and experimental needs, there has been, through the years, great interest in indices that are capable of quantifying myocardial contractility and ventricular wall strength—in the sense of the *potential* for force generation, or shortening, or both—that cardiac muscle possesses in the beating heart under any given functional state. At least 30 indices have been developed to measure contractility [21]. Myocardial and ventricular performance are related to contractility, but are not equivalent to it in meaning, since they pertain to what the muscle or heart actually does when observed under given operating conditions, e.g., end-diastolic volume or preload, total systolic load, and heart rate.

The functional capability of cardiac muscle cells or the pumping ventricle ultimately derives from the interaction of cross-bridges in sarcomeres. Nevertheless, exactly where the pumping ventricle functions within the range of possibilities available to it depends on a multitude of factors, which include not only the *potential* for force generation and shortening of the sarcomeres in the ventricular muscle, but also the heart rate, and the applying preload and total systolic load (see Section 7.9, on pp. 369 ff., and Fig. 7.27, on p. 370).

By quantifying the sensitivity of cardiac function to the applying operating conditions and defining the functional form of its dependence on them, we can delineate the capability of the integrated cardiac muscle/pump system. This is done in the practise of clinical cardiology and research. Here we are merely interested in presenting some useful indices whose evaluation enters in the assessment of contractile state. Thanks to modern advances in instrumentation, which allow high-fidelity measurements of intracardiac pressures and velocities [54,88], it is nowadays possible to learn how a given patient's heart is raising the intraventricular pressure and setting the blood in motion in the course of ejection. This allows cardiologists and experimenters alike to identify both the conditions which impair ejection, and the interventions that improve it, based on high-frequency information brought out by taking derivatives of pressure, flow velocity and work.

Indeed, clinicians daily face the need to assess the functional state of the myocardium, especially of the left ventricle, for prognosis and evaluation of the management of patients with cardiac problems, including heart failure. The ejection fraction (EF) is the most common index of ventricular functional state [21,22] and is given by $(EDV - ESV)/EDV$, where EDV denotes end-diastolic, and ESV end-systolic ventricular volume. Since the volume of blood ejected with each ventricular contraction is the product of the ejection fraction and the end-diastolic volume, it follows that the same stroke volume may result from different combinations of these variables. We can represent this by a hyperbolic function, an *isostroke* curve that sweeps up all possible combinations of ejection fraction and end-diastolic volume that result in the same value of stroke volume. As systolic performance deteriorates, an increase in end-diastolic ventricular volume associated with left ventricular enlargement moves the ventricle along the isostroke line allowing it to propel the same volume of blood albeit with reduced fiber shortening and a depressed ejection fraction (see Fig. 7.30).

Cardiac *remodeling* denotes alterations of size and shape of the cardiac chambers [132, 154], ensuing as an adaptive morphomechanic response after myocardial injury or overload. The increased chamber size and more spherical shape resulting from such remodeling enable the ventricle to maintain the same stroke volume with a reduced change in its effective radii. This mechanism is especially apparent in a large spherical ventricle with poor ejection fraction, such as typifies the dilated cardiomyopathies and heart failure. However, a dilated ventricle is capable of maintaining systolic pressure only at the cost of higher systolic wall stress levels, which initiate a myocardial hypertrophic response; this will, if left untreated, lead to multiple myocardial and fluid dynamic diastolic abnormalities, subendocardial ischemia, myocardial fibrosis and eventual decompensation [75, 76, 87, 88, 98, 105, 106, 108, 109].

Conventionally, the maximal value of ventricular dP/dt during isovolumic contraction (see Fig. 7.31) and the ejection fraction are taken as readily obtainable ventricular systolic performance indices. The minimal value of the negative dP/dt during isovolumic relaxation (see Fig. 7.31) and the time constant of pressure decay during this phase [27] are taken as useful indices of myocardial diastolic relaxation, in clinical practise. Generally, one is interested in the ability of the myocardium to augment its performance under homeometric conditions, i.e., independently of the Frank–Starling response. The rather loose (when applied to a ventricle in situ) term "contractility" refers to this ability. In

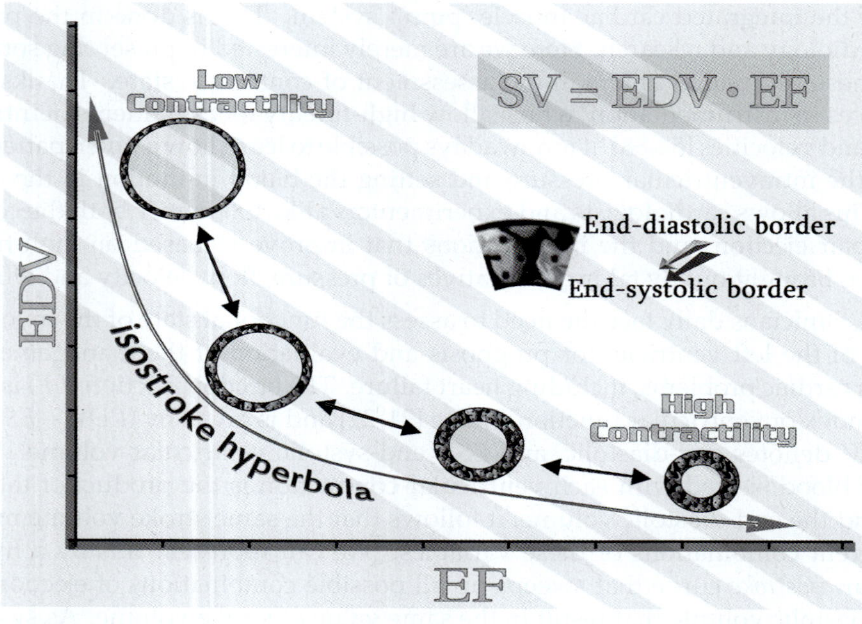

Figure 7.30: The hyperbolic relationship between the ventricular end-diastolic volume (*EDV*) and ejection fraction (*EF*), for a given stroke volume (*SV*).

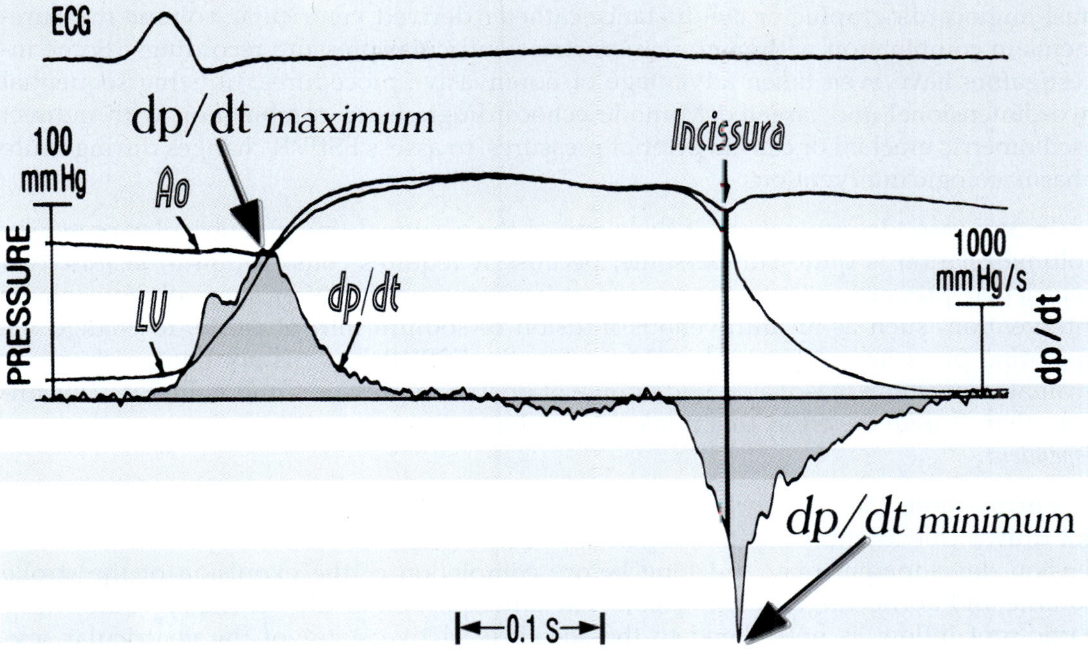

Figure 7.31: The relationships between the left ventricular (LV) and aortic root (Ao) micromanometric pressure signals obtained by multisensor catheter during elective cardiac catheterization, and the time derivative (dp/dt) obtained from the LV pressure by an analog differentiating circuit.

going from investigations of papillary muscle preparations [103] to clinical situations, one faces problems relating not only to control of dynamic conditions but to the effects of wall hypertrophy or aneurysm, valvular lesions, etc., which can underlie hemodynamic changes [76,88] not attributable to contractile state as such. Naturally then, many so-called "indices of myocardial contractility" have been proposed for clinical purposes. However, none of them can accurately measure *contractility* as an independent physiological phenomenon, or myocardial property.

The pressure-volume diagram is composed from instantaneous recordings of ventricular pressure and volume. It has been long established as a means of assessing ventricular function because it provides the interconnections between end-diastolic volume, end-systolic volume, stroke volume, and ejection fraction in a single image. The slope of an assumed to be linear left ventricular end-systolic pressure–volume relation, or ESPVR, is taken by many to be a reliable contractility index. Suga and Sagawa first proposed [138] it and designated it as *maximal LV elastance* (E_{max}). This contractility index is determined in the clinical setting by connecting, during titrated intravenous infusion of sodium nitroprusside, different LV end-systolic pressure-volume points, namely, the upper-left corners (or "shoulders") of individual pressure-volume loops. Ventricular

ESPVRs are acquired clinically by using invasive techniques; specifically, sequential contrast angiocardiographic or conductance-catheter derived ventricular volume measurements in combination with micromanometric ventricular pressure recordings. Some investigators have even taken advantage of noninvasive procedures, utilizing sequential two-dimensional and targeted M-mode echocardiograms in combination with indirect oscillometric brachial or carotid arterial pressures, to assess ESPVR changes during acute pharmacologic interventions.

In any case, determination of the slope of the assumed linear ventricular pressure–volume relation is quite cumbersome, because it requires construction of *at least* two ventricular pressure–volume loops, one at baseline and one after some pharmacologic intervention, such as an intravenous infusion of sodium nitroprusside, to change the operating pressures and volumes. Moreover, the ESPVR curve is not linear, when it is evaluated over any reasonably wide range of operating pressures and volumes. This implies that despite the effort that it takes to evaluate it properly, it is *pressure-* and *volume-dependent*.

Furthermore, *fluid dynamically and hemodynamically* it has some aspects that have not drawn due attention by its proponents. Physically, ventricular myocardial systolic tension development may end long before completion of the expulsion of the stroke volume and aortic valve closure [103]. The latter portion of the ventricular outflow, or aortic root inflow, is not related to the so-called "active state" of the ventricular myocardium [16, 17, 103]. It is due to the *momentum* that has been built-up during the *preceding phases* of systole and is carrying the blood out of the ventricle, even in the face of an *adverse* pressure gradient. The rapidity with which the adverse pressure gradient is established and its magnitude will be determined, in part, by the input impedance of the systemic and pulmonary arterial systems, for the left and right ventricles, respectively. Thus, extraventricular, specifically, *vascular* factors affect the magnitude of the stroke volume, of the end-systolic volume and, consequently, of the local slope of the ESPVR as well.

Accordingly, we will focus our main attention not to assessing the merits and defects of the various contractility indices [19], but to ventricular outflow acceleration, which has obvious fluid dynamic interest.

7.11.1 Ventricular outflow acceleration

Since the ventricle's function is to set the blood in motion, to fully understand ventricular function one will certainly need knowledge of stroke volume, as well as of the velocities and accelerations in the course of ejection. Looked at from this viewpoint, a single ejection time index of ventricular function is almost inconceivable; any single index will give evidence of only one aspect of function related to either blood displacement, velocity, or acceleration. Which of these aspects is most important will depend on the problem at hand and on how subtle are the changes that are being evaluated. The hemodynamic situation may best be explained by an analogy [88].

Suppose that one cylinder of an automobile engine is dead and the problem is to discover the resulting performance defect. Clearly, the information given by the odometer would be useless for this problem, since the car could still be driven over a long distance. Input from the speedometer would probably not reveal the weakness, since the car might still cruise at 65 *mph* on the freeway. But knowledge of acceleration will detect the weakness readily, because with one cylinder out, the pickup will certainly be impaired. From these simple considerations we can expect that ventricular dysfunction (or hyperfunction) will best be revealed by estimates of outflow *acceleration* during ejection.

Already in 1963, Rushmer et al. [122] reported that when conscious dogs, chronically instrumented with an aortic root flowmeter, were subjected to coronary occlusion, acceleration levels during ejection decreased immediately although stroke volume was maintained. In similar experiments shortly thereafter, Noble et al. [84] measured up to a 40% reduction in peak blood acceleration with no, or only minimal, stroke volume impairment. They also found that positive inotropic agents may increase peak acceleration by more than 60% from control *without* changing stroke volume.

Outflow acceleration generally attains its peak very early in the ejection phase, at a time when maybe just a few ml of blood have been injected into the aortic root (cf. Fig. 4.14, on p. 203). Inertial effects regularly dominate the ejection process in the time interval to maximum outflow acceleration, provided that there is no severe outflow tract or valve obstruction. Thus, during this time the force (f) exerted by the ventricle on the blood column that is being accelerated is

$$f = M \cdot \frac{dv}{dt}, \tag{7.5}$$

where, M is the *effective mass* of the accelerated blood column, and v is an effective blood column velocity average. Consequently,

$$\frac{dv}{dt} = \frac{f}{M}. \tag{7.6}$$

Under conditions of low end-diastolic aortic root pressure and in the absence of outflow obstruction, $\frac{dv}{dt}max$ is a useful index of myocardial force development and contractility. Note however that this index is also subject to variation with the end-diastolic volume, the "preload," which will tend to modify both the effective mass M (directly), and the ejection force f (indirectly) by the Frank–Starling response.

The peak intraventricular ejection pressure gradient, i.e., peak ejection pressure difference generated between the deep left ventricle (LV apex) and the aortic valve ring (subvalvular region) by dynamic ventricular myocardial contraction, is also related closely to the myocardial inotropic state, and, in the absence of outflow obstruction, reaches its peak very near the time of peak outflow acceleration, as is illustrated in Figure 4.14, on p. 203. It too represents a clinically sensitive index of systolic ventricular function [54, 88, 89, 101, 118, 123], and can be assessed noninvasively by postprocessing color Doppler M-mode images [163].

When assessing ejection time indices, such as ventricular outflow acceleration, one should bear in mind the implications of the inverse relation between shortening load and fiber shortening velocity and acceleration [35, 88], which is depicted diagrammatically in Figure 2.40, on p. 107. In view of this, a *negative* feedback loop is constituted between the total systolic load and the ventricular muscle fiber shortening velocity and acceleration, through the velocity and the acceleration of blood flow [14, 54, 75, 88, 94, 100, 101]. Figures 7.27 and 2.40, on pp. 370 and 107, respectively, illustrate this concept, which holds great importance for the proper evaluation of what may at times appear to be "impaired," compared to normal, acceleration and velocity patterns during ejection. Returning to the automobile analogy, for any available motor power, the pickup will depend on variables such as the car's weight and the grade and condition of the road. It has been shown [49, 54], in fact, that decreased outflow acceleration and velocity in dilated cardiomyopathy result from augmented feedback loading functions, in addition to an impaired contractile state.

In an early modern study [15], myocardial contractility was characterized using time derivatives of the left ventricular pressure signals. Power-density functions, energy-averaged power density and power-averaged rate of power-density generation were derived, in order to relate the free energy in the myocardium to systolic pressure. The phase-plane functions were shown to reflect the myocardial inotropic state and to be insensitive to volume loading. However, numerous subsequent investigations have demonstrated that the isovolumic $\frac{dP}{dt}max$, as well as the peak outflow acceleration $\frac{dQ}{dt}max$, which occurs soon after the onset of ejection, are useful but not *absolute* indices of cardiodynamic state, i.e., "myocardial contractility." The isovolumic $\frac{dP}{dt}max$ is more reliable when end-diastolic aortic root pressure is normal or high; early ejection $\frac{dQ}{dt}max$ becomes more reliable when end-diastolic aortic root pressure is low. As an extreme example, when the aortic root is clamped, outflow and outflow acceleration must fall to zero and $\frac{dQ}{dt}max$ fails, whereas $\frac{dP}{dt}max$ remains unaffected [33, 69].

Since these indices, as well as every other presently available one, are not absolute, meaning that they do not quantify contractility as an independent physiologic parameter or phenomenon, care should be taken by both clinicians and animal experimenters in using them. Under circumstances in which one of these indices is reasonably valid, it should be used in evaluating the relative effects of particular therapeutic agents on myocardial contractile state. Clearly, routine comparisons of absolute values of a given "contractility index" among different patients with dissimilar cardiac geometries and operating circulatory conditions may lead to unwarranted conclusions. Examination of the relevant literature [136] reveals several ejection phase indices of left ventricular performance and explorations of their meaning, details of their derivation, as well as specific advantages and shortcomings.

7.12 Clinically important patterns of altered cardiac cycle phase durations

Most abnormal circulatory states modify the relative duration of the cardiac cycle phases. We systematize our approach to patterns of altered phase intervals by differentiating between those arising out of abnormal myocardial contractility, and those caused mainly by other factors. The latter comprise patterns that are related to ventricular volume overload on the one hand, and to ventricular pressure overload on the other.

Volume overload states are usually associated with shortened isovolumic contraction, and prolonged ejection time. There is usually a greatly augmented $\frac{dQ}{dt}max$, and raised levels of isovolumic $\frac{dP}{dt}$, although $\frac{dP}{dt}max$ may or may not be increased. These changes are seen when there is primarily an increased ventricular "preload," associated with raised ventricular filling pressures—atrial septal defect (ASD), ruptured aneurysm of a sinus of Valsalva, etc.—or an increased ventricular diastolic filling time—complete A–V block, overdose of digitalis, etc. When the volume overload is associated with low end-diastolic aortic root pressure—patent ductus arteriosus, severe aortic regurgitation—or when there is an otherwise induced reduction of impediment to ejection—severe mitral regurgitation, early stages of a ventricular septal defect (VSD), etc.—the picture gets more complicated and unpredictable; for instance, overall $\frac{dP}{dt}$ levels and $\frac{dP}{dt}max$ may be depressed.

Pressure overload states fall into two categories:

- When the pressure overload is associated with raised end-diastolic aortic root pressure, as in systemic hypertension, they tend to be characterized by: prolonged isovolumic contraction, with possibly shortened ejection, and unchanged isovolumic overall $\frac{dP}{dt}$ levels and $\frac{dP}{dt}max$, and (greatly) depressed $\frac{dQ}{dt}max$, although the mean outflow rate may be increased.
- When the pressure overload is associated with outflow valve stenosis, there are: a prolonged ejection time with possibly abbreviated isovolumic contraction, and raised isovolumic overall $\frac{dP}{dt}$ levels and $\frac{dP}{dt}max$, with depressed $\frac{dQ}{dt}max$ as well as peak outflow rate.

The picture is more complicated in the case of a so-called "mixed" pressure overload, as exemplified by aortic coarctation: there is then both an elevation of end-diastolic aortic root pressure and an ("outflow") stenosis in a major trunk close to the aortic valve.

Augmented myocardial contractility is associated with shortened isovolumic contraction as well as ejection phases, and raised isovolumic overall $\frac{dP}{dt}$ levels and $\frac{dP}{dt}max$, with an augmented $\frac{dQ}{dt}max$ as well as peak outflow rate. Depressed contractility, as is typified in heart failure, is characterized by plolonged isovolumic contraction with an abbreviated ejection phase, and depressed isovolumic overall $\frac{dP}{dt}$ levels and $\frac{dP}{dt}max$, with a reduced $\frac{dQ}{dt}max$. Findings in individual patients with known types of predominant cardiovascular abnormalities may not conform to the patterns described here. This is attributable to counteracting effects of coexisting changes in other hemodynamic parameters, including compensatory adaptations; e.g., altered myocardial contractility in the presence of valvular disease. In fact, the encountered *inconsistency* itself may permit an assessment of the compensatory capabilities of the cardiovascular apparatus, and of the myocardium in particular. For instance, a normal isovolumic contraction time in the face of an abnormally high end-diastolic aortic root pressure, and with a normal heart size, is a strong indication of augmented isovolumic overall $\frac{dP}{dt}$ levels and $\frac{dP}{dt}max$, and implies an adequate myocardial compensation by neurohumoral compensatory mechanisms.

7.13 Fluid dynamics of cardiac valve operation

We will discuss in some detail the operation of the outflow and inflow valves of the left ventricle. No fundamentally different mechanisms enter into the operation of the corresponding valves of the right ventricular chamber.

7.13.1 Aortic valve opening

The dynamic changes that we are about to discuss can be visualized by considering an umbrella (see Fig. 7.32) whose rim is attached inside an elastic tube with an unstressed circumference that is longer than the rim, such that when a vanishingly small or no push is applied to its concave dome, the umbrella is held in its open configuration. When a significant net push is applied to its dome concavity, however, the umbrella's rim tends to collapse inward; the rim then must tug on the tube wall to which it is attached. When the net push to the dome is removed, the umbrella and the attached tube spring back into the "open" configuration.

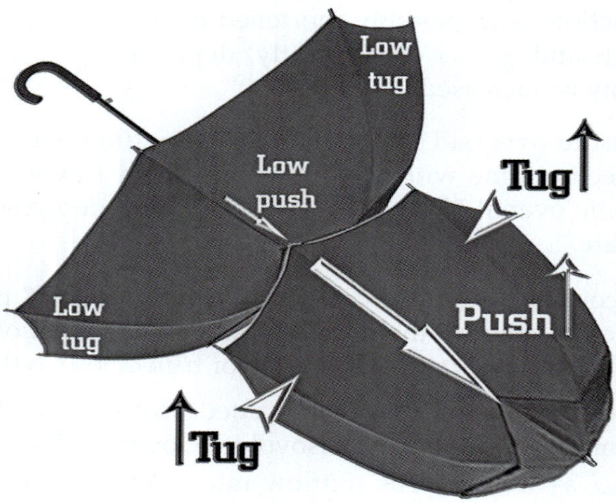

Figure 7.32: Dynamic changes illustrated by an *umbrella analogy*. When the net push on the umbrella's concave dome is high, the mechanical *interactions* between an elastic tube and the attached umbrella rim (see discussion in text) produce an *inward tug* on the tube, restraining it from dilating. As the net push on its concave dome decreases, the umbrella's rim can expand, the inward pull on the attached tube is reduced, and the tube can pop out.

In early and mid diastole, the pressure difference between the aorta and the left ventricle elicits tensile stresses on the closed valve leaflets. These stresses tug on the aortic wall at their attachments, pulling the base of the aortic root inward, toward the central portion of the aortic orifice. Additionally, the *early-* and *mid-*diastolic recoil of the aortic root walls contributes to this decrease in diameter In late diastole, the tug of the cusps on the aortic wall lessens as increasing blood volume fills the ventricle. At this time, shortly before aortic valve opening, an initial small expansion of the aortic root has been demonstrated [147]. The aortic root ascends toward the aortic arch, its walls recoiling laterally as pressure rises in the LV outflow tract. This flattens the cusps while tension across them lessens, thus diminishing overlap and apposition of their free edges. Thus, aortic root expansion induces commissure (leaflet attachment) separation, and stretching of the free edges of the elastic valve leaflets. The action of such an aortic root dilatation, which can begin leaflet opening even before any LV isovolumic contraction pressure is applied, has been confirmed recently [28,40,48]. The minimal initial opening of the aortic valve occurs without any detectable forward flow and in the absence of an elevation of aortic pressure. On account of it, the valve has an *intrinsic potential* to open.

During the phase of isovolumic[21] ventricular contraction, the aortic root pressure (P_{AR}) is higher than the pressure (P_V) on the ventricular side of the valve cusps—the transvalvular pressure difference, $\Delta P = P_V - P_{AR}$, is negative and the valve is closed. As LV pressure shoots upward, ΔP swiftly vanishes, and no tension remains within the leaflets to tug on their line of attachment to the aortic rim so as to pull the aortic root inward. The rapidly rising P_V leads to an abrupt fall in ΔP and in the pressure load stresses on the cusps, which are recoiling toward the aortic root. At the transient moment when ΔP becomes zero, the cusps cease to sustain any pressure load. Ejection practically starts as soon as ΔP becomes positive [48]; as the aortic root expands, it allows the valve to open rapidly with the onset of the main ejection surge, offering minimal interference to the outflow.

During the first part of the ejection phase proper, valve opening lags behind the aortic root flow; as the cusps are being pushed into the aortic root, blood is accelerated forward, even though the free edges of the cusps remain apposed to a large extent. The valve leaflets start to swing open only after some 8% of the total delivery time has lapsed, some 25–30 *ms* after the onset of ejection in the aortic root. By that time, the blood flow rate in the aortic root may have attained about 10–15% of its maximum value (see Fig. 7.33). The acceleration to a flow rate of, say, 30 *mL/s* (15% of a peak flow of 200 *mL/s*) is accomplished with displacement of maybe just 0.5 *mL* of blood into the root of the aorta—by the piston-like action of the forward recoiling cusps.

Figure 7.33, on p. 384, gives simultaneous plots of the time-course of valve opening and of aortic root blood flow. Representative recorded instantaneous flow rates (Q) have been normalized by dividing them by the peak outflow rate, (Q_{max}). Computed instantaneous areas (A) of the orifice bounded by the cusp free margins have been similarly normalized by dividing them by its area when the cusps are in the fully opened position (A_{max}). Although in the initial stage of the actual flow-delivery physical valve opening *lags* behind the aortic root flow rate, the cusps are subsequently swung into the fully opened position *before* the peak outflow rate is attained; complete opening precedes peak flow by, say, 50 *ms*. This slight delay in reaching Q_{max} must be attributed to the inertia of the accelerated blood column. The normal valve—and the small quantity of blood in its

---

[21] In view of the discussion in Section 7.5.7, on pp. 348 ff., this phase might best be denoted as pre-ejection time, or PET.

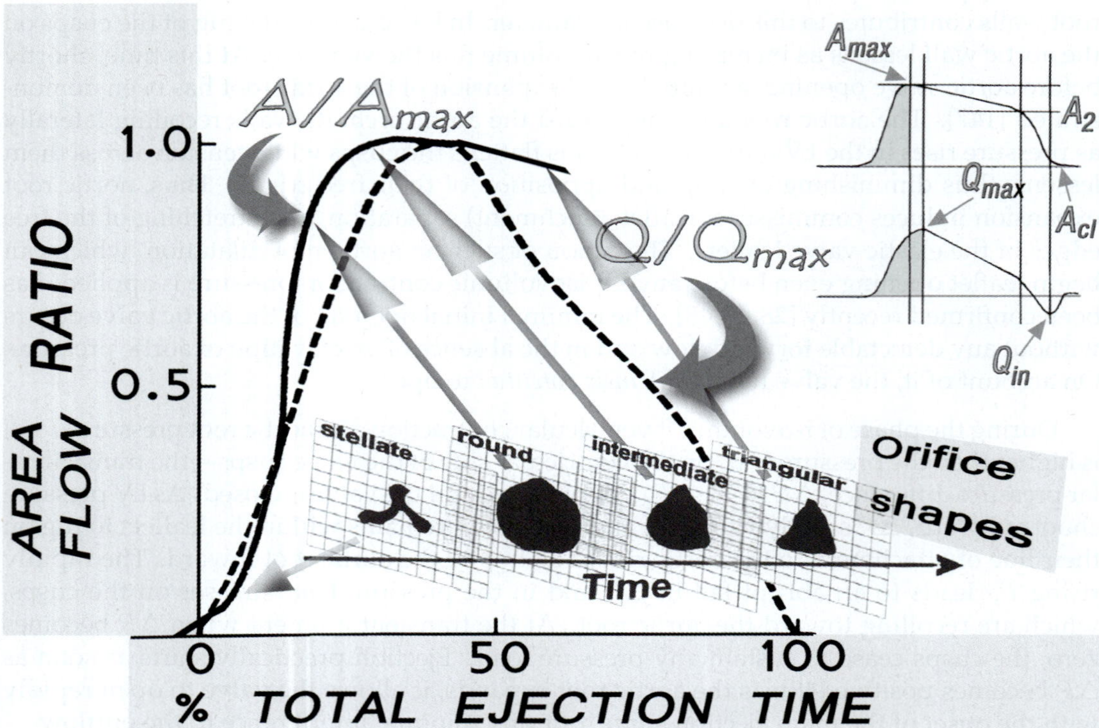

Figure 7.33: Schematic representation of the temporal relations between aortic root flow (Q) and aortic valve opening area (A)—both normalized to their peak (max) values—and the configuration of the aortic valve orifice under normal conditions, where $t = 0$ coincides with the onset of the ejection upstroke of the aortic flow. A_2: consistently present inflection point of the descending limb of $A(t)$; Q_{in}: peak of incisural backflow. [Composite drawing based on occasionally conflicting details—related to small electronic circuitry delays involving velocimetric signals, which were uncorrected in the original publications—from several sources [40, 43, 48, 52, 80, 121, 135, 141, 142, 146, 147]].

immediate vicinity that becomes displaced during opening—has negligible inertia, and normally offers negligible opposition to flow throughout ejection. The onset of maximum valve opening always precedes the onset of peak aortic root flow.

Figure 7.34, on p. 385, shows the buckling, whipping motion of a cusp with normal starting contour, in the opening process toward maximum valve opening.[22] Approximately

[22] Bending stresses arise during this motion and are important functionally because they are associated with structural fatigue of normal and prosthetic valve leaflets. Bending stresses arise from the motion of the valve cusps during the cardiac cycle [148]. During bending, individual constituents may experience compression or tension, contingent on their position within the leaflet. Bending creates internal shear as the valve leaflet tissues are deformed. Two modes of bending occur in a leaflet: First, the belly of the leaflet undergoes a reversal of its curvature during opening and closing. Second, the attachment zone acts as a hinge during leaflet motion.

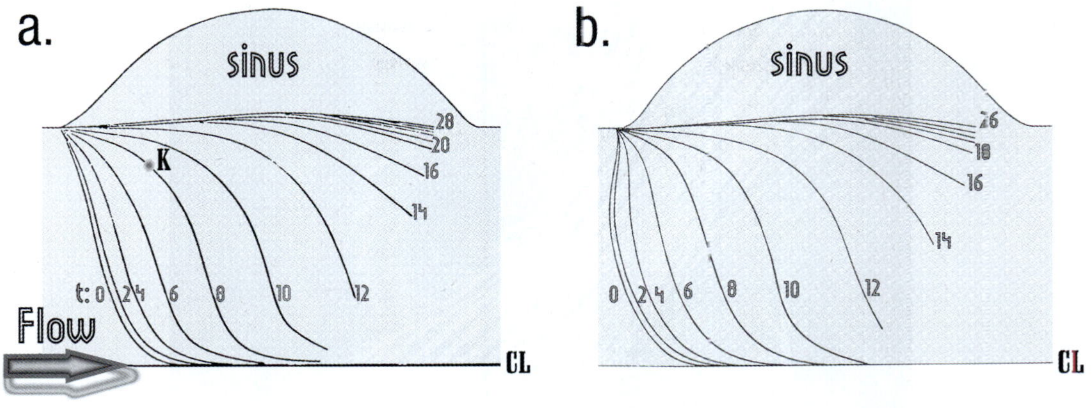

Figure 7.34: Diagramatic representation of approximate aortic cusp contours under normal conditions (a.) and after loss of normal precurved shape (b.), at successive times (t) during valve opening, expressed as percent of total ejection flow time, where $t = 0$ coincides with the onset of the ejection upstroke of the aortic root flow. Point K is the point of maximum curvature of the normally precurved cusp. (Redrawn from Swanson and Clark [141] with kind permission of the Am. Heart Assoc.)

computed (numerical-graphical fluid dynamic solution) cusp contours in a longitudinal diametral plane that bisects one sinus are plotted for 28 successive and equal time-increments. The contour $t = 0$ corresponds to the instant at which blood and cusp displacement is just about to start; $t = 28$ coincides with the instant at which the valve first attains the fully opened position (after 28% of the total delivery time, for which $t = 100\%$, has lapsed). Point K in this representation is the point of maximum curvature and thus of maximum bending stress on the cusp; another large curvature point is near the centerline where mutual coaptation of the cusps takes place. As illustrated in the diagram, there is a large change in curvature at K during opening of the cusp, but this change is normally less than the maximum curvature at K, because of the normally *precurved* shape of the cusp. For any point on the cusp, the operating bending stress is determined to a greater extent by the *change* in curvature from the starting to the maximum value, than by the maximum curvature itself.

7.13.2 Aortic valve closure

Just after the aortic valve area attains its maximum, it starts to decrease slowly toward valve closure. The initial decrease in area ($A_{max} - A_2$ slope, in the inset of Fig. 7.33, on p. 384) is slow ($4{-}5\,cm^2/s$), and the late decrease in area ($A_2 - A_{cl}$ slope) is faster ($25{-}30\,cm^2/s$) [48]. The inflection point, A_2, of the descending limb of $A(t)$ is a constant phenomenon [160] persisting in every beat. It is a striking fact that the stage is set for aortic valve closure while the cusps are *being swung out* into their fully opened position.

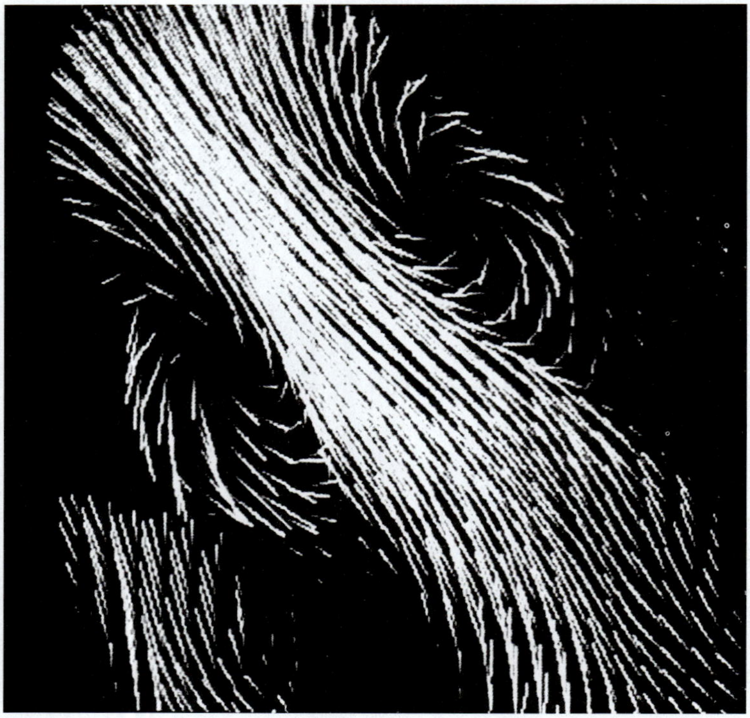

Figure 7.35: Ejection flow through the aortic valve region, mapped by magnetic resonance. This is a late systolic vector map, located through the two coronary cusp sinuses. It shows recirculating vortical flows within the sinuses of Valsalva, which contribute to efficient valve closure at end systole. (From Kilner et al. [60], with kind permission of the authors and the Am. Heart Assoc.)

In less than one-third of the ejection time they attain this position, and tend to overshoot it and to swing into the sinuses of Valsalva. The flow streamline along each cusp strikes the corresponding sinus ridge and is split into two parts: one part curls back into the sinus, generating a vortex that persists through ejection (see Fig. 7.35, and Fig. 7.36a. on p. 387); the other part flows along the aortic wall beyond the ridge.

During peak and nearly peak flow, the thrust exerted by the vortex that is trapped in the sinus maintains the corresponding cusp in a stable position, almost flush with the sinus ridge (see Fig. 7.36a). Subsequently, as the outflow decelerates, the thrust exerted by the persisting vortex on the sinus side of the cusp combines with the locally reversed pressure gradient to push the leaflet away from the sinus wall; the valve starts to close (see Fig. 7.36b.). As the aortic root outflow rate decelerates further, the effective instantaneous pressure difference between the sinus cavity and the aortic valve ring becomes even more *positive*, i.e., pressure is *increasing* distally to the valve ring. Under this pressure difference that promotes closure, the cusps move toward their closed position; they attain more than three-quarters of valve closure by the last stage of ejection. The persistence of the sinus vortices is responsible for the prevention of jet formation as the cusps

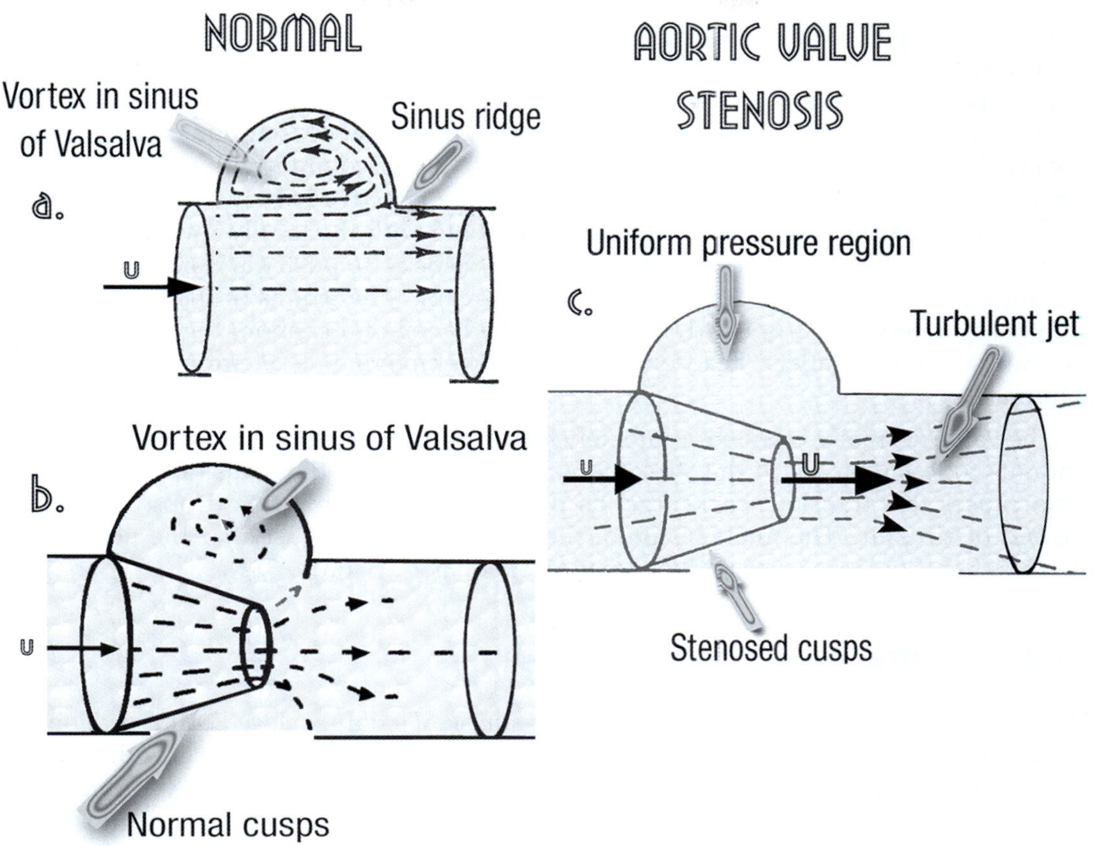

Figure 7.36: Schematic representation of vortical contribution to aortic valve closing. a. Under normal conditions, vortices form in the sinuses of Valsalva as some ejection flow strikes the middle of each sinus ridge, is deflected, enters the sinus and curls back into a recirculating pattern before exiting to join the main flow in the vicinity of the commissures. b. Streamline pattern with the valve about three-quarters into the closing process. The normal cusps approximate the curved surface shape of a truncated cone. c. Streamline pattern in a stenosed aortic valve; there is no vortical flow in the sinuses. In the region outside the turbulent jet, and including the sinuses, the pressure is approximately uniform. The velocity at the stenosed orifice is greatly increased, with a corresponding drop in pressure by the unsteady Bernoulli equation. The pressure at the coronary ostia is consequently lowered and retrograde systolic coronary flow is likely, by a venturi effect. (Redrawn slightly modified after Bellhouse et al. [11, 13], with kind permission of the authors, the Am. Heart Assoc., and CUP.)

close, and for the maintenance of a positive difference between the sinus cavity and the aortic ring pressures, which closes the cusps during the last stage of the ejection phase.

A heretofore overlooked closure mechanism may also be conceived as follows (see Section 7.6, on pp. 358 ff.): During ejection, as blood is pushed into the ascending aorta toward the head, muscular histoarchitectonic and contraction patterns act with fluid dynamic mechanisms to produce a descent of the base that contains the aortic anulus. The *ascent* of the anulus in the later stages of ejection should push the semilunar valve leaflets toward closure as they encounter the "oncoming" blood column within the ascending aorta. All that this mechanism would require to be effective is that the thrust exerted by the vortex on the sinus side of the cusps combine with the locally reversed pressure gradient during the downstroke of the aortic root velocity, to push the leaflets away from the sinus wall and into the "oncoming" blood stream. The trunks of the aorta and the pulmonary artery recoil upward, in fact, like the barrel of a cannon, tugging along the attached semilunar leaflets "head-on" onto the slower moving, decelerating central blood column.

The valve normally is sealed completely by a backsurge of blood (flow *incisura*), which amounts to less than 5% of the stroke volume. The recoil of the walls of the ascending aorta causes this transient backsurge, as the aortic root inflow rate drops abruptly at the end of ejection. The final closure of the valve is achieved just after the peak of the incisural backflow (see upper right corner inset of Fig. 7.33, on p. 384).

7.13.3 Mitral valve operation

The mitral valve cusps take less than 100 *ms* to supplant a tightly closed configuration, capable of withstanding the high atrioventricular systolic pressure difference, with a widely open arrangement, allowing the copious surge of normal early diastolic ventricular inflow (see Fig. 7.14, on p. 345). In fact, blood displacement into the ventricle begins before the mitral valve starts to open physically; the situation is akin, in part, to that described earlier for the aortic valve. The mitral cusps swing into their fully opened position very early in the rapid filling phase and mitral inflow may begin before leaflet separation [63].

Recent videofluorographic studies of the mitral leaflets and anulus in sheep, using radiopaque markers, have shown that all annular and leaflet structures start moving toward their open configuration during the rapid intraventricular pressure decay [59]. However, leaflet edge separation with valve opening in the physical sense does not occur until the left ventricular micromanometric pressure is nearly at its early diastolic *nadir*. Thus, leaflet edge separation is the last event in a cascade of changes involving the mitral valvular and subvalvular apparatus during the rapid fall of intraventricular pressure. Although physical valve opening lags behind flow in the earliest stage, peak flow is attained a few *cs* after complete valve opening.

In the fully opened position, the mitral cusps form a conical canal whose outlet orifice lies at an *oblique* plane to the mitral valve ring. During ventricular filling, two stable (laminar) surges pour into the ventricle via this canal, in more or less rapid succession depending on the heart rate, as is shown in Figures 7.10, 7.12, and 7.14 on pp. 340, 343

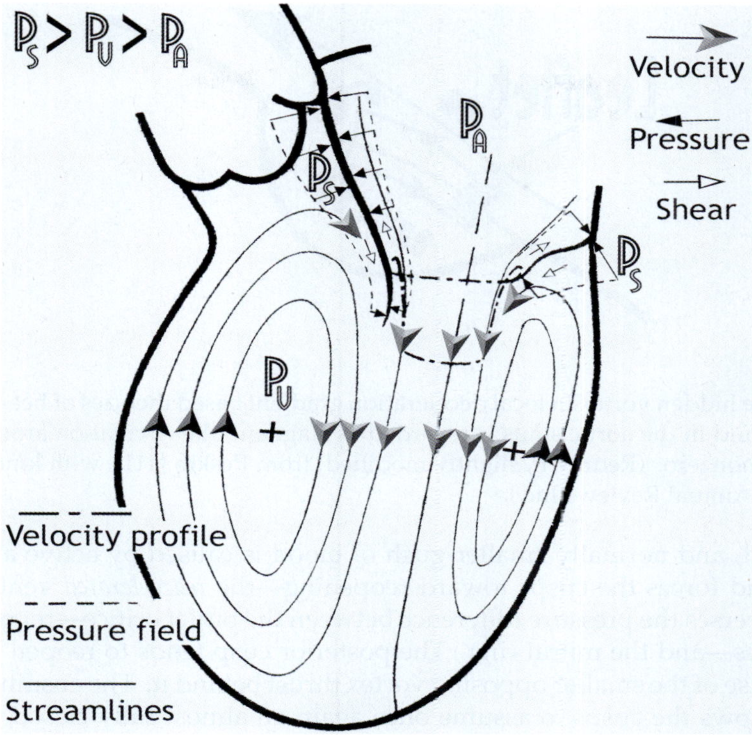

Figure 7.37: Forces causing mitral valve leaflet closure under an adverse atrioventricular pressure gradient. (Redrawn, slightly modified, from Reul et al. [120], with kind permission of the authors and Pergamon/Elsevier.)

and 345, respectively. The first and normally major gush corresponds to the *rapid filling phase*: the inflowing stream strikes the wall beyond the outlet orifice and spreads out to flow up the septal and lateral walls toward the base. There it curls again and flows behind the cusps toward the apex. A ring vortex, akin to a familiar smoke ring, is thus formed between the cusps and the expanding ventricular walls (cf. Fig. 7.37). This vortex is asymmetrical, being wider behind the posterolateral leaflet. The swirling motion is more vigorous behind the anterior cusp because of the smaller space between it and the wall (see Section 2.8, on pp. 59 f.).

Since the thrust exerted by the vortex on the anterior cusp is greater than that exerted on the posterior one, the anterior cusp is pushed toward the closed position earlier and faster than the posterior. As the inflow begins to *decelerate* after it has attained its peak value, the unsteady pressure at the outlet orifice formed by the cusp free edges exceeds that at the mitral ring. This strongly reinforces the optimizing action of the trapped vortex in pushing the cusps toward closure even while some *forward* flow persists, before the end of the filling phase. These effects are conceptually similar to those described in connection with aortic valve closure.

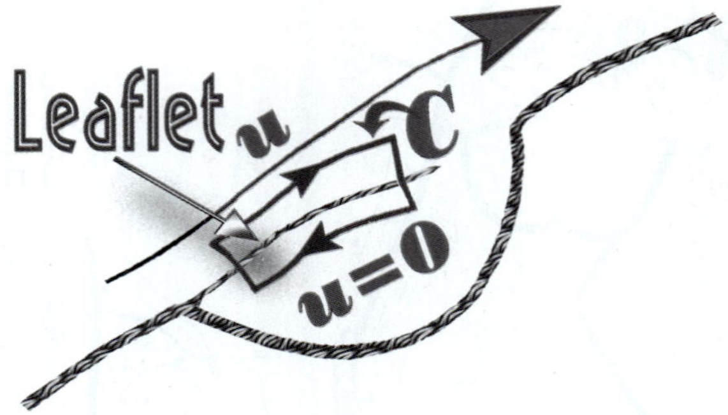

Figure 7.38: The hidden vortex in local deceleration gradient based theories of heart-valve closure. Although the fluid in the aortic sinus is regarded as stagnant, the circulation around the contour C is obviously nonzero. (Redrawn, slightly modified, from Peskin [111], with kind permission of the author and Annual Reviews Inc.)

The second, and normally smaller gush of blood is caused by active atrial muscular contraction and forces the cusps toward reopening—the *reaccelerated* ventricular inflow transiently reverses the pressure difference between the outlet orifice—represented by the cusp free edges—and the mitral ring. The posterior cusp tends to reopen more than the anterior because of the smaller opposing vortex thrust behind it. The ensuing deceleration of the flow allows the cusps to assume once again an almost fully closed position *before* the onset of the following ventricular myocardial contraction. As in the case of the aortic valve, normally negligible or no flow reversal is needed to seal off the valve completely.

Some theories of valve closure, going back to Leonardo as we saw in Chapter 3—see Section 3.3, on pp. 119 ff.—are founded on vortex dynamics: Leonardo believed that cardiac valves are closed during forward flow by the "revolving impetus" of a vortex that forms behind the valve leaflets. Other theories, namely Henderson and Johnson's alternative "breaking of the jet" theory [46], do not appear to contain a vortex at all. The concept underlying the latter theory is simply that during flow deceleration the jet of transvalvular flow is *broken*, and the surrounding fluid rushing in from the sides to fill the incipient gap then closes the valve leaflets. Bellhouse [10] is the main modern-day proponent of the central role played by large scale vortical motions in mitral and aortic valve closure; Reul et al. [120] have disputed this and emphasized the role played by local deceleration of the flow and the adverse axial pressure gradient that accompanies it.

Charles Peskin, the pioneer mathematical biofluiddynamicist, has noted [111] that there is a vortex hidden in all of the theories of valve closure, even where it is not explicitly invoked. Such theories assume a stagnant, constant-pressure region behind the valve leaflets. Consider the two-dimensional contour C that encompasses a valve leaflet, as is shown in Figure 7.38. The circulation around this contour is clearly nonzero; therefore, there is vorticity concentrated along the valve leaflets themselves. Fundamentally, a valve is an irreversible machine. As such, viscosity must play an essential role in its operation. The generation of vorticity at boundaries by the viscous shear forces is the irreversible process that is needed for efficient valve closure. In fact, vorticity is essential for deceleration to achieve cardiac valve closure. To see this, consider the alternative, namely, a *potential* flow (see Section 4.12, on pp. 208 ff.). Under a potential flow regime, the valve would keep opening for as long as forward flow was maintained. Indeed, for the potential flow to close the valve it would have to reverse its motion and *undo* what was accomplished during the forward flow phase. The net transvalvular flow volume in that hypothetical case would have to be *zero*. This follows from the *reversibility* properties (see Section 4.7.1, on p. 193) of potential flow.

The chordae tendineae-papillary muscle apparatus prevents marked prolapse, and possible eversion, of the cusps during ventricular contraction. Papillary muscle shortening and shrinkage of the mitral valve ring circumference and area during ventricular systolic emptying, assure no excessive prolapse and no regurgitation. When the mitral ring is calcified, the circumference and the area of the mitral orifice are not reduced during ventricular systole, and mild degrees of regurgitation may ensue.

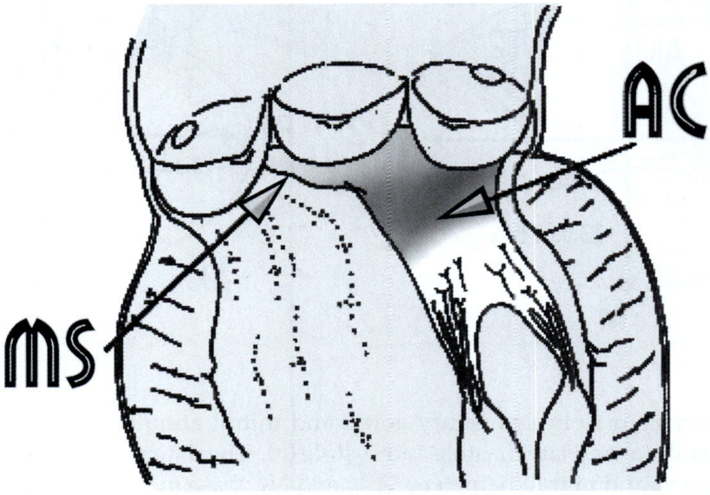

Figure 7.39: Anatomy of the aortic valve and LV outflow tract, opened through a commissure between right and left coronary cusps. The aortic and mitral valves share the so-called aortic curtain. This is fibrous tissue, anchored to the two trigones, and situated immediately below the left and the noncoronary aortic leaflets; it is in continuity with the anterior leaflet of the mitral valve. MS = membranous septum; AC = aortic curtain. (Slightly modified from Yacoub et al. [161], with kind permission of the authors and The Society of Thoracic Surgeons.)

7.14 Reciprocal transformations of mitral and aortic rings

In the foregoing sections, the aortic and mitral valves have been considered as two separate entities and studied independently, as if their operations were disconnected. Anatomically, both valves are situated in the common "roof" of the left ventricular chamber (see Fig. 7.25, on p. 366), and are separated by the aortic curtain anchored to the two fibrous trigones. Superiorly, the aortic curtain is part of the aortic root anulus, and inferiorly, it is in continuity with the anterior leaflet of the mitral valve (see Fig. 7.39, on p. 391). Both the mitral intertrigonal distance and the aortic curtain are a common structure or *mitroaortic junction* [64]. Through it, mitral anulus deformation is intimately related to aortic root dynamics, and *vice versa*. Because of this and because the mitral and aortic valves share a common myocardial pump, both valves not only work in a *coordinated* mode but must also *contribute* to each other's geometric transformations.

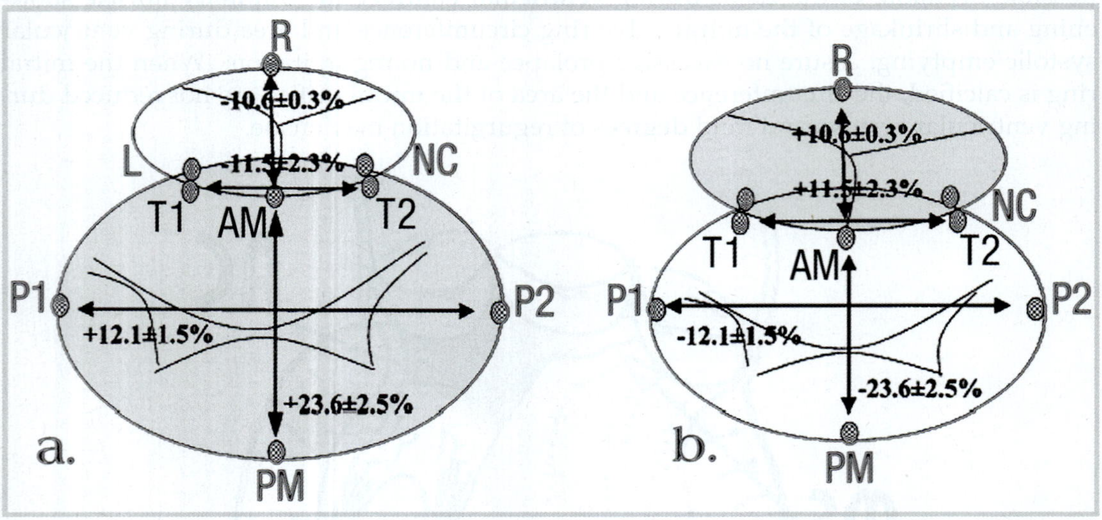

Figure 7.40: Summary of complementary aortic and mitral annular dimension changes which occur in early diastole (a) and late diastole and systole (b). The diagrams show the increase (+) and reduction (−) in aortic and mitral diameters. R, L, and NC: base of the right, left, and noncoronary sinuses of Valsalva; T1 and T2: left and right fibrous trigones; AM: midpoint between T1 and T2; PM: midpoint of posterior arch of mitral anulus; P1 and P2: widest mitral anulus diameter. Placement of the sonomicrometric crystals used for the cyclic length change measurements is also shown. (Redrawn from Lansac et al. [64] with kind permission of the authors and The American Association for Thoracic Surgery.)

The aortic root is a dynamic structure that expands during ejection to reduce shear stress on the aortic leaflets. Mitral anulus reduction has been traditionally related to its posterior contraction, whereas its anterior portion or intertrigonal distance remains fixed. Recent investigations [64] have demonstrated alternating complementary adjustments in the size and configuration of the mitral anulus and the aortic root. Analysis of the combined data from the aortic and mitral annular movements revealed their *complementary synchronicity*, as is clearly shown in Figure 7.40, on this page.

During ejection, the posterior movement of the aortic curtain allows for aortic root expansion, conducive to maximizing ejection, whereas during diastolic LV inflow, aortic root reduction is complementary to mitral anulus dilatation. During early diastole, the mitral anulus is expanded, whereas the mitroaortic junction recoils. Maximal expansion of the mitral anulus area occurs during mid-diastole. During late diastole and systole, the aortic base and the mitroaortic junction spread out while the remaining mitral anulus grows smaller. The minimal annular area comes about during the second half of ejection.

This is a very efficient coordinated mechanism to enhance ventricular filling and emptying. These functional anatomic findings should affect mitral and aortic *surgical* approaches. Correct function of one valve depends on the integrity of the other, and consequently, surgical interference with one must take into account its repercussions on the other. Mitral or aortic valve replacement with a *rigid* prosthesis must significantly *interfere* with the normal movements of the other valve. If the valve is repaired, insertion of a rigid annuloplasty ring that immobilizes not only the posterior mitral anulus but also the aortic curtain must interfere with aortic valve dynamics [64, 161].

7.15 Pathophysiology and fluid dynamics of cardiac valves

7.15.1 Functional mitral insufficiency

As we have seen, the diastolic vortex motion is less vigorous and the thrust exerted on the mural aspect of each cusp is smaller when the space in which the vortex is trapped is larger [10, 12]. Therefore, any abnormal left ventricular dilatation reduces the vortex strength behind both of the mitral cusps, and the valve is no longer almost fully closed before the onset of ventricular contraction: a functional insufficiency results. The ventricular diastolic filling vortex is dissipated by the action of blood viscosity, a process that requires a finite time interval. From dimensional analysis, the vortex would form convectively in a time of order L/U, where L and U are a characteristic ventricular length and velocity, respectively. To decay by viscous action, the ventricular vortex would take a time of order L^2/ν, where L is the characteristic ventricular chamber length and ν is the kinematic viscosity of blood. If the vortex is to form early in diastole and to then persist throughout diastole, the vortex formation time must be *short* and the decay time very *long* compared with the duration of diastole. If atrial systole is weak or absent (atrial fibrillation), and if there is also a protracted interval of slow filling, as occurs with abnormally slow heart rates, viscous dissipation may have enough time to effectively destroy the vortex. Again, the cusps will no longer be in the almost fully apposed position before the onset of ventricular contraction, and a functional insufficiency may result.

Note that the constellation of an enlarged left ventricle, atrial fibrillation, and slow average heart rate—possibly complicated by polycythemia and increased viscosity—is associated not only with functional mitral regurgitation, but also with a propensity toward mural thrombus formation (see also the discussion in Chapter 14, Section 14.15, on pp. 791 ff.).

7.15.2 Functional coronary insufficiency

Severe aortic valvular stenosis prevents vortex formation in the sinuses of Valsalva: the flow streamline along each cusp no longer strikes the sinus ridge, so that no part of it *curls into* the corresponding sinus (Fig. 7.36c. on p. 387). The turbulent systolic jet emerging from the stenotic orifice formed by the free margins of the aortic valve cusps induces, by the venturi effect (see Section 7.3, on pp. 329 ff.), a rather *uniformly distributed* low pressure in the region between the sinus walls and the cusps. By this venturi action, pressure in this annular region surrounding the jet gets depressed the most during the *peak* of systolic ejection, when $\frac{\rho v^2}{2}$ is highest. Consequently, the pressure at the coronary ostia within the sinuses of Valsalva may be lowered quite substantially during ejection, whose duration is *prolonged* in aortic valvular stenosis.

The preceding fluid dynamic factors may cause the effective systolic values of the pressure difference between the coronary ostia and the subepicardial coronary arteries to attain high negative magnitudes, especially when the cardiac output is augmented, intensifying the venturi effect. This is quite a drastic change from the normal situation in which the mean systolic pressure difference is positive, albeit low, and tends to rise with the cardiac output—an early *systolic* coronary inflow surge into the subepicardial coronary arteries is well known to occur [152], especially during exercise and high cardiac output states. Aortic valvular stenosis may therefore impede systolic coronary inflow during exertion, and may even induce abnormal *blood suction* out of the subepicardial coronaries during the ejection phase [11, 13]. This may well be a fluid dynamic reason for the syndrome of *angina on exertion*, which is a frequent complication of severe aortic stenosis with jet formation.[23]

7.15.3 Fatigue of semilunar cusps

When the aortic valve cusps lose their normally precurved shape and assume an overall convex (bulging) "closed-position" shape, a greater change in curvature and greater bending stresses are associated with the opening motion (see Fig. 7.34, on p. 385). Weakened cusps may have convex starting contours bulging toward the ventricle. Their maximum bending stress during the whip-like opening motion may amount to over two times the normally exerted stress. They are, therefore, subject to a vicious-circle process and to progressive deterioration—e.g., trileaflet prosthetic valve failure [141] in the region of point K, which is defined pictorially in Figure 7.34.

7.15.4 Arteriosclerosis and aortic root stiffening

Under normal resting conditions, the effective valve orifice area inside a stiff aortic root is not very different compared to a compliant one [133]; in fact, inside a stiff root it may

[23] Furthermore, LV hypertrophy and a rise in diastolic volume levels compensate for the raised systolic load [75, 98]. These adjustments raise subendocardial wall stresses and the mural component (intramural vessel compression) of coronary resistance, which further worsens perfusion reserves [75, 98, 152].

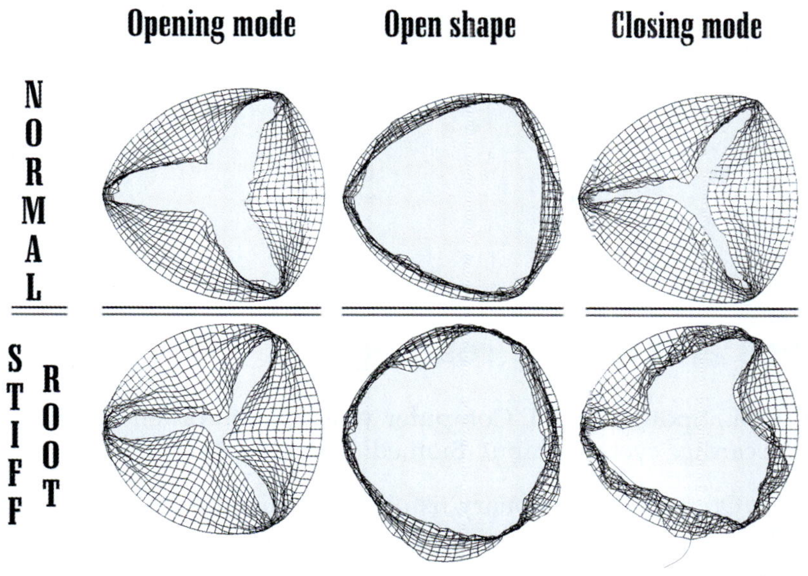

Figure 7.41: The opening and closing of the aortic valve leaflets inside a normal root and a stiff root. (Redrawn from Sripathi et al. [133] with kind permission of the authors and The Society of Thoracic Surgeons.)

be slightly higher because of the absence of triangulation of the orifice (see Fig. 7.41). A compliant aortic root contributes substantially to rapid, smooth and symmetrical leaflet opening with minimal gradients. In contrast, the leaflet opening inside a stiff root is delayed, asymmetric, and *"wrinkled."* Most importantly, normal aortic root compliance also contributes to the ability of the aortic valve to increase its effective valve orifice area in response to increased cardiac output demands, such as the physiologic demands of exercise [133]. In compliant roots, the effective orifice area can substantially increase in response to increased root pressure and transvalvular gradients. This subtle but important physiologic adjustment (cf. Murray's law discussion in Section 1.9, on pp. 20 ff.) is strikingly absent in the setting of a stiffened aortic root.

References and further reading

[1] Ahmad, R.M., Spotnitz, H.M. Computer visualization of left ventricular geometry during the cardiac cycle. Comput. Biomed. Res. 25: 201–11, 1992.

[2] Angelini, P. Questions on coronary fistulae and microfistulae. Tex. Heart Inst. J. 32: 53–5, 2005.

[3] Appleton, C.F., Hatle, L.K., Popp, R.L. Relation of transmitral flow velocity patterns to left ventricular diastolic function: New insights from a combined hemodynamic and Doppler echocardiographic study. J. Am. Coll. Cardiol. 12: 426–40, 1988.

[4] Ashikaga, H., Coppola, B.A., Yamazaki, K.G., Villarreal, F.J., Omens, J.H., Covell, J.W. Changes in regional myocardial volume during the cardiac cycle: implications for transmural blood flow and cardiac structure. Am. J. Physiol. Heart Circ. Physiol. 295: H610–18, 2008.

[5] Axel, L. Papillary muscles do not attach directly to the solid heart wall. Circulation 109: 3145–8, 2004.

[6] Baccani, B., Domenichini, F., Pedrizzetti, G., Tonti, G. Fluid dynamics of the left ventricular filling in dilated cardiomyopathy. J. Biomech. 35: 665–71, 2002.

[7] Barbetseas, J., Alexopoulos, N., Brili, S., Aggeli, C., Marinakis, N., Vlachopoulos, C., Vyssoulis, G., Stefanadis, C. Changes in aortic root function after valve replacement in patients with aortic stenosis. Int. J. Cardiol. 110: 74–9, 2006.

[8] Baumhakel, M., Janzen, I., Kindermann, M., Schneider, G., Hennen, B., Bohm, M. Images in cardiovascular medicine. Cardiac imaging in isolated noncompaction of ventricular myocardium. Circulation 106: e16–17, 2002.

[9] Becker, A.E., de Wit, A.P.M. The mitral valve apparatus: a spectrum of normality relevant to mitral valve prolapse. Br. Heart J. 42: 680–9, 1980.

[10] Bellhouse, B.J. Fluid mechanics of a model mitral valve and left ventricle. Cardiovasc. Res. 6: 199–210, 1970.

[11] Bellhouse, B., Bellhouse, F. Fluid mechanics of model normal and stenosed aortic valves. Circ. Res. 25: 693–704, 1969.

[12] Bellhouse, B.J., Bellhouse, F.H. Fluid mechanics of the mitral valve. Nature 224: 615–16, 1969.

[13] Bellhouse, B., Talbot, L. The fluid mechanics of the aortic valve. J. Fluid Mech. 35: 721–35, 1969.

[14] Bird, J.J., Murgo, J.P., Pasipoularides, A. Fluid dynamics of aortic stenosis: Subvalvular gradients without subvalvular obstruction. Circulation 66: 835–40, 1982.

[15] Bloomfield, M.E., Gold, L.D., Reddy, R.V., Katz, A.I., Moreno, A.H. Thermodynamic characterization of the contractile state of the myocardium. Circ. Res. 30: 520–34, 1972.

[16] Brady, A.J. Time and displacement dependence of cardiac contractility: problems in defining the active state and force–velocity relations. Fed. Proc. 24: 1410–20, 1965.

[17] Brady, A.J. A measurement of the active state in heart muscle. Cardiovasc. Res. 1: Suppl. 1: 1–7, 1971.

[18] Brutsaert, D.L., Sys, S.U. Relaxation and diastole of the heart. Physiol. Rev. 69: 1228–315, 1989.

[19] Burkhoff, D., Mirsky, I., Suga, H. Assessment of systolic and diastolic ventricular properties via pressure-volume analysis: a guide for clinical, translational, and basic researchers. Am. J. Physiol. Heart Circ. Physiol. 289: H501–12, 2005.

[20] Caldini, P., Permutt, S., Waddell, J.A., Riley, R.L. Effect of epinephrine on pressure, flow, and volume relationships in the systemic circulation of dogs. Circ. Res. 34: 606–23, 1974.

[21] Carabello, B.A. Cardiologists: do we have the right to call ourselves physiologists? [Editorial]. J. Am. Coll. Cardiol. Img. 1: 12–4, 2008.

[22] Carabello, B.A. Evolution of the study of left ventricular function: everything old is new again [Editorial]. Circulation 105: 2701–3, 2002.

[23] Carlhäll, C., Wigström, L., Heiberg, E., Karlsson, M., Bolger, A.F., Nylander, E. Contribution of mitral annular excursion and shape dynamics to total left ventricular volume change. Am. J. Physiol. Heart Circ. Physiol. 287: H1836–41, 2004.

[24] Chadwick, R.S., Tedgui, A., Michel, J.B., Ohayon, J., Levy, B.I. Phasic regional myocardial inflow and outflow: comparison of theory and experiments. Am. J. Physiol. Heart Circ. Physiol. 258: H1687–98, 1990.

[25] Coleman, T.G., Manning, R.D., Jr., Norman, R.A., Jr., Guyton, A.C. Control of cardiac output by regional blood flow distribution. Ann. Biomed. Eng. 2: 149–63, 1974.

[26] Condos, W.R., Jr., Latham, RD., Hoadley, S.D., Pasipoularides, A. Hemodynamics of the Mueller maneuver in man: Right and left heart micromanometry and Doppler echocardiography. Circulation 76: 1020–8, 1987.

[27] Craig, W.E., Murgo, J.P., Pasipoularides, A. Calculation of the time constant of relaxation. In: Grossman, W., Lorell, B. [Eds.] Diastolic Relaxation of the Heart. 1987, The Hague, Holland: Martinus Nijhoff. pp. 125–32.

[28] Dagum, P., Green, R., Nistal, F.J., Daughters, G.T., Timek, T.A., Foppiano, L.E., Bolger, A.F., Ingels, N.B., Miller, D.C. Deformational dynamics of the aortic root: modes and physiologic determinants. Circulation 100 Suppl II: II-54–II-62, 1999.

[29] De Hart, J., Peters, G.W.M., Schreurs, P.J.G., Baaijens, F.P.T. A three-dimensional computational analysis of fluid–structure interaction in the aortic valve. J. Biomech. 36: 103–12, 2003.

[30] DeMaria, A.N., Wisenbaugh, T. Identification and treatment of diastolic dysfunction: Role of trans-mural Doppler recordings. J. Am. Coll. Cardiol. 9: 1106–7, 1987.

[31] Devereux, R.B. Toward a more complete understanding of left ventricular afterload. J. Am. Coll. Cardiol. 17: 122–4, 1991.

[32] Dietz, J.R. Mechanisms of atrial natriuretic peptide secretion from the atrium. Cardiovasc. Res. 68: 8–17, 2005.

[33] Forwand, S.A., McIntyre, K.M., Lipana, J.G., Levine, H.J. Active stiffness of the intact canine left ventricle. With observations on the effect of acute and chronic myocardial infarction. Circ. Res. 19: 970–9, 1966.

[34] Galiuto, L., Ignone, G., DeMaria, A.N. Contraction and relaxation velocities of the normal left ventricle using pulsed-wave tissue Doppler echocardiography. Am. J. Cardiol. 81: 609–14, 1998.

[35] Gault, J.H., Ross, J., Jr., Braunwald, E. Contractile state of the left ventricle in man. Circ. Res. 22: 451–63, 1968.

[36] Gelpi, R.J., Pasipoularides, A., Lader, A.S., Patric, T.A., Chase, N., Hittinger, L., Shannon, R.P., Bishop, S.P., Vatner, S.F. Changes in diastolic cardiac function in developing and stable perinephritic hypertension in conscious dogs. Circ. Res. 68: 555–67, 1991.

[37] Georgiadis, J.G., Wang, M., Pasipoularides, A. Computational fluid dynamics of left ventricular ejection. Ann. Biomed. Eng. 20: 81–97, 1992.

[38] Gilbert, J.C., Glantz, S.A. Determinants of left ventricular filling and of the diastolic pressure-volume relation. Circ. Res. 64: 827–52, 1989.

[39] Glantz, S.A., Parmley, W.W. Factors which affect the diastolic pressure–volume curve. Circ. Res. 42: 171–80, 1978.

[40] Gnyaneshwar, R., Kumar, R.K., Komarakshi, R.B. Dynamic analysis of the aortic valve using a finite element model. Ann. Thorac. Surg. 73: 1122–9, 2002.

[41] Goetz, W.A., Lansac, E., Lim, H.S., Weber, P.A., Duran, C.M. Left ventricular endocardial longitudinal and transverse changes during isovolumic contraction and relaxation: a challenge. Am. J. Physiol. Heart Circ. Physiol. 289: H196–201, 2005.

[42] Hamilton, W.F., Rompf, J.H. Movements of the base of the ventricle and relative constancy of the cardiac volume. Am. J. Physiol. 102: 559–65, 1932.

[43] Handke, M., Heinrichs, G., Beyersdorf, F., Olschewski, M., Bode, C., Geibel, A. In vivo analysis of aortic valve dynamics by transesophageal 3-dimensional echocardiography with high temporal resolution. J. Thorac. Cardiovasc. Surg. 125: 1412–19, 2003.

[44] Hasegawa, H., Little, W.C., Ohno, M., Brucks, S., Morimoto, A., Cheng, H.J., Cheng, C.P. Diastolic mitral annular velocity during the development of heart failure. J. Am. Coll. Cardiol. 41: 1590–7, 2003.

[45] Hatle, L.K., Appleton, C.P., Popp, R.L. Differentiation of constrictive pericarditis and restrictive cardiomyopathy by Doppler echocardiography. Circulation 79: 357–70, 1989.

[46] Henderson, Y., Johnson, F.E. Two modes of closure of the heart valves. Heart 4: 69–82, 1912.

[47] Higashidate, M., Tamiya, K., Kurosawa, H., Imai, Y. Role of the septal leaflet in tricuspid valve closure. J. Thorac. Cardiovasc. Surg. 104: 1212–7, 1992.

[48] Higashidate, M., Tamiya, K., Beppu, T., Imai, Y. Regulation of the aortic valve opening: in vivo dynamic measurement of aortic valve orifice area. J. Thorac. Cardiovasc. Surg. 110: 496–503, 1995.

[49] Hoadley, S.D., Pasipoularides, A. Are ejection phase Doppler/echo indices sensitive markers of contractile dysfunction in cardiomyopathy? Role of afterload mismatch. Circulation 76: Suppl. IV-404, 1987.

[50] Hoffman, E., Ritman, E. Invariant total heart volume in the intact thorax. Am. J. Physiol. 249: H883–90, 1985.

[51] Hoffman, E.A. Interactions: The integrated functioning of heart and lungs. In: Sideman, S., Beyer, R. [Eds.] Interactive Phenomena in the Cardiac System. 1993, New York, NY: Plenum. pp. 347–364.

[52] Howard, I.C., Patterson, E.A., Yoxall, A. On the opening mechanism of the aortic valve: some observations from simulations. J. Med. Eng. Technol. 27: 259–66, 2003.

[53] Ihara, T., Shannon, R.P., Komamura, K., Pasipoularides, A.D., Patrick, T., Shen, S., Vatner, S.F. Effects of anaesthesia and recent surgery on diastolic function. Cardiovasc. Res. 28: 325–36, 1994.

[54] Isaaz, K., Pasipoularides, A. Noninvasive assessment of intrinsic ventricular load dynamics in dilated cardiomopathy. J. Am. Coll. Cardiol. 17: 112–21, 1991.

[55] Kalmanson, D., Veyrat, C., Witchitz, S., Derai, C., Chiche, P. Les dysfonctionnements tricuspidiens: une nouvelle entité physiopathologique [Tricuspid dysfunction: a new physiopathologic entity]. Ann. Cardiol. Angeiol. (Paris) 21: 433–47, 1972.

[56] Katz, A.M. Physiology of the heart. 4th ed. 2006, Philadelphia, PA: Lippincott Williams & Wilkins. xix, 644 p.

[57] Keren, G., Sonnenblick, E.H., LeJemtel, T.H. Mitral annulus motion: relation to pulmonary venous and transmitral flows in normal subjects and in patients with dilated cardiomyopathy. Circulation 78: 621–9, 1988.

[58] Khalafbegui, F., Suga, H., Sagawa, K. Left ventricular systolic pressure-volume area correlates with oxygen consumption. Am. J. Physiol. 237: H566–9, 1979.

[59] Karlsson, M.O., Glasson, J.R., Bolger, A.F., Daughters, G.T., Komeda, M., Foppiano, L.E., Miller, D.C., Ingels, N.B., Jr. Mitral valve opening in the ovine heart. Am. J. Physiol. Heart Circ. Physiol. 274: H552–63, 1998.

[60] Kilner, P.J., Yang, G.Z., Mohiaddin, R.H., Firmin, D.N., Longmore, D.B. Helical and retrograde secondary flow patterns in the aortic arch studied by three-directional magnetic resonance velocity mapping. Circulation 88: 2235–47, 1993.

[61] Kranidis, A., Kostopoulos, K., Anthopoulos, L. Evaluation of left ventricular filling by echocardiographic atrioventricular plane displacement in patients with coronary artery disease. Int. J. Cardiol. 48: 183–6, 1995.

[62] Kussmaul, W.G., Noordergraaf, A., Laskey, W.K. Right ventricular-pulmonary arterial interactions. Ann. Biomed. Eng. 20: 63–80, 1992.

[63] Laniado, S., Yellin, E.L., Miller, H., Frater, R.W. Temporal relation of the first heart sound to closure of the mitral valve. Circulation 47: 1006–14, 1973.

[64] Lansac, E., Lim, K.H., Shomura, Y., Goetz, W.A., Lim, H.S., Rice, N.T., Saber, H., Duran, C.M.G. Dynamic balance of the aortomitral junction. J. Thorac. Cardiovasc. Surg. 123: 911–8, 2002.

[65] Latham, R.D., Westerhof, N., Sipkema, P., Rubal, B.J., Reuderink, P., Murgo, J.P. Regional wave travel and reflections along the human aorta: A study with six simultaneous micromanometric pressures. Circulation 72: 1257–69, 1985.

[66] Laxminarayan, S., Sipkema, P., Westerhof, N. Characterization of the arterial system in the time domain. IEEE Trans. Biomed. Eng. 25: 177–84, 1978.

[67] Leier, C.V., Chatterjee, K. The physical examination in heart failure—part I. Congest. Heart Fail. 13: 41–7, 2007.

[68] Leier, C.V., Chatterjee, K. The physical examination in heart failure—part II. Congest. Heart Fail. 13: 99–103, 2007.

[69] Levine, H.J., Forwand, S.A., McIntyre, K.M., Schechter, E. Effect of afterload on force-velocity relations and contractile element work in the intact dog heart. Circ. Res. 18: 729–44, 1966.

[70] Lundbäck, S. Cardiac pumping and function of the ventricular septum. Acta Physiol. Scand. Suppl. 550: 1–101, 1986.

[71] Luo, J., Xuan, Y.T., Gu, Y., Prabhu, S.D. Prolonged oxidative stress inverts the cardiac force-frequency relation: role of altered calcium handling and myofilament calcium responsiveness. J. Mol. Cell. Cardiol. 40: 64–75, 2006.

[72] Maughan, W.L., Shoukas, A.A., Sagawa, K., Weisfeldt, M.L. Instantaneous pressure-volume relationship of the canine right ventricle. Circ. Res. 44: 309–15, 1979.

[73] Milnor, W.R. Arterial impedance as ventricular afterload. Circ. Res. 36: 565–70, 1975.

[74] Mirsky, I. Assessment of passive elastic stiffness of cardiac muscle: Mathematical concepts, physiologic and clinical considerations, directions of future research. Prog. Cardiovas. Dis. 18: 277–308, 1976.

[75] Mirsky, I., Pasipoularides, A. Elastic properties of normal and hypertrophied cardiac muscle. Fed. Proc. 39: 156–61, 1980.

[76] Mirsky I., Pasipoularides A. Clinical assessment of diastolic function. Prog. Cardiovas. Dis. 32: 291–318, 1990.

[77] Mirsky, I., Rankin, J.S. The effects of geometry, elasticity, and external pressures on the diastolic pressure–volume and stiffness–stress relations. Circ. Res. 44: 601–11, 1979.

[78] Murgo, J.P., Westerhof, N., Giolma, J.P., Altobelli, S.A. Aortic input impedance in normal man: Relationship to pressure wave forms. Circulation 62: 105–16, 1980.

[79] Myreng, Y., Smiseth, O.A. Assessment of left ventricular relaxation by Doppler echocardiography. Comparison of isovolumic relaxation time and transmitral flow velocities with time constant of isovolumic relaxation. Circulation 81: 260–6, 1990.

[80] Nanda, N.C., Roychoudhury, D., Chung, S., Kim, K.S., Ostlund, V., Klas, B. Quantitative assessment of normal and stenotic aortic valve using transesophageal three-dimensional echocardiography. Echocardiography 11: 617–25, 1994.

[81] Nemes, A., Galema, T.W., Geleijnse, M.L., Soliman, O.I.I., Yap, S-C., Anwar, A.M., ten Cate, F.J. Aortic valve replacement for aortic stenosis is associated with improved aortic distensibility at longterm follow-up. Am. Heart. J. 153: 147–51, 2007.

[82] Nichols, W.W., Conti, C.R., Walker, W.E., Milnor, W.R. Input impedance of the systemic circulation in man. Circ. Res. 40: 451–8, 1977.

[83] Nikolic, S., Yellin, E.L., Tamura, K., Tamura, T., Frater, R.W.M. Effect of early diastolic loading on myocardial relaxation in the intact canine left ventricle. Circ. Res. 66: 1217–26, 1990.

[84] Noble, M.I.M., Trenchard, D., Guz, A. Left ventricular ejection in conscious dogs: 1. Measurement and significance of the maximum acceleration of blood from the left ventricle. Circ. Res. 19: 139–47, 1966.

[85] Nolan, S.P., Dixon, S.H. Jr., Fisher, R.D., Morrow, A.G. The influence of atrial contraction and mitral valve mechanics on ventricular filing. A study of instantaneous mitral valve flow in vivo. Am. Heart J. 77: 784–91, 1969.

[86] Olsen, C.O., Van Trigt, P., Rankin, J.S. Dynamic geometry of the intact left ventricle. Fed. Proc. 40: 2023–30, 1981.

[87] Pasipoularides, A. On mechanisms of improved ejection fraction by early reperfusion in acute myocardial infarction: Myocardial salvage or infarct stiffening? J. Am. Coll. Cardiol. 12: 1037–8, 1988.

[88] Pasipoularides, A. Clinical assessment of ventricular ejection dynamics with and without outflow obstruction. J. Am. Coll. Cardiol. 15: 859–82, 1990.

[89] Pasipoularides, A. Cardiac mechanics: basic and clinical contemporary research. Ann. Biomed. Eng. 20: 3–17, 1992.

[90] Pasipoularides, A. Complementarity and competitiveness of the intrinsic and extrinsic components of the total ventricular load: Demonstration after valve replacement in aortic stenosis [Editorial]. Am. Heart J. 153: 4–6, 2007.

[91] Pasipoularides, A. Invited commentary: Functional imaging (FI) combines imaging datasets and computational fluid dynamics to simulate cardiac flows. J. Appl. Physiol. 105: 1015, 2008.

[92] Pasipoularides, A., Latham, R., Schatz, R. The genesis of aortic root pressure waveform patterns in man. Circulation 74: II-166, 1986.

[93] Pasipoularides, A., Latham, R. External left ventricular load during Mueller and Valsalva maneuvers in man. Circulation 74: II-441, 1986.

[94] Pasipoularides, A., Miller, J., Rubal, B.J., Murgo, J.P. Left ventricular ejection dynamics in normal man. In: Melbin, J., Noordergraaf, A. [Eds.] Proceedings of the Vlth International Conference and Workshop of the Cardiovascular System Dynamics Society. 1984, Philadelphia: University of Pennsylvania. pp. 45–48.

[95] Pasipoularides, A., Murgo, J.P. Ejection dynamics in man with and without outflow obstruction. In: Proceedings of the 20th Annual Meeting of the Association for the Advancement of Medical Instrumentation. 1985, Boston: AAMI. p. 68.

[96] Pasipoularides, A., Mirsky, I. Models and concepts of diastolic mechanics: Pitfalls in their misapplication. Math. Comput. Modelling 11: 232–234, 1988.

[97] Pasipoularides, A., Mirsky, I., Hess, O.M., Krayenbuehl, H.P. Incomplete relaxation and passive diastolic muscle properties in man. Circulation 62: Suppl. III-205, 1980.

[98] Pasipoularides, A., Mirsky, I., Hess, O.M., Grimm, J., Krayenbuehl, H.P. Myocardial relaxation and passive diastolic properties in man. Circulation 74: 991–1001, 1986.

[99] Pasipoularides, A., Moody Jr., J.M., Johns, J.P. Left ventricular isovolumic contraction period vanishes during intense exercise. J. Am. Coll. Cardiol. 13: 102A, 1989.

[100] Pasipoularides, A., Murgo, J.P., Bird, J.J., Craig, W.E. Fluid dynamics of aortic stenosis: Mechanisms for the presence of subvalvular pressure gradients. Am. J. Physiol. 246: H542–50, 1984.

[101] Pasipoularides, A., Murgo, J.P., Miller, J.W., Craig, W.E. Nonobstructive left ventricular ejection pressure gradients in man. Circ. Res. 61: 220–7, 1987.

[102] Pasipoularides, A., Murgo, J.P., Westerhof, N. Aortic input impedance and pressure waveforms in man. In: Proceedings of the 19th Annual Meeting of the Association for the Advancement of Medical Instrumentation. 1984, Washington, DC: AAMI. p. 64.

[103] Pasipoularides, A., Palacios, I., Frist, W., Rosenthal, S., Newell, J.B., Powell, W.J., Jr. Contribution of activation-inactivation dynamics to the impairment of relaxation in hypoxic cat papillary muscle. Am. J. Physiol. 248: R54–62, 1985.

[104] Pasipoularides, A., Kussmaul, W.G., Myers, B.S., Doherty, B.J., Stoughton, T.L., Laskey, W.K. Phasic characteristics of transaortic pressure gradients in valvular stenosis. J. Am. Coll. Cardiol. 17: 254A, 1991.

[105] Pasipoularides, A.D., Shu, M., Shah, A., Glower, D.D. Right ventricular diastolic relaxation in conscious dog models of pressure overload, volume overload and ischemia. J. Thorac. Cardiovasc. Surg. 124: 964–72, 2002.

[106] Pasipoularides, A., Shu, M., Shah, A., Silvestry, S., Glower, D.D. Right ventricular diastolic function in canine models of pressure overload, volume overload and ischemia. Am. J. Physiol. Heart Circ. Physiol. 283: H2140–50, 2002.

[107] Pasipoularides, A.D., Shu, M., Womack, M.S., Shah, A., von Ramm, O., Glower, D.D. RV functional imaging: 3-D echo-derived dynamic geometry and flow field simulations. Am. J. Physiol. Heart Circ. Physiol. 284: H56–65, 2003.

[108] Pasipoularides, A., Shu, M., Shah, A., Womack, M.S., Glower, D.D. Diastolic right ventricular filling vortex in normal and volume overload states. Am. J. Physiol. Heart Circ. Physiol. 284: H1064–72, 2003.

[109] Pasipoularides, A., Shu, M., Shah, A., Tucconi, A., Glower, D.D. RV instantaneous intraventricular diastolic pressure and velocity distributions in normal and volume overload awake dog disease models. Am. J. Physiol. Heart Circ. Physiol. 285: H1956–65, 2003.

[110] Paulus, W.J., Grossman, W., Serizawa, T., Bourdillon, P.D., Pasipoularides, A.D., Mirsky, I. Different effects of two types of ischemia on myocardial systolic and diastolic function. Am. J. Physiol. Heart Circ. Physiol. 248: H719–28, 1985.

[111] Peskin, C.S. The fluid dynamics of heart valves: experimental, theoretical, and computational methods. Ann. Rev. Fluid Mech. 14: 235–59, 1982.

[112] Peters, D.C., Ennis, D.B., McVeigh, E.R. High-resolution MRI of cardiac function with projection reconstruction and steady-state free precession. Magn. Reson. Med. 48: 82–8, 2002.

[113] Petersen, S.E., Selvanayagam, J.B., Wiesmann, F., Robson, M.D., Francis, J.M., Anderson, R.H., Watkins, H., Neubauer, S. Left ventricular non-compaction: insights from cardiovascular magnetic resonance imaging. J. Am. Coll. Cardiol. 46: 101–5, 2005.

[114] Pohost, G.M., Dinsmore, R.E., Rubenstein, J.J., O'Keefe, D.D., Grantham, R.N., Scully, H.E., Beierholm, E.A., Frederiksen, J.W., Weisfeldt, M.L., Daggett, W.M. The echocardiogram of the anterior leaflet of the mitral valve. Correlation with hemodynamic and cineroentgenographic studies in dogs. Circulation 51: 88–97, 1975.

[115] Prinzen, F.W., Augustijn, C.H., Allessie, M.A., Arts, T., Delhaas, T., Reneman R.S. The time sequence of electrical and mechanical activation during spontaneous beating and ectopic stimulation. Eur. Heart J. 13: 535–43, 1992.

[116] Prosi, M., Perktold, K., Ding, Z., Friedman, M.H. Influence of curvature dynamics on pulsatile coronary artery flow in a realistic bifurcation model. J. Biomechan. 37: 1767–75, 2004.

[117] Perloff, J.K., Roberts, W.C. The mitral valve apparatus. Functional anatomy of mitral regurgitation. Circulation 46: 227–39, 1972.

[118] Redaelli, A., Montevecchi, F.M. Intraventricular pressure drop and aortic blood acceleration as indices of cardiac inotropy: a comparison with the first derivative of aortic pressure based on computer fluid dynamics. Med. Eng. Phys. 20: 231–41, 1998.

[119] Rankin, J.S., McHale, P.A., Arentzen, C.E., Ling, D., Greenfield, J.C. Jr., Anderson, R.W. The three-dimensional dynamic geometry of the left ventricle in the conscious dog. Circ. Res. 39: 304–13, 1976.

[120] Reul, H., Talukder, N., Müller, E.W. Fluid mechanics of the natural mitral valve. J. Biomech. 14: 361–72, 1981.

[121] Robicsek, F., Thubrikar, M.J. Role of sinus wall compliance in aortic leaflet function. Am. J. Cardiol. 84: 944–6, 1999.

[122] Rushmer, R.F., Watson, N., Harding, D., Baker, D. Effects of acute coronary occlusion on performance of right and left ventricles in intact unanesthetized dogs. Am. Heart J. 66: 522–5, 1963.

[123] Rushmer, R.F. Initial ventricular impulse: a potential key to cardiac evaluation. Circulation 29: 268–83, 1964.

[124] Sarnoff, S.J., Mitchell, J.H. The control of the function of the heart. In: Hamilton, W.F. [Ed.] Handbook of Physiology. 1962, Washington, D.C.: Am. Physiol. Society, Sec. II. pp. 1: 489–532.

[125] Sarris, G.E., Miller, D.C. Valvular-ventricular interaction: the importance of the mitral chordae tendineae in terms of global left ventricular systolic function. J. Card. Surg. 3: 215–34, 1988.

[126] Schatz, R.A., Pasipoularides, A., Murgo, J.P. The effect of arterial pressure reflections on myocardial supply-demand dynamics. Circulation 64: Suppl. IV-324, 1981.

[127] Sengupta, P.P. Exploring left ventricular isovolumic shortening and stretch mechanics: "The heart has its reasons..." J. Am. Coll. Cardiol. Img. 2: 212–15, 2009.

[128] Shim, Y., Hampton, T.G., Straley, C.A., Harrison, J.K., Spero, L.A., Bashore, T.M., Pasipoularides, A.D. Ejection load changes in aortic stenosis. Observations made after balloon aortic valvuloplasty. Circ. Res. 71: 1174–84, 1992.

[129] Shim, Y., Pasipoularides, A., Straley, C., Hampton, T.G., Soto, P., Owen, C., Davis, J.W., Glower, D.D. Arterial windkessel parameter estimation: a new time-domain method. Ann. Biomed. Eng. 22: 66–77, 1994.

[130] Shoucri, R.M., Dumesnil, J.G. The dynamics of the ventricular wall and some observations on blood flow. Biophys. J. 23: 233–45, 1978.

[131] Spee, F. von. Bemerkungen betreffend Spannung, Bewegung, Nomenklatur der Brustorgane des Menschens. Verh. Anat. Ges. 1909. Erg. H, Anat. Anz. 34: 169–80, 1909.

[132] Spinale, F.G. Myocardial matrix remodeling and the matrix metalloproteinases: influence on cardiac form and function. Physiol. Rev. 87: 1285 – 1342, 2007.

[133] Sripathi, V.C., Kumar, R.K., Balakrishnan, K.R. Further insights into normal aortic valve function: Role of a compliant aortic root on leaflet opening and valve orifice area. Ann. Thorac. Surg. 77: 844–51, 2004.

[134] Steenhoven, A.A van, van Dongen, M.E.H. Model studies of the closing behaviour of the aortic valve. J. Fluid Mech. 90: 21–32, 1979.

[135] Steenhoven, A.A. van, Verlaan, C.W.J., Veenstra, P.C., Reneman, R.S. In vivo cinematographic analysis of behavior of the aortic valve. Am. J. Physiol. 240: H286–92, 1981.

[136] Stein, P.D., Sabbah, N.N. Evaluation of left ventricular function during ejection. Ann. Biomed. Eng. 20: 127–38, 1992.

[137] Suga, H. Total mechanical energy of a ventricle model and cardiac oxygen consumption. Am. J. Physiol. 236: H498–505, 1979.

[138] Suga, H., Sagawa, K. Instantaneous pressure–volume relationships and their ratio in the excised, supported canine left ventricle. Circ. Res. 35: 117–26, 1974.

[139] Suga, H., Goto, Y., Yaku, H., Futaki, S., Ohgoshi, Y., Kawaguchi, O. Simulation of mechanoenergetics of asynchronously contracting ventricle. Am. J. Physiol. Regul. Integr. Comp. Physiol. 259: R1075–82, 1990.

[140] Sun ,Y.C., Belenkie, I., Wang, J.J., Tyberg, J.V. Assessment of right ventricular diastolic suction in dogs with the use of wave intensity analysis. Am. J. Physiol. Heart Circ. Physiol. 291: H3114–21, 2006.

[141] Swanson, W.M., Clark, R.E. Aortic valve leaflet motion during systole. Circ. Res. 32: 42–8, 1973.

[142] Talukder, N., Reul, H., Müller, E.W. Fluid mechanics of the natural aortic valve. INSERM—Euromech. 92, Cardiovascular and pulmonary dynamics 71, pp. 335–50, 1977.

[143] Tamiya, K., Higashidate, M., Kikkawa, S. Real-time and simultaneous measurement of tricuspid orifice and tricuspid anulus areas in anesthetized dogs. Circ. Res. 64: 427–36, 1989.

[144] Thomas, J.D., Choong, C.Y.P., Flachskampf, F.A., Weyman, A.E. Analysis of the early transmitral Doppler velocity curve: Effect of primary physiologic changes and compensatory preload adjustment. J. Am. Coll. Cardiol. 16: 644–55, 1990.

[145] Thomas, J.D., Weyman, A.E. Numerical modelling of ventricular filling. Ann. Biomed. Eng. 20: 19–39, 1992.

[146] Thubrikar, M., Bosher, L.P., Nolan, S.P. The mechanism of opening of the aortic valve. J. Thorac. Cardiovasc. Surg. 77: 863–70, 1979.

[147] Thubrikar, M., Harry, R., Nolan, S.P. Normal aortic valve function in dogs. Am. J. Cardiol. 40: 563–8, 1977.

[148] Thubrikar, M. Geometry of the aortic valve. pp. 1–20; In: M. Thubrikar, [Ed.] The aortic valve (1st ed.). 1990, Boca Raton: CRC Press. 221 p.

[149] Toumanidis, S.T., Sideris, D.A., Papamichael, C.M., Moulopoulos, S.D. The role of mitral annulus motion in left ventricular function. Acta Cardiol. 47: 331–48, 1992.

[150] Tsakiris, A.G., Gordon, D.A., Padiyar, R., Frechette, D. Relation of mitral valve opening and closure to left atrial and ventricular pressures in the intact dog. Am. J. Physiol. 234: H146–51, 1978.

[151] Tsakiris, A.G., Von Bernuth, G., Rastelli, G.C., Bourgeois, M.J., Titus, J.L., Wood, E.H. Size and motion of the mitral valve annulus in anaesthetized intat dogs. J. Appl. Physiol. 30: 611–8, 1971.

[152] Vatner, S.F., Pagani, M., Manders, W.T., Pasipoularides, A. Alpha adrenergic vasoconstriction and nitroglycerin vasodilation of large coronary arteries in the conscious dog. J. Clin. Invest. 65: 5–14, 1980.

[153] Wearn, J.T., Mettier, S.R., Klumpp, T.G., Zschiesche, L. The nature of the vascular communications between the coronary arteries and the chambers of the heart. Am. Heart J. 9: 143–64, 1933.

[154] Weber, K.T., Anversa, P., Armstrong, P.W., Brilla, C.G., Burnett, J.C., Cruickshank, J.M., Devereux, R.B., Giles, T.D., Corsgaard, N., Leier, C.V., Mendelsohn, F.A.O., Motz, W.H., Mulvany, M.J., Strauer, B.E. Remodeling and reparation of the cardiovascular system. J. Am. Coll. Cardiol. 20: 3–16, 1992.

[155] Whalley, G.A., Walsh, H.J., Gamble, G.D., Doughty, R. N. Comparison of different methods for detection of diastolic filling abnormalities. J. Am. Soc. Echocardiogr. 18: 710–17, 2005.

[156] Wiggers, C.J. Studies on the consecutive phases of the cardiac cycle. I. The duration of the consecutive phases of the cycle and the criteria for their precise determination. Am. J. Physiol. 56: 415–38, 1921.

[157] Wiggers, C.J. Studies on the consecutive phases of the cardiac cycle. II. The laws governing the relative duration of ventricular systole and diastole. Am. J. Physiol. 56: 439–59, 1921.

[158] Wiggers, C.J. Circulatory Dynamics; Physiologic Studies. 1952, New York: Grune and Stratton. vii, 107 p.

[159] Wyman, B.T., Hunter, W.C., Prinzen, F.W., McVeigh, E.R. Mapping propagation of mechanical activation in the paced heart with MRI tagging. Am. J. Physiol. Heart Circ. Physiol. 276: H881–91, 1999.

[160] Yacoub, M.H., Cohn, L.H. Novel approaches to cardiac valve repair. From structure to function: Part I. Circulation 109: 942–50, 2004.

[161] Yacoub, M.H., Kilner, P.J., Birks, E.J., Misfeld, M. The aortic outflow and root: a tale of dynamism and crosstalk. Ann. Thorac. Surg. 68 Suppl. 1: 37–43, 1999.

[162] Yellin, E.L., Nikolic, S., Frater, R.W.M. Left ventricular filling dynamics and diastolic function. Prog. Cardiovas. Dis. 32: 247–71, 1990.

[163] Yotti, R., Bermejo, J., Desco, M.M., Antoranz, J.C., Rojo-Alvarez, J.L., Cortina, C., Allue, C., Rodríguez-Abella, H., Moreno, M., Garcia-Fernandez, M.A. Doppler-derived ejection intraventricular pressure gradients provide a reliable assessment of left ventricular systolic chamber function. Circulation 112: 1771–9, 2005.

[164] Zaky, A., Grabhorn, L., Feigenbaum, H. Movement of the mitral ring: a study in ultrasound cardiography. Cardiovasc. Res. 1: 121–31, 1967.

Chapter 8

Addendum to Chapters 4, 5, & 7: A Gallery of Multisensor Catheter Cardiodynamics

The true instrumental method of analysis requires no reduction of data ..., no corrections or computations,... It indicates the desired information directly on a dial or counter and if it is desired to have the answer printed on paper—that can be had for the asking.

——Ralph Müller, "Instrumentation" (January 1947) [14]

... there is a difference between seeing and seeing; ... the eyes of the spirit have to work in perpetual living connection with those of the body, for one otherwise risks seeing and yet seeing past a thing.

——Goethe, "Discovery of a worthy Forerunner" [Entdeckung eines trefflichen Vorarbeiters], 1817) In: Goethe: Die Schriften zur Naturwissenschaft, edited by G. Schmidt et al. in Aufrage der Deutschen Akadamie der Naturforscher (Leopoldina) Weimar, 1947 ff. I.9.74; trans. by Lehrs, p.89. [11]

IN CONVENTIONAL CATHETER-TRANSDUCER SYSTEMS used in cardiac catheterization laboratories the frequency response is usually quite inadequate for faithful reproduction of the hemodynamic signals, and a relatively poor representation of the pressure waveforms will be obtained, if elaborate care is not taken to eliminate, or minimize, those factors which degrade frequency response.

8.1 Signal distortion in standard catheterization systems

The greatest source of poor frequency response and signal distortion in clinical catheterization laboratories is related to the fact that the pressure pulse is converted into an electrical pulse analog at some point that is far removed from the actual measurement site, in the cardiovascular system. This is accomplished by the introduction of a long fluid-filled catheter between the site of interest in the cardiovascular system and the electrical transducer itself. The pressure pulse is delayed by the time taken for its travel through the catheter to the transducer, and it is usually changed in shape owing to a variety of complex interactions with the mass of the fluid in the catheter, the viscosity of the fluid, the mechanical properties of the catheter, and the flexibility of the diaphragm at the end of the catheter. In routine clinical practice, the frequency response of conventional fluid-catheter measurement systems may be improved by using the shortest catheter length feasible, by keeping connecting adaptors and intervening stopcocks to a minimum, and by flushing the catheter with saline, or dextrose and water, from which all air bubbles have been carefully eliminated. By convention, cardiovascular pressures are measured relative to mid-right atrial level and atmospheric pressure. Accordingly, an external strain-gauge manometer should be positioned at mid-right atrial level, and the associated amplifier should be adjusted to measure $0\,mm\,Hg$ when the manometer is exposed to atmospheric pressure.

Techniques of cardiac catheterization differ mainly in the method used to enter the vascular tree and to advance the catheter into the heart and great vessels. The procedure is usually performed on the alert, or lightly sedated, patient using local anesthesia; this allows data collection also during submaximal ergometric supine bicycle exercise. The original method for vascular access and one which is still in frequent use involves direct exposure of an artery and vein through a small incision, usually in the antecubital fossa.[1] An arteriotomy and venotomy are performed and the catheter is inserted into the vessel under direct vision, as described in the next paragraph. Upon completion of the procedure the vessels and overlying tissues are surgically repaired.

Once within the venous or arterial system, the catheters are advanced toward the heart under fluoroscopic control, and commonly with simultaneous pressure monitoring. The chambers of the right heart, the coronary sinus, the main and branch pulmonary arteries, and the pulmonary capillary wedge position can be reached by a catheter introduced into a systemic vein. The left-heart chambers are usually entered retrogradely by catheters passed across the aortic valve from the brachial or femoral arteries. Using retrograde methods, it is generally difficult to enter the left atrium; therefore the pulmonary capillary wedge pressure is regularly used as a useful approximation to the left atrial pressure.[2] Once the catheters have been appropriately positioned, the process of the fluid dynamic, hemodynamic, and angiographic data collection commences.

[1]The Seldinger technique entails percutaneous cannulation of a vessel (usually the femoral artery or vein) with use of a guidewire for suitable positioning of the catheter [29].

[2]The left-heart chambers can also be reached by a variety of less frequently used techniques, the most common of which is the transseptal approach, across the thin atrial septal membrane at the fossa ovalis into the left atrium and left ventricle.

As we saw in Chapter 5, solid-state sensors are miniaturized versions of the commonly used conventional transducers. The frequency response of micromanometers may be 500 times greater than conventional fluid-filled catheter manometer systems, and pressure pulses from within the cardiovascular system may be reproduced with great accuracy, hence the term *"high-fidelity"* pressures. To demonstrate these principles pictorially, Panel a. in Figure 8.1, on p. 411, shows a pulmonary arterial pressure tracing recorded by a high-fidelity micromanometer. In Panel b., the same beat is shown as recorded simultaneously by a conventional catheter, which transmits the pulmonary artery pressure wave through its fluid-filled lumen to a conventional external strain-gauge manometer. Exemplified here is the behavior typical of what is known as an "underdamped" catheter-manometer system. The signal recorded by the system is *delayed* in time and its *shape* is spuriously changed, with superimposed oscillations and a poor reproduction of the "incisura." The oscillations are often caused by movement of the catheter and the forced vibrations of the long fluid-filled column; in some instances they may be of such a magnitude as to significantly overestimate the true systolic pressure and underestimate the diastolic pressure. Superimposition of this pulse upon a simultaneously recorded micromanometric high-fidelity signal is shown in Panel "a. & b."

In contrast to the preceding underdamped system response, in Panel c., a pressure pulse from the same patient and measurement site was obtained with blood intentionally withdrawn into the catheter lumen, in order to produce an "overdamped" catheter-manometer system. The ensuing change in the viscosity of the catheter-fluid has brought about a significant change in the overall amplitude and shape of the pressure signal. Superimposition of this pulse upon the simultaneously recorded micromanometric high-fidelity signal is shown in Panel "a. + c." Marked distortion of the pulse is again evident with an overall loss of its characteristic features. A significant *time-delay* is again clearly visible between the micromanometric and the conventional pressure pulses, and *incorrect* values of systolic and diastolic pressures are exhibited by the latter.

The examples in Figure 8.1 demonstrate the important advantages of micromanometric over conventional pulsatile pressure measurements. Moreover, they reveal that inattention to some of the basic principles of manometry will give incorrect information, not only regarding absolute magnitudes of a recorded pulsatile pressure, but also regarding its characteristic time course and pattern of inflections that contain valuable (patho)physiologic and diagnostic information. To eliminate the aforementioned sources of distortion, the solid-state multisensor catheters have been developed, in which one or multiple pressures and flow velocity are converted into electrical signals at the site of measurement in the cardiovascular system.

8.2 Preamble to high-fidelity cardiodynamic tracings

In the following figures, normal hemodynamics (Figs. 8.6 and 8.7) and some important examples of the application of high-fidelity multisensor catheterization in several

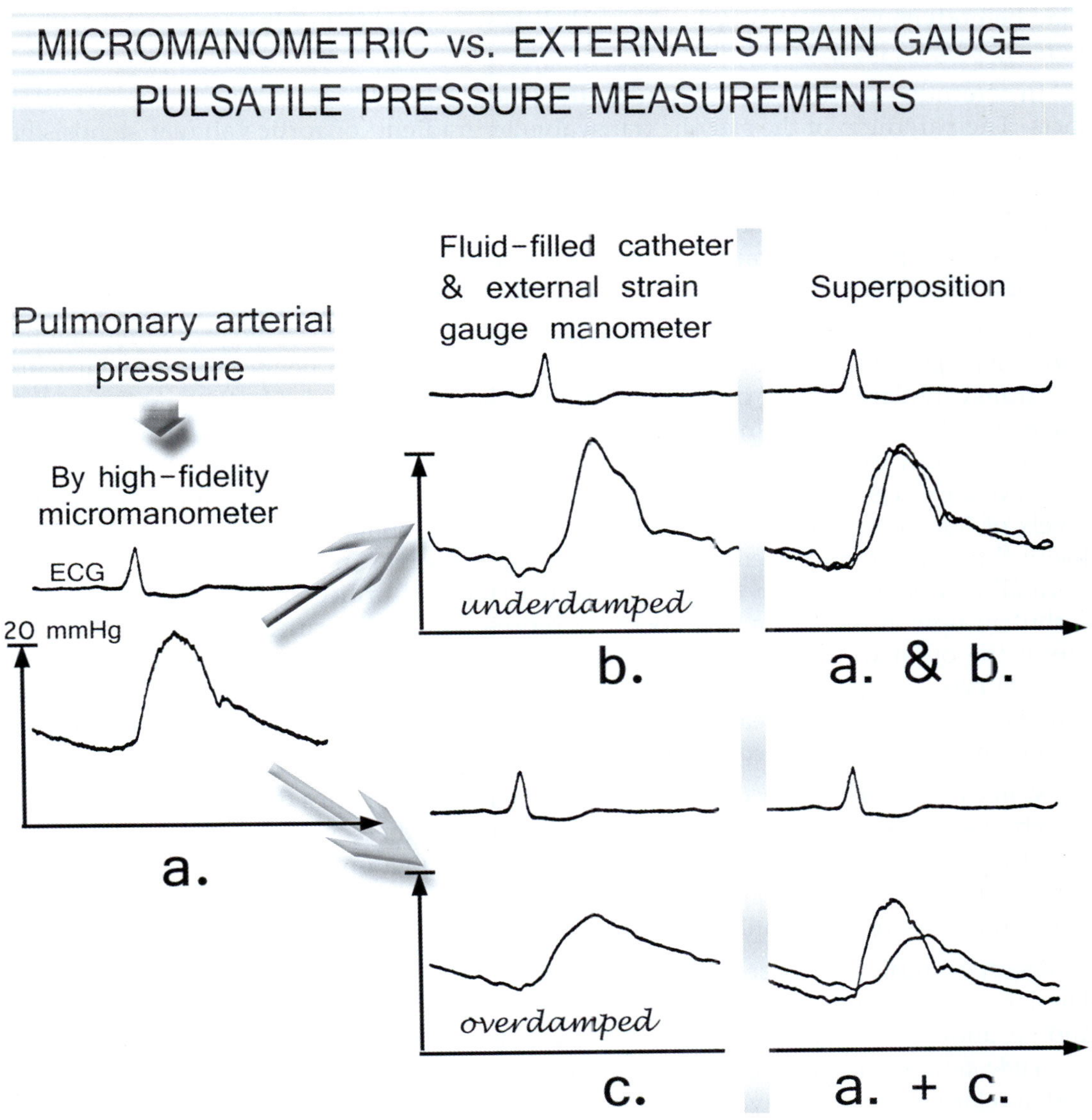

Figure 8.1: Recordings of pulmonary arterial pressure pulse. a. High-fidelity micromanometric pressure waveform. b. Pressure waveform obtained with an underdamped fluid-filled catheter and an external strain-gauge manometer. a. & b. Superimposition of tracings a. and b. c. Pressure waveform obtained with an underdamped fluid-filled catheter. a. & c. Superimposition of tracings a. and c.

common heart valve and myocardial diseases (Figs. 8.8–8.22) are shown.[3] More details and numerous additional high-fidelity multisensor catheterization recordings of cardiac hemodynamic signals in health and disease can be found in many published papers [1,3,16,17,19,22,24–26,30].

In carefully examining these figures, the reader should keep in mind some important facts. The paradigm of the systolic transvalvular gradient[4] of aortic valvular stenosis has led observers in the catheterization laboratory to invoke obstruction as the mechanism underlying prominent ejection gradients, in general. Thus, a prominent systolic gradient in wide aortic valvular insufficiency is taken as evidence for coexisting organic orifice stenosis; in hypertrophic cardiomyopathy, such a gradient is accounted for on the basis of a "dynamic" obstruction to orthograde flow, and so on.

Nonetheless, the fluid dynamic principles already discussed in the preceding chapters show that ejection should be associated with considerable gradients and intraventricular and transvalvular pressure differences, even in the absence of obstruction. At times, multisensor catheter gradients measured by micromanometers $5\,cm$ apart in normal subjects may transiently exceed $25\,mm\,Hg$ (or $5\,mm\,Hg/cm$) during submaximal supine ergometric bicycle exercise. As aortic valvular stenosis develops, the maintenance of adequate levels of left ventricular output requires progressive obligatory increases in linear velocity through the narrowed valve. Peak linear velocities in excess of $5\,m/s$ ($vs.$ $1\,m/s$ normal) can be attained in the vicinity of the stenosed orifice and beyond in the jet of turbulent flow at the aortic root. Because representative velocities in the deep chamber are of the order of $0.1\,m/s$, it follows that strong intensification of convective acceleration effects, compared with normal, takes place in the subvalvular region [1, 16, 24]. This is associated with greatly accentuated driving pressure gradients, as is indicated by the unsteady Bernoulli equation—see Section 4.5, on pp. 187 ff.

Moreover, there are not only quantitative but also *qualitative* differences between obstructive and nonobstructive ejection gradients, just as there is a fundamental dissimilarity between accelerating a fluid by means of a piston in a uniform tube and accelerating it by means of a constriction. Accordingly, proper interpretation of systolic gradients requires much more information than simply their magnitude.

As an example, consider the fluid dynamics of ventricular outflow valvular stenosis. The large obstructive micromanometric pressure gradient tends to be quite symmetric and "rounded" and closely tracks the ejection flow waveform, as does the characteristic *crescendo-decrescendo* high-frequency murmur. This large gradient is, in fact, associated with a relatively low peak volumetric outflow rate recorded simultaneously at the aortic

---

[3]I am indebted to my associates at Duke University School of Medicine, Drs. J. Kevin Harrison, and Thomas M. Bashore, and to my former associates at Brooke Army Medical Center, where I was formerly Director of Cardiology Research, Drs. Steven R. Bailey, Julio J. Bird, William R. Condos, William E. Craig, Stephen D. Hoadley, Stephen H. Humphrey, Joseph P. Johns, John R. Krouse, Ricky Latham, Jerry W. Miller, Joe M. Moody, Jr., Julio Morera, Joseph P. Murgo, Bernard J. Rubal, Richard A. Schatz, and Thomas L. Stoughton for their invaluable expert cooperation in obtaining these hemodynamic illustrations, several of which are previously unpublished. I am likewise indebted to Drs. Warren K. Laskey and William G. Kussmaul, of the University of Pennsylvania Hospital, where I was formerly a Visiting Professor.

[4]The terms pressure *drop* and *gradient* are used interchangeably by convention in cardiology. Although pressure gradient refers to the rate of change of pressure with distance, both terms emphasize that, so far as flow is concerned, it is the *differences* in pressure that matter, not the pressure itself.

root. It is the greatly augmented contribution of the convective acceleration, or Bernoulli, component to the total measured systolic pressure gradient in aortic or pulmonic stenosis [16, 22–25] that causes it to be more *in-phase* with the ejection velocity than is seen normally (see Fig. 7.20, on p. 355, and several of the Figures in the *Gallery*).

As I have previously emphasized [16,24], this is equally as important a hemodynamic *hallmark* of severe aortic stenosis as the augmentation of the magnitude of the driving pressure gradient. Moreover, it is only under conditions such that the Bernoulli component far outweighs the local acceleration, or "Rushmer," component (see Section 13.3.6, on pp. 706 ff.) that the time course of the ejection pressure gradient can be obtained directly from noninvasive measurements of Doppler outflow velocities. This point, elegantly embodied in the Euler and unsteady Bernoulli equations (see Equation 4.10, on p. 181, and Equation 4.13, on p. 187, respectively), is sometimes overlooked. This has led to some erroneous estimates in the literature of the time course of the ejection pressure gradient using the "simplified Bernoulli equation" ($\Delta P\, mm\, Hg = 4v^2$, where v is in m/s). This formula allows only for convective acceleration effects and is *not* applicable in situations where the local acceleration, or Rushmer, gradient prevails.

During the upstroke of the ventricular ejection waveform, both local and convective acceleration gradients are acting in the same direction (mutually reinforcing). On the contrary, during the upstroke of the diastolic filling E-wave, they act in opposition to each other (local acceleration $vs.$ convective deceleration). This, as I have stated previously [27,28], is what underlies the relatively small observable early maximum magnitude of the diastolic (atrioventricular) filling pressure gradient (see Section 14.13.1, on pp. 784 ff.). Because a considerable array of high-fidelity clinical measurements are now available (multisensor heart catheters, Doppler echocardiography, color blood-flow imaging, and so on), better evaluation of ventricular systolic function and improved diagnostic insights are now within reach of the clinical hemodynamicist.

As one illustrative example, consider Figure 8.12, on p. 428. In panel B., the downstream micromanometer and the velocimeter are in the vicinity of the stenosed aortic valvular orifice, and the measured pressure gradient is increased along with the velocity from its levels in panel A. Interestingly, the downstream pressure exhibits a prominent mid-systolic dip *coincident* with peak velocity in the third beat of the panel, where the velocity is highest. Such a "dip" requires meticulous effort to be demonstrated in aortic stenosis, although a large-scale counterpart is typically present in micromanometric recordings from the outflow tract or the aortic root in cases of hypertrophic cardiomyopathy with large dynamic systolic gradients (cf. Fig. 8.20, on p. 436).

It is my view, based on fluid dynamic analytic considerations and experience with micromanometric/velocimetric human catheterization data with and without outflow obstruction, that such a "dip" represents an *unmistakable* hallmark of intensified convective acceleration effects. In the aortic stenosis tracing under discussion, note that the instantaneous pressure gradient is maximum at the inscription of the mid-systolic dip, *right at the time* when the velocity and its square attain their peak values; this is exactly as required by a flow process dominated by convective acceleration effects. Alternatively, the dip can be viewed as a reflection of the transformation of ventricular flow work or "pressure energy" into the kinetic energy of the flow through the converging field of the stenosed orifice.

In panel D., the downstream sensors for pressure and velocity are in the region of turbulent flow in the "poststenotic dilatation" of the ascending aorta. Note that the downstream pressure has recovered very markedly in conjunction with the decrease in the linear velocity, and hence the kinetic energy of the flow, as is required by the Bernoulli equation. This pressure loss recovery was a new and previously unreported catheterization finding at the time of publication of my survey on *Clinical Assessment of Ventricular Ejection Dynamics With and Without Outflow Obstruction* in JACC [16]. In the case under consideration, the peak-to-peak gradient is lower by about $20\,mm\,Hg$ in panel D. than in panel C., as a result of the equal *increase* in the peak downstream pressure.

As a second example, consider the fluid dynamics of systolic ventriculoannular disproportion, exemplified in aortic valvular insufficiency (see Fig. 8.14, on p. 430) and in dilated cardiomyopathy (see Fig. 8.18, on p. 434). The ratio of aortic anulus cross-section to inner wall surface area is a major geometric determinant of intraventricular ejection gradients [16,18]. Both local acceleration and convective acceleration pressure gradient components are accentuated, the latter more so, when this area index is depressed. In view of the foregoing discussion of the fluid dynamics of ejection in the paradigm of aortic stenosis, this makes intuitive sense. After all, the essence of aortic stenosis is the diminution of the size of the outflow orifice in relation to chamber size. As seen in diverse chronic volume overload conditions, including wide aortic valvular regurgitation, and in the various dilated cardiomyopathies, left ventricular enlargement results in a relative disproportion between the size of the globular chamber and the aortic ring—a situation I have denoted as a "ventriculoannular disproportion" [16,18]—which is *functionally equivalent* to a relative outflow port stenosis.

The effects of ventriculoannular disproportion on impulse and Bernoulli gradients are exemplified in Figure 8.2. Dynamic coefficients for a normal area index of about 4% (the inner surface area of the chamber is 25 times as large as that of the aortic anulus) are compared with coefficients that pertain to an area index of 2%, characteristic of the enlarged globular ventricle in dilated cardiomyopathy. Convective gradients are given by the product of the *Bernoulli coefficient* and the square of the instantaneous radial systolic contraction velocity $(dR/dt)^2$; local acceleration gradients are given by the product of the *impulse coefficient* and the factor $R \cdot d^2R/dt^2$ that applies at any instant throughout ejection [16]. Note that the Bernoulli coefficient at the aortic ring is four times higher in the dilated than in the normovolumic chamber. Therefore, if radial contraction velocities were similar, the convective pressure gradients would be four times normal in magnitude. However, *depressed* radial contraction velocities in cardiomyopathy mitigate this effect [16]. Also notable is the intense rise of the Bernoulli coefficient in the immediate vicinity of the outflow valve ring. The impulse coefficient is much more uniformly distributed along the axis than the Bernoulli coefficient.

This relative augmentation of the convective effects is responsible for characteristic changes in the configuration of ejection pressure gradients, which are qualitatively reminiscent of the pattern that typifies aortic valvular stenosis (see Fig. 7.20, on p. 355).

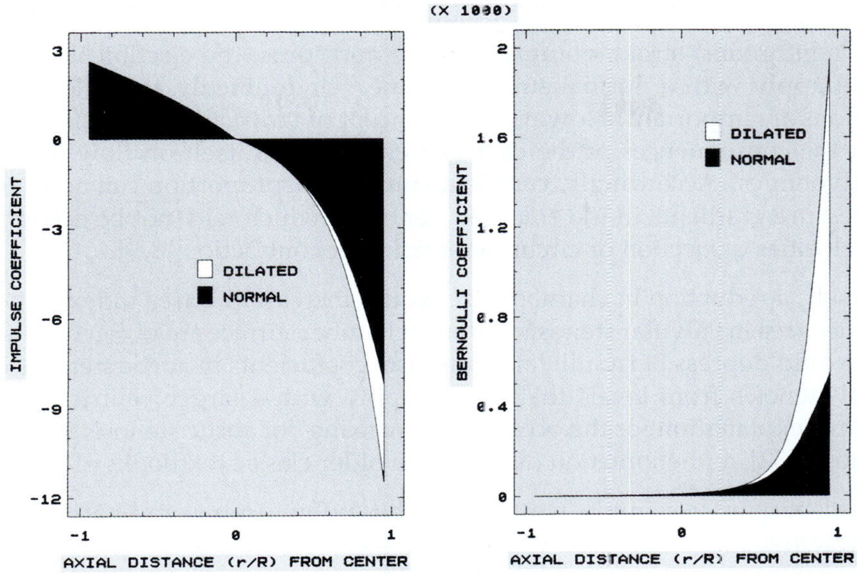

Figure 8.2: Output of computerized model for the effects of ventriculoannular disproportion in a dilated globular ventricle (cardiomyopathy) on impulse (left panel) and Bernoulli (right panel) coefficients *vs.* the normalized (as fraction of the radius) axial distance from chamber center. (Slightly modified from Pasipoularides [16], with kind permission of the American College of Cardiology.)

Consider the multisensor catheter-derived signals from the patient with dilated cardiomyopathy in Figure 8.18, on p. 434. Although small compared with that in aortic stenosis (see Figs. 8.8–8.13), the instantaneous transvalvular pressure difference is distributed quite symmetrically over the ejection interval both at rest and during exercise, and this goes along with reduced upstroke slopes in the aortic root flow signals and prolonged times to peak flow. The ejection waveforms are more symmetric than normal both at rest and during exercise. This is caused in part by the *diminished steepness* of their upstrokes and also by an *increased steepness* in their downstrokes. In other words, in the cardiomyopathic ventricle, there is both a depressed rate of ejection velocity increase *and* an enhanced rate of velocity decay. The very rapid downstroke of the ejection waveform, especially during exercise, probably reflects a high wall stress level maintained throughout ejection and the operation of the inverse force–velocity relation [9,16,17], which was considered in an early section of this book (see Fig. 2.40, on p. 107). In the dilated ventricle, the normal swift decrease in wall stress that accrues from wall thickening and radial contraction (a ventricular *"self-unloading,"* as it were) is minimized.

In aortic regurgitation, the effect of ventriculoannular disproportion in accentuating convective acceleration gradients may be amplified greatly by coexisting organic valvular stenosis. Indeed, it is well known that modest degrees of aortic stenosis can be associated with a very large transvalvular gradient in conjunction with significant aortic insufficiency. However, this has been accounted for solely by the fact that the total (forward plus regurgitant) stroke volume is larger and, thus, the ejection flow rate higher than would apply with a normal stroke volume. Undoubtedly, such flow rate-related considerations are important. However, my concept of *ventriculoannular disproportion* [16] focuses on the consequences of the chamber enlargement itself on flow-field geometry and fluid dynamics. Accordingly, ventriculoannular disproportion can account for augmented pressure gradients in the enlarged ventricle, which may not be accompanied by elevated velocities of ejection or circumferential fiber contraction [8, 9].

Conversely, a reduction in chamber size would increase the area index (ratio of aortic ring, or orifice area in valvular stenosis, to inner chamber surface area). Such a chamber size reduction would depress Bernoulli (and impulse) coefficients in aortic stenosis coexisting with mitral stenosis from levels that would apply with a larger ventricle. This is the fluid dynamic explanation for the occasional "masking" of aortic stenosis in the setting of mitral stenosis [32], a phenomenon described in older classic textbooks of cardiology.

As a third, and final, example, we consider the "polymorphic gradients" [16] of hypertrophic cardiomyopathy (HCM). Inertial forces associated with local and convective accelerations of intraventricular blood dominate the early phase of ejection in hypertrophic cardiomyopathy. This phase is characterized by increasing deep and outflow tract left ventricular and aortic root pressures, while aortic root flow velocity *briskly* attains and transiently remains near its peak (see Fig. 8.20, on p. 436). We can, therefore, analyze ejection dynamics by the Euler equation [16] and its integral, the unsteady Bernoulli equation (see Equation 4.10, on p. 181, and Equation 4.13, on p. 187, respectively) rather than the unwieldy complete Navier–Stokes equations, which encompass viscous along with pressure and inertial effects.

As in the previously examined ejection fields, it is the interaction of flow-field geometry (here, outflow tract narrowing by subaortic septal hypertrophy) with enhanced early velocities and accelerations that underlies the augmentation of the early ejection gradients. Mathematical modeling [16, 22], using ejection velocity and gradient patterns obtained by multisensor catheters and angiographic measurements, suggests that convective effects are accentuated preeminently; thus, at peak aortic root flow acceleration, they account for over half the instantaneous intraventricular gradient, whereas under normal conditions, they may contribute less than one-quarter its magnitude. This confirms that intensified Bernoulli gradients in the narrowed subaortic region may give rise to a Venturi mechanism, entraining, or *sucking*, the neutrally buoyant mitral leaflets toward the septum, in a systolic anterior motion (SAM) [31].

Whether mitral leaflet–septal contact is the cause of the enormous mid- and late-systolic intraventricular gradient remains controversial. It is noteworthy that, as highlighted in Figure 8.20, on p. 436, this gradient rises to its peak levels and maintains these levels in the face of minuscule forward, or even negative, aortic root velocities recorded by the catheter-mounted electromagnetic sensor. Such negative aortic velocities probably represent coherent turbulent flow structures, or vortices, with *recirculating* retrograde velocity components. They are also seen in the ascending aorta in conjunction with the jet issuing from a stenosed valve, as discussed in the context of the transvalvular gradients in aortic stenosis. Because of the intense turbulence, there is no significant pressure loss recovery in the wide flow area of the ascending aorta; this is easily verified by comparing the outflow tract and aortic root pressure signals in Figure 8.20. It implies negligible conversion of intraventricular flow kinetic energy into pressure; rather, there is transfer of this energy to turbulent eddies that dissipate mechanical energy into heat in the *eddy cascade* (see Section 4.14.4, on pp. 217 ff.).

The great heterogeneity of velocity contours in the ascending aorta in hypertrophic cardiomyopathy, with eddy-related secondary positive or negative (recirculating) velocity peaks, has been demonstrated in an elegant Doppler velocimetric study [31]. This study established conclusively that reliance on ascending aortic volumetric or linear velocity signals in investigations of the *mid-* and *late-*systolic intraventricular flow dynamics of hypertrophic cardiomyopathy is apt to be very misleading. Its findings suggest that augmented hydrodynamic acceleration as well as viscous shear forces are associated with the enormous mid- and late-systolic intraventricular gradients. If indeed so, this would have an important repercussion. Because viscous forces would no longer be negligible, the Euler equation and the rest of the developments predicated for inviscid behavior would be inapplicable. A solution to the complete Navier–Stokes equations encompassing pressure, inertial *and* viscous forces would be called for in analyzing these *mid-* and *late-*systolic gradients.

The continuing importance of inertial forces is obvious from the sharp local accelerations and high velocities demonstrated by Doppler recordings in the outflow tract as echocardiographic dimensions shrink [31]. To assess the importance of viscous effects, which grow rapidly with shrinking cavity size, we can estimate how thick the viscous boundary layer can grow relative to flow passageway dimensions in late systole, by evaluating the dimensionless variable $r_0^2/\nu t_0$ [16, 24]. This is the ratio of r_0^2/ν, the viscous diffusion time it would take for viscous effects to penetrate from the flow boundary throughout the central core, to the time available for this unsteady diffusion process (t_0). Taking $r_0 = 0.3\,cm$ as representative of the late systolic passageway radius, $\nu = 0.04\,cm^2/s$ for the kinematic viscosity of blood, and $t_0 = 0.2\,s$ for available late systolic time, $r_0^2/\nu t_0$ is approximately 10. This implies that viscous effects cannot be neglected, although the unsteady boundary layers and velocity profiles will remain quite undeveloped in the shrinking *late-*systolic flow passageway in hypertrophic cardiomyopathy [16]. The intraventricular flow regime has, indeed, changed from its quasi-inviscid *early-ejection* character. Accordingly, the dynamics of the flow can no longer be analyzed by using the nonviscous fluid model approximation that underlies the Euler and Bernoulli equations. This greatly complicates the analysis.

I have developed a model [16] that might provide useful insight into late systolic dynamics in HCM. The deep chamber is represented as a narrow tube (starting radius $0.3\,cm$) with contracting walls (see Fig. 8.3, on p. 418). A solution to the Navier–Stokes equations is derived using a similarity transformation [7,16], according to methods developed for nonlinear boundary layer problems. Some rather interesting results are shown in Figure 8.3, assuming a small ($20\,mL/s$) constant volumetric outflow rate. As shown in the middle panel, the cross-sectionally average linear outflow velocity increases at an increasing rate with advancing cavity shrinkage, and by the time the effective radius falls to half its

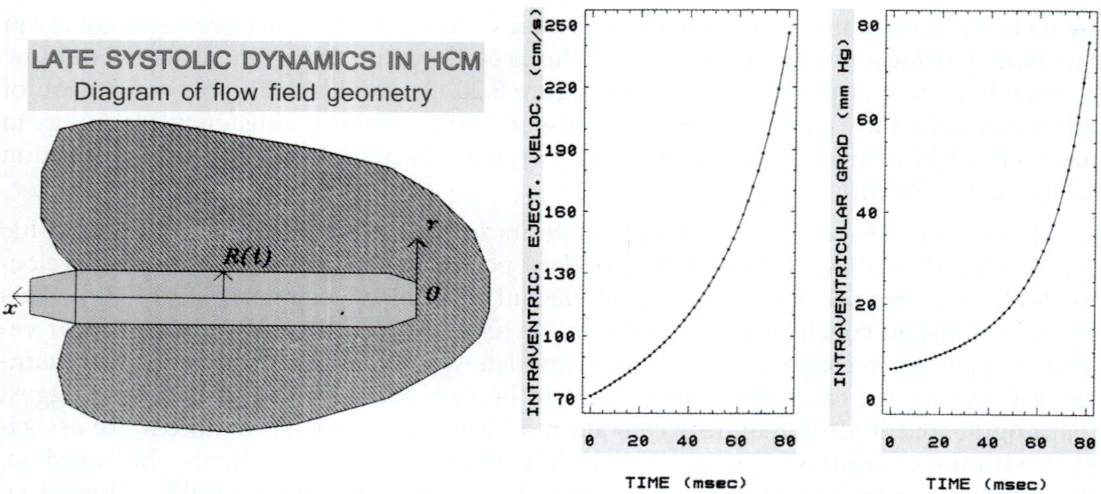

Figure 8.3: Geometry of model simulating late systolic dynamics in HCM with cavity elimination. The chamber is represented as a narrow tube with contracting walls. Local and convective (associated with wall collapse, which displaces sequentially increasing flow increments from apex to outlet) inertial as well as viscous effects are important. A schematic undeveloped, unsteady velocity profile with a thin shear layer is shown at the segment's outlet. R = instantaneous uniform radius; r and x denote the radial and axial coordinates. Output of computerized model for late systolic kinematics and pressure gradients in HCM with cavity elimination. The middle panel shows the cross-sectional average linear "outflow" (relative to the narrow tubular segment) intraventricular ejection velocity (INTRAVENTRIC. EJECT. VELOC.). The right panel shows the time course of the simultaneously developed "intraventricular" pressure gradient (GRAD). (Slightly modified from Pasipoularides [16], with permission of the American College of Cardiology.)

starting value, it attains a level of nearly $2.5\,m/s$. The agreement with the Doppler echocardiographic findings [31] is intriguing. The right panel of Figure 8.3 shows the time course of the simultaneously developed "intraventricular" gradient. Its sharp increase with elapsing time despite the low constant volumetric outflow agrees with the burgeoning mid- to late-systolic intraventricular pressure gradients in hypertrophic cardiomyopathy (see Fig. 8.20, on p. 436) in the setting of greatly reduced volumetric ejection rate levels.

The prominent ejection pressure gradients in HCM have focused attention for the most part to systole and away from important coexisting biventricular [10] diastolic function abnormalities (see Fig. 8.21, on p. 437). The relative contributions of relaxation defects [20,21], asynchrony [4,5,15], altered passive diastolic properties, and geometry [12,13,21] to the diastolic dysfunction in HCM remain open.

It should be noted that application of the "simplified Bernoulli formula" ($\Delta P = 4v^2$, where the gradient is in $mm\,Hg$ and the velocity in m/s) to the highest velocity shown in the middle panel of Figure 8.3 ($2.5\,m/s$) would predict a ΔP of $25\,mm\,Hg$, too low in comparison with the huge late gradients of HCM and the simulated gradient of nearly $80\,mm\,Hg$ in the right panel. This is a consequence of neglecting *viscous hydrodynamic shear* forces, as well as *local acceleration* effects, in the simplified Bernoulli formula, which encompasses only convective acceleration effects. This example supports the idea of having to first ascertain that a given flow problem is *amenable* to analysis by a formula that has only a circumscribed range of validity *before* using such a formula.

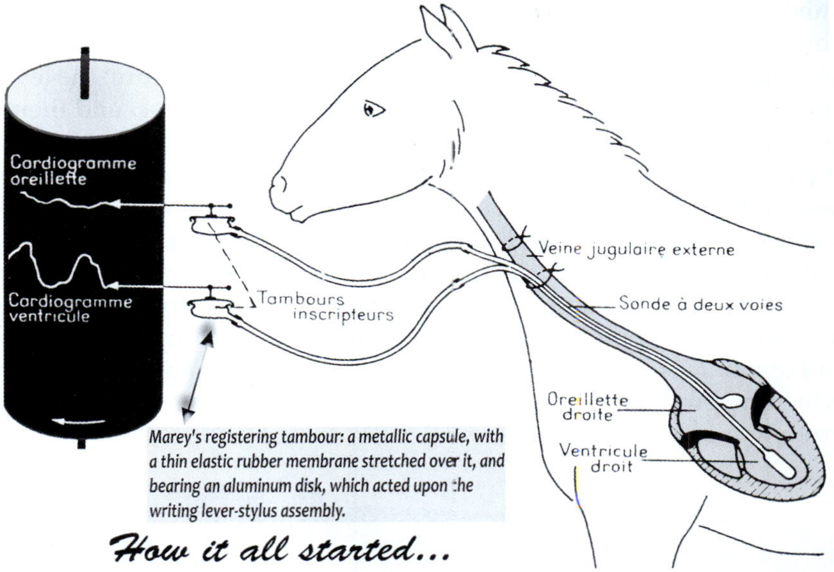

Figure 8.4: Schematic representation of the placement of cardiomanometric probes in an intact, awake horse, after Chauveau and Marey (1861). The probes comprised small rubber bulbs subjectible to elastic dynamic deformations proportional to the variations of pressure engendered within the cardiac chambers—in this illustration, the right atrium and ventricle. The probes relayed the pressure signals by means of a double-lumen catheter, introduced via the external jugular vein, to drum (*tambour*) lever styluses inscribing them continuously on a cylindrical smoked paper recorder revolving at an adjustable steady rate. (Reproduced, slightly modified, from Chauveau and Marey [2].)

8.3 High-fidelity hemodynamic/fluid dynamic tracings

For the most part in this book, images usually serve as adjuncts to the text; the images depict what is described elsewhere. In this Addendum, however, the priorities are reversed: the images of hemodynamic and fluid dynamic recordings obtained by multisensor left- and right-heart catheters from human subjects with and without cardiovascular abnormalities are the *primary objects* of the viewer/reader's attention, while words of explication in this Preamble and in the figure legends serve to bring forth and illuminate concepts that might not be apparent otherwise.[5] In this sense, the illustrations that follow are *self-authenticating*.

In choosing the word "Gallery" for this Addendum, I implicitly acknowledge the human cardiac hemodynamic/fluid dynamic recordings presented in the collection as an art form. Such recordings go back a long way, at least to the elegant "modern" tracings of Chauveau and Marey, at around 1861: as I noted in Chapter 2, they determined the duration of the dynamic events that occur within the heart, and also the intracardiac pressures (see Fig. 8.4, and Fig. 3.10, on p. 139). As is shown in the latter figure, the levels of the intracardiac pressures recorded by Chauveau and Marey were correct and their waveforms were not grossly distorted. As an experimentalist, he used elastic tubes in which he intermittently injected a liquid in order to investigate pulse wave generation and propagation under the intermittent influx of blood in the vessels [6]. He employed three manometers to measure average pressure levels and three *sphygmographs* to record the pulse waveforms at specific sites of interest. As he explained, "The graphic indications of the pulse wave shapes recorded in several places at the same time allow one to see, in one glance only, what on each curve corresponds to one given moment" [6]. Marey was also one of the first modern fluid dynamicists. He studied airflows by means of instant photography of smoke currents, which he produced in the "machine à fumée" that he devised, one of the first modern aerodynamic wind tunnels (see Fig. 3.11, on p. 140).

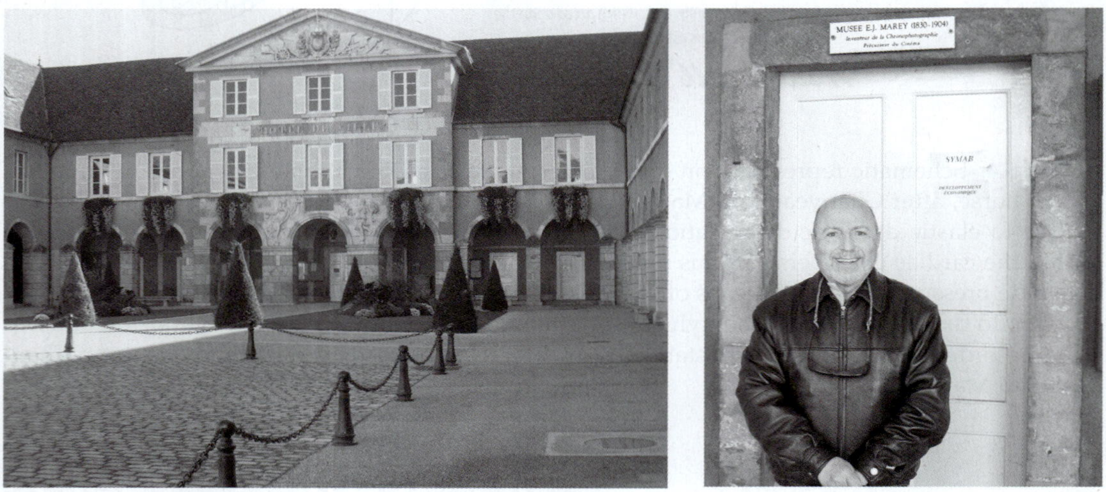

Figure 8.5: The beautiful building housing the Museum E.J. Marey in Beaune of Burgundy, his birthplace, and the author in front of the entrance to the museum, dedicated to the "Inventor of Chronophotography, Precursor of Cinema."

Marey was both a founder of modern cardiovascular physiology and an inventor of the modern art form of cinematography; in fact, the museum commemorating his

[5]Of course, further pertinent information and insights are to be found throughout this volume, particularly in Chapters 4, 5, 7, 9, 13, 14, and 16.

achievements at his birthplace, Beaune of Burgundy (Côte d'Or), bears the inscription "Museum E.J. Marey, Inventor of Chronophotography, Precursor of Cinema" (see Fig. 8.5). He built upon the trailblazing studies of Leonardo da Vinci, the archetypal Renaissance man. Leonardo's wonderful sketches (see Figs. 3.2 and 3.3, on pp. 122 and 124, respectively) provide an obvious early link between fluid dynamics and art.

Although the great Russian fluid dynamicist Lev Landau once said, "The domain of science and the domain of art are not in any way connected for me," I cannot believe that anyone can refute the claim that some of the images obtained in the course of hemodynamic/fluid dynamic investigations of the human heart and great vessels are truly artistic. Although not deliberately created within the (at best, indistinct) boundaries of a *true art form*, they may, in the future, stand as an art form in their own right. Enjoy!

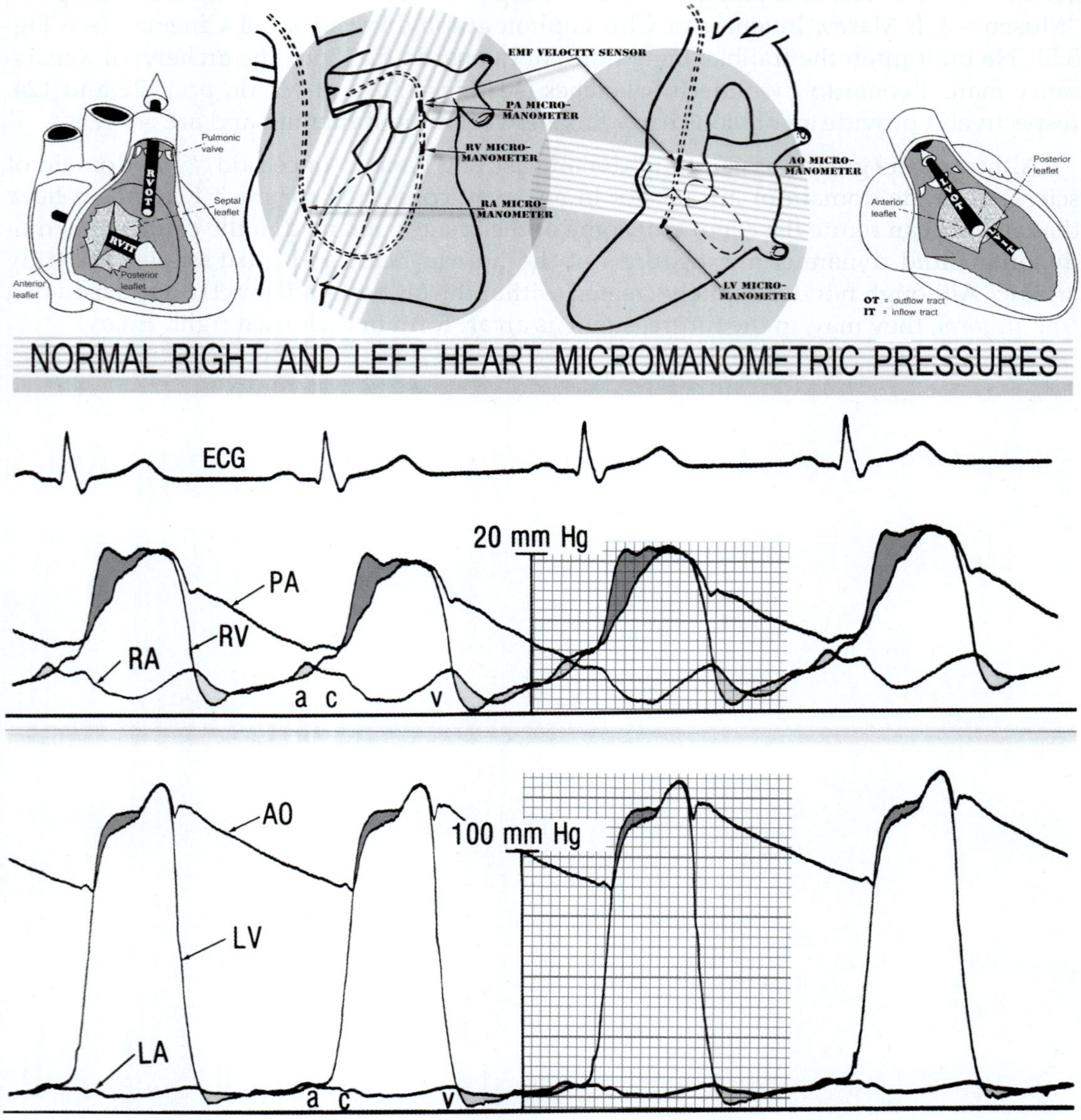

Figure 8.6: Simultaneous, high-fidelity micromanometric pressure recordings from the great arteries and cardiac chambers, demonstrating systolic ejection and diastolic filling pressure gradients. The catheter placement and sensor positioning are shown in the top panel. PA = pulmonary artery; RV = right ventricle; RA = right atrium; AO = aorta; LV = left ventricle; and LA = left atrium. For additional human cardiac multisensor catheterization examples, beyond those in the Gallery, see also Figures 4.14, 5.9, 5.10, 7.5, 7.10, 7.18, 7.19, and 7.20, on pp. 203, 246, 248, 332, 340, 352, 353, and 355, respectively.

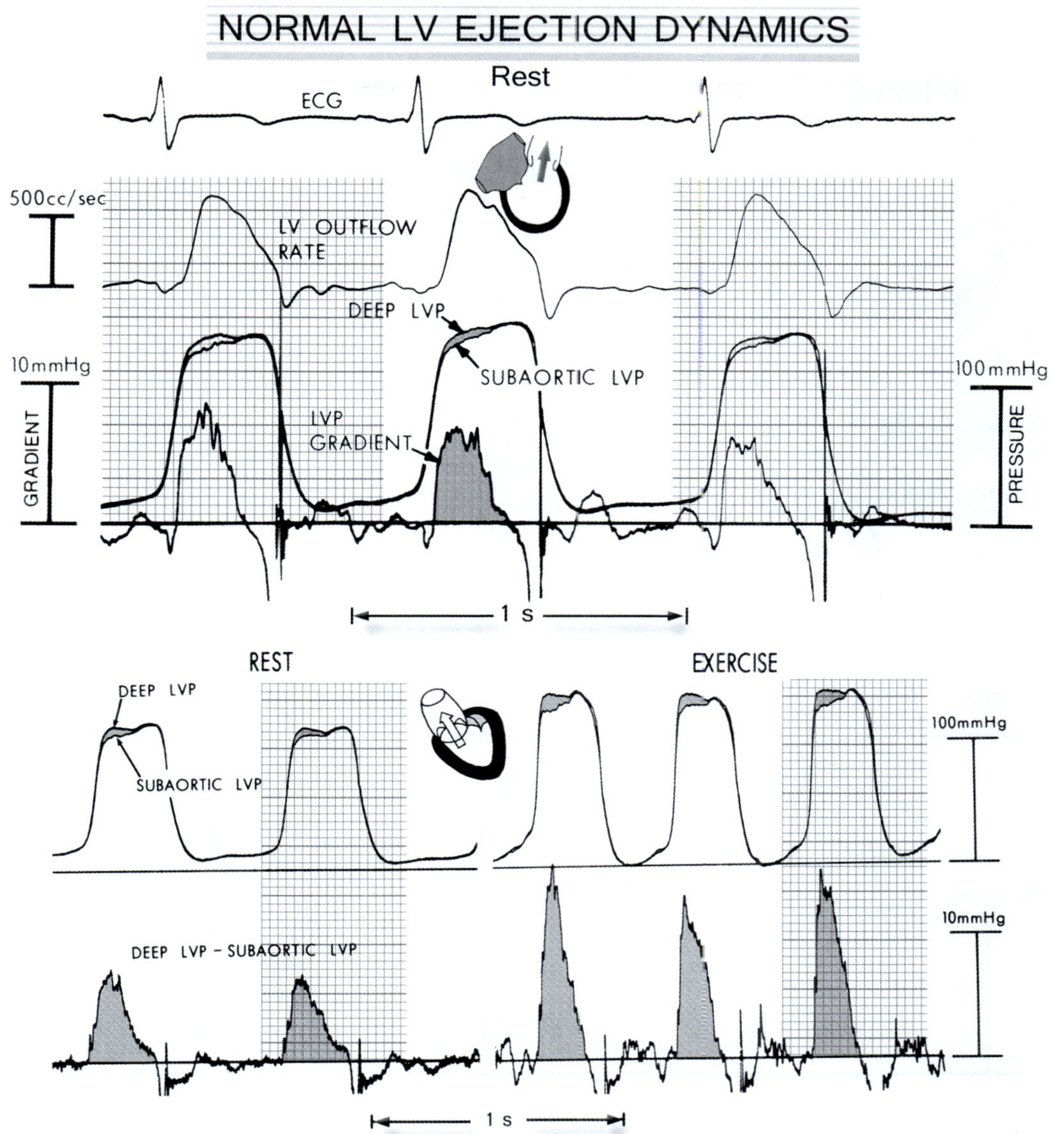

Figure 8.7: Top: Representative simultaneous LV intraventricular pressure and outflow velocity tracings, in absence of outflow obstruction. The deep and subaortic LV pressures are displayed along with their instantaneous difference on a blown-up scale. Note the prominent intraventricular pressure (IVP) difference in early ejection. (Slightly modified from Pasipoularides et al. [19], with kind permission of the Cardiovascular System Dynamics Society.) Bottom: During submaximal supine exercise (2–3 METS) the intraventricular pressure gradients rise in step with the accentuation of flow accelerations and velocities. (Adapted, slightly modified, from Pasipoularides et al. [25], with kind permission of the American Heart Association.)

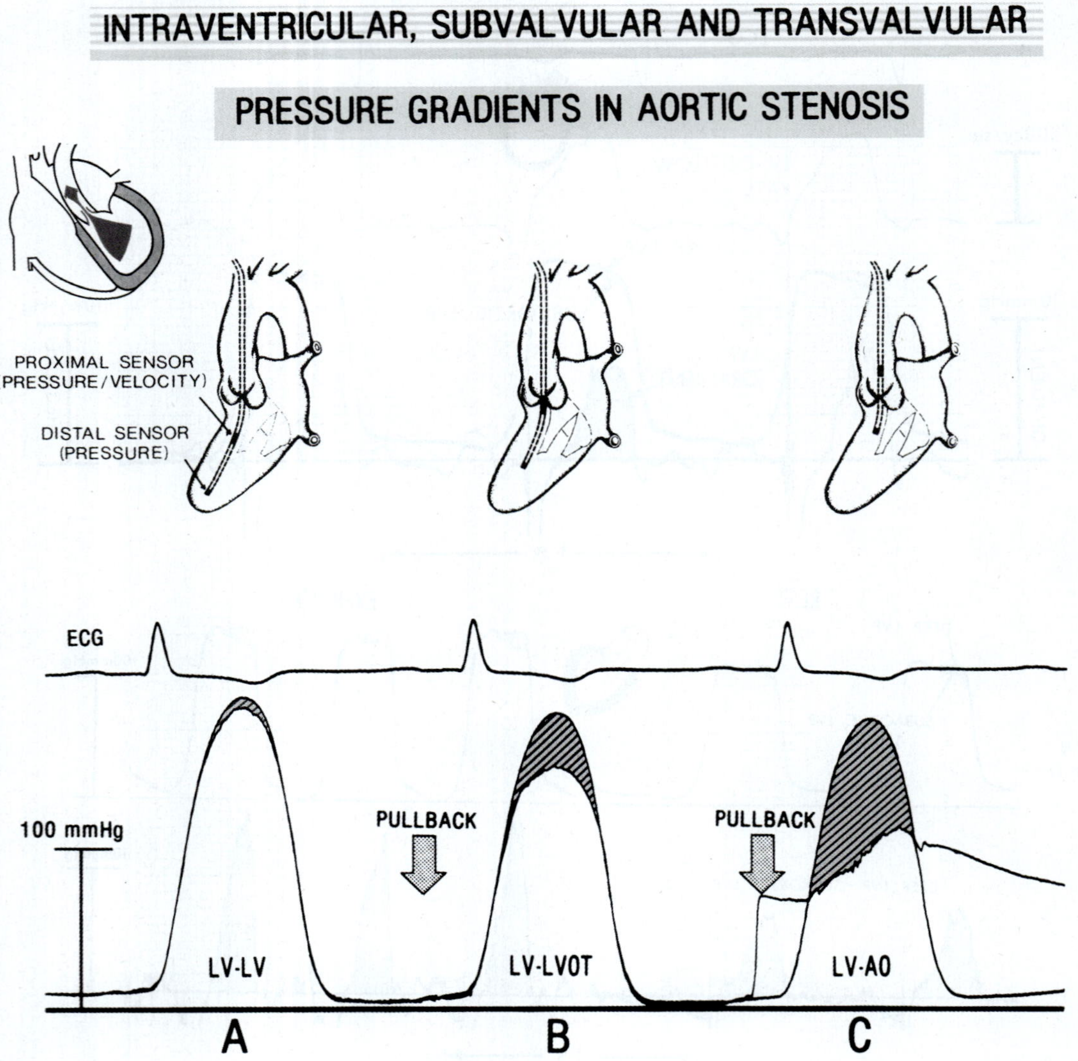

Figure 8.8: Typical simultaneous deep intraventricular (A), subvalvular (B), and transvalvular (C) LV micromanometric pressure recordings obtained by a multisensor left-heart catheter from a patient with aortic stenosis. The pressure tracings correspond to the catheter positions illustrated in the top panels. LV = deep left ventricle; LVOT = left ventricular outflow tract in the aortic subvalvular region; AO = aortic root. (Slightly modified from Pasipoularides et al. [24], with kind permission of the American Physiological Society.)

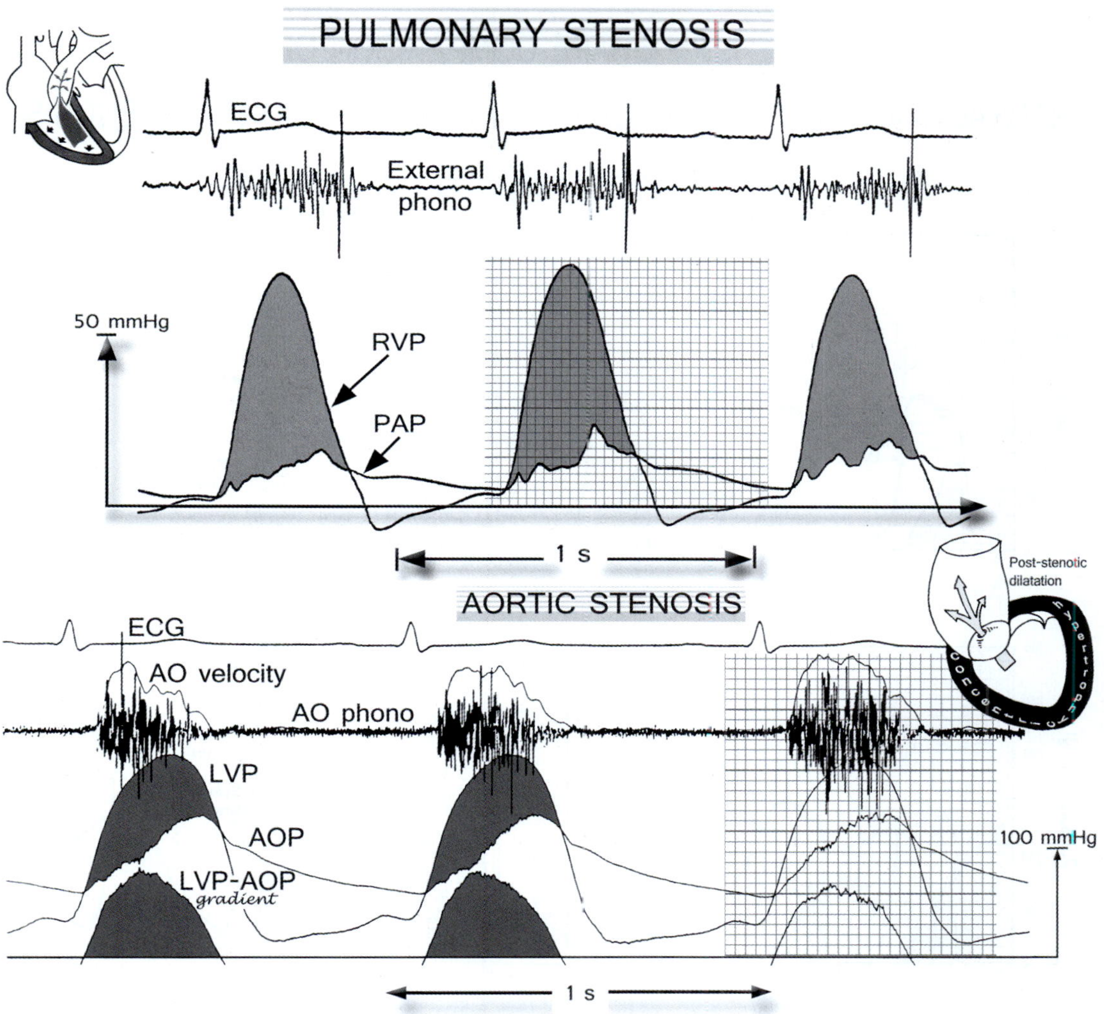

Figure 8.9: Multisensor catheterization in pulmonary and aortic stenosis. Micromanometric RV, LV, and outflow trunk pressures illustrate the high driving pressures generated by the affected ventricle. The large energy expended to convert pressure to kinetic energy across the stenotic valve is represented by the pressure gradient, and reflects the greatly increased intrinsic component of the total systolic load. In the pulmonic stenosis case, the intrinsic is by far the greatest portion of the total load, and is mostly dissipated in viscous interactions of turbulent eddies (see Section 4.14.4) in the poststenotic dilatation region. Turbulence generates sound (external phono) and pseudosound (intravascular aortic phono, demonstrating the classic diamond-shaped ejection murmur). The slow rise in the outflow trunk pressure pulses is a consequence of the pressure energy lost across the stenotic orifice; in aortic stenosis it underlies the sluggish carotid pulse. (The AS panel is slightly modified from Pasipoularides [16], with kind permission of the American College of Cardiology.)

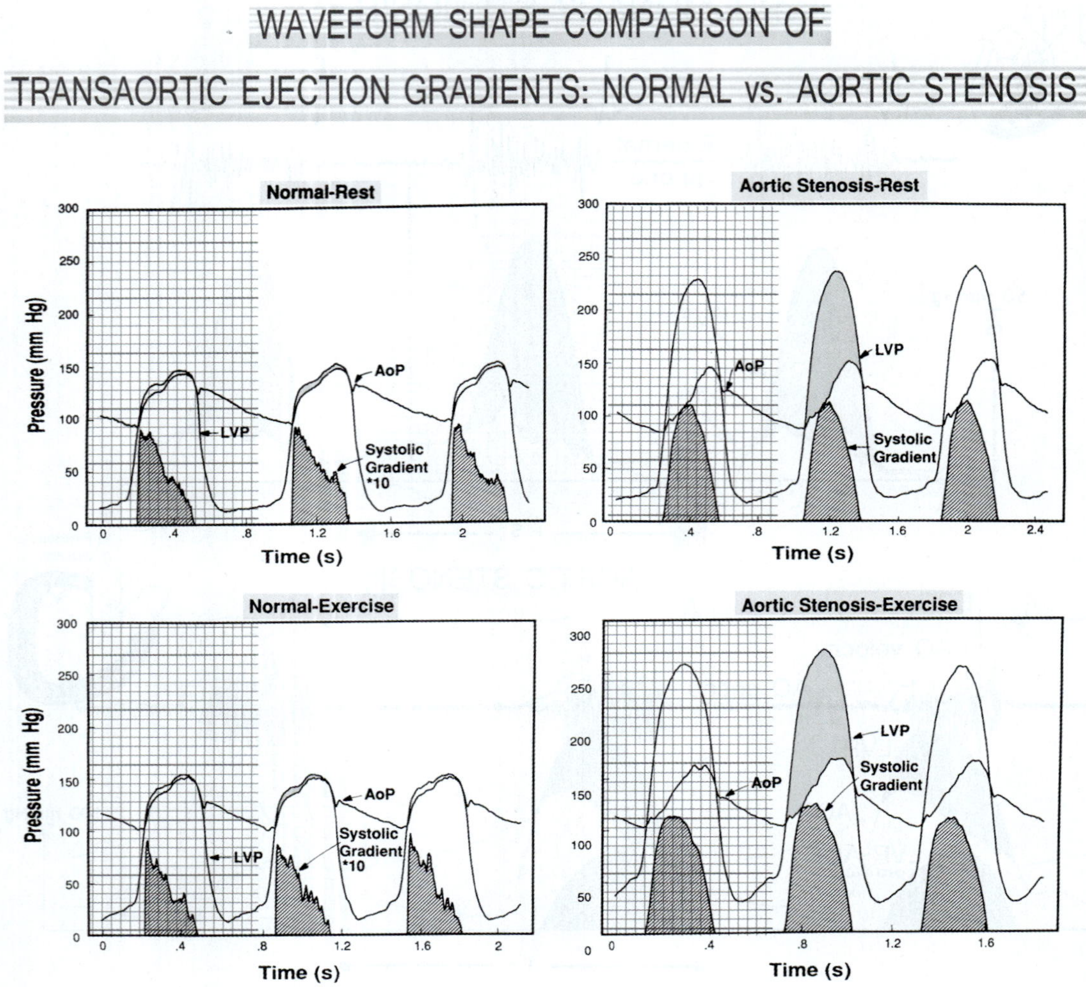

Figure 8.10: Important phasic differences distinguish obstructive and nonobstructive transaortic ejection pressure gradient and velocity waveforms, as found in aortic stenosis (AS) compared to normal. Symmetric, rounded $\Delta P(t)$'s are equally as distinctive a hemodynamic sign of AS as the increased gradient magnitudes. Time to peak gradient, time of positive gradient and their ratio are significantly higher both at rest and in exercise in patients with AS. In AS, $\Delta P(t)$ waveforms are symmetric and rounded in contrast to their nonobstructive counterparts that peak very early. In a preliminary study comparing 13 AS patients to 5 normal controls, on average, ΔP at peak ejection flow amounted to 94% of maximum ΔP at rest and 98% during submaximal exercise in AS; to 71% and 79% of maximum ΔP, respectively, in the normal subjects. Such distinctive differences need to be further investigated because they could be of great importance in estimating the severity of stenosis and in better characterizing systolic ventricular loading in AS.

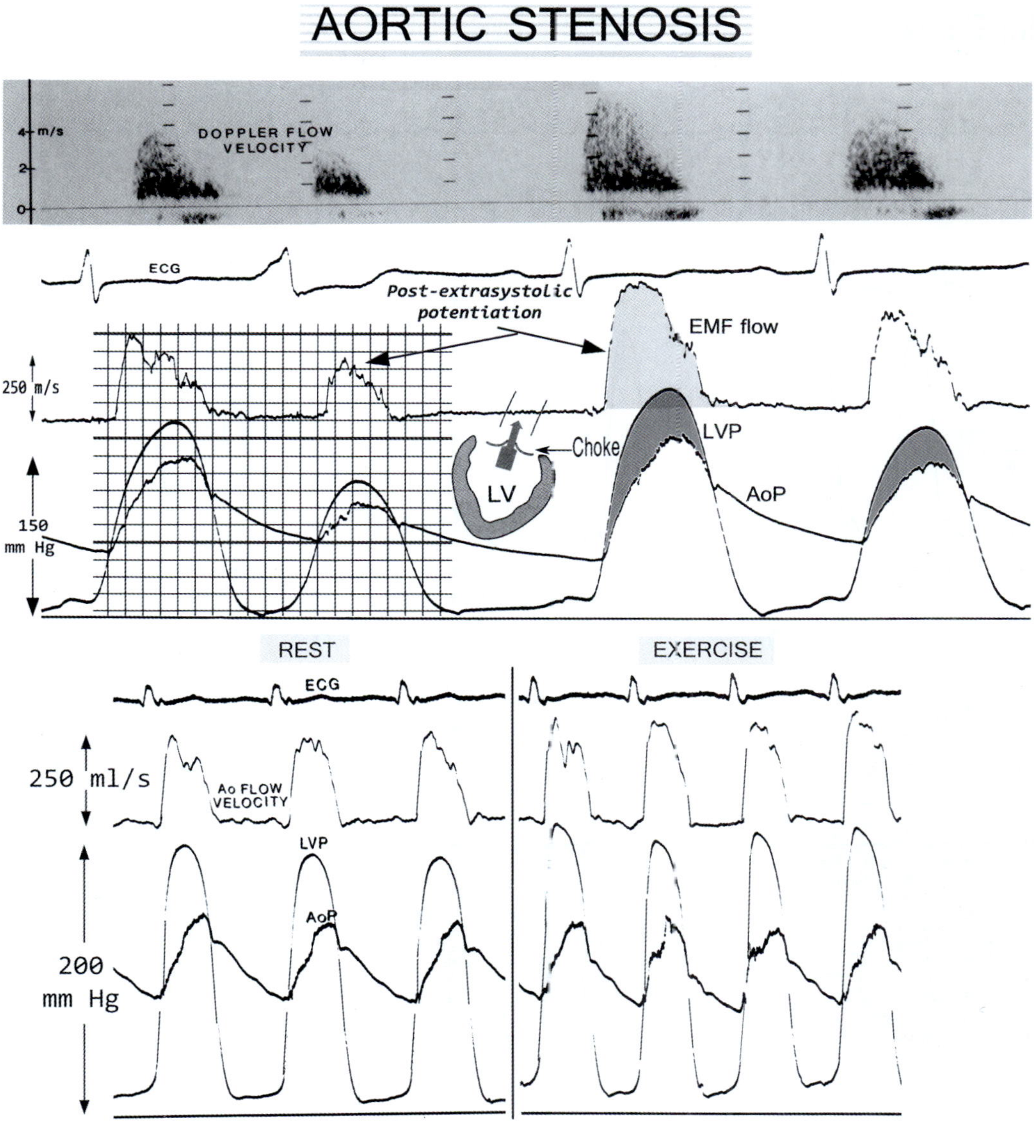

Figure 8.11: Top panels: In a patient with AS, the congruence in the simultaneously measured flow waveform shapes by transthoracic continuous wave Doppler (CWD) and by an intravascular catheter-mounted electromagnetic flowmeter (EMF) probe is striking. Bottom panels: The high-frequency fluctuations on the *downstroke* of the aortic root EMF velocity waveforms and on the aortic root pressure pulse in AS are characteristic of the inception of turbulence—decelerating flows are relatively unstable, as a rule, whereas accelerating flows (*upstroke*) tend to be more stable. These fluctuations tend to be more prominent during even a modest intensity exercise, because of the ensuing rise in turbulence intensity with the higher transvalvular ejection velocities.

MULTISENSOR LEFT-HEART CATHETER PULLBACK IN AORTIC STENOSIS

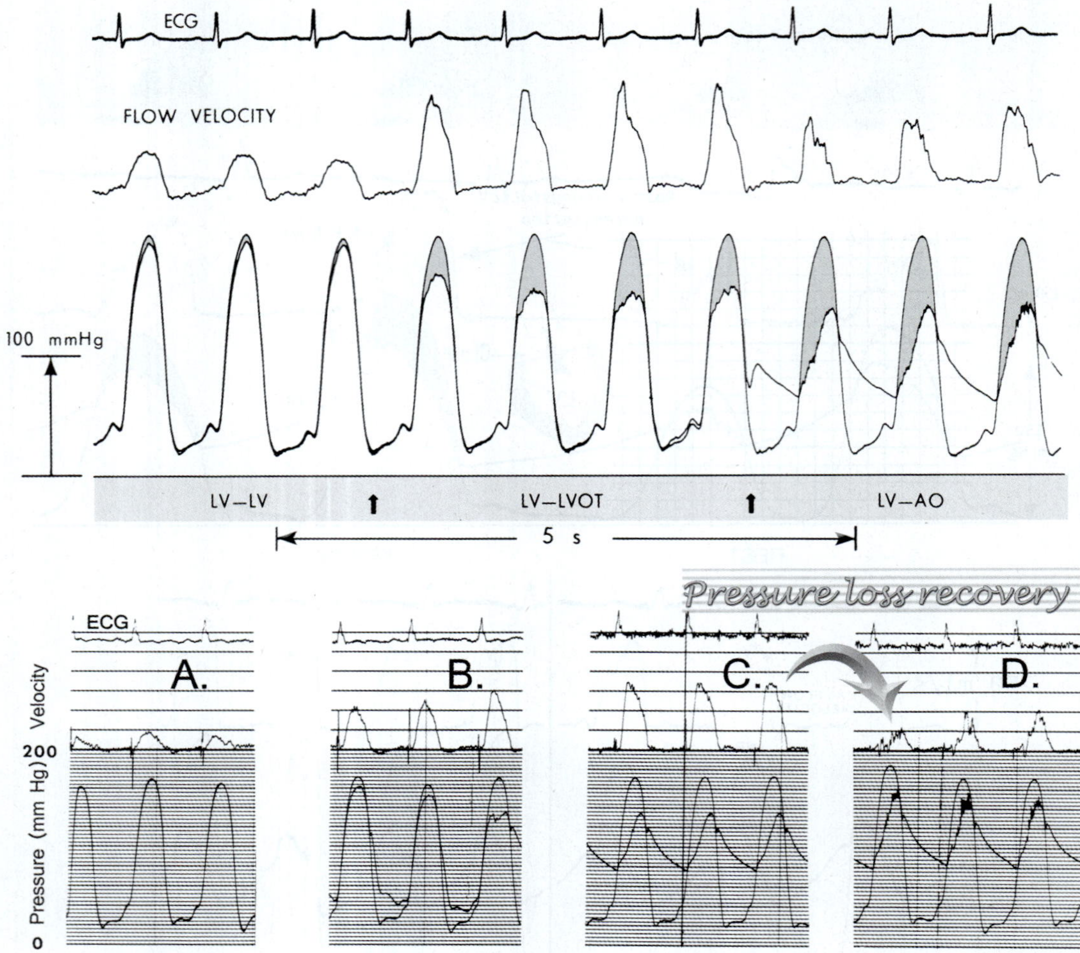

Figure 8.12: Top panel: Simultaneous flow velocity and pressure signals in a representative catheter pullback maneuver. Strong increase in the subvalvular flow velocity just upstream of stenosed orifice is associated with large subvalvular pressure gradient. Beyond stenosed orifice, the flow regime is highly disturbed. Abbreviations as in Figure 8.8. (Slightly modified from Pasipoularides et al. [24], with permission of the American Physiological Society.) Bottom panel: Multisensor catheter pullback demonstrating pressure loss recovery in the ascending aorta in aortic valvular stenosis. From top downward: electrocardiogram; linear velocity in deep chamber (panel A), subvalvular region (panel B), vena contracta (panel C) and dilated ascending aorta (panel D); distal and proximal micromanometric signals. (Slightly modified from Pasipoularides [16], with permission of the American College of Cardiology.)

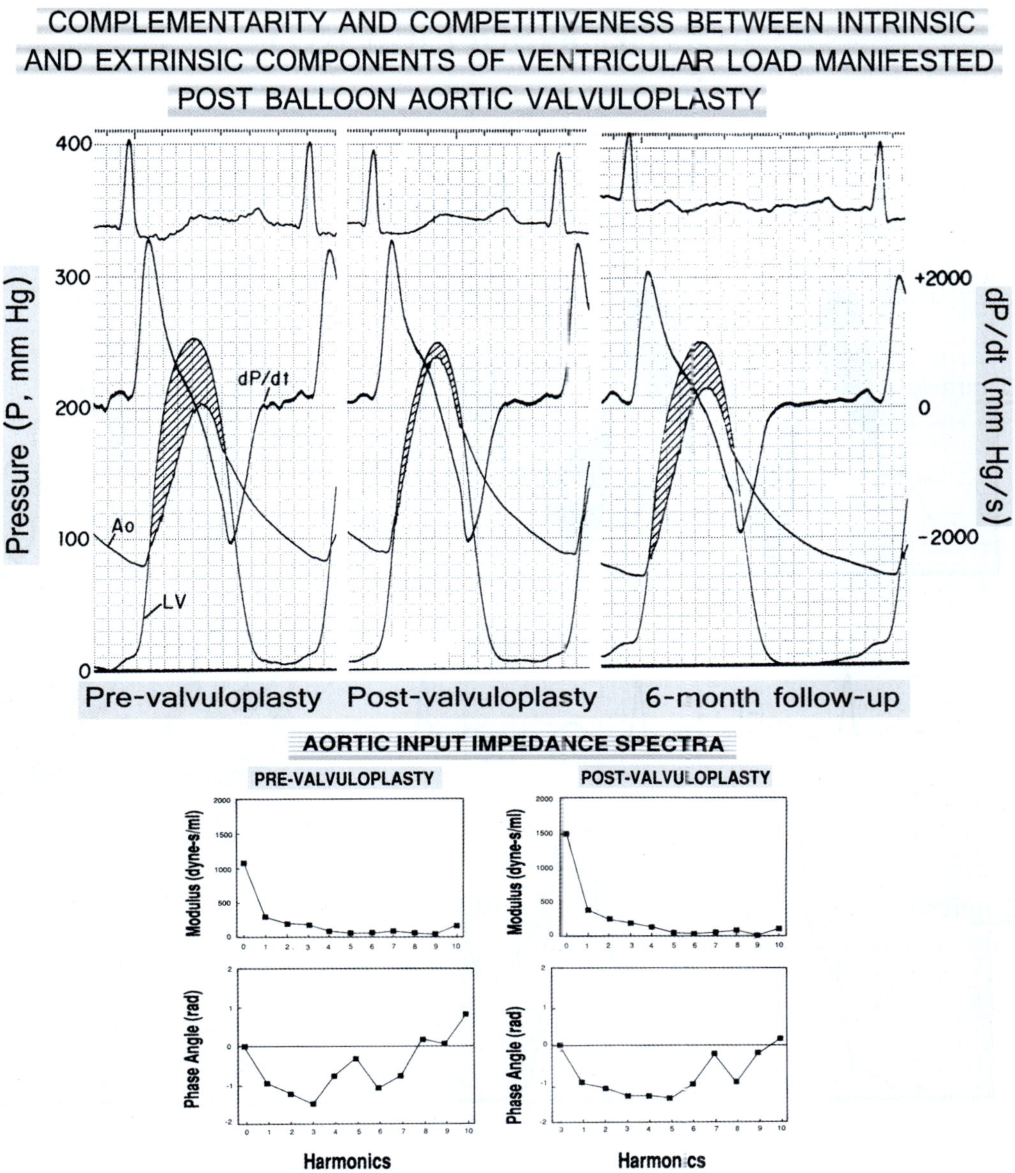

Figure 8.13: Top: Pressure waveforms of a patient with raised peak aortic pressure (Ao) after balloon aortic valvuloplasty (BAV). The decrease in the ejection pressure gradient (hatched area) after BAV is accounted for by a rise in systolic aortic pressure—the *extrinsic* component of ventricular load. LV systolic pressure—the *total* load—remains unchanged. Bottom: The input impedance spectra show that post-BAV both the steady component of the impedance and the characteristic impedance rise. (Slightly modified from Pasipoularides [18,30], with permission of the American Heart Journal (Mosby/Elsevier) and Circulation Research (AHA).)

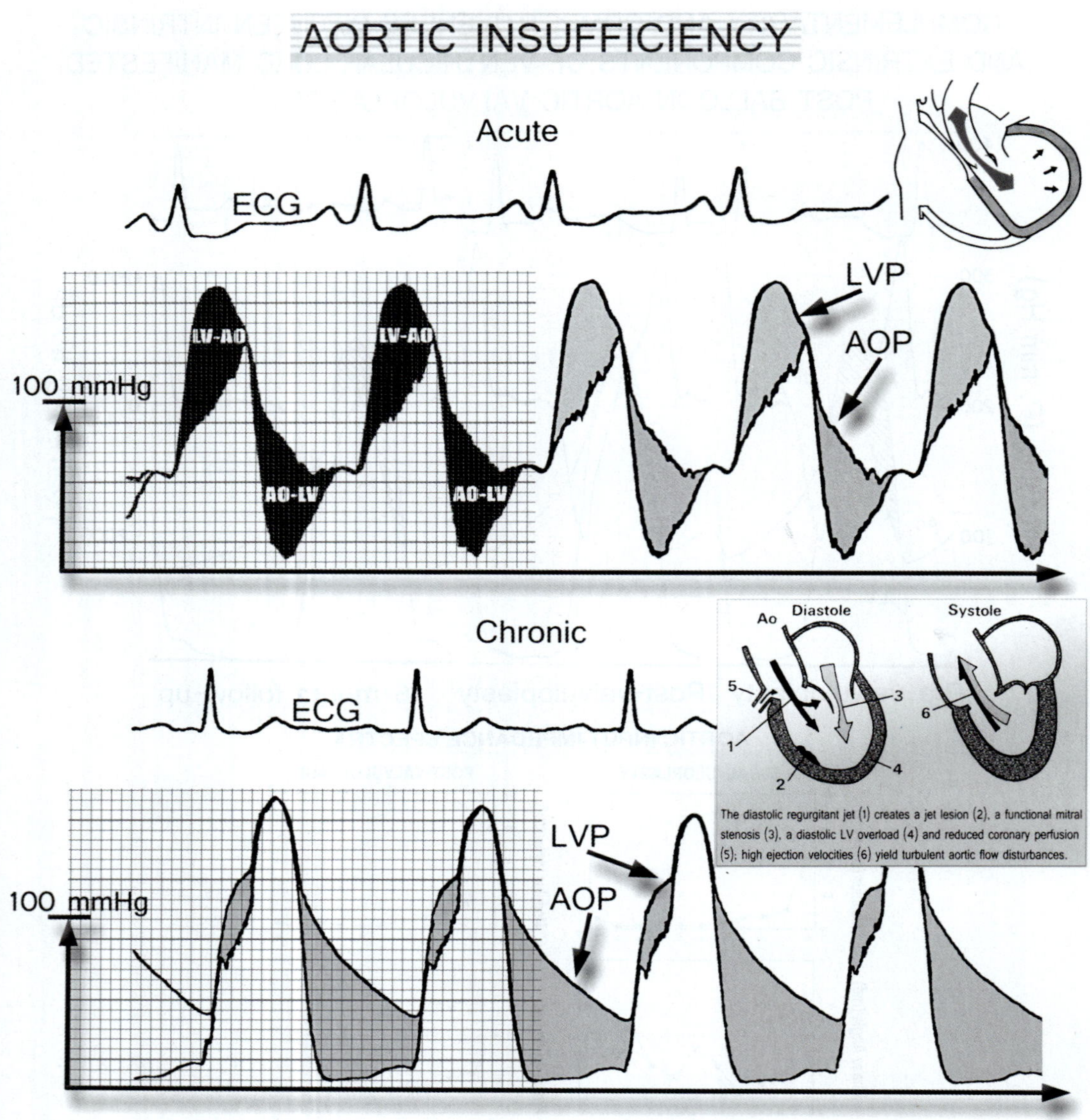

Figure 8.14: Simultaneous aortic (AOP) and left ventricular (LVP) pressure tracings from patients with acute and chronic aortic regurgitation. The very prominent systolic ejection gradient (LV–AO) in the acute case shown does not necessarily imply any coexisting stenosis; it is referable to the *ventriculoannular disproportion* and the augmented systolic outflow rate levels (net forward plus regurgitant volumes need to be ejected), and the correspondingly enhanced convective and local accelerations. Note also the large AO–LV diastolic regurgitation gradient, and the complete equalization of the AOP and LVP levels ensuing in late diastole in the acute case shown: this equalization is a hallmark of a wide regurgitant orifice.

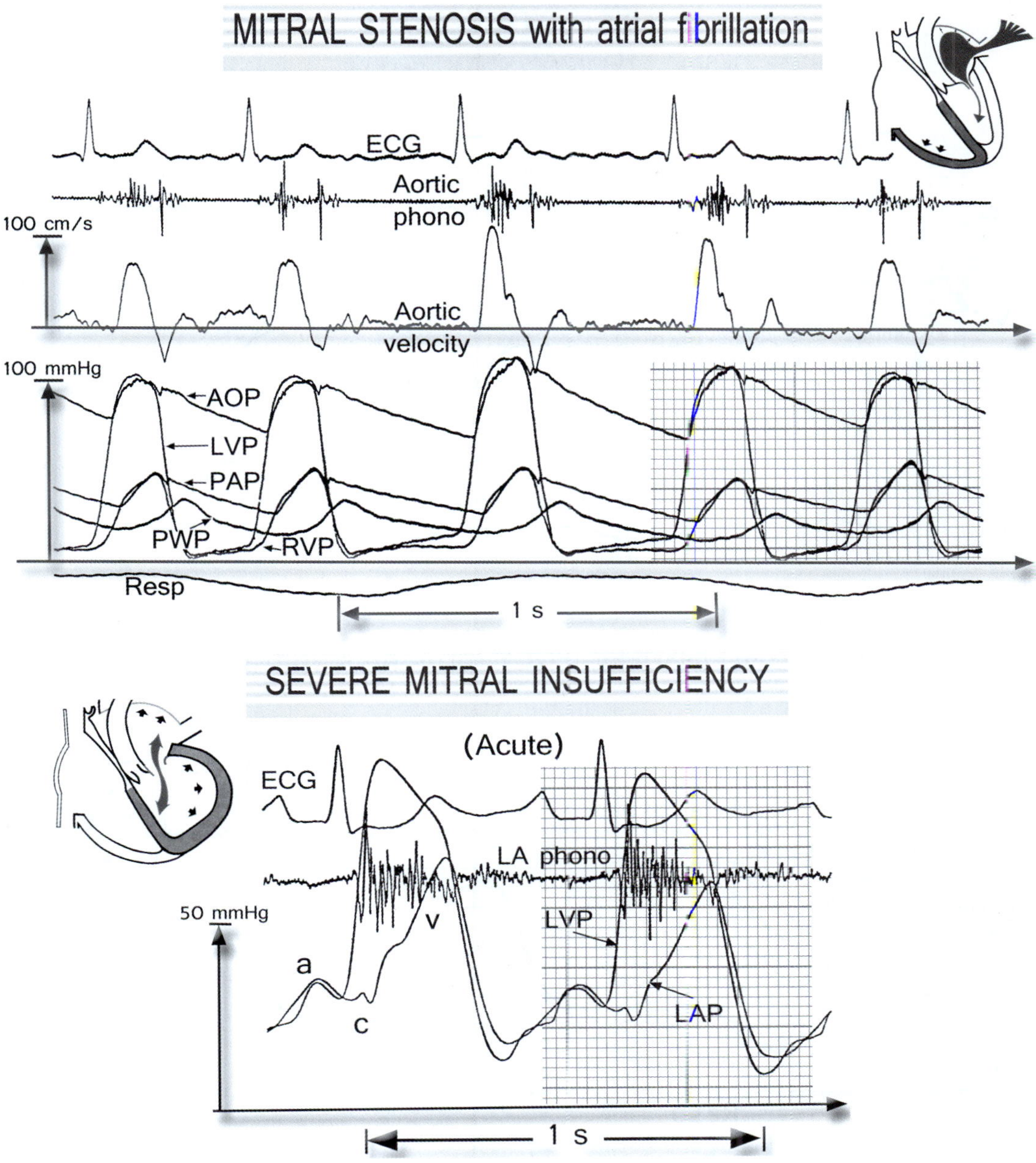

Figure 8.15: Top panels: Right- and left-heart multisensor catheterization in mitral stenosis with atrial fibrillation (abbreviations as in previous figures). The left atrial (indirect via pulmonary wedge position, PWP) and left ventricular (LVP) pressure tracings exhibit the typical pandiastolic atrioventricular gradient. Bottom panels: Simultaneous LVP and left atrial (LAP) pressure tracings in acute mitral regurgitation showing a gigantic regurgitant "v" wave in the LAP.

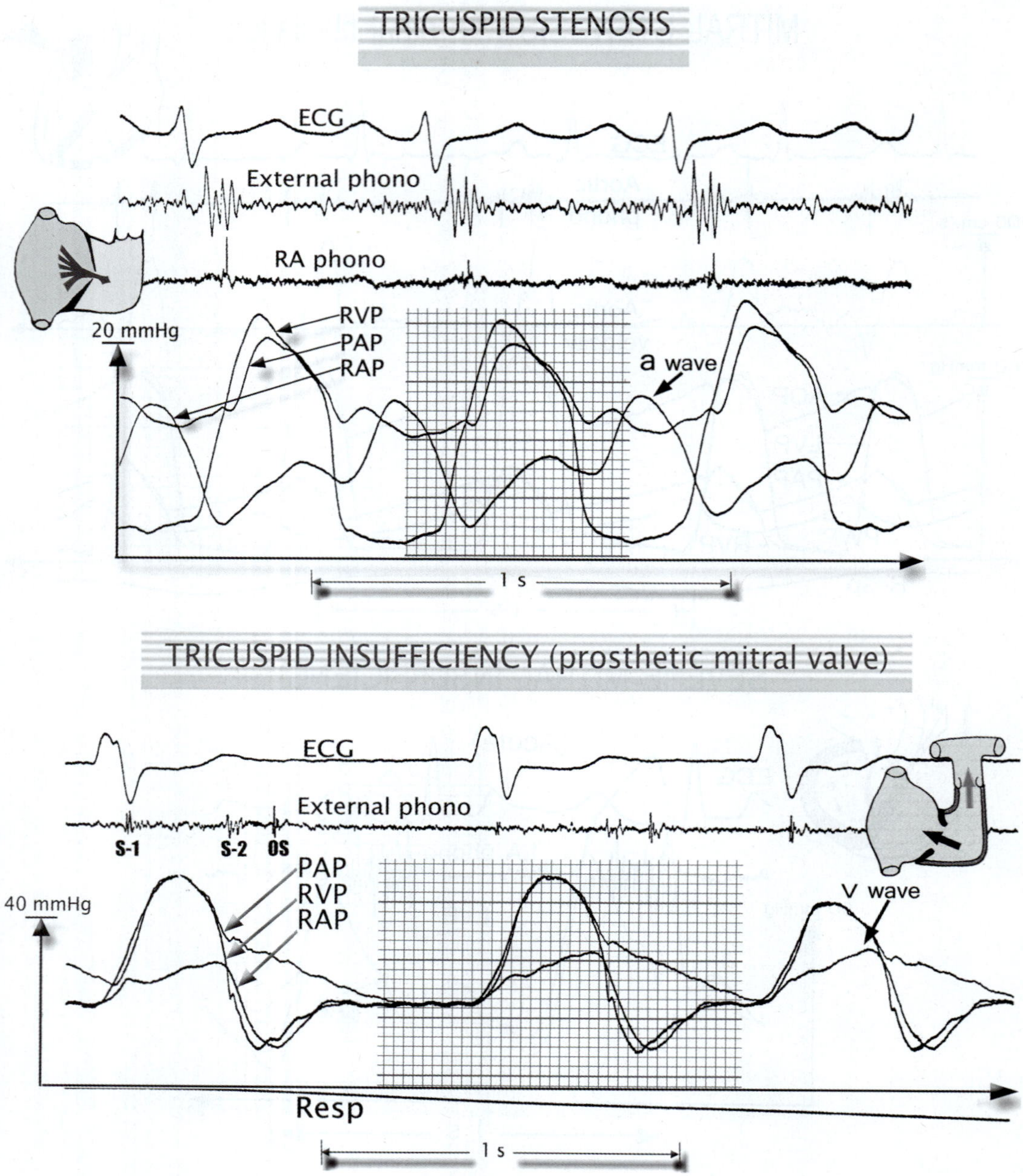

Figure 8.16: Right-heart multisensor catheterization in tricuspid stenosis (top panels) and regurgitation (bottom panels)—abbreviations as in previous figures. The findings are analogous to those shown for mitral valve disease in Figure 8.15, except for the huge *"a"* wave in the atrial pressure in tricuspid stenosis with normal sinus rhythm.

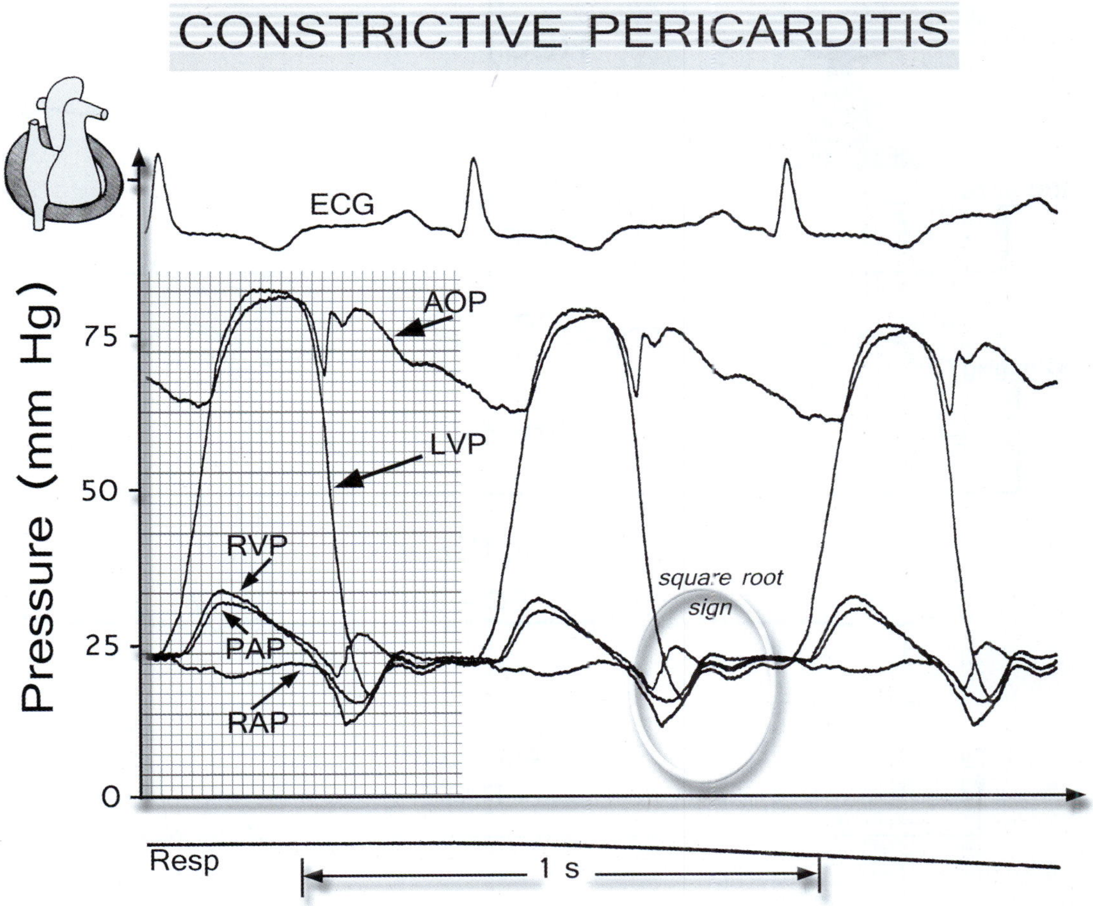

Figure 8.17: Right- and left-heart multisensor catheterization in a patient with constrictive pericarditis. In constrictive pericarditis, early diastolic filling is unrestrained, and only at the end of the first third of diastole does the stiff pericardium abruptly restrict right and left ventricular filling. As a result, RVP and LVP first fall rapidly in the early rapid filling phase and then rise abruptly to an elevated level, where they remain for the remainder of diastole until the next ventricular contraction. The resulting pattern of ventricular diastolic pressure is denoted as the "dip-and-plateau pattern" or the "square root sign," and is characteristic of constrictive pericarditis. End-diastolic ventricular pressures and mean atrial pressures are elevated and nearly equal (within few $mm\,Hg$), while end-diastolic volumes and thus stroke volume and cardiac output are restricted. Note that during inspiration, the decreased intrathoracic pressure is associated with only a muted decline in the intracardiac pressure levels (cf. Fig. 5.8, on p. 245).

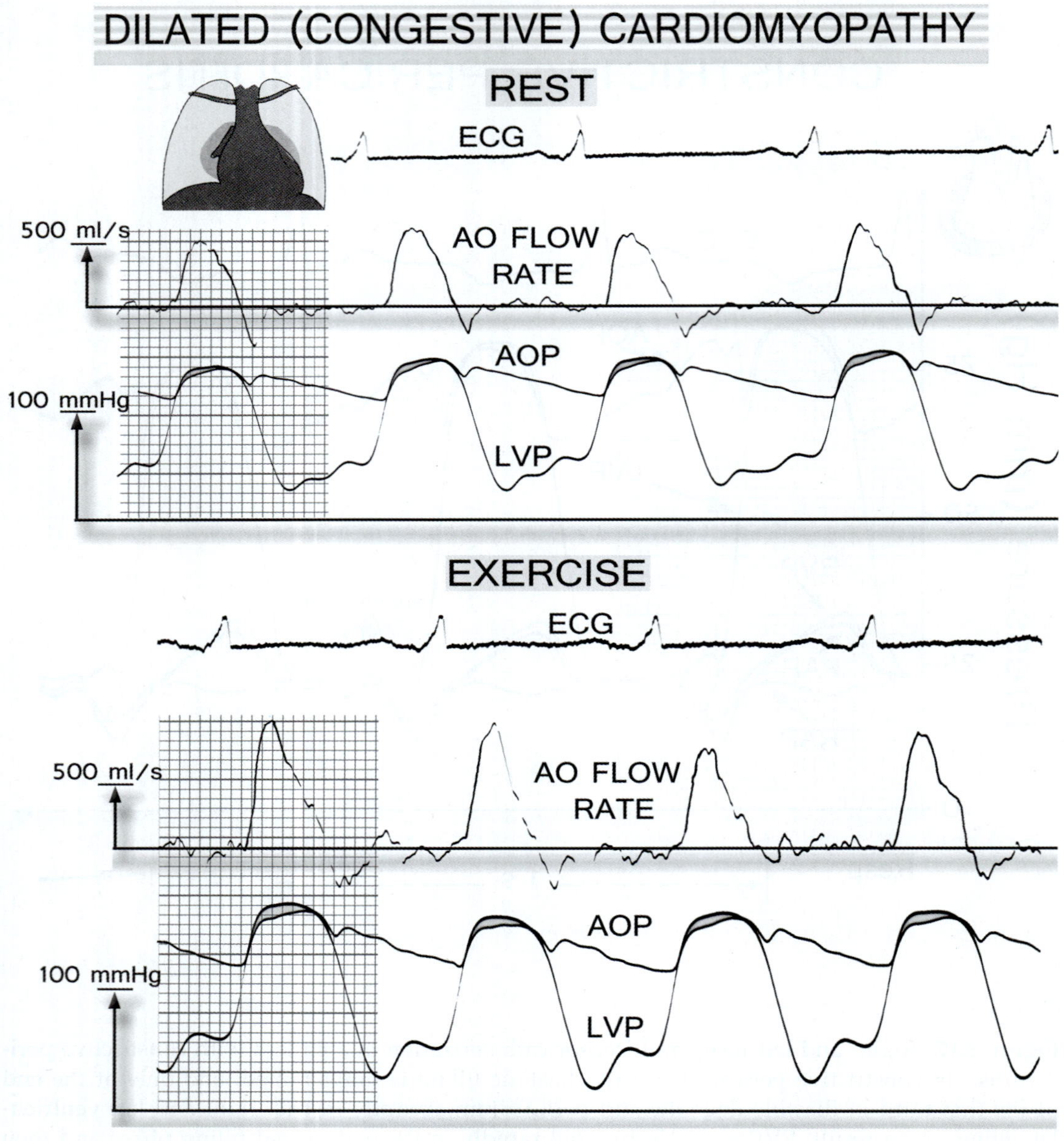

Figure 8.18: Left ventricular (LVP) and aortic (AOP) multisensor catheterization in dilated (congestive) cardiomyopathy showing elevated LV filling pressures and more rounded and symmetric than normal ejection waveforms and transaortic pressure gradients, at rest and during exercise. Note the reduced upstroke slopes in the aortic flow signals, with prolonged times to peak flow. By enhancing convective effects, ventriculoannular disproportion brings about these changes in configuration that are qualitatively reminiscent of the pattern in aortic stenosis. (Slightly modified from Pasipoularides [16], with permission of the American College of Cardiology.)

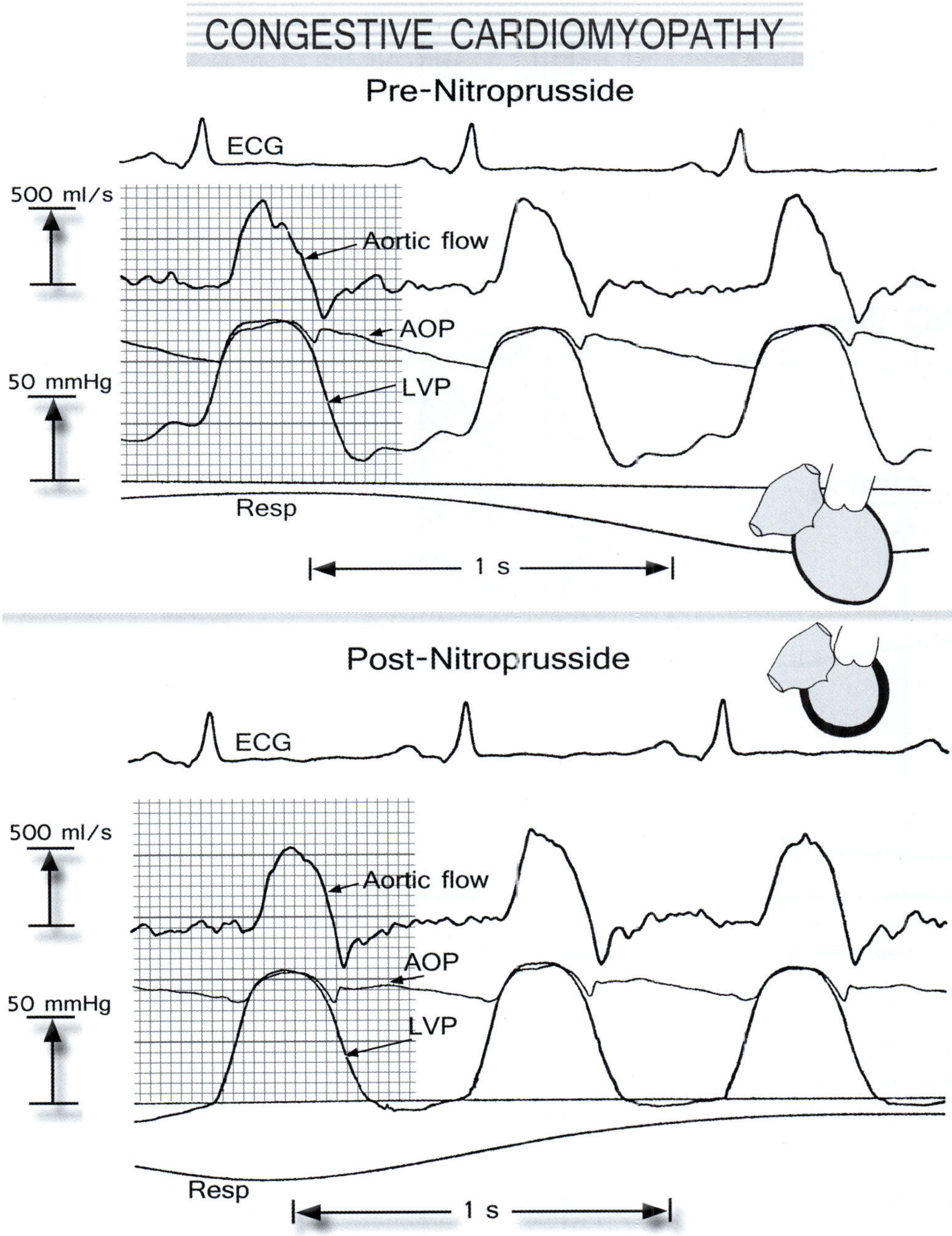

Figure 8.19: LVP and AOP multisensor catheterization tracings in congestive cardiomyopathy pre- and post-nitroprusside infusion. The vasodilator induces translocation of intrathoracic blood to peripheral capacitance vessels, with central unloading and dramatic reductions in intracardiac pressures.

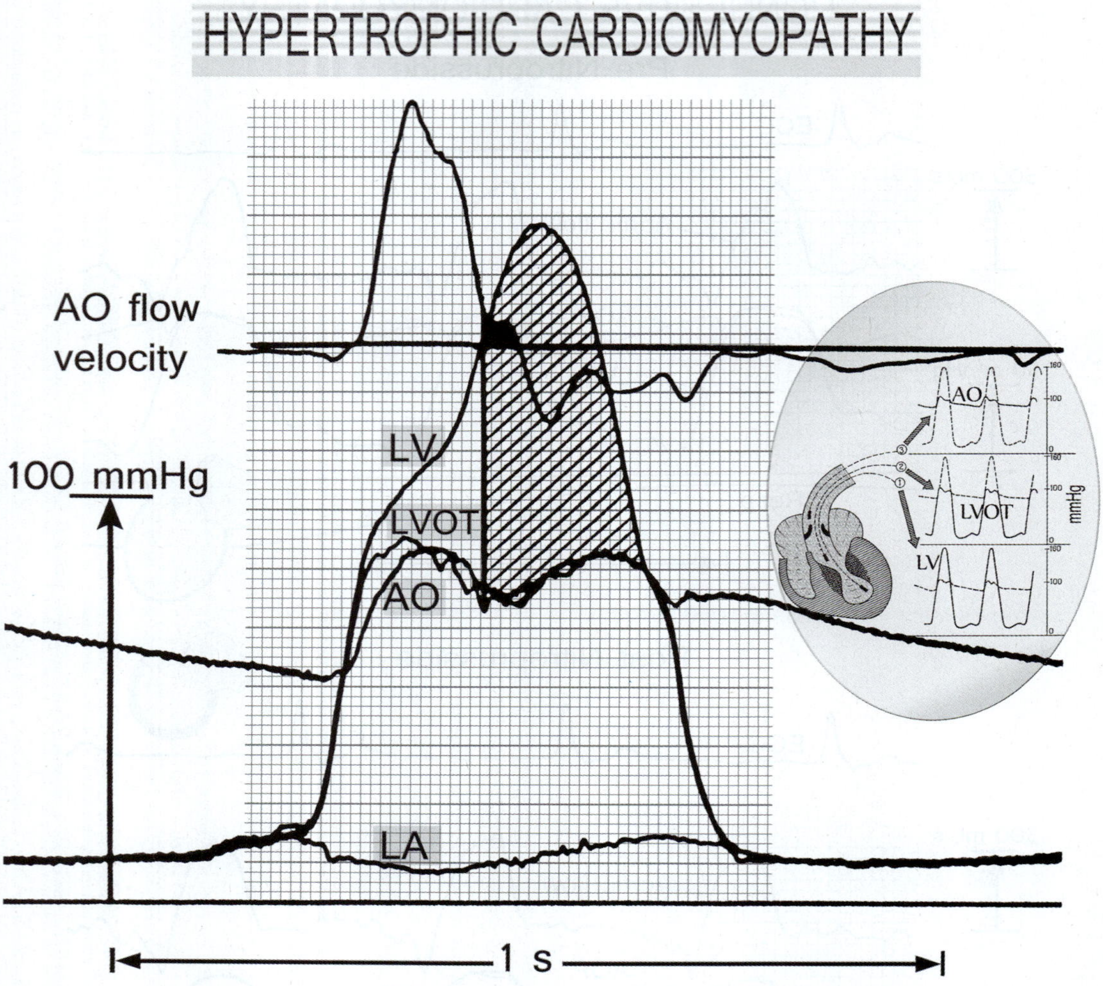

Figure 8.20: Pressure-flow relation with large early and enormous mid- and late-systolic dynamic gradients in HCM. From top downward: aortic velocity signal, and deep left ventricular (LV), left ventricular outflow tract (LVOT), and aortic root (AO) micromanometric signals, measured by retrograde triple-tip pressure plus velocity multisensor left-heart catheter. Left atrial (LA) micromanometric signal was measured simultaneously by transseptal catheter. The vertical straight line identifies the onset of SAM-septal contact, determined from a simultaneous M-mode mitral valve echocardiogram (not shown); the majority of aortic ejection flow is already completed by this time. The huge mid- and late- systolic gradient (hatched area) is maintained in the face of minuscule remaining forward or even negative aortic velocities. AO = aortic; SAM = systolic anterior motion of the mitral valve. (Modified from Pasipoularides [16], with permission of the American College of Cardiology.) Inset isolates schematically using continuous lines the individual signals from (1) LV, (2) LVOT, and (3) AO, superposed on interrupted-line tracings from the other sites.

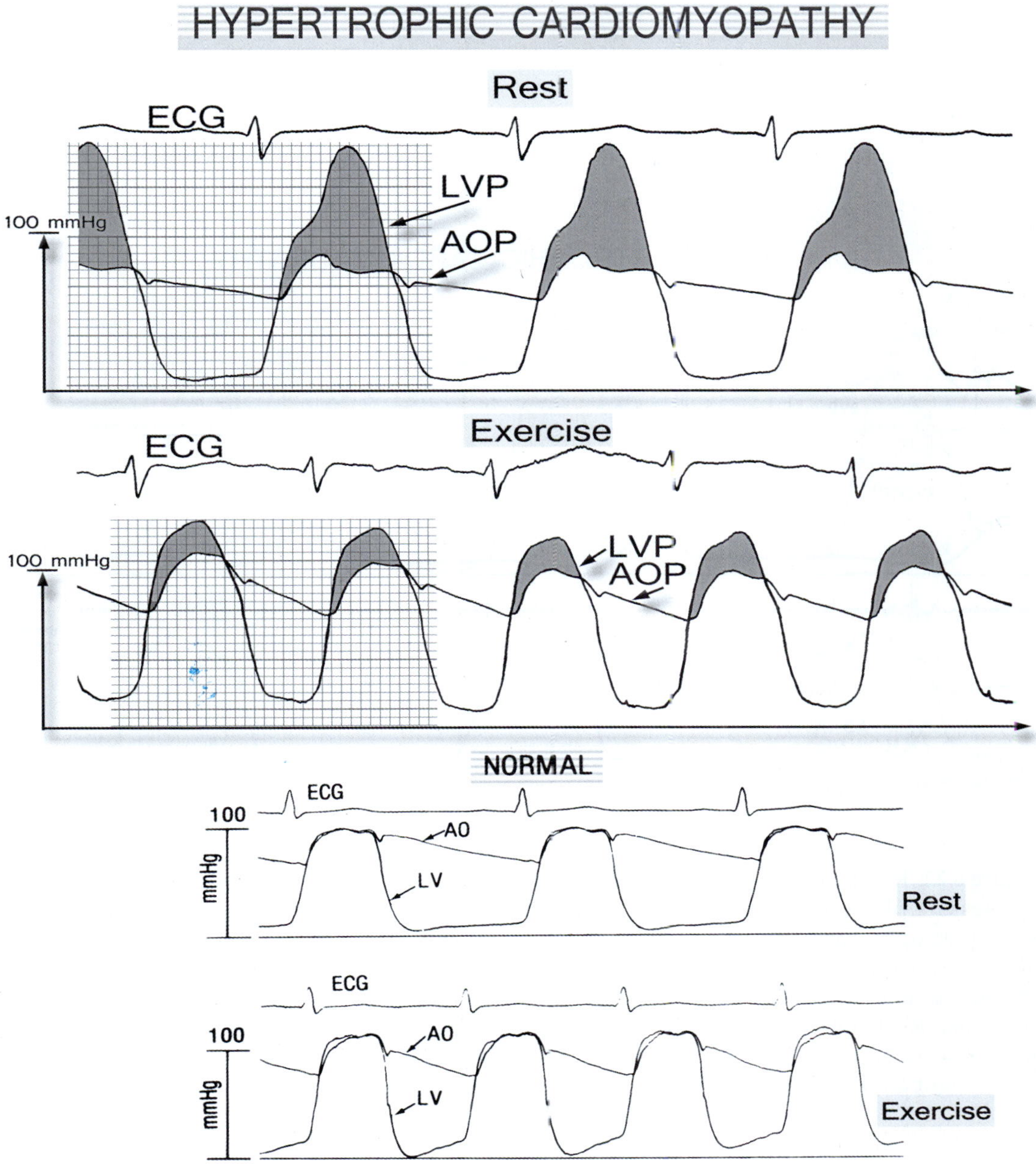

Figure 8.21: Deep left ventricular (LVP) and aortic root (AOP) pressures in hypertrophic cardiomyopathy (HCM) at rest and during supine bicycle exercise, which elicits an abnormal LVP diastolic decay, suggesting impaired ventricular relaxation; LVP decays *throughout* diastole, in sharp contrast to the normal pattern shown in the bottom panel.

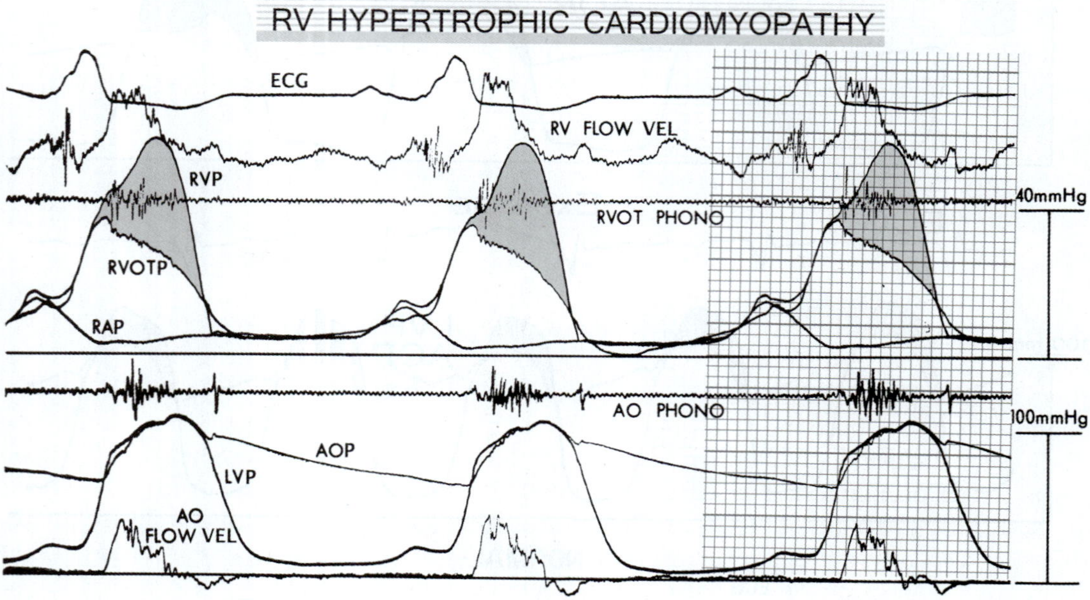

Figure 8.22: Right- and left-heart multisensor catheterization, using multisensor orthograde triple-tip pressure plus velocity right-heart catheter and retrograde left-heart catheter, in a patient with RV hypertrophic cardiomyopathy at rest. Deep right ventricular chamber (RVP) and outlow tract (RVOTP) micromanometric pressures demonstrate the enormous mid- and late-systolic dynamic pressure gradient, which is maintained in the face of minuscule remaining forward RV outflow velocities (RV FLOW VEL). Simultaneous left ventricular (LVP) and aortic root (AOP) pressure and aortic root flow velocity signals (AO FLOW VEL), shown in the bottom panel, appear normal. RAP = right atrial pressure.

References and further reading

[1] Bird, J.J., Murgo, J.P., Pasipoularides, A. Fluid dynamics of aortic stenosis: subvalvular gradients without subvalvular obstruction. Circulation 66: 835–40, 1982.

[2] Chauveau, A., Marey, É.-J. Détermination graphique des rapports du choc du coeur avec les mouvements des oreillettes et des ventricules: expérience faite à l'aide d'un appareil enregistreur (sphygmographe). Comptes rendus des séances et mémoires de la Société de Biologie 3: 3–11, 1861.

[3] Condos, W.R., Latham, R.D., Hoadley, S.D., Pasipoularides, A. Hemodynamic effects of the Mueller maneuver by simultaneous right and left heart micromanometry. Circulation 76: 1020–8, 1987.

[4] Craig, W.E., Murgo, J.P., Pasipoularides, A. Calculation of the time constant of relaxation. In: Grossman, W., Lorell, B. [Eds.] Diastolic relaxation of the heart. 1987, The Hague: Martinus Nijhoff. pp. 125–32.

[5] Craig, W.E., Pasipoularides, A. Ventricular diastolic dynamics: effects of wall asynchrony on global relaxation indices. In: Proceedings of the 21st Annual Meeting of the Association for the Advancement of Medical Instrumentation. Chicago, 1986.

[6] Debru, C. Étienne Jules Marey: l'innovation médicale. Bulletin de l'Académie Nationale de Médecine 188: 1413–21, 2004.

[7] Hansen, A.G. Similarity analyses of boundary value problems in engineering. 1964, Englewood Cliffs, NJ: Prentice-Hall. xiv, 114 p.

[8] Hoadley, S.D., Pasipoularides, A. Are ejection phase Doppler/echo indices sensitive markers of contractile dysfunction in cardiomyopathy? Role of afterload mismatch. Circulation 76: IV-404, 1987.

[9] Isaaz, K., Pasipoularides, A. Noninvasive assessment of intrinsic ventricular load dynamics in dilated cardiomyopathy. J. Am. Coll. Cardiol. 17: 112–21, 1991.

[10] Krouse, J.R., Pasipoularides, A., Bailey, S.R., Mulrow, J.P., Murgo, J.P. Right ventricular hemodynamic abnormalities in hypertrophic cardiomyopathy. J. Amer. Coll. Cardiol. 9: 231 A, 1987.

[11] Lehrs, E. Man or matter; introduction to a spiritual understanding of nature on the basis of Goethe's method of training observation and thought. 2nd ed. 1958, London: Faber and Faber. 456 p.

[12] Mirsky, I., Pasipoularides, A. Elastic properties of normal and hypertrophied cardiac muscle. Fed. Proc. 39: 156–61, 1980.

[13] Mirsky, I., Pasipoularides, A. Clinical assessment of diastolic function. Prog. Cardiovas. Dis. 32: 291–318, 1990.

[14] Müller, R. Instrumentation. Ind. Eng. Chem., Analyt. Edn. 19: 23A–24A, 1947.

[15] Pagani, M., Pizzinelli, P., Gussoni, M., Craig, W.E., Pasipoularides, A. Diastolic abnormalities of hypertrophic cardiomyopathy reproduced by asynchrony of the left ventricle in conscious dogs. J. Am. Coll. Cardiol. 1: 641, 1983.

[16] Pasipoularides, A. Clinical assessment of ventricular ejection dynamics with and without outflow obstruction. J. Am. Coll. Cardiol. 15: 859–82, 1990.

[17] Pasipoularides, A. Cardiac mechanics: basic and clinical contemporary research. Ann. Biomed. Eng. 20: 3–17, 1992.

[18] Pasipoularides, A. Complementarity and competitiveness of the intrinsic and extrinsic components of the total ventricular load: demonstration after valve replacement in aortic stenosis [Editorial]. Am. Heart. J. 153: 4–6, 2007.

[19] Pasipoularides, A., Miller, J., Rubal, B.J., Murgo, J.P. Left ventricular ejection dynamics in normal man. In Melbin, J., Noordergraaf, A. [Eds.] Proceedings of the Vlth International Conference and Workshop of the Cardiovascular System Dynamics Society. 1984, Philadelphia: University of Pennsylvania. pp. 45–8, 1984.

[20] Pasipoularides, A., Mirsky, I. Models and concepts of diastolic mechanics: pitfalls in their misapplication. Math. Comput. Modell. 11: 232–4, 1988.

[21] Pasipoularides, A., Mirsky, I., Hess, O.M., Grimm, J., Krayenbuehl, H.P. Myocardial relaxation and passive diastolic properties in man. Circulation 74: 991–1001, 1986.

[22] Pasipoularides, A., Murgo, J.P. Ejection dynamics in man with and without outflow obstruction. In: Proceedings of the 20th Annual Meeting of the Association for the Advancement of Medical Instrumentation. 1985, Boston: AAMI. p. 68.

[23] Pasipoularides, A., Murgo, J.P., Bird, J.J., Craig, W.E. Fluid dynamics of aortic stenosis: mechanisms of subvalvular gradient generation. In: Proceedings of the Sixth Annual Conference of the American Society of Biomechanics. 1982, Seattle: ASB. p. 5.

[24] Pasipoularides, A., Murgo, J.P., Bird, J.J., Craig, W.E. Fluid dynamics of aortic stenosis: mechanisms for the presence of subvalvular pressure gradients. Am. J. Physiol. 246: H542–50, 1984.

[25] Pasipoularides, A., Murgo, J.P., Miller, J.W., Craig, W.E. Nonobstructive left ventricular ejection pressure gradients in man. Circ. Res. 61: 220–7, 1987.

[26] Pasipoularides, A., Kussmaul, W.G., Myers, B.S., Doherty, B.J., Stoughton, T.L., Laskey, W.K. Phasic characteristics of transaortic pressure gradients in valvular stenosis. J. Am. Coll. Cardiol. 17: 254A, 1991.

[27] Pasipoularides, A., Shu, M., Shah, A., Womack, M.S., Glower, D.D. Diastolic right ventricular filling vortex in normal and volume overload states. Am. J. Physiol. Heart Circ. Physiol. 284: H1064–72, 2003.

[28] Pasipoularides, A., Shu, M., Shah, A., Tucconi, A., Glower, D.D. RV instantaneous intraventricular diastolic pressure and velocity distributions in normal and volume overload awake dog disease models. Am. J. Physiol. Heart Circ. Physiol. 285: H1956–65, 2003.

[29] Seldinger, S.I. Catheter replacement of the needle in percutaneous arteriography: a new technique. Acta Radiol. 39: 368–76, 1953.

[30] Shim, Y., Hampton, T.G., Straley, C.A., Harrison, J.K., Spero, L.A., Bashore, T.M., Pasipoularides, A.D. Ejection load changes in aortic stenosis: observations made following balloon aortic valvuloplasty. Circ. Res. 71: 1174–84, 1992.

[31] Yock P.G., Hatle L., Popp R.L. Patterns and timing of Doppler-detected intracavitary and aortic flow in hypertrophic cardiomyopathy. J. Am. Coll. Cardiol. 8: 1047–58, 1986.

[32] Zitnik, R.S., Piemme, T.E., Messer, R.J., Reed, D.P., Haynes, F.W., and Dexter, L. The masking of aortic stenosis by mitral stenosis. Am. Heart. J. 69: 22–30, 1965.

Chapter 9

Vortex Formation in Fluid Flow

... the middle of the blood [stream] which surges through the [aortic aperture] to a much greater height than that which surges along the sides of this [aperture]. This occurs so that the blood in the middle of the [aperture] directs its impetus straight upwards and that which surges along the sides distributes its impetus by lateral motion, and percusses against the front of the arches of the hemicycles (sinuses of Valsalva), and follows the concavity of [each] hemicycle, constantly passing downwards, until it percusses against the concavity at the base of this hemicycle (concavity of the corresponding valve cusp) and then by reflected motion turns upward [again] and continues to revolve upon itself with a circular motion until it expends its impetus.

—Leonardo da Vinci; slightly modified from Keele and Pedretti [32].

THE CHANGING PATTERNS of familiar fluid flows in the face of *nearly* unchanging conditions are a central property that fascinates those who observe them. The idea is expressed in the line: "The River flows on without cease, yet its waters are never the same."[1] In nature, nonequilibrium systems frequently form distinct patterns. In fact, when a spatially homogeneous system is driven out of equilibrium, a well-ordered pattern can form. We see neatly raked sand dunes in deserts, cloud bands overhead, and *vortical structures* in cardiovascular flows. Such patterns are created in different media by different mechanisms, on different length and time scales. Some are dynamic, even turbulent, as the eddying flow behind a large arterial stenosis, and others appear static for as long as we can wait to watch them, as many a cloud formation. The appearance of any such pattern is due to the competition between a driving force and a dissipation of energy, and hence these patterns are also known as "dissipative structures" [51].

Pattern formation is an inherently nonlinear effect: patterns form due to an instability in which small perturbations are amplified through nonlinear feedback. Systems with similar symmetries will often form similar patterns in spite of obvious differences in mechanism. Nonlinear dynamic systems theory explains, via bifurcation theory, how qualitatively new behavior and structure can arise abruptly with the smooth variation in the applying experimental conditions [26,68,69].

9.1 Symmetry and the breaking of symmetry

In current scientific language, the concept of *symmetry* includes a *commensuration*[2] of relationships among structural elements that is so extreme as to be actually unnoticeable: i.e., any difference between the designated structure or object and that obtained by applying a symmetry transformation on it, is indiscernible—e.g., think of a glass rotated around its axis. A transformation is a symmetry transformation if it leaves the structure unchanged, and symmetry is *invariance* after a transformation; it is *indiscernibility* of the change produced by a transformation. Symmetry implies the impossibility of measuring or perceiving the alteration of basic quantities, characteristic of the structure or object [60,80]. In this sense, symmetry is more like *uncertainty*, or entropy, than *order*, or correlation.

Symmetry breaking is a spontaneous process in which a spatially uniform state, subject to some perturbation, evolves into a stable nonuniform pattern as a result of the balance of forces acting within the system, which make the initial spatially homogeneous state unstable. A breaking of symmetry involves the establishing of correlations, or of order, among structural elements originally having a relationship of indifference to each

[1] Idea attributed [31] to a 13th-century Japanese hermit who built a hut for himself in the forest and wrote about it in an essay entitled "Tale of the Ten-Foot-Square-Hut."

[2] From the Greek $\sigma\upsilon\mu \cdot \mu\epsilon\tau\rho\iota\alpha$, the concept of $sym \cdot metry$ refers to a $com \cdot mensuration$ of relationships among the elements or components of a structure or object. Symmetry is also related to the concept of harmony.

other. Symmetry assumes the undetectability of transformations; accordingly, the *breaking of symmetry* implies a detectability of transformations and is therefore contemporaneous to the production of information and, in a visual context, to the *emergence of pattern* [78].

In fluid flow systems, the passing from one pattern whose elements are characterized by certain geometric or dynamic correlations, to another characterized by different geometric or dynamic correlations among the elements that compose it, is not a one-time event; rather, successive symmetry breakings may occur in a *cascade*, depending on changing flow parameters, with attendant emergence of additional recognizable geometric patterns. Many of these patterns may have a kind of haunting beauty.

9.2 Flow regime bifurcations

We have previously discussed (see Section 4.11.1, on p. 206) the Reynolds number as an index characteristic of instability and turbulence. Let us now consider hydrodynamic motion to be generally described, in addition to dynamic variables, by such a characteristic dimensionless parameter, as Re. The corresponding dynamics of the flow tend to be stable at small values of Re. However, at $Re > Re_1$, an increase in Re results in an onset of instability and the appearance of a new type of motion which, in turn, is stable at small values of $Re - Re_1 > O$. In the general case, hydrodynamic systems can have a sequence of numbers $Re_1, Re_2, ...$, at which their dynamic evolution undergoes qualitative modifications called *bifurcations*.

Mathematically, a "bifurcation" denotes a sudden qualitative (as opposed to merely quantitative) change in state that ensues in response to a very small change in applying conditions—say, a branch snaps as you are bending it progressively. Not only in fluid mechanics but also in many other fields, including embryology and physiology, there has been through the years an interest in bifurcations as successive stages of "self-organization" [15, 20, 23, 51, 55, 67]. A sequence of bifurcations in a flow system leads—because of its inherent nonlinearity—to an irregular, chaotic motion at $Re > Re_{crit}$, and generally $Re_{crit} > Re_1, Re_2, ...$ The ultimate regime is turbulent. As the Reynolds number, or the Rayleigh number (see Section 1.5, on pp. 10 ff.), or other parameter appraising the speed of a class of dynamically similar flows with a given configuration is raised, the temporal and spatial complexity of observed flows often increases in a progression of abrupt bifurcations. Each bifurcation is unveiled by the onset of instability of one flow regime and is followed by equilibration to another stable regime, which may be steady or unsteady. This notion goes back to the work of Malkus [39], who interpreted in this way his measurements of nonlinear Rayleigh–Bénard convection as the Rayleigh number increased (see Section 1.5, on pp. 10 ff.).

The preceding idea has been subsequently developed and refined by many others. Various examples of such physical flow situations can be found in the classic monograph by Monin and Yaglom [46]. The stable flow ensuing after the first bifurcation of a basic flow as the Reynolds number increases is identified as the "secondary flow" in fluid dynamic descriptions; and its instability at the second bifurcation as the Reynolds number increases further is often called "secondary instability;" subsequent successive bifurcations generally follow one another after smaller and smaller Reynolds number increments, so as to eventually become practically indistinguishable [15].

If a flow has some symmetries, then usually these are at first broken, one by one, at bifurcations as the Reynolds number increases, and may be eventually "restored" upon the onset of turbulence, such that the mean turbulent flow has all the previously disrupted symmetries [23, 67]. The Taylor–Couette flow, which we will consider shortly (Section 9.5.4, on pp. 463 ff.), is a classic paradigm of flow with a succession of bifurcations toward transition to turbulence, as the Reynolds number increases.

9.2.1 Flow-associated structures and pattern formation

We have all experienced vortices in our lives. The best examples are found in tornadoes, rivers, streams, and rugged coasts. For most people who don't often get to experience and observe rugged coasts or tornadoes, there is the experience of a stirred cup, and a draining bathtub, or sink. In all these situations, the relatively large coherent structures, or eddies, evolving in the flow-field tend to persist in space as well as in time.

A fascinating area of fluid dynamics of special interest in intracardiac flow phenomena is the study of how interacting fluid particles cooperate to produce large-scale coherent structures, such as spiraling vortical motions. There is also the emergence of the apparent randomness of turbulence as the product of the moment-to-moment application of elemental, but nonlinear, operations, involving the interplay of convective acceleration and viscous effects. Thus, coherent features are often not readily discernible because they are buried within highly disorganized flow. Velocity pattern measurements over a number of cycles must then be "ensemble averaged," as we discussed in Section 2.1, on pp. 37 ff., in order to disclose the embedded flow features. The field of pattern formation focuses on systems with many components, and attempts a level of detailed analysis of underlying mechanisms. It explains the emergence of patterns in spatial processes.

Pattern formation models have a long history that includes Alan Turing's [76] and René Thom's [73, 74] work on morphogenesis in the 1950s and 1970s, respectively, and that of Prigogine and Nicolis [50, 51, 55, 56] on dissipative structures. The concept of a *dissipative structure* [4, 14, 41, 50] indicates a structure according to which a system may organize itself, when it is removed from thermodynamic equilibrium. In such a structure, a dynamic ordered pattern (*viz.* "structure") is maintained at the cost of energy injected—at the necessary rate and in sufficient quantity—from outside the system, and then dissipated within the structure. Irreversibility, which results from energy dissipation during the evolution of a process [20], can actually have a constructive role: it can generate *form*.

The flow of energy in dissipative systems allows them to self-organize spontaneously, so that ordered patterns appear, unexpectedly and suddenly! In far-from-equilibrium conditions, such systems give rise to and maintain novel structures and new modes of behavior. They are thus seen to be "creative." The process of self-organization happens

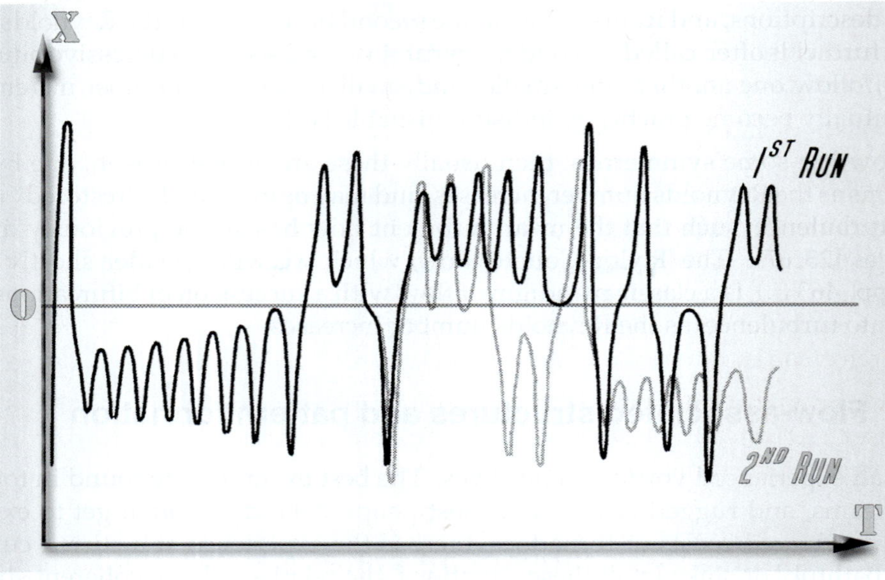

Figure 9.1: The MIT meteorologist Edward Norton Lorenz was plotting numerical solution results of a set of simplified but *nonlinear* fluid dynamic equations when he decided to rerun a portion of his output. Rather than start again from the beginning, he entered intermediate values that due to rounding were close, but not identical, to the values that had existed at that stage of the initial computational run. The second run (plotted here in gray) tracked the first one closely for a while, then began to deviate slightly from it, and then deviated more and more. This discovery affords us with a stark illustration of the concept of *sensitive dependence* on initial conditions. (Adapted from Lorenz [35], with kind permission of the American Meteorological Society.)

spontaneously, as is the case in the familiar example of a flock of migratory birds that adjust and adapt to their neighbors, unconsciously ordering themselves into a *patterned* flock. Pattern formation theory and experiment have experienced a tremendous growth in the past century [29]. They have yielded a large body of results on coherent flow structures and regimes that portend and presage the onset of turbulence in a wide range of fluid flows.

Characteristic control parameters, for each flow system studied, measure how far away the system is from the critical point of a bifurcation that leads to a dynamic instability. The control parameter is associated to dynamic instabilities between a state of equilibrium and the bifurcation to a dissipative structure, or between dissipative structures in cascade. This may be expressed (cf. Fig. 1.3, on p. 14) in terms of a difference between "gain" and "loss"; that is, between an external destabilizing action and the system's dissipative reaction, which tends to maintain it in the status quo. When the destabilizing action wins out, the critical fluctuation associated with one of the system's collective variables, instead of regressing, emerges as the order parameter, and the system organizes itself, quite abruptly, according to a new structure, or *pattern*.

9.2.2 Sensitive dependence on initial conditions

It is very notable—and counterintuitive—that a very small difference between two initial conditions of a nonlinear flow system—beyond human ability to measure—can lead to divergence, and ultimately to an absence of any correlation between the trajectories of the subsequent evolution of the system. The idea is that the small initial difference causes a change in what is encountered just beyond the "initial" moment, which yields slightly different influences, producing slightly different outcomes. Through *repeated iterations* of *small* differences, the paths diverge, eventually to form very disparate trajectories. The paths do not endlessly diverge, but after a surprisingly brief interval they no longer have any noticeable relation to one another (see Fig. 9.1, on p. 446). This idea forms the cornerstone of modern chaos theory. It was originally formulated by Henri Poincaré in his book *Science et Méthode* [54]; in it, he summarized the concept as follows: "There are situations where small differences in the initial conditions can produce very large ones in the final result: a small error in the former can lead to a huge error in the latter. In those cases, predictions become impossible."

A phrase identified with this phenomenon is the *Lorenz butterfly effect*. Interestingly, in the study of nonlinear dynamic systems, a graphical representation of a collection of states known as a "Lorenz attractor" resembles a butterfly [37]; perhaps Lorenz named the butterfly effect after this attractor.[3] The Lorenz attractor, developed by Lorenz while probing the nonrepeatability of weather patterns, is the plot of the orbit of a dynamic system consisting of three first order nonlinear differential equations. The solution to the system of differential equations is a vector-valued function of one variable [35,36]. If you think of the variable as time, the solution traces out a three-dimensional orbit as time passes. The orbit, an example of which is given in Figure 9.2 on p. 448, is made up of two oblong spirals (the butterfly wings), at an angle to each other in three dimensions.

The *butterfly effect* eponym stems from the idea that the flapping of a butterfly's wings changes local air flow conditions slightly, setting into motion a series of small, then potentially larger, changes that ultimately might result in a storm in another region of the globe. The idea may be apocryphal, but many embrace the metaphor as a way of thinking about sensitivity of nonlinear flow systems to small, perhaps random, initial condition differences. Although a complex dynamic system may have sensitive dependence on initial conditions, this does not mean that everything about it is unpredictable. Establishing what *is* in fact predictable and what *is not*, is naturally a challenge, since the divergence of the solutions, or *evolutionary paths*, depends on details of the initial conditions that are practically unknowable.

Nearly everything that is known about chaotic system behavior relates to simple mechanical systems with only a few components, or *degrees of freedom*. Almost none of the ideas pertaining to the mathematics of chaos has been put in the context of continuous fields, such as the flow-field of a fluid within a region of interest. We know only that

[3] "Does the flap of a butterfly's wings in Brazil set off a tornado in Texas?"—provocative question posed by Lorenz in a speech to the American Association for the Advancement of Science, in Washington, D.C., in December 1972.

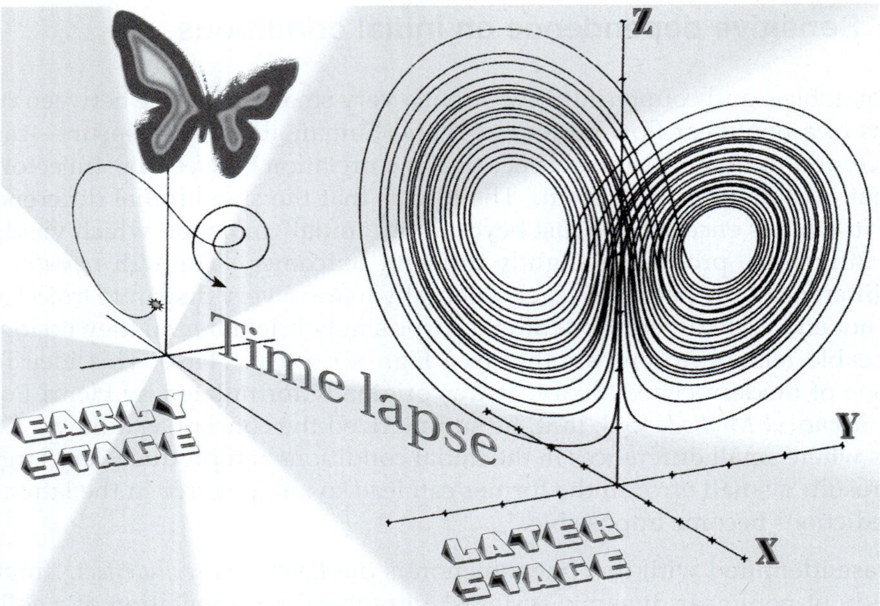

Figure 9.2: The Lorenz attractor is the plot of the orbit of a dynamic system consisting of three first order nonlinear differential equations. The orbit is described in terms of the trajectory of the nondimensional dynamic variables X, Y, and Z, which evolve in nondimensional time, T (cf. Fig. 9.1). States not on the butterfly-shaped attractor flow to it and then both diverge and converge on the attractor. The local divergence leads to sensitivity to initial conditions. If the system is released from two points that are arbitrarily close to each other on the attractor, their subsequent trajectories remain on the attractor surface but diverge away from each other. After sufficient time lapses, the two trajectories can be arbitrarily far apart on the attractor surface. (Adapted from a diagram in Holden [27], with kind permission of Princeton University Press.)

a fluid in turbulent motion is *chaotic*, e.g., as a function of time at a space point, albeit deterministic, and displays the butterfly effect [28].

9.3 Vorticity and circulation

The translation of fluid elements along *circular trajectories*, i.e., the motion of a fluid along a circular path, and the concept of *vorticity*, or local rate of spin of fluid particles around their own axis as they flow, are distinct phenomena. Particles in laminar viscous flow undergo rotation because adjacent laminae of fluid move at different velocities as determined by the applying velocity profile [16, 75]. As its name suggests, the vorticity, ζ, measures the strength of vortical spinning locally in a flow velocity field [1, 44, 62]. For an idealization, we turn to Figure 9.3, on p. 449. An imaginary wheel has been inserted into a 2-D flow-field. In case A., u, the velocity component along the x-axis, increases

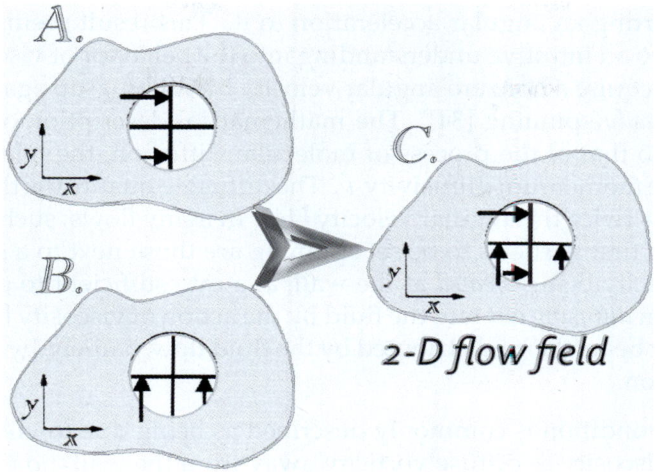

Figure 9.3: Visual explanation of the vorticity of a flow velocity field. Effectively, the vorticity at any point within a flow-field reflects how much angular velocity a fluid element acquires due to unbalanced shear stress acting on it locally.

in the y-direction, $\frac{\partial u}{\partial y} > 0$, causing the wheel to rotate clockwise. In case B, clockwise rotation is also produced, but this time due to v, the velocity component along the y-axis, decreasing in the x-direction: $\frac{\partial v}{\partial x} < 0$. To account for the total vortical spinning effect, cases A and B are combined in case C., and we arrive at the vorticity:

$$\zeta = \frac{\partial u}{\partial y} - \frac{\partial v}{\partial x} \,. \tag{9.1}$$

The vorticity is defined so that anticlockwise rotation yields positive vorticity [44,66].

For a rigid disk in a fully developed, 2-D shear flow along parallel streamlines, with an axial velocity gradient perpendicular to the flow direction, the rotational rate, or angular velocity ω_0, is related to the local velocity gradient, du/dy, as follows:

$$\omega_0 = \frac{1}{2}\frac{du}{dy} \,, \tag{9.2}$$

in other words, its angular velocity is half the magnitude of the local value of the vorticity of the flow. Equivalently, the vorticity is twice the rotation rate of the rigid spinning disk.

Figure 9.4a., on p. 451, illustrates smooth laminar flow of a viscous liquid in a straight tube. When fully developed, this familiar Poiseuille flow has a parabolic velocity distribution. Dye slowly injected in the flow moves in straight lines indicating fluid translation along straight streamlines. However, minuscule "paddle wheels" placed in the flow would also rotate as they move, indicating that the flow has vorticity, i.e., the fluid particles are *spinning* around their own axes as they move along straight streamlines. This occurs because viscous stresses vary from one side of a wheel to the other, so as to apply a net torque imparting an angular acceleration to it. This result seems entirely abstract, but it contributes to an intuitive understanding into the behavior of viscous fluids: a fluid particle can only acquire a nonzero angular velocity by rubbing-up against a neighboring particle that is *already* spinning [34]. The mathematical description of this process corresponds closely to that of the process of molecular diffusion, the relevant coefficient of diffusion being the momentum diffusivity, ν. The diffusing quantity is the vorticity, which, as we saw above, is twice the angular velocity [44]. In many flows, such as that illustrated in Figure 9.4a., the first particles to be set spinning are those next to a solid wall, and we can visualize vorticity being *created* at the wall, at a rate sufficient to enforce the no-slip condition, and then *diffusing out* into the fluid by the action of viscosity [34]. After this first step, vorticity may be further redistributed by the fluid flow, namely, by convection and by continuing diffusion.

The "no-slip" condition is commonly described as being due to viscosity. To be more precise, without viscosity to diffuse vorticity away from the wall, no effect of the no-slip condition would ever be observable. The vortex sheet would remain at the wall, affecting the velocity in only an infinitely thin region (cf. Section 4.10, on pp. 202 ff., especially Fig. 4.15, on p. 204). Figure 9.4b. illustrates a flow-field called an inviscid vortex where all fluid elements move in circular trajectories. However, small paddle wheels here do not rotate, indicating an irrotational flow with the fluid merely translating in circular paths. These two flows illustrate two extremes: one has straight pathlines but fluid element rotation; the second has circular pathlines, but fluid elements that do not rotate about their own axes, and exemplifies irrotational flow. Viscosity in the first flow produces the fluid elements' local rotation about their own axes, i.e., vorticity, which is absent in the second flow.

Nonspherical particles, such as discs, rotate in a periodic fashion so that they spend more time in certain orientations than in others. Such particles will tend to spend more time in positions aligned with the flow. An immiscible liquid droplet should simply deform into an elongated shape with its surface rotating around it like a tractor tread. Red blood cells in a shear layer combine the behavior of disc-like rigid particles and immiscible droplets, both deforming and rotating in a quasi-periodic fashion [5,17,21].

We define as circulation the line integral (see Section 2.15, on pp. 70 f.) of the velocity, v, around any loop, or closed contour, within the flow-field. We have seen (Fig. 9.4, on p. 451) how vorticity pertains to rotation in the fluid, at least in the small region around the point at which the vorticity is calculated. We can interpret vorticity in a more global way, if we integrate it over an area, to obtain the circulation around a given closed loop in the fluid [34]. For two-dimensional flow, the integral over a surface of the vorticity (component normal to the surface) equals the integral of the velocity component along the edge of the surface. This is Stokes' theorem, and applies as a vector relationship in three-dimensional space [44,62].

The flow of an incompressible fluid with no vorticity satisfies the zero divergence ($\nabla \cdot \mathbf{v} = 0$) and the zero curl ($\nabla \times \mathbf{v} = \mathbf{0}$) equations, respectively [44]. There is a solution for the flow around a cylinder when the fluid at increasing distances moves in concentric circles around the cylinder. The flow is, then, circular everywhere, as in Figure 9.4b. Such

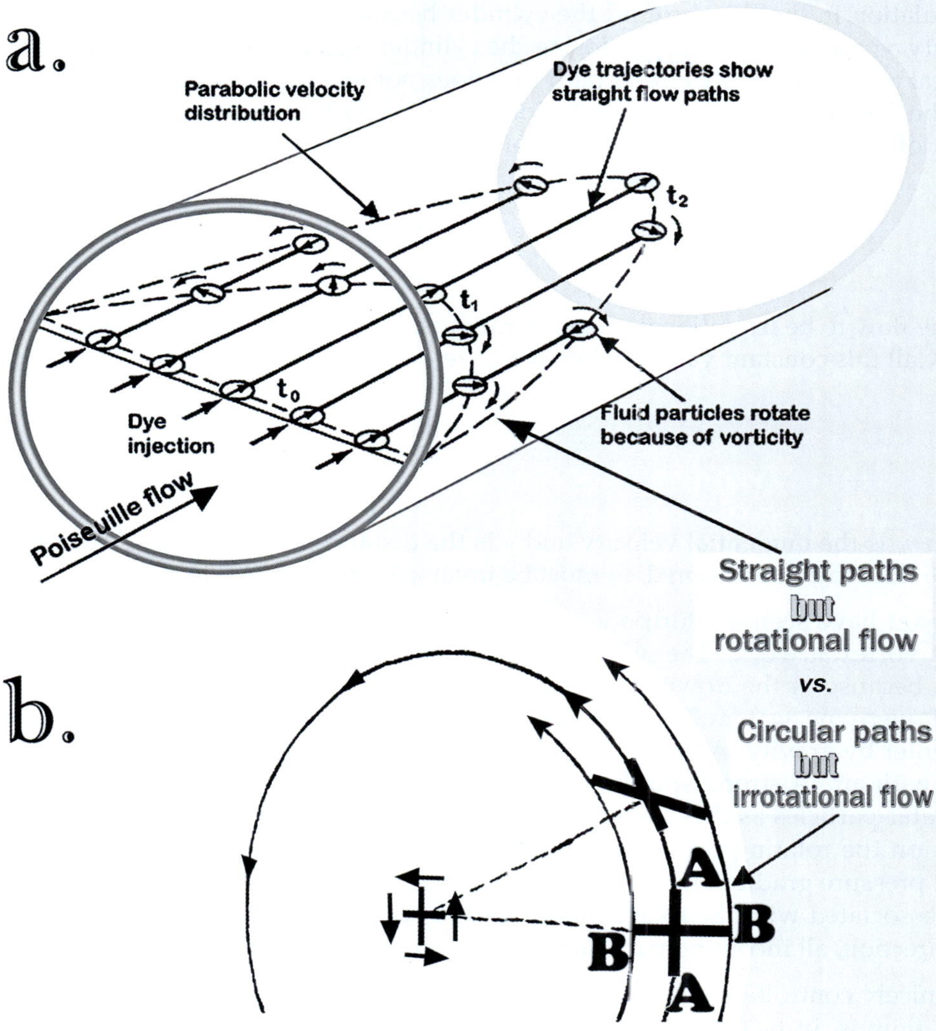

Figure 9.4: Rotation and shear each contribute to the curl of a vector field and the vorticity of a flow. a. Laminar flow of a viscous fluid along straight streamlines. The fluid particles rotate because of viscous force moments giving rise to net viscous torque actions, which are revealed by the rotation of small wheels in the flow. b. Only the paddle wheel at the central nucleus of the vortex rotates around its own axis. Fluid particles outside the nucleus undergo distortion as they slide along circular paths but without rotation, as a compass needle on a turntable. The vorticity of this flow-field vanishes despite the fact that the flow rotates around an axis (but not in rigid rotation) and that the flow has a nonzero shear. The reason that the vorticity vanishes is that the contribution of the rotation around the axis to the vorticity is equal but of *opposite* sign to the contribution of the viscous shear, so that the *total* vorticity vanishes.

a flow has a circulation around the cylinder, although $\nabla \times \mathbf{v} = 0$ in the fluid. We have a circulation in the flow around the cylinder because the line integral (see p. 70) of the velocity, $\mathbf{v}$, around any loop enclosing the cylinder is not zero. At the same time, the line integral of $\mathbf{v}$ around any closed path that does not include the cylinder is zero, showing that the flow is indeed irrotational. For a circular path of radius r with its center at the center of the cylinder, the line integral of the velocity is given by the following equation:

$$\oint \mathbf{v} \cdot d\mathbf{l} = 2\pi r v_\theta \,. \tag{9.3}$$

For the flow to be irrotational, the integral must be independent of r, as shown in Figure 9.4b. Call this constant value Γ; then we have

$$v_\theta = \frac{\Gamma}{2\pi r} \,, \tag{9.4}$$

where v_θ is the tangential velocity and r is the distance from the axis. We conclude that for the flow to be irrotational, v_θ must be inversely proportional to r.

If you have seen a whirlpool in a fairly full sink when water is draining, you have seen a vortex at work. The water goes round, spiraling into the drain. A drain's vortex forms because of the downdraft and low pressure that the suction of the drain creates in the overlying water. The water is pulled down and forced toward the drain hole in the center by gravity. As water drains fast from the central opening, a hole forms that is filled with air. A strong spiraling tendency is generated by centripetal forces acting on the water particles as they are pulled down toward the point of suction. The balance of forces on the rotating water can be represented as a dynamic antagonism between the radial pressure gradient force acting toward the center of low pressure, and a centrifugal force associated with the rotary motion pulling outward. Once the spiral starts going in one direction, all incoming particles are entrained in that same direction.

A nicely controlled experimental demonstration of the concepts pertaining to irrotational flow is, in fact, provided by water circulating around a hole. Take a large clear plastic bottle and cut off the base. Cap it and fill it with water, then stir up some circulation with a stick, and remove the cap. You get the pretty effect shown in panel a. of Figure 9.5, on p. 453. Although you put in some rotation at the beginning, it soon dies down because of viscosity and the flow becomes very nearly irrotational—although still with some circulation around the hole. This flow corresponds to that in an ideal "free vortex." It is to be distinguished from that in a "forced vortex," considered on pp. 60 ff. and Figure 2.19. As a water particle moves inward, it picks up speed. The tangential velocity here varies as $1/r$. This is different from solid-body rotation, in which tangential velocity varies as r: the spokes of a bicycle wheel move more slowly near the hub than at the rim. As Leonardo da Vinci wrote, "A vortex, unlike a wheel, moves faster toward its center." This is just a manifestation of the *conservation of angular momentum*, which is proportional to a fluid particle's tangential velocity and its distance from the center of

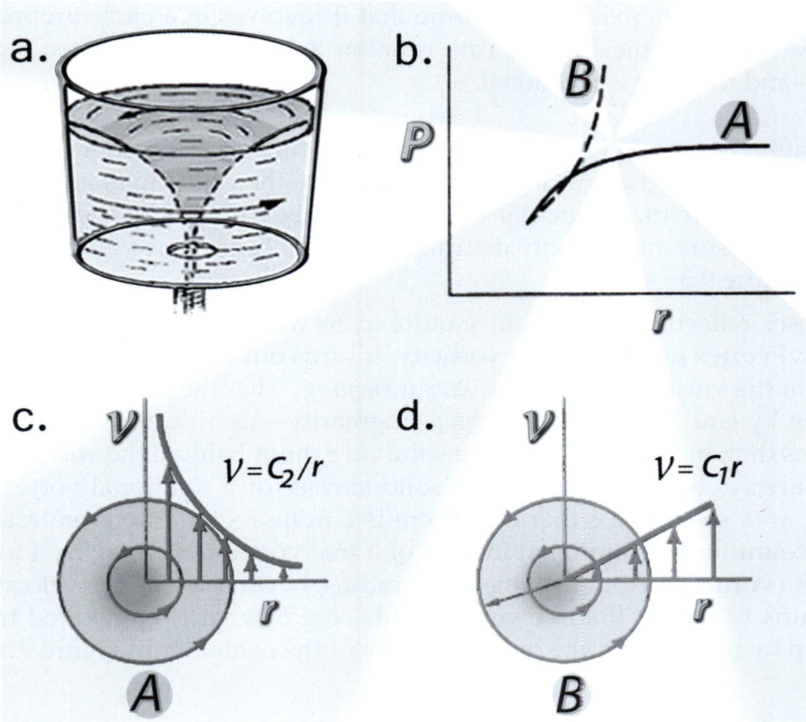

Figure 9.5: a. Water with circulation draining from a cylindrical funnel, after stirring it with a rod and unplugging the outflow orifice. b. Pressure (P) distributions along the radial (r) coordinate for irrotational (A) and rotational (B) flow-fields. c. Tangential velocity (v) distribution along r for irrotational flow. d. Tangential velocity distribution for rotational flow.

rotation. The radial velocity also varies as $1/r$. If we assume that the hole in the funnel is small compared to the diameter of the bottle, the axial velocity away from the hole is negligible, and we have water going radially inward toward the hole. Therefore, the total velocity also increases as $1/r$ and the water swirls inward along Archimedean spirals.

The distinctions of rotational and irrotational motions are fundamental. To illustrate them, we envisage a minute fluid particle that has an arrow inscribed on it and moves in a circular trajectory in a vortical flow (see Fig. 9.5). The fluid particle can, for our present purpose, exhibit two simple motions around its trajectory.

1. In the first motion, A, it moves about a circle with its arrow always pointing in one direction, e.g., West (cf. the Ferris wheel in Fig. 2.18. on p. 61, or a compass needle on a turntable). It does not rotate around its own axis and the flow is irrotational.

2. The fluid particle can also move, B, around the circle with its arrow always pointing to the center of the circle; its arrow therefore points, progressively, through all the points of the compass. In motion B, a rigid-body rotation, the fluid particle rotates

once about its own axis for each time that it revolves in a circle around the center of flow—just like the Moon in its rotation around the earth (see Fig. 2.18, on p. 61)—and the flow is rotational.

These two different motions with the same circular trajectory experience different accelerations. The pressure gradient necessary to balance the centrifugal acceleration and to keep the fluid particle on its circular trajectory will be different in these two cases. Accordingly, the pressure and velocity distributions differ radically, as is shown in panels b., c., and d. of Figure 9.5.

Upon closer reflection, one might inquire as to what is maintaining the irrotational (*zero* vorticity) vortex going without vorticity. It turns out that vorticity is indeed present somewhere in the vortex core, so as to *keep it turning*. That the irrotational velocity solution, as given by equ. 9.3 on p. 452, has a singularity—i.e., it cannot be defined—at the origin implies that, in the real world, the solution cannot hold all the way down to $r = 0$. There must always be either a spinning solid surface or a rotational vortex core in the vicinity of $r = 0$, so that in either case there is a finite region of concentrated vorticity. A way to account for the rotational motion of a free vortex is to imagine a forced vortex occupying the vortex core out to some small radius, beyond which the velocity field continuously shifts to that of the free vortex. This core is what is eliminated from explicit consideration by unplugging the outflow orifice of the container in Figure 9.5a.

9.3.1 Vortex or eddy

This is the rotating motion of a multitude of fluid particles around a common center. The paths of the individual particles do not have to be circular, but may also be asymmetric. Robinson [59] provided a more rigorous definition of a vortex:

> *A vortex exists when instantaneous streamlines mapped onto a plane normal to the vortex core exhibit a roughly circular or spiral pattern, when viewed from a reference frame moving with the center of the vortex core.*

Leonardo da Vinci described vortex motions in the sinuses of Valsalva in his Quaderni d' Anatomica in 1513 [32, 52]. Large-scale (of a size comparable with the aortic radius) vortices dissipate little energy by viscous effects. However, the interactions of these vortices with each other generate intermediate and small-scale eddies that are strongly dissipative. Thus, there is a *cascade* of energy from large through intermediate to small eddies, where kinetic energy is dissipated as heat (see Fig. 4.21, on p. 218).

9.4 Vortex dynamics

A vortex is a mass of fluid whose elements are moving in nearly circular pathlines about a common axis. As we saw in the preceding sections, vortices are to be distinguished from

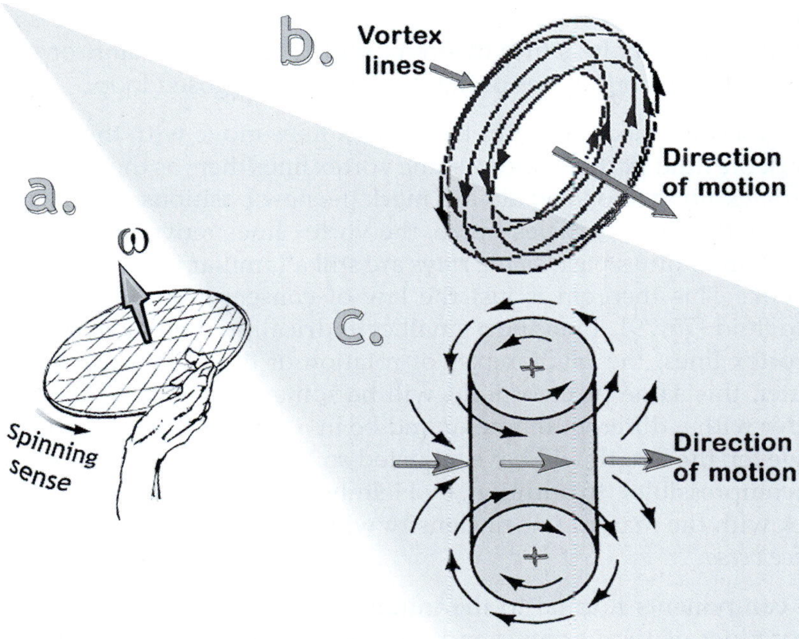

Figure 9.6: a. The *right-handed screw* rule gives the direction of the vorticity vector. b. Vortex lines in a moving vortex ring. c. A vortex ring propels itself forward.

vorticity, which is the local rate of rotation of infinitesimal[4] fluid elements about their own axes. Vorticity must be generated or annihilated by the action of nonconservative forces, such as viscous—"frictional"—forces. Moreover, vorticity can exist without vortex motion, as shown in Figure 9.4a. on p. 451, and vortex motion can exist without vorticity, as in Figure 9.4b.

The physiologist–physicist Hermann von Helmholtz (see pp. 133 ff.) in 1858 presented the famous *vorticity theorems* for the vorticity field of an inviscid fluid, coined the term "vortex motions," and remarkably extended the knowledge of the nature of fluid motion. He described the physics of vortex motions in incompressible, inviscid fluids in terms of two theorems [38]. We will next discuss the content of Helmholtz's equations in words. First, imagine that we were to draw vortex lines in the fluid, rather than streamlines. By vortex lines, we mean field lines that have the direction of the vorticity, ω, and have a density in any region proportional to the magnitude of ω [16]. Vorticity vectors take their direction according to a right-handed screw pointing in the direction of the vector ω and rotating with the fluid locally (see Fig. 9.6a.). The vorticity of the flow-field at a point is a measure of the net tangential component of the velocity along the surface of an *infinitesimal* volume surrounding the point. The divergence of ω is always zero (ω is

[4] *Infinitesimal* signifies immeasurably small; i.e., smaller than any assignable magnitude, and continuously approaching zero as a limit.

the curl of the velocity of the fluid particles, and the divergence of a curl is always zero). Thus, according to Helmholtz's first theorem, vortex lines never start or stop in a fluid; they must extend to the boundaries of the fluid, or form a closed loop.

Helmholtz's second theorem states that vortex lines move with the fluid. This means that if you mark the fluid particles along some vortex lines then, as the fluid moves and carries those particles along, they will always mark the new positions of the vortex lines [66]. In whatever way the fluid particles move, the vortex lines move with them [62]. Albeit less abundant than in times past, *smoke rings* are still a familiar illustration of Helmholtz's second theorem. This theorem is just the law of conservation of angular momentum applied to the fluid [75,79]. Imagine a small cylindrical fluid element whose axis is parallel to the vortex lines, the pivotal axes of rotation of the fluid particles in the vortex. Some time later, this same piece of fluid will be somewhere else. Generally, it will occupy a cylinder with a different diameter and be in a different place. If the diameter has changed, however, the length will have adjusted so as to keep the volume constant (since the fluid is incompressible). In addition, by Helmholtz's second theorem, since the vortex lines are stuck with the material, their density will go up as the cross-sectional area goes down, and *vice versa*.

If the $\boldsymbol{\omega}$ components normal to the initial and subsequent areas A_1 and A_2 are ω_1 and ω_2, the product of the vorticity and area of the cylinder will remain constant, so according to Helmholtz, we should have $\omega_1 A_1 = \omega_2 A_2$. The vortical cylinder may also acquire a different orientation. Generally, an increase in the vorticity component in one direction will be accompanied by a complementary decrease in some other direction(s), and conversely. Note that with zero viscosity (as required for a strict applicability of Helmholtz's Theorems) all the forces on the surface of the cylinder (or any volume) are normal to the surface. The pressure forces can cause the volume to move from place to place, or can cause it to change shape; but with no tangential (viscous shear) forces, the magnitude of the angular momentum of the material inside *cannot change*. Therefore, Helmholtz's second theorem stems physically from the simple fact that in the absence of viscosity the angular momentum of an element of the fluid cannot change.

Vorticity relates to the local rate of rotation of fluid elements. The angular momentum, L, of a small material element that is instantaneously spherical is $L = (1/2)\ I\ \boldsymbol{\omega}$, where, I is its moment of inertia. The angular momentum will change at a rate determined by the tangential surface stresses alone, which are zero for an inviscid fluid. Consider an initially spherical blob of vorticity in an inviscid flow-field consisting of converging streamlines. The blob stretches out into an ellipsoid by the converging flow. The moment of inertia of the element about an axis parallel to $\boldsymbol{\omega}$ decreases, and consequently $\boldsymbol{\omega}$ must rise to conserve the angular momentum. It is possible, therefore, to *intensify* vorticity by *stretching* fluid blobs. Intense rotation can result from this process; the familiar bathtub vortex being just one example. In general, the rate of rotation of a fluid blob may increase or decrease due to changes in its moment of inertia (see Section 2.8, on pp. 59 f.), or because viscous stresses spin it up or slow it down.

A smoke ring is a torus-shaped bundle of vortex lines [79], as shown in Figure 9.6b., on p. 455. These vortex lines represent also a circulation of v as shown in Figure 9.6c.

We can understand intuitively the forward motion of a vortex ring in the following way: The circulating velocity around the bottom of the ring extends up to the top of the ring, having there a forward motion. Since the lines of ω move with the fluid, they also move ahead with the velocity v. Of course, the circulation of v around the top part of the ring is similarly responsible for the forward motion of the vortex lines at its bottom.

Helmholtz's second theorem implies that if ω is initially zero, it will always be zero—it is impossible to produce any vorticity under any circumstances. Yet, we know that we can start some vorticity in a teacup with a spoon. Moreover, inviscid fluid flow theory supposes that the fluid can slide along the surface of a solid boundary and does not allow for any friction between the fluid and the solid. It is an experimental fact, however, that the velocity of a real fluid always goes to zero relative to the velocity of the surface at the surface of a solid boundary. Clearly, to get a comprehensive understanding of the behavior of a fluid [30], we must allow for the effects of viscosity and incorporate viscous fluid dynamics in the analysis (see pp. 190 ff.).

9.5 Interesting vortical patterns

We have already introduced, in Section 9.4, an example of flow where vorticity is concentrated along a line, the vortex ring. Smoke rings are well-known to be emitted from circular openings; e.g., from the mouth of a skilled cigarette smoker. We might also recall the formation of vortical patterns in the Rayleigh–Bénard instability seen previously in Figure 1.2, on p. 12, and in Section 1.5, on pp. 10 ff. In this section we will consider a few other interesting vortical patterns.

9.5.1 The Helmholtz–Kelvin instability

Hermann von Helmholtz studied the dynamics of two fluids of different densities when a small disturbance such as a wave is introduced at the boundary connecting the fluids. The Helmholtz–Kelvin instability is an important instability in fluid dynamics. Helmholtz–Kelvin instability can occur when velocity shear is present within a uniform fluid, or when there is sufficient velocity difference across the interface between two stratified fluids moving at different velocities in plane parallel streams, a so-called free shear flow. Transverse velocity gradients develop in both fluids, and these serve as a source of free energy that feeds perturbations at the interface, causing them to grow (see Fig. 9.7). For short enough wavelengths, and if surface tension can be ignored, the two fluids in parallel flow with *different* velocities and densities will yield an *interface* that is unstable for all speeds. However, the existence of surface tension stabilizes the short wavelength instability and theory predicts stability maintenance until a *velocity threshold* is reached.

The importance of the surface instability relates to its role as a vortex formation mechanism (see Section 9.6, on pp. 473 f.) and in the production of turbulence. The theory can be used to predict the onset of instability and transition to turbulent flow in fluids of different densities moving at various speeds. In addition to cloud shapes in the sky, the

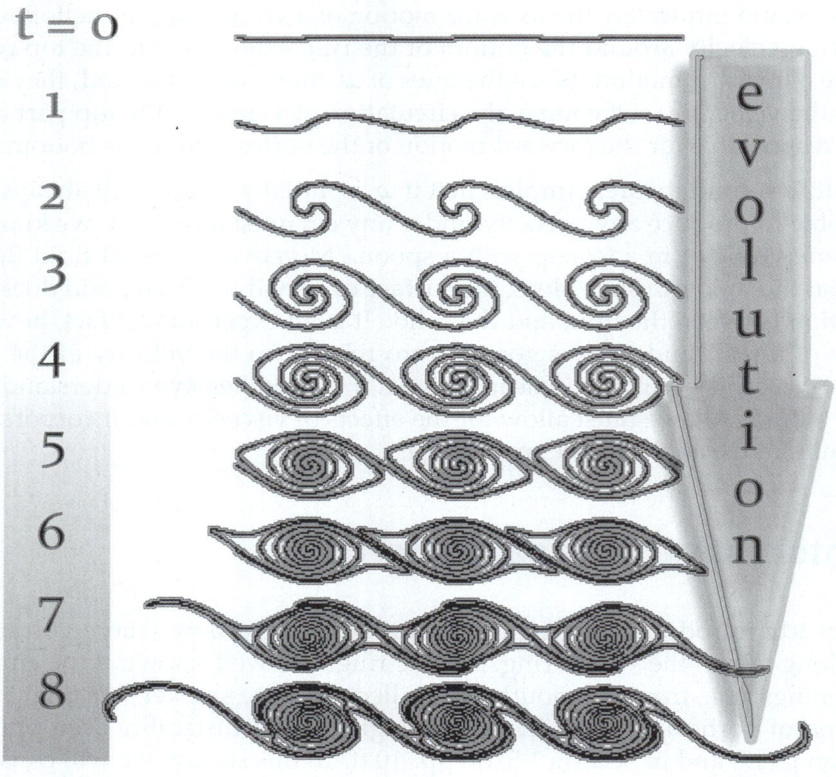

Figure 9.7: CFD simulation of the evolution of the Helmholtz–Kelvin instability at the interface between two stratified fluids moving at different velocities in plane parallel streams, a so-called free shear flow.

Helmholtz–Kelvin instability can be observed in sand dunes, in rising cigarette smoke, and in water waves. Nonlinear development leads to turbulent mixing in a free shear layer. The monumental study by Chandrasekhar [9] contains a good exposition of this instability, as well as references to some of the specialized literature.

9.5.2 Flow past a cylinder

We explore first, qualitatively, the evolution of the incompressible flow of a viscous fluid around a cylinder. When the velocity is very low or, equivalently, when the viscosity is very high, then the inertial terms are negligible and the Reynolds number is very small, $Re < 1$. The flow is steady, that is, the velocity is constant at any place, and the flow goes around the cylinder by dividing ahead of it only to reunite immediately behind it. As a fluid particle flows toward the leading edge of the cylinder, the pressure on the particle rises from the free stream pressure to the stagnation pressure, P_s in Figure 9.8. The high fluid pressure near the leading edge impels flow about the cylinder, as boundary

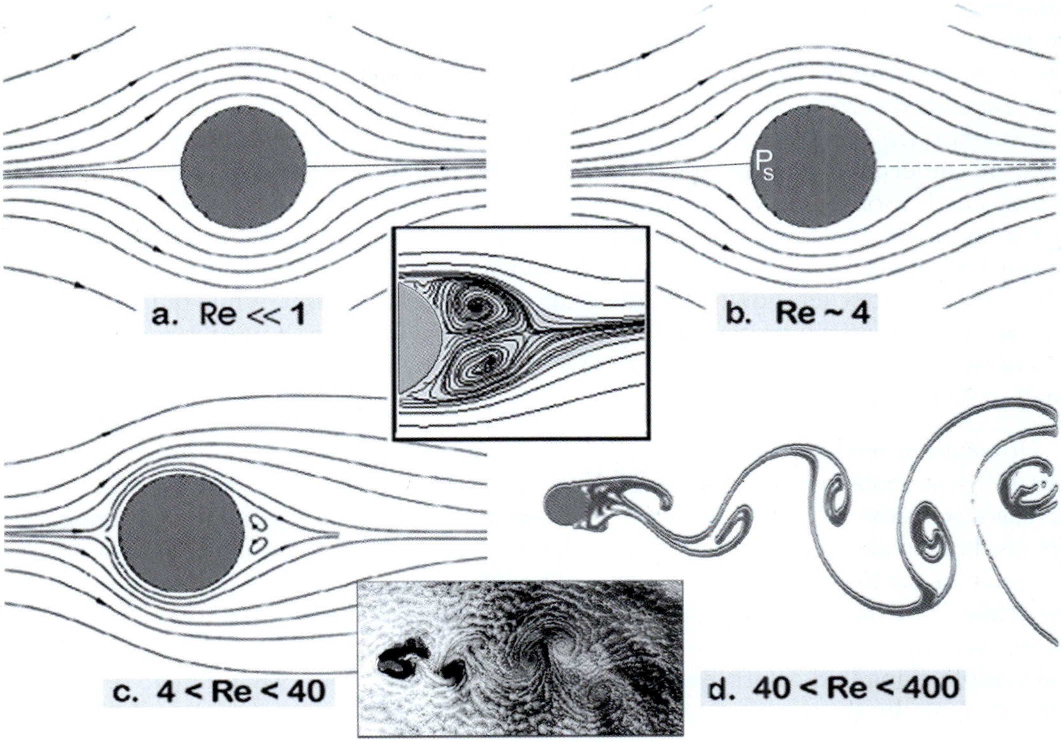

Figure 9.8: Flow past a circular cylinder for various Reynolds numbers, as shown, defined in terms of the approach velocity and the cylinder diameter. As the stream is flowing from left to right past the cylinder, the separating boundary layers from the upper and lower sides roll up into discrete vortices. A "Kármán" vortex street consists of a sequence of alternate-signed vortices, arranged in two rows and traveling downstream in the wake, as shown in panel d. The vortices in the upper row are rotating clockwise, and the lower counterclockwise. These vortices are laminar in the case of low Reynolds numbers ($Re < 250$), whereas they are turbulent for higher Reynolds numbers. P_s = stagnation pressure. (Based on photographs by S. Taneda [70], with kind permission of the Physical Society of Japan.) *Lower inset*: Kármán street downstream of an islet in the Aegean. (Photographed by author.)

layers develop about both sides. Figures 4.16, on p. 205, and 9.8a., illustrate the actual distribution of the streamlines.

There are remarkable symmetries in the flow pattern: top–bottom, front–rear halves, along the cylinder's axis. This is Stokes' "creeping flow" solution and is available in standard texts [64]. The streamlines would look exactly *the same*, with just a *reversal* of flow direction.[5] If we increase the fluid speed to get a $Re \approx 4$, the front–rear symmetry is broken,

[5] This does not imply thermodynamic reversibility. Thermodynamically, creeping flows are as irreversible as can be imagined, because all of the work done to drive such flows is dissipated by viscosity, rather than going into kinetic or gravitational potential energy.

reflecting an increasing influence of convective inertial effects on the flow dynamics. If we increase the fluid speed further to get a $Re > 4$, we find that the flow is different. The high pressure is not sufficient to force the flow about the back of the cylinder and, near the widest section of the cylinder, the boundary layers separate from each side of the cylinder surface and form two shear layers that trail aft in the flow and bound the wake. Since the innermost portion of the shear layers, which is in contact with the cylinder, moves much more slowly than the outermost portion of the shear layers, which is in contact with the free flow, the shear layers roll into the near wake, where they fold on each other and coalesce into two discrete swirling vortices. Thus, there is a circulation behind the cylinder, as shown in Figure 9.8c. and the center inset, while the flow remains stationary and tends to preserve the top-bottom half symmetry. It used to be thought that the circulation grew continuously, i.e., that there is always a circulation there even at the smallest Reynolds number.

However, a newer postulate is that the circulation may appear suddenly at $Re > 4$, because of a more pronounced front–rear symmetry breaking, and it is certain that it increases with the Reynolds number. The trigger for this decisive symmetry breaking is the onset of instability in the more symmetric solution [67]. In any case, there is a different character to the flow for $Re \approx (4 - 40)$. There is a pair of vortices behind the cylinder. The wake is completely laminar, and the vortices act effectively like rollers over which the main stream flows; these eddies get progressively longer as Re is increased, coming to resemble elongated caterpillar treads (cf. central inset in Fig. 9.8, on p. 459). The flow changes again by the time we get to $Re > 40$. There is suddenly a complete change in the character of the motion, as the flow becomes time-periodic. Here, there is a break in the time symmetry and the wake undergoes a transition to a time-dependent state, characterized by a *periodic* shedding of vortices.

What happens is that one of the vortices behind the cylinder gets so long that it breaks off and travels downstream with the fluid. Then the fluid curls around behind the cylinder and makes a new vortex. The vortices peel off *alternately* on each side, so that an instantaneous view of the flow looks roughly as sketched in Figure 9.8d. The top–bottom symmetry is not broken insofar as, *after half a period*, the upper eddies are mirror images of the lower ones [33]. The stream of vortices, which always appear for $Re > 40$, marks out a "Kármán vortex street."[6] The wake develops a slow oscillation, and the amplitude of the oscillation increases with downstream distance [64,77]. As shown in Figure 9.8d., the oscillating wake rolls up into two staggered rows of vortices with opposite sense of rotation, reminiscent of the pair of rows of trees astride a city street. The forces exerted by the flow on the cylinder also alternate in direction periodically.

Upstream of the cylinder, fluid elements possess linear momentum, but no angular momentum. On the other hand, in the Kármán street, fluid elements have both linear and

[6]Theodore von Kármán (1881–1963) was born in Budapest, Hungary, and was an engineer and physicist who was active primarily in the field of aerodynamics during its seminal era, the 1940s and 1950s. He was a student of Ludwig Prandtl at the University of Göttingen, and received his doctorate in 1908. He is known for many key advances in aerodynamics. His many contributions include the theories of unsteady wakes in the cylinder flow under discussion here, stability of laminar flow, turbulence, and boundary layers [22].

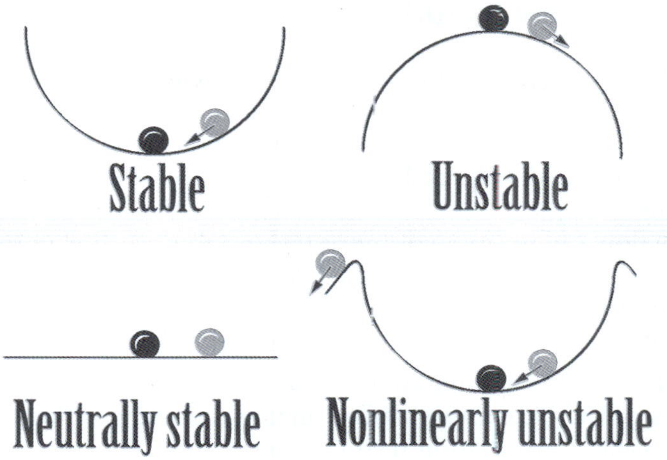

Figure 9.9: Gravitational analog of instabilities and possible equilibrium states of a flow system. Note how a nonlinearly unstable flow is stable for small disturbances but unstable for large ones.

angular momentum. We can get an intuitive perception of how these vortices come into existence.

We know that the fluid velocity must be zero at the surface of the cylinder and that it increases rapidly away from that surface. This large local variation in fluid velocity creates vorticity (see pp. 473 f.). Now, when the mainstream velocity is low enough, there is sufficient time for this vorticity to diffuse out of the thin region near the solid surface and to grow into a large region of vorticity [33]. However, as the velocity increases further, there is less and less time for the intensely concentrated vorticity to diffuse into a larger region of fluid. By the time that we reach $Re \approx 100$, the vorticity begins to fill in a thin band, in which the flow is chaotic and irregular. This irregular flow region, where the fluid is subjected to intense shearing forces, works its way upstream on the curved cylinder surface as Re is increased. The angular momentum of the vortices in the Kármán vortex street appears to have come from this boundary layer. In the turbulent region, the velocities are very irregular; also, the flow is no longer two-dimensional but twists and turns in all three dimensions. There is still an orderly alternating motion superimposed on the turbulent one.

However, at very high Reynolds numbers, there appears a tendency inside the wake far from the boundaries to restore the symmetries in a statistical sense. For such fully developed turbulence, it is necessary that the flow should not be subject to any constraint, such as a strong large-scale shear, which would prevent it from accepting all possible symmetries. This is one reason why *nothing even approximating* fully developed turbulence can occur in flows of cardiovascular, or physiological, interest [52], regardless of how high the instantaneous Re might be.

9.5.3 A note on flow disturbances and instabilities

The complex and shifting character of the flow past a cylinder is not exceptional; on the contrary, a rich variety of flow-regime possibilities is a general occurrence [16]. Fluid flows can be *stable* or *unstable*. When critical thresholds are crossed, small disturbances introduced in the flow-field will tend to grow. The growth could be at any point with respect to time (an example of *absolute* instability), or with respect to a fluid particle as it travels with the flow (an example of *convective* instability). It is in the sense of growth of small disturbances that the evolution of a prevailing flow regime to other regimes, via *successive* transition stages, can be thought of as a *process of instability* of the flow system. The notion of stability can be explained by a simple example.

Consider a ball placed in a gravitational field, as in Figure 9.9, which depicts possible equilibrium states of the ball, as a stability analog modeling a flow system. A flow is *unstable* if even a small perturbation results in a different flow-field. If a flow is *stable*, and we perturb it slightly, the flow-field returns to its original state. If this occurs only for small perturbations (i.e., disturbances with velocities much smaller than those present in the original flow-field), then the flow is *linearly stable* but *nonlinearly unstable*. If it occurs for large perturbations as well, then the flow is *neutrally* or *unconditionally stable*. It is a somewhat unappreciated fact that flow instability phenomena have subtle, and unexpected, nonlinearities.

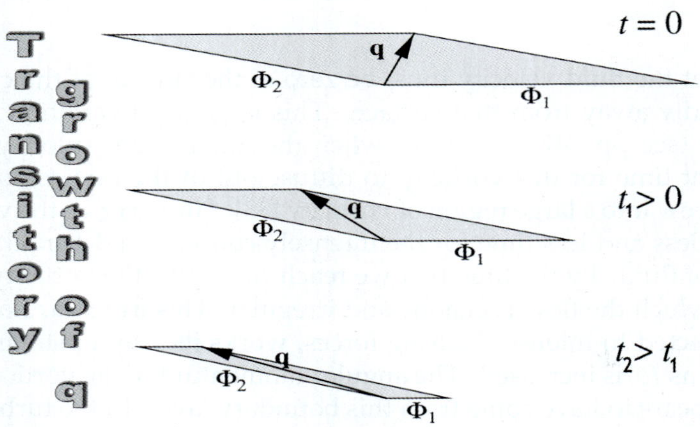

Figure 9.10: Sketch illustrating a transitory *growth* of a disturbance, **q**, due to nonorthogonal superposition of its two *continuously decaying* component vectors, Φ_1 and Φ_2, that decay *at different rates* as time evolves—the component Φ_1 decays much faster than Φ_2.

As an example, a flow regime may transiently appear to become unstable in response to a disturbance, only to regain its stability after an interval of time. I propose a simple geometric model involving a nonorthogonal modal representation in two dimensions to help the reader understand the evolution of such a *transient* growth [65]. Let us assume that we expand a disturbance **q**, initially of *unit* length, in a nonorthogonal (two-dimensional) basis, as is shown in Figure 9.10. Note that the expansion coefficients are not of order one, as is reflected in the magnitudes of the component vectors Φ_1 and Φ_2, relative to the magnitude of $\mathbf{q}$. This is a characteristic of nonorthogonal expansions. Let us further assume that the components, Φ_1 and Φ_2, are associated with exponentially decaying modes, but that the component in the first direction decays *more rapidly* than the component in the second. After a short time, the subtle cancellation of the nonorthogonal vectors Φ_1 and Φ_2 at time $t = 0$ ceases to be present, giving rise to a transient *growth*, reflected in the length of the vector $\mathbf{q}$. Since we assumed exponentially decaying components Φ_1 and Φ_2, the length of $\mathbf{q}$ will *eventually* decay to zero, and stability will be regained.

In light of the above discussion, as a consequence of instability, an initially stable flow state undergoes successive transitions to a series of intermediate states, leading ultimately to turbulence. Consider a physical system consisting of a viscous fluid and rigid bodies not subjected to any external action. This system will be in a state of rest. As the system departs from equilibrium, a parameter N can be conceived, which quantifies external action. In unstable situations, small perturbations grow spontaneously and frequently equilibrate as finite amplitude disturbances. On raising further the parameter N, the new state can become unstable to more complicated disturbances, and the system eventually can reach a chaotic state. Generally, as N increases, new phenomena occur as follows:

1. A steady motion is initiated.
2. The motion alters its symmetry pattern.
3. The motion becomes periodic.
4. The motion becomes quasi-periodic and may display chaotic patterns.
5. For sufficiently large N, the motion becomes irregular and turbulent.

Steps 1 to 5 define transition as a flow evolves, toward turbulence. Some instructive examples of flow patterns undergoing transition are presented here.

9.5.4 Taylor–Couette flow

Flow instabilities produced by thermal buoyancy were considered in the Rayleigh–Bénard horizontal layer of a fluid heated from below (see Section 1.5, on pp. 10 ff.) That naturally occurring flow pattern arises because the fluid is from place to place lighter (tending to rise), or heavier (tending to sink), because the temperature, and thus its mass density, are not uniform. Hydrodynamic instability is readily accessible to study in axisymmetric configurations. Foremost among axisymmetric fluid systems is the Taylor–Couette system of flow between differentially rotating cylinders [4, 13], which has become aprincipal example for *pattern formation* in nonlinear fluid dynamics. The Taylor–Couette[7] system, which

[7] The name of M. Couette, alone or hyphenated with another, is applied as an eponym to a variety of flows that are driven by differential tangential motion of enclosing walls [12], just as the more familiar one of the physician J. L. M. Poiseuille is to steady, rectilinear flows that are driven by a pressure gradient in conduits with cylindrical or planar geometry.

is depicted pictorially in Figure 9.11, on p. 465, is the quintessential example of fluid flow exhibiting successive instabilities and transitions (mathematical "bifurcations") with spontaneous formation of rich, new, dynamic flow structures. More precisely, it exhibits, in discrete steps, a variety of time independent patterns with periodic spatial structure. Each time it reaches the next critical speed and transition, the flow gets one-step closer toward becoming turbulent.

The Taylor–Couette experiment [71, 72] consists of a fluid (oil) in the gap between two *very long* (to achieve an approximate homogeneity of the flow regimes in the axial direction) concentric cylinders, one or both of which are rotating along their common axis.[8] If we put a fine aluminum powder as a suspension in the oil, the flow is easy to see [63]. If we turn the outer cylinder slowly, nothing startling happens. If the outer cylinder is rotating and the inner cylinder is stationary, the velocity increases outward in a near-linear manner. The centrifugal force on the fluid particles tends to move them outward and that force is counteracted by the pressure gradient acting inward. Since the outer fluid particles have greater velocity, the centrifugal force on those particles is greater and they tend to stay in the outer part of the motion, a tendency that leads to stability. Alternatively, if we turn the inner cylinder slowly, nothing extraordinary occurs and no flow structures are discernible [Fig. 9.11a.]. It is a featureless, smooth flow that looks the same at all points of the cylinder. As such, it exhibits both rotational symmetry *around* its axis and translational symmetry *along* its axis.

However, if we turn the inner cylinder at a higher rate, a bewildering phenomenon snaps the dullness of the viscometric Couette flow: the fluid breaks into a horizontal stack of *car tire* or *rope-like bands* [see Fig. 9.11b.]. Clearly, if the inner cylinder is rotating and the outer cylinder is stationary, the effect is opposite and the flow tends toward *instability*. This effect is produced by centrifugal forces which push fluid from the inner cylinder toward the outer. When the inner layers of the fluid are moving more rapidly than the outer, they tend to move outward because the centrifugal force is *greater* than the pressure holding them in place. When a stability threshold is overcome, the inertial toroidal roll cells appear. A whole layer cannot move out uniformly, because the outer layers are in the way, and so it breaks into cells that *circulate*. Their outermost diameter is roughly equal to the width of the gap between the cylinders. The term "instability" must be accepted with a qualification; it only means that there is some secondary effect superimposed on the main stream. These secondary roll cells are stable in both time and space. Obviously, the flow pattern is now less symmetric than before [67]: it remains *axisymmetric*, i.e., it still preserves its rotational symmetry around its axis; however, it has lost its translational symmetry *along* its axis.

To understand this process, it helps to consider a quickly stirred cup of coffee. The spoon acts as the inner cylinder. The stirring generates a coffee "annulus" having an angular velocity, which—through viscous wall shear—diminishes, as the wall of the cup is

[8] Sir Isaac Newton (1642–1727) in 1687 considered the circular motion of fluids, in Book II of the Principia, Section IX. In Corollary 2 of Proposition 51, Newton says, [49] "If a fluid be contained in a cylindric vessel of an infinite length, and contain another cylinder within, and both the cylinders revolve about one common axis,... " This must be one of the earliest references discussing flow in the annulus between rotating cylinders.

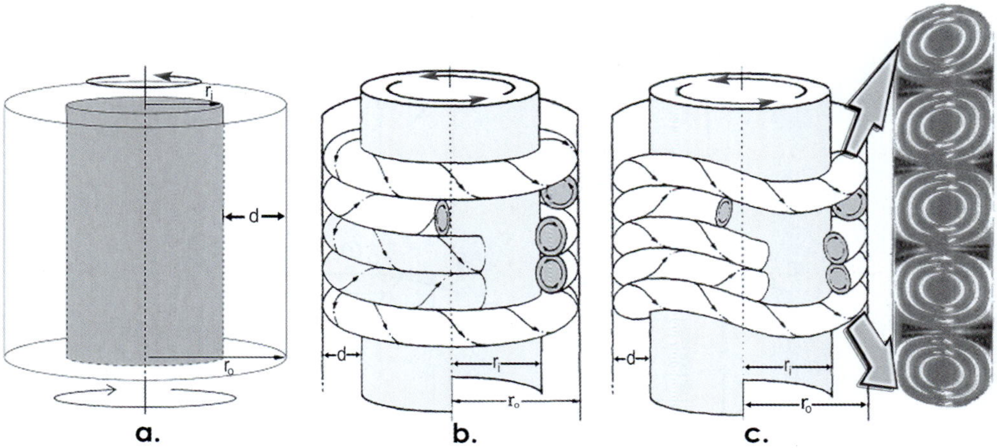

Figure 9.11: Some fluid flow patterns in the gap (d) between two rotating cylinders with radii r_o and r_i. In Couette flow a liquid of kinematic viscosity ν is contained in the gap between the two concentric cylinders, one of which has an angular velocity ω with respect to the other. At low Reynolds number, $Re = \frac{r_i \cdot \omega \cdot d}{\nu}$, the flow is azimuthal, as in a. As Re increases, flow symmetry is lost and toroidal vortices develop, as in b. A further increase of Re causes harmonic oscillations of the vortices in the axial direction, producing transverse waves along the toroidal vortex lines, as in c.

approached. In the rotating fluid, the centrifugal force is added to gravity and the resultant of the two determines that the coffee surface conforms to a paraboloid. The faster the stirring, the more forcefully is the coffee pressed against the wall by the centrifugal force,[9] which is forcing it to ascend. Thus, there is an elevation (axial extension) of the coffee at the wall of the cup, produced by the radial centrifugal motion of the fluid. In the closed Taylor–Couette apparatus, such an axial displacement cannot take place, and this generates compressional axial stresses. *Fluid structuring* on the concave surface of the outer cylinder relieves these stresses. This results in evenly spaced, annular rings—the Taylor vortices—if the energy of the system is sufficient.

The transition at hand illustrates a symmetry breaking pattern attendant to a flow instability. When a solution of the Navier–Stokes equations for a flow system loses stability because of changes in applying conditions, other solutions bifurcate [67]. Generally, a system undergoes a bifurcation if its global behavior—which depends on a parameter,

[9] For a solid body or a fluid particle to move in a curved path, some force must be applied. The force restraining bodies that move in curved path is the centripetal force; it points continually toward the center of rotation. When we swirl a rock around on a string, the centripetal force is exerted by the tension of the string. Equal and opposite in direction to the centripetal force is the centrifugal force, the reacting force directed outward from the center of rotation. As you know, a bucket of water can be swung over your head at a rate of revolution that allows the water to remain in the bucket. This is an example of both centrifugal and centripetal force. Your arm swinging the bucket applies centripetal force, while the water is held against the bucket by the centrifugal force tending to shove it outward.

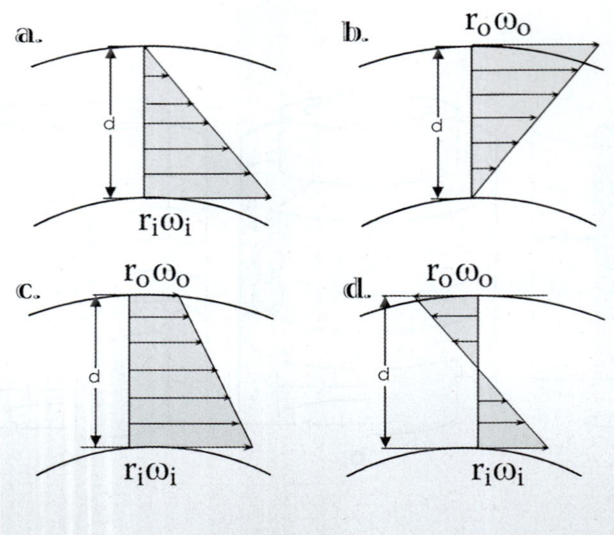

Figure 9.12: Fully developed azimuthal velocity ($v = r\omega$, where $r = radius$, and $\omega = angular\ velocity$) profiles for concentric rotating cylinders prior to the onset of any instability. a. The inner (subscript i) cylinder rotating and the outer (subscript o) cylinder at rest. b. The inner cylinder at rest and the outer cylinder rotating. c. Both cylinders rotating in same direction but at different speeds. d. Cylinders rotating in opposite directions.

such as the spinning rate of the cylinders—changes as the parameter undergoes critical changes.[10] A bifurcation is usually a *sudden*, rather than a slow and gradual, change of a nonlinear system to a *qualitatively new* dynamic pattern. Bifurcation of solutions to flows in general, including *intracardiac flow fields*, stems from the nonuniqueness of the solutions, which is due to the convective nonlinearity—$\mathrm{v} \cdot \nabla \mathrm{v}$—in the velocity vector in the equations of motion (see Fig. 4.4, on p. 177, and Section 4.6, on pp. 190 f.).

When the outer cylinder rotates at a similar rate with the inner one at rest (cf. Fig. 9.12a., on p. 466), no such effect occurs. How can it be that there is a difference between rotating the inner or the outer cylinder? We can get the answer by considering the azimuthal (tangential) velocity profiles prior to the onset of any instability in Figure 9.12, and the cross-sections in Figure 9.11, on p. 465. When the inner layers of the fluid are moving more rapidly than the outer [see Fig. 9.12 a., c., d.], they tend to move outward (see Fig. 9.11a.) because the centrifugal force is greater than the pressure force holding them in place. This introduces the flow instability. A whole layer cannot move out uniformly because the outer layers are in the way. It must *break into cells* and *circulate* like the convection currents in a room that has hot air at the bottom. Thus, the instability appears in the form of the counter-rotating toroidal vortices that are illustrated in Figure 9.11. We call these,

[10]The customary bifurcation parameter is the Reynolds number $Re \equiv \Omega r_1(r_2 - r_1)/\nu$, where Ω is the inner cylinder angular frequency, ν is the kinematic viscosity of the working fluid, and r_1 and r_2 are the inner and outer cylinder radii respectively.

"Taylor vortices," in honor of Sir Geoffrey Taylor (grandson of George Boole, the inventor of modern logic and "Boolean" algebra [2]) whose analysis of the problem is arguably a classic masterpiece of fluid dynamics, both experimentally and theoretically.[11]

In Taylor's findings [72], it is shown that the increase of fluid viscosity can delay the instability. Generally, the energy loss due to viscosity in shear flows is helpful in *delaying* the flow instability when subjected to a perturbation, such as found in Taylor–Couette flows and demonstrated by Taylor. The Taylor cell streamlines are in the form of helices, with axes wrapping around the annulus, somewhat like the stripes on a barber's pole. When the outer cylinder has a high velocity, the centrifugal forces build up a pressure gradient that keeps everything in equilibrium, as in a room with hot air on top.

As the speed of the inner cylinder is increased, there is a progressive *loss of degrees of symmetry* in the Taylor–Couette system, resulting in an *increase in pattern*. A whole range of remarkable *flow patterns* are generated [11, 67]. At first, the number of bands increases. Then suddenly the bands become wavy, and waves move around the cylinder [Fig. 9.11c.]. This infringes on the *rotational symmetry* as well. If we now start rotating the outer cylinder also, but in the opposite direction, the flow pattern starts to break up. Wavy regions start alternating with apparently quiet regions making a spiral pattern. In these deceptively quiet regions, however, the flow is actually strongly turbulent. The wavy regions also begin to show irregular turbulent flow. If the cylinders spin faster still, the whole flow becomes chaotically turbulent, an unexpected *reestablishment* of rotational and translational symmetry, but on a *coarser scale* than in the viscometric Couette flow. This is an instance of a *symmetry-increasing* bifurcation. Increasing the cylinders' spin further, ushers in a series of successive symmetry-breaking patterns all over again.

Contemporary advances in flow imaging technologies allow detailed experimental studies of hydrodynamic instabilities, and elucidation of the spatiotemporal coherent structures associated with flow transition. For instance, by tagging and tracking the evolution of Cartesian grids in water, MRI allows the noninvasive visualization of 3-D Taylor–Couette flow patterns, by providing sectioning on multiple arbitrary visualization planes [47, 48]. The findings from such studies validate direct numerical simulation insights on symmetry-breaking instabilities and flow pattern transitions (see Fig. 9.13), which have consequences for hydrodynamic mixing in complex flow regimes [57]. Generally, the symmetry-breaking instabilities result in the emergence of *more complex* from simpler (more symmetric) streamline patterns and structures.

In such simple experiments, we see many interesting flow regimes, which are quite different, and yet *are all contained* in the governing Navier–Stokes equations for various values of one parameter: the Reynolds number. With the rotating cylinders, we can see many of the effects that occur in the flow past a cylinder: On rotating the inner cylinder while keeping the outer cylinder stationary, Couette flow becomes unstable to motion in the axial direction, and this gives rise to Taylor vortex flow at a critical value of the rotational speed. Increasing the latter further, gives rise to secondary instabilities in the form

[11]In his postdoctoral *(habilitation)* paper [24], Görtler showed the instability of flow along a *concave* wall, which gives rise to longitudinal Görtler vortices, analogous to the Taylor vortices between rotating cylinders.

of wavy vortex flow, where a wave-like disturbance propagates around the Taylor vortices; the flow varies in time but in a regular, smooth way. Finally, rotating both cylinders can give rise to a variety of other nonaxisymmetric flows, for example spirals, ribbons and twisted vortices, as the flow becomes completely irregular.

Polymorphic flow patterns, which may be observed arising and dissipating unpredictably in a chaotic flux of randomly colliding currents, have for centuries attracted the interest of scientists from many disciplines; they are intrigued by the paradox of their shifting states of *order* and *disorder* that seem all but impossible to describe, determine, and predict.[12] You have seen such shifting patterns in a column of smoke rising in still air. There is a smooth steady column followed by a series of twirls as the smoke stream begins to break up, ending finally in an irregular churning cloud.The main point from

[12] Less apparent but equally fascinating has been a very ancient tradition of fluid turbulence imagery, involving symbolic representations of whirling spirohelical and vortical phenomena, that originates in ancient times and develops across the ages into the modern era [45].

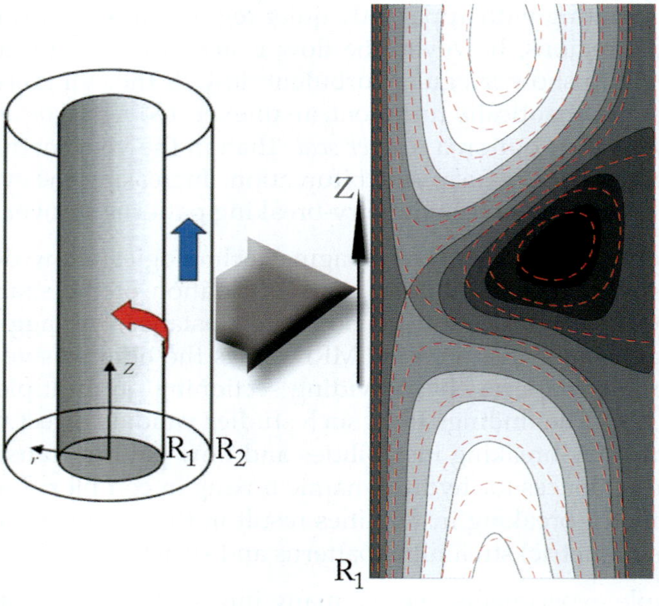

Figure 9.13: A Taylor–Couette–Poiseuille (TCP) flow is produced when an axial pressure gradient (blue arrow) is added to a Taylor–Couette flow arrangement (red arrow)—left panel. The main TCP flow pattern is a stationary helical vortex (SHV) structure, consisting of a pair of asymmetric counter-rotating helical cells in a double helix structure. Comparison of SHV flow streamlines for one axial wavelength in the $r-Z$ plane obtained via an MRI velocimetric reconstruction (solid contours) with numerical simulation results (dashed lines)—right panel. (Montage adapted from slightly modified Figs. 1 and 7 in Raguin and Georgiadis [57], with permission of the authors and Cambridge University Press.)

all of this is that the same Navier–Stokes equations and boundary conditions can encompass *a tremendous variety* of flow patterns. All the flow regimes are solutions for the *same* equations, only with different values of *Reynolds number*! That we have "written an equation" does *not* remove from fluid flow its charm, or mystery, or its surprise! It is an intrinsic and characteristic feature of fluid dynamics that many different physical processes are involved, and that although each of them separately may be regarded as well understood, in combination they can produce *unexpected* effects!

It is one thing to know that the Navier–Stokes equations describe the motion of a fluid, and quite another to know, for instance, that thin boundary layers form on the upstream side, but not on the downstream side, of a cylinder placed in a stream. Ability to predict what will happen in a given situation, in broad outline if not in detail, is an essential part of knowledge. The motion of a given body of fluid is only weakly constrained by the shape and nature of the flow-field boundaries. Many possible flow regimes are *consistent* with the more obvious requirements, namely, conservation of mass, of momentum, and of energy for the flow field that will actually be apparent in a given situation. These constraints are not sufficiently strong to generate analytically a *unique* flow-field.

It is perhaps the basic feature shared by all fluids, of yielding to shear stress, that makes fluid motions extremely rich, colorful, and complicated. For example, if a viscous flow has a solid boundary, a strong shear must occur there since the fluid ceases to move on the boundary. A boundary layer is thereby formed, whose *separation* from the solid boundary is the source of various free shear layers that roll into concentrated vortices that evolve, interact, become unstable, and break to turbulence, finally to dissipate into heat. The phenomena of fluid motions are sensitive to the circumstances giving rise to them, and exhibit a wide variety of patterns [42, 43, 63]. The Navier–Stokes equations probably contain all of *intracardiac* blood flow patterns. Yet it would be foolish to try to guess what their "consequences" are without looking at clinical and experimental *facts*. The phenomena are almost as varied as the *innumerable* phenomena in the realm of life; and they have many secret, valuable messages that need to be discerned and understood by clinicians and researchers alike.

9.5.5 Secondary flows

Stability is influenced by rotation, and the curvature of streamlines changes the stability characteristics of flows, in general. Phenomena analogous to the Taylor vortices exemplify secondary flows [1, 3], because they are overlain on a primary flow, such as Couette flow along circular streamlines, in the case just examined. The same considerations hold for concave and convex walls as were discussed for the concentric cylinders. The fluid following a convex wall—analogous to the stationary inner cylinder—tends to be more stable than the fluid following a concave wall. There are other situations where a combination of curved streamlines (which give rise to centrifugal forces) and viscosity result in instability and secondary flows in the form of vortices [10, 19]. The secondary flows are generally streamlined on planes perpendicular to the direction of the main flow and are the result of *inertial instability* of flow.

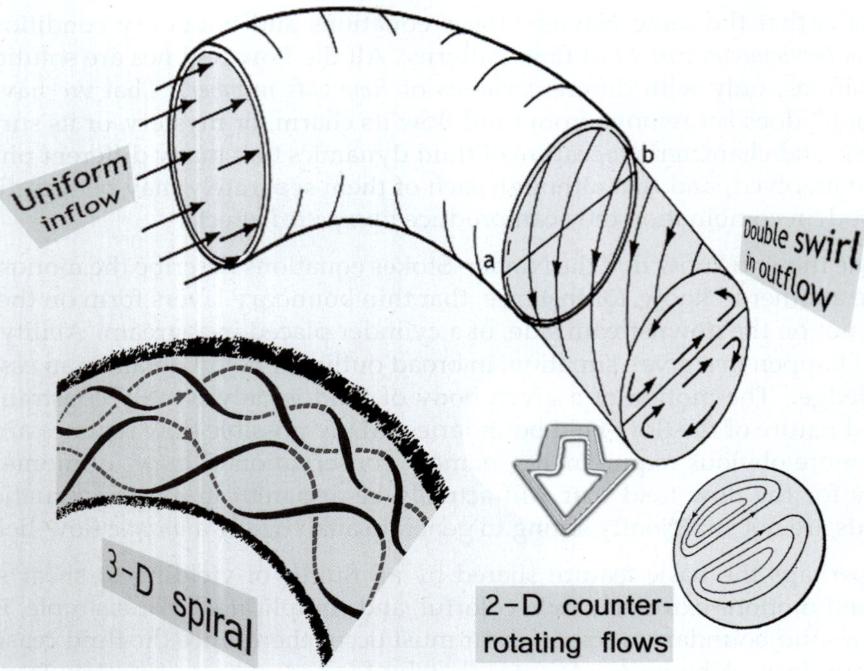

Figure 9.14: Secondary motion of a Newtonian fluid in a curved circular tube. The fluid moves centrifugally across the vessel diameter with respect to the center of curvature of the bend. Note the resulting spiral 3-D flow pattern, which is caused by the two secondary revolving currents that are superposed on the main downstream flow.

One example is the flow through a curved conduit, driven by a pressure gradient. As was pointed out in the previous section, the possibility of secondary flows signifies again (see Section 9.5.4) that the solutions of the Navier–Stokes equations are *nonunique*, in the sense that more than one solution can prevail under the *same* boundary conditions [42,45,63]. Secondary flows augment mixing and mass and heat transfer operations, both in the cardiovascular system and in artificial organs, e.g., blood oxygenators. Secondary flows commonly occur in connection with unbalanced centrifugal effects and with vortex stretching, and by other mechanisms. In a sense, the term "secondary" represents a human significance judgment, rather than an absolute distinction in fluid behavior. This is especially true in the case of the Taylor vortices laying over the circular streamlines of Couette flow. Another example of secondary flow of great cardiovascular interest is flow in curved vessels.

9.5.6 Flow in curved vessels

When a fluid is driven through a vessel or duct by a pressure gradient in the direction of flow, the fluid develops a more or less blunt velocity profile across the vessel, with

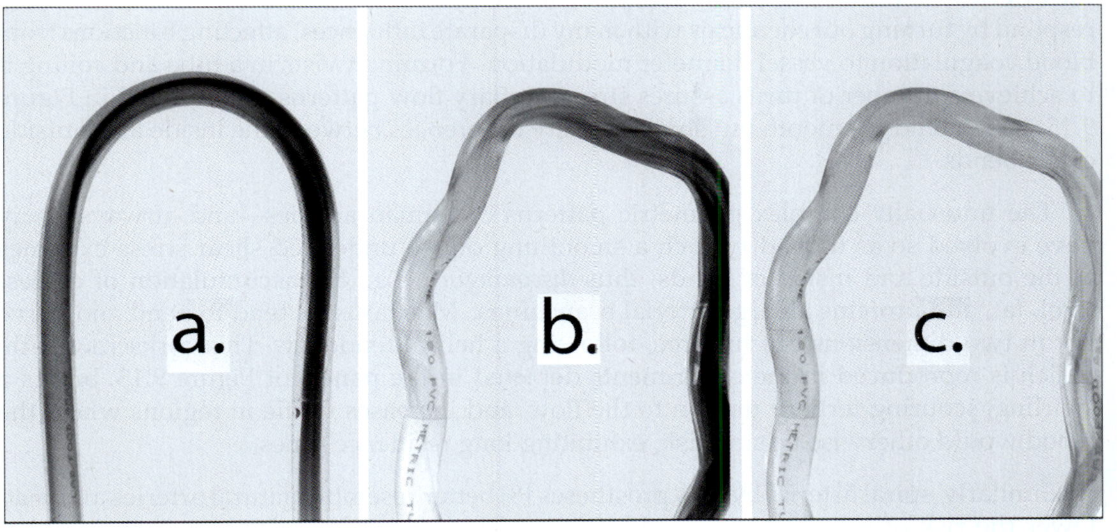

Figure 9.15: Bolus injection of 0.5 mL ink (black color) into water flowing (Reynolds number 550) in 0.8 cm internal diameter (D) pvc U-tubes, tube radius/radius of curvature approximately 0.1. a. Conventional tube; b. and c. helical tube, amplitude ratio and pitch approximately $0.5D$ and $6D$, respectively. In a., axial dispersion is seen of the indicator, which has a long residence time in the inlet tube and at the inner wall of curvature of the U-bend. In b. and c., sequential images of flow in the helical tube, axial dispersion of the indicator is diminished, as reflected in its retention in the inlet tube and at the inner wall of curvature of the U-bend. The natural *corkscrew flow* through helical conduits and vessels is a complicated, 3-D phenomenon, which, in the snapshots of panels b. and c., is made visible by the dark streaks of ink-marked fluid particles. (Adapted from Caro et al. [8] by kind permission of the Royal Society of London.)

zero velocity at the walls and a more or less localized maximum in the central region [66,75]. If the vessel or duct is curved, the flow becomes asymmetrical. Higher-momentum fluid in the central region experiences a greater centrifugal stress than fluid at the wall on the outside of the tube curvature, a situation favorable for penetration of fluid from the tube center toward the outside edge [64]. Continuity of fluid requires that there be a compensating inflow from the other edge. A secondary motion develops with sequential displacements of adjacent fluid, as illustrated in Fig. 9.14 for a circular pipe. This motion does not require the achievement of a critical flow velocity to begin. However, the speed of the secondary motion does depend upon the arc of curvature.

Depending on the applying conditions, leading to predominance of inertial or viscous effects, secondary flows cause faster or slower primary flow and corresponding higher or lower shear stress near the inside or outside of vascular bends (cf. Fig. 4.9, on p. 188), respectively. Fatty deposits that obstruct arteries accumulate where the flow is most sluggish. But fast-moving blood imposes high shear stresses on the endothelial cells lining the arteries. Too much hydrodynamic shear is *also* detrimental for blood vessels. They respond by turning out chemicals with many disparate influences, affecting functions from blood coagulation to vessel diameter modulation. Forming twists in a tube and coiling it to achieve a number of turns assures strong tertiary flow patterns, exemplified in Figure 9.15, which tend to smooth out sharp velocity differences between the inside and outside of the bends.

The unusually complex geometric patterns of human arteries—and airways—may have evolved so as to lead to such a smoothing out of undesired shear stress extremes at the outside and inside of bends, thus *discouraging*, e.g., the accumulation of cholesterol, fat, and proteins at large arterial branchings. Most arteries tend to bend and curve not in two dimensions but in three, following a helical tendency. This corkscrew path, which is reproduced in the experiments depicted in the panels of Figure 9.15, brings a swirling, scouring tertiary motion to the flow, and increases traffic in regions where the blood would otherwise be sluggish, exhibiting long residence times.

Similarly, spiral arterial bypass prostheses [8] better resemble natural arteries and may lower the risk of two common modes of arterial graft failure: plaque accumulation at the stagnation point where the blood stream in the graft meets the primary artery, and excessive muscle cell *hyperplasia* in the arterial wall, which is thought to be triggered by high hydrodynamic *shear stress* levels on endothelial surfaces. In fact, the geometry of almost every large bend and branch in the circulatory system is helical or *nonplanar*.

Thanks to their sensitive endothelial lining [25,40], cardiovascular organs can "sense" the blood flowing, and respond to how hard it impinges, rubs, and shears their inner surfaces [53]. The endothelial and endocardial cells that line them can move, change shape, and switch genes on and off [61] in response to changes in hydrodynamic shear and pressure [6,7]. They are so sensitive to the mechanical stresses of blood flow that the arterial system has evolved fluid dynamic means that help to smooth out and moderate the hydrodynamic forces, avoiding dangerous extremes—high or low—of shear stress.

By thinking of arteries as sensitive and responsive *living* vessels rather than as passive inert pipes, we can discover how their complex interactions with the blood flow forces produce cardiovascular disease. In the present context, it seems plausible, indeed likely, that different individuals may be more or less susceptible to cardiovascular disease simply because of the *shape* of their arteries [18], which may be more or less conducive to secondary and tertiary flow motions. Bringing to mind how pebbles and mud build up under the forces of secondary flow on the inside banks of curving streams, one can accept that the particular geometry of blood vessels has the capacity to produce *pathology*. Fatty deposits that obstruct arteries were shown decades ago to accumulate where the flow is most sluggish.

A recent multidisciplinary paper illustrates how computational fluid dynamics together with computer visualization form a useful complement to physical flow model experiments and, when broader knowledge of fluid dynamics is also capitalized on, help to make the interpretation of complex, but clinically important, secondary and tertiary fluid flow motions in the circulatory system orderly and systematic [58].

9.6 Vortex formation mechanisms

Vortices always originate [30] in the surfaces of contact between elements moving at different velocities (see Section 9.5, on p. 457) in a viscous flow field. To understand this basic concept, we begin by considering how fluid moves over a surface [66, 75]. Since fluid adheres to any surface with which it is in contact, in order to move past the surface the fluid must *roll* forward. This rolling is called vorticity. A vortex is concentrated vorticity [62].

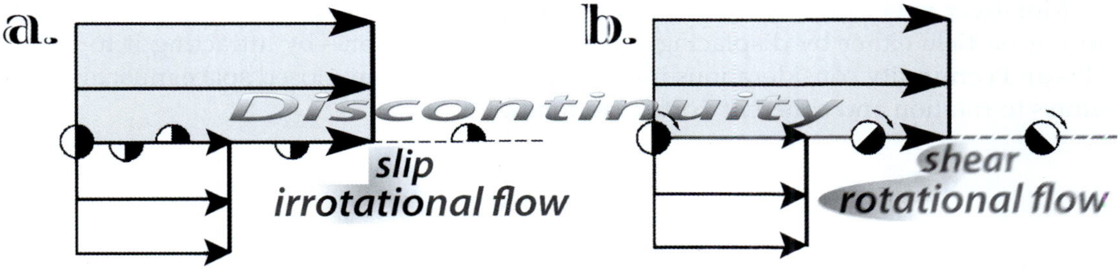

Figure 9.16: Tangent velocity discontinuity. a. Step-change in velocity at the surface of discontinuity, in strictly inviscid flow; b. concentrated vorticity in infinitely thin vortex sheet, at the surface of discontinuity.

Generally, wherever any qualitative differences in a flowing medium come together, vortices form. Such differences may be: slow, and fast; solid, and liquid; warm, and cold; and so on. At the surfaces of discontinuity, there is always a concentrated difference in velocity akin to the representation in Figure 9.16: there ensues a tendency for the particles of the faster of the adjoining layers to *slip by* [ideal fluid, irrotational flow, panel a.] or to *spin* and *roll over* the slower-layer particles [viscous fluid, rotational flow, panel b.]. In particular, the flow naturally occurring at a solid bounding surface, such as, e.g., the inner surface of the cardiac outflow tracts during ejection, consists of the familiar boundary layer, comprising a shear layer through which the velocity changes progressively from zero on the wall surface to its mainstream value at the outer edge of the layer. Vorticity is continuously created at the wall within the boundary layer and, once created, is free to undergo convection, under all surrounding influences, and diffusion, under the action of viscosity.

At increasing Reynolds numbers, the boundary layer will shrink in thickness to the limiting case of an infinitely thin vortex sheet, across which the velocity increases from zero beneath the sheet to its value just outside the sheet. The infinite Reynolds number flow of a real fluid thus approaches the ideal flow situation [44], but with the crucial difference that the boundary surface is "clothed," as it were, in an infinitely thin *vorticity sheet*.[13] However, the vorticity sheet is not bound to the body surface but convects,

[13]Mathematically, the infinite Reynolds number limit leads to an analytical *singularity*, because the order of the Navier–Stokes equations changes from second to first.

rolling freely along the surface—see Figure 4.15, on p. 204. If the difference in speed between neighboring layers reaches a certain degree, macroscopic vortex formations, or "eddies" occur [59]. Vortices can also come into existence when a stream is stalled against its boundaries—as happens in forming the diastolic filling vortex in the right and left ventricles of the heart (see Chapter 14). The stalled stream breaks up and rolls over on itself [10, 19]. At increasing distances from the boundary, the flow moves with higher velocities and the difference in velocities causes the stream to curl around on itself; the faster layers of fluid overshoot the slower ones and the fluid particles fold over to form a circular vortex motion.

Moreover, every movement of a fluid particle in a flow field must influence its neighboring particle either by displacing it or—by viscous action—by attracting it to follow. This and continuity considerations imply that flow in a finite, closed space must also lead *always* to rotation and coherent vortex motions [30].

References and further reading

Here are some useful references, mostly about less familiar topics of Fluid Dynamics. These references are cited in the text. It may help to read parts of some of them, in order to find different accounts of concepts presented in this chapter. This should further develop your understanding of the physics involved with complicated aspects of flow that underlie intracardiac flow patterns.

[1] Batchelor, G.K. An introduction to fluid dynamics. 2nd pbk. ed. 1999, Cambridge, UK; New York: Cambridge University Press. xviii, 615 p., 24 of plates.

[2] Batchelor, G.K., Taylor, G.I. The life and legacy of G.I. Taylor. 1996, Cambridge [England]; New York: Cambridge University Press. xv, 285 p.

[3] Batchelor, G.K., Moffatt, H.K., Worster, M.G. Perspectives in fluid dynamics: a collective introduction to current research. 2000, Cambridge, UK: Cambridge University Press. xii, 631 p.

[4] Bestehorn, M. Hydrodynamik und Strukturbildung mit einer kurzen Einführung in die Kontinuumsmechanik. 2006, Berlin: Springer. xiv, 392 p.

[5] Bitbol, M. Red blood cell orientation in orbit C = 0. Biophys J. 49: 1055–68, 1986.

[6] Caro, C.G., Fitz-Gerald, J.M., Schroter. R.C. Arterial wall shear and distribution of early atheroma in man. Nature 223: 1159–61, 1969.

[7] Caro, C.G., Fitz-Gerald, J.M., Schroter. R.C. Atheroma and arterial wall shear: observation, correlation and proposal of a shear dependent mass transfer mechanism for atherogenesis. Proc. R. Soc. Lond. B 177: 109–59, 1971.

[8] Caro, C.G., Cheshire, N.J., Watkins, N. Preliminary comparative study of small amplitude helical and conventional ePTFE arteriovenous shunts in pigs. J. R. Soc. Interface. 2: 261–6, 2005.

[9] Chandrasekhar, S. Hydrodynamic and hydromagnetic stability [1961]. 1981, New York: Dover. 704 p.

[10] Chang, P.K. Separation of flow. International series of monographs in interdisciplinary and advanced topics in science and engineering; v. 3. 1970, Oxford, New York: Pergamon Press. xviii, 777 p.

[11] Chossat, P. Iooss, G. The Couette–Taylor problem. 1994, New York: Springer-Verlag. ix, 233 p.

[12] Couette, M. Études sur le Frottement des Liquides. Ann. Chim. Phys. 21: 433–510, 1890.

[13] Criminale, W.O., Jackson, T.L., Joslin, R.D. Theory and computation in hydrodynamic stability. 2003, Cambridge, UK; New York: Cambridge University Press. xxii, 441 p.

[14] Cross, M.C., Hohenberg, P.C. Pattern formation outside of equilibrium. Rev. Mod. Phys. 65: 851–1112, 1993.

[15] Drazin, P.G. Introduction to hydrodynamic stability. Cambridge texts in applied mathematics. 2002, Cambridge, UK; New York: Cambridge University Press. xvii, 258 p.

[16] Faber, T.E. Fluid dynamics for physicists. 1995, Cambridge, UK; New York: Cambridge University Press. xxvi, 440 p.

[17] Fischer, T.M., Stöhr-Lissen, M., Schmid-Schönbein, H. The red cell as a fluid droplet: tank tread-like motion of the human erythrocyte membrane in shear flow. Science 202: 894–6, 1978.

[18] Friedman, M.H., Deters, O.J., Mark, F.F., Bargeron, C.B., Hutchins, G.M. Arterial geometry affects hemodynamics: a potential risk factor for atherosclerosis. Atherosclerosis 46: 225–31, 1983.

[19] Gersten, K. Deutsche Forschungsgemeinschaft. Physics of separated flows: numerical, experimental, and theoretical aspects: DFG Priority Research Programme 1984–1990. Notes on numerical fluid mechanics; v. 40. 1993, Braunschweig: F. Vieweg. ix, 293 p.

[20] Glansdorff, P., Prigogine, I. Thermodynamic theory of structure, stability and fluctuations. 1971, London; New York: Wiley-Interscience. xxiii, 306 p.

[21] Goldsmith, H.L., Marlow, J. Flow behaviour of erythrocytes. I. Rotation and deformation in dilute suspensions. Proc. Royal Soc. 182: 351–84, 1972.

[22] Goldstein, S. Theodore von Kármán, 1881–1963. Biographical Memoirs of Fellows of the Royal Soc. London 12: 335–65, 1966.

[23] Golubitsky, M., Stewart, I. The symmetry perspective: from equilibrium to chaos in phase space and physical space. 2002, Basel; Boston: Birkhäuser. xvii, 325 p.

[24] Görtler, H. Über eine dreidimensionale Instabilität laminaren Grenzschichten an konkaven Wänden. Habilitation. Univ. Göttingen. Nachr. Ges. Wiss. Göttingen 1941: 1–26.

[25] Henderson, A.H. Endothelium in control. Br. Heart J. 65: 116–25, 1991.

[26] Hirsch, M.W., Smale, S., Devaney, R.L. Differential equations, dynamical systems, and an introduction to chaos. 2nd ed. 2004, San Diego, CA: Academic Press. xiv, 417 p.

[27] Holden, A.V. Chaos. 1986, Princeton, NJ: Princeton University Press. vi, 324 p.

[28] Holmes, P., Lumley, J.L., Berkooz, G. Turbulence, coherent structures, dynamical systems, and symmetry. 1996, Cambridge, UK; New York: Cambridge University Press. xviii, 420 p.

[29] Hoyle, R. Pattern formation. An introduction to methods. 2006, Cambridge, UK; New York: Cambridge University Press. 422 p.

[30] Hunt, J.C.R., Vassilicos, J.C. Turbulence structure and vortex dynamics. 2000, Cambridge, UK: Cambridge University Press. xiii, 306 p.

[31] Kamo, C. The ten foot square hut, and Tales of the Heike; being two thirteenth-century Japanese classics, the "Hojoki" and selections from the "Heike monogatari." Tut books. L. 1972, Rutland, Vt.: C. E. Tuttle xii, 271 p.

[32] Keele, K.D., Leonardo, Pedretti, C. Leonardo da Vinci, corpus of the anatomical studies in the collection of Her Majesty the Queen at Windsor Castle. 1978, London [New York]: Johnson Reprint; Harcourt Brace Jovanovich. 3 v.

[33] Koumoutsakos, P., Leonard A. High resolution simulations of the flow past an impulsively started cylinder using vortex methods. J. Fluid Mech. 296: 1–38, 1995.

[34] Lighthill, M.J. An informal introduction to theoretical fluid mechanics. IMA monograph series; 2. 1986, Oxford [Oxfordshire]; New York: Clarendon Press; Oxford University Press. xi, 260 p.

[35] Lorenz, E.N. Deterministic nonperiodic flow. J. Atmosph. Sci. 20: 130–41, 1963.

[36] Lorenz, E.N. The problem of deducing the climate from the governing equations. Tellus 16: 1–11, 1964.

[37] Lorenz, E.N. The essence of chaos. 1993, Seattle: University of Washington Press. xii, 227 p.

[38] Majda, A., Bertozzi, A.L. Vorticity and incompressible flow. Cambridge texts in applied mathematics; 27. 2001, Cambridge, UK; New York: Cambridge University Press. xii, 545 p.

[39] Malkus, W.V.R. Discrete transitions in turbulent convection. Proc. Roy. Soc. Lond. A 225: 185–95, 1954.

[40] McCann-Brown, J.A., Webster, T.J., Haberstroh, K.M. Vascular cells respond to endothelial cell flow- and pressure-released soluble proteins. Chem. Eng. Commun. 194: 309–21, 2007.

[41] Manneville, P. Dissipative structures and weak turbulence. 1990, Boston: Academic Press. xvii, 485 p.

[42] Merzkirch, W. Flow visualization. 2nd ed. 1987, Orlando: Academic Press. x, 260 p.

[43] Meyer-Spasche, R. Pattern formation in visous flows: the Taylor–Couette problem and the Rayleigh–Bénard convention. International series of numerical mathematics; v. 128. 1999, Basel Boston: Birkhäuser. xi, 209 p.

[44] Milne-Thomson, L.M. Theoretical hydrodynamics. 5th ed. 1968, New York: Macmillan. xxii, 743 p.

[45] Minahen, C.D. Vortex/t: the poetics of turbulence. 1992, University Park, PA: Pennsylvania State University Press. xi, 205 p.

[46] Monin, A.S., Yaglom, A.M. Statistical fluid mechanics; mechanics of turbulence. English updated, augmented and rev. ed. 1971, Cambridge, MA: MIT Press. 2 v.

[47] Moser, K.W., Georgiadis, J.G., Buckius, R.O. On the use of optical flow methods with spin-tagging magnetic resonance imaging. Ann. Biomed. Eng., 29: 9–17, 2001.

[48] Moser, K.W., Raguin, L.G., Georgiadis, J.G. MRI Tomographic study of helical modes in bifurcating Taylor–Couette–Poiseuille flow. Phys. Rev. E 64: 16319-1–5, 2001.

[49] Newton, I., Cajori, F., Motte A. Mathematical principles of natural philosophy and his system of the world. 1946, Berkeley: University of California Press. xxxv, 680 p.

[50] Nicolis, G., Prigogine, I. Self-organization in nonequilibrium systems: from dissipative structures to order through fluctuations. 1977, New York: Wiley. xii, 491 p.

[51] Nicolis, G., Prigogine, I. Exploring complexity: an introduction. 1989, New York: W.H. Freeman. xi, 313 p.

[52] Pasipoularides, A. Clinical assessment of ventricular ejection dynamics with and without outflow obstruction [Review]. J. Am. Coll. Cardiol. 15: 859–82, 1990.

[53] Pasipoularides, A., Shu, M., Shah, A., Womack, M.S., Glower, D.D. Diastolic right ventricular filling vortex in normal and volume overload states. Am. J. Physiol. Heart Circ. Physiol. 284: H1064–72, 2003.

[54] Poincaré, H. Science et méthode. 1908, Paris: E. Flammarion. 2 p. l., 314 p., 1 l.

[55] Prigogine, I. From being to becoming: time and complexity in the physical sciences. 1980, San Francisco: W. H. Freeman. xix, 272 p.

[56] Prigogine, I., Stengers, I. Order out of chaos: man's new dialogue with nature. 1984, Toronto; New York: Bantam Books. xxxi, 349 p.

[57] Raguin, L.G., Georgiadis, J.G. Kinematics of the stationary helical vortex mode in Taylor–Couette–Poiseuille flow, J. Fluid Mech. 516: 125–54, 2004.

[58] Richardson, P.D., Pivkin, I.V., Karniadakis, G.E., Laidlaw, D.H. Blood flow at arterial branches: complexities to resolve for the angioplasty suite. Lecture Notes in Computer Science (LNCS) 3993: 538–45, 2006.

[59] Robinson, S.K. Coherent motions in the turbulent boundary layer. Ann. Rev. Fluid Mech. 23: 601–39, 1991.

[60] Rosen, J. A symmetry primer for scientists. 1983, New York: Wiley. xiv, 192 p.

[61] Rosenfeld, M.G., Lunyak, V.V., Glass, C.K. Sensors and signals: a coactivator/ corepressor/ epigenetic code for integrating signal-dependent programs of transcriptional response. Genes Dev. 20: 1405–28, 2006.

[62] Saffman, P.G. Vortex dynamics. Cambridge monographs on mechanics and applied mathematics. 1992, Cambridge, UK; New York: Cambridge University Press. xi, 311 p.

[63] Samimy, M., Breuer, K.S., Leal, L.G., Steen, P.H. A gallery of fluid motion. 2003, Cambridge, UK; New York: Cambridge University Press. x, 118 p.

[64] Schlichting, H., Gersten, K. Boundary-layer theory. 8th rev. and enl. ed. 2000, Berlin; New York: Springer. xxiii, 799 p.

[65] Schmid, P.J. Henningson, D.S. Stability and transition in shear flows. 2001, New York: Springer. xiii, 556 p.

[66] Shapiro, A.H. Shape and flow; the fluid dynamics of drag. Science study series; S21. 1961, Garden City, NY: Anchor Books. 186 p.

[67] Stewart, I., Golubitsky, M. Fearful symmetry: is God a geometer? 1992, Oxford, UK; Cambridge, MA: Blackwell. xix, 287 p.

[68] Strogatz, S.H. Nonlinear dynamics and Chaos: with applications to physics, biology, chemistry, and engineering. 1994, Reading, Mass.: Addison-Wesley Pub. xi, 498 p.

[69] Strogatz, S.H. Sync: the emerging science of spontaneous order. 2003, New York: Hyperion. viii, 338 p.

[70] Taneda, S. Experimental investigation of the wakes behind cylinders and plates at low Reynolds numbers. J. Phys. Soc. Jpn. 11: 302–7, 1956.

[71] Taylor, G.I. Experiments with rotating fluids. Proc. Camb. Phil. Soc. 20: 326–9, 1921.

[72] Taylor, G.I. Stability of a viscous liquid contained between two rotating cylinders. Phil. Trans. Roy. Soc. A 223: 289–343, 1923.

[73] Thom, R. Structural stability and morphogenesis; an outline of a general theory of models. 1st English ed. 1975, Reading, MA: W. A. Benjamin. 348 p.

[74] Thom, R. Mathematical models of morphogenesis. Ellis Horwood series in mathematics and its applications. 1983, Chichester; New York: Ellis Horwood; Halsted Press. 305 p.

[75] Tritton, D.J. Physical fluid dynamics. 2nd ed. 1988, Oxford [England]; New York: Clarendon Press; Oxford University Press. xvii, 519 p.

[76] Turing, A.M., Millican, P.J.R., Clark, A. The legacy of Alan Turing. Mind Association occasional series. 1996, Oxford; New York: Clarendon Press; Oxford University Press. 2 v.

[77] Van Dyke, M. An album of fluid motion. 1982, Stanford, CA: Parabolic Press. 176 p.

[78] Waldrop, M.M. Complexity: the emerging order at the edge of order and chaos. 1992, New York: Simon & Schuster. 380 p.

[79] Whitehead, K.D. The generation and development of a viscous vortex ring. 1968, Atlanta: Georgia Institute of Technology, School of Aerospace Eng., Rep. 68-4. xxv, 375 p.

[80] Weyl, H. Symmetry. 1952, Princeton, NJ: Princeton University Press. 168 p.

Part II

Visualization of Intracardiac Blood Flows: Methodologies, Frameworks, and Insights

Chapter 10

Cardiac Computed Tomography, Magnetic Resonance, and Real-Time 3-D Echocardiography

As all the information on the body is stored in three dimensions, it is possible therefore to display the object at any angle. This allows it to be examined by rotating it around on the screen. The views seen around the organ to be examined may reveal information that hitherto could have been missed, when it was viewed normally in one fixed plane, normal to the axis of the body.—Sir Godfrey N. Hounsfield, Nobel Lecture, December 8, 1979.

——From *Nobel Lectures, Physiology or Medicine 1971–80,* World Scientific Publishing Co., Singapore, 1992.

FOLLOWING HOUNSFIELD AND CORMACK'S invention (see Section 3.11.1, on pp. 149 ff.), cardiac computed tomography (CT), magnetic resonance imaging (MRI), and other tomographic imaging modalities, including live 3-D echocardiography, have developed rapidly. These techniques share basic unifying features, as follows:

1. They are sectional and reveal internal structure *slice-by-slice*, in the way in which the slices of a loaf of bread expose its internal structure.[1] Imaging successive thin, axial cross-sections of the body (cf. Fig. 10.1, on p. 484) avoids the "collapse" of superposed 3-D structures onto a planar 2-D representation, which is the problem with conventional projection radiography (see Panel III. of Fig. 11.5, on p. 590). To illustrate the notion of tomographic scanning, we will consider the geometry of space by constructing and visualizing a 3-D cube. We proceed to build a cube from geometric primitives in lower dimensions. This method will allow us successively to build a geometric element in the next higher dimension using the one constructed in the previous dimension. Notice that we will expand dimensionality sequentially, as is indicated in Figure 10.1 to which we refer now:

   The 0-D primitive is pretty easy: it is just a *point*. We now ink up this 0-D geometric primitive and drag it one unit in a new (x) direction. This dragging produces a *line*

[1] This feature they share with 2-D echocardiography, for which the term ultrasono*cardio*tomography had actually been used [71] before Dr. Harvey Feigenbaum's term became accepted universally.

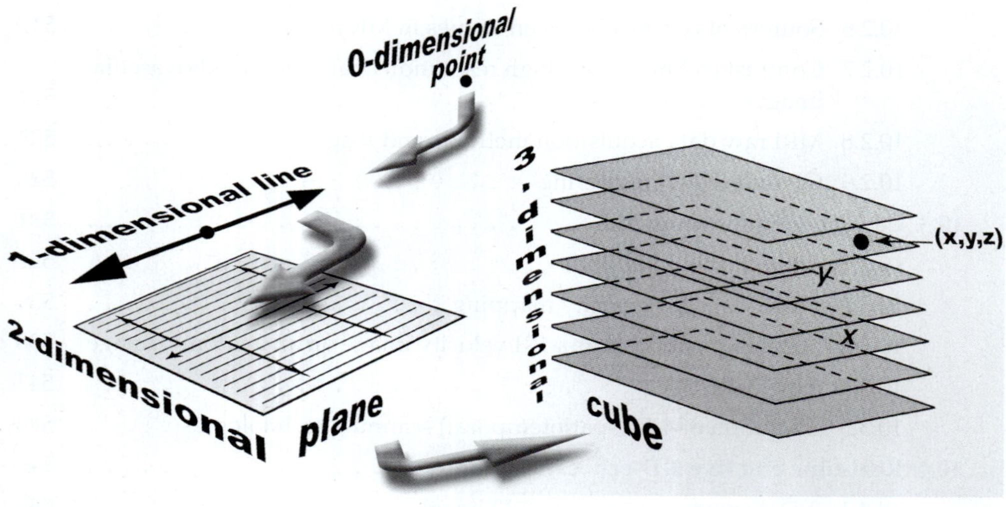

Figure 10.1: Dragging the inked-up 0-D point in a fixed direction produces the 1-D *line*. Dragging the inked-up line vertically, yields the 2-D *plane*. Dragging the inked-up 2-D plane vertically, sweeps out 3-dimensional *space*. Tomographic scans correspond to juxtaposed 2-D plane "cuts" through 3-D body regions and organs.

segment that is actually a 1-D geometric primitive. If we ink up the line segment and drag it one unit in a direction (y) perpendicular to the previous one, we get a 2-D geometric primitive, the familiar *square*. If we ink up the entire 2-D square and drag it one unit in a direction (z) perpendicular to the previous ones, we construct the 3-D geometric primitive that is easily recognized as a *cube*.

2. All tomographic techniques depend on high performance workstations, or computers, to reconstruct sectional or other images from complex datasets. These are massive computational tasks.[2]

10.1 Computed tomography—CT

Figure 10.2 provides a simplified overview of the tomographic process, as it pertains to x-ray computed tomography, or CT. To appreciate the approach of the computed tomographic methods, including CT, MRI, and live 3-D echo, it helps to consider the body as being embedded into a grid comprising a vast but finite number of minuscule volume elements, or *voxels*. Roughly speaking, this corresponds to a wireframe comprising discrete, narrow, imaginary slices in the transverse, sagittal, and coronal plane directions.

[2] Other imaging technologies (e.g., digital subtraction angiography) also use computer image processing but do not yield sectional data.

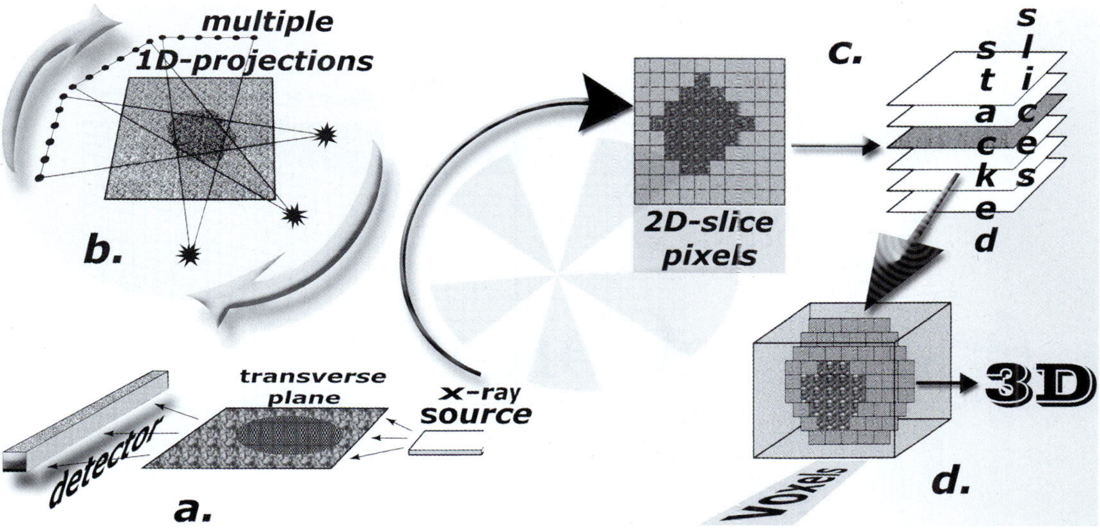

Figure 10.2: In tomographic systems, 3-D imaging information is sampled from parallel stacks of thin, transverse plane *slices*. These systems collect data in such sets of planes according to some particular property, such as the x-ray attenuation coefficient at each point in the plane (panels a.–c.). Typically, the characteristic resolution within a plane (512×512) is much greater than the resolution between planes. The gaps of missing data between the acquired tomographic images are filled through interpolation of the values of adjacent images. In this way, a solid cube of data is obtained. The entire stack of planes is then considered as volume data, from which voxel values are inferred (panels c.–d.), and is rendered accordingly to give 3-D organ reconstructions.

Medical images are typically displayed in three main planes (see Fig. 10.3, on p. 486): (i) *coronal planes*, which divide an organ, or the body, into front and back regions, (ii) *sagittal planes*, which separate the organ or body into left and right parts, and (iii) *transverse planes*, perpendicular to the organ or body's long axis, which divide the body into upper and lower domains. In approaching tomographic examinations of the heart, it is important to bear in mind that a 3-D object may have an infinite number of 2-D projections. As shown in Figure 10.3, *transverse* slices (oriented along the $x-y$ plane) correspond to a series of axial circumferential sections—like slicing the body into a series of thin pancakes and stacking them atop one another. *Sagittal* sections (along $x-z$ plane) are juxtaposed sequentially from one side of the body to the other, i.e., left-to-right. *Coronal* sections (along $y-z$ plane) are juxtaposed vertically from front to back, as though cutting through a halo (*L.,= corona*) around the head. For CT images obtained without gantry tilt, the reconstructed image (transverse plane) is perpendicular to both sagittal and coronal planes. Any planes that are not parallel to any of these three principal planes represent oblique planes.

Computed tomography (CT) is a diagnostic procedure that uses special x-ray equipment to obtain cross-sectional images of regions and organs inside the body [22, 50], as in looking inside a loaf of bread by slicing it. The essential element in CT is mapping out quantitatively, point-by-point, how readily contiguous tissues contributing to the

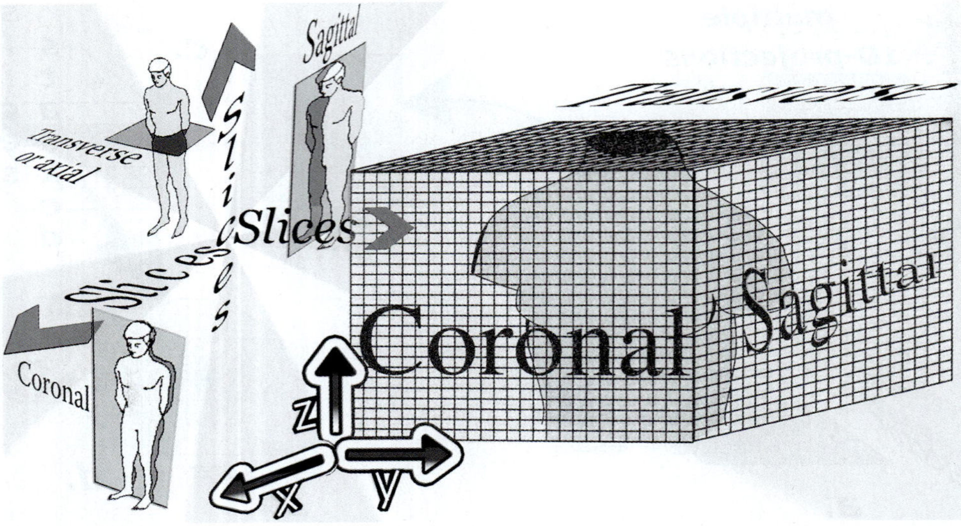

Figure 10.3: Transverse (or, axial), sagittal, and coronal planes. Slices are stacked along each coordinate direction; they correspond to juxtaposed cross-sections forming sets of 2-D images. The gaps of missing data between the acquired tomographic images are filled through interpolation of the values of adjacent, nearest neighbor, images (see also Fig. 11.10, on p. 600). A solid 3-D cube of data is obtained. The gray-scale value of an array element is the value of the corresponding voxel.

topographic anatomy of an organ or body region *remove energy* from an x-ray beam. The only way to produce such a map, in practice, is from measurements made outside the body. As opposed to conventional x-rays, in CT an x-ray source and detector, situated $180°$ across from each other, move $360°$ around the patient, continuously sending and detecting information on the attenuation of x-rays as they pass through the body. The inventors of CT and its subsequent developers have devised efficient hardware and software processes for generating such tissue mappings [9]. In principle, they entail acquisition of a great deal of data on the amounts of energy removed as an x-ray beam systematically traverses sequentially numerous different specific paths through the body region of interest.

The CT scanner consists of a circular *gantry*, or rotating circular goniometric[3] frame, through which is passed the platform upon which is placed the patient. Within the gantry is a rotating ring with an x-ray source opposite a linear array of detectors. The basic principle of CT is that a fan-shaped, thin x-ray beam passes through the body from many angles to allow for complete cross-sectional images. The corresponding x-ray transmission measurements are accumulated by a detector array. The x-ray source is *collimated* so that the x-rays form a flat fan beam with a given thickness. During image acquisition, the source–detector ring is rotated around the patient. In effect, narrow x-ray beams are

[3]From the Greek *goniometrikon*; an adjective signifying that an instrument either *measures angles* or allows an object to be *rotated* accurately to a precise *angular position*; it is derived from the words $\gamma\omega\nu\iota\alpha$, meaning angle and $\mu\epsilon\tau\rho o\nu$, meaning measure.

pointed at the body organ or region of interest from various directions and the reduction in their intensities as they come out from the far side is measured. The collimated x-ray beam generates thin sections conveying tissue topographic information to the detector array; collimation also minimizes blurring, by avoiding unnecessary photon scatter. Once a body slice is formed, the table is advanced and then another slice is acquired. In other words, the gantry rotates $360°$ in one direction and acquires an image, and then rotates $360°$ back in the other direction to obtain the next slice. In between each successive slice, the gantry comes to a complete stop and then reverses direction, while the patient table is moved forward by an increment equal to the slice thickness.

Conventional CT scanners can generally acquire one slice within 1–5 s. A complete exploration usually represents 30–40 slices, with a total study time of 3–15 min. Because of the rapid pulsations of the heart and great vessels and the limitations in scan speed, temporal resolution and volume coverage, cardiac imaging with CT scanners has been a challenging area of research and development. The radiation dose from a CT scan is comparable to that of a series of traditional x-rays.

The output from a CT scanner is the series of the acquired transverse slices of the patient's body region or organ. Each transaxial slice represents a body slab with a thickness set by the collimation for the slice (typically, 1–10 mm). The transmission measurements recorded by the detector array are digitized into pixels with known dimensions by a computer that manipulates and integrates the acquired data, and assigns numerical values based on the subtle differences in x-ray attenuation. For most CT scanners, each slab has 512×512 pixels. The size of a pixel can be varied within certain limits—typically, 0.5-2 mm. The between-slice gap is also variable. Each pixel represents the absorption characteristics of the corresponding volume element. Complex mathematical procedures, requiring millions of mathematical operations to be carried out in seconds, translate the set of measurements of beam attenuation into the desired imaging slice. A gray-scale axial image is generated that can distinguish between topographic anatomic details with even small differences in density. The gray-scale information assembled in each individual pixel is reconstructed according to the attenuation of the x-ray beam along its path using a standardized filtered back-projection algorithm, as is discussed below in Section 10.1.3, on pp. 490 ff. It is truly astonishing that recent-generation multislice (MSCT) systems, acquiring 64 slices per rotation, enable a whole body CT angiography with 1,500 mm scan range and an isotropic resolution of down to 0.4 mm in only 22–25 s [76]. 128- and 256-slice multidetector CT (MDCT) will probably be widely available before too long. Reconstruction algorithms, software capability, and acquisition protocols are also being steadily enhanced. Unfortunately, because of the relatively long rotation time, the temporal resolution (165–400 ms per image) is still insufficient to allow sampling intervals (2–10 ms) of detailed dynamic geometric boundary condition measurements suitable for the assessment of patient-specific intracardiac blood flow patterns by CFD simulations.

Nonetheless, the remarkable ongoing evolution of fast CT scanners in terms of both speed and image quality continuously challenges investigators and clinicians to test their limits by designing and identifying novel applications for analysis of cardiac anatomy and function. Currently, these techniques are already able to assess functional parameters related to the function of the cardiac pump (systolic and diastolic), the cardiac walls

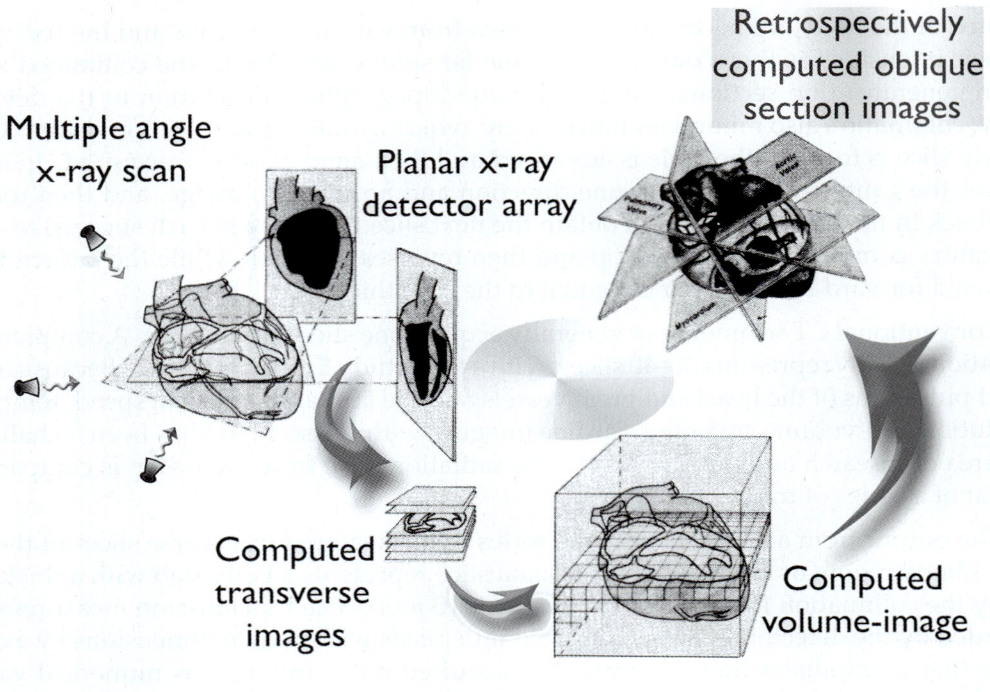

Figure 10.4: Schematic flow diagram of the sequence of procedures performed by the Dynamic Spatial Reconstructor (DSR) system for generation of volume images which could be viewed following mathematical *virtual sectioning* in arbitrary orientations and locations. X-ray images of the chest and its anatomic contents (e.g., heart) were recorded from many angles of view around the patient or experimental animal. This information was used to generate the data ("stack" of images of parallel transverse sections) required for a volume image using a reconstruction algorithm. Synthesis from up to 240 parallel, 1-*mm* thick, cross-sections of the chest and its contents resulted in a 3-D array of voxels (little cubic volume elements) each with a gray-scale value. The final panel illustrates the possibility of sectioning this volume-image in arbitrary orientations and locations, according to specific visualization needs. (Redrawn, slightly modified, from Ritman et al. [123], with kind permission of the authors and the American Physiological Society.)

(myocardial viability and motion), and the cardiac vasculature (vascular endothelial function, perfusion, and permeability).

10.1.1 DSR – the dynamic spatial reconstructor

An early generation x-ray CT system was the dynamic spatial reconstructor (DSR), developed at the Mayo Clinic in Minnesota. It was a high temporal resolution cylindrical, volumetric scanning, computerized, x-ray tomographic system; it could record 1,680 multiple view x-ray video images of the chest (encompassing in excess of 300 million 8-bit voxels) per second [124, 125]. This allowed computation of "stop-action" and 60 *frame/s* instant replay video clips of the dynamic 3-D geometric changes of the full anatomic extents of the internal and external surfaces of the heart chambers. The synchronous volumetric scanning capabilities of the DSR allowed nondestructive mathematical selection and removal of any subvolume of interest from a reconstructed volume, as is shown in Figure 10.4.

The use of a 3-D volume image to calculate a projection image with a reproducible angle of view is a particularly powerful attribute of 3-D image reconstruction. The additional abilities to "zoom in" and "section" this subvolume, so as to examine its dynamic structure, allowed "noninvasive vivisection" and direct visualization *in detail* of the internal anatomy and function of the *beating* heart within the body.

The DSR project served as a stimulus for the early development of many 3-D image display and analysis techniques [46,48,49]. Technical issues such as the roles of CT imaging variables, including tomographic image slice thickness [55] and the maximum acceptable duration of the scan aperture during the various phases of the cardiac cycle, were identified. However, although the DSR provided a temporal resolution high enough for cardiac imaging, its signal-to-noise characteristics were not adequate for most applications. Furthermore, the computing power that the DSR demanded was hard to meet at that time and, together, these important limitations resulted in discontinued use of this scanner. Nevertheless, before being dismantled in 1998, nearly 20 years after being installed, the DSR provided data to settle important physiologic issues, such as whether the total heart volume changes during the cardiac cycle [54].

10.1.2 How imaging projections yield topographic information

Consider a body made up of a uniform interior surrounded by a dense shell and containing a small dense structure S (see Fig. 10.5A., on p. 490). The density distribution of the body is to be mapped, using a visualization modality based on projections. The attenuation value of the horizontal projection (right panel) at a point H equals the line integral of density along the ray R. The higher attenuation values at the end regions of the projection, for example at H′, build up because there the ray, in this instance R′, passes through a greater width of the denser shell. For this same reason, the vertical projection (lower panel) has higher peaks, but it is less extended; nonetheless, the two projections have *equal* areas, because each area represents the attenuation accumulated by the total mass of the body. A peak H due to the small dense structure S tells us that S lies on a certain ray, and the corresponding peak V in the vertical projection places S at the site of intersection. Two projections thus suffice to pinpoint an interior object. Of course, the two attenuation humps at H and V that are accounted for by S have equal areas, corresponding to the total mass of the small dense structure.

How many projections would be needed to similarly map the density distribution of a body in full? In this context, any density distribution can be thought of as made up of numerous enclosed compact structures of different mass; consequently, we can consider two objects, three objects, and so on. If there are two different small interior dense structures, at S_1 and S_2, two attenuation humps will be distinguished (see Fig. 10.5B.) at H_1 and H_2 in the horizontal projection and at V_1 and V_2 in the vertical. Two projections will still suffice to detect them, but there may be an uncertainty if the masses of S_1 and S_2 are

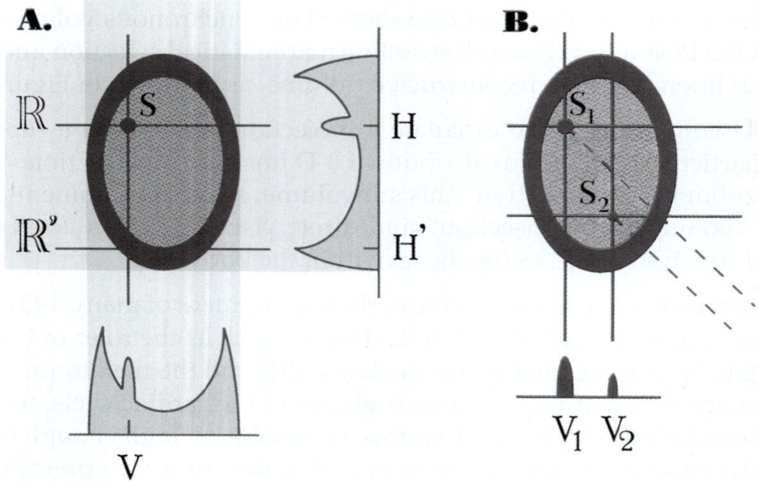

Figure 10.5: A. Density distribution of a body and two imaging projections. B. Density distribution of a body containing two small dense structures—only the attenuation peaks accounted for by them are diagrammed, for clarity. (See discussion in text.)

similar, because there are now *four* intersections at the vertices of a rectangle. S_1 and S_2 might be at the undotted vertices; the ambiguity could be settled by a third projection, whose back-projected peaks are intimated by the interrupted lines in Figure 10.5B.

Some reflection along these lines suggests that two projections would be sufficient if the masses of the compact dense structures were different. Two projections would also be adequate for three, or for any small number, of unequal masses. With limited measurement accuracy as to location or attenuation amplitude, a third projection would then settle the correct identification of each peak. Needless to say, as the number of distinct structures grows larger, accidental three-way intersections rapidly become a confounding factor, and measurement noise introduces further uncertainty. Nevertheless it is encouraging that in the preceding, somewhat contrived simplified circumstances, a very *small* number of projections may yield a great deal of hidden structural topographic information; it is certainly gratifying to be already acquainted with *how* this is accomplished.

10.1.3 What is measured in CT?

The probability of x-ray interaction with matter, and thus the absorption of the imaging x-rays is a function of tissue electron density, which depends on tissue density and the atomic numbers of the constituent atoms, tissue thickness, and x-ray photon energy [158]. Figure 10.6, on p. 491, summarizes pictorially the dependence of the absorption of the imaging x-rays by bodily tissues and regions on these factors. The absorption of a monochromatic x-ray beam depends linearly on the thickness of the specimen and on its effective mass density. Air-containing organs (airways and lungs) are well demarcated from contiguous soft tissues and blood-filled organs (heart and blood vessels) as well as bony structures (ribs), because the density of air is three orders of magnitude smaller than those of water, soft tissues, and bone. The strong dependence of absorption on the effective atomic number of various tissues, which arises from the varying relative amounts of their constituent chemical species, underlies the differing amounts of contrast corresponding to different tissues. It also underlies the effectiveness of compounds containing high-atomic number species, such as iodine and barium as contrast agents.

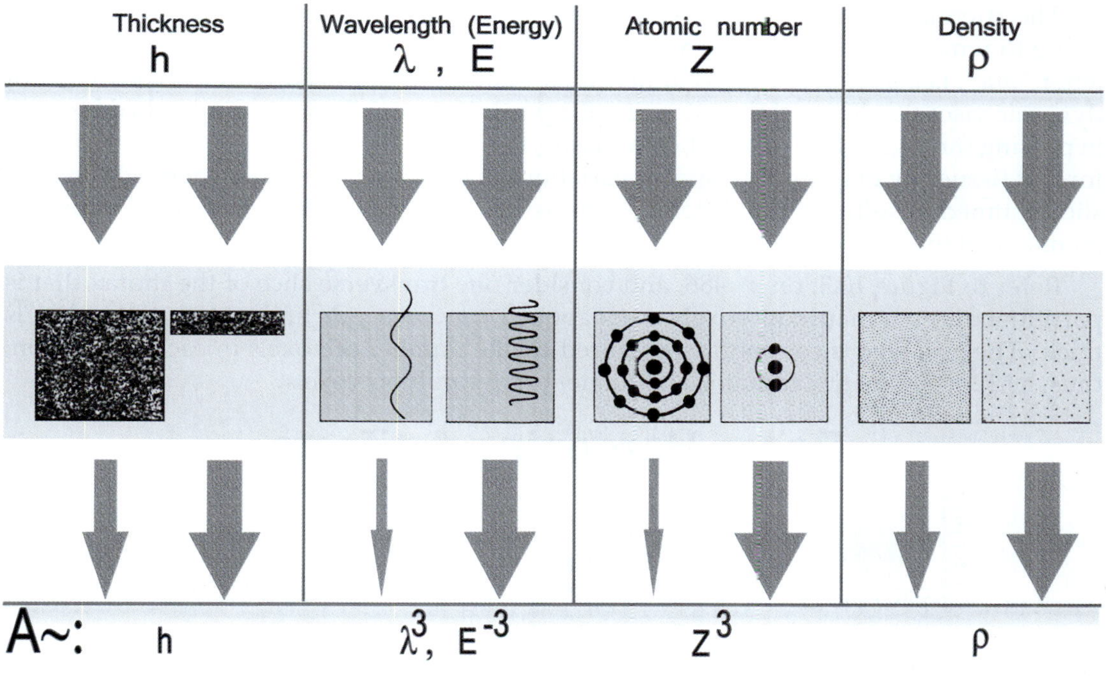

Figure 10.6: Schematic representation of the action and the effectiveness of the main factors involved in the absorption (A) of x-rays by tissues, and in the accruing attenuation of the beam emerging beyond. The power of the emerging x-rays is indicated by the width of the corresponding arrows.

The proportionality of the absorption on the wavelength raised to the third power (inverse proportionality to photon energy raised to the third power) is notable. Nonuniform attenuation of different energies results in the preferential depletion of polychromatic x-rays in energy ranges with higher attenuation coefficients. Viewed as particles, x-rays are called *photons*, and these photons have energies proportional to their frequencies, when viewed as waves. The relationship between energy and frequency for electromagnetic waves, including x-rays, is

$$E = h \cdot f, \tag{10.1}$$

where E is energy in kilo electron volts (keV), h is Planck's constant ($4.13 \cdot 10^{-18}\ keV \cdot s$, or $6.63 \cdot 10^{-34} J \cdot s$), and f is the frequency, in Hz. In general, x-rays in energy ranges that are more easily attenuated are denoted "soft" x-rays, while those in ranges that are more penetrating are referred to as "hard" x-rays.

As a consequence of this nonlinear *beam hardening* effect and the polychromatic x-ray sources used in medical CT, the attenuation is not a linear function of absorber thickness; accordingly, the effective attenuation *coefficient* (not just the attenuation) of a material depends on the thickness of material traversed. If this effect is not compensated, the reconstructed images will be corrupted by so-called cupping artefacts (see Fig. 10.7).

The attenuation coefficient, or spatial rate of attenuation, quantifies the tendency of a tissue to remove energy from an x-ray beam, and is usually represented by μ, the Greek letter "*mu*"; i.e., as $\mu(x, y)$ in two dimensions—not to be confused with the coefficient of dynamic viscosity. Thus, if the intensity of a particular x-ray beam is diminished by 3.0% in passing through $0.1\ cm$ of a particular tissue, then μ has the value ($0.03/0.1\ cm =$) $0.3/cm$ for that tissue. By mapping out spatial variations in the attenuation coefficient within each slice scanned, resulting from differences in tissue density and composition, CT provides an image of the cross-sectional topographic anatomy.

Refer to Figure 10.3, on p. 486, and consider one transverse slice of the thorax that is partitioned into a matrix of voxels, each about $1\ mm$ on a side and as tall as the slice is thick. The grid size is commonly measured by the number of voxels in each dimension; thus, a 512×512 matrix contains about one-quarter million voxels.

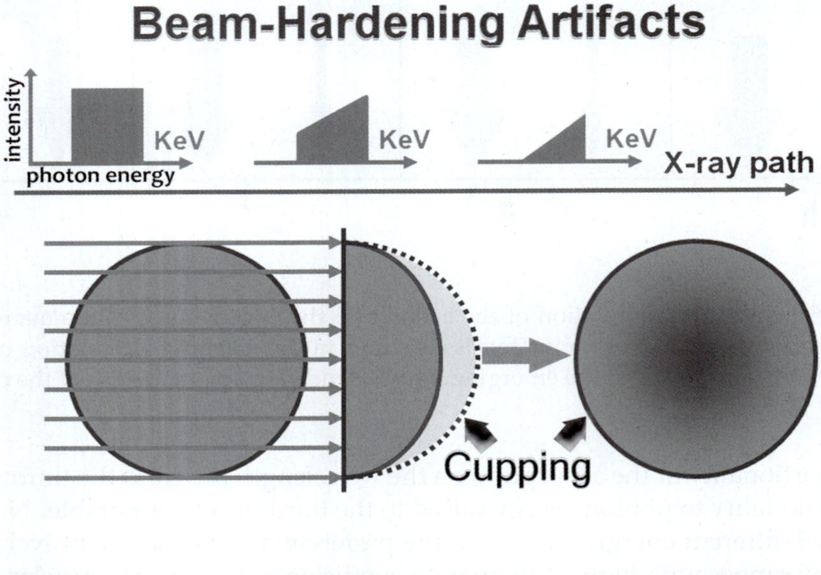

Figure 10.7: The beam from an x-ray source is not mono-energetic and the lower-energy photons will be more attenuated than the higher-energy ones.

In up-to-date CT machines, a beam of x-rays sweeps through $360°$ while detectors on the opposite side of the subject's body provide a digital readout of the amount of radiation, and hence the degree to which the beam has been attenuated. Electron dense materials, such as bone and contrast dye, attenuate the x-rays more than less dense materials (muscle, fat, or air). The differential rate of this interaction provides the contrast

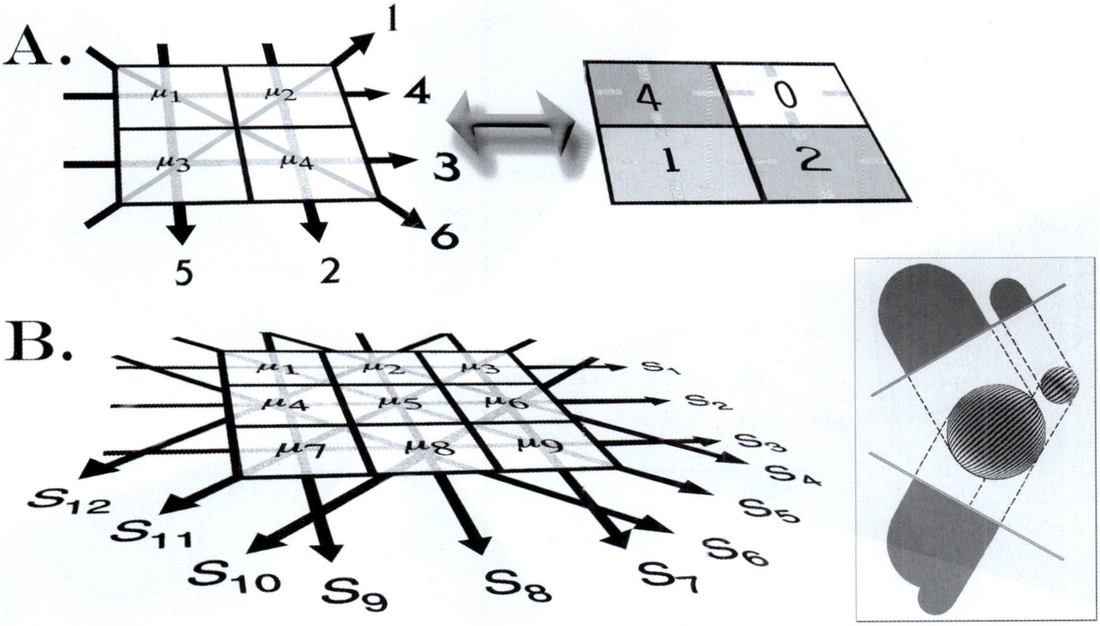

Figure 10.8: Algebraic reconstruction technique (ART). A. The amounts of x-ray beam attenuation across the four voxels of the illustrative CT scan depicted on the left are mutually consistent only with the calculated distribution of individual voxel attenuation values shown on the right. B. Generalization of A.: The N^2 unknown attenuation coefficient values, $\mu(i,j)$, of an $N \times N$ image matrix can be derived from the x-ray beam attenuation measurements by the solution of an *overdetermined (here, 12 equations for 9 unknowns)* linear equation system in μ, in the least squares sense. In the inset, two projections are shown of an object consisting of a pair of spheres.

that forms the image. From the linear attenuation in multiple projections (*"pluridirectional tomography"*), a digital plot of values of the 2-D attenuation coefficient function $\mu(i,j)$ is obtained for every sectional sweep, in the form of a 2-D matrix—i and j denote row and column numbers identifying individual pixels. From this matrix, it is possible to reconstruct a sectional display of body structure in terms of electron density, through application of advanced mathematical methods, involving the inverse *Radon transform*[4] in two or three dimensions.

CT image reconstruction involves back-calculating, from the results of thousands of x-ray transmission measurements on each tissue slice, the 2-D distribution of the attenuation coefficient, namely, the values of μ, for every voxel within the slice. The computed $\mu(i,j)$ distribution is then displayed as a raster image of pixels (or, image locations) with

[4]Projections can be computed along any angle ϕ. In general, the Radon transform [118] of a 2-D function $f(x,y)$ is the line integral of f parallel to the y'-axis, where y' is the direction of the y-axis after rotation by the particular value of the rotation angle ϕ. The desired $f(x,y)$ is obtained by applying the inverse Radon transform.

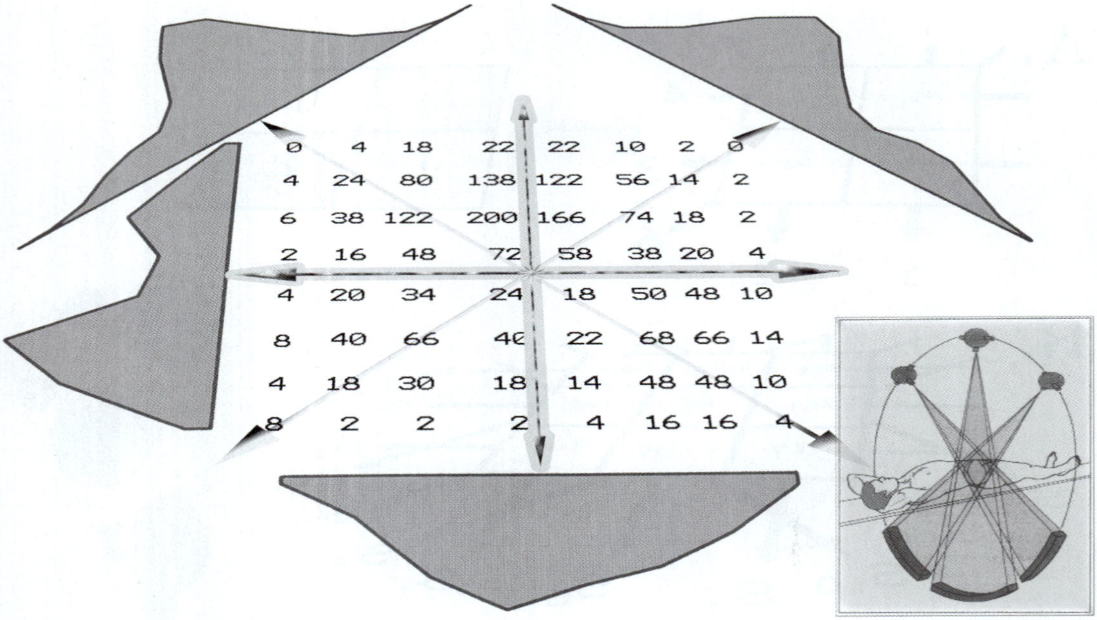

Figure 10.9: A 64-element digital map and four equispaced projections; the projections all have the same area.

an assortment of shades of gray, or in pseudo-color[5] coding on a video monitor. Usually a single pixel in the image corresponds to each voxel in the tissue slice.

To understand the basics of the CT procedure, it will be found expedient to start out not in terms of the Radon transform, but to consider instead the solution to the problem posed as follows: The image may be considered as a plot of the distribution of absorbed x-ray (photon) energy. We desire the values of N^2 unknown attenuation coefficients, $\mu(i, j)$, for the $N \times N$ pixels of the individual slice. These $\mu(i, j)$ values can be obtained in principle by an algebraic reconstruction technique (ART), such as that illustrated in Figure 10.8, on p. 493.

Figure 10.9 illustrates the projection of a digital map along four directions that are spaced at $45°$. Although different numbers of elements enter into the various scanning sums, and the spacing of contributing elements changes, the projections all have the same area. After a set of separate, adjacent transverse CT slices is obtained, the computer locates topographic landmarks in each, and then stacks the resulting curves in three dimensions—if needed, the gaps of missing data between the acquired tomographic

[5] Pseudo color pertains to a class of color mapping in which a pixel value indexes the color map entry to produce independent red, green, and blue values. That is, the color map is viewed as an array of triplets (RGB values). Gray scale can be viewed as a degenerate case of pseudo color, in which case the red, green, and blue values in any given color map entry are kept *equal*, thus producing *shades of gray*, darker or lighter depending on the intensity. The RGB and the gray values can be changed dynamically.

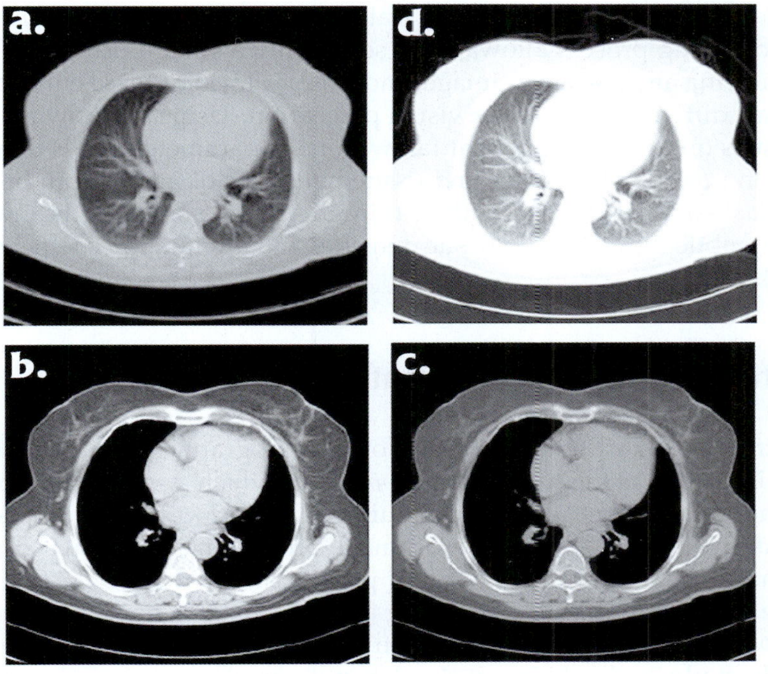

Figure 10.10: Gray-scale windowing adjusts the relationship between the different shades of gray of the image pixels and the different amounts of x-ray attenuation in the tissue voxels. A transverse CT image through the chest (a.) and three gray-scale windows, specific for soft tissue (b.), bone (c.), and lung (d.).

images can be filled through interpolation of the values of adjacent, *nearest neighbor*, images. It then tiles over the areas between adjacent contours and performs 3-D surface rendering for display. It should be recognized that interpolation does not *create* information; rather, it increases the *number of points* with which this information is represented.

Gray-scale values for pixels within the reconstructed tomogram are defined with reference to the value for water and are called *CT numbers* or *Hounsfield Units (HU)*, for Sir Godfrey Hounsfield. Air attenuates the x-rays less than water, and bone more than water, so that in a given case the HU scale may extend from −1,000 HU (air) through 0 HU (water) to approximately +1,000 HU (compact bone). A range of 2,000 gray-scale HU values represents various hard and soft body tissue densities between these two extremes. *Gray-scale windowing* and contrast adjustment help optimize subjective image quality. Images can be stored at 8, 10, 12, 16 bit, or higher gray-scale resolutions. A typical CT image consists of a 1,024 × 1,024 pixel matrix with a 12-*bit* gray-scale depth, which encompasses 4,096 shades of gray.[6] Human vision can discern differences among about

[6]Most radiographic films can make available about 256 gray levels of contrast resolution. However, computed imaging modalities with digital detectors can acquire at least 1,024 distinct levels of gray. There

128 levels (0−127; i.e., 7 bits) of the gray scale. Because of this limitation, the so-called gray-scale windowing process allows us to select only a small portion of the gray scale spectrum in viewing any particular image, and to *expand* it in order to enhance small topographic contrast differences for easier visual perception. Using windowing we can focus on certain tissues on the CT image that fall within set parameters, as is demonstrated in Figure 10.10, on p. 495. The tissues and tissue interfaces of interest can be assigned the full range of blacks and whites, rather than a circumscribed portion of the gray scale. With this technique, subtle differences in tissue densities and attenuation coefficient values can be maximized.

10.1.4 The backprojection operation

Image reconstruction algorithms for CT, and other tomographic imaging systems, usually employ what is known as the *backprojection operation*, which arises from a formula for inverting the Radon transform. The data acquired by CT represents the Radon transform of the scanned image—i.e., a collection of image projections at various scan angles. We let $S(\phi, s)$ denote any particular x-ray beam projection, at an angle ϕ. $S(\phi, s)$ is the line integral of the image intensity, $I(x, y)$, along a line, l, that is a distance s from the origin and at angle ϕ off the x-axis. The attenuation data (originating at the x-ray source, passing through the body, and arriving at the detector array) are recorded and transformed through a filtered backprojection algorithm into the CT image. The spatial filter employs convolution[7] to remove artifacts inherent in backprojection that distort the reconstructed image and blur it. This step is common to every CT modality.

Physical insight into the concept underlying the standard method of backprojection can be obtained by referring to Figure 10.11, on p. 497. Mathematically, the image reconstruction problem reduces to the problem of inverting the Radon transform. The most notable reconstruction methods are *Fourier-based* relying on the slice-projection property of the Radon transform, and *filtered backprojection* (FBP) algorithms [3]. The slice theorem states that the 1-D Fourier transform of the projection function $S(\phi, s)$ is equal to the 2-D Fourier transform of the image, evaluated on the line, l, that the projection was taken on. After determining what the 2-D Fourier transform of the image looks like (at least what it looks like on certain lines, and then interpolating), we can compute the 2-D inverse Fourier transform, to derive the desired image.

In the FBP approach, each of the projections in the Radon transform is filtered with a windowed ramp filter and then backprojected to reconstruct the image. In this way, the magnitudes of the existing higher-frequency samples in each projection are *scaled up* to compensate for their lower amount at the Fourier transform periphery, where the

is a wealth of dynamic range within digital images. This great disparity between imaging sensor resolution and human discrimination (128 shades of gray) has motivated the development of image-processing methods [82], which can *data mine* digital radiographic images and exhibit information within the range of gray-scale levels discernible by humans.

[7]A convolution is an integral that expresses the amount of overlap of one function, as it is shifted over another function. It therefore "blends" one function with another.

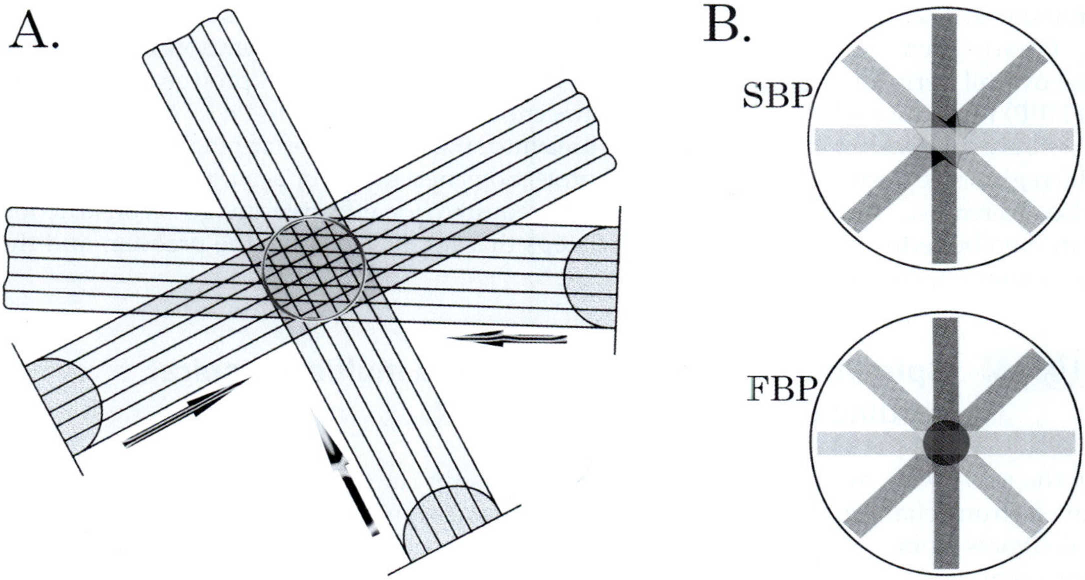

Figure 10.11: A. In the basic procedure of backprojection without further processing, every scanned profile is projected back over the image area at the same angle at which it was obtained, and any attenuation of the x-ray beam is assumed to have occurred uniformly along the entire ray path. Every projection contributes not only to the locations that originally attenuated the profile, but uniformly to all points in its path. Tomographic reconstruction of anatomic structures accrues by linear superposition of backprojections. This unfiltered technique produces *star-shaped* displays and blurring, as is schematically exemplified here; the correct *circular* outline of the hypothetical organ is sketched in to emphasize this point. B. This blurring and distorting artefact of simple backprojection (SBP) can be suppressed mathematically using filtering techniques, and the overall reconstruction method is then called filtered backprojection (FBP).

spectrum is only sparsely sampled. The filters are referred to as *convolution filters* but, in practice, the filtering is done in the frequency domain, to reduce computing cost. After completion of the filtration step, the inverse Fourier transform is applied to the data for each attenuation profile; then the backprojection procedure with linear superposition of all the filtered backprojections is carried out.

The backprojection is a computationally intensive stage in the reconstruction process with $O(M^3)$ operations,[8] M being the image size in pixels. For comparison, commonly used Fourier transform methods require at most $O(M^2 \log M)$ operations, and by appropriate strategies many fewer operations. This is discussed, in the context of the fast Fourier

[8] An order of magnitude—$O(q)$, *or* $O \propto (q)$—estimate for a variable q whose exact value is unknown is an approximation rounded to the nearest power of ten; e.g., an order of magnitude estimate for a quantity between about 5 and 20 is 10. The big O, standing for "order of," is the capital letter O, and not the digit *zero*. It refers to an asymptotic upper bound for the magnitude of a function in terms of another, simpler, function.

transform, and its application to 2-D and 3-D data fields, in Section 2.20.3, on pp. 94 f. Clearly then, efficient implementation of the backprojection operation is crucial for the overall performance of the algorithm. The fast hierarchical backprojection algorithm (FHBP) [3] reduces the cost of the backprojection asymptotically to $O(M^2 log M)$, by successively subdividing the reconstruction area into smaller nonoverlapping subregions. As the region size decreases, the number of projections necessary for accurate reconstruction also decreases. The number of projections required for effective image reconstruction can then be reduced, which reduces the steps that it takes to solve the problem and the computational difficulty.

10.1.5 Spiral/helical, electron beam, and multislice spiral cardiac CT

In the mid-1980s, an innovation called the power slip ring was developed. A *slip ring* is an electromechanical device that allows the transmission of electrical power and electrical signals from a stationary to a rotating structure without requiring a "rewinding" of any components.[9] Also called a rotary electrical joint, a slip ring can be used in any electromechanical system that requires unrestrained, continuous rotation while transmitting bidirectionally electric power and data. It allows electric power to be transferred from a stationary power source onto a continuously rotating x-ray gantry. This enabled a new type of CT scanning, called spiral or "helical," CT; the term conjures up a tracing of the spiral path of the x-ray beam along the patient, due to the gantry rotating continuously while table and patient are sliding through.

During helical scanning, data acquisition is accomplished with continuous motion of the acquisition system. The path of the x-rays can be described as a spiral or a helix, as is drawn in Figure 10.12. The scanner rotates continuously as the patient table glides, and as many as one thousand x-ray pictures may be recorded in one rotation [66,67]. Obviously, these scanners can acquire a very large volume of imaging data very fast. The speed of helical CT scanning is advantageous for several reasons: (*i*) most patients can hold their breath for the entire study, thus reducing motion artifacts; (*ii*) the technique allows for a more optimal use of intravenous contrast enhancement; and (*iii*) the imaging data acquisition process is a lot quicker than conventional CT. Furthermore, some scanners permit the performance of not only one preprogrammed helical scan, but of *multiple*, sequential helical scans, separated by short interposed breathing intervals, which allows even patients with diminished breath-holding capacity to undergo helical CT [6].

As is indicated in Figure 10.12, current spiral, or "helical," CT scanners for cardiac imaging employ a rotating x-ray source with a circular, stationary detector array [81]. Helical scanners can image entire anatomic regions like the thorax in a 20–30 s breath-hold. Instead of acquiring a stack of individual slices that may be misaligned due to intervening slight patient motion or breathing movement, spiral CT acquires a volume of data with the patient anatomy in a specified position and combines fast and high resolution data acquisition from every organ, including the heart. In spiral CT, the volume

[9] A slip ring is a component of rotatory implantable ventricular assist devices, or VADs.

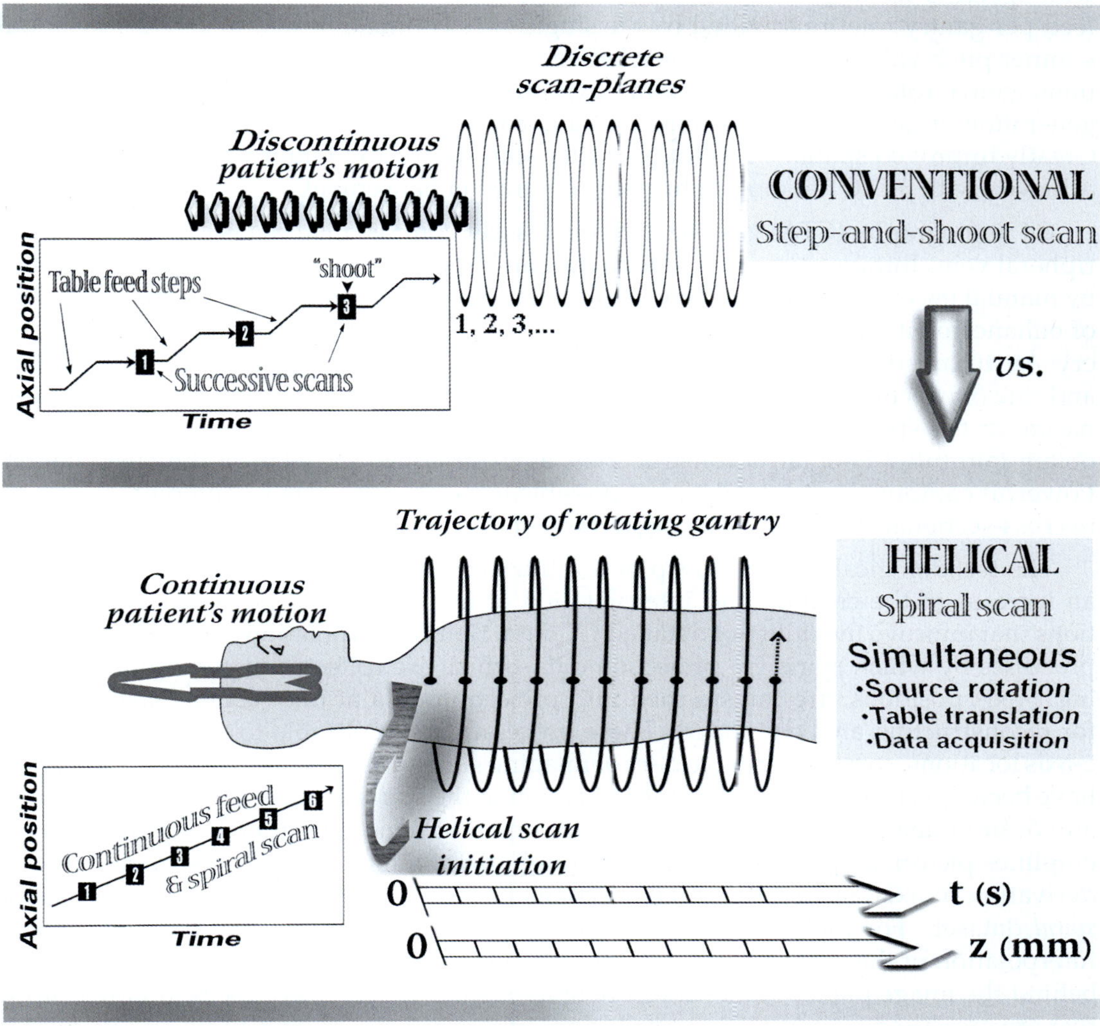

Figure 10.12: In conventional CT, the patient table traverses the x-ray gantry in short discontinuous steps, a predetermined axial distance apart; successive, juxtaposed imaging-plane, slices of a body region are obtained discretely, in the interposed pauses, as shown in the top inset. In spiral/helical CT, scanning is performed while the patient is being glided slowly but *continuously* through the rotating gantry in the axial (z) direction. A single detector arc is used and, if there were no table movement, a single CT slice would be obtained during one gantry rotation, of thickness determined by the collimation used. The continuous scan (bottom inset) allows for *nonstop* volumetric data acquisition, as data are gathered on a 3-D volume in a *helical* fashion; viewed by a fixed point on the patient, the traveling path of a point on the rotating gantry is a *helix*. Images are reconstructed from the data volume. (Montage based, in part, on pictorial elements adapted from refs. [53, 64], and [101].)

scan speed is usually described by the *spiral pitch*, which is determined by the table-feed per gantry rotation divided by the single-slice collimation width; single-slice spiral scanner pitch values commonly vary between 1 and 3 [89]. Spiral scanning with continuous gantry rotation, table-feed, x-ray exposure and data acquisition have allowed the generation of genuine volume imaging data, based on overlapping axial imaging slices. Greatly improved spatial z-resolution, faster scan speed, and larger volume coverage are achieved with 3-D CT angiography using contrast enhancement.

CT angiography (CTA) visualizes blood vessels; contrast material is injected into a peripheral vein. Intravenous contrast material can be administered with a power injector or by manual injection. The benefits of power injection over manual injection are uniformity of enhancement and ability to determine precisely the timing of contrast material delivery. An automatic power-injector machine is always used to accurately control the timing and rate of injection, which may continue during image recording. The quasi-continuous nature of the spiral CT images means that the data can be assembled by computer to obtain faithfull 3-D organ reconstructions, as is described in detail in the next chapter. Powerful computer software makes it possible to display the data in different ways, e.g., in cross-sectional slices, or as 3-D organ *casts* of the heart and blood vessels.

The technological quantum leap of multidetector row CT has, in recent years, led to an increase in the creation and interpretation of images, and to powerful 3-D applications that improve the utility of detailed CT data. Spiral interpolation algorithms embody processes by which spiral CT projection data, which are collected at continuously varying z-axis positions, are transformed into projection data at one *specific* z-axis location for reconstructing an axial image. These processes are applicable to *multiple* successive z-axis locations, corresponding to a set of imaging slices. Various interpolation algorithms have been developed for the efficient utilization of the spiral acquisition data in obtaining any desired imaging slice through the body organ or region examined. Figure 10.13 exemplifies pictorially a simple $360°$ linear longitudinal interpolation (LI) scheme. For the derivation of axial slices, *planar* data sections have to be generated from the measured *spiral* dataset. For each image plane, a set of projections can be computed by a linear interpolation of the individual x-rays measured for each projection angle in front of and behind the image plane. For a nearest neighbor $360°$ LI, the rays of the beam projections that are measured in consecutive revolutions at the same projection angle are used. This procedure results in a widening of each slice-profile to an effective slice width that is larger than the collimated slice width. A related point to stress again is that interpolation does not *create* information; rather, it increases the *number* of points with which the available information is represented. Similar considerations apply for the use of data for the creation, interpretation, and quantification of images in planes other than the traditional axial plane.

Aiming at the achievement of very short image-acquisition times for virtually "freezing" cardiac motion, another ingenious modality of CT systems has also been developed, with nonmechanical movement of the x-ray source. Whereas a traditional CT scanner has an x-ray tube that mechanically revolves around the patient, these *electron beam* computed tomography (EBCT) scanners have no mechanical motion of the x-ray source and a stationary detector array. An electron beam is generated and electromagnetically

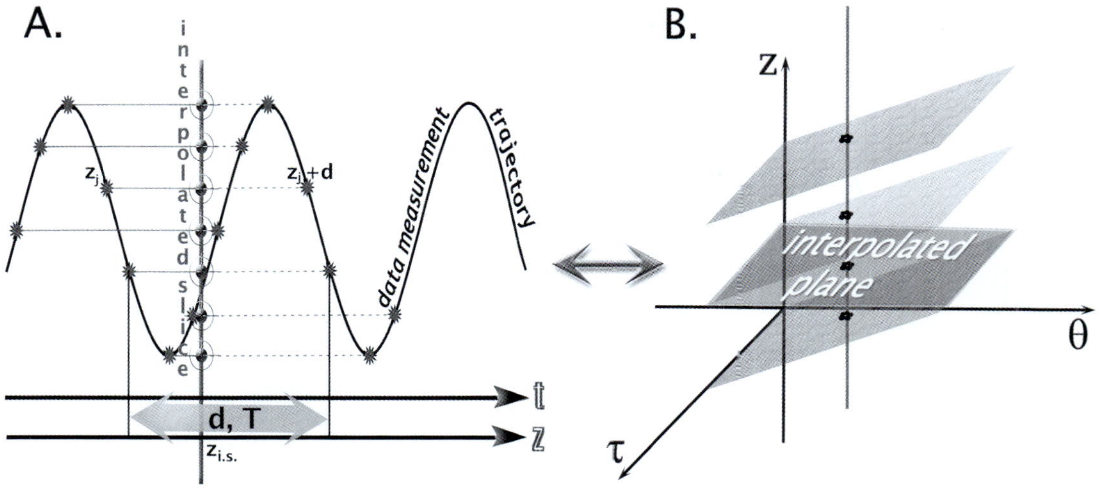

Figure 10.13: A. Simple data interpolation, linearly-weighted by axial distance: using the nearest actual data measurements (z_j, z_{j+d}) that lie astride (*above* and *below*, in panel B.) the interpolated voxel on any desired slice at axial position $z_{i.s.}$, such interpolation yields the appropriate gray-scale intensity for that or any other voxel on each successively estimated slice; d denotes the distance along the z-axis that is traversed by the patient table during the period, T, of one 360° revolution of the gantry. B. Data from each rotation of the x-ray tube gantry are specific to an angled plane of section; τ denotes an index to position in the detector array, z the axial position of the imaging planes, and θ the projection angle, which is dependent on the z-position of the detector.

swept around to be focused on an array of tungsten x-ray anodes that are positioned circularly on a stationary gantry encircling the patient. The hit anode emits x-rays that are collimated and detected as in conventional CT, and x-ray production can be triggered by the ECG. EBCT with prospective ECG triggering can acquire one slice in every heartbeat with 50–100 ms temporal resolution. Resorting to an electron beam allows for much abbreviated scanning times because the rotation of the source is provided by the sweeping motion of the electron beam, instead of mechanical motion of the x-ray tube [102]. Thus, an entire slice scan can be completed in 50–100 ms, i.e., 20 times faster than can be achieved using conventional CT scanners. This allows acquisition of a complete multi-slice imaging set of the heart during a single breath-hold. However, the high temporal resolution is associated with a somewhat limited spatial resolution.

To improve the signal-to-noise ratio, however, multiple scans are commonly averaged to generate the final image. Multi-row detectors and reconstruction algorithms common to both EBCT and helical CT permit accurate volumetric[10] imaging, and multiple high-resolution reconstructions of various volumes (*viz.*, 3-D regions) of interest are possible either prospectively or retrospectively, using ECG triggering [93]. In either case, the

[10]The term *volumetric* implies a data domain of three independent variables.

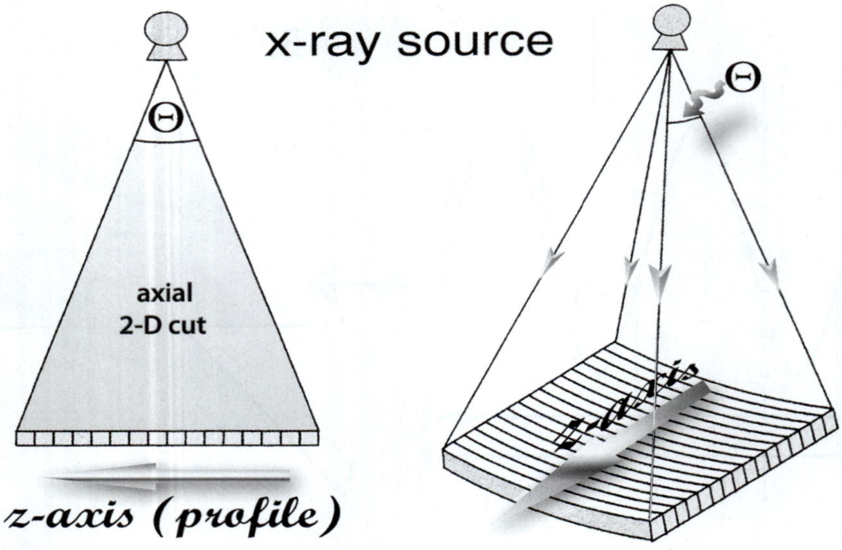

Figure 10.14: In MDCT, the single detector row of a single-slice spiral CT scanner along the z-axis is replaced by a multiple-row detector array that enables simultaneous acquisition of multiple axial slices during one gantry rotation. Sixteen detector rings are illustrated in the diagrams. The size of the *cone angle*, Θ, is magnified for clarity; actually, it amounts to only about $1°$.

patient's ECG signal is monitored during image acquisition and is used to trigger data acquisition (or *selection*, if retrospective) at particular phases of the cardiac cycle.

Because the cardiac cycle is repetitive, an image for each phase can be built up over many cycles to improve image quality. Although voluntary or imposed (end-expiratory) breath-holding acquisition techniques have been proposed to reduce, or eliminate, the respiratory motion artifacts during x-ray CT (and cine-MRI cardiovascular imaging studies with fast gradient echo sequences—see Section 10.2.5, on pp. 514 ff.), many patients cannot tolerate holding their breath. Respiratory gated volumetric CT may therefore improve examination comfort and data quality.

In cardiac studies, ECG triggering results in a series of images representing cardiac chambers during ventricular filling and then ejection throughout the cardiac cycle. Continuous scanning spiral CT with multi-detector/multi-slice (MDCT/MSCT) enhancements [120] allow for image acquisition windows that are shorter than 200 ms with brief inter-scan delay. Continuous data acquisition and retrospective reconstruction of slices allows images to be reconstructed from any given cardiac phase. At present, 64-slice MDCT scanners provide enhanced scan modes of temporal resolution as low as 165 ms (6 Hz) and, in multisector mode [57], a temporal resolution as low as 100 ms. Improved temporal resolution leads to reduced cardiac motion artifacts and less blurring. However, even a temporal resolution as low as 100 ms per image is still insufficient to allow sampling intervals (2–10 ms) of detailed dynamic geometric boundary condition measurements, such as would be directly applicable to the assessment of patient-specific intracardiac blood flow patterns by CFD simulations that we will consider in subsequent chapters.

The principal difference between MDCT/MSCT scanners and their immediate predecessors, i.e., single slice spiral or helical scanners, lies in the detector-array design. Regardless of the x-ray beam collimation, a single-slice spiral CT scanner has a single tube source that irradiates only one row of detectors along the z- or long axis [62]. As is shown in Figure 10.14, on p. 502, in MDCT this is replaced by a multiple row of detectors called a detector array that enables simultaneous acquisition of 4, 16, 64, or more, slices during one gantry rotation. Three types of detector-array matrices are available in multislice scanners: fixed, adaptive, and mixed. Fixed detector arrays have all matrix elements of the same size, while in adaptive matrix arrays the detector elements are wider away from the center; mixed arrays have a matrix of the same-size detector elements with the exception of a number of thinner detectors at the central region.

Modern multislice CT using four or more detector rows allows rapid isotropic (*cubic* voxels) volumetric imaging by utilizing multiple side-by-side detectors simultaneously. This isotropic voxel acquisition capability of MSCT provides identical resolution of an organ's structure in *all* dimensions and is of primary importance in 3-D imaging [63]. The advantage of using cubic voxels is in the avoidance of a serrated appearance of structures in multiplanar reconstructions (see Chapter 11) and an improved contour smoothness in the rendered image. If the raw data do not consist of cubic voxels, these can be derived using linear interpolation [47], to form additional slices, thus enabling a division into cubes. The most recent scanners use up to 64 detector rows, with 128, and even 256 rows, in the horizon. Advances in CT technology have led to the development by a number of manufacturers of CT scanners capable of acquiring 64 slices of image data in about one-third of a second, allowing incredible 3-D images of the heart and the coronary vessels.

The LightSpeed *VCT*, meaning *"Volume CT,"* is a state-of-the-art multislice CT scanner. The hallmark of this imaging system is the new V-Res^{TM} (GE Healthcare, General Electric Company, Fairfield, CT, USA) detector, with the ability to deliver wide anatomical coverage at high resolution. Specifically, it covers $4\,cm$ of axial patient length per rotation, gathering 64 slices at $0.625\ mm$ (about the thickness of a credit card) spacing. Gantry rotation period is $<375\ ms$, yielding 2.5–3 rotations$/s$. The high coverage speed allows capture of the heart in 5 beats. With submillimeter spatial resolution ($<0.75\ mm$), improved temporal resolution (50–200 ms), and ECG gating, the current generation of CT scanners with 16–64 row detectors makes dynamic cardiac imaging possible, and has the potential to accurately characterize *representative* heart chamber and valve geometries that apply during successive phases of the cardiac cycle.

Other tomographic imaging modalities, such as gated single photon emission computed tomography (SPECT) can be utilized to evaluate cardiac function. However, gated SPECT is affected by variations in background activity and injected dose, which can lead to overestimation of ventricular chamber volumes. Positron emission tomography (PET) appraises myocardial metabolism. It can play an important role when cardiac viability is assessed, and functional PET images can be fused to structural x-ray CT [61], or MRI, images.

10.1.6 Recent advances in cardiac CT and dynamic ventriculography

Recent advances in CT technology and acquisition protocols, which have succeeded in improving both speed and image quality, are opening new horizons for clinically useful dynamic studies of the cardiovascular system. To wit, improved speed has relaxed the until recently applying constraint that cardiac CT imaging was only feasible if the patient's heart rate was sufficiently low and stable. Additional developments in computing power for complex data manipulations and display may make CT-supported CFD studies of intracardiac flows feasible in the not too distant future. Taking into consideration contrast media application, radiation exposure, and limited temporal resolution, MDCT *solely* for patient-specific evaluations of cardiac fluid dynamics seems inappropriate at the present time. However, because the dynamic cardiac chamber data is *already obtained* during coronary evaluation, the combination of noninvasive coronary artery imaging and assessment of cardiac function with MDCT may, in the not too distant future, become a suitable approach to a conclusive cardiac workup in patients with suspected coronary artery disease [17, 103] . Given the radiation dose and contrast requirement, referring a patient to MDCT only for evaluation of cardiac fluid dynamic function is not reasonable; however it can add important clinical information to the *already acquired* volume data during retrospective triggering for noninvasive MDCT coronary angiography.

Indeed, thanks to its technical versatility, CT has marked potential for becoming central in providing dynamic geometry data for patient-specific CFD simulations. Nowadays, with dual source CT (DSCT) that equips a single rotating gantry with two x-ray tubes and two corresponding detector assemblies, mounted with an angular offset of 90°, cardiac imaging is effectively *twice* as fast as with the fastest single source CT. DSCT allows the simultaneous imaging of two fan-beam angles in the same imaging slice at any given time, effectively increasing the heart rate-independent temporal resolution by a factor of two compared to conventional single-tube systems. The current dual source 64-MSCT, Somatom Definition™ produced by Siemens Medical Solutions, Forchheim, Germany, has a gantry rotation time of 330 ms, which yields a heart rate-independent temporal resolution of 83 ms, to complement its spatial resolution of 0.33 mm. Preliminary results, in beating cardiac phantoms, suggest that with sophisticated reconstruction techniques a mean temporal resolution of 60 ms can be attained [32].

Concurrently with DSCT, the natural proliferation of detector elements in CT scanners has advanced rapidly and, with each new scanner generation, the number of detector rows along the z-axis has grown. Additionally, the number of channels along the radial coordinate has increased. A prototype 256-detector row CT scanner, developed in Japan by Toshiba Medical Systems, Inc., became available for research applications in 2005. The 256-MSCT has a detector assembly consisting of 256 segments along the z-axis with 0.5 mm collimation and 912 total channels along the radial coordinate [59]. This prototype system has undergone several modifications, primarily to increase gantry rotation speed, which in the current (*"second specification"*) model has a rotation period of 500 ms. Compared to 4-MSCT (2 cm) and 64-MSCT (4 cm), the 256-MSCT prototype provides 12.8 cm of coverage along the z-axis, meaning that 360° evaluation of the whole heart is effectively accomplished by a single gantry rotation. The 256-MSCT allows for comprehensive dynamic anatomic imaging of the entire heart. It also allows for ventricular volumes and ejection fraction, regional wall motion, and systolic thickening, to be obtained in a slightly longer time than required for a single gantry rotation. In fact, by further expanding detector coverage to a wide array containing 320 detectors in the z-axis direction it has become feasible to obtain full cardiac coverage in one gantry rotation [59,128,137].

10.2 Magnetic resonance imaging—MRI

William Gilbert, physician to Queen Elizabeth I of England, published his widely acclaimed *De Magnete* in 1600. This led on to electromagnetism, and ultimately to MRI. How contented Gilbert would be to see magnetism come back to medicine by the discoveries (summarized in a historical context in Chapter 3) of Paul Lauterbur and Sir Peter Mansfield! On the way came the towering geniuses of von Helmholtz, Michael Faraday, and James Clerk Maxwell. MRI has evolved over the last few decades to emerge as an important, and rapidly developing, noninvasive imaging modality for cross-sectional scanning.

Different MRI imaging approaches and techniques contribute to a variety of physiological and pathological morphomechanical insights [15]. MRI has many advantages over other imaging modalities, including higher spatial resolution of soft tissue differences than x-ray CT, excellent temporal resolution, and highest-quality soft tissue contrasting capabilities, as well as lack of ionizing radiation.

10.2.1 MRI in a nutshell

As is the case with all imaging modalities, MRI requires an energy source, an interaction of an energy beam with body tissues, and reception of the energy emerging from the body to form an image. The energy source in MRI is a radio frequency (RF) transmitter; the tissue interaction involves resonance between RF signals and oscillations in the magnetic field of spinning protons in the nuclei mainly of hydrogen in body water or fat molecules. Since the RF field is applied at the same frequency as the precession of tissue protons, the protons absorb energy. When the excitation RF pulse is turned off, the excited protons return to equilibrium and release their absorbed energy at the same resonant frequency, producing an MR signal. The signal receiver is an RF aerial, which can pick up the signals emitted by the protons relaxing back to their unexcited state.

Medical MRI is based on the *magnetization* that is induced in the human body when it is placed in the main magnetic field of the MRI scanner [22,50,51]. Once the patient is positioned on a table inside the scanner, a high intensity magnetic field is created by the magnet. This causes the magnetic moments (which are also referred to simply as *spins*) of mainly the hydrogen atom nuclei, i.e., *protons* within the body, to become aligned. Their magnetization is aligned with the main field of the scanner (the z, or axial, direction), just like a compass needle in the Earth's magnetic field. Deflecting an aligned proton from side

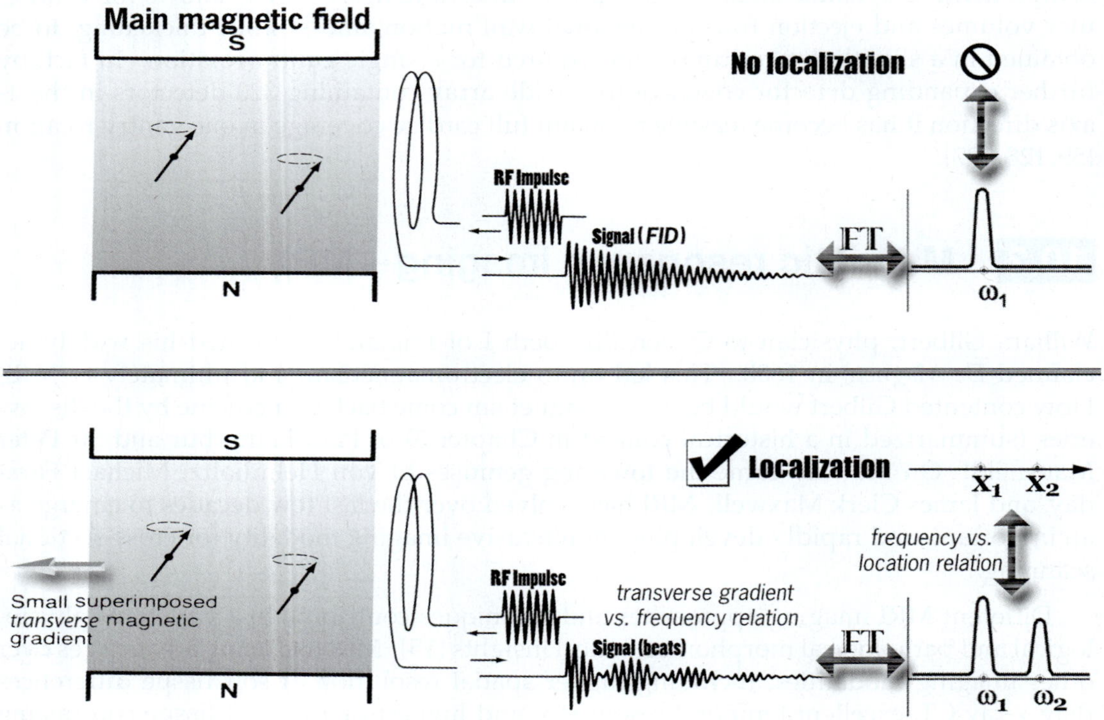

Figure 10.15: Top panel: A transverse electromagnetic pulse of the proper radio frequency (RF) will deflect a group of nuclei aligned in a main magnetic field and start them moving in a gyrating fashion, or *precessing*, at the same frequency. They will progressively get out of step and will also fall back into alignment with the main field, thus attenuating the output signal (FID) induced into the coil from which was sent the original deflecting signal. Bottom panel: If a minute magnetic field gradient in space is superimposed upon the main field, then protons at any two different locations will respond with two different corresponding frequencies, which will interfere with each other to give rise to periodic and repeating fluctuations of the type shown in the output signal. A Fourier transform (FT), or frequency analysis, of this signal converts the amplitude as a function of time into amplitude that is a function of frequency, to indicate the relative amounts of protons at the two locations.

to side can be brought about by applying a brief alternating magnetic field impulse crosswise to the main field, as is shown in the top panel of Figure 10.15. Likewise, when thus deflected nuclei are sweeping around in synchronism *transversely* to the main magnetic field, a small alternating electromagnetic signal can be picked up externally by a coil with axis pointed across the main field (top panel, Fig. 10.15); however, the nuclei will gradually get out of synchronism in their precessing due to magnetic interactions between them and, as shown, the signal in the coil will decay exponentially with time.

The radio signal, emitted while the deflected nuclei are returning to equilibrium, is at the frequency of precession; it is recorded and can then be processed to generate images. The decaying "echo" signal is known as the *free induction decay* (FID), and is further discussed below, in the context of Figure 10.16. At the top of Figure 10.15, all protons are seen acting together to return the monotonically decaying FID signal. The crux of MRI is in understanding two points: a.) If all protons (or other activated nuclei) in the scanned object act together, there is no information about the spatial distribution and density of these nuclei. b.) However, if the magnetic field is *not* everywhere of the same strength, then a given type of nucleus will respond at a different frequency at different locations. Therefore, by introducing small magnetic field gradients, superposed to the large main magnetic orienting field, the spatial location of the nonuniformly distributed nuclei emitting signals, in response to the RF impulse, can be determined.

At the bottom of Figure 10.15, a small magnetic field is superimposed, so as to make the overall field slightly stronger on the right than on the left. A short alternating current pulse applied to the coil will, in fact, contain many frequencies and stimulate nuclei everywhere. The two shown will continue to precess at slightly different frequencies, appropriate to their local magnetic fields, and will induce into the coil an outgoing signal consisting of two different frequencies. Just as listening to two slightly differently tuned tuning forks causes one to hear a beat note, so the resulting signal here will cyclically change its amplitude. An analysis of this out-coming signal will reveal the presence of two frequencies and hence indicate the presence of nuclei at two distinct positions corresponding to these particular spatial (location-encoding) frequencies.[11]

With many nuclei situated at many different values of magnetic field there will be many frequencies in the output, but a frequency analysis of this signal will show which frequencies are present, and the relative amounts of each, and thus indicate the relative number of nuclei at different positions. Nuclear magnetic resonances in liquids are so sharp that frequencies differing by as little as 1 part in 108 are resolved—responses from solids are *broader* [10]. Thus, a given frequency corresponding to one place in a magnetic gradient should be localized to less than the resolvable distance of the system and this should not impose any resolution limitation. Spatial resolution does not depend on frequency as such, but does depend on gradient field strength and overall field uniformity.[12]

A transverse magnetic field gradient projects the nominally 2-D density of nuclear spins in a slice onto the coordinate direction line along which the gradient is applied. Other projections can be collected without mechanical movement by (electrically) shifting the gradient of the magnetic field. The process of evaluating the relative amounts present of different frequencies, that is, of converting a signal of amplitude *vs.* time into one of amplitude *vs.* frequency, entails taking the Fourier transform of the signal—see Section 2.18, on pp. 82 ff.

[11]A rudimentary sort of *spatial encoding* under a magnetic field gradient can be thought to occur when two persons with initially synchronized, perfectly accurate, watches enter the MRI room for a short while. A third observer should then be able to tell who had been closer to the magnet, by observing whose watch had been thrown off more from the correct time.

[12]There is a relationship between frequency and magnetic field strength, the latter also affecting signal strength and detail for a given examination duration.

10.2.2 Spins and the MR phenomenon

Consider a volume of body tissues containing hydrogen atoms, i.e., protons. Each proton has a spin vector of the same magnitude, and the spin vectors for the collection of protons in the volume are randomly oriented. A vector addition of these spin vectors turns out a zero sum and no net tissue magnetization is observed. If the tissue volume is placed inside a magnetic field B_o, the individual protons start to rotate perpendicular to, or to *precess about*, the magnetic field. Every proton acts like a rapidly rotating body and, as a moving charge, it produces its own magnetic field, which can couple with the external magnetic field; this interaction results in a *torque* on the proton, perpendicular to its spin axis. Because of its spin and this torque, the proton's spin axis will *precess* in the external magnetic field. Thus, the protons are tilted slightly away from the axis of the field, but their axis of rotation is *parallel* to B_o. This precession is at a constant frequency, the *Larmor frequency*, named after the Irish physicist and mathematician Sir Joseph Larmor (1857-1942), Lucasian Professor of Mathematics (Newton's Chair) at Cambridge.

By convention, B_o and the axis of precession are defined to be oriented along the z-direction of a Cartesian coordinate system. The motion of each proton can be described in Cartesian coordinates perpendicular (x, y) and parallel (z) to B_o. The transverse coordinates are nonzero and vary with time as the proton precesses, but the z-coordinate is constant with time. The frequency of precession is proportional to the magnetic field strength and is given by the so-called *Larmor equation*:

$$\omega_o = \frac{\gamma \cdot B_o}{2\pi}, \tag{10.2}$$

where, ω_o is the Larmor frequency in MHz, B_o is the magnetic field strength in Tesla (T), and γ, in $[s^{-1} \cdot T^{-1}]$, is a constant for each nucleus known as the *gyromagnetic ratio*. This equation describes the relationship between the frequency of energy that a proton absorbs and the magnetic field strength that it experiences. It shows that, in an MR experiment, a measurement of the frequency of precession of the magnetization gives information on the field experienced by that group of spins. It follows that, by manipulating the spatial variation of the field in a known way, this frequency information can yield spatial information on tissue topography. The strength of the magnetization is proportional to the *proton density* (PD) of the tissues, which depends on the number of hydrogen atoms in the tissues. Fluids have the highest PD (over 95%), but water- and fat-based tissues have very similar PDs (typically 60–85%), because both water and lipids contain many hydrogen atoms.

For a population of protons in a voxel, we consider the dynamics of the net magnetization, rather than the behavior of individual protons, and represent the net magnetization with the *magnetization vector*, **M**. We have seen in the preceding paragraphs that **M** will trace out the surface of a cone in an external magnetic field and that the Larmor equation gives the frequency of its precession. Consider now an RF coil that generates a weak magnetic field perpendicular to the strong, external magnetic field. If the RF energy being generated is of a frequency much above or below the Larmor frequency, **M** simply continues to precess about the vertical external field. But if the RF radiation happens to be in resonance with the Larmor frequency, it will cause the net magnetization to undergo *nutation*, as is illustrated in Figure 10.16.

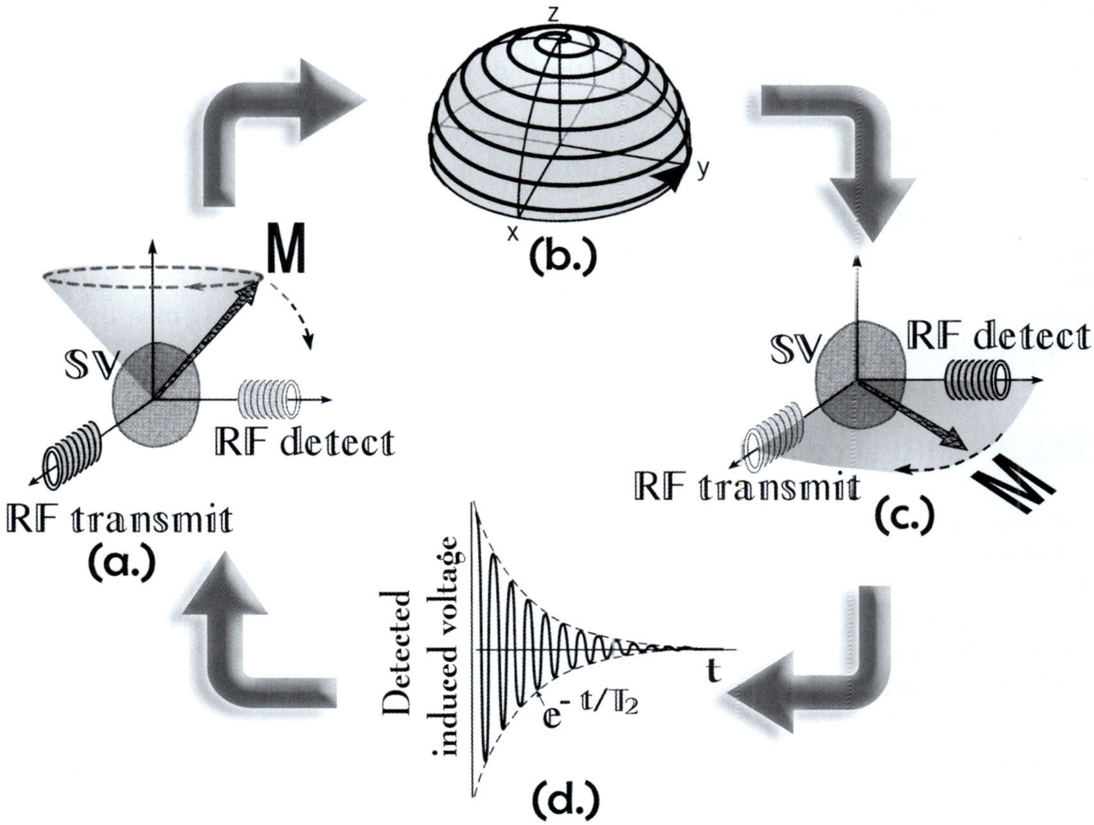

Figure 10.16: (a.) Application of a 90° pulse causes **M** for the sample volume (SV) to tip down into the transverse $x-y$ plane, (b.) along a spiral path. (c.) In the transverse plane **M** precesses at the Larmor frequency and, by Faraday's law, induces a signal voltage at this frequency in the RF coil; (d.) this so-called FID signal decays exponentially with time (t), at a rate corresponding to the relaxation time constant T_2—or, more precisely $T_2{}^*$. If the spins in a single voxel do not experience exactly the same magnetic field, then the coherence of their magnetizations will be reduced, an effect which increases with time. Field inhomogeneities erode the transverse magnetization in the same way that spin–spin relaxation does. The *combined* effects of spin–spin relaxation and an inhomogeneous field on the decay of the transverse magnetization signal is quantified by the time constant $T_2{}^*$—see also the discussion on pp. 516 f.

How can we detect that such nuclear magnetic resonance is actually occuring? The magnetization cannot be measured while it is lined up along z, which is why we use a pulse sequence. Suppose we drive Larmor frequency power into the RF coil, exactly long enough for the net magnetization **M** to nutate 90° through a spiral path from along the *vertical* z-direction down into the *transverse* $x-y$ plane, and then switch it off (see Fig. 10.16). Following application of this so-called *90° pulse*, **M** will be precessing at the

Larmor frequency in the transverse plane. Each time **M** sweeps by, the RF coil, now acting as an RF receiver antenna, will experience the rapidly changing magnetic field of **M**. This changing magnetic field cutting through the RF coil will *induce* a voltage in it, which is known as FID, or *free induction decay.*[13] So, the induction of the FID signal at the Larmor frequency in the RF coil following application of a 90° pulse reveals the magnetic resonance phenomenon, as is indicated pictorially in Figure 10.16.

In sum, excitation low-level RF microwave pulses cause some of the magnetic moments of the protons of body molecules in the scanner to oscillate and re-emit microwaves after each pulse. The RF signal is turned on and off; subsequently, the energy that is absorbed by different body atoms is echoed. These echoes are continuously measured and stored digitally.

10.2.3 MRI slice selection and signal localization

MRI uses the field dependence between the frequency of energy that a proton absorbs and the magnetic field strength that it experiences to localize these proton frequencies at different regions of space. The magnetic field is made to vary in space through the application of small gradients superimposed on the main field B_o—a typical imaging gradient introduces a total field variation of less than 1%. Three magnetic gradients are used, one in each of the x-, y-, and z-directions, and MRI is inherently 3-D, allowing resolution of voxels in 3-D space. This is called *spatial encoding*.

The scan plane selected establishes which of the three gradients performs slice selection during the excitation pulse (see Fig. 10.3, on p. 486). The z-gradient modulates the field strength and thus the nuclear precessional frequency along the z-axis of the magnet, and as a result it offers a means of distinguishing *axial* slices. The x-gradient alters the field strength and the precessional frequency along the x-axis of the magnet, and therefore selects *sagittal* slices. The y-gradient alters the field strength and the precessional frequency along the y-axis of the magnet, and thus it selects *coronal* slices. Oblique slices can be selected by using the two gradients *in combination*.

Imaging is usually carried out in 2-D planes, with typical in-plane voxel dimensions $\leq 1\,mm$, and a slice thickness of 1–2 mm, or more. Conceptually, spatial localization can be understood by considering spin distribution along one coordinate, e.g., x. Under a linear field gradient along the x-direction, all the spins which lie at a particular value of x will precess at the *same* frequency. The FID signal from such a sample will contain components from each of the sequential x-values represented by the sample, and the frequency spectrum will therefore represent the number of spins that lie along that plane, on either side of the particular value of x, as is shown schematically in Figure 10.17, on p. 511.

[13] Despite the diagrammatic representation in Figure 10.16, because the resonance frequency pertaining to the FID signal is of the order of 100 MHz, the individual oscillations are not in fact discernible in the oscilloscope tracing of a real FID from an MR scanner, but the exponentially decaying envelope is readily apparent.

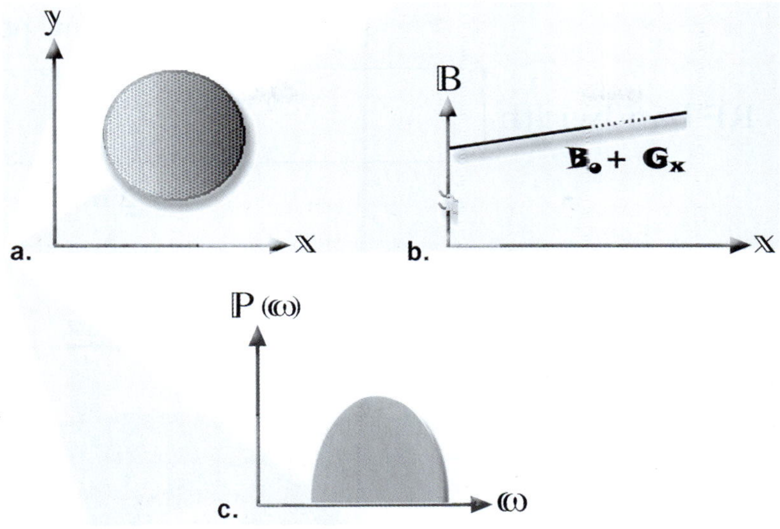

Figure 10.17: a. A cylindrical object aligned along the z-axis (perpendicular to the plane of the page). b. A linear magnetic field gradient applied along the x-axis, which causes spins in different sequential strips along the x-axis to precess at different frequencies. c. The apportionment of proton spins $P(\omega)$ as a function of frequency ω along the x-axis, which represents the 1-D NMR spectrum along the x-axis.

Gradient magnetic fields are small, linearly varying, fields applied collectively and sequentially in addition to the large static field B_o by three paired orthogonal current-carrying coils within the magnet. Their strength and direction change during the scan, allowing every voxel within the scanned volume to resonate at a different frequency. In this fashion, selective spatial excitation and encoding of the imaging volume can occur since the total magnetic field depends linearly on location inside the magnet. Each localizing gradient is assigned, through the scan control software, to one or more of the three functional gradients required to obtain an image: slice selection (G_{ss}), phase encoding (G_y), and frequency encoding, or "readout" (G_x).

Figure 10.18 illustrates the gradient-dependent slice selection process. Individual slices can be selectively excited by transmitting RF with a band of frequencies coinciding with the Larmor frequencies of spins in a particular slice as defined by the slice selection gradient, G_{ss}. Resonance of nuclei within the slice occurs because RF appropriate to that position is transmitted. On the other hand, nuclei positioned in other slices along the gradient do not resonate, because their precessional frequency is *different* due to the presence of the G_{ss} (see Fig. 10.18). The slice thickness is governed by the following equation:

$$T_s = \frac{BW_{\text{transm}}}{\gamma_0 \cdot \omega_0 \cdot G_{ss}}, \tag{10.3}$$

where, T_s is the slice thickness, BW_{transm} is the RF transmit bandwidth (the range of frequencies it covers), γ_0 is the gyromagnetic ratio, and G_{ss} is the magnitude of the

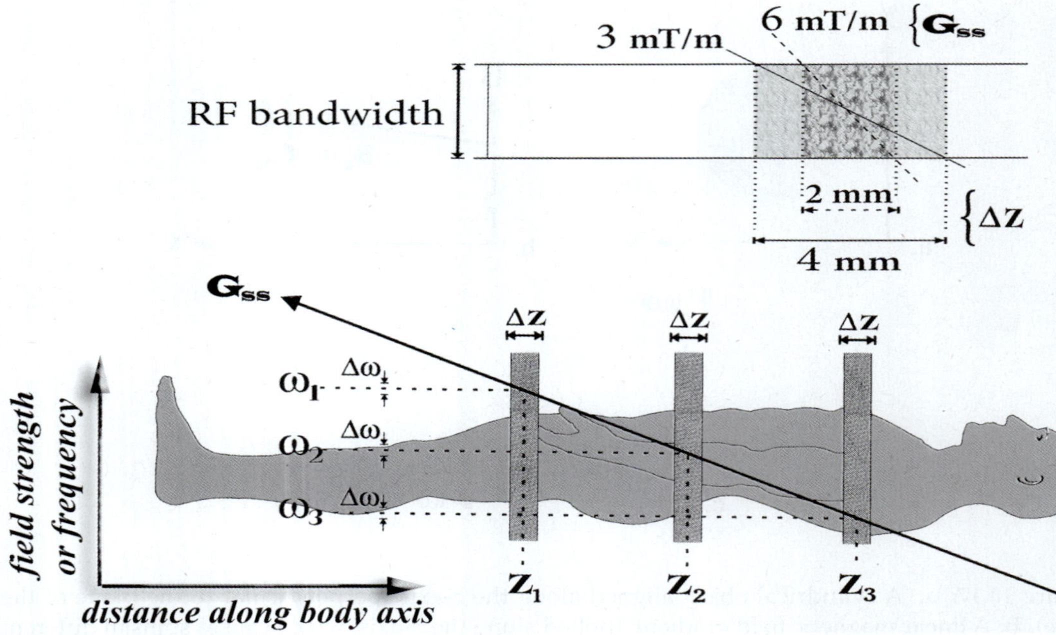

Figure 10.18: *Bottom*: In the presence of G_{ss}, the slice selection gradient, the total magnetic field experienced by a proton and its resulting resonant frequency depend on its position. Tissue located at position z_i will absorb RF energy broadcast with a unique center frequency ω_i. *Top*: Variation of slice thickness is brought about by increasing or decreasing the amplitude of G_{ss}, the slice selection gradient, as appropriate. The slice thickness Δz is determined by the amplitude of G_{ss}, and by the transmitted RF bandwidth. (Adapted and redrawn, slightly modified, from Brown and Semelka [7], with kind permission of the authors and John Wiley & Sons, Inc.)

slice selection magnetic field gradient. To achieve thin slices, a steep G_{ss} slope and/or narrow RF transmit bandwidth is applied, and for thick slices, a shallow slice selection gradient slope and/or broad RF bandwidth. The scan control software of the MRI system automatically applies the appropriate G_{ss} slope and RF transmit bandwidth according to the required slice thickness.

Gradients are also used to apply excitation and, in some fast imaging techniques, reversal pulses. Gradients are applied for short periods of time during a scan and are labeled *gradient pulses*. Protons are effectively fiddled with—energized by RF pulses and tuned and retuned by magnetic field gradients. The specific pairing of physical and functional gradients depends, *inter alia*, on the acquisition parameters and patient placement. The assemblage of RF pulses, gradient pulses, data sampling periods, and relative timing among them during an image acquisition is identified as an MRI *pulse sequence*. Pulse sequences are the basis of tissue-specific contrast generation in MRI. A very simplified pulse sequence is a combination of RF pulses, signals, and intervening periods of recovery, as is exemplified in Figure 10.19, on p. 513.

10.2.4 Slice selection, phase and frequency encoding in MRI sequences

The timing diagrams of MRI pulse sequences [4] comprise slice selection, phase encoding and frequency encoding modules. Each module occurs at a specific time during the sequence, and employs gradients along a particular coordinate axis. There are no restrictions as to which gradient axis is used for which of the three encoding modules; this allows ample leeway in defining the direction from which the image is viewed. Images in the usual tomographic planes, namely, transverse, coronal, sagittal or oblique, are simply obtained by making the appropriate axis designation for the various gradient pulses.

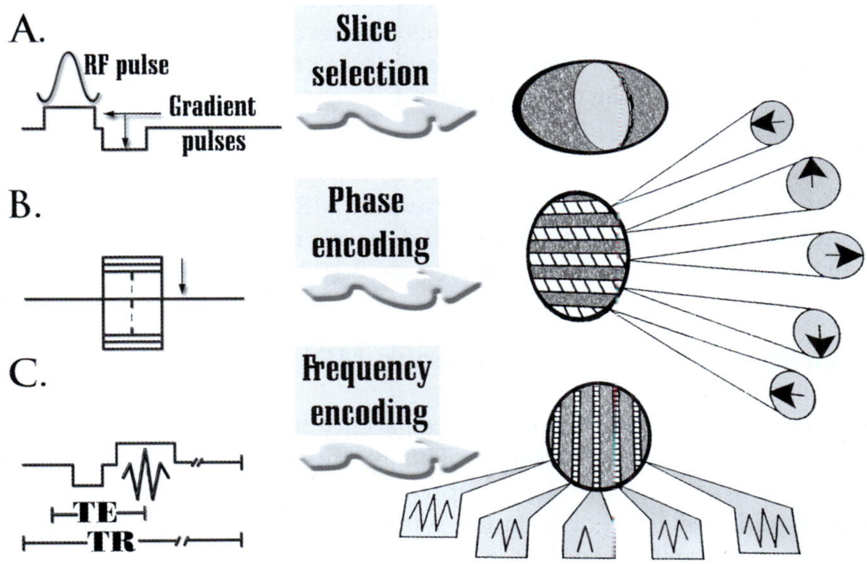

Figure 10.19: Magnetic field gradient pulses of slice selection, phase encoding, and frequency encoding modules, are shown on the left. The exploitation of each module for selecting and coding an axial slice through an oval-shaped, illustrative organ is displayed on the right.

The slice selection module involves applying the G_{ss} gradient simultaneously with the RF pulses, designed to excite the nuclear signal in only a narrow RF band. The selective excitation of an axial slice through an illustrative oval-shaped "organ" is shown in Figure 10.19A. In the 2-D Fourier imaging formalism which is outlined in Section 10.2.8, on pp. 523 ff., the 2-D spatial distribution of the tissue protons, $P(x, y)$, is mapped by rendering their precession frequencies spatially dependent. The phase-encoding and frequency-encoding modules, illustrated in panels B and C of Figure 10.19, are used to sample the spins in the two directions orthogonal to the direction of slice selection. Acting together, they partition the chosen slice into a *grid of pixels*, so that a 2-D image of the selected slice can be acquired.

The phase-encoding gradient pulse, G_y, makes the phase of the transverse magnetization different in each of the rows shown on the right side of panel B of Figure 10.19.

Magnetization from tissues within each *row* has the same phase. Frequency encoding is based on sampling the transverse plane magnetization in the presence of the gradient G_x. This gradient gives transverse magnetization a frequency that depends on the *column* in which it is located. The precession frequency is identical within any single column. The MR echo forms at time TE, the *echo time*. TE is the time, measured in ms, from the application of the RF pulse to the peak of the signal induced in the coil. It determines how much decay of transverse magnetization is allowed to occur. The TE thus controls the amount of T_2 relaxation that has occurred when the signal is read.

The *repetition time*, TR, also measured in ms, is the time from the application of one RF pulse to the application of the next RF pulse for each slice. Consequently, it determines the amount of relaxation that is allowed to occur between the end of one RF pulse and the application of the next. The TR determines, in effect, the amount of T_1 relaxation that has occurred when the signal is read. After a time TR, the three procedures are repeated in the same way, except that the G_y assumes a different amplitude.

The MR image is displayed on a 2-D device such as a video screen, with the x- and y-coordinates of the various pixels representing topographic detail within the scanned region, and the brightness at each pixel representing MR signal intensity.[14] The intensities are usually stored as 32-bit words with a 16-bit dynamic range, and are displayed on either a 16-bit or an 8-bit gray-scale monitor (see Section 2.16.1, on pp. 71 f.).

10.2.5 Gradient echo and spin echo MRI sequences

MRI possesses excellent *contrast resolution*, i.e., ability to discern differences between arbitrarily similar but not identical tissues. This requires a wide collection of MRI pulse sequences, each of which is optimized to provide image contrast based on a particular MR property of body tissues. For instance, with certain values of the echo time, TE, and the repetition time, TR, an MRI sequence will take on the property of T_2 weighting, which will render water and fluid-containing tissues bright. The typical MRI examination may encompass a number of different sequences, each of which can provide a particular type of information about the subject tissues. There is, in fact, a very broad variety of MRI pulse sequences that generate diverse types of images. Their appearance may reveal not merely tissue density, as does x-ray CT, but also functional aspects pertaining to bulk blood flow phenomena in cardiac chambers and large vessels, microcirculatory perfusion, and so on.

Mastery of the range of MRI techniques is beyond our present purposes, but can provide the MRI "artist" with a broad palette of physiological sensitivities, to exploit or reject as the image is formed. Different imaging sequences may be also used to encode velocities of flow in different directions. This is another physiologically important aspect of the versatility of MRI, that it can provide visualization of 3-D velocity vector components in *complex* flow fields (cf. Fig. 9.13, on p. 468), such as those of cardiovascular organs.

[14] The "dynamic range" of an image quantifies the contrast between its brightest and darkest parts. A plate of evenly-lit mashed potatoes is low-dynamic range; the interior of an ornate cathedral with light streaming in through stained-glass windows is high dynamic range.

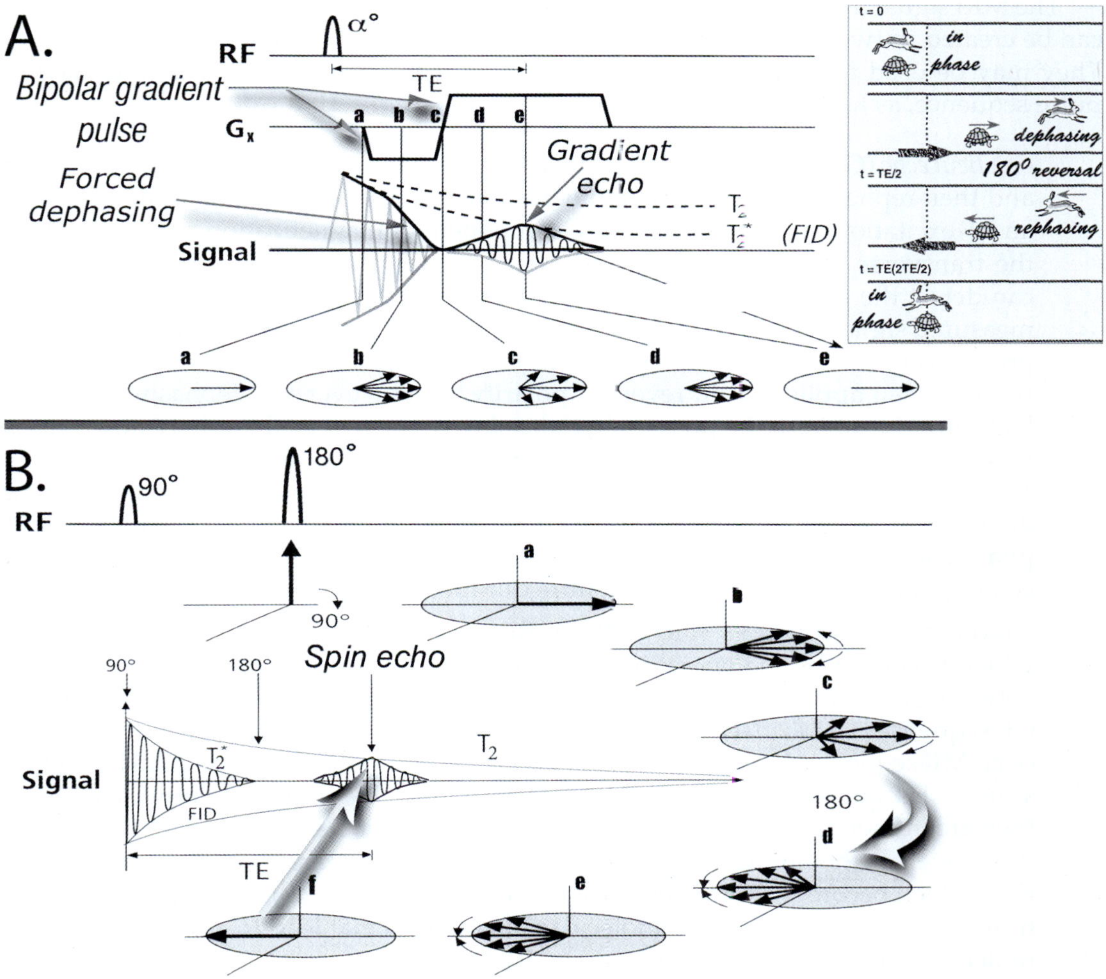

Figure 10.20: A. *Gradient echo* imaging. Following an RF excitation pulse, the transverse component of magnetization precesses about the transverse plane with phase coherence. Thereafter, the signal decays as the magnetic moments start to dephase. A gradient (G_x) is applied during this process to force an *accelerated* dephasing—gradients always cause dephasing. A second gradient pulse with reversed polarity is then applied. It causes slower precessing protons to precess faster, and *vice versa*, bringing the magnetic moments back in phase (cf. analogous situation in inset). The interval between the peak of the RF pulse and the point of maximal signal is the echo time (TE). The MR signals generated with gradient echo imaging are $T_2{}^*$-weighted: the echo amplitude is governed by $T_2{}^*$ decay (FID). B. *Spin echo* imaging. With a *90°* RF pulse, longitudinal magnetization tips into the transverse plane. Subsequently, slight differences in precessional frequencies bring about a phase shift between protons. A *180°* refocusing RF pulse then flips the slower protons *ahead* of the faster protons. When the faster protons *catch up* with the slower protons, there is spin phase coherence and a spin echo is produced; from then on, phase shift reaccumulates.

The MRI signal from the patient is collected by the scanning antenna as an echo; echoes can be created in two distinct ways, as is depicted pictorially in Figure 10.20, on p. 515. They may be used to best advantage individually or in combination, in any particular pulse sequence, as follows:

1. *Gradient echo* (GE) imaging (see Fig. 10.20A., on p. 515) relies on controlled dephasing and then rephasing of magnetic moments [56, 84, 156]. As we have seen, following an RF excitation pulse, the transverse component of magnetization precesses about the transverse plane with phase coherence. Once the RF pulse ends, an RF coil can detect the signal. However, the magnetic moments begin to dephase, and the measured signal decays. With gradient echo imaging, a gradient applied during this process causes *accelerated* dephasing. To generate a gradient echo, a second gradient pulse is then applied, with reversed polarity.[15] Wherever the dephasing gradient had caused protons to be precessing more slowly, the reversed gradient now causes them to precess faster, whereas those that had been faster will now be slower. As a result, the rephasing gradient reverses the dephasing caused by the preceding dephasing gradient and brings the magnetic moments back in phase. At maximum phase coherence, the peak of the gradient echo is produced. Typically, the gradient echo signal is acquired during the entire duration of the reversed gradient.

   Gradient echo sequences start with an RF pulse producing a flip angle α ($<90°$), which is chosen by the operator.[16] As for SE sequences *(vide infra)*, TR is the time between successive $\alpha°$ RF pulses, and TE is the time from the $\alpha°$ pulse to the echo. GE sequences use *shorter* TR and TE than SE sequences and, since the total scan time of an MR sequence depends on TR, they can be acquired much more quickly than SE scans. GE sequences can also produce images with T_1, T_2, or PD weighting. However, they are influenced by the quality of the main magnetic field (called the *inhomogeneity*) as well as the timing parameters. This affects the apparent spin–spin relaxation time which becomes shorter, because two distinct factors contribute to the decay of transverse magnetization: a.) molecular interactions that lead to a so-called *pure* T_2 molecular effect; and b.) variations in B_o that lead to an *inhomogeneous* T_2 effect. The combination of these two factors is what actually results in the observed decay of the transverse magnetization. The overall time constant is denoted $T_2{}^*$, enunciated "T2 star" and is always shorter than T_2. With modern high-quality magnets, GE T_2-weighted images have very similar contrast to SE T_2-weighted images.

2. *Spin echo* (SE) [56,84,156] is the most common sequence used in MRI [see Fig. 10.20B.], and starts with an RF excitation pulse with a 90° flip angle. Following this RF pulse, dephasing occurs and the transverse magnetization decays rapidly, governed by the $T_2{}^*$ relaxation time (FID). To make a spin echo, a 180° refocusing RF pulse is applied after the 90° pulse. How does the 180° refocusing pulse reverse the dephasing? Dephasing occurs because of B_0 heterogeneity and intrinsic T_2 decay. The B_0 heterogeneity means that some protons are exposed to slightly stronger local magnetic

[15] By convention, these gradient pulses are applied in the x-direction.

[16] This angle $\alpha°$ is the angle to which the net magnetization is rotated by the RF excitation pulse relative to the main magnetic field direction. It is also denoted *tip angle*, or angle of *nutation*.

fields and therefore, according to the Larmor equation, precess slightly *faster*, while others are exposed to slightly weaker fields and therefore precess slightly *slower*. The 180° RF pulse flips the magnetic moments within the transverse plane, so that the relationship of the protons is reversed. The faster protons are *transposed* behind the slower protons. Over time, the fast protons catch up and, with this rephasing, net transverse magnetization grows to form a measurable echo of the original FID and a spin echo is formed. The spin echo decays once again in step with the ensuing dephasing of the protons. TE is the time between the 90° RF pulse and the *peak* of the echo. Because the time taken to rephase protons equals the time to dephase, the 180° pulse takes place at time TE/2. This implies that we can effectively control exactly when the spin echo arises, by applying the 180° RF pulse at one-half the desired time interval after the 90° pulse.

SE imaging has limited temporal resolution. Shorter acquisition times are attained with Fast, or *Turbo*, Spin Echo (FSE) pulse protocols . Numerous modifications to the basic FSE sequence have also been made, including the application of one or more inversion pulses, increased echo train length, half-Fourier reconstruction, and echo-planar imaging (EPI) techniques [25].

10.2.6 Sources of contrast between tissues in MR images

By introducing magnetic field gradients, the spatial location of a re-emitted microwave can be determined. An image representing various characteristics about the molecular emissions at *discrete samples* throughout the scanned object is then reconstructed. The contrast in an MR image is strongly dependent upon the way the image is acquired. By modifying the frequency and timing characteristics of the excitation pulse, and the delay time before measurement of the emitted energy, it is possible to image particular types of molecules, motion (blood flow), and many other characteristics. The degree to which nuclear magnetic resonance interactions at tissue level can be controlled and manipulated by external magnetic gradients and imaging parameter selection is, in fact, *unique* with magnetic resonance compared with all other imaging techniques.

Contrast is due to differences in the acquired MR signal, which depend on magnetic properties of the tissues and on sequence parameters. The basis of contrast is the proton spin density in the contiguous tissues. If there are no spins present in a region, it becomes impossible to get an MR signal. Proton spin densities depend on water content.[17] Because there are only small differences in proton spin density between most soft tissues, other suitable contrast mechanisms must be employed. These are based on the variation in the values of T_1 and T_2 for the different tissues of the body. Differently timed imaging sequences, consisting of RF pulses, readout, and magnetic gradient switches, result in *different contrast* between tissues. The preceding distinctive properties of different tissues provide two principal ways to create MR signal contrast in MRI scan slices in cardiovascular applications. By controlling some characteristics of the pulse sequence parameters,

[17] The low water content, and the concomitant low proton spin density, of bone makes MRI less suitable for skeletal imaging than x-rays.

TE	TR	Image Weighting
Short	Long	Proton
Short	Short	T_1
Long	Long	T_2 (T_2^*)

Figure 10.21: Different MRI tissue parameter weighting depends on the timing characteristics of the time of repetition (TR) and the time to echo (TE).

e.g., the timings of the RF excitation pulses and the MR signal *readout* from the tissues, we can make the contrast depend mostly on just one of them. Images whose contrast depends mainly on T_1 are called T_1-weighted images, or just T_1 images. Similarly, T_2-weighted images, or T_2 images, have contrast that depends mainly on T_2.[18]

In the descriptions that follow it is assumed that the particular MRI method used is the so-called spin echo (SE) imaging (see Section 10.2.5, on pp. 514 ff.); however, similar methods can be used with the other MR imaging techniques. When a scanning sequence starts, an initial RF pulse forces ("excites," "tips," or "flips") the magnetization out of its vertical alignment and into the $x-y$, or *transverse* plane. This creates a signal, at the same frequency as the initial RF pulse, which fades away, just as the sound from a tuning fork dies down after being struck. This signal can be manipulated by subsequent gradient and RF pulses in the sequence.

Depending on the choice of characteristic MRI sequence parameters, TR and TE, SE can produce T_1, T_2, or PD-weighted images with different contrast characteristics between tissues, as is demonstrated pictorially in the panels of Figure 10.22, on p. 519. As we discussed on p. 514, TR is the *repetition time* or the time between successive 90° excitation RF pulses, and TE is the time from the 90° pulse to *"readout"* of the echo, or collection of the MR signal from the tissues.

TR and TE are operator-selectable parameters on the MRI scanner. By adjusting them appropriately, contrast differences in an MRI image due to T_1 and/or T_2 *disparities* among adjacent tissues can be manipulated to advantage, as is shown in Figure 10.22. For instance, by reinforcing differences in signal intensity coming into view as a result of differences in the T_1 of tissues, a shorter TR achieves T_1-*weighting* (cf. the tabulation in Fig. 10.21). To maximize contrast between two tissues, the TR should have an *intermediate* value between their T_1s. On the other hand, to minimize T_1 differences across tissues, long TR sequences are used—typically about 1,500–2,000 ms. Because, a long TR implies a longer acquisition time, typically TR does not go beyond 2,000 ms.

To minimize the effect of T_2 differences while maximizing the amount of signal, short TE times, generally less than 50 ms, are used (see Panel I. of Fig. 10.22). In an analogous

[18]Images where the contrast depends mainly on PD are identified as PD-weighted images, or just PD images.

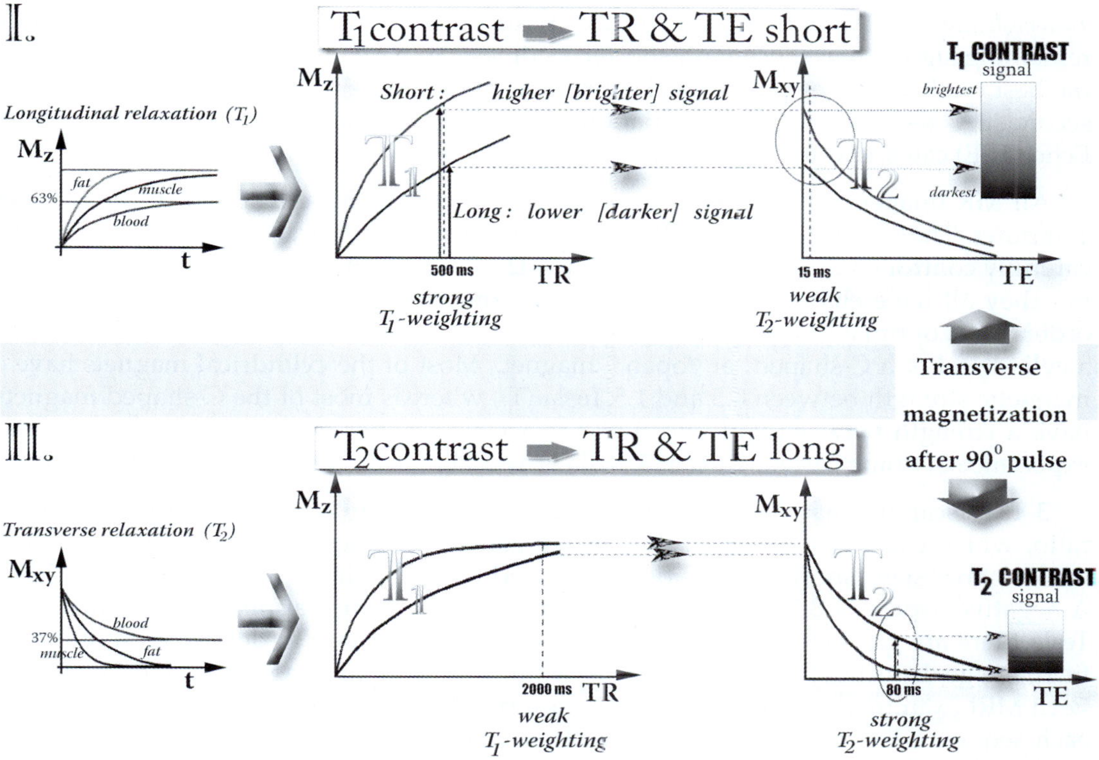

Figure 10.22: *Left insets*: T_1 and T_2 are magnetic timing parameters (measured in ms) which differ among different tissues. T_1 is a relaxation time constant that describes the recovery of the M_z (longitudinal) component and T_2 is a relaxation constant that describes the decay of the M_{xy} (transverse) component of the net magnetization vector, **M**. M_{xy} decays away faster than the regrowth of M_z: $T_2 < T_1$; typically, $T_1 \approx 5 \cdot T_2$. They can be used as a source of *contrast* between tissues in MRI images, by applying T_1- and T_2-weighting, as is displayed pictorially in the main panels. *Panel* I. The lopsided recovery of longitudinal magnetization between RF pulses separated by short RTs determines the amount of image contrast in T_1-weighting. *Panel* II. The disparate T_2 values cause lopsided decay of transverse magnetization measured with long TEs. Longer TEs are needed for T_2-weighting and image contrast.

way, optimal T_2 contrast occurs at a TE that is *intermediate* between the T_2 times of the tissues of interest. A very short TE will cause minimal image contrast, because transverse magnetization will not have decayed substantially enough to reveal signal differences between the tissues. A very long TE will make for a marginal signal, because magnetization and signal amplitude from all the tissues will have decayed a great deal. Selection of an appropriate TE depends on the T_2 times of the tissues to be imaged.

Because most tissues have T_2 times between 20 and 250 ms, T_2-weighted sequences have TE times of at least 80–100 ms—generally denoted as "long TEs." Using a longer TE, i.e., allowing a longer time interval to elapse before measuring the signal, achieves

T_2-weighting (see Panel II. of Fig. 10.22). Tissues with longer T_2 times then have more remaining signal than those with shorter T_2 times. Spin Echo images generally produce the best quality images but they take a relatively long time, several *minutes* rather than seconds. As we saw on p. 517, a variation of SE, called Fast Spin Echo (FSE) or Turbo Spin Echo (TSE) can speed up image acquisition.

All MR images are formed using a pulse sequence, which is stored in the scanner computer. The sequence contains RF pulses and magnetization gradient pulses which have carefully controlled durations and timings.[19] There are many different types of sequence, but they all have characteristic timing values and intervals, which can be modified in order to get optimal image contrast. The main component of most MRI systems is either a cylindrical or a C-shaped, or "open," magnet. Most of the cylindrical magnets have a magnetic strength between 0.5 and 1.5 Tesla (T), whereas most of the C-shaped magnets have a strength between 0.01 and 0.35 T.[20] 3-Tesla scanners are a recent advance, and experience in doing cardiac MRI at 3-Tesla is available in the literature [84,97].

3-Tesla scanning has a number of benefits, accrueing from an enhanced signal-to-noise ratio, which can translate into better image contrast, higher spatial resolution (with a *reduced* voxel size), shorter acquisition times, and various judicious combinations of these. A negative aspect of 3-Tesla imaging, particularly for cardiac applications, is that at 3-Tesla there are greater susceptibility artifacts, which can result in deformation of the B_0 field, image distortion, and signal loss or "void," in the rapid imaging modalities [52,97]. Each MRI examination usually comprises a series of two to six imaging sequences, with each sequence lasting 2–15 min. An MRI sequence, during which the patient must lie completely still, is an acquisition of data that yields a specific image orientation and a specific type of image.

The simplest RF pulse to examine is the so-called *90° pulse,* which is called so because it pushes the magnetization from a longitudinal (z) orientation exactly by *90°* into the transverse $x-y$ plane. After the 90° RF pulse, the magnetization reverts back to its equilibrium position along z via two *relaxation processes*, called *spin–lattice* and *spin–spin* relaxation:

1. Spin-lattice relaxation controls the recovery of the magnetization along z and has a characteristic time constant called the spin-lattice relaxation time, T_1. T_1s are different for the various tissues: fluids have long T_1s (e.g., 1500–2000 ms), water-based tissues are usually mid-range (e.g., 400–1200 ms), and fatty tissues generally have short T_1s (e.g., 100–150 ms).

2. Spin-spin relaxation controls the decay of the signal in the transverse plane; its characteristic time constant is identified as the spin–spin relaxation time, T_2, and is illustrated in Figure 10.16(d.) on p. 509. Fluids have the longest T_2 (700–1200 ms), while water-based tissues usually tend to have longer T_2s than fatty tissues (40–200 ms

[19] The gradient pulses make the characteristic "knocking" noise when the imager is acquiring a scan.
[20] A Tesla is equivalent to 10,000 Gauss. The earth's magnetic field is roughly 0.00005 T, so that a 1.5 T scanner has a static field that is approximately 30,000 times stronger than the earth's magnetic field.

and 10–100 ms, respectively). The two relaxation processes are independent of each other, and T_2s are always shorter than T_1s in tissues.

10.2.7 Contrast techniques for high resolution anatomical cardiovascular images

Although high spatial and temporal resolutions are desirable in cardiovascular imaging, high contrast resolution is also essential. The key contrast is between the blood and the cardiac and vessel walls that contain it. MRI techniques achieve contrast differentiation between the bounding walls and blood by employing two generic methods, black blood (dark blood/bright background tissue) and white blood (bright blood/dark background tissue) imaging [37]. MRA uses these methods to differentiate flowing blood from surrounding stationary or relatively slow-moving structures, and to generate images (angiograms) depicting vasculature based on flow phenomena

MRA methods manipulate variables in RF pulse patterns, including timing and rates of change, to generate signals from flowing blood, while signals from stationary tissue are subtracted, or suppressed, in a manner analogous to that used with conventional digital subtraction angiography [24]. In effect, MRA angiograms are physiologic studies in which moving blood, as the contrast agent, is displayed as high-signal intensity [69]. The nature of the magnetic resonance signal from flowing blood is complex and partially depends on the spin density and relaxation properties of the blood, plus the dynamics of blood flow, and the axial thickness of the imaged section. Signal intensity is determined by their combined effects.

With *white blood* imaging, the aim is to make the blood pool bright and the surrounding stationary tissues relatively dark. White blood imaging, typically gradient echo based, generates high signal intensity for blood and, because multiple consecutive images are acquired that can be viewed dynamically to depict cardiac motion, it can be used for cine-MRI images of a small number of slices in each breath-hold. Therefore, bright blood acquisitions allow both morphological and functional geometric assessment of time-dependent cardiac chamber anatomy. 4-D images with white blood are becoming available to provide approximately isotropic resolution. These sequences usually have inferior temporal resolution and contrast to 2-D dynamic sequences.

With *black blood* imaging, the aim is to *eliminate* signal from the blood pool. Since the lumen is then black and the walls are bright, black blood imaging allows for excellent imaging of the walls. A limitation of black blood techniques is the lengthy acquisition time required by the protocol, so that black blood imaging is essentially a single slice sequence for each breath-hold. As changes in scanner hardware and software are made, and as new information on optimal imaging parameters becomes available, new protocol sequences for multislice black blood imaging are being developed to address this [68,77]. Methods for reducing the acquisition time are desirable, not only because they use precious scanner time more efficiently, but also because subject discomfort is reduced.

MR black blood imaging protocols for cardiovascular imaging improve segmentation of the bounding walls from blood. Black blood techniques, usually spin echo based, are

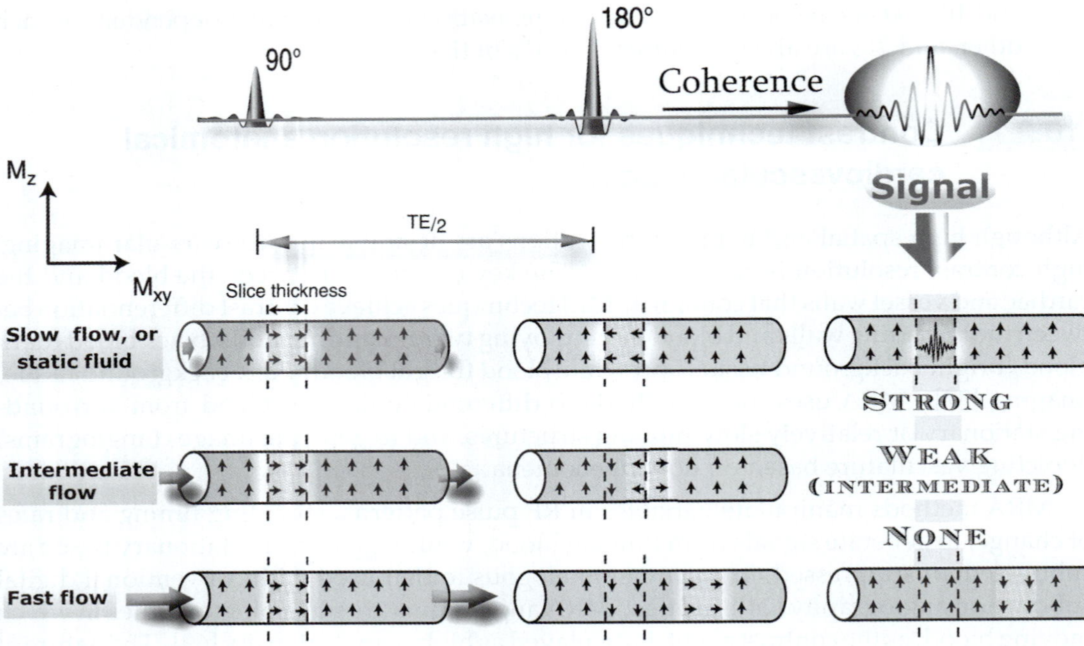

Figure 10.23: Effect of flow on spin echo formation. Small arrows within the vessels indicate the net orientation of proton spins in the flowing blood. Only protons that are tilted into the transverse plane by the 90°pulse and then are refocused within the transverse plane by the 180°pulse can turn out an echo.

characterized by the suppression of the signal from flowing blood. This gives a good visualization of the myocardium, which is of great interest for *CFD modeling* of intracardiac blood flow based on patient-specific dynamic geometry and boundary conditions.They decrease the signal from blood with reference to the walls and, by enhancing the contrast of the *demarcation* between blood and endocardium, they facilitate cardiac chamber segmentation.

The loss of signal in moving blood on spin echo imaging occurs because to generate a spin echo, protons must receive *both* the 90° and 180° pulses, both of which are slice selective. Blood which transits rapidly through the slice of interest in the time interval between the two RF pulses, will not experience both of the RF pulses and for that reason it will not generate any signal (see Fig. 10.23). Whether a complete signal void is produced by flowing blood depends on the applying velocity, the slice thickness, and the time between the 90° and 180° pulses, or TE/2.

Conditions favorable for producing a signal void are, obviously, thinner slices and longer TE. Slice orientation should be perpendicular to flow direction; if images are acquired in the flow plane, then despite rapid flow some protons may still experience both the 90° and the 180° pulses, and complex patterns of signal intensity may ensue.

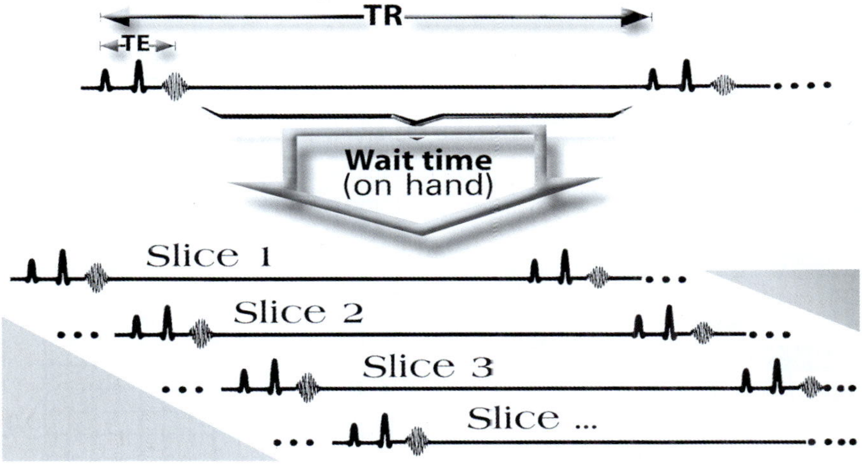

Figure 10.24: MRI multislice acquisition is feasible because of the *wait times* intervening between echo formation and the next repetition of the RF sequence. (Adapted and redrawn, slightly modified, from [27] with kind permission of the authors and the Mosby Co., a division of Elsevier.)

10.2.8 MRI raw data acquisition methods and *k*-space

The magnetic field at each position of any given MRI slice is varied in such a way that, over the course of the entire scan, each unique location in the slice experiences a *unique* combination of magnetic field variations. This leads to an unambiguous encoding of the MR signals, since tissues are encoded by the magnetic gradients to send out signals with phases and frequencies that are a unique function of position. These MRI signals can be represented as functions of spatial frequency, or of space. Essentially then, acquisition of an MRI image entails first sampling the spatial frequency content of the image directly, and then performing an inverse Fourier transform to reconstruct the image. The Fourier transform is a lossless transformation, and thus the representations in each domain—spatial frequency, or space—have the *same* information content. It is the formal representation of that content that differs between the two domains (cf. the equivalence of *frequency* and *time* domain representations depicted pictorially in Fig. 2.29, on p. 84).

Clearly, there are many different ways to acquire MRI data. The requirement is simply that enough of spatial frequency space, or *k–space,* be sampled to allow an image to be reconstructed. A common way to sample k–space is with a rectilinear raster scan. This is known as a 2-DFT acquisition, because the 2-D Fourier transform of the image is directly acquired. Image reconstruction is performed with a simple 2-D fast Fourier transform. This method is also known by the colorful name "spin-warp" [150]. In 2-DFT imaging, each slice is individually excited and its MR signal separately recorded and stored. Multislice acquisition is possible because of the "wait times" within the structure of the majority of MR imaging sequences. As is shown in Figure 10.24, this interlude between echo

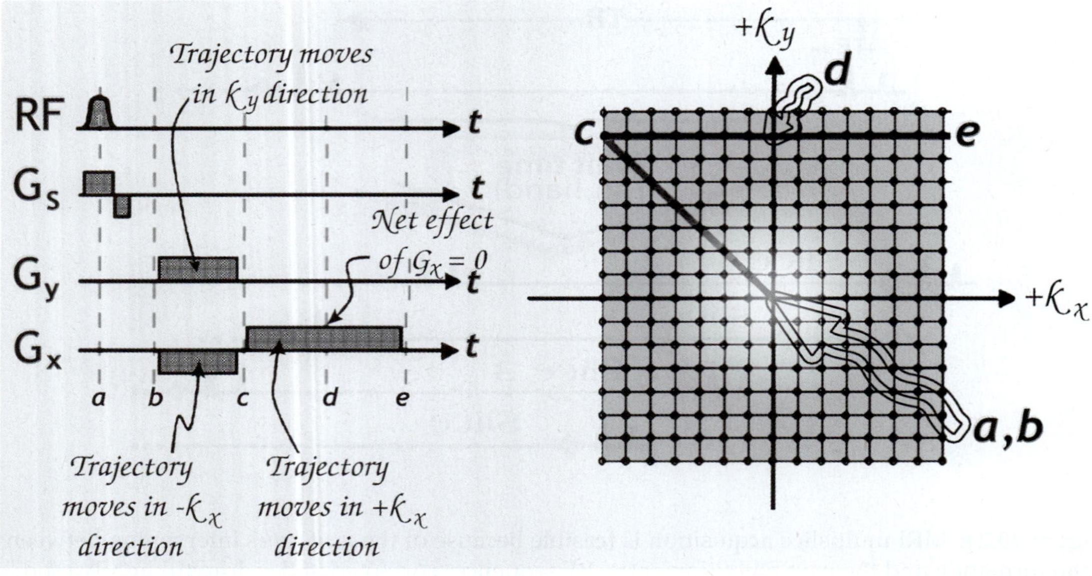

Figure 10.25: Gradient echo pulse sequence and corresponding k-space trajectory. The slice-select gradient, G_S, is assumed to be along the z-direction, and is followed by a *phase-rewind* pulse, of opposite sign as G_S and appropriate duration to cancel the phase across the slice profile, as is necessary in order to reset the stage for slice selection in the next pulse sequence. G_x and G_y gradient events, along the x- and y-directions, respectively, lead to changes in k-space coordinates, according to the time integral of the applied gradient(s). Letters (a, b,...,e) indicate data collection times in one repetition of the pulse sequence; it is customary to designate as time reference the center of the initial RF pulse that creates transverse magnetization. Note the correspondence between the pulse sequence events (left panel) and the k-space trajectory (right panel).

collection and the next 90° pulse can be put to good use by stimulating and obtaining MR signals from other slices during its passage.

MRI acquisition methods are most often described by pulse sequence diagrams, which show the timing and amplitudes of the application of the gradient fields along different coordinate axes, as well as the timing of the RF pulses. A summary representation for a 2-D Fourier transform pulse sequence is shown in Figure 10.25. Two basic elements of the pulse sequence are identified by interrupted lines. The first is the slice-selective excitation, G_S, which prepares the magnetization in a slice for imaging. The second element are the magnetic field gradients, G_x and G_y, for the 2-D Fourier transform acquisition. The k-space position is the integral of the gradient waveforms. This means, quite simply, that the net strength and duration of the gradient events determine how far and in what direction from the origin of k-space ($k_x = 0, k_y = 0$) a data point belongs.

The 2-D Fourier transform acquisition consists of two stages. First, gradient lobes move the k-space position to the beginning of one of the raster lines. A fixed area negative x-gradient lobe, called a dephaser, moves the k_x position to the same initial value for each line. A variable area y-gradient lobe, called the phase-encode, moves the k_y

position to a specific line in k-space. Then a constant gradient is applied to the x-gradient to scan along this line in k-space, while the raw MRI data is acquired. This is repeated typically 128 or 256 times, until enough data has been acquired to reconstruct an image. The number of points collected along any axis in k-space is always a power of 2 (e.g., 64, 128, or 256), because the MRI computers use the fast Fourier transform, or FFT, that requires $2N$ points to perform the reconstruction (see Section 2.20.3, on pp. 94 f.). The FFT can only process a sampled waveform where the number, N, of sampled data points is a power of 2. If the number of data points does not meet the power of 2 requirement, one may interpolate the dataset to satisfy this requirement.

It is important to note that MRI does not map spatial data linearly with respect to time. The gradients of an MR scanner make tissues at different locations resonate at different frequencies, giving off a time signal measured by the *receive* coil that might look like the graph in panel d. of Figure 10.16, on p. 509. The computer then performs the FT to reveal an image of the relative signal strength of each tissue location, analogous to the elementary data graphs in Figure 2.33, on p. 90 of Section 2.18 of Chapter 2.

Because k-space itself maps spatial frequencies rather than spatial data, the k–space data do *not* directly correspond to image space. Instead, different parts of k–space data determine different image *features*. For example, the central region (see "illuminated" round area in the right panel of Fig. 10.25, on p. 524) of k-space, or "low" spatial frequencies, dominate image *contrast*, whereas the periphery of k-space, or "high" spatial frequencies, contribute more to fine details, such as edges. Most image information, including contrast and general shape, is contained in the low spatial-frequency data mapped to the center of k-space. The farther data collection extends from the origin of k-space, the better the spatial resolution of our image. Thus, adding the high-spatial-frequency and progressively more peripheral data in the k-space improves the spatial resolution of the image, but does not modify contrast or the general shapes in the image (see Fig. 10.26, on p. 527). This has important implications regarding image contrast and effective echo times.

The coordinates of k-space are spatial frequencies with units of reciprocal distance, such as mm^{-1}. Spatial frequency (see Section 2.18, on pp. 82 ff.) describes the rate at which image features change as a function of position. Low-amplitude and/or short-duration gradient events encode low spatial-frequency information. Conversely, high-amplitude and/or long-duration gradient events encode high spatial-frequency information; this information is mapped to the periphery of k-space. Edges, such as the endothelial border of a blood vessel or the endocardial lining of a cardiac chamber, are represented by high spatial frequencies. Usually, phase encoding is performed "sequentially" such that central k-space is acquired at the mid-point of the scan. Alternative ways to perform phase encoding in k-space have various advantages and disadvantages. With 3-D MR imaging, the entire 3-D *Fourier* or *k-space* dataset is collected before individual slices are reconstructed.

The action of the magnetic field gradients causes a continuous change of the k_x and k_y coordinates, but the MR signal is sampled at discrete instants of time for digital computer processing. Given that unambiguous encoding of tissue signals requires changes in the magnetic field at each spatial position over the course of the entire scan, to successfully capture these unique combinations of field variations, the MR signal must be digitized at appropriately high spatial sampling rates. Otherwise, encoding is ambiguous and *aliasing* results in the image. The lowest sampling frequency is defined by the Nyquist criterion (see Section 2.17.2, on pp. 79 ff.). The Nyquist theory states that to fully represent the rate of brightness change or details in an original image we must sample it at a rate at least twice as high as the highest spatial frequency of the spatial feature details. In practice, deviations from this theorem may be necessary because of hardware limitations. Most computer video capture (frame grabber) hardware provides for 512×512 or 640×480 spatial resolution. The two numbers define the size of the monitor image matrix, namely, the number of pixels and the number of lines contained in the digital image, as vertical columns and horizontal rows.

Motion presents major challenges in MRI. To avoid blurring, k-space must be filled with little or no difference in the position of every tissue sample in the slice when each data point is acquired. One way to achieve this is to attempt to acquire the entire dataset in a time that is very short relative to the motion, e.g., by developing ultra fast gradient echo scans. Another option is to eliminate the motion, through breath-holding. Finally, data acquisition can be synchronized with cyclic motions such as cardiac contraction or respiration. This is the basis of cardiovascular cine-MRI.

Through prospective or retrospective gating, data are only written to any given k–space array when the heart returns to the same position within the cycle. The time window over which data for one image are collected within one cardiac cycle is kept narrow enough that, effectively, "no motion" occurs. To reduce total scan time, so-called *segmented scans* acquire a segment (i.e., several lines) of k-space using multiple excitations within one motion cycle. Variations in the *pattern* of k-space filling can increase imaging speed; some techniques apply more frequent updates of the central (i.e., lower spatial-frequency) lines of k-space while sharing the peripheral (i.e., higher frequency) lines of k-space.

10.2.9 Cardiac (ECG) triggering

MRI scanners were originally designed for use on the central nervous system, which is relatively free of motion. Thus, image acquisition times of several minutes duration were appropriate and presented no problem. However, the heart, great vessels, and blood are in rapid motion, and MRI is too slow to image the heart in real-time with adequate spatial and temporal resolution. Rather, average images over particular short intervals, or segments, at successive stages in the cardiac cycle are built up from MR data acquired over multiple cardiac cycles. Accordingly, synchronization with the cardiac cycle is needed in order to resample the same subinterval of the cycle and to effectively "freeze" cardiac motion. Imaging may be synchronized, or gated, with a pulse oxymetry trace (*peripheral gating*) or, more optimally, with a high-quality ECG signal [41].

Similarly, motion artefacts caused by *breathing* create difficulties in the acquisition of cardiac MR images. It has been estimated that the movement of the diaphragm and heart

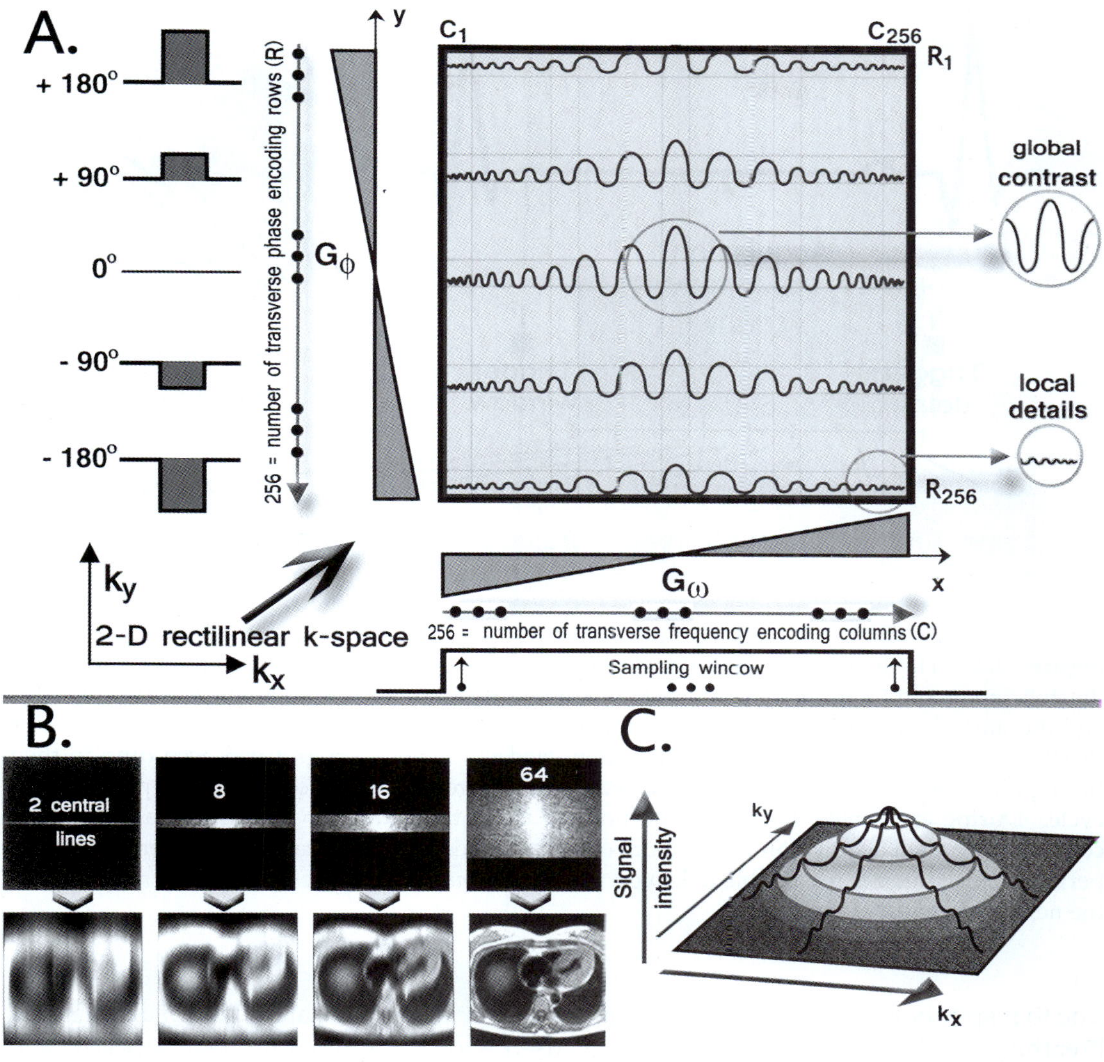

Figure 10.26: A. The central part of k-space represents high contrast characteristics of the image and comprises the lower frequencies of the MRI signal (larger "waves"); the periphery represents the higher resolution fine details of the image and comprises the higher frequencies (smaller "ripples"). B. Transverse "cut" of the thorax reconstructed by means of 2, 8, 16, and 64 k-space lines, astride the center. The two most central lines already form a vague image, but the spatial resolution is enhanced greatly with the progressive addition of more and more peripheral lines. C. Representation of the signal in the k-space by introducing as third dimension the signal *amplitude*. The 3-D k-space signal describes concentric circles undulating in amplitude while decreasing toward the periphery, as their spatial frequency increases and their spatial wavelength decreases. The central part contains the highest signal amplitudes, i.e., the strongest contrast levels, while the periphery contains the highest spatial frequencies, i.e., the finest spatial resolution components of the corresponding image.

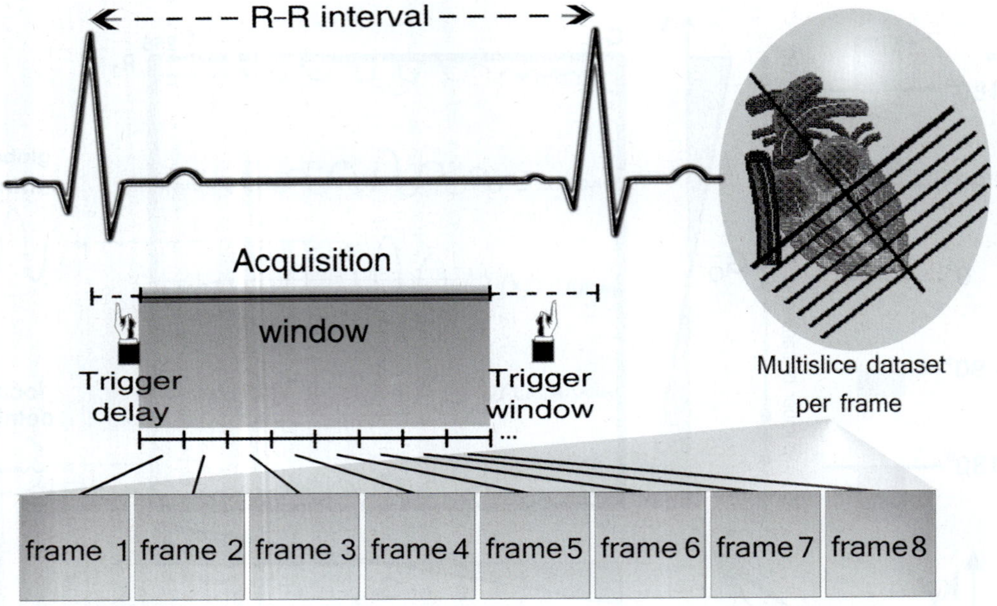

Figure 10.27: The R wave initiates conventional *ECG-triggered* MR pulse sequences. To obtain diastolic images, a *trigger delay* of at least 150–250 ms is interposed between the R wave detection and the start of imaging; for systolic imaging, this delay is zero. The total data sampling duration (85–90% of the R–R interval) is the *acquisition window*. Echoes are grouped according to their timing after the R wave, so that consecutive images correspond to successive time points of the cycle. During each cycle, only small portions of the data needed for each image are collected; consequently, data acquisition is continual over many heartbeats. Because R–R intervals are not perfectly constant, it is reasonable to leave a *trigger window* between the end of data sampling and the next projected R wave.

due to respiration in a human in the supine position is approximately 15 mm during tidal breathing [36, 155]. Breath-hold imaging is used widely for avoiding respiratory-related displacements of the heart. Right and left ventricular filling show normal respiratory variations [14, 111]. With inspiration, systemic venous return into the right atrium increases, and peak right ventricular diastolic filling volumes are 20% greater than end-expiratory values. Left atrial filling does not increase with inspiration, because pulmonary venous return is not influenced significantly.

All imaging data should be acquired at the same end-expiratory phase to minimize the changes produced by respiratory movements. Respiratory motion can be monitored by either an elastic band or a pneumatic bellows wrapped around the abdomen, or by MRI navigator echoes that image the position of the diaphragm or heart. MRI systems with respiratory navigator-guided sequences [104] reduce the number of artefacts resulting from chest wall motion and may eliminate the need for breath-holding.

The respiratory navigator approach [2, 18] relies on the excitation of a narrow beam of tissue along the axis of primary motion. Similarly to M-mode echocardiography (see Section 5.8, on p. 279), data sampling then ensues along the axis of this beam. If the beam traverses tissues with different MR-specific properties, a sharp demarcating interface within this beam can be detected, corresponding to the *tissue interface*. With sampling at consecutive time points, the successive positions of the interface can be measured by comparing with a predefined reference. If, e.g., a navigator is positioned through the dome of the right hemidiaphragm, a sharp interface can be detected between lung and liver. During breathing this interface *oscillates* caudally, during inspiration, and cranially, during expiration. Any kind of respiratory gating prolongs scan times substantially, since image data are only accepted during a short segment of the respiratory cycle.

ECG gating provides a means for synchronizing cardiac imaging at preset intervals during the cardiac cycle (see Fig. 10.27, on p. 528). Data are gated, i.e., collected in time-windows at synchronized intervals, to turn out *gated images* throughout the successive phases of the cardiac cycle [43]. Sequential images can be played back as a *cine loop*, which represents an ensemble averaged cardiac cycle, typically acquired over several heartbeats during a single breath-hold.

Prospective cardiac gating was developed for cardiac synchronization of MR data acquisition and can be used for any type of MRI sequence. The duration of image acquisition must be less than or equal to the duration of the shortest R–R interval; this implies that the last 10–15% of diastole is usually not usable for the ensemble averaging. *Retrospective* gating was developed for synchronization of rapid repetitive cine acquisition to the heart cycle. In retrospectively interpolated gated cine-MRI, images are acquired continuously while the ECG is recorded, and are afterward sorted according to their position in the cycle, thus allowing the entire cardiac cycle to be effectively imaged [29].

Because prospective as well as retrospective gating require data acquisition over multiple heart beats, markedly irregular heart rhythms may diminish image quality substantially [136]. *Arrhythmia rejection* is a method that is valuable, when the heart rate is very irregular. It commands the system to reject a beat, if its R-peak is not within the *predefined* RR-window [104]. Improved resolution in cardiac MRI scans in the time dimension is achieved by gating at a series of progressively shorter time intervals. As the patient is placed within the magnet, however, an electrical current termed magnetohydrodynamic effect (which underlies the operation of the electromagnetic flowmeter [159]) is induced in flowing blood, which results in distortions of the ECG signal. With imperfect synchronization, acquired images can become blurred. In the event that such problems due to ECG gating arise during an MR imaging study, troubleshooting techniques may be used [37].

Flowing ionic fluids, such as blood, where the velocity vector is perpendicular to that of the magnetic field, will be subjected to charge separation owing to Faraday's law, and hence to the development of an electric field. It has been estimate that a magnetic field of 5 T will only furnish a current density of roughly 100 mA/m^2 at the sinuatrial node [74], a value of the order of 10% of the naturally occurring maximum current density.

The ECG can detect the electric field caused by flow in the aorta; flow in the proximal aorta is at its peak during the T wave of the ECG. Accordingly, the ECG trace will be dis-

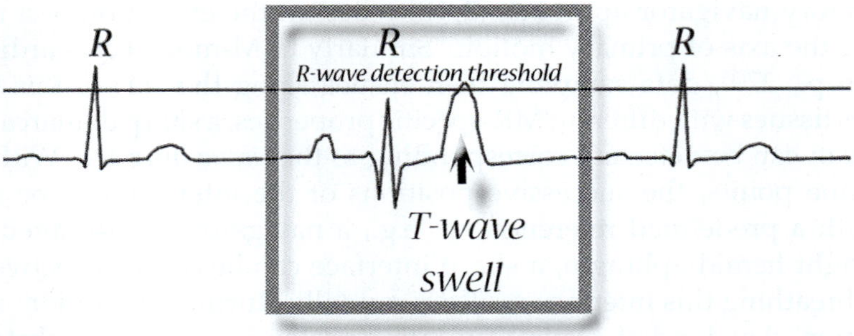

Figure 10.28: The magnetohydrodynamic effect can interfere with reliable R wave initiation of conventional ECG-triggered gating, because the induced *T wave swell* artefact can cause T wave peaks to exceed the R wave detection threshold, vitiating true R–R interval detection.

torted at this time, giving a *T wave swell*. This reversible phenomenon makes it extremely difficult to obtain reliable ECG-gating with increasing magnetic field, as is suggested by Figure 10.28. Furthermore, in the process of charge separation, a current will flow until the electrical field resulting from the charge accumulation is sufficiently strong to prevent it. This current produces a force retarding the flow; the cardiac pump will consequently have to perform additional work to overcome this force. Even for an external field of 10 T, however, the (nominal) increase in vascular pressure is less than 0.2% [70]. The practical effect of these forces in major blood vessels can therefore be neglected, aside from the magnetohydrodynamic effect interfering with reliable ECG-gating. The magnetohydrodynamic interference may be minimized by applying the ECG electrodes relatively *close together* on the chest wall.

The spectra of the QRS complex of the ECG and MR-related interference overlap enough to render filtering approaches to enhance the R wave difficult. Vectorcardiography (VCG) is a classical approach for representing the electrical activity of the heart in 4-D (x, y, z, and $time$). In recent years, *vectorcardiographic gating*, a sophisticated method of using the electrical signal from the heart, has emerged as a superior means of synchronization, which minimizes the interference from the B_o magnet field and RF and gradient-switching noise, and reduces the distortions of the ECG in the magnetic field that are due to the magnetohydrodynamic effect [31, 84]. The additional information content of the VCG, as compared with a single lead ECG under MR conditions, can be used to improve the accuracy of R wave detection and therefore to enhance the quality of gated MR scans. The VCG approach functions well under most circumstances and prior knowledge of the electric heart vector and flow artefact are not required in order to apply it [31].

Even more intriguing are new "self-gated" (SG) acquisition techniques, which can extract the motion synchronization signal directly from the same MR signals used for image reconstruction. Several strategies have been proposed for deriving the SG signal from data acquired using radial k–space sampling [83]. Because the SG signals are derived from MR signal changes that result from cardiac motion, SG techniques may be unable to provide cardiac cycle synchronization in cases of severely depressed cardiac function, with little ventricular wall motion. Otherwise, the SG techniques provide cine image series with no significant differences in quality, compared to conventional ECG gating.

10.3 Cardiac MRI techniques

In recent years, rapid technical developments are rendering MRI the imaging procedure of choice for assessment of cardiac structure and function [1], including simulation and detailed evaluation of intracardiac blood flow phenomena. MR angiography (MRA) is an MRI blood vessel study without using any contrast material, although contrast agents, such as *gadolinium*,[21] may be given by intravenous injection, linked with a chelating agent such as DTPA (diethylenetriamine pentaacetate), to make the MR images even clearer. Because of its high magnetic moment, gadolinium reduces the T_1 relaxation time constant of blood (approximately to 50 ms, shorter than that of the surrounding tissues) and enhances MR signal intensity.

Similarly to x-ray angiography, the images obtained by contrast enhanced MRA delineate the lumen of vessels and cardiac chambers, which appear bright (white), while the surroundings tissues produce a very hypo-intense signal (black). Thus, **Gd** highlights heart chambers and blood vessels making them stand out from surrounding tissues. The quality of images depends on the strong magnetic effect induced on blood hydrogen nuclei by the high concentration of **Gd**-based contrast media within the lumen [87].

As we have seen, several tissue-specific parameters affect the MR signal: proton density, T_1, and T_2 relaxation time constants. There is enough variation in these parameters between different tissues to permit acquisition of organ images with great contrast between the different constituent soft tissues. Furthermore, the effect on the contrast in an MR image of the tissue-specific parameters can be *selectively* suppressed or enhanced. Drastic manipulation of MR images of the same organ is possible, in order to provide different kinds (i.e., *morphological*, *functional*) of information.

The techniques that have given most information are:

- Wash-in/wash-out flow and time-of-flight methods, which provide some basic information about the presence of flow and bright blood angiographic anatomic details. However, the flow information is only qualitative because the signal intensity of flowing blood has a complicated dependence on sequence parameters, flow direction, and relaxation times [156].

[21] Gadolinium, **Gd**, is a metallic chemical element (a *Lanthanide*) that is paramagnetic and is used as a contrast agent because of its effect of strongly decreasing the T_1 relaxation times of the tissues to which it has access. When injected during MRI, gadolinium will tend to change signal intensities by shortening the T_1 time in its surroundings. The gadolinium ion cannot be used in its chloride, sulfate, or acetate forms because of poor tolerance and low solubility in water in the neutral pH range. Although toxic by itself, gadolinium can be given safely in a chelated form that still retains much of its strong effect on relaxation times.

- MR phase-contrast velocity mapping, which permits quantitative calculation of intracardiac blood flow velocities in *any* spatial direction. It measures blood flow in any selected direction by obtaining two complete sets of raw MR data using different gradient parameters in the direction of flow [8], and creates an image in which pixel intensity depends on the average velocity of the spins inside each pixel.

- Cine-MRI, where moving images of the heart are obtained throughout the entire cardiac cycle in *any* desired orientation. Cine-MRI using short repetition time (TR) gradient echo sequences and cardiac gating can be used for imaging the evolution of time dependent processes. By combining phase-contrast velocity mapping and cine-MRI [99], a technique for depicting pulsatile cardiac chamber wall motion and intracardiac blood flow throughout the cardiac cycle can be produced.

Both time-of-flight and phase-contrast MRA can be acquired in 2-D slices (individual stacked sections) or as a 3-D volume acquisition. The slice thickness in 2-D TOF techniques is generally on the order of 2–4 mm. In 3-D TOF MRA, signal is acquired from a 3–6 cm thick slab as a 3-D volume set rather than individual slices. This both increases the signal-to-noise (S/N) ratio (compared to the 2–4 mm thick slice of 2-D TOF) and decreases the obtainable slice thickness, improving the spatial resolution in the derived images. Accordingly, the 2-D technique is typically chosen in applications requiring *screening* of a large area, while 3-D techniques provide *finer resolution* of a smaller region of interest. In the following sections, we will provide an overview of these MRA techniques.

10.3.1 Time-of-flight methods

Time-of-flight (TOF) used to be a widely used MRA technique [85], but it has now been replaced by contrast-enhanced MR angiography for many applications [143]. It images slices perpendicular to the direction of blood flow using short TR sequences, as is shown in Figure 10.29, on p. 533. If stationary spins within a region experience only an *incomplete* T_1 *relaxation*[22] between the repetitive RF excitation pulses, their longitudinal magnetization decreases progressively (see Fig. 10.30, on p. 534); *pari-passu*, their transverse magnetization and thus their potential MRI signal intensity become depressed to distinctly lower levels compared to those of the completely relaxed spins within newly arriving blood. The applying short TR period saturates the stationary tissue spins. On the other hand, the flow-related enhancement (FRE) yields a high signal from continuously "new" blood moving into the slice, and makes the blood–wall interface stand out bright against a dark gray stationary tissue background (see Fig. 10.29). The FRE provides positive contrast (bright blood) demarcation of anatomic topographic details in time-of-flight MRA. It is important to bear in mind, however, that MR angiography is a *map of flow*, and not of true anatomy. It is therefore prone to artifacts related to flow disturbances or other complex fluid motion phenomena.

[22] The dynamics of incomplete relaxation here are mathematically analogous to those of incomplete myocardial diastolic τ relaxation (see Chapter 7 and refs. [107–110]).

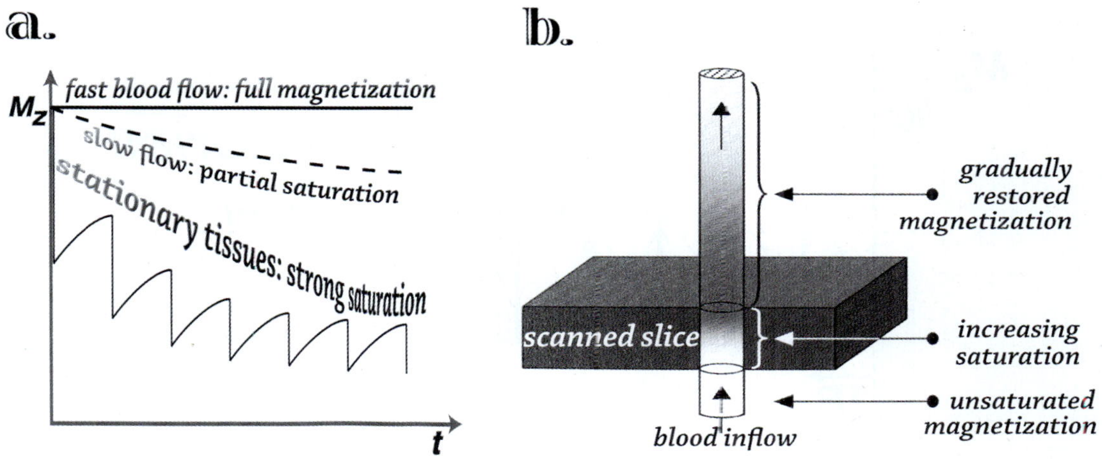

Figure 10.29: Time-of-flight is based on the principle that flowing blood entering an MR imaging slice or volume will have a higher MR signal intensity than the background tissues whose protons have been "saturated" by the recurring, closely-spaced RF excitation pulses. Since the protons within the blood have not been exposed to the repetitive RF pulses to the same extent as the background tissues, flowing blood has a higher signal intensity. a. Slowly flowing blood has longitudinal magnetization and signal levels intermediate between those of rapidly flowing blood and stationary tissues. b. The gray scale reflects the intensity of the longitudinal magnetization and the MRI signal (cf. Fig. 10.30.)

When imaging is performed one 2-D slice at a time, each slice will show flow-related enhancement. On the other hand, when multiple slices or an entire 3-D volume are imaged in a single acquisition, the FRE is most prominent at the first, or "entry," slice. The effect is moderated deeper into the imaging stack or volume, where even the moving protons will have been subjected to RF excitations before reaching the specific imaging slice. To decrease this entry slice phenomenon, the imaging order should be *countercurrent* to the flow, so that more slices will show flow-related enhancement, and *vice versa* [84]. With the 2-D technique, multiple thin, sequential sections are acquired. The acquired sections are either viewed individually or are reformatted with the MIP technique (see Fig. 11.9, in Section 11.5.2, on pp. 596 f.) so as to obtain a 3-D image.

The degree of the flow related enhancement is proportional to the blood flow velocity and inversely proportional to the applied repetition time. Maximum MR signal intensity is achieved when the imaging slices are positioned at a right angle to the direction of flow, and when a totally new column of blood enters each slice every TR period, i.e., when flow velocity equals or exceeds (slice thickness/TR). Clearly, TR and slice thickness must be appropriate to the anticipated flow velocities, and even small changes in slice thickness can affect the performance of the MRA sequence.

Saturation prepulse bands can be placed adjacent—proximal or distal—to the slices to selectively destroy MR signal from blood flowing in from one side of the stack of slices

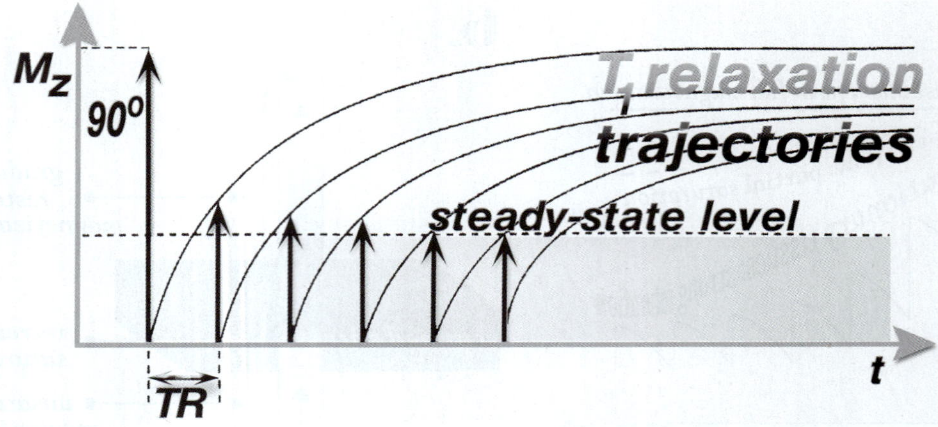

Figure 10.30: A short repetition time (TR) between consecutive RF excitations prevents a complete relaxation with return of protons to alignment with the external field B_o following each RF excitation. There ensues a steady state that is characterized by a greatly depressed longitudinal magnetization, M_z, and attendant reductions in transverse magnetization and MR signal.

of interest. The technique can thus be rendered *flow-direction* sensitive, and capable of acquiring selectively arteriograms (distal band) or venograms (proximal band) [56,84,156]. For TOF sequences, the presaturation bands may also be sequentially repositioned, so as to travel with the acquisition slices, keeping the same position relative to each transverse imaging-slice in a series. The set of slice images can either be viewed as individual sections or be processed by the maximum intensity projection (MIP) computer algorithm (see Section 11.5.2, on pp. 596 f.) to interactively create projection angiograms in a range of views; for complete analysis, the base slices should also be examined individually and with multi-planar reconstruction (MPR) software (see Section 11.5.1, on pp. 595 f.).

10.3.2 Phase-contrast velocity mapping

Magnetic resonance velocimetry is capable of 3-D flow velocity measurements [88]. The velocity field is measured across the entire vascular cross-section, and it can be measured in deep vessels that cannot be explored by Doppler techniques. Several methods have been proposed for imaging flow phenomena. Wash-in/wash-out flow and TOF methods provide some information about the presence of flow. However, this information is only *qualitative* because the signal intensity of the flowing blood has a complicated dependence on sequence parameters, flow directions, and relaxation times.

The most successful general methods for intracardiac blood flow measurement in investigative and clinical applications involve velocity phase-encoding, or "phase-contrast velocity mapping" (PCVM), which employs the signal from blood-conveyed protons stimulated by specially designed magnetic field gradients. Conveniently, the output phase shift is proportional to flow velocity, and the velocity-encoded, or phase-contrast

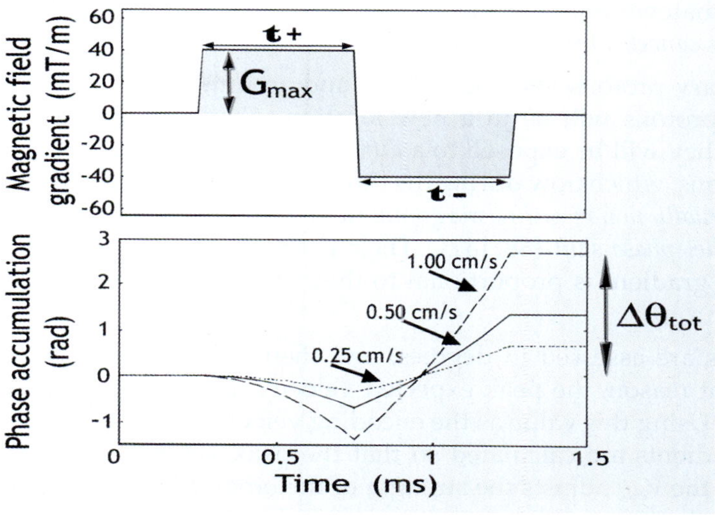

Figure 10.31: Phase accumulation due to flow through a magnetic field gradient. *Top panel*: Bipolar symmetric magnetic field gradient ($\pm G_{max}, t+ = t-$), with a total area of zero, applied to encode velocity. *Bottom panel*: Phase accumulated by blood flowing at constant velocity during the application of a bipolar gradient. Moving precessing spins experience a velocity-induced phase shift due to the presence of the balanced bipolar gradient. At the end of the gradient operation, the net accumulated phase change, $\Delta\theta$ is *proportional* to the flow velocity. Above a critical velocity, the aliasing velocity, a phase greater than π radians will accrue, and will make blood appear to move in the opposite direction. Such aliasing can be averted by using shorter or weaker velocity encoding gradients.

techniques, are based on these phase shifts. Phase-contrast techniques supplement, or can be used instead of, TOF sequences for situations, such as evaluations of intracardiac blood flow phenomena, in which *quantitative* and *directional* velocity information are desired.

The flow-encoded phase shifts result from application of *bipolar* magnetic field gradients [88], which are composed of two lobes with *opposite* signs, as shown diagrammatically in Figure 10.31.[23] A magnetic field gradient is briefly applied. When the first lobe is applied, the spins of the stationary and moving tissues begin to accumulate phase. Phase differences develop at different locations along the gradient because the rate of proton precession is proportional to the *local* magnetic field strength. For linear field gradients, the amount of this phase shift is proportional to the velocity of the flowing spins in the gradient-encoded direction. Immediately after the first lobe, the second lobe is applied. The polarity is *reversed*, so that the gradient has the same profile (equal magnitude and duration) but opposite polarity, as is depicted in Figures 10.31 and 10.32, on p. 537. In

[23]Generally, *bipolar gradients* are gradients that are either positive or negative during a specified time interval and are followed by a gradient of the opposite sign that is maintained during an equal time interval. The amplitude of these opposite gradients is the same, as is exemplified in Figure 10.31.

view of that, whatever phase change was induced in *stationary* tissue protons by the first gradient lobe is *canceled* by the second.

The stationary protons lose their phase and accumulate a net phase of zero. However, flowing protons will be in a new location when the second gradient is applied and therefore they will be exposed to a *different* gradient strength. Consequently, blood-conveyed protons, which flow during the time intervening between the two gradient lobes experience *mutually nonoffsetting* magnetic field gradients, and, consequently, end up accumulating a *net phase shift* [88, 141]. Their net phase shift that is accumulated during such a bipolar gradient is proportional to their effective velocity in the *gradient-encoded* direction.[24]

Phase shifts are assessed in degrees, and their values should be within a range of ±180°. For that reason, the peak expected velocity must be selected before starting the measurement. Using this value as the encoding velocity, V_{enc}, the amplitudes of the flow-sensitizing gradients are calculated so that the peak velocity corresponds to a shift of 180°. In effect, the V_{enc} adjusts the strength of the bipolar gradient, so that the maximum velocity selected corresponds to a 180° phase shift in the data. Velocity encoding, in cm/s, specifies the highest and lowest measurable velocities encoded by a phase-contrast sequence and is inversely proportional to the area of the flow-encoding gradients. Therefore, for the imaging time to remain unchanged, stronger gradient amplitudes are called for in order to encode smaller velocity magnitudes.

Since only the transverse component of spin magnetization can accumulate a phase shift in response to motion, it is obligatory to *first* induce a transverse magnetization by an RF pulse, before the flow-gauging magnetization gradients are applied. Since the frequency of spin precession is directly proportional to the strength of the magnetic field, when precessing spins move in a magnetic field gradient, they undergo a frequency shift that is related to their velocity along the gradient direction. This frequency shift multiplied by the time duration of its occurrence gives the accumulated phase angles gained or lost with respect to unshifted magnetic moments, depending on whether the flowing spins move *in* or *against* the gradient direction. The relative angle accumulation is called the phase shift, and will be proportional to the velocity component in the direction of the gradient.

Thus, the protons in flowing blood will accumulate a net phase shift relative to stationary protons that is dependent on their velocity and direction as is shown in Figure 10.32, on p. 537. If the direction of flow is reversed, the phase shift will become reversed, as well. The amount of phase shift that a precessing spin undergoes in flowing through a magnetic field is, in fact, proportional to the applying gradient, to the flow velocity, and to the *square* of the time throughout which the gradient is acting. Because of this quadratic dependence of the phase shift on gradient duration, the longer the TE interval, the much more intense becomes the flow-related dephasing.

[24] Unintended phase shifts may also be induced by other factors, such as magnetic field inhomogeneity. Such effects can be counteracted by acquiring a second set of phase data without velocity encoding or with a different velocity-encoding gradient. Subtraction of the two sets of phase data from each other leaves only the flow signal, and the phase difference that remains after subtraction is used for a voxelwise calculation of velocities.

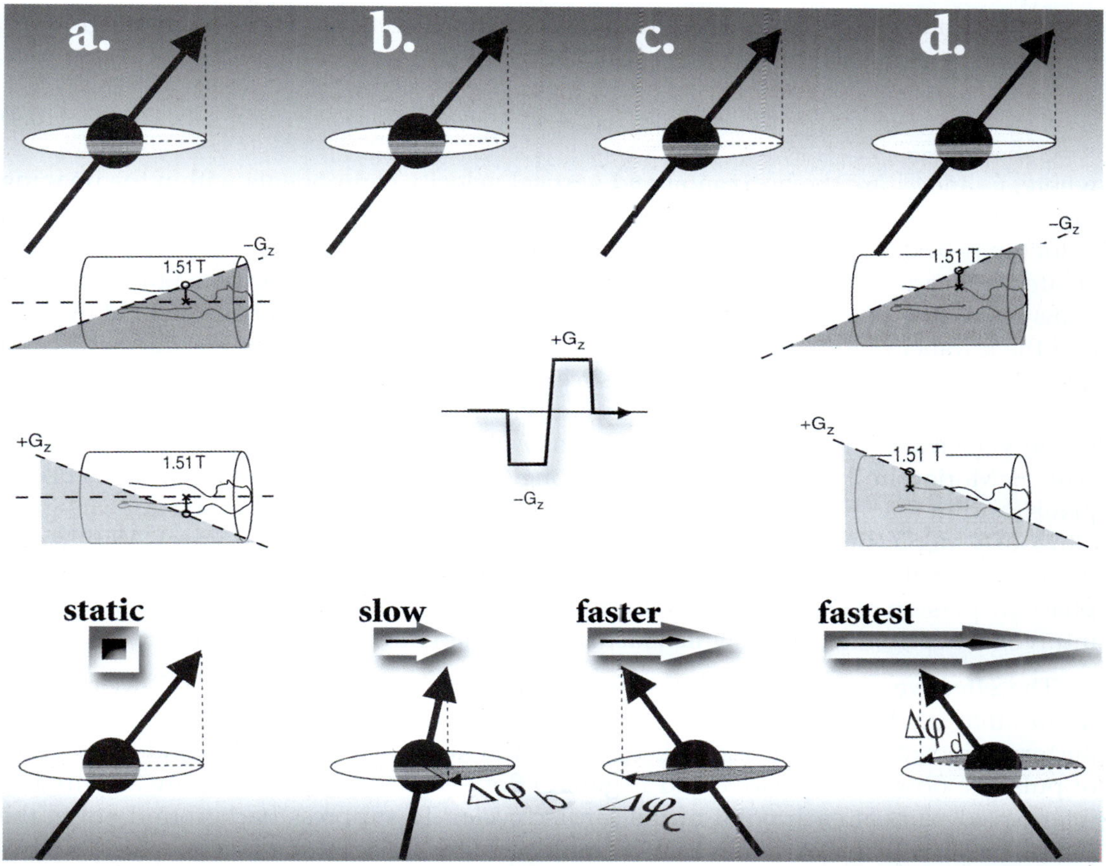

Figure 10.32: When the areas under the positive and the negative gradient lobes are equal, a motionless proton will obviously not experience a *net* phase shift, but a flowing one will. Consider that, as shown in a., the flowing proton starts in a region of the magnetic field gradient that produces a positive phase shift. By the time of gradient reversal, it will have moved closer to the feet and as a result it will again experience a positive shift. Therefore, with the bipolar (*dephasing* and *rephasing*) gradient, a flowing proton experiences a *net* positive phase shift. The amount of phase shift experienced as a result of moving through the field is proportional, *inter alia*, to the velocity of flow—cf. b., c., and d.

If a proton is flowing from the heart to the feet (arterial flow), the net phase shift will be positive; while if a proton is moving in the opposite direction (venous flow), it will accumulate a negative net shift; the gradients exemplified in Figure 10.32, are along the body axis, but the same pattern applies to gradients in any direction. Thus, MR signal changes can be used to obtain information about the flow direction as well as the speed. Not only is the sign of the phase shift contingent on the flow direction, but the amount of phase shift is directly proportional to the blood flow velocity in the frequency-encoding direction. PCVM uses the phase information to determine detailed intracardiac blood flow-field velocities [72, 95, 96].

Velocity encoding is performed in all three spatial directions. The velocity magnitude, V, in each pixel in each time-frame is calculated as:

$$V = (v_x^2 + v_y^2 + v_z^2)^{1/2}, \tag{10.4}$$

where, v_x and v_y are the horizontal and vertical velocity components within the imaging plane, and v_z is the velocity component *through* the measurement plane. The calculated values may be displayed as gray-scale maps for each time frame. Thus, the PCVM method creates an image in which pixel intensity depends on the mean velocity magnitude of the spins inside the pixel (in 2-D) or voxel (in 3-D). The size of the transverse field of view and the number of data points in the acquisition matrix determine pixel dimensions and the *in-plane spatial* resolution; the axial slice thickness determines the axial dimension of the voxels and *through-plane* spatial resolution. The phase shift, which is proportional to the velocity, is displayed as pixel intensity on the phase map image of the monitor screen. Motion in the positive direction along the flow-encoding axis appears as bright pixels, and in the opposite direction as dark pixels, while stationary tissue appears gray. Obviously, dephasing because of flow effects may occur also *within* a voxel. Within any finite voxel, different blood-conveyed protons may have varying velocities, which lead to phase dispersion of the protons within the voxel with attendant signal loss, the so-called intravoxel dephasing [84], to which factors other than flow may also contribute.

The effective temporal resolution is determined by the number of PCVM imaging frames that can be obtained during a representative (average period) heart cycle. When performing cardiac gating, which is clearly mandatory for visualization and assessment of pulsatile flow, two (positive and negative) flow-encoded acquisitions are acquired as interleaved pairs at each point of the cardiac cycle. To suppress background noise, the phase-encoded pixel intensities may be multiplied by a magnitude image, which is a by-product of the interleaved phase difference technique. The resulting images are called "flow" images [141].

It should be borne in mind that *in vivo* detailed quantitative validation of PCVM 3-D velocity field measurements is extremely challenging, because there are no in vivo gold-standard measurement methods. Several studies have compared MR velocity fields to theoretical predictions of relatively simple steady flow and pulsatile flow velocity profiles [35,78,126], and others have compared MR velocity fields to those acquired by different modalities, including ultrasonic flow probes [13,161], and other *in vitro* experimental velocimetric methods, such as laser-Doppler anemometry [133], and particle image velocimetry [23,28]. In the absence of turbulence, these studies have demonstrated a very good agreement between MRI velocity measurements and the other modalities *in vitro*.

10.3.3 Superimposition of an MRI velocity image on an anatomic image

Every data acquisition ascertains information about the MRI signal's magnitude as well as its phase at each voxel. Signal intensities are processed into an anatomic image: the *magnitude* image. In conventional MRI sequences, the phase information is of no value because the phase in the individual voxels is disorganized. In phase-contrast MRI velocimetry, phase accumulations are processed into a *phase* or *velocity* image, because they determine the velocity in each voxel (see discussion above and Section 2.19, on pp. 88 ff.). A most valuable capability is the simultaneous *blending* of the phase and magnitude MRI images, so as to generate flow velocity snapshots colocalized with images of cardiac anatomy, thus improving the diagnostic and research utility of MRI procedures.

By applying a bipolar gradient in an image sequence it is possible to record the velocity of the blood in each voxel. The bipolar gradient can be applied in any chosen direction, or in all three spatial directions to obtain 3-D velocity information. As we have seen, finite phase shifts can have other causes than flow velocity, e.g. magnetic field inhomogeneities. Consequently, it is necessary to record a flow-compensated background image. Through the use of flow-compensated gradients it is possible to record a phase image, where phase effects stem only from unwanted deviations. This flow-compensated image can then be subtracted from the phase velocity map, leaving a phase image that is the result of only the phase shifts accruing from the flow velocity. The entire procedure is summarized pictorially in Figure 10.33, on p. 540.

Clearly, phase velocity mapping requires acquisition of *several images per slice*: one image for each of the three components of the velocity *vector* and one velocity-compensated image. Therefore, it increases the total scan time. Velocity images with in-plane velocity components shown as vectors are of limited value when examined on their own, but they are very revealing when they are *superimposed* on the corresponding anatomic (modulus) images. This combination is a powerful imaging technique when intracardiac blood flow phenomena and their modifications brought about by various physiological and pathophysiological operating conditions are evaluated. These overlayed, colocalized, MRI images are completely analogous to those color Doppler flow images obtained using *duplex* color ultrasound scanners, capable of displaying both B-mode and Doppler blood flow data simultaneously in real time, which are discussed in Section 5.9.5, on pp. 288 f.

In duplex color ultrasound, the Doppler shift of the reflected signal is encoded in color and the magnitude of the reflected signal is encoded in gray scale. With color-flow MR imaging, at multiple instants during the cardiac cycle, a phase image and a corresponding magnitude image, representing the transverse magnetization measured by the sequence, are constructed. Thus, the signal magnitude images delineate the specified cardiac chamber anatomy. On the phase images, the intensity of each voxel within the intracardiac flow field corresponds to the velocity of blood flow at that location. Motion along the velocity-encoding direction is displayed as bright or dark voxels, depending on direction, and stationary tissue appears mid-gray. Colorization can be used too.

Just as the color Doppler ultrasound technique has advantages, including low cost, high temporal resolution, and good spatial resolution, the MRI method has advantages of its own: It is not limited to anatomic areas that have "acoustic windows," as is the case with Doppler ultrasound. With MR imaging, flow velocity component encoding can be along any *arbitrary* directions, whereas with ultrasound the only measurable velocity component is (nearly) orthogonal to the transducer face. Moreover, both the degree of the

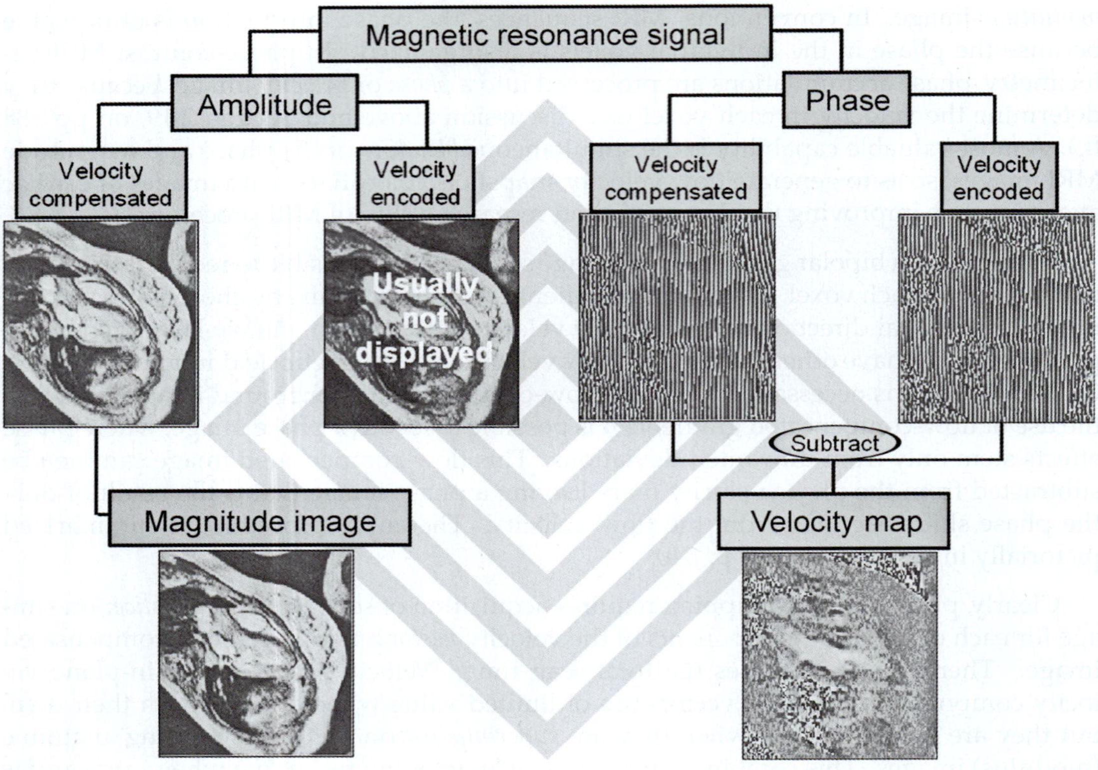

Figure 10.33: Schematic diagram summarizing PCVM. Pairs of velocity compensated (reference) and velocity encoded datasets are acquired. The latter datasets are subtracted to yield a velocity or phase map with pixel values linearly related to velocity. (Adapted, modified, from Chai and Mohiaddin [12], with permission of the authors and Taylor & Francis.)

MRI flow encoding and the field of view are adjustable [122], whereas ultrasound has no such interactive capabilities. Finally, with MRI, one can interactively fine-tune the spatial resolution, with a proportionate change in the acquisition time.

In order to produce a veritable *color* overlaid image, each pixel's density and velocity needs to be quantized to one byte coding, and then passed though a color map template to assign different colors to different velocity levels: an adapted version of a Doppler ultrasound color map ensues through such a pixel-by-pixel overlay. A major concern in such an overlay process is the accuracy of velocity maps. When there is little signal in a pixel, its phase is more prone to noise, and thus the velocity estimate becomes less reliable. To prevent this from appearing in overlaid images, minimum density criteria can be used. Coloring is *restricted* to pixels that have signals of sufficient density to yield reliable velocity estimates. This limits the *colored* areas of the displayed image [98]. In the case of pulsatile flow the velocity calculated is, obviously, an average of the flow over the data acquisition period for each image frame.

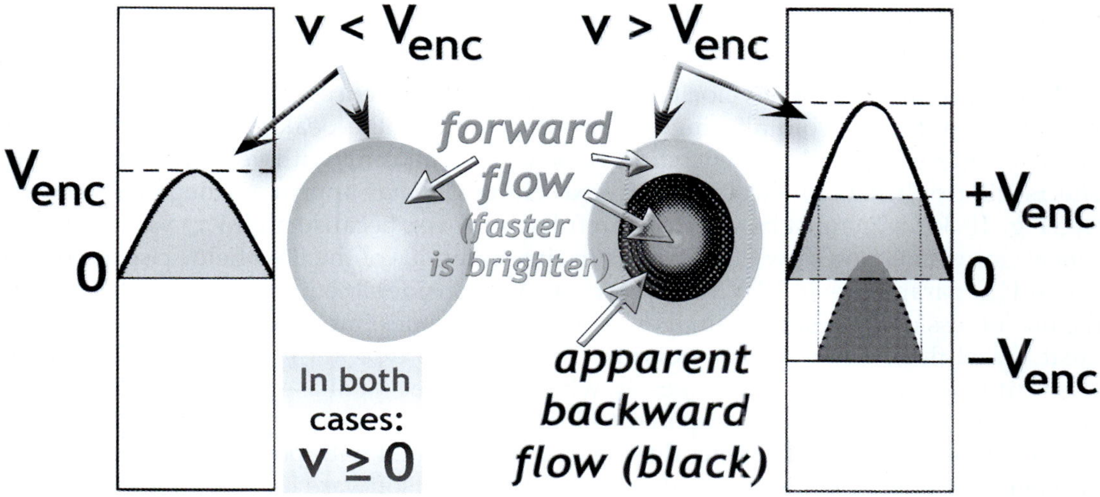

Figure 10.34: Aliasing is typically clear-cut to detect in PCVM images, in which the voxels of aliased peak velocities exceeding V_{enc} have an inverted signal intensity, corresponding to flow in the reverse direction, compared to that of the surrounding voxels and the velocity profile appears irregular.

MR phase-contrast velocity mapping can quantify the flow rate through the cardiac valves and large deep intrathoracic arteries and veins [94], because it allows time-resolved simultaneous measurements of both vascular area and blood velocity within the area; it is becoming indispensable in studying flow patterns using *multidirectional* and *multidimensional* measurements of blood flow.

The phase information is determined within each imaging plane pixel and is used to construct velocity maps [1, 5, 12, 13, 73, 95, 96, 153]. At each "point" (pixel) on the map, the velocity is functionally displayed by using a gray scale and can be read out numerically. The direction of velocity can be measured in 3-D, but routinely MRI velocimetry is obtained through-plane with the imaging plane perpendicular to the direction of flow. Pixel-wise integration of velocities (cm/s) distributed over the cross-section of a vessel and multiplied with vessel cross-sectional area (cm^2) yields "instantaneous" flow-rate (mL/s). Volumetric flow rates in the great vessel outflow trunks of the right and left ventricles at each "instant" may be calculated. By a subsequent temporal integration over the cardiac period, the net blood flow volume per cardiac cycle, i.e., the stroke volume (mL) is obtained. Then, multiplication by the heart rate provides the mean flow rate per minute, namely, the cardiac output.

In such determinations, flow measurements are most reliable if the imaging plane is orthogonal to the main direction of flow and *through-plane* flow encoding is used. For assessment of left ventricular output from phase-contrast data, the imaging plane in the ascending aorta should be at the level of the bifurcation of the pulmonary trunk [160]. Generally, velocity mapping is used to quantify the velocity of flowing blood, but it can also be applied to determine the velocity of the contracting or dilating myocardium.

It is important to set the velocity sensitivity of the sequence above the expected peak velocity, in order to avoid aliasing (phase-wrapping). If the peak velocity in the vessel or site of interest exceeds the encoding velocity, V_{enc}, aliasing with velocity wraparound effects will result; e.g., a forward velocity exceeding V_{enc} may appear as a negative velocity (see Fig. 10.34). V_{enc} must be selected carefully, however, because high V_{enc} values are *not suitable* for visualizing slow flow regions or time-intervals of the flow field. Use of appropriate V_{enc} parameters in PCVM acquisitions has considerable influence in determining the usefulness of the resulting images. This issue becomes important in intracardiac and great vessel flow, where highly pulsatile velocities are typical. Fortuitously, aliasing is clear-cut to detect in velocity images, in which the voxels of aliased peak velocities have an inverted signal intensity compared to that of the surrounding voxels, as is shown in Figure 10.34. To a limited extent, aliasing can be remedied with postprocessing software packages, by offsetting the range of V_{enc} on the display software [38, 160]. However, it is generally prudent and more efficient [88] to repeat the flow measurement with a modified V_{enc} than to adjust the aliased dataset.

Another similarity to Doppler flow imaging is the need to suppress the small motions of background cardiac chamber wall and adjoining structures that may mimic low-velocity blood flow field regions. This is accomplished with a reduced phase-difference threshold [122] that is analogous to the "wall filter" used in Doppler ultrasound (however, see Section 14.4, on p. 742); for MR imaging, a threshold on magnitude is also used.

To map *in-plane* flow patterns in an imaged slice through a cardiac chamber or a vessel, we must note that the *in-plane* complex velocity at each pixel is essentially a 2-D vector. Thus, it is usually necessary to make separate measurements of two orthogonal components of the velocity vector, unless the direction of flow is known *a priori*. Similar considerations apply for the *through-plane* flow velocity component. Flow details through 3-D flow velocity fields are measured, in principle, by acquiring PCVM sequences associated with particular flow-field planes and with velocity encoding in the directions defined by orthogonal Cartesian coordinates: in this fashion, all three orthogonal components of the intracardiac vectorial velocity distribution can be measured [95, 142].

Although only one velocity component can be measured at a time, with three acquisitions (plus generally an additional acquisition to correct for other possible sources of phase shift) we can reconstruct the full velocity vector at each location within the 3-D image dataset. Acquiring such flow images throughout the cardiac cycle permits evaluation of the temporal evolution of flow patterns in the cardiac chambers or the great vessels [117]. Complete acquisition of complex intracardiac and great vessel flows requires cine phase-contrast in three *directions* and three *dimensions* [5,39,72,95,96,142]. In practice, considerable difficulties are encountered.

The sensitivity of the PCVM velocity imaging must be adjusted to the estimated range of velocities to be measured, as there will be an *ambiguity* beyond $\pm 180°$ of phase change. Within regions of fine-scale turbulent disturbances, the phenomenon of *intravoxel dephasing* can cause inconsistencies in the data; such inconsistencies may just result in the loss of signal or possibly in artifacts propagating across the image in the direction of the phase-encoding gradient. This type of signal loss can be seen in the proximity of rapidly moving heart valves or at sites where flow is strongly accelerated and nonuniform. Jets of signal loss are *indicative* of valvular stenosis or incompetence. The extent of the signal loss region depends on the combination of both physiological and technical parameters, and is thus at best only a semiquantitative measure of the severity of valvular defects.

The presence of high-shear flows, as occur within thin, unsteady boundary layers, which result in a large range of phases within the corresponding pixel of the image, may also result in such a loss of signal. Even with uniform intravoxel velocities and phases, when in principle the phase of a single pixel, and thus its velocity, can be measured with high precision, in practice, signal-to-noise ratio limits will generally require averaging of the signal from multiple adjacent pixels; this will tend to limit the accuracy of the determination of the phase and the effective spatial resolution of the technique.

As the case is often with MR imaging, not all of the most powerful techniques are easy to understand or to master, and many—nonspecialists and specialists alike—are challenged to stay abreast. This reemphasizes that clinical diagnosis and physiological investigation of intracardiac blood flow phenomena by MRI methods is a dynamic *interdisciplinary* field, and the hope is that sufficient information and insight are provided here to stimulate the motivated reader to take his or her interest to the next level [11,21,26,30,39,51,80,84,88,121,141,142,144].

10.3.4 Cine-MRI

Conventional cine-MRI imaging required several minutes of acquisition time per slice, but with the introduction of new, more efficient raw data matrix acquisition techniques, in combination with phased-array surface coils, high quality cine-loops can now be obtained within breath-holds of generally 10–16 heart beats [44,157]. The spatial resolution is in the order of 1 mm and temporal resolution around 20 ms. Shorter acquisition times can be attained, up to real-time imaging, but only at the expense of concomitant reductions in spatial resolution and signal-to-noise ratio.

Ventricular chamber geometry and function can be dynamically displayed using ECG-gated gradient echo techniques allowing acquisition of cine-loops of the heart in any orientation, and providing sharp contrast between flowing blood and the endocardial boundaries, valuable in the assessment of wall motion and dynamic ventricular volumes (see Fig. 10.35). Complete short-axis coverage of the ventricular chambers allows calculation of changing ventricular volumes *without* any geometric model assumptions. However, cardiac image registration is a complex problem, because the heart exhibits few accurate anatomical landmarks, and also because of the nonrigid and mixed motions of the heart and the intrathoracic structures, even during breath-hold intervals.

The same slice is acquired at successive time "points" of the cardiac cycle. Nevertheless, due to the motion of the heart, we do not observe exactly the same anatomical short-axis region along the long axis of the heart within the same slice. Correction of through-plane motion in real-time cardiac imaging is feasible using *"slice-following"* [60,129]. Moreover, several cardiac cycles are required to reconstruct slices. Also, because of the constraints

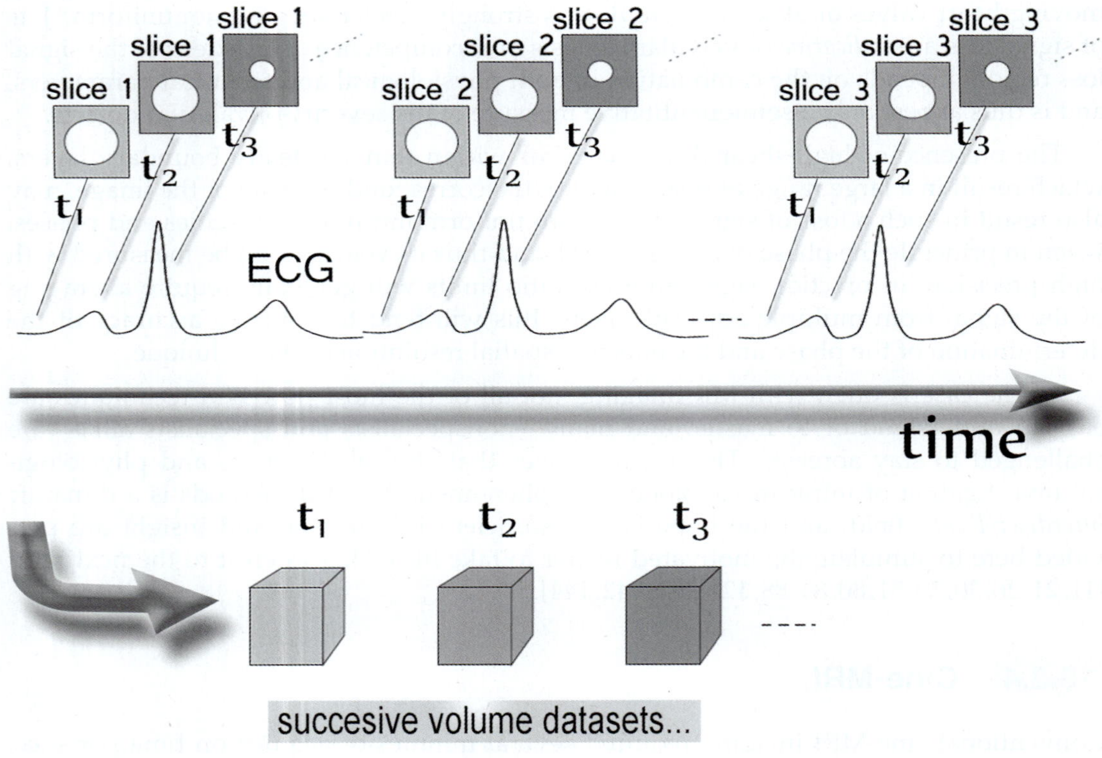

Figure 10.35: ECG-gated tomographic techniques allow acquisition of time-dependent volumetric datasets of the heart, from which cine-loops of cardiac chambers with intersecting planes in any orientation can be derived, providing sharp contrast between the flowing blood and the endocardial boundaries.

involved in 4-D spatiotemporal acquisitions, cardiac images have lower resolutions than attainable with static organs. These are problems entailed by the spatiotemporal image acquisition from a *dynamic structure* that need to be recognized.

From the discussion in Section 10.2.8, on pp. 523 ff., it follows that the *particular* contrast applying when the central portion of k-space is filled will effectively determine the *overall* image contrast. This is pertinent when passage of a bolus of contrast agent, used to delineate better the blood-endocardium interphase, occurs in the course of a scan. One might then make use of a delay between contrast injection and central k-space data acquisition, to derive an image dominated by the effects of peak contrast agent concentration [105]. Tracing of endocardial and epicardial contours is needed in quantifying ventricular volumes, myocardial mass, and wall kinematics.

In recent years, thanks to technological advances, MR image acquisition times have been driven down and image quality has improved [44, 157]. Determination of dynamic ventricular volumes by manual planimetry from multislice, multiphase MR imaging avoids geometric assumptions, necessary with 2-D echocardiography or angiocardiography, and has been in use for some time. It has been shown to be reproducible and give good agreement with other methods [42, 116]. In a research environment, quantitation still depends on manual segmentation, which is time consuming and tedious. A typical study comprises 20–25 time phases over the cardiac cycle, at each of 10–15 short-axis slice locations through the heart from base to apex [127], plus a number of long-axis cross-sections, adding up to about 200 or more images per cardiac acquisition. In this situation, analyzing all these images becomes a formidable task and segmentation may take several hours. Accordingly, there is an extensive literature on algorithms with the potential for automatic or semiautomatic MR image analysis [42]. These include schemes based on thresholding, edge detection, deformable models [92], active contour models [42, 119], and theory based on *a priori* knowledge [139].

Cine-MRI, using short repetition-time gradient echo sequences and ECG gating, can be used for imaging dynamic processes. By combining PCVM and cine-MRI, *fusion* images depicting simultaneous wall motions and intracardiac blood flow velocities throughout the cardiac cycle can be produced.

To display the time-varying 3-D data encountered in cardiac imaging, we must accumulate each volume of the study as a separate 3-D texture. For 3-D texture-based rendering methods, it is then sufficient to bind each texture in a cyclic manner. This can provide excellent frame rates and visual quality. However, for 2-D texture-based rendering methods a slightly different approach must be employed because, in this rendering mode, three sets of textures must be stored in memory. Storing large 3-D volume datasets in texture memory would not be feasible on most current video cards. For the typical size of a cine gated cardiac dataset, the high data rates required for real-time display ($512 \times 512 \times 8$ *bits* at 30 *frames/s*, i.e., around 2 *GB/s*), this is beyond the video memory storage capabilities of most general purpose graphics cards. Therefore, for 2-D texture based rendering, each set of textures must be loaded from main memory during the process of cine or video loop 3-D display.

The latter approach can provide interactive frame rates for small- to medium-sized studies; nevertheless, large studies can strain the interface between *main memory* (also known as RAM, or Random Access Memory) and the video card. To generate sufficiently high frame rates (>20 *fps*) regardless of volume size or technique used, we need to cache each rendered frame in a series of 2-D textures. This allows for fast cyclic rendering of quadrilateral polygons that are textured with these images. Such cached textures must be prepared every time that the orientation or appearance of the rendered volume is changed.

10.3.5 Evolution of 4-D (spatiotemporal) scanning technologies

The driving force behind the rapidly improving capability of noninvasive 3-D flow measurement and dynamic geometry reconstruction technologies, such as CT and MRI, are the multifaceted advances in computational technologies encompassing hardware and software, including computational fluid dynamics (CFD) modules. To wit, it requires massive computational ability to build the high resolution, 3-D images from the raw x-ray or magnetic resonance tomographic patterns that CT or structural MRI scanners produce. It is these high resolution 3-D images that we seek in order to provide the 4-D spatiotemporal[25] geometric data for the patient-specific boundary conditions, which are required in the investigation of intracardiac blood flow phenomena by CFD, as we discuss in subsequent chapters. Here, we should note that intracardiac flow processes from such CFD simulations can then be recovered by high-dimensional visualization algorithms and analyzed using vector field operators, to produce a variety of visualization maps. These maps can be designed to reflect the magnitude and principal directions of pulsatile chamber wall contraction and dilatation with corresponding rates of strain, and local shear, curl, and gradient values of intracardiac flow-field variables, as recovered by the CFD simulations.

The visualization maps can be displayed side-by-side or superimposed to allow improved interpretation. The color overlay of Doppler flow information over anatomical information has of course had a long history in ultrasound and other, newer, cardiac imaging modalities [75]. Combining *multimodality* data, derived from complementary imaging modalities, with 4-D (spatiotemporal) CFD simulation maps can result in comprehensive representations of structure-function relationships and their intricate interactions, and can help elucidate subtle pathophysiologic processes that are difficult to appreciate by structural imaging in isolation.

Table 1 Performance characteristics[a] of CT in a comparison from 1974 to 2004

	1974	1984	1994	2004
Minimum scan time	300 s	5–10 s	1–2 s	0.33–0.5 s
Data per 360° scan	57.6 kB	1 MB	1–2 MB	10–100 MB
Data per spiral scan	–	– —	24–48 MB	200–4000 MB
Image matrix	80 × 80	256 × 256	512 × 512	512 × 512
Power	2 kW	10 kW	40 kW	60–80 kW
Slice thickness	13 mm	2–10 mm	1–10 mm	0.5–1 mm
Spatial resolution	3 Lp/cm	8–12 Lp/cm	10–15 Lp/cm	12–25 Lp/cm
Contrast resolution	5 mm/5 HU/ 50 mGy	3 mm/3 HU/ 30 mGy	3 mm/3 HU/ 30 mGy	3 mm/3 HU/ 30 mGy

[a] Typical values for high performance scanners

[25] Spatiotemporal signals are of the form $f(x, y, z, t)$, where x, y, and z are the three spatial dimensions, and t is time.

As the table on the preceding page so aptly demonstrates, the evolutionary process of technology seeks to improve capabilities in an exponential fashion. This is so because inventive innovators seek to improve things by multiples and independent innovations, each of which is a linear addition to knowledge, tend to increase the power of a particular technology in a *multiplicative*, rather than an additive way. For instance, one independent innovation might be an algorithmic discovery that yields the same result with half the computation; another might be a circuit advance that yields twice the transistor circuits in a given space. Each of a number of such *concomitant* increments of knowledge more or less multiplies synergistically the effect of all of the others and, therefore, technology tends to grow exponentially in their number.

Consequently, innovation is multiplicative, not additive; thus, technology, like any evolutionary process, builds on itself. This characteristic will continue to accelerate as technology itself takes full control of its own progression. In these early years of the twenty-first century, we are at the inflection region, or "knee," of the accelerating exponential rise in computational power. The exponentially increasing computational ability provided by the accelerating evolution of technology will enable us, more rapidly than most might expect, to continue to improve the resolution and speed of these powerful, noninvasive, scanning technologies.

10.4 Real-time and live 3-D echocardiography

Ultrasound technology has improved strikingly in the past 15 to 20 years, allowing us to extend its use in studying not only cardiac structure but also function [90, 91, 112, 113, 131, 154, 162, 163]. New ultrasound equipment and techniques provide superior image quality, greater accuracy, and expanding capabilities. Accordingly, more and improved ultrasound imaging modalities are available for evaluating cardiac anatomy, ventricular function, and blood flow velocity fields. 3-D echocardiography improves and expands the capabilities of cardiac ultrasound, which we examined in Chapter 5. The echocardiographic signal is generated as a response to the distribution of acoustic impedances in the scanned region of the body. The ultimate goal of echocardiographic imaging is to develop real-time 3-D scanners that can obtain any desired view, or cross-section, of the beating heart and its chambers. Several general approaches have been developed over the years.

10.4.1 3-D reconstructions from 2-D images

Freehand probes use an electromagnetic location system. Computer-controlled, electronic or mechanized, *parallel plane* or *rotational*, probes rely on 1-D linear phased arrays. They capture multiple 2-D images in 3-D space and perform interpolation between the acquired slices to create a 3-D volume, as is summarized in Figure 10.36. As is detailed in Chapter 5 (see, in particular Sections 5.5–5.7), to acquire each 2-D image a pulse is sent out, ultrasound is reflected, and a B-mode line is built up from the reflected signals. This means that as each successive pulse is sent out, the transducer has to wait for the returning echoes, before it sends out a new pulse to generate the next line in the image.

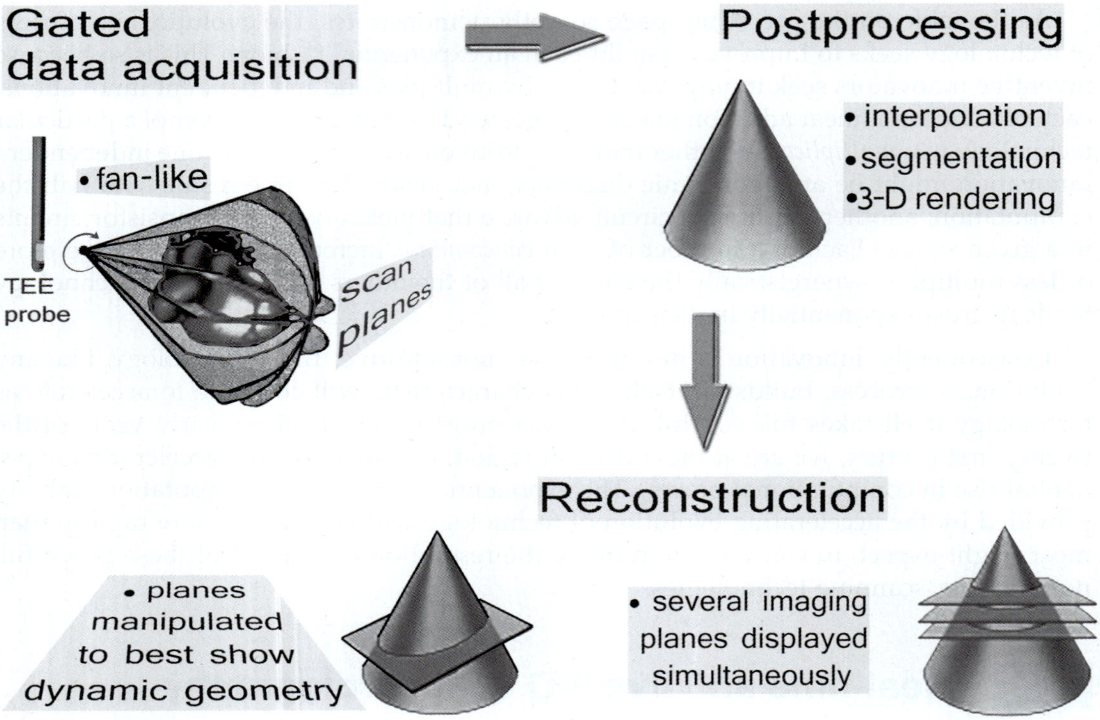

Figure 10.36: Schematic of the transthoracic or transesophageal (TEE) acquisition of a fan-like family of 2-D, B-mode scan planes, and the postprocessing of this dataset, which allows multiple reconstruction and 3-D organ visualization options.

By making the ultrasound beam sweep over a sector, the scanning process can build up a 2-D echocardiographic image made up of *multiple* B-mode lines. In principle, the image is built up line by line, by emitting the pulse, waiting for the reflected echoes and then tilting the beam a bit further and emitting the next pulse. After the complete sector is scanned, a 2-D frame or image will have been acquired. Completion of each frame takes an interval equal to the time for transmitting and receiving the total number of pulses, which corresponds to the number of B-mode lines in the image. Multiple such 2-D images in 3-D space must be acquired, and interpolations between the acquired slices must be performed in order to create a cardiac 3-D volume scan.

These approaches for 3-D reconstructions from 2-D images are relatively simple to implement, but they are subject to errors that are primarily related to the interpolations in the reconstruction and to inaccuracies in the tracking of the exact transducer location relative to the beating heart during acquisition. Because with mechanized transducers the intervals and angles between the 2-D images are defined, a 3-D coordinate system can be derived from the 2-D images in which the volume is more uniformly sampled than with the freehand scanning approach. The data acquisition can be done by either the transthoracic or the transesophageal approach. Sequential data acquisition is used to reconstruct dynamic 3-D geometry; accordingly, to minimize reconstruction artifacts, sequential images are gated to both ECG and respiration [58].

For transthoracic acquisition, various types of motorized carriage devices are mounted on the ultrasound probe, which are controlled by a computer connected to the ultrasound machine. The transducer is made to scan in a linear mode, a fan-like tilting mode, or a rotational mode. These techniques produce 3-D datasets in the form of a prism, a pyramid, or a cone. With the transesophageal approach, special software in the echo unit allows the acquisition of 2-D multiplane images directly, by operating the probe in a rotational mode. After the data acquisition phase, the acquired 2-D images are realigned and are digitally reformatted into rectangular pixels [19].

The third category, real-time 3-D echocardiography, is different from the first two because it uses 2-D instead of 1-D arrays and is capable of capturing volume data all at once. This ensures that the transducer location is the *same* during the examination.

10.4.2 Real-time 3-D echocardiography

As the name implies, real-time 3-D echocardiography takes place "on the fly," with reconstruction accomplished simultaneously with imaging by a computer that is attached to the ultrasonography machine. Real-time 3-D echocardiography (RT3D) was first developed in the 1990s at the Duke University Center for Emerging Cardiovascular Technologies. A key point to 3-D ultrasound imaging is the fact that rather than frames/s, as in 2-D echocardiography, volumes/s are acquired. This gives the ultrasound image depth for a 3-D perspective in looking into the beating heart and its chambers. Standard ultrasound systems transmit and receive ultrasound waves in 2-D, and are described in Chapter 5. These systems are limited to producing sequences of flat, circle sector (or pizza slice) shaped 2-D images.

A major disadvantage of 2-D ultrasonography is its inability to measure accurately the irregular 3-D volumes of body organs, such as the cardiac chambers. Real-time 3-D offers more information in less time, which improves the spatial conception of cardiac 3-D dynamics. This version of real-time 3-D imaging never made an impact on clinical practice because spatiotemporal image resolution was limited, although it is still useful for animal research studies, e.g., in conjunction with simultaneous sonomicrometric measurements [113]. In recent times, a more highly developed version of real-time 3-D echocardiography was introduced by Philips Medical Systems, and is characterized as "live 3-D." Because of improved *spatiotemporal* image resolution, this variety of 3-D imaging is at the present time becoming adopted in both the research and clinical cardiovascular settings.

The RT3D transthoracic echocardiography probe developed at Duke University [134, 148] contained a 2-D matrix transducer array, which allows a pyramidal volume (see Fig. 10.37), rather than a single slice, to be scanned without physically moving the transducer, and to be displayed in real time. This transthoracic probe, which steers and focuses the ultrasound beam in three dimensions, contained 512 piezoelectric elements (256 nonsimultaneously firing *transmit* and 256 *receive*) configured in a "sparse" array pattern [86]

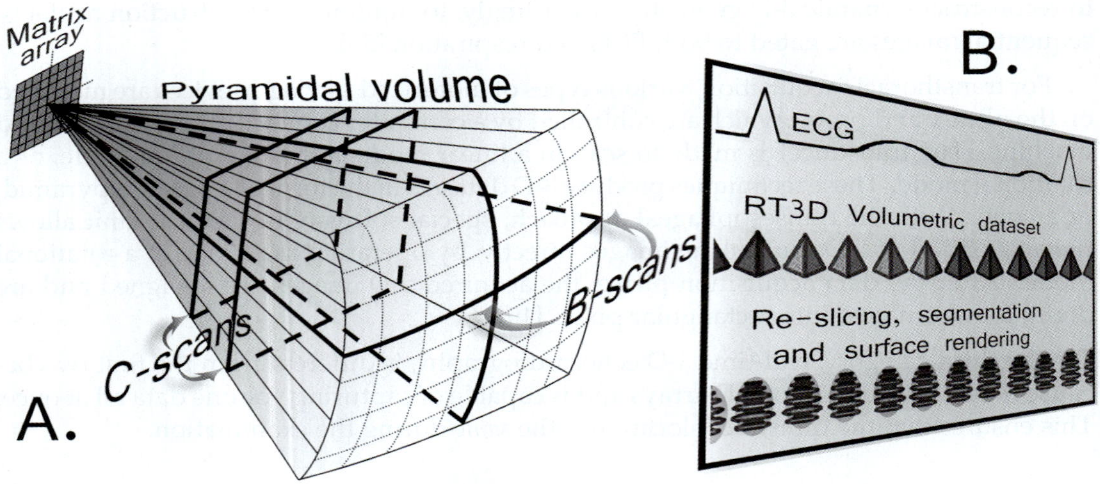

Figure 10.37: A. Schematic of the pyramidal scan from the matrix phased-array probe of an RT3D system. Bold lines indicate possible display planes: two simultaneous orthogonal B-mode image planes (one meridional and one azimuthal, see Fig. 10.38, both perpendicular to the transducer array) and two C-mode planes (parallel to the transducer array) are depicted; alternatively, each C-scan plane may be inclined at any desired angle. B. By means of the matrix phased-array probe and data processing by 16 parallel processors, the RT3D systems provided real-time scanning of pyramid-shaped volumes at a depth-dependent rate of 17–40 volumes$/s$.

and transmitting at a frequency of 2.5 or 3.5 MHz. *Sparse arrays* are so named because either the transmit and receive elements are positioned strategically so that, in conjunction with parallel processing, they can capture the necessary angles to create a dynamic image of the heart, or because only certain array subsets are turned on at any one time. The 2-D transducer array allows beam steering in the azimuthal (θ) and the meridional (ϕ) ("elevation") directions. At this juncture, it should be noted that RT3D ultrasound data is in spherical coordinates (see Fig. 10.38, on p. 551) and requires resampling to be visualized in Cartesian coordinates.

In a phased array all elements are used simultaneously, while in a linear array only a subset of the total array elements is used. Using a smaller number of elements in a linear array increases the time to image a given field of view. A phased array is different; because of its pie shape a very small transducer can image a large area in the far field. That is why phased-array transducers are the transducers of choice in applications like cardiac imaging where one has to deal with the narrow intercostal spaces between the ribs, through which the much larger heart needs to be scanned.[26]

[26]Unlike CT or MRI, there are relatively limited transthoracic windows for acquiring the data. Transesophageal imaging overcomes this to some degree (particularly for basilar cardiac structures), but has the disadvantage of requiring a semi-invasive procedure.

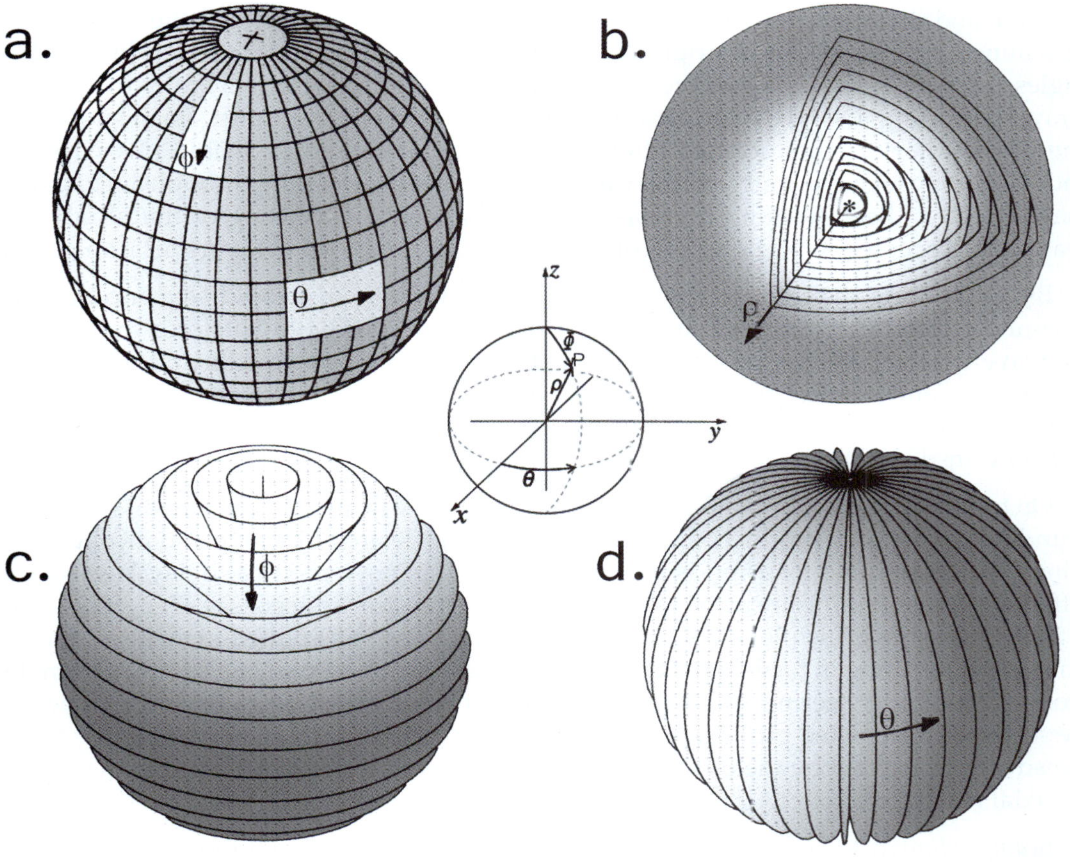

Figure 10.38: The spherical coordinate system uses three coordinates, two of which are visible on the spherical surface in panel a. They are: the radial distance (ρ) of a point from a fixed origin ($\rho = 0$), the meridional angle (ϕ) from the positive z-axis, and the azimuthal angle (θ) from the positive x-axis. The three coordinates (ρ, ϕ, θ) are defined as: $\rho \geq 0$ is the distance from the origin to a given point P, as shown in panel b.; $0 \leq \phi \leq 180°$ is the angle between the positive z-axis and the line formed between the origin and P, as shown in panel c.; $0 \leq \theta \leq 360°$ is the angle between the positive x-axis and the line from the origin to the P projected onto the xy-plane, as shown in panel d. To plot a point from its spherical coordinates, go ρ units from the origin along the positive z-axis, rotate ϕ about the y-axis in the direction of the positive x-axis and rotate θ about the z-axis in the direction of the positive y-axis, as is shown in the inset. Successive small (*differential*) increments—$d\rho$, $d\phi$, $d\theta$—of each of the three spherical coordinates are visualized in panels, b., c., and d., respectively.

In order to achieve a probe footprint sufficiently small and with a sufficiently wide far field to image the heart from the intercostal spaces, the scanning beams must each emanate and diverge from virtually the same "point." This implies that the image must be scanned by a single beam originating from the same array but deflected in different angles, so as to build up a complete sector image. This can be achieved by the phased array by sending a single beam that is stepwise rotated electronically. Each successive line in the image is then formed after a slight angular rotation. Such a phased array with electronic focusing and steering can generate a beam sweeping through a pizza slice shaped sector. Beamforming by phased array also enables focusing of the ultrasound beam as is discussed in Section 5.5.1, on pp. 261 ff., and is shown in Figure 5.23, on p. 265.

By stimulating the transducers of a phased-array probe in a rapid sequence, the ultrasound will be sent out in an interference pattern. According to Huygens' principle,[27] the wavefront will behave as a single beam; thus, the beam is formed by all transducers in the array, and its direction is determined by the applying time sequence. In this way, phased arrays use electronic focusing and steering to derive a circle sector shaped B-scan *without* transducer movement.

On transmit, a directed beam is achieved by timing the firing of each element so that the sound wave that each produces adds coherently in the desired direction and incoherently otherwise. Electronic focusing is achieved by applying symmetrical delay laws to the different elements of a linear or annular phased-array transducer (see Fig. 5.23A., on p. 265). The same principle of electronic phase steering can be applied to make a concave wavefront, resulting in focusing of the beam with its narrowest part at a distance from the probe. Combining steering and focusing will result in a focused beam that sweeps across the sector, as is depicted pictorially in Figure 5.23B. Axial resolution, perpendicular to the transducer face, is set by the ultrasound pulse duration; the shorter the pulse, the higher the axial resolution.

Beamforming in 3-D is similar to beamforming in 2-D; however, unlike traditional linear phased arrays, the 2-D phased arrays can implement steering delays for any scan mode plane perpendicular to the transducer face. Consequently, linear arrays allow for 2-D beam steering, while matrix arrays allow for 3-D beam steering in any direction within a pyramid of tissue underneath the scan head. In this way, arbitrary sectors can be obtained directly at any desired orientation. The images obtained with the original Duke system were not volume-rendered online; instead, they consisted of computer-generated 2-D cut planes derived from the 3-D volume dataset. This allows a compelling view of cardiac chambers and structures, but is critically dependent upon the quality of the raw data. Furthermore, simply reslicing the 3-D data in arbitrary 2-D slices is easy to implement and visualize, but negates much of the purpose of 3-D echocardiography itself. Alternatively, the volumetric datasets can be segmented to distinguish dynamic endocardial

[27] In 1678, the great Dutch physicist Christiaan Huygens (1629–95) wrote a treatise titled *Traité de la Lumiere* on the wave theory of light; in it he stated that the wavefront of a propagating wave at any instant conforms to the envelope of spherical wavelets emanating from every point on the wavefront at the prior instant. Huygens' Principle applies equally to any locus of constant phase, and not just to the leading edge of the wave [130].

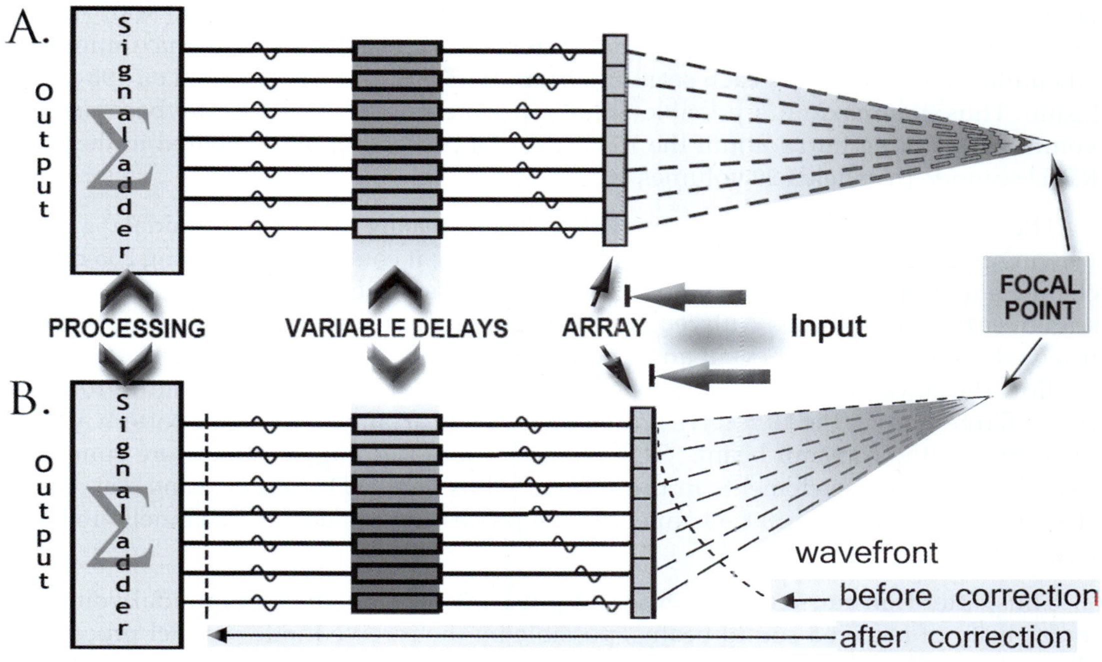

Figure 10.39: Principle of *delay-and-sum* beamforming with linear phased arrays. The received ultrasound pulses reflected from a particular focal point along a beam are stored for each channel, then aligned in time, and coherently summed. In the diagrams, the ultrasound echoes are represented by the wavy squiggles on the horizontal time lines emanating from the array—with time increasing horizontally from the array surface.

boundaries, with surface rendering then applied to the segmented images. Such semiautomated chamber reconstructions facilitate the accurate quantification of dynamic chamber geometry [58]; they are considered at some length in the next chapter.

On receive, the array is made direction-sensitive by delaying the received signals and summing them coherently. The depth of scatterers generating echo signals during reception increases with time. For a coherent summation of the echo signals of different transducer elements, the received signals have to be delayed individually according to the distance from the scatterers. In this way, the beamformer calculates a so-called scan line, and an image can then be reconstructed from a set of adjacent scan lines, as is depicted pictorially in Figure 10.39, on p. 553.

In view of the physical constraint imposed by the finite speed of sound in soft body tissues (1,540 m/s), image quality (beam spacing), field of view (pyramidal scan volume), and volume update rate (volumes/s) are strongly *interdependent* with one another in determining the performance of the 3-D ultrasound scanner. The higher the demands on one or two of these three performance determinants, the worse will be the performance of the other(s). An example should make this clear: Consider that the pyramidal scan volume is $64° \times 64° \times 15\ cm$. The $1°$ beam spacing demands $4,096$ beams. The maximum time taken for the round trip of each scanning beam is $15\ cm \cdot 2/154000\ cm/s$, i.e., $195\ \mu s$ per beam. Thus, the maximum possible volume-update rate (3-D frame rate) becomes 1.25 volumes$/s$. Taking into account the $16 : 1$ parallel processing implemented in the Duke RT3D scanner, this yields 20 volumes$/s$.

Thus, the RT3D system could scan with $1°$ beam spacing up to 23 pyramidal ($64° \times 64°$ viewing pyramids) volumes$/s$ at $13\ cm$ depth of field; it could do so by using 256 receive channels with the $16 : 1$ receive mode parallel processing schema to write the $4,096$-line scan over the 3-D volume. With receive mode parallel processing, multiple beams can be received for each transmit event and multiple scan lines can be processed *simultaneously*, to allow the efficient acquisition of echocardiographic data. As shown in Figure 10.40, on p. 555 (large arrow), the 16 receive line elements were arranged in a 4×4 pattern around the center of the transmit beam. Each of these beam-forming systems were connected to each of the receive elements in the system. Thus an RT3D scanner using 256 receive elements would have a $4,096$-channel receive processing system (256 channels $\cdot 16$ beam formers).

Thus, after transmission of each sound pulse into a wide-angle pyramidal volume, a multiplicity of received sound beams, possible by the receive mode parallel processing, allowed sampling the volume *"in one go."* As noted, the resulting 16-fold improvement in the data acquisition rate allowed the beamforming system to form $4{,}096$ lines of image in real time. Thus, each pyramidal volume contained $4,096$ scan lines, with a spatial line density (step size) of $1° \times 1°$ in the azimuthal (θ) and the meridional (ϕ) coordinate directions, as is shown in Figure 10.37, on p. 550. Using $16 : 1$ receive mode parallel processing, the scanner could generate the corresponding $4{,}096$ B-mode image lines at up to 20–30 volumes$/s$, depending on scan depth.

The RT3D probe was mounted in a hand-held case with a circular aperture, $16\ mm$ in diameter. At the site of skin contact the transducer and casing measured $18\,mm$ in diameter. The hand held transducer was free to be moved by the operator in any direction, so as to optimize images. RT3D volumetric echocardiography allowed real-time or reconstructive imaging of freely definable 2-D image planes from a single volume dataset, independently of the acquisition window. The system could turn out so-called *C-plane* images; these are arbitrary cross-sections that are perpendicular or oblique with respect to the scanning axis at various levels of the 3-D viewing pyramid, as is diagramed in Figure 10.37 and exemplified in Figure 10.40, on p. 555. By integrating and spatially filtering echoes between two user-selected planes (e.g., C-mode planes), the system could also display 3-D rendered images in real-time.

Images could be viewed in real time or in a 3-second captured volume. The RT3D system was capable of storing several consecutive cardiac cycles of volumetric data, which could be stored on a removable optical disk to be processed further for visualization and analysis. Image display comprised several simultaneously steerable, intersecting B-scan sector arcs with multiple C-scan planes, parallel to the transducer face, or inclined so as to maximize chamber dimensions; the relation between B- and C-scan planes is shown

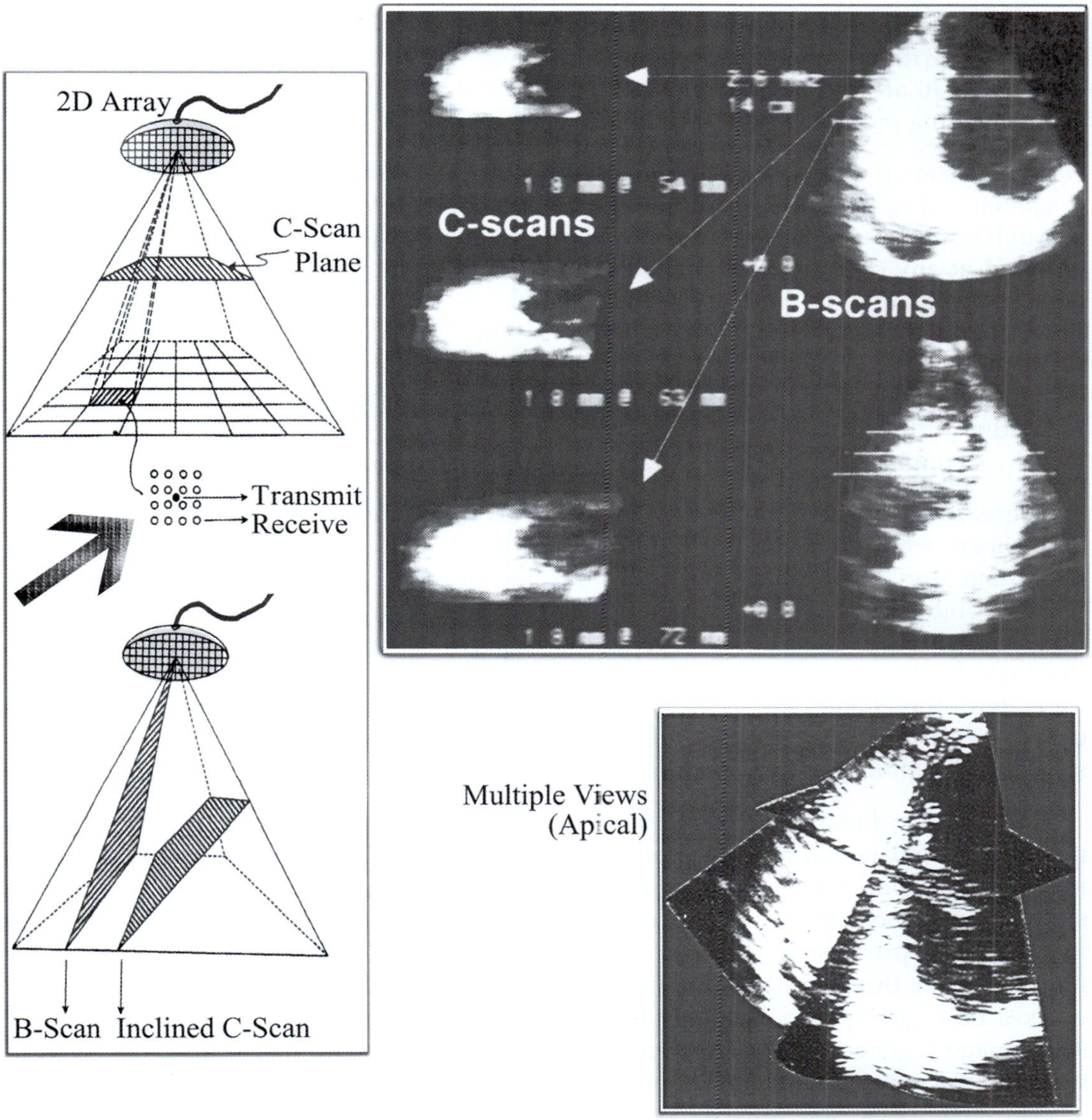

Figure 10.40: RT3D imaging illustrating B- and C-scan simultaneous planes within the pyramidal scanned volume. Such cross-sectional cuts within the scanned volume could be steered anywhere in the pyramid and were simultaneously displayed on a multipanel screen in real-time motion. Stop-frame simultaneous RV images are shown here, after intraluminal contrast medium injection for endocardial border enhancement before image segmentation. (Reproduced, slightly modified, from Pasipoularides et al. [113], with kind permission of the Am. Physiol. Soc.)

in Figures 10.37 and 10.40. These plane cuts through the heart and its chambers were adjustable in depth anywhere in range within the scan volume, in *real time* or in *playback* mode, with no image degradation. Although the system could simultaneously display up to 16 arbitrary planes from the pyramidal volume, because of the limited size of the imaging monitor, only 4 or 5 planes were displayed at one time, as in Figure 10.40.

That system provided a fast means of collecting 3-D ultrasound data, but it was limited in spatial and in temporal resolution by, *inter alia*, the finite speed of sound propagation through body tissues. Real-time display options included not only multiple image planes oriented at any desired angle and depth within the pyramidal scan, but also real-time 3-D rendering, and, in the most recent versions of the commercial RT3D system,[28] real-time 3-D pulsed-wave and 3-D color flow Doppler[29] [145]. The real-time 3-D rendering mode allowed the reconstructed 3-D image to be animated and moved in space and to be examined from different perspectives. For off-line analysis using semiautomated software preloaded in the Duke-VMI system, real-time "captured volume" datasets of 3-second length, encompassing 2–3 cardiac cycles, could be stored on magneto-optical disk.

A great advantage of the VMI RT3D system was that, using it, an anatomic dissection of the heart, while it was beating in real time on the display screen, could be accomplished from data stored on optical disk, both on- and off-line in playback mode. The result was the ability to view multiple planes and more cardiac anatomy *simultaneously* than were available with standard 3-D echocardiography. It is important to recognize that all the data, displayed or not displayed, are contained within the scanned 3-second dataset. Thus, with the Duke-VMI RT3D system, capture of a scanned volume provided all the data necessary for *complete* volumetric interrogation of cardiac chamber and anatomic structure dynamic geometry, simply by adjusting plane locations during playback.

On the other hand, an obvious disadvantage of that archetypal RT3D system is that it acquired a sparse volume dataset, providing comparatively poor image quality. The maximum possible number of transmitted ultrasound pulses were dispersed over a considerable volume rather than concentrated in a single plane. In spite of 16 : 1 receive mode parallel processing, this wide scatter reduced the information density in the volumetric dataset, thus reducing the spatial resolution and image quality. One consequence of reduced image quality was a systematic underestimation of volumes. Moreover, the slow image regeneration rate lowered the time resolution, and the narrow, 64°, field of view did not generally include all of the ventricular walls, especially in large hearts.

The application of sophisticated image processing techniques [16] to ultrasonographic data allowed a semiautomatic segmentation of heart chambers, regularizing their shapes and improving endocardial edge fidelity, despite the presence of endocardial edge gaps that were common in RT3D ultrasound data. This allowed reconstruction of, e.g., left ventricular shape and evaluation of LV volume in the course of the cardiac cycle, as is exemplified in Figure 10.41, on p. 557.

[28]This RT3D system was marketed by Volumetrics Medical Imaging, VMI, Durham, NC.

[29]The main problem with the conventional estimation of blood flow velocities using linear arrays is that it is not able to estimate velocity components perpendicular to the transducer.

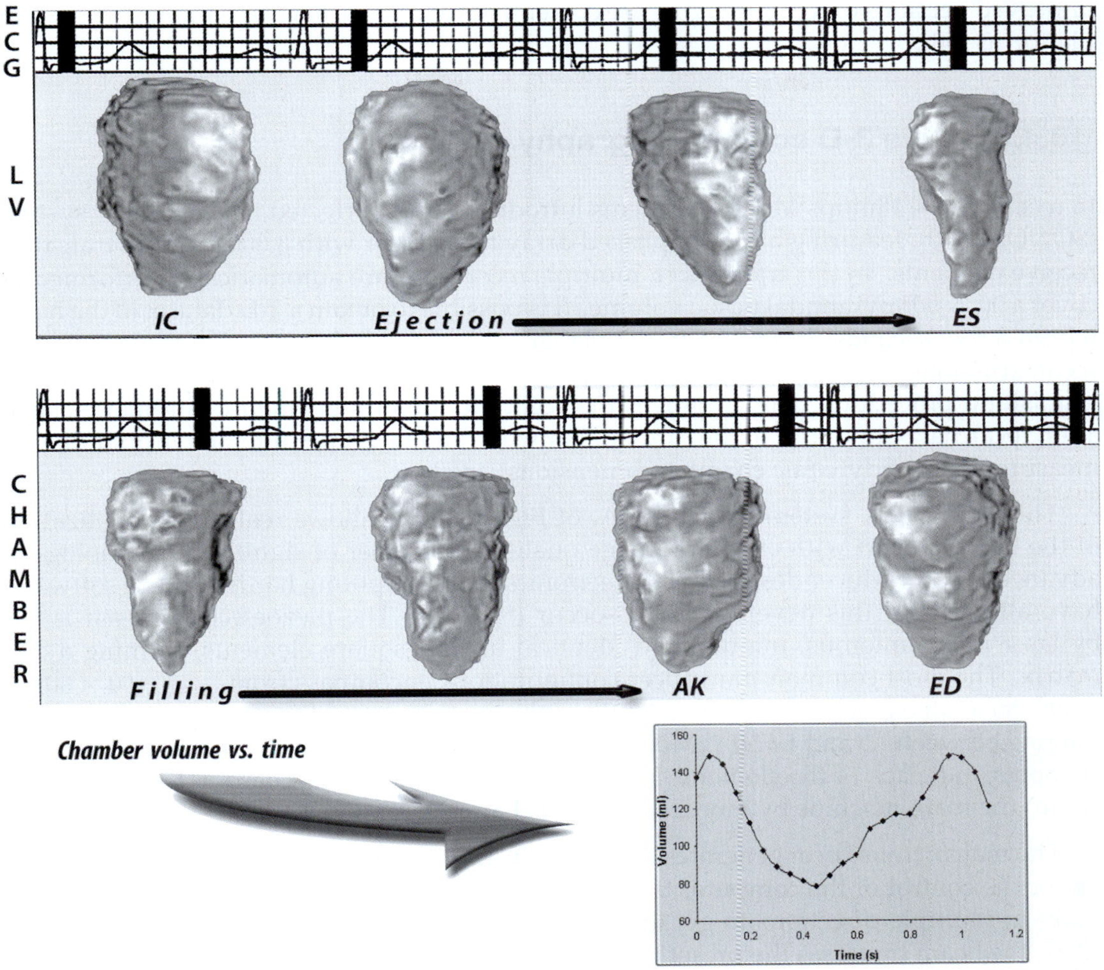

Figure 10.41: LV surface detection on RT3D echocardiography data of a normal subject; the phase of the cardiac cycle corresponding to each successive surface is indicated by the black bar on the ECG signal. IC = isovolumic contraction; ES = end-systole; ED = end-diastole. (Adapted and modified from Corsi et al. [16], with kind permission of the authors and the IEEE.)

The Duke RT3D paradigm was a quantum jump in the quantitative ventriculographic capabilities of ultrasonography, analogous to the jump from M-mode to 2-D echocardiography. In recent years, advances in the methodology embodied in the Duke RT3D paradigm have evolved rapidly. Lately, the development of very large matrix-array transducers incorporating well over 3,000 imaging elements (see below), has transformed RT3D echocardiography by making available markedly improved image resolution. Further advances have resulted in better penetration, less artifact, and a smaller transducer *"footprint,"* and have also incorporated harmonic imaging. In fact, different greatly improved versions of RT3D imaging are currently available on several commercial system platforms [58].

10.4.3 Live 3-D echocardiography

In recent years, Phillips Medical Systems introduced and perfected its *"live 3D"*[30] system (SONOS 7500), featuring a matrix phased-array transducer with $3{,}000$ or more transmit-receive elements. In this transducer, multiple recordings are automatically performed to cover a $90° \times 90°$ pyramidal tissue volume. It is possible to obtain a 3-D dataset of the heart within a few seconds, from which 2-D planar images can be extracted, and various 3-D reconstructions can be performed and displayed in real time, or near real-time, during the acquisition procedure. This improves the ability to identify geometric landmarks, such as endocardial boundaries of the cardiac chambers, and facilitates interactive quantitative measurements of dynamic chamber dimensions.

This full matrix system (see panel A. of Figure 10.42) allows real time visualization of the beating heart with excellent image quality. A number of significant technological advances, in transducer design, microelectronics, and computing hardware and software, have allowed for this development to occur [58, 154]. The piezoelectric crystal is cut by laser into numerous, minute, and identical in size, square elements, forming a 2-D matrix. The most common transducer configurations encompass from $3,600$ (60×60) to $6,400$ (80×80) elements, housed in the tip of the transducer, and operating at frequencies ranging between 1.6 and 4 MHz. More than 150 mini-circuit boards are placed between the elements, and each of the elements is connected to a mini-circuit board in the transducer and to the main machine by more than $10{,}000$ channels.

The matrix transducer generates ultrasonic beams in a phased array manner, such that under the control of the computer the emitted ultrasound beam can be steered automatically in multiple directions to get to any targeted area. Referring to Figures 10.38 and 10.37, the beam traverses the preset ρ-axis to turn out a 1-D display scan line from near to far; then the scan line is steered (phased-array technique) along the azimuthal θ-direction to sweep a 2-D sector image; finally, the 2-D sector image carries out the elevation steering (phased-array technique) along the meridional ϕ-direction to end up with the pyramidal 3-D image dataset [132].

To overcome the technical bottleneck of inadequate scanning speed, the researchers at Philips Corporation have built upon Duke University's RT3D $16:1$ receive-mode parallel processing approach to implement more powerful $(32:1$, or even higher) parallel processing. This technology allows numerous ultrasound beams to be emitted simultaneously. With increasing pulse repetition frequency, the interval between successive pulses can increase in proportion to the parallel processing ratio; this expands the *depth* of the scanned pyramidal body region over which the ultrasound beams can perform azimuthal and meridional steering. Therefore, larger overall pyramidal volumes can be scanned and a *live 3D* image with line density equivalent to that of a 2-D echocardiographic image can

[30]The qualifiers *"live"* and *"real-time"* are sometimes used interchangeably [154].

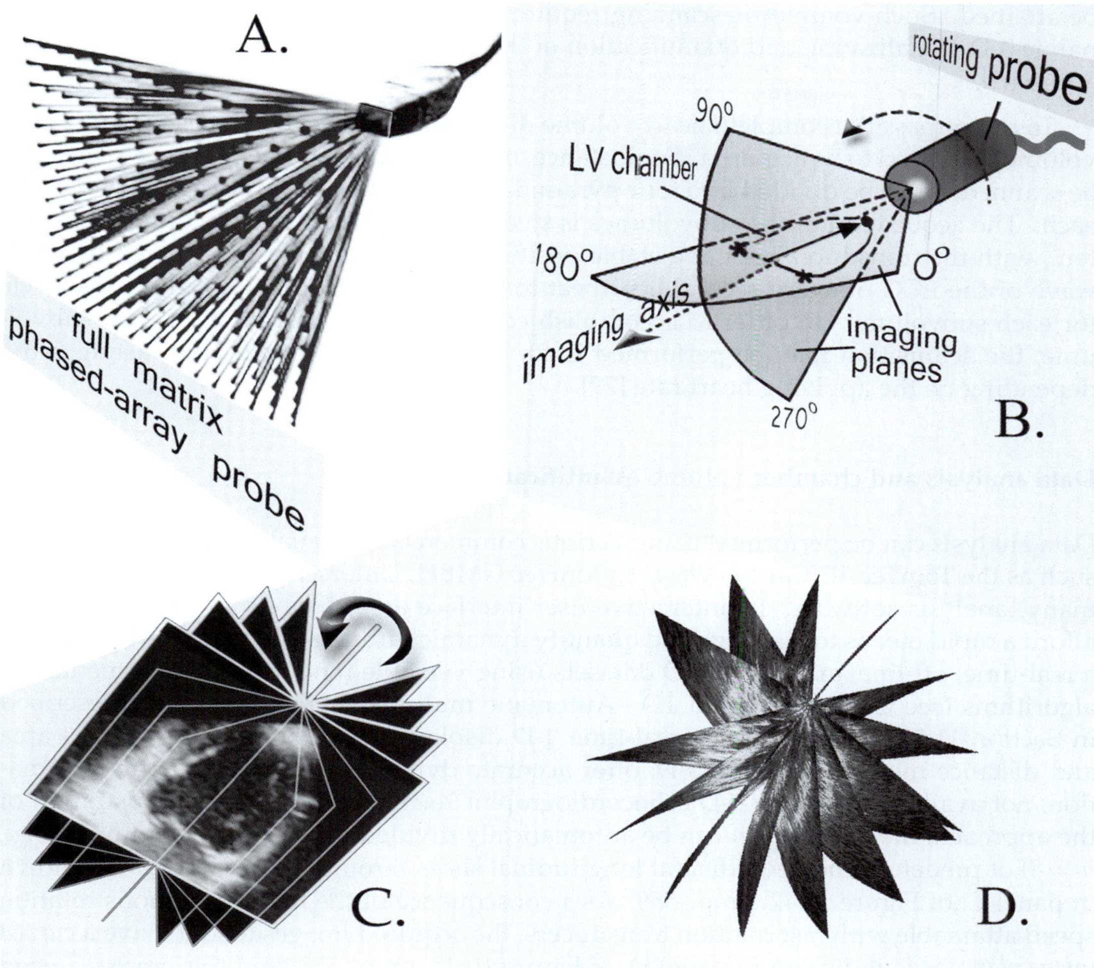

Figure 10.42: A. A full matrix phased-array probe allows acquisition and rendering of full volume data with excellent isotropic voxel resolution and at real-time 3-D frame rates; currently, matrix-array transducers incorporate several thousand imaging elements. B. The *conceptually different* rotating probe rotates in a 180° arc about its imaging axis acquiring multiple cross-sectional cuts for 3-D reconstruction. The terminal 180° placement of the imaging plane scans a mirrored image of the initial 0° position. In the transthoracic approach, for complete reconstruction of the left ventricle (LV), the probe is positioned close to the apex of the heart. The left ventricular (LV) apex and mitral valve (MV) ring are earmarked by a black dot and asterisks, respectively. The conventional long axis of the LV chamber is defined by the center of the MV ring and the LV apex, and may not be parallel to the imaging axis. C. A stack of eight rotated long-axis images of the LV chamber acquired at sequential, equidistant (22.5° apart) rotation points between the 0° and 180° azimuthal locations. D. As a consequence of the high continuous rotation speed with fast rotation transducers, the acquired images tend to have a *curved* image plane, requiring special acquisition and image processing techniques.

be attained. Such volumetric scanning requires no off-line reconstruction, enabling dynamic 3-D visualization and quantification of the heart in real time using a transthoracic approach.

To encompass the complete heart volume of interest into the 3-D dataset, a large scan volume may need to be acquired. For instance, if a pyramidal volume of $90° \times 80°$ needs to be scanned, it can be divided into four pyramidal subvolumes of approximately $90° \times 20°$ each. The acquisition of the subvolumes is steered electronically by the ultrasound system, with the transducer kept at a stable position. The acquisition is triggered by the R wave of the ECG of every second heartbeat to ensure acquisition of a full cardiac cycle for each subvolume. In order to accomplish correct spatial registration of each subvolume, the acquisition may be performed in an end-expiratory breath-hold lasting 6–8 s, depending on the applying heart rate [79].

Data analysis and chamber volume quantification

Data analysis can be performed using various commercially available software packages, such as the TomTec 4D Cardio-View™ (TomTec GMBH, Unterschleissheim-Munich, Germany) analysis software. Its interactive user interface as well as its powerful 3-D tools afford a rapid means to visualize and quantify dynamic cardiac structures in 3-D. It allows a real-time, off-line analysis of 4-D datasets using versatile rendering and segmentation algorithms (see Chapters 11 and 12). Automatic multiplanar reconstruction (described in Section 11.5, on pp. 594 ff.), real-time 4-D display, and volumetric as well as area and distance measurements in 3-D, offer accurate dynamic cardiac geometric information, not available with any 2-D echocardiographic technology. As a brief illustration of the approach, the 3-D dataset can be automatically divided into a variable number (e.g., $n = 8$) of predetermined equidistant longitudinal slices through the LV apex, as is shown in panel C. of Figure 10.42, on p. 559. As a consequence of the high continuous rotation speed attainable with fast rotation transducers, the acquired images tend to have a *curved image plane*, as is indicated in panel D. of Figure 10.42, on p. 559, and this creates a need for specialized acquisition and image processing techniques [147].

A recent study [151] has demonstrated that accurate LV chamber volume quantification is possible with 8 randomly selected equiangular long-axis images. Appropriate landmarks are identified. In each of the longitudinal slices a semiautomatic border detection algorithm is then used to track the endocardial borders throughout the cardiac cycle to obtain a dynamic *virtual cast* of the LV chamber, as well as instantaneous global and regional LV volume *vs.* time curves [79,138].

An alternative method of calculating ventricular chamber volumes from a real time 3-D cardiac volume dataset is using the Simpson's rule or disc summation method (see Section 2.14.3, on pp. 68 f.). With this method, many short-axis cut planes are obtained from base to apex using a predefined axial interval. In each short-axis slice, endocardial borders are detected and the summation of their volume contributions is used to calculate instantaneous ventricular chamber volume. For endocardial border detection, several semiautomatic, interactive methods are available, e.g., a *spline curve* fitting algorithm may be applied [20], allowing the definition of a smooth, closed contour by setting points on the endocardial border. Commercial software such as the Q-lab™ (Philips Company, Andover, MA) is available for the automated off-line calculation of ventricular volume, by implementation of the *summation disk* method [45].

Fast-rotating ultrasound transducer

Variable plane (multiplane) transducers using linear phased arrays driven by mechanical means have also been introduced for real-time data acquisition by several firms, including Hewlett Packard, Acuson, Toshiba, and others. The miniature transducer array is rotated mechanically (see panel B. of Fig. 10.42, on p. 559, and panel B. of Fig. 5.27, on p. 273), by means of a micro motor, inside the tip of the probe. It is either rotated backward and forward yielding volumetric information at 10–15 volumes/s, or continuously rotated at a speed of 8 rotations/s, which produces conical 3-D datasets at 16 volumes/s. If the transducer is rocked like a fan ("pivoted") in the elevation plane, the datasets will have a pyramidal structure. Both panels B. and C. in Figure 10.42, on p. 559, exemplify the propeller-like [100] geometry, in which the images intersect along the scanning axis. Rotation can be controlled either manually, by using forward and reverse buttons on the probe handle, or by system software. The latter generally allows incremental step setting and ECG gating regulation. Although originally not designed for 3-D image acquisition, this technology can be used for rapid, automated 3-D image collection, thanks to the incorporated software control.

The fast-rotating ultrasound (FRU) transducer developed at the Thorax-center of Erasmus University in Rotterdam, Holland [149, 151, 152], comprises a high precision rotary drive, a slip ring device,[31] and a 64-element phased array. The slip ring device consists of a rotating and a static part; it has 76 conducting slip ring connectors. Rotation, generated by the motor, is transferred to the rotating part of the slip ring and to the phased-array transducer. Key features of the transducer are its wide bandwidth, allowing harmonic imaging, and a feedback regulation for a highly constant rotation speed, which can be controlled manually. The harmonic imaging capability allows for improved endocardial border detection of the ventricular chambers (see Section 5.6, on p. 268 ff.). For acquisition of a 3-D dataset, the rotation speed is usually set at 4–8 rotations per second (*Hz*), corresponding to 240–480 *rpm*. 8 *Hz* results in 16 3-D datasets/s. Assuming a heart rate of 60 beats per minute, it is possible to acquire real-time 3-D data of the cardiac cycle with a temporal resolution of 16 3-D frames per beat, because a complete volumetric dataset can be obtained with a rotation of only $180°$.

The sector angle, number of scan lines per sector, scanning depth, the number of parallel beam formers, and the rotation speed, determine the spatiotemporal resolution that is attainable. The transducer is rotationally mounted in a TTE scanning device. At a certain scan depth, increasing the step angle will reduce the acquisition time but will at the same time increase the gaps between consecutive scan planes, resulting in *less dense* sampling of the volume. Moreover, since the scan lines *spread out*, distortions occur that must be

[31]See footnote on p. 498.

appropriately corrected by hybrid hardware–software means, and the resolution is poorer for deeper structures.

Since the beam width depends on the scan depth and scan angle, the image resolution will degrade at points *farther away* from the transducer and at larger scan angles (see Fig. 5.27B. on p. 273). Advanced parallel beamforming technology, however, improves the performance by a factor 2 to 4. The transducer is connected to a Vivid 5^{TM} platform (General Electric, VingMed, Horten, Norway) like a conventional phased array, but it can be used with any platform, as no special interfacing is required. In fact, the probe can be easily integrated in state-of-the-art 2-D echo systems because of its versatile and cost-effective design. The Vivid 5^{TM} platform allows accurate motor control, image synchronization, and fast 3-D dataset processing.

The acquisition time is approximately $10\,s$. After the real-time data acquisition, 3-D reconstruction takes less than $4\,s$. 4-D imaging is performed by showing a 3-D rectangular voxel space as function of time. The original dataset is conical and nonequidistantly sampled in space, as noted in the preceding paragraph. Furthermore, the scan planes are curved in space, an effect brought about by the continuous *rotation* of the transducer. Interpolation schemes have been developed for optimal 4-D image representation. 3-D reconstruction with volume and surface rendering can be performed off-line using various commercial software packages, such as the MassPlus^{TM} and EchoPAC Dimension^{TM} 3-D (GE Healthcare), and the TomTec 4D Cardio-View^{TM} (TomTec GMBH, Unterschleissheim-Munich, Germany) [79,151,152]; typical rendering times are less than $1\,min$.

The combination of short acquisition times, good spatiotemporal resolution characteristics, advanced quantification software, and the general advantages of ultrasonography make live 3-D echocardiography suitable for rapid determination of dynamic cardiac chamber geometry and function in the clinical and basic research settings, as well as in daily clinical practice [154]. This is true irrespective of whether the particular live 3-D echocardiography system employed involves an *electronic* real-time approach using 3-D matrix array transducers, or a *mechanical* real-time approach using a linear phased-array rotational transducer driven by mechanical means.

10.4.4 3-D Doppler echocardiography

A real-time 3-D color Doppler imaging system, was also developed, in conjunction with the RT3D, at the Duke University Center for Emerging Cardiovascular Technologies [135], and was marketed by Volumetrics Inc., Durham, NC. It utilized a 2-D matrix phased-array probe allowing electronic multidirectional steering and focusing for scanning of 3-D space in real time; the analogous *delay patterns* for a linear phased array in a 2-D situation are depicted schematically in Figure 10.43, on p. 563. To obtain reasonable volumetric frame rates, $16:1$ receive parallel processing was used with a spatial line density (step size) of $1° \times 1°$ in the azimuthal (θ) and the meridional (ϕ) coordinate directions (see Figures 10.37 and 10.38, on pp. 550 and 551, respectively). Using a 2.5-MHz probe with an aperture size of $14\,mm$, the axial and lateral resolutions were around $12\,mm$ and 34 mm, respectively.

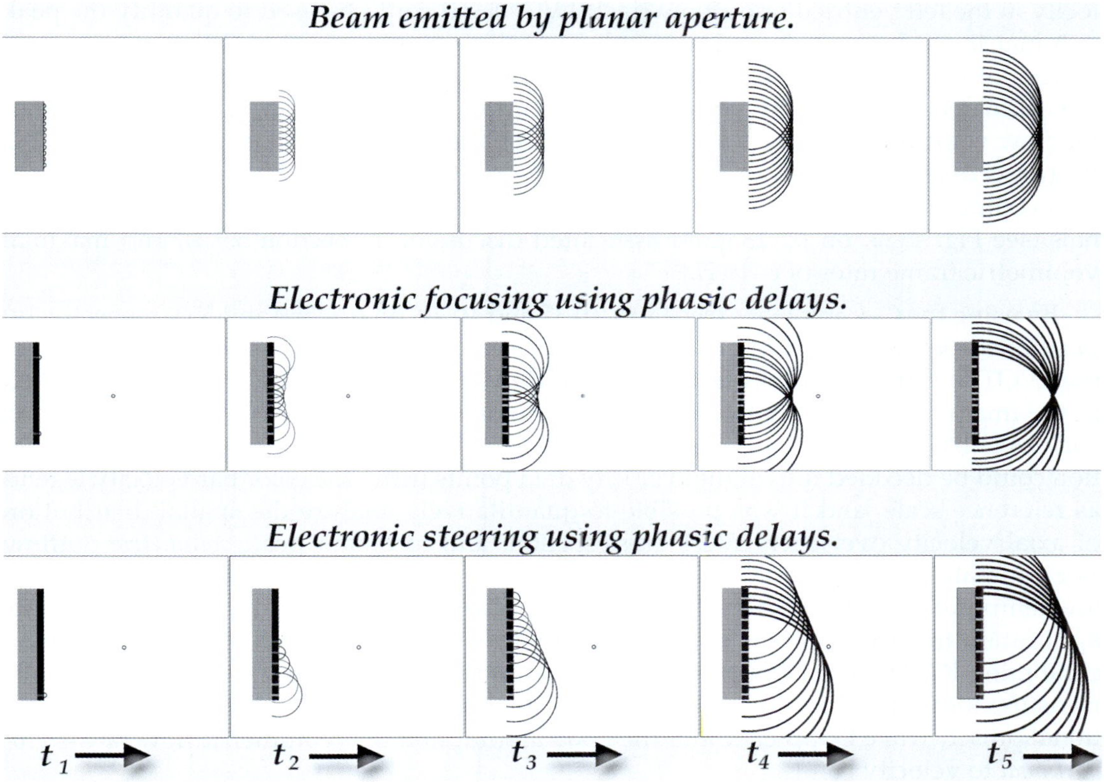

Figure 10.43: The front face of the transducer through which the ultrasound passes on its way to the body can be thought of as an *aperture* through which the ultrasound waves emerge. The physical principles of diffraction at an aperture apply here. Obviously, with too long an *aperture*, the beam would be too wide making the lateral resolution in localizing echo sources imprecise. With a narrow transducer (small in diameter compared to the wavelength, λ, of the ultrasound), the effects of diffraction as the ultrasound emerges from the narrow aperture would give a beam of expanding diameter. Doppler echoes could come from anywhere within the scope of this beam and their source would again be very imprecisely located. Top panels: A wider transducer (compared to λ) gives a directed beam, suffering less from the effects of diffraction. The resolution of ultrasound imaging is not as good as λ (0.1-1 mm), but with additional focusing mechanisms it is better than determined by the aperture alone. Middle panels: In a linear phased-array transducer, by firing off the individual array elements at different times (t_1, t_2, etc.), the wavefront of the beam can be shaped so that it focuses at any distance from the transducer array (i.e., any depth inside the patient). Bottom panels: Similarly, in a linear phased-array transducer, by firing off the individual array elements with appropriate electronically implemented delays, the wavefront of the beam can be steered in any desired direction.

The RT3D Doppler system could determine the 2-D spatial distributions of axial velocity in the left ventricular outflow tract (LVOT) and could be used to quantify the peak volumetric outflow rate by using simultaneously acquired real-time 3-D cross-sectional images of the LVOT. The Doppler interrogation angles had to be kept within 10° from the estimated axial velocity vector direction, implying less than 2% underestimation of the flow velocity due to the *cosine effect* (see Sections 5.9 and 5.9.3, on pp. 280 f. and 282 ff., respectively). Instrumental settings for the color Doppler were typically optimized for maximum gain without random noise, maximum wall filter to eliminate clutter signals (see Fig. 5.33, on p. 285 and associated discussion in Section 5.9.3), and maximal volumetric frame rates of 6–10 *Hz*.

By using the C-scan planes (see Figs. 10.37 and 10.40, on pp. 550 and 555, respectively) positioned perpendicular to the axial velocity vector, dynamic cross-sectional images of the LVOT at different depths from the LV apex to the base could be acquired and stored in the image memory buffer of the system. By using custom and commercial software, such as LabView™ (National Instruments, Austin, TX), color-encoded velocity information could be decoded into digital velocity data points using the color bar velocity legend as reference scale, and it was possible to quantitatively analyze the spatial distribution of axial velocity over each LVOT cross-section, and to obtain peak *volumetric* outflow rate estimates by commonly used numerical integration methods [145]. However, the low temporal resolution of the RT3D color Doppler system (6–10 frames/*s*) precluded its application to stroke volume measurements. This limitation could be circumvented by combining RT3D color Doppler-derived peak outflow rate estimates with simultaneous measurements of the outflow velocity-time integral and the peak velocity using conventional pulsed-wave Doppler, under the good assumption that volumetric flow rate is *proportional* to velocity [146].

The "live 3-D echocardiography" developments, which are described in the preceding section, have improved substantially the spatiotemporal resolution of 3-D Doppler echocardiography. The Philips "live 3D" system, which generates volumetric images "instantaneously," incorporates a Doppler modality that enables it to depict blood flow inside the heart in three dimensions. 3-D Doppler datasets can be acquired at up to 28−30 frames/*s*. The ability to extract hemodynamic information derived from 3-D color Doppler ultrasonography is currently being investigated [58]. To capture and analyze color flow imaging in 3-D, the area of interest should be obtained within the 3-D dataset, with the angle of the ultrasound beam aligned as parallel as possible to the direction of blood flow. Extraneous flows should be cropped to display only the flow region of interest, and depth and sector settings should be optimized for best *spatiotemporal* color Doppler resolution. The color Doppler flow patterns should be analyzed in multiple views to provide a comprehensive assessment of the data.

Limitations of 3-D Doppler echocardiography

It should be recognized that, despite the implications of the term "3-D Doppler," the method cannot actually provide measurements of the distribution of the 3-D velocity vectors in unsteady 3-D flow fields, such as those within the LV and RV chambers during

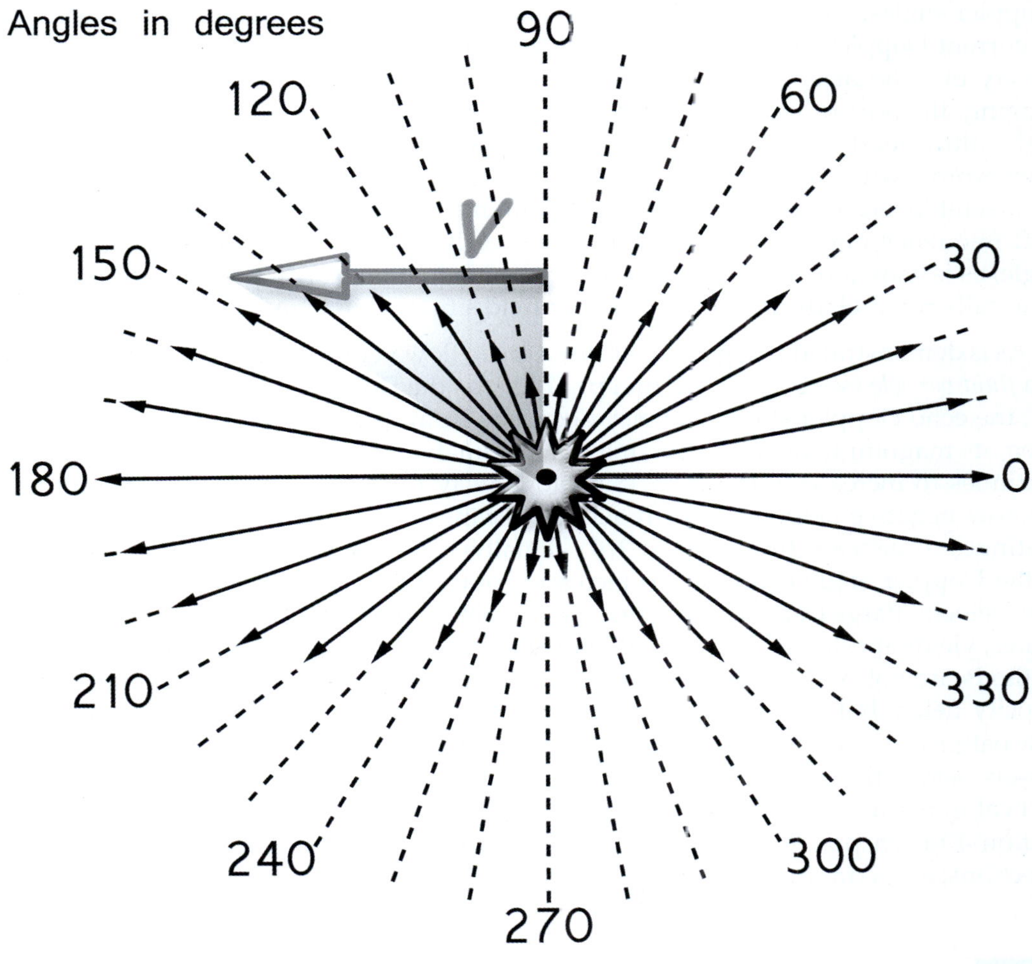

Figure 10.44: The instantaneous Doppler angle, i.e., the angle between the direction of the sound beam sent from a Doppler probe and the direction of the velocity of the red blood cells (ultrasound reflectors or "scatterers"), is shown in degrees (°) in the diagram for a relatively simple 2-D flow-field situation. The direction of the black arrows indicates the ultrasound beam direction. The length of the arrows indicates the magnitude of the measured Doppler shift for a given instantaneous flow velocity v (large translucent arrow) of a fluid particle (see discussion in text).

diastolic filling. The 3-D flow field of the LVOT considered in the preceding paragraphs is well-behaved in that the velocity vectors over the flow cross-section are *aligned* along the axial direction. The instantaneous 3-D velocity vectors in the diastolic vortical flows of the filling ventricles can generally be expected to be directed in different directions (Doppler angles, see Fig. 10.44, on p. 565) and to defy accurate quantitative measurement by current Doppler methods. In fact, the current position statement from the American Society of Echocardiography [58] is that: "To capture and analyze 3-D color Doppler imaging, the area of interest should be obtained within the 3-D dataset, with the angle of the ultrasound beam aligned as parallel as possible to *the direction* of blood flow." In other words, with current Doppler methods, imaging must be parallel to the direction of the instantaneous flow velocity vectors, to minimize the angle of insonation. The Doppler shift frequency depends strongly and nonlinearly (cosine dependence) on the Doppler angle, as is shown by the Doppler equation (see equation 5.3, on p. 280), and is depicted pictorially for a relatively simple 2-D flow-field situation in Figure 10.44.

As is demonstrated in Figure 10.44, for a given flow velocity v (large translucent arrow) of a *fluid particle* (see Section 4.3, on pp. 173 f.), as the Doppler angle increases from $0°$ to $90°$, the echo Doppler shift frequency decreases from its maximal positive value to zero. Then, its magnitude increases again to its maximal negative value, as the Doppler angle continues to increase from $90°$ to $180°$ (flow away from the probe). The magnitude of the now negative Doppler shift frequency declines to zero again, as the Doppler angle continues to increase from $180°$ to $270°$. Finally, it rises again to its positive maximum, as the Doppler angle continues to increase from $270°$ to $360°$ (or $0°$). Clearly, the same flow velocity (large translucent arrow, v) at a point of the flow field, insonated at different angles, yields spectacularly different Doppler shifts. Accordingly, current "3-D Doppler" methods are not only unsuitable for quantitative spatiotemporal evaluation of vectorial velocity fields, but are also prone to *misinterpretation* of complicated intracardiac blood flow patterns, as well as those coming about in curves, branches, bifurcations, and tortuous vessels, where the direction of the instantaneous flow velocity vectors may be helical or vortical in nature.[32] In addition, the presence of diseases and associated turbulence (see Section 4.14, on pp. 212 ff.) cause the blood to move in many different and tortuous directions, e.g., eddying motions.

10.5 Functional Imaging of unsteady, 3-D intracardiac flow patterns

The time-dependent, multidimensional, and multidirectional nature of intracardiac blood flows imposes overwhelming challenges not only in the acquisition and the presentation of velocity data, but also in the *conceptualization* of flow patterns. Relatively few medical researchers have the fluid dynamic background and understanding necessary in order

[32]To overcome these problems, various techniques for measuring 2- or 3-D velocity vectors (true velocity) in different settings have been proposed. These techniques fall into three main categories: speckle tracking, multiple transceivers, and projection computed velocimetry. They all have important limitations.

to observe and evaluate the significance and the multifaceted functional *implications* of multidirectional patterns of flow in health and disease. It is easier to conceptualize flow as linear and unidirectional, as is approximately admissible, e.g., for ejection flow along the LVOT.

As we saw in the preceding section, use of so-called 3-D Doppler ultrasound, able to measure the distribution over any flow cross-section of components of the velocity vector directed to or from the transducer, may have tended to foster *oversimplified* conceptions of intracardiac and great vessel flow fields. In fact, in common usage the term "flow pattern" generally connotes a *temporal* rather than a *spatial* distribution of blood flow velocities. 3-D color Doppler flow mapping is a technique that has provided more extensive information on intracardiac flow fields. But the unidirectionality of velocity acquisition and limited spatiotemporal resolution and quantitative accuracy compromise the effectiveness of the approach.

In many respects, magnetic resonance velocity mapping has capabilities beyond those of Doppler echocardiography, being capable of measuring velocities in voxels *throughout* a plane or volume of acquisition. Data can be acquired at any depth, unrestricted by windows of access. It also allows selection of the *direction* in which velocities are measured, either in or through the image plane, or both. At the present stage of development, magnetic resonance velocity mapping is the only imaging modality with the potential to acquire 4-D (3-D space and time) and 3-*directional* (the 3 orthogonal components of the velocity vector) velocity information. Even magnetic resonance phase-contrast velocity mapping, which is the most comprehensive available approach for investigation of spatiotemporal patterns of flow in the heart and great vessels is limited by constraints of acquisition times, and temporal and spatial resolution. Both hardware advancements, leading to faster and stronger gradients, and sequence optimizations, are still required in order to improve quantification of intracardiac flows.

Thus, at present, gaining relatively comprehensive information on velocities and local and convective velocity changes of blood within the intracardiac blood flow fields is a goal that can be achieved only through the application of computational fluid dynamics (CFD) methods to *simulations* of intracardiac flows, as is shown in Chapters 12-14 and 16. In the process, questions pertaining to the dynamics of these flows associated with the changing spatiotemporal velocity patterns in health and disease can be answered, and their implications on cardiac function and pathophysiology, as well as embryology and epigenetics (see Chapter 15), appreciated.

The imaging methods examined in this chapter provide the data which define the dynamic geometry of the cardiac chambers. To allow for accurate CFD simulations, it is necessary to prescribe the movement of the endocardial surface of the LV at a higher temporal resolution than that which can be acquired using the various currently available imaging techniques. For this purpose, various interpolation methods, and/or sonomicrometric implanted crystal techniques in animal experiments [113], can be used to create intermediate meshes. Following postprocessing of the raw imaging datasets and rendering of organ surfaces of interest, such as endocardial surfaces of cardiac chambers, the discretization, or *mesh generation* step then takes place; these processes are described in subsequent chapters. Mesh generation entails the placement of points that indicate subdivision locations on the curves and surfaces of flow fields that are to be simulated by CFD [40, 113]. These points, and information about how they are connected, define the various boundaries of the computation. The discretized flow-governing equations are then solved numerically on powerful computers, as is detailed in Chapters 12, 13, and 14. Then, special scientific visualization methods [40, 113–115] are applied to showing quantitatively the measured vector field (see Fig. 7.35, on p. 386). Such methods may display with shaded unity vectors the *directions* of the computed local velocities and can represent the velocity *magnitude* by a color or gray-scale coded map, as is used for color Doppler and MRI velocity mapping, but with high spatiotemporal resolution and accuracy.

A major advantage of the combined utilization of modern imaging, CFD and scientific visualization methods (see Fig. 2.38, on p. 103), which constitutes what I have previously termed the "Functional Imaging method," or FI [106, 113], is that much more extensive information can be extracted compared with clinical or experimental invasive or noninvasive imaging and hemodynamic measurements; FI yields values of the intracardiac and great vessel flow-field variables at literally *thousands of discrete points in space and time.* From this high-density information, we can extract informative snapshots of instantaneous velocity vector and pressure distributions [40, 113–115]. Even high-fidelity catheterization measurements obtained through multisensor (micromanometric/velocimetric) catheters, on the other hand, traditionally have been limited to global quantities (e.g., chamber "pressure" values) or to values at a small number of points in space and time. Thus Functional Imaging can reveal information on important intracardiac dynamic blood flow patterns and flow behavior that was previously *inaccessible.*

The Functional Imaging approach is already shifting the main thrust within cardiology from the assessment of disease through demonstration of changes in structure to assessing disease through changes in the fluid dynamics of cardiac pumping function [106,113–115]. The body of knowledge within cardiac pathology has largely provided the basis for the conventional anatomic approach. The new developments in imaging, particularly the use of computers in image acquisition and processing, and in CFD have fostered the emergence of the FI approach [113]. This new functional approach should not be viewed as competing with anatomic cardiac imaging but, rather, as *complementary*, because it allows visualization of cardiac function combining intracardiac flow information with the already proven benefits of anatomic imaging. At a time of increasing cost restraint within health care, FI also benefits from potentially fulfilling both approaches within one cardiac imaging examination and without the need of additional equipment, once the CFD simulation resource is in place.

Functional Imaging has come at a time when CFD has emerged as a major topic within cardiovascular investigations. Rather than being merely coincident, CFD and Functional Imaging are connected by the fact that alterations in cardiac muscle pumping activity are primarily expressed with changes in intracardiac (encompassing the roots of the great vessels) blood flow phenomena, which affect, e.g., endocardial/endothelial surface receptors and can be transduced into cellular and (global) cardiac shape and functional changes, through two *cooperating pathways*: by direct mechanical action on the cell structure, intermediated by a spatial reorganization of the *cytoskeleton*, and by chemical signaling (see Section 1.10, on pp. 23 ff.). This is a paradigm of *phenotypic plasticity*, an emerging powerful concept in biology that has stimulated a recent boom in research [33].

Phenotypic plasticity (see discussions in Sections 1.9 and 1.10, on pp. 20 ff., on p. 569, and in Section 15.6, on pp. 835 ff.) describes the capacity of a genotype to exhibit a range of phenotypes in response to variation in the environment [34]. In my view, this new concept of phenotypic plasticity has broad significance and appeal because it underscores and explains in a straightforward manner the importance of intracardiac blood flow phenomena for many normal and abnormal cardiac structural and functional adjustments, or *"adaptations,"* and for possible transitions to disease and heart failure [113–115]. Phenotypic plasticity in this context embraces genetics and development, and in its application to the heart, it ought to include fluid dynamics, computational physics, and physiology. This view reflects contemporary, new understanding that phenotypic plasticity is a powerful means of adaptation. Alternative alleles or their products react *differently* to the internal environment, which encompasses blood flow-related hydrodynamic shear stress patterns; this leads to adaptations that may or may not be *beneficial*. This mechanism produces flexible organisms that respond to environmental shifts with phenotypic changes; some of these phenotypic changes may *transition* to abnormal adaptations and disease; indeed, a well known example of cardiac phenotypic plasticity is the so-called *"cardiac remodeling."*[33] In other words, phenotypic plasticity can also be a liability. If a single phenotype is best in all circumstances, then environmentally induced deviation away from the best phenotype only reduces cardiac fitness and physical condition.

[33] *Remodeling* qualifies changes that result in a rearrangement of normally existing structures. Although remodeling does not necessarily define a pathological condition, myocardial remodeling is reversible up to a point and is commonly restricted to diseased conditions [140].

References and further reading

[1] Axel, L. Biomechanical dynamics of the heart with MRI. Ann. Rev. Biomed. Eng. 4: 321–47, 2002.

[2] Barry, R.L., Menon, R.S. Modeling and suppression of respiration-related physiological noise in echo-planar functional magnetic resonance imaging using global and one-dimensional navigator echo correction. Magn. Reson. Med. 54: 411–8, 2005.

[3] Basu, S., Bresler, Y. $O(N^2 \log N)$ filtered backprojection reconstruction algorithm for tomography. IEEE Trans. Image Process. 9: 1760–73, 2000.

[4] Bernstein, M.A., King, K.F., Zhou, X.J. Handbook of MRI pulse sequences. 2004, Burlington, MA: Elsevier Academic Press. xxii, 1017 p.

[5] Bogren, H.G., Buonocore, M.H., Valente, R.J. Four-dimensional magnetic resonance velocity mapping of blood flow patterns in the aorta in patients with atherosclerotic coronary artery disease compared to age-matched normal subjects. J. Magn. Reson. Imag. 19: 417–27, 2004.

[6] Brink, J.A., Heiken, J.P., Wang, G., McEnery, K.W., Schlueter, F.J., Vannier, M.W. Helical CT: principles and technical considerations. RadioGraphics 14: 887–93, 1994.

[7] Brown, M.A., Semelka, R.C. MRI: basic principles and applications. 3rd ed. 2003, Hoboken, NJ: Wiley-Liss. xiv, 265 p.

[8] Bryant, D., Payne, J., Firmin, D., Longmore, D. Measurement of flow with NMR using gradient pulse and phase difference techniques. J. Comput. Assist. Tomogr. 8: 588–93, 1984.

[9] Buzug, T.M. Computed tomography: from photon statistics to modern cone-beam CT. 2008, Berlin: Springer. xiii, 521 p.

[10] Canet, D., Boubel, J.-C., Soulas, E.C. La RMN: concepts, méthodes et applications. 2002, Paris: Dunod. x, 235 p.

[11] Castillo, E., Bluemke, D.A. Cardiac MR imaging. Radiol. Clin. North Am. 41: 17–28, 2003.

[12] Chai, P., Mohiaddin, R.H. How we perform cardiovascular magnetic resonance flow assessment using phase-contrast velocity mapping. J. Cardiovasc. Mag. Res. 7: 705–16, 2005.

[13] Chatzimavroudis, G., Oshinski, J., Franch, R., Walker, P., Yoganathan, A., Pettigrew, R. Evaluation of the precision of magnetic resonance phase velocity mapping for blood flow measurements. J. Cardiovasc. Mag. Res. 3: 11–9, 2001.

[14] Condos, W.R., Jr., Latham, R.D., Hoadley, S.D., Pasipoularides, A. Hemodynamics of the Mueller maneuver in man: right and left heart micromanometry and Doppler echocardiography. Circulation 76: 1020–8, 1987.

[15] Constantine, G., Shan, K., Flamm, S.D., Sivananthan, M.U. Role of MRI in clinical cardiology. Lancet 363: 2162-71, 2004.

[16] Corsi, C., Saracino, G., Sarti, A., Lamberti, C. Left ventricular volume estimation for real-time three-dimensional echocardiography. IEEE Trans. Med. Imag. 21: 1202-8, 2002.

[17] Cury, R.C., Nieman, K., Shapiro, M.D., Nasir, K., Cury, R.C., Brady, T.J. Comprehensive cardiac CT study: evaluation of coronary arteries, left ventricular function, and myocardial perfusion—is it possible? J. Nucl. Cardiol. 14: 229–43, 2007.

[18] Danias, P.G., Manning, W.J. MR navigators and their use in cardiac and coronary imaging. Chapter 2. In: Duerinckx, A.J. [Ed.] Coronary magnetic resonance angiography. 2002, New York: Springer. xv, 342 p.

[19] De Castro, S., Yao, J., Pandian, N.G. Three-dimensional echocardiography: clinical relevance and application. Am. J. Cardiol. 81(12A): 96G–102G, 1998.

[20] Dempski, K. Focus on curves and surfaces. 2002, Indianapolis, IN: Premier Press. 280 p.

[21] Di Carli, M.F., Kwong, R.Y. [Eds.] Novel techniques for imaging the heart: cardiac MR and CT. 2008, Chichester, West Sussex, UK; Hoboken, NJ: Wiley-Blackwell. xvi, 360 p.

[22] Dowsett, D.J., Kenny, P.A., Johnston, R.E. The physics of diagnostic imaging. 2nd ed. 2006, London: Hodder Arnold. xii, 725 p.

[23] Draney, M.T., Taylor, C.A. Experimental validation of computational simulation and magnetic resonance imaging of flow through a tapered tube. Proc. Am. Soc. Mechan. Engin., Bioengin. Div.(ASME-BED) Summer Bioeng. Meeting, Big Sky, MT, 42: 209–10, 1999.

[24] Dumoulin, C.L., Cline, H.E., Souza, S.P. Three-dimensional time-of-flight magnetic resonance angiography using spin saturation. Magn. Reson. Med. 11: 35–46, 1989.

[25] Earls, J.P., Ho, V.B., Foo, T.K., Castillo, E., Flamm, S.D. Cardiac MRI: recent progress and continued challenges. J. Magn. Reson. Imag. 16: 111–27, 2002.

[26] Edelman, R.R. Contrast-enhanced MR imaging of the heart: overview of the literature. Radiology 232: 653–68, 2004.

[27] Elster, A.D., Burdette, J.H. Questions and answers in magnetic resonance imaging. 2nd ed. 2001, St. Louis: Mosby. xiv, 333 p.

[28] Ensley, A., Ramuzat, A., Healy, T., Chatzimavroudis, G., Lucas, C., Sharma, S., Pettigrew, R., Yoganathan, A.P. Fluid mechanic assessment of the total cavopulmonary connection using magnetic resonance phase velocity mapping and digital particle image velocimetry. Ann. Biomed. Eng. 28: 1172–83, 2000.

[29] Feinstein, J.A., Epstein, F.H., Arai, A.E., Foo, T.K., Hartley, M.R., Balaban, R.S., Wolff, S.D. Using cardiac phase to order reconstruction (CAPTOR): a method to improve diastolic images. J. Mag. Res. Imag. 7: 794–8, 1997.

[30] Finn, J.P., Nael, K., Deshpande, V., Ratib, O., Laub, G. Cardiac MR imaging: state of the technology. Radiology 241: 338–54, 2006.

[31] Fischer, S.E., Wickline, S.A., Lorenz, C.H. Novel real-time R-wave detection algorithm based on the vectorcardiogram for accurate gated magnetic resonance acquisitions. Magn. Reson. Med. 42: 361–70, 1999.

[32] Flohr, T.G., McCollough, C.H., Bruder, H. Petersilka, M., Gruber, K., Süss, C., Grasruck, M., Stierstorfer, K., Krauss, B., Raupach, R., Primak, A.N., Küttner, A., Achenbach, S., Becker, C., Kopp, A., Ohnesorge, B.M. First performance evaluation of a dual-source CT (DSCT) system. Eur. Radiol. 16: 256–68, 2006.

[33] Flück, M. Functional, structural and molecular plasticity of mammalian skeletal muscle in response to exercise stimuli. J. Exp. Biol. 209: 2239–48, 2006.

[34] Fordyce, J.A. The evolutionary consequences of ecological interactions mediated through phenotypic plasticity. J. Exp. Biol. 209: 2377–83.

[35] Frayne, R., Steinman, D.A., Ethier, C.R., Rutt, B.K. Accuracy of MR phase contrast velocity measurements for unsteady flow. J. Magn. Reson. Imaging 5: 428–31, 1995.

[36] Fredrickson, J.O., Wegmüller, H., Herfkens, R.J., Pelc, N.J. Simultaneous temporal resolution of cardiac and respiratory motion in MR imaging. Radiology 195: 169–75, 1995.

[37] Gaba, R.C., Carlos, R.C., Weadock, W.J., Reddy, G.P., Sneider, M.B., Cascade, P.N. Cardiovascular MR imaging: technique optimization and detection of disease in clinical practice. RadioGraphics 22: e6–6e, 2002.

[38] Gatehouse, P.D., Firmin, D.N. The cardiovascular magnetic resonance machine: hardware and software requirements. Herz 25: 317–30, 2000.

[39] Gatehouse, P.D., Keegan, J., Crowe, L.A., Masood, S., Mohiaddin, R.H., Kreitner, K.F., Firmin, D.N. Applications of phase-contrast flow and velocity imaging in cardiovascular MRI. Eur. Radiol. 15: 2172–84, 2005.

[40] Georgiadis, J.G., Wang, M., Pasipoularides, A. Computational fluid dynamics of left ventricular ejection. Ann. Biomed. Eng. 20: 81–97, 1992.

[41] Geva, T., Sahn, D.J., Powell, A.J. Magnetic resonance imaging of congenital heart disease in adults. Prog. Pediatr. Cardiol. 17: 21–39, 2003.

[42] Graves, M.J., Berry, E., Eng, A.A., Westhead, M., Black, R.T., Beacock, D.J., Kelly, S., Niemi, P. A multicenter validation of an active contour-based left ventricular analysis technique. J. Magn. Reson. Imag. 12: 232–9, 2000.

[43] Greenberg, S.B., Sandhu, S.K. Ventricular function. Radiol. Clin. North Am. 37: 341–59, 1999.

[44] Greil, G.F., Germann, S., Kozerke, S., Baltes, C., Tsao, J., Urschitz, M.S., Seeger, A., Tangcharoen, T., Bialkowsky, A., Miller, S., Sieverding, L. Assessment of left ventricular volumes and mass with fast 3D cine steady-state free precession k-t space broad-use linear acquisition speed-up technique (k-t BLAST). J. Magn. Reson. Imaging 27: 510–5, 2008.

[45] Grison, A., Maschietto, N., Reffo, E., Stellin, G., Padalino, M., Vida, V., Milanesi, O. Three-dimensional echocardiographic evaluation of right ventricular volume and function in pediatric patients: validation of the technique. J. Am. Soc. Echocardiogr. 20: 921–9, 2007.

[46] Harris, L.D., Robb, R.A., Yuen, T.S., Ritman, E.L. Display and visualization of three-dimensional reconstructed anatomic morphology: experience with the thorax, heart and coronary vasculature of dogs. J. Comput. Assist. Tomogr. 3: 439–46, 1979.

[47] Hemmy, D.C., Lindquist, T.R. Optimizing 3D imaging techniques to meet clinical requirements. National Computer Graphics Association, Conference Proceedings, Technical Sessions, pp. 69–80, 1987.

[48] Herman, G.T., Liu, H.K. Display of three dimensional information in computed tomography. J. Comput. Assist. Tomogr. 1: 155–60, 1977.

[49] Herman, G.T. Image reconstruction from projections: the fundamentals of computerized tomography. 1980, New York: Academic Press. xiv, 316 p.

[50] Higgins, C.B., Roos, A.d. [Eds.] MRI and CT of the cardiovascular system. 2nd ed. 2006, Philadelphia, PA: Lippincott Williams & Wilkins. 656 p.

[51] Higgins, C.B., Roos, A.d. [Eds.] Cardiovascular MRI and MRA. 2003, Philadelphia, PA: Lippincott Williams & Wilkins. x, 496 p.

[52] Hill, J.M., Dick, A.J., Raman, V.K., Thompson, R.B, Yu, Z., Hinds, K.A., Pessanha, B.S.S., Guttman, M.A., Varney, T.R., Martin, B.J., Dunbar, C.E., McVeigh, E.R., Lederman, R.J. Serial cardiac magnetic resonance imaging of injected mesenchymal stem cells. Circulation 108: 1009–14, 2003.

[53] Hofer, M. CT-Kursbuch, Ein Arbeitsbuch für den Einstieg in die Computertomographie. 5th ed. 2006, Düsseldorf: Didamed-Verlag. 224 p.

[54] Hoffman, E.A., Ritman, E.L. Invariant total heart volume in the intact thorax. Am. J. Physiol. 249: H883–90, 1985.

[55] Hoffman, E.A., Ritman, E.L. Shape and dimensions of cardiac chambers: importance of CT section thickness and orientation. Radiology 155: 739–44, 1985.

[56] Hombach, V. Kardiovaskuläre Magnetresonanztomographie: Kursbuch und Repetitorium. 2006, Stuttgart; New York: Schattauer. 196 p.

[57] Horiguchi, J., Nakanishi, T., Tamura, A., Ito, K., Sasaki, K., Shen, Y. Technical innovation of cardiac multirow detector CT using multisector reconstruction. Comput. Med. Imag. Graph. 26: 217–26, 2002.

[58] Hung, J., Lang, R., Flachskampf, F., et al. 3D echocardiography: a review of the current status and future directions (ASE position paper). J. Am. Soc. Echocardiogr. 20: 213–33, 2007.

[59] Hurlock, G.S., Higashino, H., Mochizuki, T. History of cardiac computed tomography: single to 320-detector row multislice computed tomography. Int. J. Cardiovasc. Imag. Jan. 15, 2009.

[60] Ibrahim, el-S.H., Stuber, M., Fahmy, A.S., Abd-Elmoniem, K.Z., Sasano, T., Abraham, M.R., Osman, N.F. Real-time MR imaging of myocardial regional function using strain-encoding (SENC) with tissue through-plane motion tracking. J. Magn. Reson. Imag. 26: 1461–70, 2007.

[61] Kajander, S., Ukkonen, H., Sipila, H., Teras, M., Knuuti, J. Low radiation dose imaging of myocardial perfusion and coronary angiography with a hybrid PET/CT scanner. Clin. Physiol. Funct. Imag. 29: 81–8, 2009.

[62] Kalender, W.A. Principles and applications of spiral CT. Nucl. Med. Biol. 21: 693–9, 1994.

[63] Kalender, W.A. Thin-section three-dimensional spiral CT: is isotropic imaging possible? Radiology 197: 578–80, 1995.

[64] Kalender, W.A. Computer-tomographie. Grundlagen, Geratetechnologie, Bildqualitat, Anwendungen. 2000, Munchen: Publicis MCD Verlag. 216 p.

[65] Kalender, W.A. CT: the unexpected evolution of an imaging modality. Eur. Radiol. 15 Suppl. 4: D21–4, 2005.

[66] Kalender, W.A., Seissler, W., Klotz, E., Vock, P. Spiral volumetric CT with single-breathhold technique, continuous transport, and continuous scanner rotation. Radiology 176: 181–3, 1990.

[67] Kalender, W.A., Polacin, A. Physical performance characteristics of spiral CT scanning. Med. Phys. 18: 910–5, 1991.

[68] Karaus, A., Merboldt, K.-D., Graessner, J., Frahm, J. Black-blood imaging of the human heart using rapid stimulated echo acquisition mode (STEAM) MRI. 26: 1666–71, 2007.

[69] Keller, P.J., Saloner, D. Time-of-flight flow imaging. In: Potchen, E.J., Haacke, E.M., Siebert, J.E., Gottschalk, A. [Eds.] Magnetic resonance angiography: concepts and applications. 1993, St. Louis: Mosby Year Book. pp. 146–59.

[70] Keltner, J.R., Roos, M.S., Brakeman, P.R., Budinger, T.F. Magnetohydrodynamics of blood flow. Magn. Reson. Med. 16: 139–49, 1990.

[71] Kikuchi , Y. Present aspects of "ultrasonotomography" for medical diagnostics. In: Stroke, G.W. [Ed.] Ultrasonic imaging and holography: medical, sonar, and optical applications. 1974, New York, London: Plenum Press. pp. 229–86.

[72] Kilner, P.J., Yang, G.Z., Wilkes, A.J., Mohiaddin, R.H., Firmin, D.N., Yacoub, M.H. Asymmetric redirection of flow through the heart. Nature 404: 759–61, 2000.

[73] Kim, W.Y., Walker, P.G., Pedersen, E.M., Poulsen, J.K., Oyre, S., Houlind, K., Yoganathan, A.P. Left ventricular blood flow patterns in normal subjects: a quantitative analysis by three-dimensional magnetic resonance velocity mapping. J. Am. Coll. Cardiol. 26: 224–38, 1995.

[74] Kinouchi, Y., Yamaguchi, H., Tenforde, T.S. Theoretical analysis of magnetic field interactions with aortic blood flow. Bioelectromagnetics 17: 21–32, 1996.

[75] Klipstein, R.H., Firmin, D.N., Underwood, S.R., Nayler, G.L., Rees, R.S., Longmore, D.B. Colour display of quantitative blood flow and cardiac anatomy in a single magnetic resonance cine loop. Br. J. Radiol. 60: 105–11, 1987.

[76] Kohl, G. The evolution and state-of-the-art principles of multislice computed tomography. Proc. Am. Thorac. Soc. 2: 470–6, 2005.

[77] Krasinski, A., Chiu, B., Fenster, A., Parraga, G. Magnetic resonance imaging and three-dimensional ultrasound of carotid atherosclerosis: mapping regional differences. J. Magn. Reson. Imag. 29: 901–8, 2009.

[78] Ku, D., Biancheri, C., Pettigrew, R.I., Peifer, J., Markou, C., Engels, H. Evaluation of magnetic resonance velocimetry for steady flow. J. Biomech. Eng. 112: 464–72, 1990.

[79] Kühl, H.P., Schreckenberg, M., Rulands, D., Katoh, M., Schäfer, W., Schummers, G., Bücker, A., Hanrath, P., Franke, A. High-resolution transthoracic real-time three-dimensional echocardiography: quantitation of cardiac volumes and function using semi-automatic border detection and comparison with cardiac magnetic resonance imaging. J. Am. Coll. Cardiol. 43: 2083–90, 2004.

[80] Kupari, M., Jarvinen, V., Poutanen, V.P., Hekali, P. Skewness of instantaneous mitral transannular flow-velocity profiles in normal humans. Am. J. Physiol. Heart Circ. Physiol. 268: H1232–8, 1995.

[81] McCollough, C.H., Zink, F.E. Performance evaluation of a multi-slice CT system. Med. Physics 26: 2223–30, 1999.

[82] Laine, A.F. Wavelets in temporal and spatial processing of biomedical images. Annu. Rev. Biomed. Eng. 2: 511–50, 2000.

[83] Larson, A.C., White, R.D., Laub, G., McVeigh, E.R., Li, D., Simonetti, O.P. Self-gated cardiac cine MRI. Magn. Reson. Med. 51: 93–102, 2004.

[84] Lee, V.S. Cardiovascular MRI: physical principles to practical protocols. 2006, Philadelphia, PA: Lippincott Williams & Wilkins. xiv, 402 p.

[85] Lewin J.S., Laub G., Hausmann R. Three-dimensional time-of-flight MR angiography: applications in the abdomen and thorax. Radiology 179: 261–4, 1991.

[86] Light, E.D., Davidsen, R.E., Fiering, J.O., Hruschka, T.A., Smith, S.W. Progress in 2-D arrays for real-time volumetric imaging. Ultrason. Imag. 20: 1–16, 1998.

[87] Lombardi, M., Aquaro, G., Favilli, B. Contrast media in cardiovascular magnetic resonance. Curr. Pharm. Des. 11: 2151–61, 2005.

[88] Lotz, J., Meier, C., Leppert, A., Galanski, M. Cardiovascular flow measurement with phase-contrast MR imaging: basic facts and implementation. RadioGraphics 22: 651–71, 2002.

[89] Mahesh, M. The AAPM/RSNA physics tutorial for residents: search for isotropic resolution on CT from conventional through multiple-row detector. RadioGraphics 22: 949–62, 2002.

[90] Marabotti, C., Bedini, R., L'Abbate, A. Right ventricular volume determination: not a matter for echocardiography. J. Appl. Physiol. 104: 1547, 2008.

[91] Marabotti, C., L'Abbate, A., Bedini, R. Cardiac changes after SCUBA diving: the evasive shape of right ventricle. J. Physiol. (Lond.) 583: 405, 2007.

[92] McInerney T., Terzopoulos D. Deformable models in medical image analysis: a survey. Med. Image Anal. 1: 91–108, 1996.

[93] Mochizuki, T., Murase, K., Higashino, H., Koyama, Y., Doi, M., Miyagawa, M., Nakata, S., Shimizu, K., Ikezoe, J. Two- and three-dimensional CT ventriculography: a new application of helical CT. Am. J. Roentgenol. 174: 203–8, 2000.

[94] Mohiaddin, R.H., Gatehouse, P.D., Henien, M., Firmin, D.N. Cine MR Fourier velocimetry of blood flow through cardiac valves: comparison with Doppler echocardiography. J. Magn. Reson. Imag. 7: 657–63, 1997.

[95] Mohiaddin, R.H., Yang, G.Z., Kilner, P.J. Visualization of flow by vector analysis of multidirectional cine magnetic resonance velocity mapping. J. Comput. Assist. Tomogr. 18: 382–92, 1994.

[96] Mohiaddin R.H. Flow patterns in the dilated ischaemic left ventricle studied by magnetic resonance imaging with velocity vector mapping. J. Mag. Reson. Imag. 5: 493–8, 1995.

[97] Moser, E., Trattnig, S. 3.0 Tesla MR Systems [Editorial]. Invest. Radiol. 38: 375–6, 2003.

[98] Nayak, K.S., Pauly, J.M., Kerr, A.B., Hu, B.S., Nishimura, D.G. Real-time color flow MRI. Magn. Reson. Med. 43: 251–8, 2000.

[99] Nayler, G., Firmin, D., Longmore, D. Blood flow imaging by cine magnetic resonance. J. Comput. Assist. Tomogr. 10: 715–22, 1986.

[100] Nelson, T.R., Downey, D.B., Pretorius, D.H., Fenster, A. Three-Dimensional Ultrasound. 1999, Philadelphia, New York, Baltimore: Lippincott Williams & Wilkins. xii, 252 p.

[101] Ohnesorge, B.M., Flohr, T.G., Becker, C.R., Reiser, M.F. Multi-slice CT in cardiac imaging: technical principles, clinical application, and future developments. 2002, Berlin; New York: Springer. vi, 120 p.

[102] O'Rourke, R.A., Brundage, B.H., Froelicher, V.F., Greenland, P., Grundy, S.M., Hachamovitch, R., et al. American College of Cardiology/American Heart Association Expert Consensus document on electron-beam computed tomography for the diagnosis and prognosis of coronary artery disease. Circulation 102: 126–40, 2000.

[103] Orakzai, S.H., Orakzai, R.H., Nasir, K., Budoff, M.J. Assessment of cardiac function using multidetector row computed tomography. J. Comput. Assist. Tomogr. 30: 555–63, 2006.

[104] Paelinck, B.P., Lamb, H.J., Bax, J.J., Van der Wall, E.E., de Roos, A. Assessment of diastolic function by cardiovascular magnetic resonance. Am. Heart J. 144: 198–205, 2002.

[105] Paschal, C.B., Morris, H.D. K-space in the clinic. J. Cardiovasc. Magn. Reson. 19: 145–59, 2004.

[106] Pasipoularides, A. Invited commentary: Functional imaging (FI) combines imaging datasets and computational fluid dynamics to simulate cardiac flows. J. Appl. Physiol. 105: 1015, 2008.

[107] Pasipoularides, A., Mirsky, I., Hess, O.M., Krayenbuehl, H.P. Incomplete relaxation and passive diastolic muscle properties in man. Circulation 62: Supplement III-205, 1980.

[108] Pasipoularides, A., Mirsky, I., Hess, O.M., Grimm, J., Krayenbuehl, H.P. Myocardial relaxation and passive diastolic properties in man. Circulation 74: 991–1001, 1986.

[109] Pasipoularides, A., Mirsky, I. Models and concepts of diastolic mechanics: pitfalls in their misapplication. Math. Comput. Modelling 11: 232–4, 1988.

[110] Pasipoularides, A., Palacios, I., Frist, W., Rosenthal, S., Newell, J.B., Powell, W.J., Jr. Contribution of activation-inactivation dynamics to the impairment of relaxation in hypoxic cat papillary muscle. Am. J. Physiol. 248: R54–62, 1985.

[111] Pasipoularides, A.D., Shu, M., Shah, A., Glower, D.D. Right ventricular diastolic relaxation in conscious dog models of pressure overload, volume overload and ischemia. J. Thorac. Cardiovasc. Surg. 124: 964–72, 2002.

[112] Pasipoularides, A., Shu, M., Shah, A., Silvestry, S., Glower, D.D. Right ventricular diastolic function in canine models of pressure overload, volume overload and ischemia. Am. J. Physiol. Heart Circ. Physiol. 283: H2140–50, 2002.

[113] Pasipoularides, A.D., Shu, M., Womack, M.S., Shah, A., von Ramm, O., Glower, D.D. RV functional imaging: 3-D echo-derived dynamic geometry and flow field simulations. Am. J. Physiol. Heart Circ. Physiol. 284: H56–65, 2003.

[114] Pasipoularides, A., Shu, M., Shah, A., Womack, M.S., Glower, D.D. Diastolic right ventricular filling vortex in normal and volume overload states. Am. J. Physiol. Heart Circ. Physiol. 284: H1064–72, 2003.

[115] Pasipoularides, A., Shu, M., Shah, A., Tucconi, A., Glower, D.D. RV instantaneous intraventricular diastolic pressure and velocity distributions in normal and volume overload awake dog disease models. Am. J. Physiol. Heart Circ. Physiol. 285: H1956–65, 2003.

[116] Pattynama P.M., Lamb H.J., van der Velde E.A., van der Wall E.E., de Roos A. Left ventricular measurements with cine and spin echo MRI: a study of reproducibility with variance component analysis. Radiology 187: 261–8, 1993.

[117] Pelc, N.J., Herfkens, R.J., Shimakawa, A., Enzmann, D.R. Phase contrast cine magnetic resonance imaging. Magn. Reson. Q. 7: 229–54, 1991.

[118] Radon, J. Über die Bestimmung von Funktionen durch ihre Integralwerte längs gewisser Mannigfaltigkeiten. Berichte über die Verhandlungen der Königlich Sächsischen Gesellschaft der Wissenschaften zu Leipzig, Mathematisch-Physikalische Klasse 69: 262–77, 1917.

[119] Ranganath S. Contour extraction from cardiac MRI studies using snakes. IEEE Trans. Med. Imag. 14: 328–38, 1995.

[120] Reiser, M.F., Takahashi, M., Modic, M., Becker, C.R. [Eds]. Multislice CT. 2nd edn. 2004, Berlin; Heidelberg; New York: Springer-Verlag. x, 280 p.

[121] Rerkpattanapipat, P., Mazur, W., Link, K.M., Hundley, W.G. Assessment of cardiac function with MR imaging. Magn. Reson. Imag. Clin. N. Am. 11: 67–80, 2003.

[122] Riederer, S.J., Wright, R.C., Ehman, R.L., Rossman, P.J., Holsinger-Bampton, A.E., Hangiandreou, N.J., Grimm, R.C. Real-time interactive color flow MR imaging. Radiology 181: 33–9, 1991.

[123] Ritman, E.L., Harris, L.D., Padiyar, R., Chevalier, P.A., Robb, R.A. Non-invasive visualization and quantitation of cardiovascular structure and function. Physiologist 22: 39–43, 1979.

[124] Ritman, E.L., Kinsey, J.H., Robb, R.A., Harris, L.D., Gilbert, B.K. Physics and technical considerations in the design of the DSR: a high temporal resolution volume scanner. Am. J. Roentgenol. 134: 369–74, 1980.

[125] Ritman, E.L., Kinsey, J.H., Robb, R.A., Gilbert, B.K., Harris, L.D., Wood, E.H. Three-dimensional imaging of heart, lungs, and circulation. Science 210(4467): 273–80, 1980.

[126] Robertson, M., Kohler, U., Hoskins, P., Marshall, I. Quantitative analysis of PC MRI velocity maps: pulsatile flow in cylindrical vessels. Magn. Reson. Imag. 19: 685–95, 2001.

[127] Roussakis, A., Baras, P., Seimenis, I., Andreou, J., Danias, P.G. Relationship of number of phases per cardiac cycle and accuracy of measurement of left ventricular volumes, ejection fraction, and mass. J. Cardiov. Mag. Reson. 6: 837–44, 2004.

[128] Rybicki, F.J., Otero, H.J., Steigner, M.L., Vorobiof, G., Nallamshetty, L., Mitsouras, D., Ersoy, H., Mather, R.T., Judy, P.F., Cai, T., Coyner, K., Schultz, K., Whitmore, A.G., Di Carli, M.F. Initial evaluation of coronary images from 320-detector row computed tomography. Int. J. Cardiovasc. Imag. 24: 535–46, 2008.

[129] Sampath, S., Prince, J.L. Automatic 3D tracking of cardiac material markers using slice-following and harmonic-phase MRI. Magn. Reson. Imaging. 25: 197–208, 2007.

[130] Serway, R.A., Jewett, J.W. Physics for scientists and engineers. 7th ed. 2006, Belmont, CA, Thomson Brooks/Cole. 1 v. (various pagings).

[131] Shiota, T. [Ed.] 3D echocardiography. 2007, London, Boca Raton, FL: Informa Healthcare, CRC Press. ix, 166 p.

[132] Shung, K.K. The principle of multidimensional arrays. Eur. J. Echocardiog. 3: 149–53, 2002.

[133] Siegel, J., Oshinski, J., Pettigrew, R., Ku, D. The accuracy of magnetic resonance phase velocity measurements in stenotic flow. J. Biomech. 29: 1665–72, 1996.

[134] Smith, S.W., Pavy, H.E., von Ramm, O.T. High speed ultrasound volumetric imaging system—Part I. Transducer design and beam steering. IEEE Trans. Ultrason. Ferroelec. Freq. Control 38: 100–8, 1991.

[135] Smith, S.W., Trahey, G.E., von Ramm, O.T. Two-dimensional arrays for medical ultrasound. Ultrason. Imaging 14: 213–33, 1992.

[136] Sondergaard, L., Stahlberg, F., Thomsen, C. Magnetic resonance imaging of valvular heart disease. J. Mag. Res. Imag. 10: 627–38, 1999.

[137] Steigner, M.L., Otero, H.J., Cai, T., Mitsouras, D., Nallamshetty, L., Whitmore, A.G., Ersoy, H., Levit, N.A., Di Carli, M.F., Rybicki, F.J. Narrowing the phase window width in prospectively ECG-gated single heart beat 320-detector row coronary CT angiography. Int. J. Cardiovasc. Imag. 25: 85–90, 2009.

[138] Sugeng, L., Weinert, L., Lang, R.M. Left ventricular assessment using real time three dimensional echocardiography. Heart 89(Suppl III): iii29–36, 2003.

[139] Suh D.Y., Eisner R.L., Mesereau R.M., Pettigrew R.I. Knowledge based system for boundary detection of four-dimensional cardiac MR image sequences. IEEE Trans. Med. Imag. 12: 65–72, 1993.

[140] Swynghedauw, B. Phenotypic plasticity of adult myocardium: molecular mechanisms. J. Exp. Biol. 209: 2320–7, 2006.

[141] Szolar, D.H., Sakuma, H., Higgins, C.B. Cardiovascular applications of magnetic resonance flow and velocity measurements. J. Mag. Res. Imag. 6: 78–89, 1996.

[142] Tan, R.S., Mohiaddin, R.H. Cardiovascular applications of magnetic resonance flow measurement. Rays 26: 71–91, 2001.

[143] Tatli, S., Lipton, M.J., Davison, B.D., Skorstad, R.B., Yucel, E.K. From the RSNA refresher courses: MR imaging of aortic and peripheral vascular disease. RadioGraphics 23: S59–78, 2003.

[144] Thompson, R.B., McVeigh, E.R. Flow-gated phase-contrast MRI using radial acquisitions. Magn. Reson. Med. 52: 598–604, 2004.

[145] Tsujino, H., Jones, M., Shiota, T., et al. Real-time three-dimensional color Doppler echocardiography for characterizing the spatial velocity distribution and quantifying the peak flow rate in the left ventricular outflow tract. Ultrasound Med. Biol. 27: 69–74, 2001.

[146] Tsujino, H., Jones, M., Qin, J.X., et al. Combination of pulsed-wave Doppler and real-time three-dimensional color Doppler echocardiography for quantifying the stroke volume in the left ventricular outflow tract. Ultrasound Med. Biol. 30: 1441–6, 2004.

[147] Van Stralen, M., Bosch, J.G., Voormolen, M.M., Van Burken, G., Krenning, B.J., Van Geuns, R.-J.M., Lancée, C.T., de Jong, N., Reiber, J.H.C. Left ventricular volume estimation in cardiac three-dimensional ultrasound: a semiautomatic border detection approach. Acad. Radiol. 12: 1241–9, 2005.

[148] von Ramm, O.T., Smith, S.W., Pavy, H.E. High speed ultrasound volumetric imaging system—Part II. Parallel processing and display. IEEE Trans. Ultrason. Ferroelec. Freq. Control 38: 109–15, 1991.

[149] van Stralen, M., Bosch, J.G., Voormolen, M.M., et al. Left ventricular volume estimation in cardiac three-dimensional ultrasound: a semiautomatic border detection approach. Acad. Radiol. 12: 1241–9, 2005.

[150] Talagala, S.L., Lowe, I.J. Introduction to magnetic resonance imaging. Conc. Magn. Reson. 3: 145–59, 1991.

[151] Voormolen, M.M., Krenning, B.J., van Geuns, R.-J., et al. Efficient quantification of the left ventricular volume using 3-dimensional echocardiography: the minimal number of equiangular long-axis images for accurate quantification of the left ventricular volume. J. Am. Soc. Echocardiogr. 20: 373–80, 2007.

[152] Voormolen, M.M., Krenning, B.J., Lancee, C.T., et al. Harmonic 3D echocardiography with a fast rotating ultrasound transducer. IEEE Trans Ultrason Ferroelectr Freq Control 53: 1739–48, 2006.

[153] Walker, P.G., Cranney, G.B., Grimes, R.Y., Delatore, J., Rectenwald, J., Pohost, G.M., Yoganathan, A.P. Three-dimensional reconstruction of the flow in a human left heart by magnetic resonance phase velocity encoding. Ann. Biomed. Eng. 24: 139–47, 1996.

[154] Wang, X.-F., Deng, Y.-B., Nanda, N.C., Deng, J., Miller, A.P., Xie, M.-X. Live three-dimensional echocardiography: imaging principles and clinical application. Echocardiography 20: 593–604, 2003.

[155] Wang, Y., Riederer, S.J., Ehman, R.L. Respiratory motion of the heart: kinematics and the implications for the spatial resolution in coronary imaging. Magn. Reson. Med. 33: 713–9, 1995.

[156] Weishaupt, D., Köchli, V.D., Marincek, B. How does MRI work? An introduction to the physics and function of magnetic resonance imaging. 2nd edn. 2006, Berlin; New York: Springer. x, 169 p.

[157] Wintersperger, B.J., Reeder, S.B., Nikolaou, K., Dietrich, O., Huber, A., Greiser, A., Lanz, T., Reiser, M.F., Schoenberg, S.O. Cardiac CINE MR imaging with a 32-channel cardiac coil and parallel imaging: impact of acceleration factors on image quality and volumetric accuracy. J. Magn. Reson. Imaging 23: 222–7, 2006.

[158] Wolbarst, A.B. Physics of radiology. 1993, Norwalk, CN: Appleton & Lange. xiii, 461 p.

[159] Wyatt, D.G. Blood flow and blood velocity measurement in vivo by electromagnetic induction. Trans. Inst. Meas. Control 4: 61–78, 1982.

[160] Yang, G.Z., Burger, P., Kilner, P.J., Karwatowski, S.P., Firmin, D.N. Dynamic range extension of cine velocity measurements using motion-registered spatiotemporal phase unwrapping. J. Magn. Reson. Imag. 6: 495–502, 1996.

[161] Zhang, H., Halliburton, S., Moore, J., Simonetti, O., Schvartzman, P., White, R., Chatzimavroudis, G. Accurate quantification of steady and pulsatile flow with segmented k-space magnetic resonance velocimetry. Exp. Fluids 33: 458–63, 2002.

[162] Zhong, L., Tan, R.-S., Ghista, D.N., Ng, E.Y.-K., Chua, L.-P., Kassab, G.S. Validation of a novel noninvasive cardiac index of left ventricular contractility in patients. Am. J. Physiol. Heart Circ. Physiol. 292: 2764–72, 2007.

[163] Zhong, L., Sola, S., Tan, R.-S., Le, T.-T. , Ghista, D.N., Kurra, V., Navia, J. L., Kassab, G.S. Effects of surgical ventricular restoration on left ventricular contractility assessed by a novel contractility index in patients with ischemic cardiomyopathy. Am. J. Cardiol. 103: 674–9, 2009.

Chapter 11

Postprocessing Exploration Techniques and Display of Tomographic Data

[...] We shall not cease from exploration
And the end of all our exploring
Will be to arrive where we started
And know the place for the first time.

—From the Quartet No. 4, *Little Gidding.*
——Eliot, T. S. *Four quartets.*, Harcourt Brace Jovanovich, A Harvest book, New York, 1971.

The Allegory of the Cave can be found in Book VII of Plato's best-known work, *The Republic*, a lengthy dialog on the nature of justice [42].

11.1 Plato's cave and modern 3-D imaging modalities

In the present context, Plato envisaged our perceptions as being like those of prisoners confined since their childhood in shackles deep within a cave, unable to directly see the world of light beyond. The chains immobilized their limbs; their heads were chained in one direction as well, so that their gaze was fixed on the cave's back wall. These prisoners viewed all real 3-D objects only via the 2-D shadows that they cast on the cave's back wall. To them, who had no other experience, the shadows themselves represented the *real* objects.

Behind the prisoners was an enormous fire, and between the fire and the prisoners a raised walkway, along which puppeteers moved along various animals, plants, and other things. The 3-D objects cast 2-D shadows on the wall, just as radio-opaque bodily organs do on conventional x-ray film, and the prisoners watched these shadows (see Fig. 11.1, on p. 584). When one of the puppet-carriers spoke, an echo against the cave's back wall caused the prisoners to believe that the words came from the shadows.

When Socrates was asked, in Plato's dialog, how one could overcome the limitations that confound the true nature of reality, his response was particularly telling, especially in light of our current 3-D digital imaging perspective. The answer involved the study of abstractions—in particular, arithmetic, the science of numbers. As Socrates put it, "Number, then, appears to lead toward the truth." Only through the study of abstractions of the mind—as he viewed the mathematical disciplines—could one perceive nature's truth. Plato's entreaties now appear hauntingly modern. If his own abstraction—via the 2-D shadows of 3-D objects—might open the minds of his contemporaries to the infinite possibilities of reality, what knowledge might modern mathematical applications unveil? All the wonders of *computed tomography*, *magnetic resonance imaging*, computational fluid dynamics, and the other *3-D digital imaging* modalities.

Spectacular improvements in x-ray computed tomographic imaging modalities, with fast and high resolution imaging, increase the overall amount of imaging information in terms of raw data and source images. Tomographic methods encompass a host of sensing techniques and mathematical algorithms, which reconstruct 3-D body region and organ images, and fields (see Section 4.2, on pp. 170 f.) of various properties of interest, by processing multiple 1-D scans of the body. Volume data comprise discrete sampling points of a scanned *in situ* cardiovascular structure or a simulated flow field, usually as a sequence

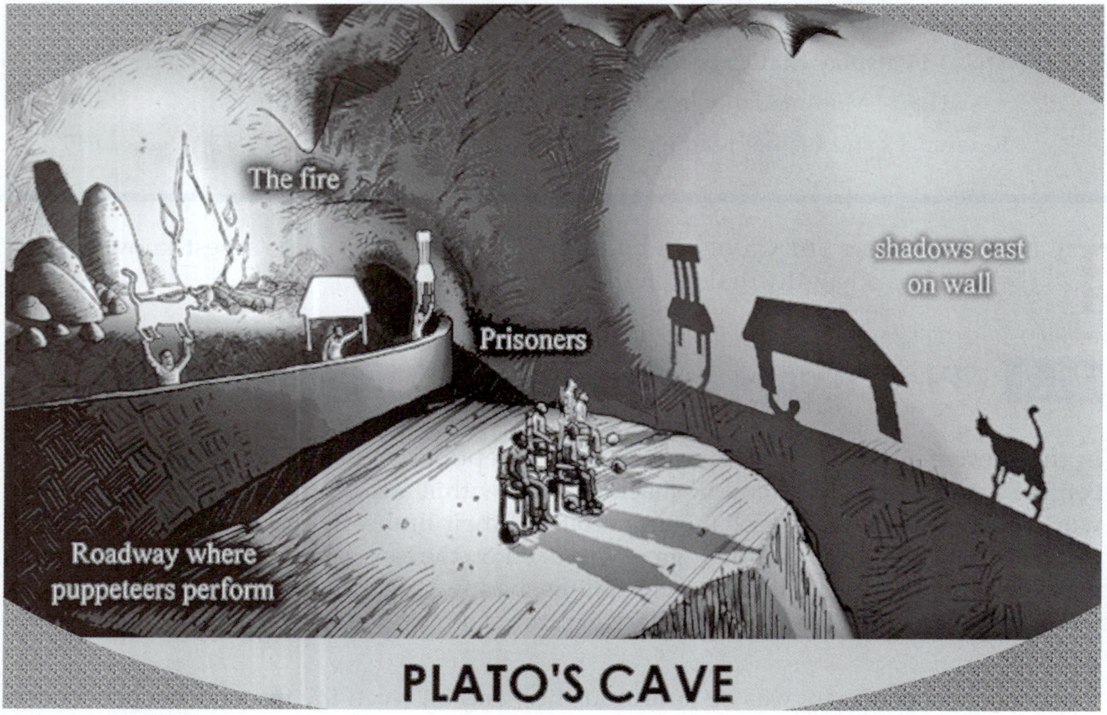

Figure 11.1: *Socrates*—Behold! human beings living in a underground cave, which has a mouth open toward the light and reaching all along the cave; here they have been from their childhood, and have their legs and necks chained so that they cannot move, and can only see before them, being prevented by the chains from turning round their heads. Above and behind them a fire is blazing at a distance, and between the fire and the prisoners there is a raised way; and you will see, if you look, a low wall built along the way, like the screen which marionette players have in front of them, over which they show the puppets. ... *Glaucon* You have shown me a strange image, and they are strange prisoners. *Socrates* Like ourselves, I replied; and they see only their own shadows, or the shadows of one another, which the fire throws on the opposite wall of the cave? ... *Glaucon* True, he said; how could they see anything but the shadows if they were never allowed to move their heads? *Socrates* To them, I said, the truth *("reality")* would be literally nothing but the shadows of the images. *Glaucon* That is certain. (English translation adapted, slightly modified, from Jowett [43].)

of cross-sectional 2-D scans or matrices. Such volume datasets are preprocessed by 2-D image-processing techniques and are then 3-D reconstructed into corresponding 3-D volumetric datasets, by *stacking* the cross-sections and interpolating between them—see Figure 11.10, on p. 600; see also Chapter 10, and Figures 10.1, 10.2, and 10.3, on pp. 484–486. Following rendering of organ surfaces of interest, such as endocardial surfaces of cardiac chambers, the discretization, or mesh-generation step can occur. Mesh generation typically entails the placement of points that indicate subdivision locations on the curves and surfaces of flow fields that are to be simulated numerically. These points, and information about how these points are connected, define the various boundaries of the computation. Furthermore, mesh generation also includes the placement of points and connectivity information between the flow region boundaries, such that the flow phenomena may be approximated within the internal volumes or areas that form the geometric model.

As we saw in Chapters 5 and 10, a great variety of digital sensing techniques are employed in current medical scanners, based on absorption, refraction, scattering, and emission of various forms of radiation and sonic waves. Among the many commonly used tomographic methods are positron emission tomography (PET), nuclear magnetic resonance (NMR), magnetic resonance imaging (MRI), and computerized axial tomography (CAT, or CT) methods; some currently evolving 3-D echocardiographic methods that employ transthoracic and transesophageal rotational probes are also tomographic, in principle. MRI, CT, and 3-D echocardiographic methods are of special angiocardiographic interest, and are therefore considered at length in Chapter 10. Typically in CT, a sensor records the cumulative effect of property change along a linear path across the object, a number of such records along intersecting paths on the same plane are obtained simultaneously or sequentially, and the multiple records are processed by a mathematical algorithm capable of reconstructing the local values of the desired property over a planar section of the object. The 3-D field of the property can be also reconstructed, with high soft-tissue contrast in MRI scans, by processing multiple planar sections.

In fluid mechanics research too, tomographic methods are used for 3-D flow-field visualization and for the measurement of velocity, temperature, and concentration. Although the resolution and the accuracy of such methods are generally inferior to those of other fluid dynamic measurement methods [21], such as laser velocimetry, they are valuable in revealing 3-D patterns, especially of transient and unsteady phenomena. Simulated data are generated by a powerful computer that runs a simulation, e.g., of a CFD model of intracardiac blood flow. The data produced are generally a scalar, vector, or tensor field of the 3-D spatial grid, or a sequence of 2-D planar slices. Both the underlying flow phenomenon and the computer simulation may generate 3-D or multidimensional lattices of tensor fields. A *tensor field* of rank zero is a scalar field, in which every voxel has a single value (magnitude); a tensor field of rank one is a vector field, in which each voxel has a magnitude as well as a direction.

11.2 Volume visualization in a nutshell

Volume visualization encompasses an array of techniques that provide the mechanisms which make it possible to reveal and explore the inner, or unseen, structures of volumetric data[1] and allow visual insights into opaque or complex datasets. Techniques used to produce 3-D views of volumetric data differ in their computational complexity and in the image quality that results [11]. 3-D medical imaging has been the pioneering and primary application of volume visualization and a driving force in its development. The 3-D volumetric imaging datasets occupy a 3-D discrete *voxel space*, which is a 3-D integer

[1]Volumetric data is data with a domain of three independent variables.

grid of unit volume cells or elements, called voxels. An individual voxel is commonly depicted as a unit cube centered at a grid point (see Figure 1.7, on p. 27). Alternatively, it is represented as a 0-D point located at the grid coordinates. The aggregate of voxels tessellating the volume forms the *volumetric dataset*. The dataset is commonly stored in a cubic frame buffer, which is a large 3-D array of voxels.

Both the synthesis and analysis of voxel representations require a considerable mathematical and theoretical foundation, pertaining to the field of discrete 3-D space and its topology,[2] as well as the use of 3-D discrete geometry to develop voxelization algorithms. *Voxelization* is the process of converting geometric objects from their continuous geometric representation into a set of voxels that best approximates the continuous object. The process mimics the scan-conversion process that pixelizes (rasterizes) 2-D geometric objects; accordingly, it is also referred to as 3-D scan-conversion [27]. In 2-D rasterization the pixels are directly drawn onto the screen to be visualized and filtering is applied to reduce the aliasing artifacts causing *jaggedness*, or *stair-steps*, in edges (cf. Fig. 5.16, on p. 256). However, the voxelization process does not render the voxels but merely generates a database of the discrete digitization of the continuous scanned object. Theoretical studies have been conducted to characterize the 3-D discrete space. Their primary goal is to devise a framework for discrete space that is a close analog of continuous space, in which case the discrete space is labeled as *"well behaved"* [30]. An interest in well-behaved spaces is related to 3-D scan-conversion and to surface-tracking algorithms. A variety of algorithms to voxelize various geometric objects—e.g., 3-D lines, planar polygons, polyhedra, surfaces and volumes—have been developed.

The generated digital representations must conform to fidelity and connectivity requirements. Once the 3-D voxel image has been reconstructed and voxelized, it is then enhanced by 3-D image-processing techniques, such as filtering [4,58], in order to reduce the staircase artefacts, and by applying image processing operators to improve contrast. Next follows the process of classification of the voxelized volume. *Classification* is the process of assigning an opacity to each voxel by applying classification algorithms in which the user chooses a transfer function to compute the opacities from the scalar values. An alternative method is to partition the volume into specific structures and organs (using a segmentation algorithm [41]) and then to assign opacities to each structure. Proper choice of the classification function is crucial. A good classification function reveals the structures in the volume or highlights some subregion of the volume in an informative way.

Experimentation with different classification functions is often necessary to produce an informative visualization. After classifying the data comes the application of a shading function. The *shading function* specifies the illumination model and a rule for determining the shade of gray or color of each voxel. Shadows and depth cueing can greatly improve the effectiveness of a visualization. Finally there is the choice of *viewing parameters* [37]: the viewpoint, the type of projection (parallel or perspective), clipping planes, and so on. With this information and the shaded classified volume, the rendering algorithm

[2]Topology, a modern branch of geometry, focuses on the properties of geometric objects that remain unchanged upon continuous deformation, i.e., shrinking, stretching, and folding, but not tearing.

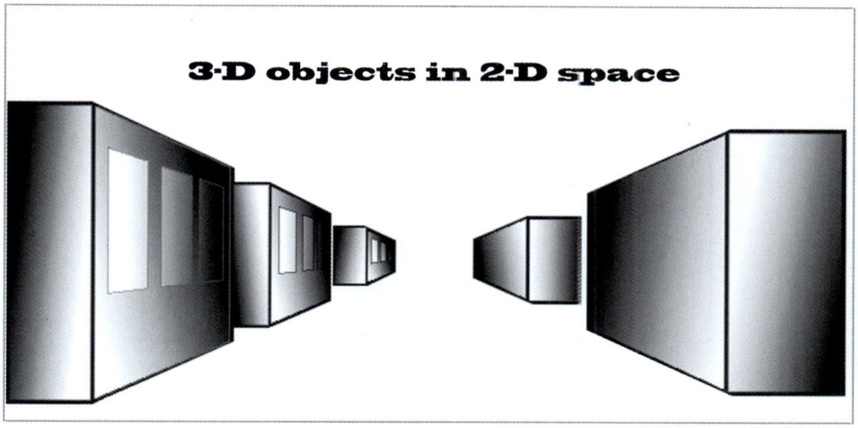

Figure 11.2: The illusion of three-dimensionality and depth on a 2-D plane, using primarily linear perspective, and secondarily shading and surface hiding by overlying objects.

produces an image. Because of the subjective choices involved in classification and shading, it is difficult to decide a priori on a set of optimal parameters; accordingly, the user must rely on *"trial-and-error"* to produce a good visualization. With the introduction of hardware accelerated volume rendering [50], 3-D imaging datasets can be rendered and explored at interactive rates.

There are two technical aspects to exploring, analyzing, and visualizing volume imaging information of internal organs: *data reduction*, and *data rendering* and *presentation*. Broadly speaking, methods for reducing the data dimensionality include slicing the data, projecting the data along one or more axes, and accumulating features along any specified dimension. In many applications, techniques are required for data enhancement, segmentation, modeling, and statistical analysis, in addition to rendering. Data presentation methods entail using the spatial domain, temporal sequences, color and texture, as well as various specialized iconic forms.

11.3 Visualizing 3-D on a monitor screen

To understand the challenge that visualizing 3-D on the monitor screen plane entails (see Fig. 11.2), we must first examine briefly how we see 3-D space [8,18,35]. We perceive three dimensions because our brain combines the slightly different images that are acquired by each of our eyes (see Fig. 11.3, on p. 588). When the two images arrive simultaneously in the visual cortex, the brain processes and interprets them, and makes all the calculations needed to determine the relative position of the objects in the scene using information from them. The two images are combined into one picture, matching up the similarities and integrating the small divergences that add up to a big difference in the final representation.

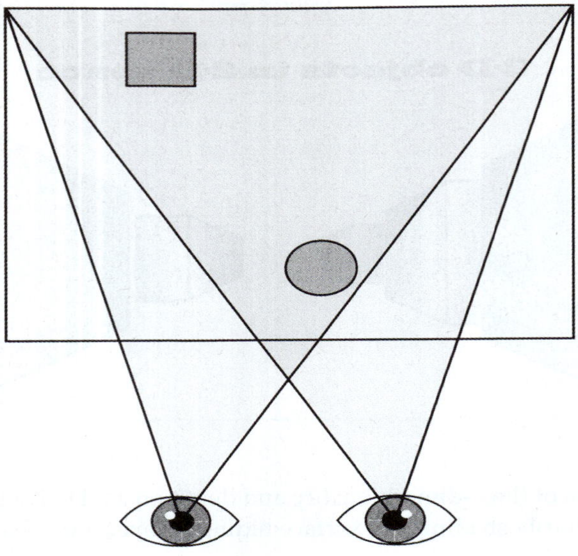

Figure 11.3: The basis of 3-D vision lies in using two independently captured images from slightly separated points of view, corresponding to left and right eye frustrums. The brain processes and interprets these images to determine the relative position of the objects in space using information from the images.

The connecting path between the eye and the perception of 3-D is not simple. A subtle interplay of psycho-optical illusions, eye-muscle tension, image focus and overlap, and head motion augment the two incoming images with information our brain brings into play to construct the perception of depth. The combined image is more than the sum of its constituents; it is a 3-D "stereo" [Gk. *stereon*, meaning *solid*] picture.

Missing from all unadjusted 2-D displays are the physical clues that guide our brains in processing 3-D views. The small lack of correspondence in the images seen by each of our eyes is called binocular disparity. It forces our eyes to perform two other actions that are crucial to seeing in 3-D: our eyes must both converge toward a common viewing location where the images from both overlap, and must focus at that depth.[3] In addition, head movements, allowing us to see previously obstructed parts of the 3-D image, give our brain vital data for the 3-D image it constructs. That movement-engendered sense of depth is refer to as motion parallax. A lot of what goes into a good 3-D display is skillful use of psychological cues, which essentially trick our minds into seeing flat 2-D images as 3-D. We can now proceed to examine the shape of 3-D objects seen on a flat monitor screen.

[3]If the images on the retinas are too disparate, we get double vision. To see this, hold two fingers in front of you, one behind the other. Now fixate on the front one. If the second is not too far behind, it will appear as single. But as you move the second finger away from the first, it will appear double. The visual system can tolerate only a certain amount of disparity without getting double vision.

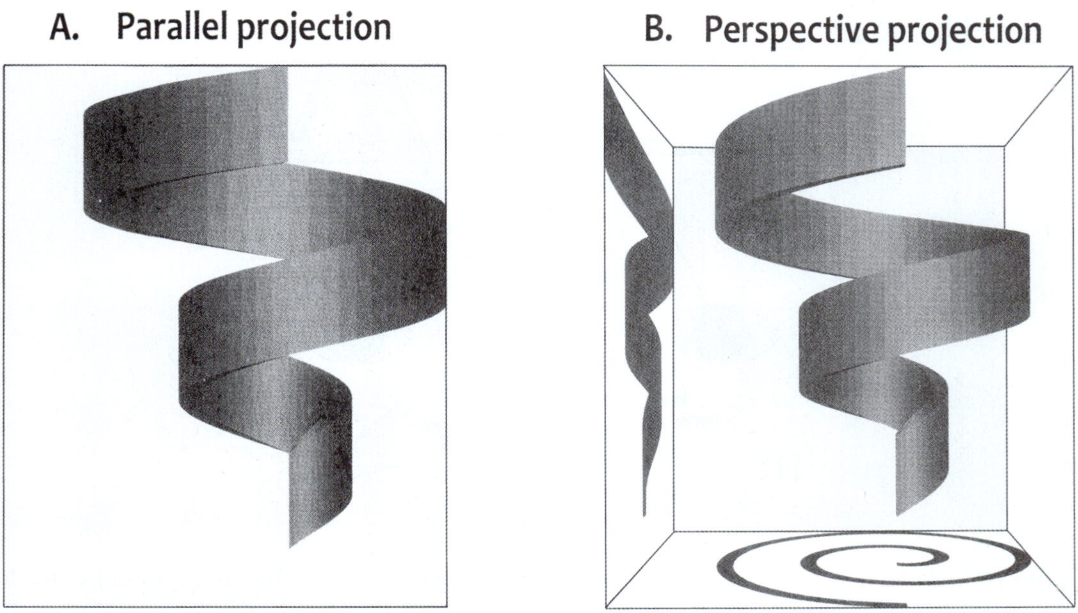

Figure 11.4: A 3-D helix and two projections on the left and bottom walls of the bounding cube. The two projections are not visible in Panel A., due to the parallel-ray orthographic projection method used for the whole scene. The two projections are visible in Panel B., due to the perspective projection method that is used for the whole scene.

11.4 Translating 3-D into 2-D

Before we examine the shape of objects seen on a screen, we must gain a basic understanding of perspective. Linear perspective has a history going back at least to the classic age of Greece (see Section 3.1, on pp. 116 ff.). If we can learn to deal with the illusions of perspective [8, 18, 35], we can use them to good advantage to help us understand complicated 3-D organ structures. Exactly what is perspective and how does one bring it forth on a monitor screen? In projections or shadows of objects cast by parallel rays of light, the images of parallel lines appear as parallel lines, and parallel segments of the same length have images that are segments of the same length, as is seen in orthographic[4] projections (cf. Panel A. of Fig. 11.4).

As is demonstrated in Figure 11.4, however, this is not what we actually see when we take in a large view. To wit, parallel railroad tracks appear to converge to a point on

[4]Orthographic drawings are views (front, side, top, and so on) of an object based on the assumption that the light rays reaching our eyes are parallel, similar to seeing objects from a great distance. House plans are a form of orthographic projection. An orthographic view is only one side. It takes several such views to show all the object.

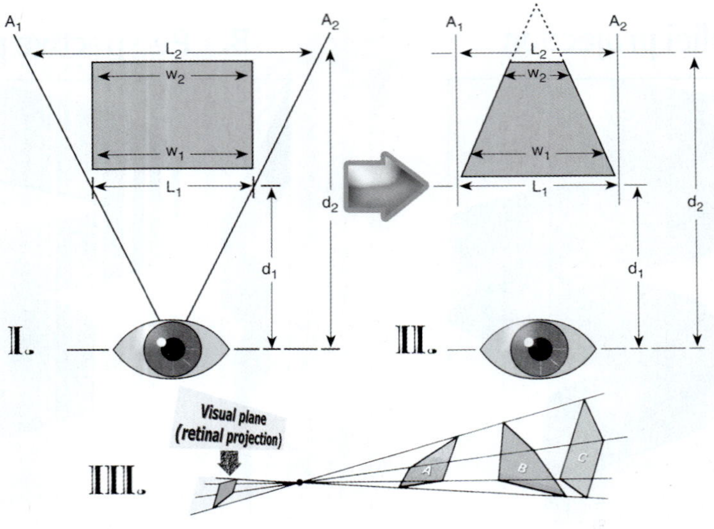

Figure 11.5: Panel I. The field of view and perspective vision. The farther away an object is, the smaller it appears because it occupies less of our field of view. Panel II. A 2-D representation of the 3-D view in panel I. Making the lines A_1 and A_2 parallel, effectively flattens out the representation—see discussion in text. Panel III. Very different shapes in 3-D space can have the same 2-D retinal projection.

the horizon. The railroad ties may look to be parallel to the horizon, but they get shorter and closer together as they recede into the distance, as happens with the distant face of the bounding cube in Panel B. of Figure 11.4. The reason why a distant railroad tie looks smaller is that the rays from its endpoints to the observer's eye form a smaller angle than do the rays of an equal-length tie that is closer to the eye. In a perspective drawing, any collection of parallel lines will appear either as parallel lines or as lines converging to a vanishing point. A cube has *three* sets of parallel edges, and the image can have one, two, or three vanishing points.

Each of our eyes sees in a conical field of view. Panel I. of Figure 11.5, shows the difference in the apparent dimensions of an object as a function of its distance from us. W_1 is equal to W_2 and they both correspond to the width of the rectangle. L_1 and L_2 are of different lengths and stand for the width of our field of view at distances d_1 and d_2, respectively. To our brain, which inherently knows nothing of 3-D, the lengths L_1 and L_2 are identical, because they both embody the maximum field of view. In fact, W_2 would look as if it were much shorter than W_1. Effectively, the brain tries to make the lines A_1 and A_2 parallel, which gives rise to an image as represented by Panel II. of Figure 11.5. If you look straight ahead, you get no feeling of seeing in a conical field. You just see straight ahead. The difference is that Panel I. of Figure 11.5 actually represents a 3-D view and Panel II. is a 2-D representation of that view. Making the lines A_1 and A_2 parallel actually *flattens out* the representation. The additional changes (e.g., W_2 appearing as shorter than W_1) ensue in order to compensate for this flattening.

If we reverse the preceding conceptual paradigm, we get 3-D to 2-D projection, which loses shape characteristics in the third dimension (see Panel III. of Fig. 11.5, on p. 590). When we look at a 3-D object, such as a cube, the closer parts will have larger images and the parts farther away will have smaller ones. The front face of a cube viewed head on will be larger than the back face. This *"square-within-a-square"* is a familiar representation of our view of a cube from in front of one face. Images of vertical and horizontal edges appear as vertical or horizontal segments, but the edges heading away from us appear to converge toward the center (see Fig. 11.5). The closest and farthest faces appear to be squares, and the images of the other four faces are trapezoids. From *experience* we know that the six faces of the cube are squares of the same size and shape, even though they do not appear that way in any single view.

In panels a. and c. of Figure 11.6, on p. 592, x, y, and z represent the coordinate axes, and the viewing plane coincides with the projection plane. If we draw straight lines from each important point on the object to our eye, or center of projection, as is shown in panel a., the point where they pass through the projection plane forms an image which we call a *one vanishing point perspective* projection. Compare Panel I. and Panel II. of Figure 11.5 once again: In Panel I., the lines that define the sides of the box are parallel, but A_1 and A_2 come to a point. In Panel II., the lines A_1 and A_2 are parallel, and if we extend the lines that coincide with the sides of the box out beyond the box, they converge at the vanishing point. This is identified as a one vanishing point perspective because only those lines which are parallel to the z-axis converge at the vanishing point. If the lines parallel to the z-axis only converge at infinity, we then have a *parallel* projection.

Perspective projections carry a label that declares how many axes converge. Following the paradigm of the one vanishing point perspective that converges on one axis, a two-point perspective must then converge on two axes. In panels b. and d. of Figure 11.6, *both* the x-axis lines and the z-axis lines converge, as is shown explicitly in panel b. This type of representation is more realistic than one vanishing point perspective because, usually, objects that we view are not completely aligned with their projection plane. In the real world, all three coordinate axes converge, and this is exemplified in panel e. Three-point perspective is very difficult to draw, however, for more complicated shapes than a cube, and for life-like 3-D organ reconstructions in medical imaging we employ specialized 3-D programs, which generate perspective images automatically. All the complications of drawing are executed using a mathematical perspective projection transformation inside the computer. By feeding sets of scanned volume data into appropriate formulas, the computer can generate the 2-D projections for monitor viewing speedily and with near-perfect accuracy.

The perspective projection transformation can be modeled by simulating the viewer's eye as the convergence point for all rays reflected from objects in virtual space—not a big stretch from what is happening in reality. Each ray, before being caught by the eye, would intersect a plane located in front of the viewer. By finding the intersection and plotting a point there on the display, the viewer observing it can be deceived into thinking that the ray from the plotted point was actually coming from the original position *in space*. Perspective always causes some distortion, but we are able to accommodate the distortions by relying subconsciously on our *experiences* of viewing objects. When we see

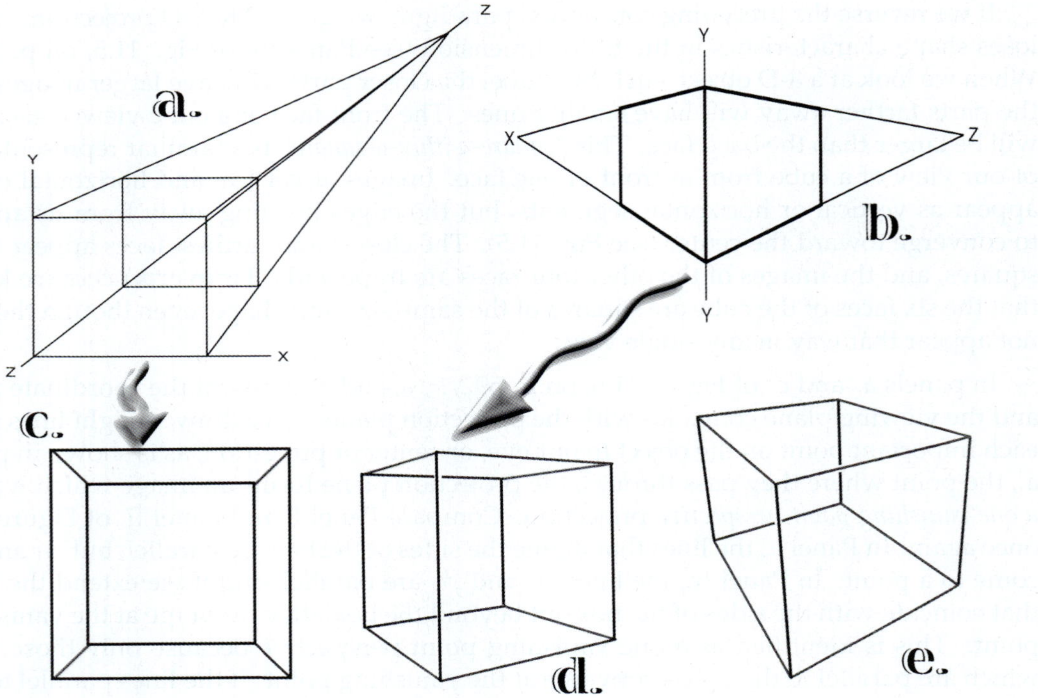

Figure 11.6: Viewing in perspective. Panels a. and c.: views of a cube with one vanishing point. Panels b. and d.: views of a cube with two vanishing points. Panel e.: view of a cube with three vanishing points.

a rotating cube, we think about a cube, not the varying sequence of squares, trapezoids, and more complicated four-sided figures. The more aware we become of the way we visualize shapes in 3-D-space, the better we can apply the principles of perspective to help us visualize scanned 3-D *organ shapes*, such as the cardiac chambers, projected on the monitor screen.

3-D reconstruction programs [7] operate on volume datasets obtained by various imaging modalities. We call these *volume datasets*, because they typically represent the values of a physical quantity, such as gray-scale intensity, throughout a volume of space. Generating a 2-D image from such a set is called volume rendering. These cubical scan datasets typically comprise just lists of coordinates in x, y, z space, similar to the examples in Figure 11.6. One at a time, the program goes down the list and applies the appropriate transformation formula to generate a projection to our viewing plane, i.e., the monitor screen, then draws the object by turning on the corresponding screen pixels.

There are many other procedures used along the way, to help make the image easier to view, with less clutter. One of these is backplane removal (see Fig. 11.7A., on p. 593). *Backplane removal* means that any part of the object viewed that is hidden by the front, or by overlying structures in general, should not be projected.

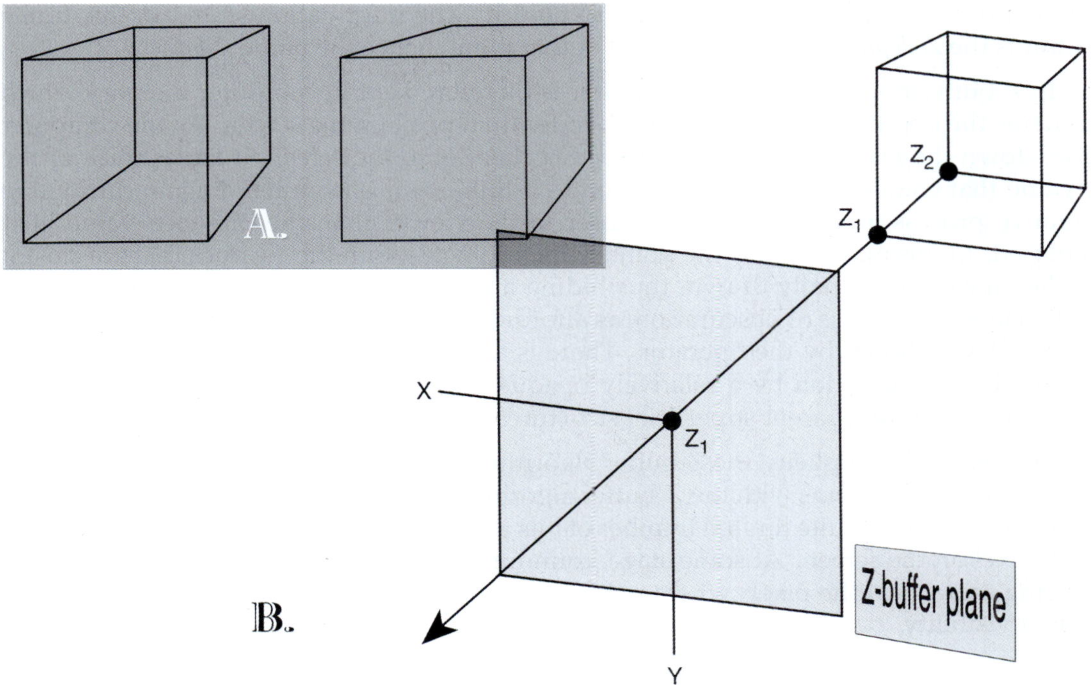

Figure 11.7: Viewing 3-D on a plane screen. Panel A. shows a wireframe model of a cube before and after backplane removal. Panel B. illustrates how a point on the screen is kept in a Z-buffer in computer memory.

11.4.1 Z-buffering

Z-buffering is one of many procedures for backplane removal, and it is quite effective. It is an example of *obscuration*, a display technique whereby structures close to the observer obscure the view of more distant structures. Clearly, if two opaque objects were projected to the same point on the screen, the closer one to the eye is the visible one.

There are many techniques for backplane removal, but the simplest to understand is Z-buffering. The name comes from using a frame buffer to store some information instead of a picture. *Frame buffers* are large pieces of computer memory that can hold numbers: one number for each pixel on the screen. The number may be a gray-scale or color number from a 2-D projection; it may represent the gray-scale or the RGB components of the color at that pixel, or it may be something else. This "something else" turns out to be extremely useful when we want to generate 2-D projections of objects or organs within 3-D volume imaging datasets, and special techniques have been developed to take advantage of this. The basic idea is that if you want to store information about a picture on a pixel-by-pixel basis, a frame buffer is a natural place to hold it. The information stored in this frame buffer is the *Z-depth* of the visible object at that point, hence the name *Z-buffer*.[5]

In Z-buffering, a separate screen buffer is therefore kept in computer memory which contains the depth (z-axis) value of each individual pixel on the screen. As the computer goes down the list of coordinates, projecting them onto the screen, it keeps track of the z value that coincides with each x, y point. If this x, y is encountered again during the iterative process and the z value is closer to the viewer than the previous value, it is replaced. In this manner, only the points which coincide with the z values that are closest to the viewer are actually drawn, thus hiding all previous points (see Fig. 11.7B., on p. 593). The effectiveness of obscuration, as afforded by Z-buffering, is closely related to the opacity level chosen by the operator. There is a *trade-off* between the depth perception afforded by obscuration by a relatively opaque structure and the medical necessity of seeing through transparent superficial structures to appreciate deeper ones.

Because of its simplicity, the Z-buffer algorithm is the one often implemented in imaging hardware. Problems with the Z-buffer algorithm usually arise from the fact that there is a finite and often quite limited number of bits available to represent the z-coordinate for each pixel on the screen. At some stage, rounding or truncating the z values may ensue, causing artifacts at the pixels where reduction of bits brought about a wrong determination of visibility.

11.5 Postprocessing techniques for tomographic data

With an average of 400–1,000 tomographic images in each volumetric dataset, 3-D postprocessing is crucial to volume visualization. Nowadays there are workstations available commercially that provide capabilities for evaluation of such enormous datasets by using a range of software programs and processing tools. Performing the proper data reduction and choosing the correct presentation to visualize dynamic vascular and cardiac anatomy and intracardiac blood flow phenomena, in particular, takes training and experience. In some instances, viewing the raw data is simply overwhelming, but reducing it to a comprehensible image requires knowing something about the data and how to extract its relevant parts. Each diagnostic or research application may, in fact, call for the data to be reduced and presented in a different manner, especially within the broad area of clinical and basic science investigations of intracardiac flows.

Axial tomographic datasets can be viewed for interpretation and geometric measurements, or used to create multiplanar or 3-D images. 3-D reconstruction techniques allow a condensed representation of imaging information for research and clinical applications. These 3-D reconstructions make more "palpable" the information that is fragmented in multiple axial slices. In addition, they can eliminate problems caused by the standard transverse slice orientation, and bring out the spatial relationships between shape, orientation, and scan plane.

[5]The Z-buffer is also known as the *depth-buffer*. The z-coordinate of a point is equal to its distance from the eye (*viz.*, its *depth*.)

The ability to acquire high-density information volume data has paved the way for the development of 3-D image processing and rendering techniques [38,40], which have become a vital component of medical imaging today. Thus, with the current advances in imaging modality technologies, an increasing part of the research, or clinical, data examination is committed to postprocessing. Consequently, 3-D reconstruction techniques are becoming a part of the standard imaging data acquisition for investigations of ventricular function and of intracardiac blood flow phenomena. There are four main postprocessing techniques available for the display of a discretely sampled 3-D tomographic measurement set, typically comprising x-ray CT, MRI, or 3-D echocardiographic systems. The following sections provide an overview of these methods, which comprise multiplanar reformations, maximum intensity projections, surface shaded displays, and volume-rendering techniques.

11.5.1 Multiplanar reformation

Volume image display methods, termed *projection imaging*, involve the numerical projection of the voxels of the 3-D reconstruction of the scanned volume onto a plane to form a 2-D projection image [31]. For x-ray CT, these projections are analogous to, and appear like, conventional radiographs.

Multiplanar reformatting or reformation (MPR) is an example of such voxel projection methods, which can display any cross-section of a volumetric reconstruction [5]. This is a technique that uses axial reconstruction data to create nonaxial 2-D images. MPR allows display of blood vessels in a 2-D format that is similar to that of conventional angiograms. The data are processed after, e.g., a helical CT acquisition has been performed with intravenous contrast enhancement, as is required in a routine CT examination. MPR images are coronal, sagittal, oblique, or curved plane images constructed from a 1-voxel thick plane as it transects a stack of axial CT images [6]. For time-varying cardiac images, the reformatted plane should be animated to show the beating of the cardiac chambers [52,60], because important dynamic geometric research information and clinical diagnostic cues can be thus derived [23].

MPR images can be banded together into slabs, by combining the data encountered by a ray passing through the stack of reconstructed sections along the line of sight toward the viewer's eye, according to one of several algorithms discussed below, including MIP, MinIP, AIP, ray sum, and volume rendering, which are then referred to as "multiplanar volume reformations" [47]. MPR is a useful technique as it allows a study to be viewed in multiple arbitrary planes that can be determined by the viewer, as is shown in Figure 5.18, on p. 258, and explained in the associated discussion. The values of pixels forming the reformatted plane can be obtained through interpolation from the closest voxels. If more distant voxels contribute to the final picture, the result is a so-called thick slab.

Curved planar reformation (CPR) is similar to MPR, but exploits the idea that it is also possible to sample a 3-D stack of CT images along a *curved* plane, as is indicated schematically in Figure 11.8, on p. 596. It allows creation of a single-voxel thick tomogram that enables an uninterrupted visualization of a curved structure by fixing points manually along the structure of interest, so that the *"display-plane"* curves along it, as needed. The manually

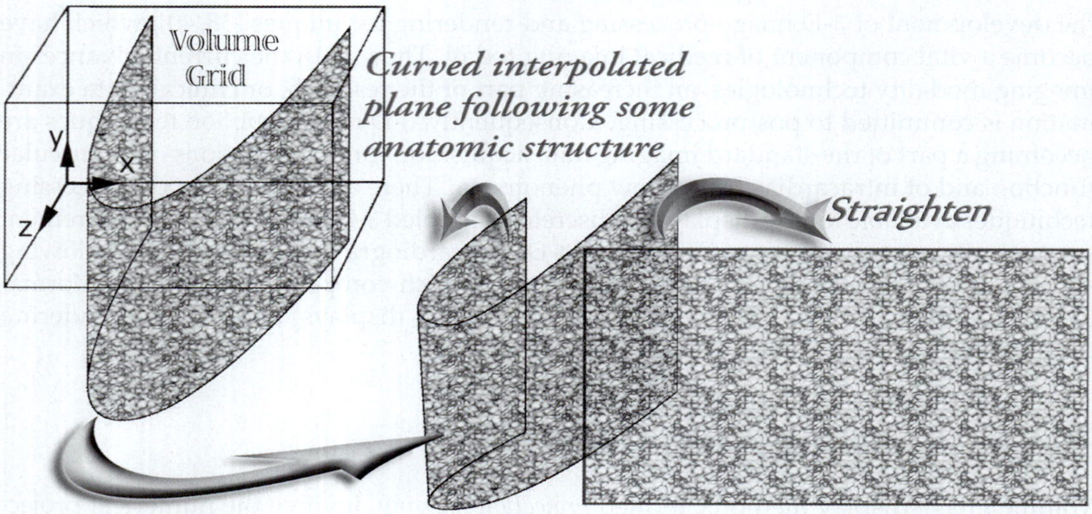

Figure 11.8: Diagram shows how data acquired in a stack of axial CT slices can be sampled along a curved plane. The whole length of a curved wall structure can be displayed within a single image, showing its lumen, wall, and surrounding tissue in a curved plane. Subsequently, the curved plane may be straightened (flattened) and displayed as a 2D, composite image, through the application of appropriate transformation software.

created points are positioned over the particular structure of interest as viewed on transverse sections, or any other projection method. The points are connected to form a 3-D curve that is then extruded through the volume perpendicularly to the desired view to create the CPR [25,26].

CPR is useful for displaying an entire hollow or tubular structure on a single image. An important application of this visualization method is in CT angiography (CTA). The disadvantage of CPR is that it is highly dependent on accurate selection of the 3-D curve. Automated methods for generating curved planar reformations have been shown to decrease the number of artifacts and user interaction time, while maintaining image quality [46]. Clearly, a single curve cannot adequately display nonaxisymmetric geometry; therefore, two curves that are *orthogonal* to each other should always be created when using CPR, to provide a more complete depiction of the geometry of cardiac chambers, vessels, or other nonaxisymmetric organs [51].

11.5.2 Maximum intensity projection

Maximum intensity projection (MIP) is a useful technique for computer visualization of vascular structures. MIPs are created when a specific projection (e.g., anteroposterior) is chosen and then mathematical rays are transmitted perpendicular to it through the scan volume formed by a stack of reconstructed sections (see Fig. 11.9, on p. 598). In effect, an array of rays is projected along the dataset in a user-selected direction and the highest voxel value along each individual ray becomes the pixel value of a 2-D MIP image. Only the *maximum intensity* voxel value (in Hounsfield units) encountered by each ray as it traverses the volume is projected onto the output image plane [28], hence the name, MIP. This leads to the entire volume being collapsed with only the highest attenuation structures being visible. Blood vessel attenuation is maximized by injection of a contrast medium, but physical limitations preclude obtaining attenuation higher than that of bone and other calcified structures. On the other hand, the higher attenuation of bone and its spatial connectivity, make possible its *selective removal* from the data during preprocessing.

Multiplanar images can be thickened into slabs with diverse projectional techniques such as maximum, minimum (MinIP), and average (AIP) intensity projection. AIP images represent the *average* of each component attenuation value encountered by a ray cast through a body region toward the viewer's eye (Fig. 11.9). This can be useful for characterizing the internal structures of a solid organ or the walls of hollow structures, such as cardiac chambers or blood vessels. Finally, MinIP images are multiplanar slab images produced by displaying only the lowest attenuation value encountered along an x-ray beam cast through a body region toward the viewer's eye (Fig. 11.9).

An advantage of MIP over MPR is that it allows immediate visualization of structures that do not lie in a single plane in their entirety; however, it does not provide for an appreciation of spatial 3-D relationships. MIP, as well as AIP and MinIP, are computationally fast, but as images obtained by all these techniques contain no shading information whatsoever, any depth suggestion is lost. Structures with higher data values lying behind a lower-valued object will seem to be in front of it. The most common way to improve the sense of 3-D and facilitate the interpretation of such images is to *animate the viewpoint* while viewing. MIP frames are computed from several view angles in which the viewpoint is slightly changed from one to the other, and can be displayed as animations in a cine or video loop creating the illusion of *rotation* (interactive frame-rates are essential here), in order to convey 3-D structure. This approach helps the viewer's perception to find the relative 3-D positions of the components of the imaged volumes. The depth cues than can be provided by such a "rotating" of an object are referred to as a *kinetic* depth effect. Real time *volume rendering* (see below) provides a higher level of interactivity, which enhances the 3-D depth cues by allowing the user to alter the perspective and display parameters in real time. Real time rendering has the significant advantage of allowing viewing from any angle, *without* the constraints imposed by the precomputed *cine-* or *video-*loop display.

Ray sum is another postprocessing algorithm [31] that is similar to AIP. Rather than averaging the data along each projected ray, ray sum may simply add all values [28]. Generally, the display is accomplished either by summing all voxel values along virtual rays of light (summed projection) or by computing only voxels of a certain maximum value range along virtual rays (maximum intensity projection). For this reason, ray sum images may have an appearance similar to that of conventional radiographs. Ray tracing techniques are frequently used, particularly for MRI data.

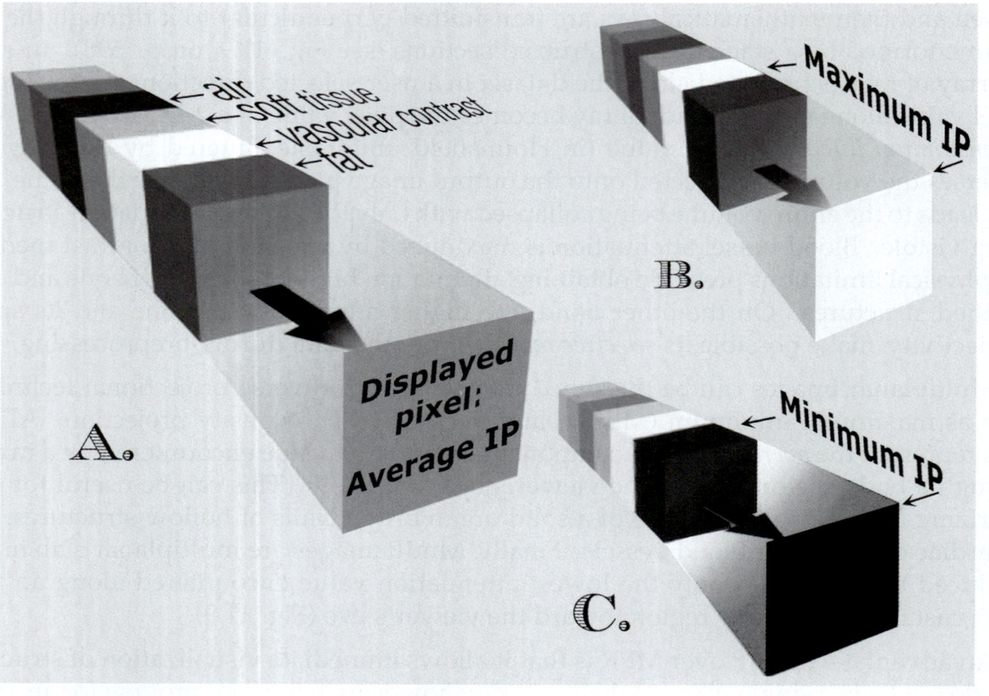

Figure 11.9: Projections reconstructed from data encountered by a ray traced through the body region of interest to the viewer. The included data contain attenuation information ranging from that of air (black) to that of a contrast medium (white). A. The average intensity projection (AIP) uses the average attenuation of the data to calculate the gray-scale projected value (mid-level gray). B. The maximum intensity projection (MIP) projects only the maximum gray-scale brightness value (white) encountered. C. The minimum intensity projection (MinIP) projects only the minimum gray-scale brightness value (black) encountered.

Within angiographic datasets, MIP exploits the fact that the data values of contrast-enhanced, blood-containing structures are *higher* than the values of the surrounding tissues [19]. It is commonly used to evaluate contrast medium-filled structures for CT angiography; by depicting the maximum data value seen through each pixel, the geometry of the vessels contained in the data is captured.

11.5.3 Shaded surface display

Shaded surface display (SSD), or surface rendering, provides 3-D representations of the surfaces of anatomic structures using gray scale or color [1]. Apparent surfaces are determined within the volume of data, and images representing the derived surfaces can be revealed. The voxels located on the edge of an anatomic structure are delineated, usually by intensity thresholding that is most likely aided by morphologic filtering, and these voxels are displayed.

Morphologic filtering is a type of processing in which the spatial form, or structure, of objects within an image is modified. Morphologic filters are nonlinear filters suited to diverse filtering tasks. First, because most image interpretation techniques and measurements are hindered by noisy data, a morphological filter must be used to touch up images degraded by some type of noise. A noisy image must be filtered prior to any further processing, such as edge detection, segmentation, and gray-scale measurements. Contrary to nonlinear morphologic filters, ordinary linear filters usually fail to preserve edges. Secondly, a morphologic filter may be used to selectively remove some image structures or objects while preserving others. The selection is based on the geometry and local contrast of the image objects. In this sense, application of a morphological filter can be interpreted as a step toward the *quantitative interpretation* of the image [54].

In SSD, each voxel intensity within the volumetric scan dataset is determined to be within some user-defined range of attenuation values. The fidelity of the resulting images to the actual anatomy depends, naturally, on the value range selected. In applying *intensity thresholding* to display edges and interfaces, the threshold value has to be chosen so that the boundary voxels of the organ of interest, such as the endocardial surface of a cardiac chamber, are selected. With the surface determined, the remainder of the data can be discarded. Surface contours are typically tessellated as a collection of polygons (see Fig. 2.37, on p. 102) and displayed with surface shading. Surface rendering is a fast image manipulation method, since computation is accomplished with only a subset of the entire 3-D data; the remaining voxels in the image are usually invisible. In the ray-casting method, hidden part removal is done by stopping at the first voxel encountered along each ray that satisfies the threshold criterion [20]. A voxel threshold is selected allowing efficient exclusion of irrelevant structures.

In transitioning from the volumetric dataset to a curved 3-D surface (or surfaces), a large portion of the available data is effectively forfeited in exchange for faster, easier computation. While this can be an advantage, by allowing real-time rendering and thereby enhancing user interactivity, the usefulness of surface rendered medical images may be limited by issues pertaining to image accuracy. More advanced surface generation techniques, such as *"marching cubes"* [34], use simple thresholding to select voxels, but also use voxel values to generate surfaces that are placed and oriented more accurately.

The thresholding assignment of the voxels that will be visible is obviously critical. Organ surface renditions can be created *interactively* directly from the imaging data as the threshold is changed. Different combinations of principles are employed for the *detection of the surface* to be displayed (gray-value threshold, gradient threshold, and zero-crossing of the second derivative), the *localization of this surface* in space (including both grid-point accuracy and subvoxel accuracy), and the *estimation of the direction* of the surface normal (from the gradient in the 2-D depth image and from the gradient in the 3-D volume). Disadvantages of this technique are that it can be affected by noise and artefacts.

Surfaces can be represented using various small triangles or rectangles (i.e., the polygonal tiling or directed contour method) or as a uniform matrix of anisotropic (noncubic)

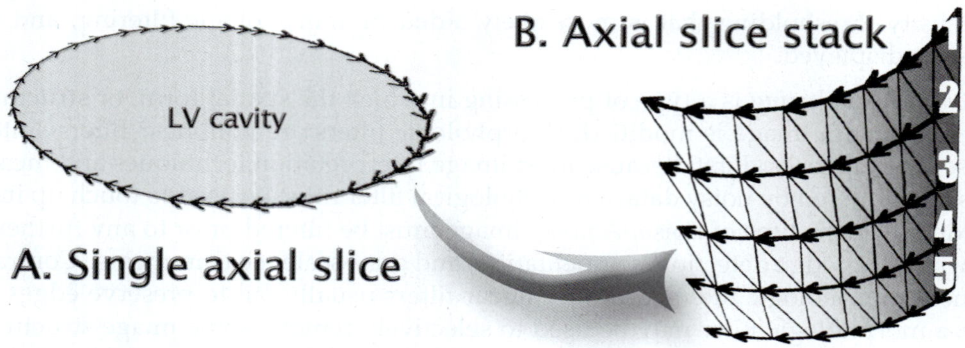

Figure 11.10: A. Contour-based representation of inner surface of LV chamber in an axial slice of imaging data. B. Tiled representation, or *"facetization"* of a portion of the surface prescribed by five juxtaposed slices.

or isotropic (cubic) voxels. The goal of *tiling techniques* is to determine the surface that encloses a given set of slice contours, and then represent the surface with a set of 2-D primitives. As a preliminary step, tiling requires the extraction of the contours of the object of interest in each slice, using, e.g., intensity thresholding. The extracted contours are then smoothed, and geometric primitives, typically triangles, are fitted to these contours to approximate the surface of the object in the interslice space. This approach is common because tiled surfaces furnish realistic representations of the objects, e.g., adjacent cardiac chambers selected for display, especially when they are differentiated with color.

Because of the data reduction inherent in going from the input imaging data to a tiled surface representation, the computational cost of displaying and manipulating the objects of interest to obtain geometric measurements is low. The disadvantages inherent in this approach are the time required to extract the surface, and the difficulty in performing the tiling. The right panel of Figure 11.10 contains a tiled depiction of a portion of the endocardial surface of the LV defined by five adjacent axial slices; the raw data for each slice is similar to that in the left panel. A contour description represents each slice; the interslice portion of the volume is delineated by triangles. A specified contour surface (with a constant surface shading value) can be algorithmically approximated and meshed into a set of triangular facets, and rendered using standard graphics engines [55], as was done here to confer a better 3-D quality to the stacked data.

The directed contour methods have the advantages of a very short computation time and considerably reduced storage requirements. This enables geometric structure reproductions of cardiac chambers, vessels, and other organs to be rotated in real time on a monitor screen around several axes. The voxel representation method yields the best results if cubic voxels are employed. If the raw data are not composed of cubic voxels, these can be created using linear interpolation. This forms additional slices, enabling a division into cubes. The advantage of cubic voxels in an improved object contour smoothness of the rendered image. Identification of different objects in a stack of images is accomplished by segmentation techniques.

Different methods of *segmentation* are available. Thresholding can be used if the anatomic boundary occurs between high-contrast regions. Otherwise, boundary detection using automatic or manual tracking is used for segmentation. Due to the complexity found in the typical cardiac image, automatic methods commonly require operator assistance to extract the boundaries of the organ structures accurately. Using thresholding as a segmentation procedure, a certain limit of voxel values is defined as a selection criterion. Voxels are differentiated by an intensity threshold: only voxels with a certain attenuation, or signal intensity value, are used for reconstruction. All voxels within the given range are allocated to the structure of interest, with the rest being excluded. Tracking is a method of drawing lines around certain regions, either completely or partially by hand, by laying down seed-points, which are subsequently connected automatically. Region growing uses a process that is able to identify the boundary of a given anatomic structure with signal similarities and delineate it automatically.

Surface representation of 3-D imaging datasets results in a significant reduction in data storage and can exploit commercial software and geometry engines for fast manipulation and display. However, in surface representation, the information inside the segmented 3-D objects is no longer available for visual exploration. Volume rendering and representation, on the other hand, will maintain the entire dataset; thus any constituent, including parts interior to larger structures, can be viewed subsequently.

11.5.4 Volume rendering

As the name implies, volume rendering (VR) renders the entire volume of scanned data rather than just surfaces or voxels of specified intensity; accordingly, it should be expected to encompass more information than a surface model. VR is often described as a direct rendering method because it directly maps sample points from the volume dataset to the viewplane, via some optical model and a transfer function that controls the extent to which the data values are transparent or opaque. With proper control of the opacity transfer function, direct rendering thus enables data exploration without the need to make firm assumptions about the boundaries between adjacent objects [29].

Essentially, volume rendering converts a scalar function on a 3-D volume into varying colors (or shades of gray) and opacities, and creates an image by integrating the color and opacity effects along viewing rays through each pixel [39]. Thus, volume rendering techniques sum the contributions of each voxel along a line from the viewer's eye through the 3-D dataset. This is done repeatedly to determine each pixel value in the displayed image. Because the information from the entire dataset is included into the resulting image, much more powerful computers are required than with other methods, in order to do volume rendering at a reasonable speed. Volume techniques are the most advanced form of 3-D rendering available for creating accurate, clinically useful cardiovascular organ reconstructions. With general availability and continued increases in computer power, it is rapidly becoming the most important rendering technique for 3-D imaging, especially for

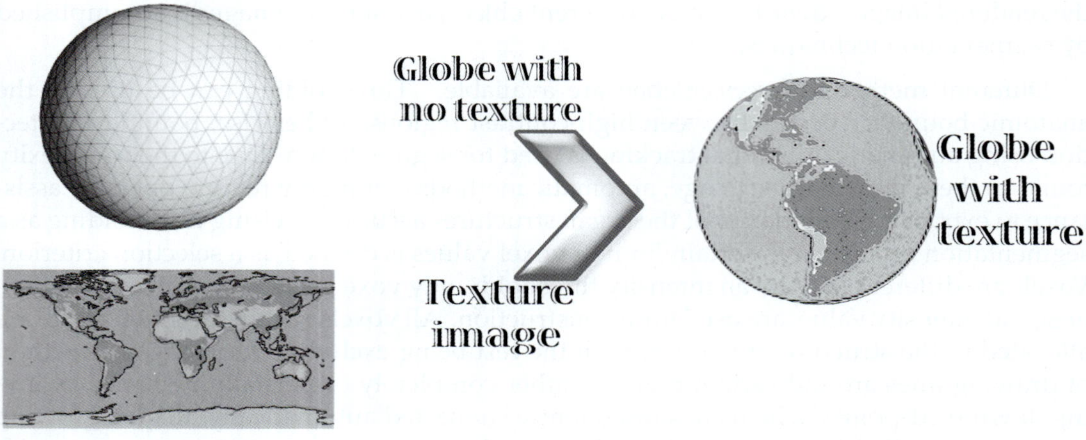

Figure 11.11: A texture map (image) is applied to the surface of a shape when building, or rendering, a 2-D representation of a 3-D structure. The Earth image shown on the right was created by mapping the flat rectangular picture of Earth on the lower left onto the ordinary sphere shown above it. Equally well the texture mapping could have been applied onto a cube, a cone, or any arbitrary 3-D model.

angiographic applications. One of the greatest advantages of VR is *perspective* or depth information (see Sections 11.3 and 11.4, on pp. 587 ff.).

Bilinear, trilinear, and sophisticated nonlinear interpolations, or even shape-based interpolations [48], are available and can be used for a better-quality reconstructed 3-D voxel image. Alternatively, slices may be replicated (zero-order interpolation) to fill in the *gaps* between successive acquired slices. Replication does not introduce artificial data and is efficient in memory use and reconstruction time, but the derived 3-D image shows stronger staircase artefacts. As expected, both interpolation and replication strive to create a 3-D isotropic dataset whose three axes are correctly proportioned.

Trilinear interpolation (TI)

The term *trilinear* in TI refers to the performing of interpolations in 3-D (horizontal, vertical and depth dimensions). TI is a texture mapping technique that produces most realistic images but requires the most computations. A texture is a pattern that is mapped to a polygon through the process of texture mapping [12]. Viewed differently, textures are simply rectangular arrays of data—e.g., color data, luminance (i.e., perceived brightness) data, or color and alpha data.[6]

[6]An alpha channel, representing transparency, or degree of opacity, information on a per-pixel basis, can be included in gray-scale and true-color images. An alpha value of zero represents full transparency, and a value of $[(2^{bitdepth}) - 1]$ represents a fully opaque pixel. Intermediate values indicate partially transparent pixels that can be combined with a background image to yield a composite image. The color values stored for a pixel are not affected by the alpha value assigned to it.

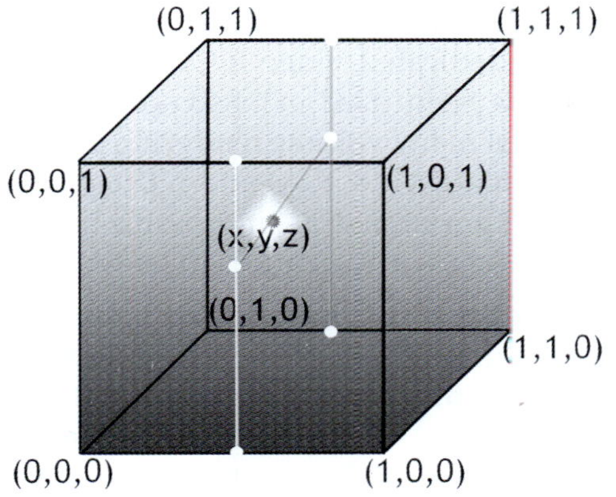

Figure 11.12: In 3-D, there are 8 grid points surrounding any point (x, y, z) in a box; they are exemplified in the diagram along with possible coordinates. To combine their respective influences requires a trilinear interpolation (linear interpolation in each of three dimensions). It takes seven linear interpolations to yield the final result. Each linear interpolation requires one multiplication procedure. The six white dots are the results of the first six interpolations, chosen here as follows: four in the left-to-right direction, followed by two in the bottom-to-top direction. Finally, a seventh interpolation in the back-to-front direction gives the final result to be assigned to point (x, y, z).

The individual values in a texture array are often called texels. A *texel*, or texture element (also *tex*ture pix*el*), is the fundamental unit of texture space [15], used in computer graphics and visualization. Textures are represented by arrays of texels, just as pictures are represented by arrays of pixels. When texturing a 3-D surface, a process known as texture mapping maps texels to appropriate pixels in the output picture, as is exemplified in Figure 11.11, on p. 602; this operation is akin to applying gift wrapping paper to a plain white box and is accomplished on the graphics card of a visualization workstation.

Common dimensions for textures are 1-, 2-, and 3-D. A 1-D texture is a line of color. A 2-D texture is an image. A 3-D texture is a stack of images and is similar to a volume of medical imaging data. In order to map a texture to a polygon, one must first define texture coordinates at each vertex of that polygon. Texture coordinates are then interpolated across the face of the polygon, applying the texture smoothly to the entire surface of the shape. The texture coordinates of each vertex must be specified in the same number of dimensions as the texture itself. Texture mapping rendering packages may use trilinear interpolation hardware to extract a parallel set of oblique slices from a 3-D dataset, and use rasterization and compositing hardware to combine the slices in a way that models the passage of a scanning beam through the examined object. This hardware-accelerated approach is much faster than traditional ray-tracing methods.

Using software and the CPU of most modern workstations, to perform accurate interactive visualization of currently obtainable volumetric cardiac datasets and to analyze cardiac images spatially and temporally at high resolutions, is difficult because the task is memory access-limited. The difficulty is mitigated by using hardware-accelerated

3-D texture mapping capabilities of commercially available high-end graphics boards, with at least 512–1,024 *MB* of dedicated video RAM. Since its introduction in the early 1990s [3], texture mapping has been used extensively for accelerating volume rendering [56], and has been the basis of many volume rendering packages, including the *OpenGL Volumizer™* library (SGI, Mountain View, CA) and *NIHmagic* [13]. Enhancements to the basic volume rendering algorithm aimed at improving both speed and voxel shading quality continue to be made, along with advances in texture mapping hardware [49].

Trilinear interpolation is the process of interpolating points within cells of a volumetric dataset and it is actually *not a linear operation* because the weighting factors used in the interpolation are volumes rather than lines, as is indicated in the successive RHS terms of Equation 11.1 that follows below. Of the commonly used techniques, this is the texture mapping algorithm that produces the most realistic images and requires the most computations. The target quality level and performance mode for RealityEngine2™(SGI, Mountain View, CA) is trilinear interpolation. This is also the highest quality texture function available on any of the newer high-end image generators for visual simulations. Of the commonly used interpolation schemes (nearest neighbor, trilinear, and high-order interpolations), trilinear interpolation represents a good trade off between accuracy and computational demands. This should not come as a surprise, since quality usually comes with a price: the higher the quality, the more time it takes to generate the image. Trilinear interpolation interpolates a point based on the weighted average of the eight data points of the cube surrounding the data point. Nearest neighbor assigns a value based solely on the nearest data value.[7] As a result, trilinear is much more accurate and nearest neighbor is much faster. Correspondingly, aliasing is quite prevalent when using nearest neighbor interpolations, but is present to a much lesser extent in trilinearly interpolated datasets. However, trilinear interpolation does have the effect of *squashing* the peaks (high brightness intensities) and *raising* the valleys (low intensities).

In a nutshell, TI involves interpolating points within a box (3-D) given values at the vertices of the box. Consider a unit cube with the lower, left, base vertex at the origin as is shown in Figure 11.12, on p. 603. The values at each vertex are denoted V_{000}, V_{100}, V_{010}, ..., V_{111}, as is implied in the diagram. Then, the value at an arbitrary position (x, y, z) within the cube is generally denoted Vxyz and is given by the following equation:

$$\begin{aligned} V_{xyz} = \; & V_{000}(1-x)(1-y)(1-z) + \\ & V_{100} \cdot x \cdot (1-y) \cdot (1-z) + \\ & V_{010} \cdot (1-x) \cdot y \cdot (1-z) + \\ & V_{001} \cdot (1-x) \cdot (1-y) \cdot z + \\ & V_{101} \cdot x \cdot (1-y) \cdot z + \\ & V_{011} \cdot (1-x) \cdot y \cdot z + \\ & V_{110} \cdot x \cdot y \cdot (1-z) + \\ & V_{111} \cdot x \cdot y \cdot z \, . \end{aligned} \tag{11.1}$$

[7] In 1-D, there are seldom good reasons to choose this one over linear interpolation, which is almost as cheap, but in higher dimensions, in multivariate interpolation, it can be a favorable choice when speed and simplicity are paramount considerations.

This process is repeated for each pixel forming the object being textured. The result of trilinear interpolation is independent of the order of the successive interpolation steps. Ordinarily, the box will not be of unit size nor will it be aligned at the origin. Simple translation and scaling (possibly of each axis independently) can be used to transform into, and then back out of, this simplified situation.

The VR algorithm produces a 2-D display image that can convey 3-D spatial information inherent in, e.g., a 3-D spiral MSCT volume dataset. Volume rendering displays a sampled 3-D data field directly, without first fitting geometric primitives to the sampled data. The original volume rendering algorithm used ray tracing to construct the 3-D image [10]. A number of specific implementations are based on ray tracing. The first step in the VR process assigns a color and opacity to each voxel in the volume dataset. The *ray-tracing* approach sequentially computes the values for each pixel displayed in the 3-D image by calculating a weighted sum of all voxels encountered along a line (or ray) projected from the chosen viewing perspective through the data volume. This process is replicated for each displayed pixel by projecting a new parallel ray through the data.

Each pixel in the final 3-D image represents the computed sum of the voxels along a ray projected through the dataset in a specific orientation. In order to generate a 512×512 3-D image, this technique entails 262,144 sequential ray tracing calculations—one for every pixel of the display screen. Additional calculations are required to incorporate surface shading into the image. Without specialized graphics hardware, this scheme can be very slow to implement.

Dedicated computer graphics hardware is commercially available which allows all of the pixel values in a 3-D image to be computed *in parallel* rather than by the serial sequential approach that is ordinarily used by ray tracing programs. This approach affords dramatic improvements in rendering speed. Volume rendered 3-D images can be rendered at real-time rates (better than 20 frames/s), depending on the size of the viewing object. Real-time rendering allows true user *interactivity* with the dataset. New lower-priced parallel architecture video cards and image processing workstations such as multicore/multiprocessor PC computers and the O2 from Silicon Graphics (Silicon Graphics, Inc., Mountain View, CA) are bringing this computer intensive technique into widespread clinical and research use. Volume rendering has extraordinary potential to become a core part of *cardiac imaging* and visualization.

The color, opacity, and position of the voxel within the volume are integrated into the computation. Volume-averaged voxels containing more than one tissue type are displayed with shades of gray. The 3-D relationships of structures are conveyed in the final 2-D image and can be interactively enhanced with perspective and stereo options [24]. Although specific implementations of the volume rendering algorithm by various manufacturers share important features, differences in the interpolation algorithms and other features may produce very different results in terms of accuracy and image appearance.

By assigning a full spectrum of opacity values and applying scale of gray or color coding to the blood and tissue classification system, volume rendering provides a robust and versatile dataset for advanced cardiac imaging applications. It is a technique that allows an accurate visualization of the *cardiac chambers and vasculature* as well as the maintenance of the all-important 3-D geometric relationships. It allows some of the advantages of SSD and MIP. Viewing the data as a 3-D field rather than as individual planes confers the immediate advantage that the information can be viewed from any vantage viewpoint. These scanning systems provide 3-D information that is represented by a set of discrete scalar values $D(i, j, k)$ defined on a 3-D grid with indices i, j, and k.[8] The scalar values $D(i, j, k)$ represent some physical property of the body tissues, like x-ray absorption, at 3-D spatial locations.

Isosurfaces are the 3-D analog of 2-D isocurves (see Fig. 2.16, in Section 2.7, on pp. 57 f.). An isosurface in a continuous 3-D field $F(x, y, z)$ is defined as the set of 3-D points that satisfy the equation $F(x, y, z) - v = 0$, for a certain value v. The selection of different isovalues v, i.e., different tissues, can be done interactively, and several tissues can be rendered simultaneously at interactive frame rates. Isosurfaces and isocontours are defined on continuous domains. If we want to define arbitrary isosurfaces in discrete data fields, we obviously need first to convert the discrete into a continuous data field. A reconstruction function $R(x, y, z)$ can be used to extend $D(i, j, k)$ to a continuous function $C(x, y, z)$, for which arbitrary isosurfaces can be defined.

11.5.5 Shading

A 3-D object in computer memory is made up of faces. *Faces* are polygons that are defined by the edge points of an object, or by the vertices. In Figure 11.10, on p. 600, the faces are spaces between the contours in the stacked slices of the dataset. Notice that the number of faces is definitive of how detailed we want the image to appear. Because computers are not infinitely fast, we must impose some limits on the definition of the image. In the case of the LV chamber of Figure 11.10, more faces will make its inner surface look smoother. With the various *shading models*, however, this is not necessary.

Flat (or constant) shading means that the computer will calculate the normal vector of each face (the vector which points *away* from the face in a direction perpendicular to its surface plane), compare it to the angle of the light hitting it, and shade it with an intensity that is representative of the angle between the angle of incidence and the surface normal. This sounds complicated, but what it really means is that if a line drawn perpendicular to the face is parallel to and opposite in direction to the light ray, it will be illuminated at full intensity. As this angle grows, the intensity is reduced. If the surface normal and the light ray are parallel and in the same direction, it means that the surface is facing directly away from the light and, therefore, no light falls on it. The results of flat shading are shown in Figure 11.13, on p. 607.

The biggest drawback of flat shading is that the edges between faces are harsh because there is no smooth gradation between intensities. In the example of Figure 11.13, this could be alleviated by making the faces smaller and smaller until they were only single pixels on the screen. But if we did that, the number of points (and thus, the calculation time) would be so big that the computer would take too long to render the image. Shading

[8] Mathematically, $D(i, j, k)$ is the result of a convolution of the point spread function of the particular acquisition device with an object at discrete sampling locations.

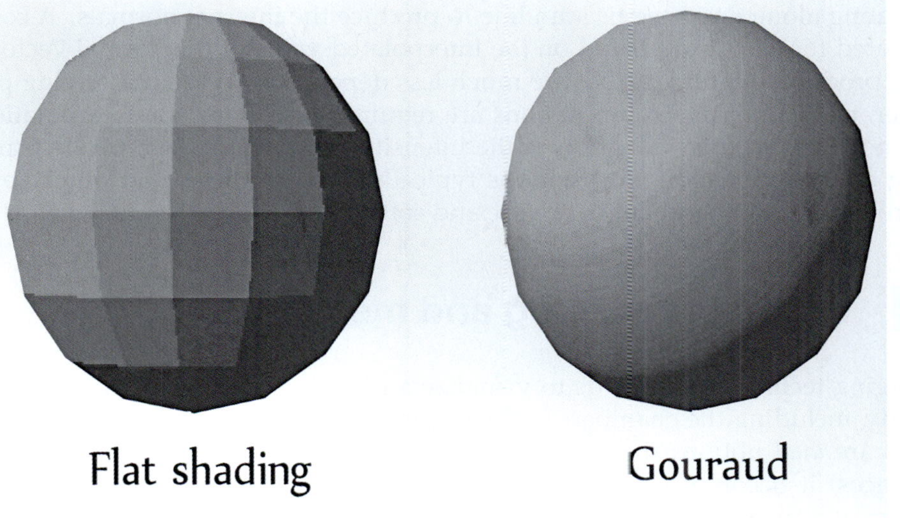

Figure 11.13: The same ellipsoidal object with flat and Gouraud shading applied. Notice that the ellipsoid with Gouraud shading appears much smoother than the flat shaded one. Both ellipsoids have the exact same number of polygons as you can ascertain by looking closely at their outlines.

computations can also be quite costly, and several methods have been devised to speed up the process. They are based on computing the shade only at the vertices of a polygon and *interpolating* the values in the interior.

Gouraud shading, named after H. Gouraud who applied it to arbitrary polygons, solves some of the problems of flat shading, as indicated in Figure 11.13. It is a very simple and effective method of adding a "curved feel" to a polygon that would otherwise appear flat. In this technique, the shading information is linearly interpolated across a face from gray-scale or color values determined for its vertices [17]. In contrast to flat polygon shading, the technique allows one to specify a different shade for each vertex of a tessellating polygon; the rendering engine of the imaging device then smoothly interpolates the shade across the entire tessellated surface. It can be implemented very quickly with integer mathematics. A point to keep in mind, however, is that it is best to restrict Gouraud shading to three-sided polygons. Sometimes polygons may not look quite as one might expect, when they have more than three vertices with *very different* shades.

Phong shading [45], also known as "normal-vector interpolation-shading," interpolates the surface normal vectors, **N**, rather than the gray-scale or color intensity. It interpolates the vertex normals across the surface of a polygon, or triangle, and illuminates the pixel at each point. At each pixel, one needs to compute the normal vector and also the reflection vector. The interpolated vectors give an indication of the local curvature of the smooth surface that every flat tessellating polygon, or triangle, is approximating. The interpolation is implemented by first calculating the vertex normals, then using these as the basis for interpolation along the polygon edges, and finally using these as the basis for interpolating along any specific scan line to produce the internal normals. A color value is calculated for each pixel based on the interpolated value of the normal vector. Phong shading produces highlights that are much less dependent on the underlying polygons. However, more intensive computations are required, involving the interpolation of the surface normal and the evaluation of the intensity function for each pixel. Current 3-D imaging and visualization workstations typically support these, and other approaches [12], through a combination of hardware and software.

11.6 Image processing and meshing

3-D imaging techniques allow us to visualize anatomical regions and organs of the human body, including the chambers of the beating heart. If we consider that surfaces and volumes are *dual* notions (i.e., cardiac chamber volumes are bounded by inner chamber surfaces) it becomes clear that surface and volume rendering are not as different as they may appear at first glance. In terms of spatial complexity, surfaces are represented by $O(N)^2$ (see footnote on p. 284) elements and volumes are represented by $O(N)^3$ elements—although both surfaces and volumes may be defined in terms of more elegant available mathematical representations, so as to be representable *parsimmoniously*, i.e., by a lot fewer elements. Considering the redundancy of volume representations and the compactness of free-shape surface representations, we may state that the two approaches are *complementary*, in the sense that volume approaches allow us to analyze numerical volume datasets and surface approaches allow us to structure the results of the analyses.

Many research and clinical applications rely upon a geometric modeling of organ structures, using efficient and reliable algorithms for constructing common tessellations of the surfaces of interest. Although shaded surface rendering (see Section 11.5.3, on pp. 598 ff.) and volume rendering (Section 11.5.4, on pp. 601 ff.) of 3-D images are gaining widespread use, multiplanar reformatting or reformation (see Section 11.5.1, on pp. 595 f.) remains a valuable visualization mode. Shaded surface rendering requires segmentation of the structures of interest, which is a challenging task. Especially with real-time 3-D (RT3D) ultrasound images, which are noisy and lack a direct correlation between voxel intensity and tissue type, opacity curves are hard to define based solely on intensity values. This makes good-quality volume rendering difficult without extensive preprocessing. Simultaneous display of several intersecting reformatted planes is a handy visualization tool, allowing exploration of time-varying 3-D geometry and important anatomic structures by smoothly varying the orientation of the displayed reformatted planes.

Inner cardiac chamber surface meshes for CFD simulations of intracardiac blood flows must match requirements related both to the accuracy of the surface approximation and to the element shape and size that are suitable for the computations. Mesh generation is a process of spatial subdivision of a generally complex domain into simple shaped subvolumes of predefined topology. These subvolumes are denoted as *mesh elements* or cells. Elements of a mesh are connected but do not intersect with each other, and cover the entire domain. The success of mesh generation algorithms and the accuracy of the numerical analyses and simulations often depend on the quality of the surface mesh. Detailed considerations of computational grid generation, and of various mesh varieties that are currently used in CFD and intracardiac blood flow simulations, are given in the following three chapters. Here, we conclude this introduction to postprocessing exploration techniques and display of tomographic data, with an initial *overture* to this field from our present imaging perspective, focusing on unstructured meshing technology.

Strictly speaking, a structured mesh can be recognized by the so-called *node valence* requirement, namely, that all of its interior nodes have an equal number of adjacent elements. Normally, the mesh generated by a structured grid generator is all quadrilateral or hexahedral. Algorithms are employed which generally involve complex iterative smoothing techniques and aim at aligning elements with flow boundaries. When complicated boundaries are at hand, "block-structured" techniques can be employed, allowing the user to break the domain up into several constituent topological blocks. As we shall see in the next three chapters, structured grids are most commonly used in CFD, where strict alignment of elements can be required by the analysis code.

Conversely, unstructured mesh generation relaxes the node valence requirement, allowing any number of elements to meet at a single node. Triangle and tetrahedral meshes are most commonly thought of when referring to unstructured meshing, although quadrilateral and hexahedral meshes can also be unstructured. While there is some overlap between structured and unstructured mesh generation methods, the main feature that distinguishes the two is to be found in the unique iterative smoothing algorithms of the structured grid generators. Three main steps lead to unstructured mesh generation, as applied in finite element CFD cardiac flow-field simulations:

- In a first stage, volumetric datasets are processed, as described in the preceding sections, to reconstruct the cardiac chamber inner surface; this is commonly associated with a triangulation step. A triangulation is a surface discretization, or *facetization*, which is not necessarily composed only of triangles since it may produce polygonal surface meshes.[9] Moreover, the initial triangulation is, most often, not suitable for numerical simulations.

- A second stage is needed in order to eliminate surface artefacts (e.g., holes, etc.), to simplify the surface reconstructed from the possibly too large set of discrete data points to a suitable number of triangles, and to ensure a computation-suited mesh. Procedures have been developed to optimize polygonal surface meshes by repositioning nodes in a series of steps. The repositioning of nodes is directed by a numerical optimization procedure, which is designed to improve the geometric shape of mesh faces while keeping the modified mesh as close as possible to the base mesh [14]. Such procedures can improve mesh quality while minimizing changes to the surface characteristics. This step provides a 3-D geometrical model.

- During the third stage, the computational mesh is generated and adapted for efficient numerical simulations of intracardiac blood flow. The procedure includes a method for improving the quality of mesh faces on the boundaries while preserving

[9]General polygons can be considered to be made up of triangular facets.

the original inner chamber surface definition, and thereby maintaining the essential characteristics of the surface. The overall procedure consists of iterations involving node repositioning on the boundary, followed by node repositioning in the interior with the boundary nodes fixed. It improves mesh quality of tetrahedral and hexahedral meshes while minimizing changes to the mesh characteristics and to the discrete boundary surfaces [16].

To provide the reader with an intuitive understanding of the process, presentation of some important approaches to unstructured mesh generation is appropriate at this point.

11.6.1 Delaunay tessellation

To ensure continuity (conservation of mass) of the discretized flow-field approximation, the tessellation model of a flow region (e.g., a cardiac chamber) has to be *topologically compatible*, which implies that its cells or volume elements do not intersect each other but they cover the full region. Popular among the triangle and tetrahedral meshing techniques are those that utilize the Delaunay criterion [9], which was formulated by the Russian mathematician Boris Delone[10] The Delaunay optimization criterion is sometimes designated as the *empty sphere* (*la sphère vide*, cf. [9]) property; it requires that vertices of neighboring *simplices*[11] not be contained within the circumcircle or circumsphere of individual simplices within the mesh[12] (see Fig. 11.14, on p. 611). The Delaunay triangulation criterion yields triangles which are closest to equilateral ones (Fig. 11.14).

The Delaunay criterion yields optimization criteria for connecting a set of existing points in space. The usual approach is to first mesh the boundary of the geometry to provide an initial set of nodes. The boundary nodes are then triangulated according to the Delaunay criterion. Nodes are subsequently inserted incrementally into the existing mesh, redefining the triangles or tetrahedra locally as each new node is inserted, so as to uphold the Delaunay criterion. It is the method that is chosen for defining where to locate the interior nodes that distinguishes one Delaunay algorithm from another.

One particular algorithm is the so-called boundary constrained Delaunay triangulation. In most Delaunay approaches, before internal nodes are generated, a 3-D tessellation of the nodes on the bounding surface is produced. In this process, there is no guarantee that the surface triangulation will be satisfied. In many implementations, the approach is to tessellate the boundary nodes using a standard Delaunay algorithm without regard for the surface facets. A second step is then employed to recover the surface triangulation. By doing so, the triangulation may no longer be strictly "Delaunay;" hence the term *boundary constrained Delaunay triangulation* [57].

[10]Various spellings of the name, transliterated from the Russian, are encountered in the literature.

[11]For our purposes, *simplices* comprise *triangles* in planar surfaces, and *tetrahedra*, their 3-D generalizations, in space.

[12]A circumcircle or circumsphere can be defined as the circle or sphere passing through all vertices of the corresponding *simplex*.

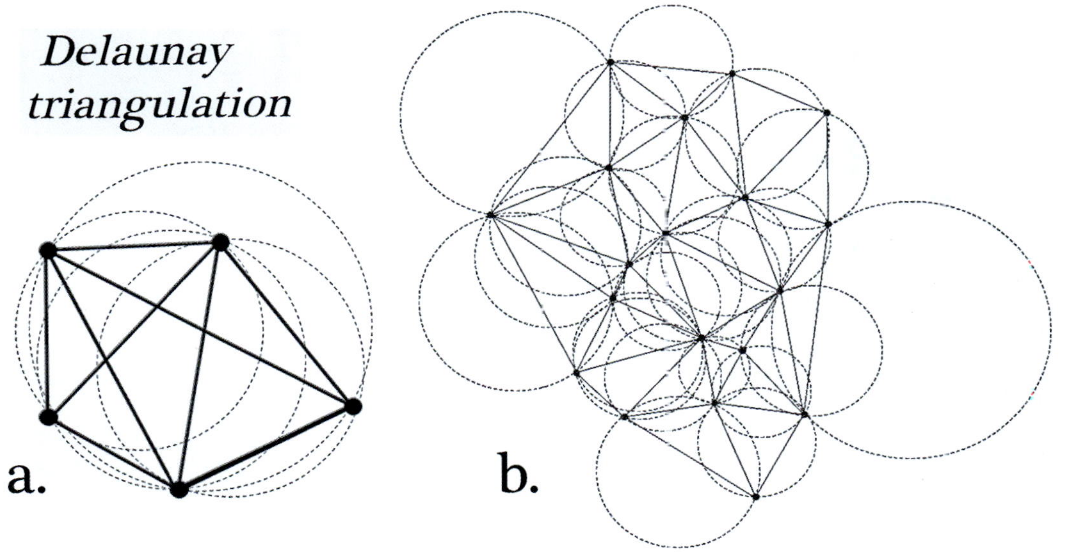

Figure 11.14: Delaunay tessellation: a. The empty circle (sphere) property prescribes that no other vertex is contained within the circumcircle (circumsphere) of any triangle (tetrahedron) of a Delaunay tessellation. b. A Delaunay triangulation (tetrahedralization) obeys the empty-circle (sphere) property.

11.6.2 Plastering

Another very popular family of triangle and tetrahedral mesh generation algorithms is the *advancing front*, or moving front approach [33]. In this approach, tetrahedra are built progressively inward from the triangulated surface (initial front), and an active front is maintained where new tetrahedra are formed. The front (boundary between the gridded and ungridded regions) is advanced into the field in an irregular manner with no predetermined, orderly structure while introducing new grid points in the field. The process is continued until the entire domain is filled with contiguous cells. Thus, in the aptly named "plastering method," hexahedral elements are first placed starting with the bounding surface and advancing into the interior of the computational domain, toward the center of the volume, as is shown schematically in Figure 11.15, on p. 612.

A heuristic set of procedures for determining the order of element formation and element placement on the bounding surface must be delineated; thus, in an advancing front approach for arbitrary 3-D surfaces, surface normals and tangents must be computed in order to compute the direction of the advancing front. With the "plastering" algorithm, a current front is defined consisting of all quadrilaterals. Individual "quads" are then projected toward the interior of the volume to form hexahedra. In addition, plastering must detect intersecting faces and determine when and how to connect to pre-existing nodes or to seam faces. As the algorithm advances, complex interior voids may result, which in some cases are impossible to fill with all-hexahedral elements. Existing elements,

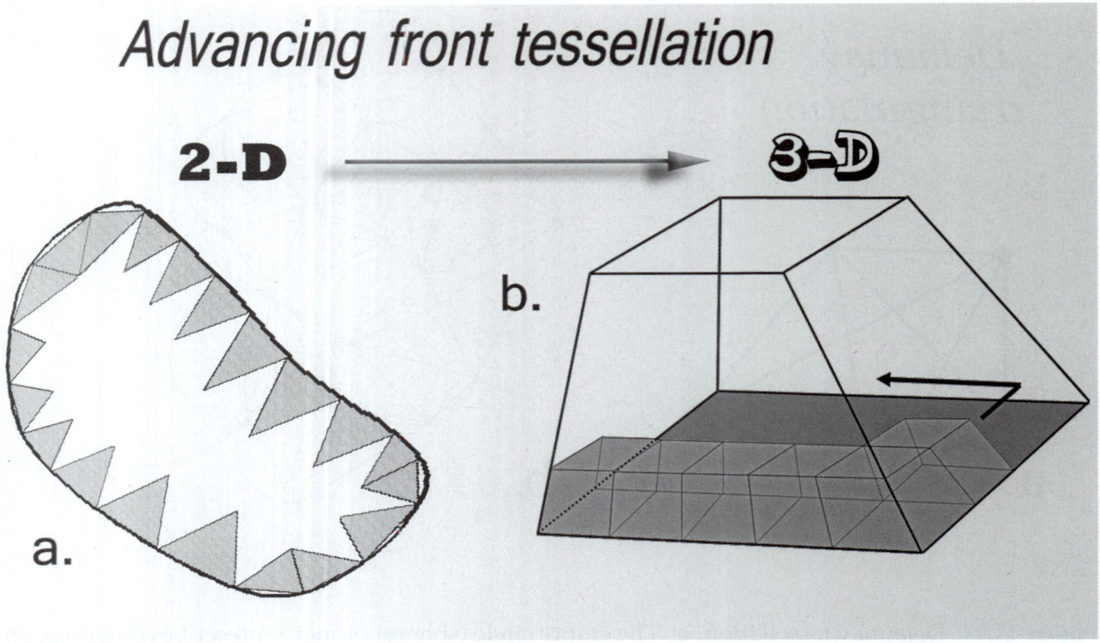

Figure 11.15: The *advancing front* approach. a. A 2-D example ("paving") of the plastering method, an advancing front approach, where one layer of triangles has been placed along the bounding curve. b. Plastering is a 3-D extension of paving; the tessellation again advances element-by-element or row-by-row.

already placed by the plastering algorithm must sometimes be modified, so as to facilitate placement of hexahedra toward the interior. It should be noted that, although several layers of hexahedral elements may be successfully placed on the boundary of a volume, intersection and closure procedures are sometimes difficult to implement effectively.

A variant of the advancing front method, sometimes called "advancing layers," is also used for generating boundary layers for CFD, Navier–Stokes applications [44]. This method lends itself well to control of element sizes in the hydrodynamic boundary layer near the flow boundary. A conventional advancing-front technique can be applied to the generation of regular, equilateral cells in the inviscid-flow region. The method is applicable to 2-D (e.g., triangular, quadrilateral grids) and to 3-D (e.g., tetrahedral, hexahedral grids) viscous flow grid-generation problems.

The viscous layers are generated by a tangential refinement of the cells that are adjacent to the solid walls, as is shown in Figure 11.16. This refinement process is performed in a number of steps [36], and enables the generation of a sufficient number of anisotropic cell layers, which are highly stretched tangentially along the walls of the computational domain, so as to satisfy the resolution requirements of the flow problem. The vertices of these cells are redistributed in the direction normal to the wall according to a specified first cell size and the desired stretching ratio.

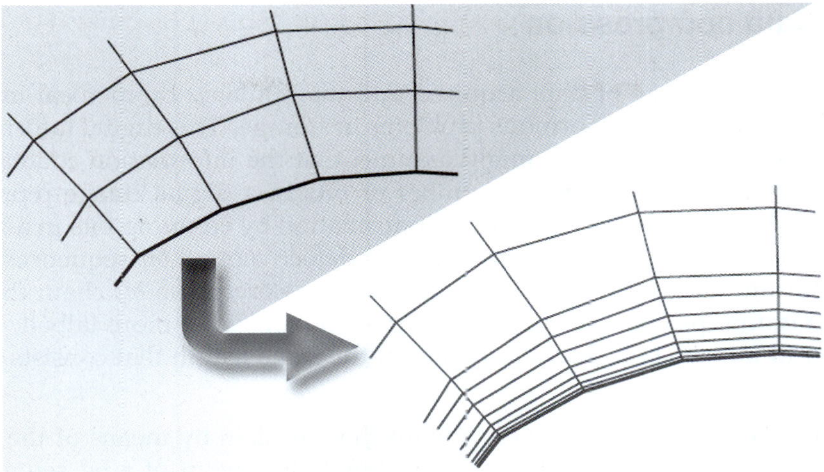

Figure 11.16: Viscous layer cell insertion.

11.7 Dynamic mesh deformation

Intracardiac blood flow simulations are part of a wide class of flow-phenomena modeling which requires flow analysis in domains of shapes that change during the computation. This class encompasses multiple coupled unsteady state problems with moving or deforming interfaces, fluid–structure interaction problems, and many others. By the Courant–Friedrichs–Lewy condition, as the spatial resolution of the simulation increases, its timestep must be shortened too (see Section 12.8.2, on pp. 665 ff.) and more computational time is required to complete the simulation. Solving such problems demands that the computational mesh follow the dynamic deformation of the boundaries of the flow domain. Accordingly, two principal possibilities exist.

The first one is to deform the existing mesh according to the transpiring deformation of its boundary. Thus, for neighboring timesteps during which relative deformation of the mesh boundary may be small, full re-meshing appears to be too costly. Instead, *deforming* the already existing mesh can be a "quick" and reliable technique, provided that appropriate algorithms are available. The methodology should be optimized to preserve mesh topology and should modify only the positions of vertices, preserving high mesh quality. The second possibility is to fully *regrid* the domain every time its shape is modified significantly.

These two approaches can be applied separately, or *in combination*, alternating with each other throughout the time encompassed by the entire simulation. Highly unsteady intracardiac blood flow problems involving moving cardiac chamber boundaries during ejection and filling can be accommodated using such a parsimmonious approach to mesh deformation. This allows regridding to only take place after several computational timesteps, e.g., every 3rd or 4th timestep.

11.7.1 Data compression

Clearly, the large amounts of data acquired and manipulated by medical imaging and analysis methods can create enormous problems in storage. This digital information consists of sequence of bits, and, one might assume, that the information content might be quantifiable by simply counting the number of bits in a digital image representation. However, although the idea of quantifying information by counting bits in a sequence is simple and conceptually useful, it has a serious defect: not all *bit* sequences of a given length contain the same amount of information. For example, a *bit* chain that is determined by a random process, such as a coin-toss, contains a lot more (albeit, admittedly not very useful) information than a sequence of the same length that consists of all zeros or all ones.

Algorithmic information theory deals with this problem by means of the concept of *compression* of information. It defines the information content of a *bit* sequence as the number of bits in the smallest computer program that will generate that sequence. Any *bit* sequence reproducible by a computer program that is shorter than the sequence itself is, therefore, compressible by definition. A conservation law, very similar to conservation of energy in classical physics, governs compressed information. Just as the quantity of energy is unchanged under physical operations, the quantity of compressed information is unchanged under any sequence of logical operations. Conservation of compressed information implies that the quantity of information output from any computer program must be less than or equal to the information input.

The design goal of image compression is to develop computer algorithms to represent images with as few bits as possible, according to some fidelity criterion, in order to save storage and transmission channel capacity. All image compression techniques try to get rid of the inherent redundancy, which may be spatial (neighboring pixels), spectral (pixels in different spectral bands in a color image), or temporal (correlated images in a sequence, e.g., video clips).

The widespread, consumer-market use of information in the form of images has contributed much to the development of data compression techniques. There are lossless methods, which are reversible, i.e., they do not sacrifice any information, and lossy methods which may be used if the quality of a compression-decompression sequence is judged by general criteria, like unchanged quality for ordinary human visual perception. Thus, in image processing jargon, "lossless" is sometimes used in the sense of "no visible loss". Compression of digital images and video is readily accomplished using a wide variety of compression algorithms, including JPEG, MPEG, CMP, LZW, G3/G4, Huffman, run-length, and many more. Using the JPEG algorithm, image compression up to approximately 3:1 is lossless.

The application of transform methods (see footnote on p. 2.18) to image compression was introduced in Section 2.19, on pp. 88 ff. The fundamental property of lossy image compression is the *similarity* of *different* resolutions of the same image. Lossy compression means that we assign the same output representation to multiple, similar input representations. The basic similarity relation for images is resolution, or scale, invariance: If we

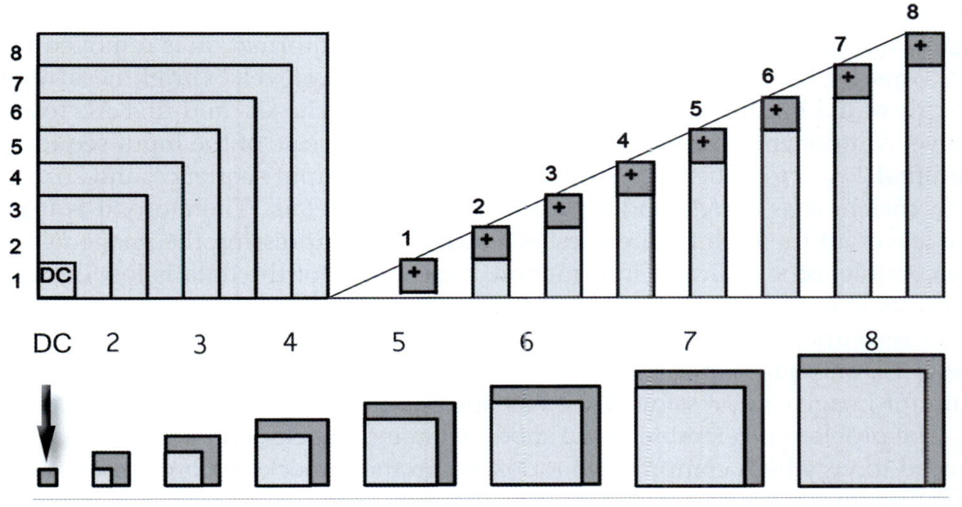

Figure 11.17: DCT block resolution bands and additive resolution progression.

see the same image in different resolutions (scales, sizes), then we talk about *the same* image. The discrete cosine transform (DCT) provides the best resolution separation property for digital images. The 8-point DCT gives 8 linearly increasing resolution representations from 8 spatial sample values. Other transforms, such as the *wavelet transform*[13] used in JPEG2000, do not provide such optimal resolution separation.

As was indicated on p. 88, DCT is very closely related to the discrete Fourier transform (DFT). It is actually possible to compute DCT using DFT. The main difference between DCT and DFT, which involves complex exponentials (see Section 2.18, on pp. 32 ff.), is that DCT has only real values and it is comparatively easier to compute. In DCT, an image is broken into blocks—8×8, or 16×16, or bigger—bigger blocks take quite longer times to do the processing. Typically $8 \cdot 8$ blocks are applied. The procedure effectively divides the image like a checkerboard into square patches of 8×8 pixels. These blocks, which constitute the complete image, are each transformed into 64 DCT coefficients [2], which represent all possible spatial frequencies and phases along the x- and y-axes. Any eight-by-eight patch of the original image can be reconstructed by adding up various weighted combinations of these basic frequency elements, or *basis functions*.

Considering the DCT further, it has a strong "energy compaction" property: most of the signal information tends to be concentrated in a few low-frequency components of the DCT [32], because image features do not normally change rapidly with distance in any

[13]The mathematical theory of *ondelettes* (wavelets) was originally developed by French mathematicians and engineers and was designed for the approximation of possibly irregular functions and surfaces; it has been successfully applied in data compression, image and signal processing, and turbulence analysis [22]. Making a small change in the wavelets only causes a small change in the original signal. In data compression, a variable number of wavelet coefficients are changed to zero to progressively allow for more compression, and when the signal is recomposed the new signal is only slightly different from the original.

direction. Accordingly, many DCT coefficients are either zero or very small and become negligible during compression, so that only redundant information is removed from the image. Thus, the DC term (proportional to the average gray level, or brightness) represents a 1/8 scale of the input sequence (*thumbnail*[14] version). The DC and first AC (oscillatory gray-level component) together represent a 2/8 (or 1/4) scale of the input sequence. The DC and first 2 ACs together represent a 3/8 scale of the input sequence, and so on. Every DCT coefficient *adds* corresponding higher resolution detail. Therefore, it is feasible to simply leave out the high frequencies as a means of compressing the image *without* losing perceptible, or significant, information. Since some of the data is lost or neglected, DCT results in *lossy* compression. This fundamental DCT property, i.e., the similarity of different resolution (zoom) levels of the same image, is demonstrated schematically in Figure 11.17, on p. 615, and is the key to understanding why the DCT is an optimal algorithm for image compression. DCT has one possible problem, namely, the "blocking" effect. The problem is referable to the subdivision into blocks, and arises when an image is reduced to very high compression ratios, when these blocks become discernible. This problem becomes more prominent when the compression ratios are higher and also when the block sizes are smaller.

11.8 3-D display challenges

Visualizing complex 3-D objects within the human body has always been difficult and, in dynamic cardiac chamber geometry or intracardiac blood flow visualizations [59], is exacerbated by the fact that the geometric or flow structures are continually evolving, and may increase in complexity with time. In dealing with 3-D visualizations, it seems to be essential to be able to rotate and zoom with ease, so that the best view of a given structure or a field variable can be obtained. Wire-frame images are a first step in visualizing 3-D objects but are quickly becoming unsatisfactory. As we have seen in this chapter, tools from solids modeling are now being used to bring out organ structure in greater detail. The merit of these techniques is that they appeal directly to the processing used by the human eye and brain.

Experience suggests that rendering of organ surfaces can make the viewer think that considerably greater resolution is available than is actually the case. The process of volume and surface rendering appears to compensate for the lack of resolution of the computer-generated image in medical imaging applications, as well as in many others. After rendering, dynamic cardiac chamber surfaces, for instance, appear continuous and to be known to high resolution. Of course, there is the danger that such an extrapolation can lead to some unfounded conclusions, but this is not really an issue, because one has not forfeited any information by improving the visual sensation of the computer-generated image through rendering, and because one can always return to the conventional "low-resolution" image set and extract whatever information is available directly from it. The rendering procedures are thus seen as an *additional* feature of potential usefulness that supplements conventional imaging procedures. Both approaches should be

[14]Thumbnails are small downscaled versions of the original image.

used to obtain accurate dynamic flow-field geometry for mesh generation in CFD simulations of intracardiac blood flows.

Standard 2-D representations of 3-D data have well known shortcomings. Among them, each different view of the data must be recalculated by the processing unit, so that it is often difficult to preview a series of views to see the relative parallax motion of parts of an image at different depths. 2-D projections also fail to engage most of the 3-D vision capabilities of the observer. An intriguing option for capturing 3-D structure in a single image is the production of a computer-generated hologram. Computer-generated holography (CGH) [53] is the process of computing the pattern needed to holographically represent stored 3-D data and then transferring that pattern directly onto a recording material. In CGH there is no need for a physical object, or for a precisely aligned coherent imaging system, to do the recording. The hologram is a completely portable *hardcopy* containing *all* 3-D views. Various fluid flow research groups are, in fact, using holograms for the representation of data. Medium resolution holograms can be recorded using standard film recorders that are already in use for production of high-resolution 2-D images.

The richness and beauty of the images acquired by evolving medical imaging modalities for visualization of dynamic cardiac geometries and for intracardiac blood flow studies is sure to increase, as it has for the past couple of decades. As medical researchers, cardiologists, surgeons, and radiologists, learn more about the available commercial graphics software and develop some of their own, images are going to increase in detail, quantitative information content and accuracy, diagnostic value, and esthetic appeal.

11.8.1 Multimodality imaging data integration

Computed tomography, live 3-D echocardiography, and magnetic resonance data are digital. Other traditional modalities such as radiography, angiography, nuclear medicine, positron emission tomography (PET), and conventional ultrasound, acquired analog information that could not be integrated with other imaging data without significant manipulation and digitization of the data. The goal of image integration is to enable clinicians and researchers alike to view *integrated images* and visualize a patient in 3-D, combining anatomical, functional and physiological descriptive and quantitative information. This will enable, e.g., better surgical planning and therapy delivery through the inclusion of a more complete information package. The advent of digital imaging technology in these traditional modalities is allowing improved visualization of comprehensive sets of information. To truly benefit from this digital data acquisition, technologies must be developed and software created that will allow the integration of functional, anatomical and physiological information in a format that will enable users to rapidly verify the integrated datasets and display and analyze them quantitatively in a useful manner.

As computer graphics technology continues to expand to meet such increasing demands, the ability to acquire the speed necessary to permit clinically relevant usage will improve and further enhance the scope of multimodality imaging data integration and visualization. More and more often, we should witness that novel image analysis techniques will tend to incorporate knowledge from other disciplines, like computational fluid dynamics, to yield physically sound approaches where the final quantitative analysis that one is pursuing is taken into account from an early phase. New (patho)physiologic insights and clinical indices will stem from the fact that such novel techniques exploit better the dynamic information provided from modern 3-D spatiotemporal imaging techniques and from the fusion of information from multiple modalities. Finally, image-analysis techniques should no longer be seen only as a postprocessing step providing no feedback to image acquisition. More and more often, image-processing and analysis techniques are driving the acquisition itself, e.g., to *prospectively* compensate for image artifacts or to obtain optimal spatiotemporal datasets for CFD simulations. All of the previous considerations provide clear evidence that cross-fertilization with other fields is essential in medical image analysis.

References and further reading

[1] Addis, K.A., Hopper, K.D., Iyroboz, T.A., Kasales, C.J., Liu, Y., Wise, S.W. Optimization of shaded surface display for CT angiography. Acad. Radiol. 8: 976–81, 2001.

[2] Ahumada, A.J., Jr., Peterson, H.A. A visual detection model for DCT coefficient quantization. AIAA Computing in Aerospace Conference, 9th, San Diego, CA, Oct. 19–21, 1993, Technical Papers. Pt. 1 (A94-11401 01-62), 1993, Washington, D.C.: American Institute of Aeronautics and Astronautics, pp. 314–18.

[3] Akeley, K. Realityengine graphics. In Proceedings of the ACM SIGGRAPH'93 Conference on Computer Graphics, pp. 109–16, 1993.

[4] Andreopoulos, A., Tsotsos, J.K. Resampling 4D images using adaptive filtering. In: Proceedings of the 2nd Canadian Conference on Computer and Robot Vision (CRV 2005). 2005, IEEE Computer Society Press, pp. 18–26.

[5] Bradshaw, K.A., Pagano, D., Bonser, R.S., McCafferty, I., Guest, P.J. Multiplanar reformatting and three-dimensional reconstruction: for pre-operative assessment of the thoracic aorta by computed tomography. Clin. Radiol. 53: 198–202, 1998.

[6] Brink, J.A., Heiken, J.P., Balfe, D.M., Sagel, S.S., DiCroce, J., Vannier, M.W. Spiral CT: decreased spatial resolution in vivo due to broadening of section-sensitivity profile. Radiology 185: 469–74, 1992.

[7] Calhoun, P.S., Kuszyk, B.S., Heath, D.G., Carley, J.C., Fishman, E.K. Three-dimensional volume rendering of spiral CT data: theory and method. RadioGraphics 19: 745–64, 1999.

[8] Cyganek, B., Siebert, J.P. An introduction to 3D computer vision techniques and algorithms. 2009, Chichester, U.K.: J. Wiley & Sons. xx, 483 p.

[9] Delaunay, B.N. Sur la sphère vide. Izvestia Akademia Nauk SSSR, IIV seria, 7: 793–800, 1934.

[10] Drebin, R.A., Carpenter, L., Hanrahan, P. Volume rendering. Comput. Graph. 22: 65–74, 1988.

[11] Elvins, T.T. A survey of algorithms for volume visualization. Comput. Graph. 26: 194–201, 1992.

[12] Foley, J.D., van Dam, A., Feiner, S.K., Hughes, J.F. Computer graphics: principles and practice. 2nd ed. 1995, New York: Addison-Wesley. xxiii, 1175 p., [36] p. of plates.

[13] Freidlin, R.Z., Ohazama, C.J., Arai, A.E., McGarry, D.P., Panza, J.A., Trus, B.L. NIHmagic: 3D visualization, registration and segmentation tool. In: Proc. SPIE, 3905: 194–201, 2000.

[14] Garimella, R.V., Shashkov, M.J. Polygonal surface mesh improvement. Eng. Comp. 20: 265–72, 2004.

[15] Glassner, A. S. An introduction to ray tracing. 1989, London; San Diego: Academic. xiii, 327 p., [16] p. of plates.

[16] Golias, N.A., Tsiboukis, T.D. An approach to refining three-dimensional tetrahedral meshes based on Delaunay transformations. Int. J. Num. Meth. Eng. 37: 793–812, 1994.

[17] Gouraud, H. Continuous shading of curved surfaces. IEEE Trans. Comput. 20: 623–8, 1971.

[18] Hartley, R., Zisserman, A. Multiple view geometry in computer vision. 2003, Cambridge, UK ; New York: Cambridge University Press. xvi, 655 p.

[19] Heath, D.G., Soyer, P.A., Kuszyk, B.S., Bliss, D.F., Calhoun, P.S., Bluemke, D.A., Choti, M.A., Fishman, E.K. Three-dimensional spiral CT during arterial portography: comparison of three rendering techniques. RadioGraphics 15: 1001–11, 1995.

[20] Herman, G.T., Udupa, J.K. Display of 3-D information in 3-D digital images: computational foundations and medical application. IEEE Comput. Graph. Appl. 3: 39–46, 1983.

[21] Hesselink, L. Digital image processing in flow visualization. Ann. Rev. Fluid Mech. 20: 421–85, 1988.

[22] Jaffard, S., Meyer, Y., Ryan, R.D. Wavelets: tools for science and technology. 2001, Philadelphia, PA: Society for Industrial and Applied Mathematics. xiii, 256 p.

[23] Johnson, G.A., Godwin, J.D., Fram, E.K. Gated multiplanar cardiac computed tomography. Radiology 145: 195–7, 1982.

[24] Johnson, P.T., Fishman, E.K., Duckwall, J.R., Calhoun, P.S., Heath, D.G. Interactive three-dimensional volume rendering of spiral CT data: current applications in the thorax. RadioGraphics 18: 165–87, 1998.

[25] Kanitsar, A., Fleischmann, D., Wegenkittl, R., Felkel, P., and Gröller, M.E. CPR: curved planar reformation. In: Proceedings of the Conference on Visualization '02 (Boston). 2002, Washington, D.C.: IEEE Computer Society Press, pp. 37–44.

[26] Kanitsar, A., Wegenkittl, R., Fleischmann, D., Gröller, E. Advanced curved planar reformation: flattening of vascular structures. In: Proceedings of the Conference on Visualization '03 (Seattle). 2003, Washington, D.C.: IEEE Computer Society Press, pp. 43–50.

[27] Kaufman, A. Efficient algorithms for 3D scan-conversion of parametric curves, surfaces, and volumes. In: M. C. Stone [Ed.] Proceedings of the 14th Annual Conference on Computer Graphics and Interactive Techniques, SIGGRAPH '87. 1987, New York: ACM Press, pp. 171–9.

[28] Keller, P.J., Drayer, B.P., Fram, E.K., Williams, K.D., Dumoulin, C.L., Souza, S.P. MR angiography with two-dimensional acquisition and three-dimensional display. Work in progress. Radiology 173: 527–32, 1989.

[29] Kniss, J., Kindlmann, G., Hansen, C. Interactive volume rendering using multi-dimensional transfer functions and direct manipulation widgets. In: Proceedings of the Visualization 2001, pp. 255–62, 2001.

[30] Kong, T.Y., Roscoe, A.W. A continuous analog of axiomatized digital surfaces. Comput. Vision Graph. Image Proc. 29: 60–86, 1985.

[31] Levoy, M. Display of surfaces from volume data. IEEE Comp. Graph. Appl. 8: 29–37, 1988.

[32] Lim, J.S. Two-dimensional signal and image processing. 1990, Englewood Cliffs, NJ: Prentice Hall, Prentice Hall signal processing series. xvi, 694 p.

[33] Lohner, R. Progress in grid generation via the advancing front technique. Eng. Comp. 12: 186–210, 1996.

[34] Lorenson, W.E., Cline, H.E. Marching cubes: a high resolution 3D surface reconstruction algorithm. Comput. Graph. 21: 163–9, 1987.

[35] Ma, Y. An invitation to 3-D vision: from images to geometric models. 2004, New York: Springer. xx, 526 p.

[36] Mavriplis, D.J. Adaptive meshing techniques for viscous flow calculations on mixed element unstructured meshes. Int. J. Numer. Meth. Fluids 34: 93–111, 2000.

[37] McConnell, J.J. Computer graphics: theory into practice. 2006, Boston: Jones and Bartlett Publishers. xvi, 519 p.

[38] Möller, T., Haines, E., Hoffman, N. Real-time rendering. 3rd ed. 2008, Wellesley, Mass.: A.K. Peters. xviii, 1027 p.

[39] Nelson, M. Optical models for direct volume rendering. IEEE Trans. Visualiz. Comp. Graph. 1: 99–108, 1995.

[40] Nikolaidis, N., Pitas, I. 3-D image processing algorithms. 2001, New York: John Wiley. x, 176 p.

[41] Pham, D.L., Xu, C., Prince, J.L. Current Methods in Medical Image Segmentation. Ann. Rev. Biomed. Engin. 2: 315–37, 2000.

[42] Plato, Waterfield, R. Republic. 2003, London: Folio Society. lxxiii, 515 p.

[43] Plato, Jowett, B. The Republic: the complete and unabridged Jowett translation. 1991, New York: Vintage Books. 397 p.

[44] Pirzadeh, S. Unstructured viscous grid generation by advancing-layers method. AIAA-93-3453-CP, AIAA, pp. 420–34, 1993.

[45] Phong, B-T. Illumination for computer generated pictures. Comm. ACM 18: 311–17, 1975.

[46] Raman, R., Napel, S., Beaulieu, C.F., Bain, E.S., Jeffrey, R.B. Jr., Rubin, G.D. Automated generation of curved planar reformations from volume data: method and evaluation. Radiology 223: 275–80, 2002.

[47] Ravenel, J.G., McAdams, H.P., Remy-Jardin, M., Remy, J. Multidimensional imaging of the thorax: practical applications. J. Thorac. Imag. 16: 269–81, 2001.

[48] Raya, S. P., Udupa, J. K. Shape-based interpolation of multidimensional objects. IEEE Trans. Med. Imag. 9: 32–42, 1990.

[49] Rezk-Salama, C., Engel, K., Bauer, M., Greiner, G., Ertl, T. Interactive volume rendering on standard PC graphics hardware using multitextures and multi-stage rasterization. In: Proceedings of the 2000 Eurographics/SIGGRAPH Workshop on Graphics Hardware, pp. 109–18, 2000.

[50] Roettger, S., Guthe, S., Weiskopf, D., Ertl, T. Smart hardware-accelerated volume rendering. In: Proceedings of the Visualization Symposium '03. 2003, IEEE Computer Society Press, pp. 231–8.

[51] Rubin, G.D. Data explosion: the challenge of multidetector-row CT. Eur. J. Radiol. 36: 74–80, 2000.

[52] Shekhar, R., Zagrodsky, V. Cine MPR: interactive multiplanar reformatting of four-dimensional cardiac data using hardware-accelerated texture mapping. IEEE Trans. Inform. Technol. Biomed. 7: 384–93, 2003.

[53] Slinger, C., Cameron, C., Stanley, M. Computer-generated holography as a generic display technology. Computer 38(8): 46–53, 2005.

[54] Soille, P. Morphological image analysis: principles and applications. 2002, Berlin; New York: Springer. xvi, 391 p.

[55] Udupa, J.K., Herman, G.T. 3D imaging in medicine. 2000, Boca Raton: CRC Press. 366 p., [16] p. of color plates.

[56] Westermann, R., Ertl, T. Efficiently using graphics hardware in volume rendering applications. In: Comput. Graph., Proc. SIGGRAPH'98, pp. 169–77, 1998.

[57] Weatherill, N.P., Hassan, O. Efficient three-dimensional Delaunay triangulation with automatic point creation and imposed boundary constraints. Int. J. Num. Meth. Eng. 37: 2005–39, 1994.

[58] Westin, C.F., Richolt, J., Moharir, V., Kikinis, R. Affine adaptive filtering of CT data. Med. Image Anal. 4: 161–72, 2000.

[59] Yang, G.Z., Kilner, P.J., Mohiaddin, R.H., Firmin, D.N. Transient streamlines: texture synthesis for in vivo flow visualisation. Int. J. Card. Imag. 16: 175–84, 2000.

[60] Zhang, Q., Eagleson, R., Peters, T. Dynamic real-time 4D cardiac MDCT image display using GPU-accelerated volume rendering. Comput. Med. Imag. Graph. 33: 461-476, 2009.

Chapter 12

Computational Fluid Dynamics, or "CFD"

Oh Menander, oh life, so which of you has imitated the other?

——Comment of Aristophanes of Byzantion on Menander, the great Greek playwright of the Hellenistic era—ca. 342 –291 B.C. (In Hermog. 2.23.10–11 Rabe).

The purpose of computing is insight, not numbers.

——Richard Hamming [20].

INTRACARDIAC BLOOD FLOW phenomena are difficult to study and their simulations extremely challenging both under normal and under pathological states. The geometrically complicated boundaries of the intracardiac flow are not rigid but undergo continuous dynamic changes, and have a pronounced effect on the flow, which rules out approaches using rigid wall approximations. Therefore, driven by clinical needs accompanying the emergence of powerful digital imaging modalities (see Chapters 5, 10 and 11), a multidisciplinary approach is called for, using digital imaging combined with computational fluid dynamics, or "CFD," and encompassing complementary techniques adapted to the distinctive difficulties encountered in intracardiac blood flow simulations.

In this and the next two chapters, we will consider the application of CFD to the investigation of intracardiac blood flow phenomena. Over the past several decades, many books on CFD have discussed numerical algorithm, grid generation, and boundary condition procedures. For more exhaustive treatments of CFD methods in general, introductory books are available that provide fairly extensive formulations, numerical methods, and solutions to fundamental fluid dynamics problems [1–3,9,14,17–19,23,29,30,45,47,50,52,60–63,67]. Used together, with catheterization and imaging data providing key anchor points to assess and understand the accuracy of the computational method, significant advances in CFD approaches to basic and clinical cardiovascular research have been demonstrated in recent years. Thus, advanced computational cardiac fluid dynamics is truly an area where Hamming' s adage, "the purpose of computing is insight, not numbers" is true.[1] Significant technology development resources are being directed toward improving the capability of CFD, and we can expect that in the near future we will be relying much more heavily on CFD results both in the laboratory and in the clinical setting.

As is shown in Figure 12.1, given a flow field to examine, we start with a physical problem, and then represent the physical situation with a mathematical model. We then obtain a solution for the mathematical problem and use that solution to deduce important understanding about the flow problem. Skill and experience are required to carry out this sequence of steps.

1. Start with the real intracardiac flow.
2. Create a physical model of the flow field.
3. Create the simplified mathematical model(s) to be solved.
4. Carry out the numerical solution.

[1]This quotation is the frontispiece of his book, cited above.

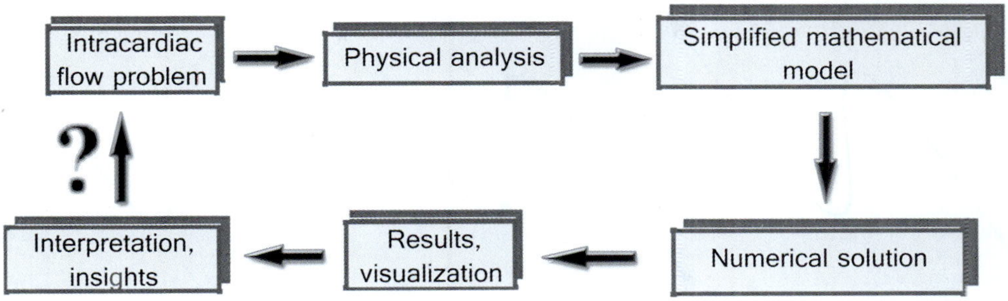

Figure 12.1: Steps in applying CFD to intracardiac blood flow phenomena.

5. Examine the results.

6. Interpret the sequence of physical model, mathematical model, and numerical solution, together with the computed results to provide the answers to the questions raised, and/or new knowledge and insights.

Notice here that the numerical solution of a computational problem is a small part of the total process. Successful intracardiac blood flow investigators must master the entire sequence of steps.

At each step in the numerical progression of a flow simulation, we use discretized transformation equations derived from the equations of motion, to make a prediction about the (approximate) evolution of a fluid dynamic process, such as an intracardiac velocity trajectory, over some small interval of process time. We can adjust the timestep size to obtain either higher temporal resolution when the trajectory is varying rapidly up-and-down or lower resolution when it fluctuates less rapidly. If the trajectory behaves very unsteadily, then we want to use a very short timestep size; but when the trajectory is changing slowly, we may increase the timestep size, so as to obtain more information in a shorter time. The process of running iterative numerical integrations with varying initial conditions and parameters in order to characterize an intracardiac flow phenomenon is comparable to a physical experiment, except that instead of testing hypotheses or theory predictions on a physiological or physical system, we try to follow the evolution of the true mathematical solution of a set of differential equations.

Since every digital computer must perform its calculations in discrete steps rather than continuously, the numerical simulation procedure is discrete also. We map from one state of the flow system to the next via the prediction that is derived from fitting a continuous curve or straight line to some of the previous discrete states, and projecting forward. We assume that the system evolves continuously, but we cannot represent that change without these intervening discrete approximations.

As the diagram in Figure 12.2 shows, we regain the impression of continuity by conceptually supplying a smooth curve fit to the pure progression of consecutive snapshots of the system—each successive state being a field, or set of numbers, calculated from the

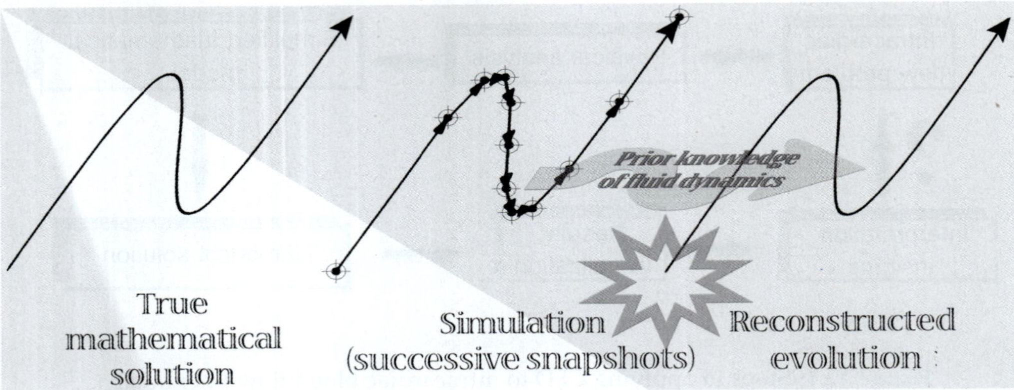

Figure 12.2: Computer simulation with visualization of flow forms a useful complement to physiological and physical flow model experiments and, when broader knowledge of fluid dynamics is also capitalized on, helps us understand the evolution of complex, but clinically important, intracardiac blood flow phenomena.

previous set of numbers. We must obviously exercise caution when we assume continuity between the discrete successive states of the numerical simulation procedure. The necessarily discrete underlying approximation may bring about a potential *divergence* between the true and the simulated solutions, a pitfall which may be allayed only by applying a sound knowledge of fluid dynamics, gained through relevant prior study and experience. CFD together with computer visualization form a useful *complement*—but are not a *substitute* for—physiological and physical experiments and for clinical measurements when it comes to making reliable, orderly and systematic interpretations of complex intracardiac blood flow phenomena.

12.1 Burgeoning computing power for CFD

The growing complexity of the CFD simulation tasks has been raising drastically the demands made on computing power, as well as on scientific visualization systems. Hence, new computers are being developed with enormous performance capabilities [48]. As is discussed later on, the Finite Element method (FEM) is often used in CFD applications for finding the solution to sets of partial differential equations. As the granularity of the computational grid of finite elements becomes finer, the approximation comes closer to the true solution of the flow-governing equations. High performance computers are useful, in that greater memory resources, greater computational power, and faster speed of computation allow for finer finite element grids, systems with a larger number of elements, and hence more accurate solutions. Their massive power reduces computing times considerably, while enabling extremely complex tasks to be solved accurately [8,60].

FLOPS is an abbreviation of *FL*oating point *O*perations *P*er *S*econd and is the yardstick used as a measure of a computing power, especially in fields that make heavy use of

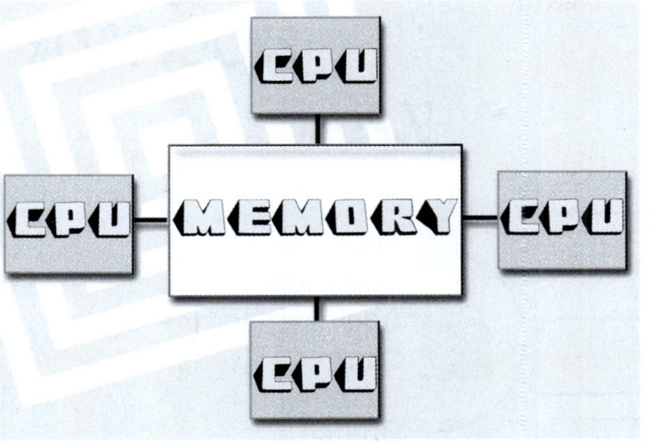

Figure 12.3: Parallel computers with shared memory vary widely, but generally have in common the capability for a collection of multiple processors to access all memory as a global address space, so that they can operate independently but share the same memory resources. Moreover, changes in a memory location brought about by one processor are visible to all others.

floating point calculations.[2] Measuring floating point operation speed does not predict accurately how the processor will perform on just *any* problem, because for ordinary non-scientific applications, integer operations (measured in *MIPS*, *M*illions of *I*nstructions *P*er *S*econd) are far more common. However, for many scientific applications such as analysis of data and CFD, a *FLOPS* rating is effective. Computing devices exhibit an enormous range of performance levels in floating-point applications, so units larger than the *FLOPS* have been introduced. The standard *SI* prefixes result in such units as the mega*FLOPS* (MFLOPS, 10^6 *FLOPS*), the giga*FLOPS* (GFLOPS, 10^9 *FLOPS*), the tera*FLOPS* (TFLOPS, 10^{12} *FLOPS*), and the peta*FLOPS* (PFLOPS, 10^{15} *FLOPS*).

The original supercomputer, the Cray-1, set up at Los Alamos National Laboratory in 1976, was capable of about 100 MFLOPS. A cheap but modern desktop computer using, e.g., the Intel Core 2 Quad and Core 2 Extreme CPU platforms, or the AMD quad-core "Phenom" CPU platform, typically runs at a clock frequency of around 3 *GHz* and provides computational performance in the range of scores of GFLOPS. The fastest general purpose computer in the world is the Lawrence Livermore National Laboratory's IBM Blue Gene/L massively parallel supercomputer (cf. Fig. 12.3); in the summer of 2007, it could deliver 478 TFLOPS. In June of 2006, a powerful computer was announced by the Japanese research institute, RIKEN, the MDGRAPE-3. That computer's performance tops out at one PFLOP—a thousand trillion operations per second. MDGRAPE-3 is a special purpose ultra-high performance supercomputer built for molecular dynamics simulations. In a little over 30 years since the Cray-1, the computational speed of supercomputers has jumped by over a *million-fold!* Electronic calculators are at the other end of the

[2] One should speak in the singular of a *FLOPS* and not of a FLOP, since the final S stands for second and does not indicate a plural.

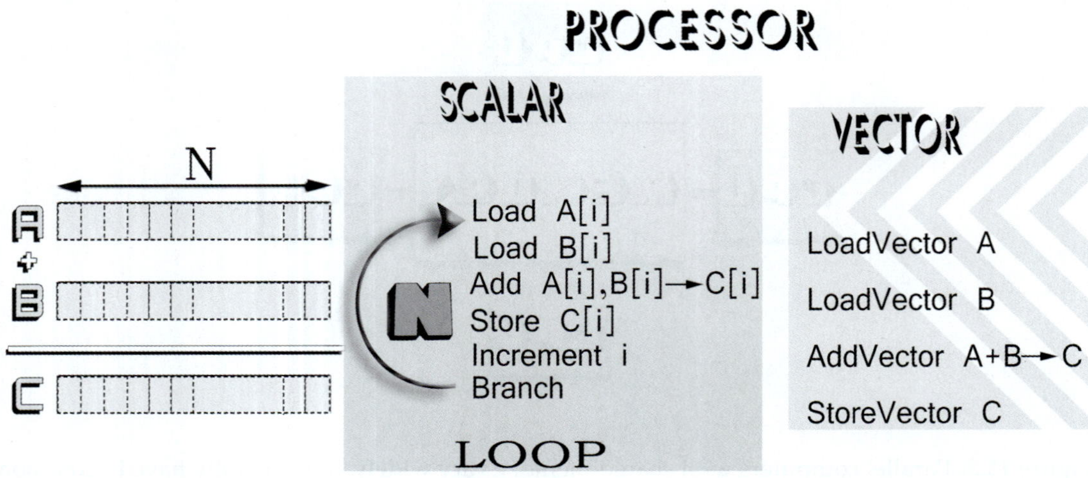

Figure 12.4: A vector processor is a processor design that runs mathematical operations on multiple data elements simultaneously; this is in contrast to a scalar processor which handles data sequentially, one element at a time, in a loop. A vector processor actually operates on entire vectors (arrays) with *one* instruction, i.e., the operands of some instructions specify complete vectors. In both scalar and vector machines the add instruction, $C = A + B$, means "add the contents of A to the contents of B and put the sum in C." In the scalar machine the operands are numbers, but in the vector processor the operands are vectors and the instruction directs the machine to compute the pair-wise sum of each pair of vector elements. A processor register, the *vector length register*, tells the processor how many individual additions to perform when it adds the vectors.

spectrum; any calculator's response time below *0.1 s* is deemed instantaneous by a user, and a simple calculator operates at about *10 FLOPS*. Humans are even worse floating-point processors, calculating in the milli*FLOPS* range. However, this purely mathematical criterion may not measure a human's overall *FLOPS* properly, because a human may concurrently be processing many other brain processes and tasks.

In a numerical intracardiac blood flow simulation, a computer is expected to generate up to several hundred timesteps of unsteady flow data. Each timestep may require tens to hundreds of megabytes of disk storage, and an entire unsteady flow dataset may amount to scores or hundreds of gigabytes. Interactive visualization and exploration of unsteady flow data of this magnitude requires powerful hardware capabilities. Interestingly, very high *FLOPS* figures are often quoted for computer video adapters and scientific visualization workstations. Most of the *FLOPS* performance for visualization consoles or video adapters comes from their *GPU*s (*G*raphics *P*rocessing *U*nits), which are deeply pipelined vector processors (cf. Fig. 12.4) specialized for graphics operations, with only limited programmability.[3] This is possible because 3-D graphics operations are a classic example of

[3] As an example, the Silicon Graphics Prism® family is capable of scaling up to 256 processors, 16 graphics pipelines, and 6.1 TB of memory, and offers an enormous visualization capability.

a highly parallelizable problem that can easily be split between different execution units and pipelines, allowing a high speed gain to be obtained from scaling the number of logic gates, rather than clock speed alone.

Admittedly, *FLOPS* in isolation are not a complete benchmark for high-performance modern computers. There are other factors in computer performance than raw floating-point computation speed, such as I/O performance, interprocessor communication, cache coherence, and the memory hierarchy. Accordingly, supercomputers are normally capable of only a variably small fraction of their theoretical peak *FLOPS* throughput. Even when operating on large, highly parallel problems, their performance will be *"bursty."*

12.2 Basic ideas in CFD analysis of flow fields

Except for a few special cases, no closed-form solutions have been found to the Navier–Stokes equations, and this fact was one of the motivations John von Neumann provided for the development of electronic computers following World War II. CFD is concerned with obtaining numerical solution to fluid flow problems governed by the Navier–Stokes equations by using computers [2,3,23]. The equations that we endeavor to solve in CFD are too complicated to solve analytically. One of the reasons for this is commonly that an equation contains many terms which make the problem simply too unwieldy. However, many of these terms may effectively be very small. Ignoring them can *unclutter* the problem to such an extent that it can be solved analytically. Furthermore, by crossing out relatively minor terms we can focus on the terms that are dominant and contain the relevant physics. This may allow better physical insights into the processes that really matter.

One caveat must be kept in mind, however: *chaos* in nonlinear dynamic systems. In a chaotic system small changes in the initial conditions lead to a change in the time evolution of the system that grows exponentially with time, as is discussed in Section 9.2.2, on p. 447. Deleting small terms from the equation of motion of such a system can have a similar effect; namely, it can lead to changes in the system that may grow exponentially with time. This means that for nonlinear dynamic systems one must be wary of omitting small terms from the flow-governing equations.

The advent of high-speed and large-memory computers has enabled CFD to obtain solutions to many complicated but important flow problems including intracardiac flow, by a sequence of steps encapsulated in the bird's-eye-view diagram in Figure 12.5. The first step of a CFD simulation is the evaluation of the possible flow-field characteristics, including *laminar*, *separated* and *turbulent* flow regimes; this is aided by geometric and flow imaging studies and by physical arguments—guided by assessments of dimensionless parameters such as the Reynolds number—of the relative importance of local, convective, and viscous effects. Then, appropriate *approximations* may be introduced by admissible simplifications of the complete Navier–Stokes equations—to wit, if viscous effects are negligible compared to the inertial (local and/or convective acceleration) effects, the

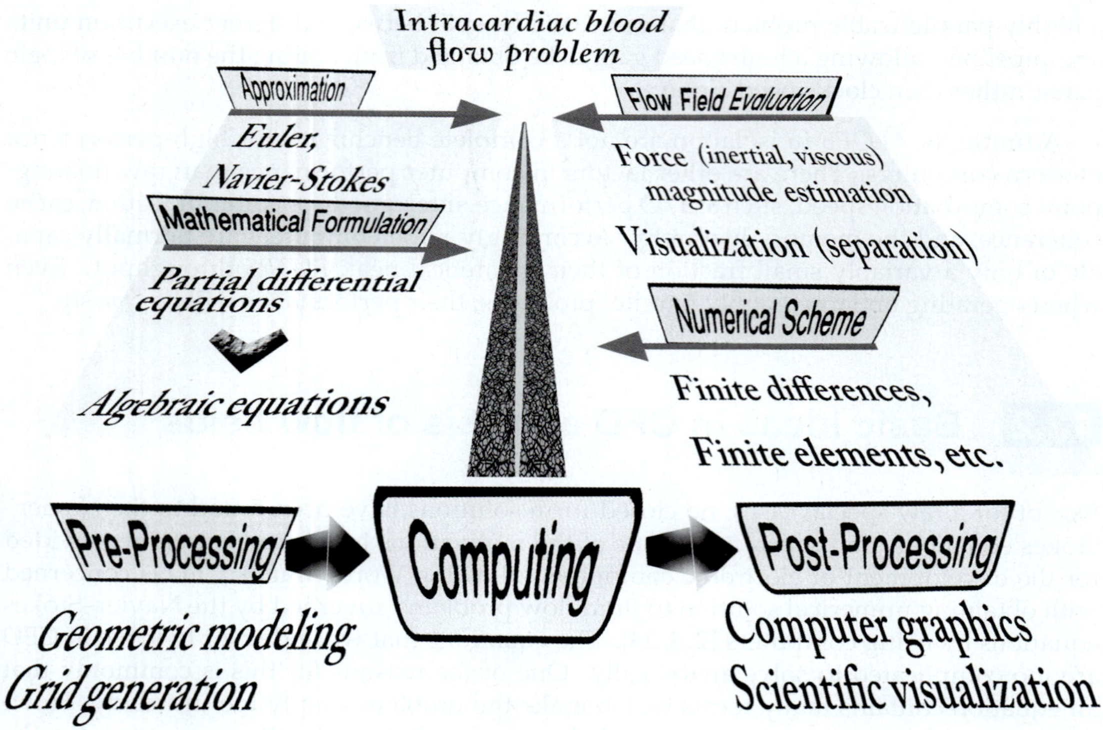

Figure 12.5: The major steps of the *CFD* procedure, as applied to intracardiac blood flow-field studies.

complete Navier–Stokes equations reduce to the much easier to integrate Euler equations, which involve only *first order* space derivatives.[4]

Based upon appropriate approximations and modeling, we compose the flow-field governing partial differential equations. Since the formulated partial differential equations are for continuous variables, we need to *discretize* them for numerical simulation on a computer. In carrying out the discretization, we make use of various methods called *numerical schemes*. By these processes, we finally obtain *algebraic* equations (cf. Fig. 12.7 on p. 633), which can be applied to the numerical models of the flow field. A computer program called "preprocessor" can be employed to define computational models and to set necessary initial and boundary conditions.

[4]The full Navier–Stokes equations are also an approximation, because they are based on the continuum hypothesis and a Newtonian fluid—the scale of the heart chambers is such that blood can in fact be treated as a Newtonian fluid, thus neglecting some behavioral aspects. The word *approximation* here is, however, not used in this sense. Further adjustments to the full Navier–Stokes equations, such as reducing them to the Euler equation by dropping viscosity, two-dimensionalization, etc., is what is meant in the present context.

The detailed numerical simulation model for an intracardiac flow field is a program that is executed, or "run," on a computer. A computer program that performs the main body of CFD computation is usually called a "solver," and it produces numerical results [2,3]. A numerical simulation does not necessarily solve the equations that make up the mathematical model directly. The words *advance* and *integrate* might be more appropriate within the context of a simulation than the word *solve*. As the general intracardiac flow problem varies in time, we solve a set of time-dependent Navier–Stokes equations, which have been converted into a set of discretized algebraic equations in the computational model, to advance the overall simulation in successive steps. Thus, the simulations that we are concerned with "integrate," or "advance," the approximate time-evolution equations of our flow model from an initial time, t_i, to a final time, t_f, in successive timesteps, Δt. Algorithms are substituted for the various mathematical terms, for their interactions, and thus for the underlying physical phenomena. The resulting equations that are then solved numerically yield a complete picture of the evolving flow field down to the resolution of the grid.

The result of an intracardiac flow-field CFD simulation itself is just a list of numbers which represents the spatiotemporal distribution of computed fluid mechanical parameters, such as velocity, pressure, and other variables of interest. The timestep used is generally smaller than the shortest characteristic times characterizing the evolution of the flow variables that we need to resolve in the calculation. The advancing simulation defines the changing state of the system at a sequence of discrete times. The usual assumption is that the state of the system at any time within a timestep can be approximated by interpolating between the state of the system at the beginning and at the end of the timestep. Typically, it takes hundreds of thousands to many millions of numbers to specify the state of the flow field at any particular time. The final accuracy and detail that we can expect depends on the interplay of a number of factors, including the availability of accurate dynamic geometric input data of high spatiotemporal resolution, high-speed computer hardware, specialized software and numerical CFD algorithms, and fast interactive visualization hardware and software. In any event, it is wise to keep in mind that, just as the clinical or animal experimental measurements that are required in their implementation, numerical results are only approximate. Beyond the unavoidable measurement inaccuracies in the geometric and boundary condition input data, there are several causes of differences between the computed results and "reality," i.e., errors arise from each process used to produce the numerical solution:

- The differential equations usually contain some approximations or idealizations.
- Approximations are made in the discretization process.
- In solving the discretized algebraic equations, iterative methods are used. Unless they are run for a very long time, the exact solution of the discretized equations is not attained.

When the governing equations are known accurately, as in the case of the Navier–Stokes equations for incompressible Newtonian fluid flow, CFD solutions of any desired accuracy can be achieved, in principle, conditioned always by the limited accuracy of the input measurements; however, the cost may be prohibitive and the accuracy nominal only, due to uncertainties in "real world" dynamic geometry and boundary condition data.

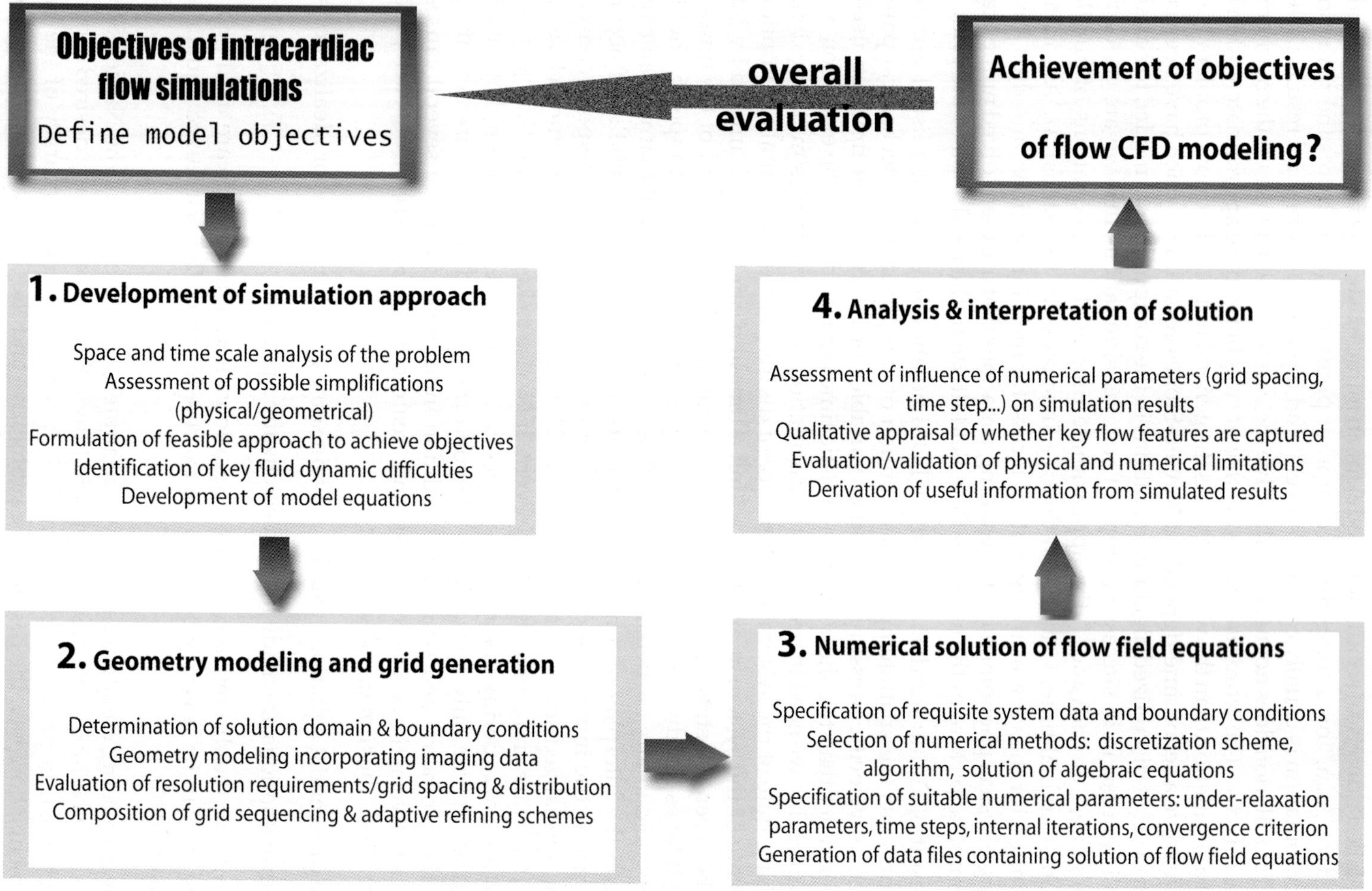

Objectives of intracardiac flow simulations
Define model objectives
overall evaluation
Achievement of objectives of flow CFD modeling ?
1. Development of simulation approach
Space and time scale analysis of the problem
Assessment of possible simplifications (physical/geometrical)
Formulation of feasible approach to achieve objectives
Identification of key fluid dynamic difficulties
Development of model equations
2. Geometry modeling and grid generation
Determination of solution domain & boundary conditions
Geometry modeling incorporating imaging data
Evaluation of resolution requirements/grid spacing & distribution
Composition of grid sequencing & adaptive refining schemes
3. Numerical solution of flow field equations
Specification of requisite system data and boundary conditions
Selection of numerical methods: discretization scheme, algorithm, solution of algebraic equations
Specification of suitable numerical parameters: under-relaxation parameters, time steps, internal iterations, convergence criterion
Generation of data files containing solution of flow field equations
4. Analysis & interpretation of solution
Assessment of influence of numerical parameters (grid spacing, time step...) on simulation results
Qualitative appraisal of whether key flow features are captured
Evaluation/validation of physical and numerical limitations
Derivation of useful information from simulated results

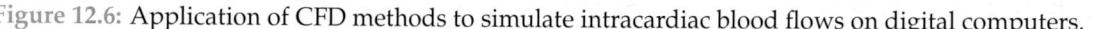

Figure 12.6: Application of CFD methods to simulate intracardiac blood flows on digital computers.

The performance-to-cost ratio of computers and CFD software, typically hundreds of thousands of lines in length, has increased at a spectacular rate since the 1950s. It requires little imagination to see that computers might fill the need for more detailed understanding of intracardiac blood flow phenomena, that has been intensified by the progress in cardiac diagnostic instrumentation and imaging modalities.

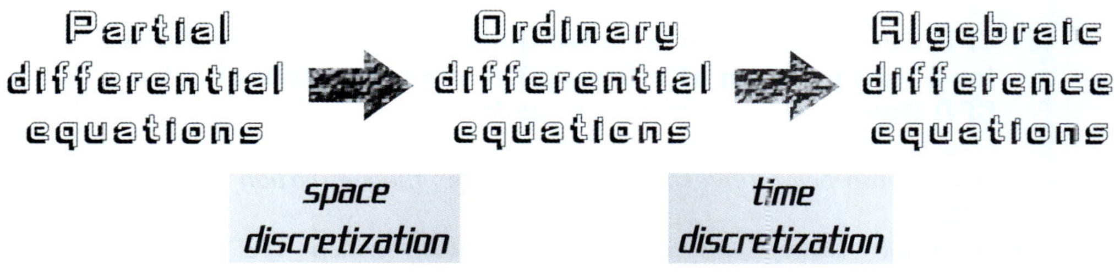

Figure 12.7: The logical steps of the *discretization* procedure, which converts a set of partial differential equations into a set of algebraic difference equations that can be solved on a digital computer.

12.3 Practical implementation of CFD to intracardiac flows

As we have seen, CFD uses a computer to solve the mathematical equations for any flow problem at hand. The main components of a CFD simulation are summarized in the tabulation on the next page. What follows in this section is an introductory overview of the specific processes [9,12,13] that are involved in any practical implementation of CFD [15,41] to the study of intracardiac flow phenomena (see Fig. 12.6 on p. 632):

1. First off, there must be identification of the key processes controlling the fluid dynamics, to allow the formulation of clear objectives for the CFD flow simulation. Accumulated conventional hemodynamic knowledge about the flow problem under consideration must be used to get whatever helpful information can be obtained, before deciding on the flow-governing equations for rigorous CFD modeling.

2. Cardiac chamber dynamic geometry representation, specification of boundary conditions, and grid generation come next. CFD works by dividing the region of interest, namely, the inside of a cardiac chamber, into a large number of cells or volume elements, the *mesh* or *grid*, by using various "gridding methods." Thus, gridding is the process of partitioning a region of interest into a more or less dense set of small cells. Numerical grid generation is a branch of applied mathematics that is essential for conducting computer-implemented simulations of fluid flow problems. The objective of gridding methods is to turn a system of partial differential equations into

a corresponding system of algebraic difference equations. Associated with each cell, there are values of the dependent flow-field variables (e.g., velocity vector components, pressure, etc.), usually representing some type of local average.

How does CFD make predictions?

CFD uses a computer to solve the mathematical equations for a flow problem of interest. The main components of a CFD flow field simulation are as follows:

- *the human being (investigator) who states the simulation problem to be solved;*
- *scientific knowledge (models, methods), which are expressed mathematically;*
- *the computer code (software), which embodies the scientific knowledge and provides detailed instructions (algorithms) for*
- *the computer hardware, which performs the actual calculations of the simulation; and*
- *the human being who inspects and interprets the simulation results, using visualization hardware and software.*

CFD is a highly interdisciplinary research area which lies at the interface of fluid dynamics, applied mathematics, and computer science.

It enables investigators to conduct *numerical experiments* (i.e., computer simulations) in a *virtual flow laboratory.*

Numerical algorithms generating discretized approximations to the flow-field governing equations of mass, momentum, and energy can then be used to compute these variables in each cell. As shown in Figure 12.7, this task is accomplished in two steps: first the partial differential equations are converted into ordinary differential equations via discretization of the spatial variables, and then the ordinary differential equations are converted into algebraic difference equations via time discretization.

Some CFD schemes employ *Lagrangian* grids, which deform to follow the motion of the fluid; others use fixed *Eulerian* grids. A combination of Lagrangian-Eulerian grids may be used to prevent moving grids from becoming excessively distorted. The number of grid cells may amount to many million. Advanced software can adaptively optimize the mesh as needed, to concentrate analysis on points and subregions of interest. Fast and efficient dynamic mesh adaptation is an important feature in the CFD analysis of unsteady intracardiac flows.[5] It is essential to

[5] However, mesh adaptation on parallel computers can cause serious load imbalance among the processors. With unbalanced loads, some processors will remain idle while others are over-burdened. This

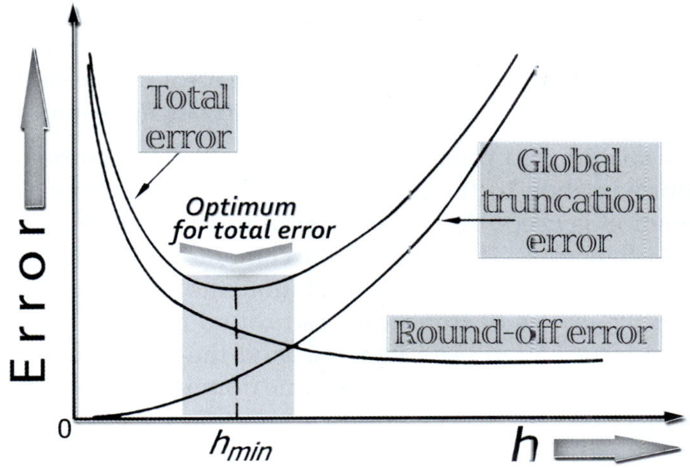

Figure 12.8: Schematic diagram showing the total error, which is produced by round-off and truncation, as a function of timestep size, h. The global truncation error decreases as h decreases for a fixed integration interval, but the maximum round-off error increases. Round-off error can contribute significantly to the global error when very short timesteps are used. Thus there is an optimal step size, shown as h_{min}, where truncation and round-off errors are comparable.

formulate grid sequencing and adaptive refinement strategies, and to understand the influence of grid spacing and cell distribution on the simulated results.

Most real flow problems involve infinite sets of values in every variable, each of which can in turn require an infinite number of digits for its exact representation. Digital CFD computation is, by its very nature, finite: it involves a finite set of numerical values, each of which is represented through a finite set of digits. These two approximations of *inestimable* quantities by *finite* ones lead to two types of error, *truncation* and *round-off* error, respectively. These are the two sources of local error.

The round-off error is the error which arises from the fact that, in implementing numerical methods, digital computers only calculate results to a fixed precision—typically between seven and 15 decimal digits. Round-off errors depend only on the number and type of arithmetic operations per step, and are therefore independent of the integration step size, h. The truncation error of a numerical procedure results from the approximation of an infinite-dimensional object, such as a *continuous* function, by a *discrete* one. This is illustrated by the approximation of a smooth graph of a function by a series of straight lines (a piecewise-linear approximation), or by a truncated Taylor series expansion[6] at successive discrete points on the graph.

is equivalent to introducing a serial component into the parallel computation, causing the power of some processors to be underutilized. Dynamically balancing the processor loads at runtime is a complex task.

[6]A Taylor series expresses the value of a function $f(x)$ at any point x in terms of its value at a nearby point a, the distance $(x-a)$ between the points, and the derivatives of the function with respect to x. It is $f(x) = f(a) + f'(a)\cdot[(x-a)/1!] + f''(a)\cdot[(x-a)^2/2!] + f'''(a)\cdot[(x-a)^3/3!] + HOT$, where the primes indicate

The truncation error is machine independent, depending only on the algorithm used and the step size, h. It often turns out that the truncation error is the dominant error source. Whereas the *local* truncation error is the error in one step, the *global* error is the accumulated error over all the steps of the advancing solution.

More closely spaced grid points and shorter timesteps can be used to get a more accurate approximation to the true solution, but the additional points mean that more information is used. As the amount of information increases, the total error due to round-off increases, because it is the combined effect of an increasing number of round-off errors. In the overall computation, the total error in the answer, which is the sum of the effects of truncation and round-off errors, initially decreases as the amount of information used increases and the truncation error decreases, but then increases as the round-off errors become dominant, as is depicted pictorially in Figure 12.8, on p. 635.

3. Next comes the specification of fluid properties such as blood's dynamic viscosity, density, etc., and selection of flow-governing mathematical equations with appropriate dynamic boundary conditions applied over the inner cardiac chamber surfaces. Solution of the discretized flow-field equations proceeds on the generated grid by a selected numerical scheme, with suitable implementation specifications (under-relaxation parameters, timestep, convergence criteria for the iterations, and so on [1–3,9,14,60]).

   Numerical methods such as the Finite Element method are an irreplaceable means of simulating a wide variety of physical phenomena in scientific computing. They place particularly difficult demands on grid generation. In each of the cells of the grid, the partial differential equations describing the fluid flow (the Navier–Stokes equations) appear as nonlinear algebraic equations that relate the pressure, velocity, and possibly other dependent variables, to the values in the neighboring cells. The number of unknowns is the product of the number of grid nodes and the number of dependent variables. In addition to the treatment of flow equations in the so-called "primitive variables," namely, velocity and pressure, representation with streamfunction and vorticity as the unknown flow-field quantities is also used [15]. Detailed intracardiac flow simulations are often highly resource demanding, in terms of CPU time and memory requirements. Memory requirements may become rather prohibitive at higher grid granularity levels, since with each halving of the internodal spacing along each coordinate direction memory requirements will rise as 2^3. The number of iterations required to reach a certain convergence will increase approximately linearly with the grid size (number of nodes). Since the time per iteration will rise as the cube of this parameter, the amount of computation will thus increase at about the fourth power of the grid size. Because the computer representation uses discrete numbers rather than continuous variables, the resolution in time is also broken up into discrete intervals. These intervals are denoted as *timesteps* and provide convenient increments over which to advance the numerical solution

differentiation with respect to x, and HOT means "higher order terms." The definition can be extended by analogy to a function of more than one independent variable.

of the flow-field equations. If one can generate grids that are completely satisfying for numerical techniques like the FEM, the other applications fall easily in line.

It is amusing to note that the *continuum* flow-field equations were invented in the first place in order to simplify the *discrete* equations of particle dynamics. In CFD, the continuum approach is reformulated so that we can use digital computers to solve the flow-field equations. Nevertheless, the discretized set of equations is considerably smaller (even if in the tens of millions) and "infinitely easier" to solve than the simultaneous equations of particle dynamics would be if applied to individual molecules in blood. Once the mesh is complete, there is input of the initial and boundary conditions that pertain to the flow. Powerful computers can then solve the equations for each cell numerically, until an acceptable convergence is at hand. This can be a time-consuming process, but fast CFD codes can exploit parallel processing. The results of the simulation call for numerical and for *graphical* analysis.

4. This is followed by the analysis and interpretation of the CFD simulation results, and the intracardiac blood flow-field phenomena revealed. CFD solutions generate huge amounts of data about the simulated intracardiac blood flow-field phenomena. Without appropriate tools for scientific visualization, one may become lost in a sea of numbers. Most commercially available CFD software provides a powerful, comprehensive set of *postprocessing tools* to create visualizations ranging from simple line plots and 2-D graphs to 3-D representations of particle trajectories, vectors and contour plots, yielding a complete picture of the flow down to the resolution of the grid [35, 59]. From the fluid dynamics point of view, we are interested in the physiological and pathophysiologic interpretations of the computed result. A "postprocessor" is a program to convert for us the computed results into physically or physiologically meaningful data and to display them in vivid fashion. Appropriate ways of identifying and displaying key flow features, such as vortices, are useful for qualitative evaluation of simulation results. Methods for error analysis and for validation are also indispensable and can point out the need for further studies, which may be necessary to better meet the objectives of the CFD simulation.

12.4 Solving intracardiac flow problems with computers

In order to create a computer program to solve a particular problem we must first abstract a concise description or mathematical model of the flow field, omitting details irrelevant to solving it; then, we must create an appropriate algorithm for solving the mathematical model.[7] An algorithm is a systematic, step-by-step, procedure for solving a problem. The

[7] The word *algorithm* is named for Muhammad ibn Musa *al-Khowarizmi,* a ninth century Persian mathematician who is among those who worked in the "House of Wisdom" in Baghdad to translate Greek scientific manuscripts. In addition to others, he wrote a book on the treatment of equations, basing it on the work of Greek mathematicians. Algebra is a corruption of part of the title of al-Khowarizmi's great work.

set of steps that define an algorithm must be unambiguous and the algorithm must have a clear stopping point. The ultimate goal of all numerical algorithms and simulations is to produce the most accurate answer in the least amount of time. Therefore, the implementation of elegant algorithms that are as simple as is admissible by the difficulties of the flow field at hand, and require the *fewest steps* possible, is a principal attribute of a good computer code.

12.5 Dynamic intracardiac flow-field geometry

Modern digital imaging technologies such as ultrasound, CT and PET scanning, and especially magnetic resonance imaging, provide detailed, high resolution information on dynamic cardiac chamber geometry throughout the cardiac cycle. As faster and more powerful noninvasive digital imaging modalities, computers, and software tools, have become available and more affordable, so too has grown the accessibility to CFD for the study of intracardiac flows [15,41]. This is resulting in new ideas and challenging issues, involved in developing a "virtual catheterization" approach in the near future.

A difficult part in the representation of an intracardiac blood flow field, is figuring out how to tell the computer where a large enough number of points defining the 3-D heart chamber endocardial surface are located. Because a computer does not operate in the analog, but in the digital mode, a problem arises when we try to transfer to it flow-field geometry information. Just as our fingers are digits, or separate units, computers store information in digital units. If you draw a circle on paper with a pencil, the information about the circle is in analog format.

If you form a circle with your fingertips, the information about the circle is in digital format. Obviously, the circle shape formed by your fingertips is not nearly as informative as the drawn circle. If you press your fingertips together in a circular shape, the form is more recognizable, but the circle is much smaller. To accomplish the same semblance of a circle in an enlarged size, you would need more digits. The pencil-drawn circle includes an *infinite* number of points (the pieces of lead on the paper), while the finger-demarkated circle has only five *discrete* points. To approximate the penciled circle, a digital circle will need *thousands* of points.

Similarly, the computer cannot represent a shape that looks like a real heart chamber contour unless a multitude of points on the inner surface are input into the computer's memory storage locations. To input any such point manually, you must calculate its three coordinates in three dimensions. When the computer knows the three coordinates, it can represent a dot in the corresponding location. It sounds like a long process by hand, and it certainly is. The rapidly evolving digital 3-D imaging hardware and software tools eliminate much of the work required. These systems calculate the necessary coordinates

---

He chose five Arabic words for its title, *al jabr w' al muquabalah*, "the reunion and the opposition." These words referred to the two main processes employed in solving "equation" problems: *reunion*, bringing together terms involving the unknown quantity, and *opposition*, the final stage when a "reunited" unknown quantity faced some number [24].

for each point semi-automatically and interactively for quality control, and translate the numbers into a computer compatible format. Automated methods are available that are useful in interpolations of irregularly sampled data. The *Delaunay triangulation* [46] is the creation of triangular tiles with vertices at each of the points that cover the region over which the geometric data points are contained (see Fig. 11.14, on p. 611), such as the inner surface of a cardiac chamber. It has the property that the circumscribing circle for each triangle contains no other vertices of the triangulation within it. Admittedly, a fully automated analysis of cardiac images still entails many difficulties. Noise, variation in anatomical shape, varying imaging characteristics, and incomplete endocardial target boundaries make the identification of the dynamic chamber geometry arduous. By performing manual traces of endocardial target boundaries, it becomes readily apparent how simplistic most computer segmentation routines are compared to human capabilities for image analysis. Multiple clues are employed during the manual tracing, beyond what the human operator is explicitly aware of, in identifying the complete boundary outline. The human brain remains far more sophisticated, flexible, and reliable for this type of task than the machine, but artificial intelligence research in this area may change this in the not distant future.

12.5.1 Edge detection

Endocardial edge detection entails manual and interactive semiautomatic cardiac chamber contour tracking. It is a problem of fundamental importance in heart image motion analyses for endocardial velocity field determinations that are required in intracardiac blood flow simulations. In typical images, edges characterize object boundaries and are therefore useful for registration, identification, and segmentation of cardiac chambers. An edge is a jump in intensity. An ideal edge is a discontinuity (i.e., a ramp with an infinite slope), but the cross-section of a real edge has the shape of a more or less smooth ramp function. Since much of the visual information in any real scene is conveyed by the edges, our eye-brain system has evolved exquisite abilities to extract edges. Here we are concerned with some elementary aspects of edge detection.

A little reflection on the one-dimensional situation hints that a strong slope, or large value of the derivative, is indicative of an edge. In fact, the first derivative assumes a local maximum at an edge. Thus, local maxima of the gradient magnitude of a function $F(x, y)$, defined for a 2-D image can help identify edges within the image. When the first derivative achieves a maximum, the second derivative is zero. For this reason, an alternative edge detection strategy is to locate zeros of the second derivatives of $F(x, y)$. The differential operator used in these so-called *zero-crossing* edge detectors, is the Laplacian, which was discussed in Section 2.11 on p. 62. It can be shown that the zero-crossings are independent of the steepness of the transition, while the gradient magnitude is directly related to the edge slope. But if the ordinates are reduced by a factor, thus yielding weaker slopes, we would not want the edges to change. For that reason, absolute slope alone is not a sufficient gauge. Using *slope / ordinate* neutralizes the effect of reduction or magnification on absolute slope and will correct for this, just as taking $(dP/dt)/P$ corrects for different levels of ventricular isovolumic contraction pressure when assessing contractility. Effectively, we are now locating steep slopes in the *logarithm* of the image gray-scale values.

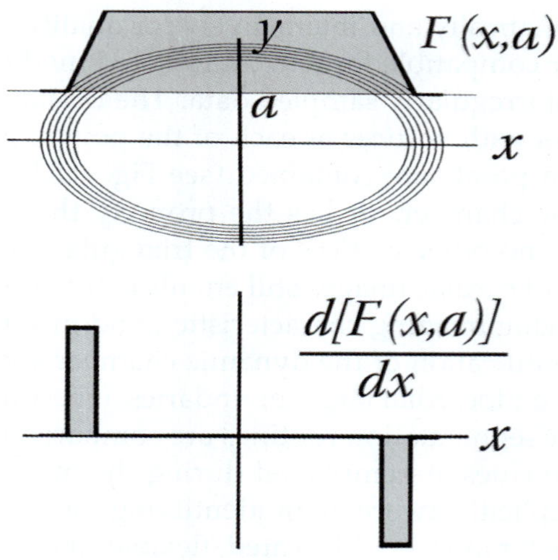

Figure 12.9: Contour diagram of an upside-down bucket of top radius $a-\tau$ and and bottom radius a, a cross-section at constant y, and the derivative of this cross-section with respect to x plotted below—see discussion in nearby text.

The strength of the response of the derivative operator is proportional to the degree of discontinuity of the image at the point at which the operator is applied. Thus, image differentiation enhances edges—such as the endocardial boundary of the cardiac chambers—and other discontinuities (noise), whereas it deemphasizes areas with slowly varying gray-level values. When we consider an image function of two or three variables, we must obviously employ partial derivatives along the two or three spatial axes. To illustrate the derivative-based approach, we consider a function that is equal to zero outside the circle $r = a$, equal to unity inside the circle of radius $a-\tau$, and equal to the height of the cone forming a continuous surface between the two circular rims of radius a and $a-\tau$, as is sketched out in Figure 12.9. We differentiate this function with respect to x and consider the successive results as $\tau \rightarrow 0$. Along each line $y = const.$, the derivative produces two unit-area rectangles of width τ and heights $1/\tau$ and $-1/\tau$, respectively, representing so-called *delta functions* of strength 1 and -1, and situated on the locus $r = a$. They demarcate the bucket wall at any given elevation y unequivocally. This differentiation technique is applicable to other edge detection situations, where partial differentiation in two or three dimensions is feasible.

If a change in base level of brightness is produced, however, the logarithmic derivative could be diminished. Thus, different brightness levels in different areas might imply that a perfectly perceptible edge, such as the endocardial boundary, running across a continuous structure but subject to space-varying brightness will not be detected in places, if a preset threshold for slope/ordinate is adopted. A way out might be as follows: We begin by dividing the image into portions, within each of which the sort of problem associated with different brightness levels is not of consequence. We then determine the absolute gradient by adding the squares of the first derivatives in the two coordinate directions. We make a *histogram*, namely, a bar graph depicting frequency data, of these gradients and determine the gradient that is exceeded by, e.g., only 10% of all values. Then we single out the points having these large values. Where they exhibit continuity, rather than appearing in isolation, we have candidates for edges. The missing factor here is intelligent *judgment*; to locate edges by computer requires artificial intelligence software. There may, however, be applications for simpler procedures in special circumstances, where the same kind of image has to be reduced to a line drawing repetitively, as is the case of the detection of pulsating endocardial edges.

By comparing the gradient to a threshold, we can detect an edge whenever the threshold is exceeded. We can thus find the edge, but the edge may be too "thick" due to the thresholding approach. A straightforward operation that is then useful rests on the observation that, as noted above, on a steep slope, not only the gradient has a large peak centered around the edge, but the curvature changes sign as well. Hence, a locus of zero curvature is interesting, especially the curvature in the direction of the local gradient. Since we know that the edge occurs at the peak, we can localize it by computing the Laplacian—in one dimension, the second derivative with respect to distance—and finding the zero crossings. In practise, the locus of zero curvature does not necessarily coincide with a steep slope; all the same, a normalization with respect to the ordinate is generally a useful operation. Perceptible edges may also be seen even in the absence of a sharp change in function value, when changes in texture occur with only a small or no change in gray-level.

The quality of edge detection is limited by what is in the image [4]. Obviously, edge detection is difficult in noisy images, because both the noise and the edges contain high-frequency content. Attempts to reduce the noise can bring about blurred and sometimes distorted edges. Not all edges involve a step change in intensity. Moreover, effects such as poor or suboptimal focus can result in objects with boundaries defined by a gradual change in intensity.

Edge detection is admittedly a somewhat subjective task [31]. A user of an edge detection software should not expect the software to automatically detect all of the edges that he or she wants and nothing more, because a program cannot possibly know what level of details the human operator has in mind. Usually it is easy to detect those obvious edges, or those with high S/N ratio. But what about those not very distinct? If a program detects all the pixel intensity discontinuities in an image, the resulting image may be little different from a field of noise. Sometimes the human operator knows that there should be a definite edge in the image but it is not shown in the result. So he or she adjusts the parameters of the program, trying to get the edge detected. However, if the edge the user has in mind is not as obvious to the program as some other undesirable or *confounding* features, the latter may give rise to "noise" before the desired edge is detected. Edge detecting programs process the image "as it is." As a human being, an experimenter knows where there is an edge because he or she is using knowledge in addition to what is unequivocally contained in the image. How to use such knowledge about the real world in the process of general edge detection is a huge topic in quantitative image processing [16].

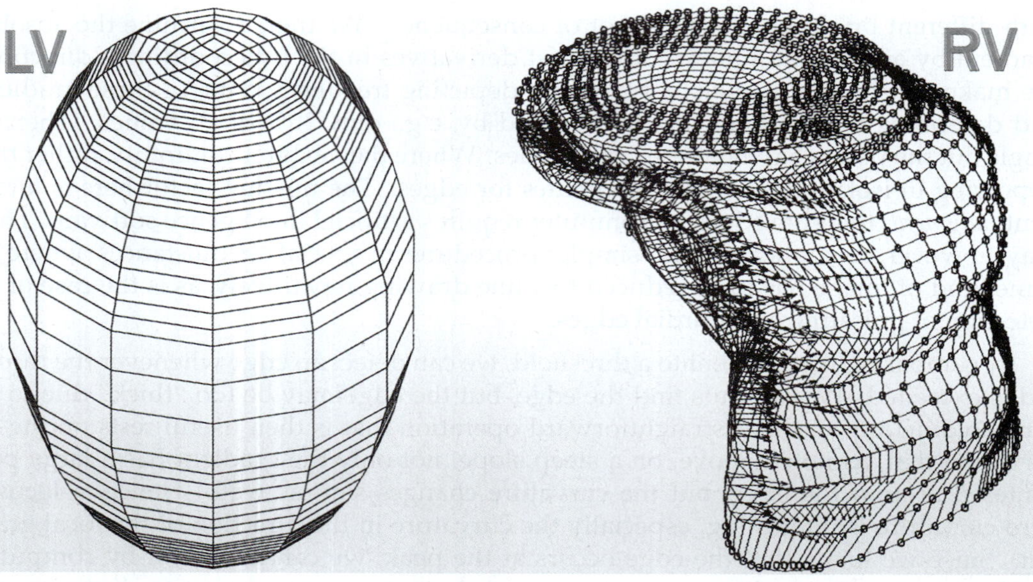

Figure 12.10: Left panel: An instantaneous boundary-fitted grid of the surface of the ejecting left ventricle. (Adapted from Hampton et al. [22], with kind permission from the IEEE). Right panel: An instantaneous boundary-fitted grid of the surface of the right ventricle during diastolic filling. The instantaneous velocity boundary conditions are indicated by arrows only for the septal portion of the grid. (Modified from Pasipoularides et al. [41], with kind permission from the American Physiological Society.)

12.5.2 Image segmentation: the first step in CFD simulations

Segmentation describes processes involved in automated or interactive computer-aided analysis of images to find their component parts. In the analysis of objects in sequences of dynamic images, it is essential to differentiate between the objects of interest, e.g., the dynamic cardiac chamber boundaries, and "the rest," or background. The techniques that are used to find the objects of interest comprise various segmentation techniques—segmenting the foreground from background. In a sense this is similar to edge detection, where the edge closes to define a structure. The edge detection algorithms are followed by linking procedures to assemble edge pixels into meaningful border lines.

A basic task in 3-D image processing is the segmentation of an image or series of images, which classifies voxels/pixels into objects or groups. 3-D image segmentation makes it possible to create 3-D rendering for organs of interest, such as the cardiac chambers of the beating heart, and to perform quantitative analysis for their changing dynamic size and shape.

A raw 3-D image, whether it is CT, MRI or live 3-D echocardiography image, comes as a 3-D array of voxels or pixels. Each voxel has a gray-scale range from 0 to 65, 535 in the 16-*bit* pixel case or 0 to 255 in the 8-*bit* pixel case. Most medical imaging systems generate images using a 16-*bit* gray-scale range. A 3-D imaging dataset typically has a large number of voxels and is very computer intensive for processing, such as segmentation and use in CFD flow simulations. A segmented image, on the other hand, provides a much simpler description of objects that allows the creation of 3-D dynamic surface models or display of volume data.

While the raw image can be readily displayed as 2-D slices, 3-D analysis and visualization requires explicitly defined organ boundaries, especially when creating 3-D surface models. For example, to create a 3-D rendering of a heart chamber from an MRI dataset, the chamber needs to be identified first within the 3-D dataset and then its endocardial boundary marked and used for 3-D rendering. The pixel detection process is the image segmentation process, which identifies the attributes of pixels and defines the boundaries for pixels that belong to the same geometric group. Additionally, measurements and quantitative analysis for parameters such as area, perimeter, volume and length, can be obtained easily when organ boundaries have been defined.

Because of the importance of identifying objects from a 3-D imaging dataset, there have been extensive research efforts on image segmentation for the past several decades. A number of image segmentation methods have been developed using fully automatic or semi-automatic approaches for medical imaging and other applications. At the outset, it must be acknowledged that, no matter whether 2- or 3-D imaging frames are involved, parts of the endocardial border are not adequately visualized in all of the frames of the cardiac cycle. For this reason, accrual of knowledge within *local time intervals* can be very beneficial in dealing with such incomplete, or "corrupted," contour data. To this end, various methods for establishing local correspondences between shapes have been applied on sets of endocardial imaging frames acquired throughout the cardiac cycle. Such methods can lead to accurate segmentation of the endocardial contours on the collection of imaging frames spanning a complete cardiac cycle.

The current trend in computational intracardiac fluid dynamics is to employ realistic dynamic cardiac chamber geometries derived from in vivo imaging [6]. Such studies typically produce a series of images at each timestep of the simulation through the heart cycle, or time phase thereof. From this series of images the endocardial boundaries of one or more cardiac chambers must first be individually extracted (i.e., 2-D segmentation), and then serially reconstructed at each successive timestep, in order to produce the 3-dimensional inner surface geometry [41], as is exemplified pictorially in Figure 12.10. There are also rapid segmentation techniques that combine these two steps, based on the idea of an expanding-contracting shape primitive—a virtual balloon in 3-D [55,56], or an ellipse in 2-D [40]—that is fitted in a statistical sense to the inner surface of the cardiac chamber of interest at each timestep. Figure 12.11, on p. 645 demonstrates the geometric consistency and coherent tracking that are attainable with this type of minimally interactive approach in segmenting several LV short-axis echocardiographic clips. In order to anchor the segmentation process in such automatic approaches, we need to compare it to some standard. One way to do this is by the so-called "ground truth," which is a part of the calibration process. This is where a trained person makes a measurement of the same border that the software is trying to measure at the same time. The two answers can then be *compared* to help evaluate how well the segmentation algorithm is performing. The term originated in satellite photography, where we believe the *ground truth* more than the satellite, because we have more experience making measurements on the ground.

It is implicitly recognized in such endocardial border segmentation undertakings that, since the heart is confined within the generally snugly-fitting pericardium, its moving about in relation to the adjoining organs is limited. Moreover, the phasic passive and active endocardial border displacements, brought about by the pumping activity of the walls of its individual chambers, are typically so sizeable that global cardiac movement remains *negligible* in comparison. Consequently, the coordinate of the center, as well as the orientation, of the dynamic endocardial contour-modeling geometric shapes can be considered constant over short successions of imaging frames, in certain applications. Accordingly, the exact form of the 2- or 3-D geometric figures approximating the endocardium varies relatively little and scale factors quantifying size can be considered as the only temporal variable.

Cardiac chamber segmentation techniques mostly work in a *semi-automatic* fashion: Approaches requiring a large degree of interactivity include *intelligent scissors* and *live-wire* techniques, where the human operator specifies points lying on the endocardial boundary that are then automatically connected by the segmentation algorithm. However, in order to increase work efficiency, manual interaction in the segmentation process has to be minimized. A widely used method for cardiac chamber segmentation entails so-called "deformable model" techniques [34]. The idea behind these deformable models, or "active contours," for image segmentation is quite simple: at the outset, an initial guess for the deformable contour is initialized by the user; then, by applying an assortment of image driven forces, it is aligned with significant gradients in the image. Thus, the contour is moved to the boundaries of the desired objects.

In such segmentation models, two types of forces are considered: the internal forces, defined within the contour curve, are designed to keep the model smooth during the deformation process; the external forces, which are computed from the underlying image data, are designed to move the model toward the desired object boundary within the image. Such techniques typically require the initialized endocardial border line to be positioned very close to the estimated final result, which amplifies the level of manual interaction. Popular deformable models include so-called *"snakes,"* which are energy-minimizing splines [28,36]. The snakes method detects the edges in the image under the constraints that the boundaries formed from the edges should be smooth and continuous. Jones and Metaxas [27] have exploited *pixel-affinity*, a measure of probability that two neighboring pixels belong to the same object, to initialize a deformable model; the cardiac chamber boundary is initialized in the middle of the cavity and iteratively inflated into all directions until pixels of low affinity are made contact with.

Segmentation techniques yield raw data in the form of pixels along a boundary, or pixels contained in a region; these data sometimes are used directly to obtain elegant (compact) descriptors of the features of interest. Standard techniques are used to compute such descriptors from the raw data, in order to decrease the size of the dataset. Thus, the Fourier coefficients of the outline of the endocardial border in a tomographic section of the heart are its Fourier descriptors. Other methods of segmentation invoke the prior

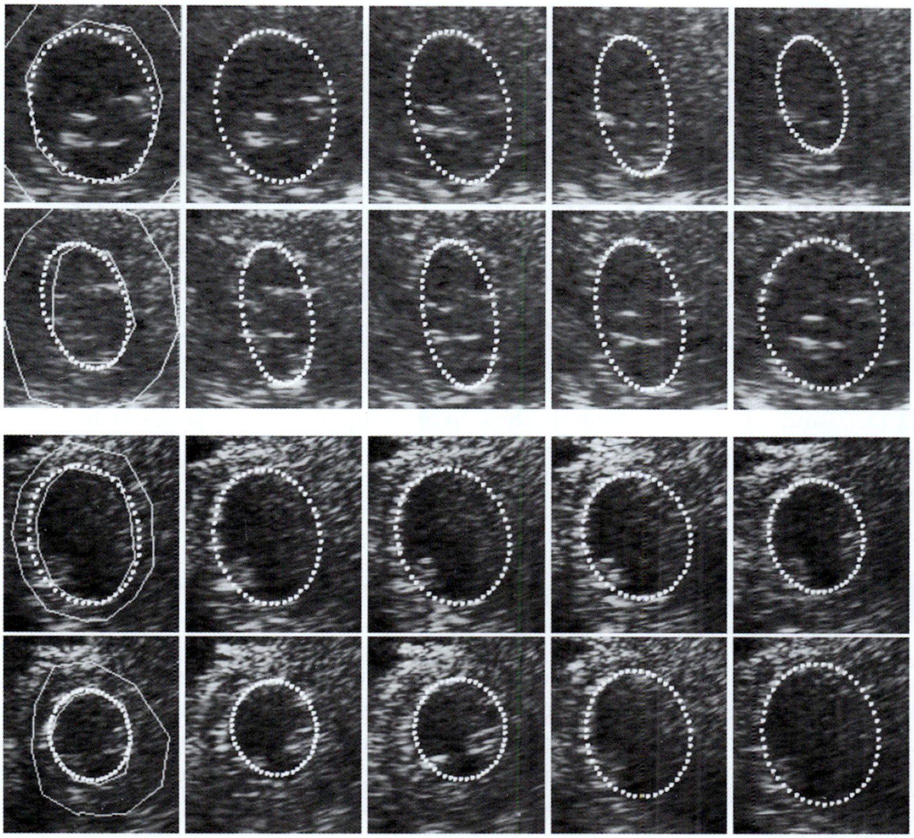

Figure 12.11: Segmentation using a 2-D ellipse model on a complete cardiac cycle for two different patients. The dotted ellipse shows the recovered endocardial contour on each frame. The thin lines show the "ground truth" for both endocardium and epicardium, as drawn by an expert on two frames in each patient. (Reproduced from Taron et al. [57], with kind permission of the authors and Springer.)

knowledge of shapes and the use of templates, prior information on absolute dimensions, prior familiarity with distinctive textures or gray-levels, and other descriptors. This type of approach is completely automatic and efficient, and it can be used with large 2- or 3-D training anatomical datasets of cardiac chambers and structures [26, 66]. The compact statistical representations (prior models) thus built can be used in a similar manner to the active contour models for primitive model search in image segmentation and endocardial boundary tracking applications [40].

After the dynamic chamber contours have been derived for each timestep from the clinical or experimental animal imaging data, the CFD software can in turn manipulate the data interactively, to prescribe dynamic endocardial geometry and flow-field boundary conditions, as is indicated in Figure 12.10, on p. 642.

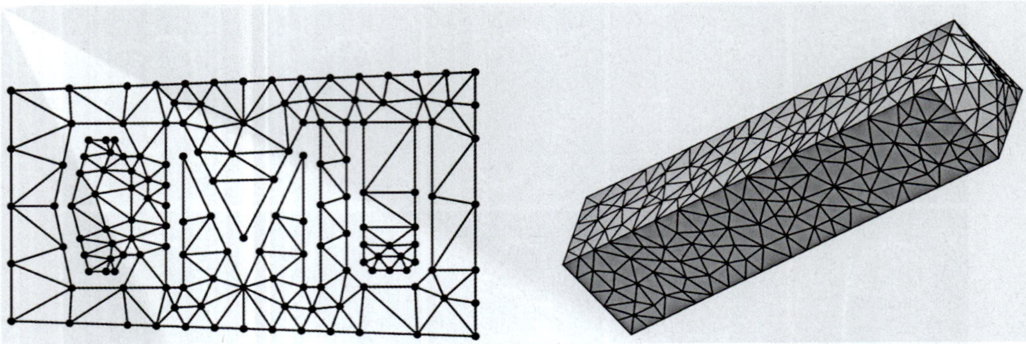

Figure 12.12: 2- and 3-D finite element meshes. In the left panel, each triangle is an element; in the right panel, each tetrahedron is an element.

12.6 Flow-field discretization

Computational modeling of blood flow and obtaining the solution to a particular problem generally requires the division of time into discrete intervals, or *timesteps*, and the discretization of the flow-governing partial differential equations over the entire 3-D flow field. The latter is accomplished by subdividing the computational domain into a mesh, or grid, of discrete cells. Large sets of discrete variables are defined on the computational cells to approximate flow variables, such as velocity [45, 61]. This discretization is straightforward for very simple geometries, but is a difficult problem for more complicated objects. Various CFD methods are available, including the finite difference method, which may be claimed to better represent the differential equations [19], finite spectral methods, the finite volume method, and the FEM, which provides the best accuracy in irregular geometric domains [1, 14, 19, 47].

The process of discretization associates a field variable with each of a finite number of points in the problem domain, comprising the surface and the interior of the domain. For instance, to simulate blood flow through the heart, velocity values are associated with a number of points, called nodes, in the flow field. It is not enough to choose a set of points to act as nodes; the problem domain must be partitioned into small pieces of simple shape. In particular, the FEM subdivides the computational domain into nonoverlapping cells. These cells are the "elements," and the nodes are the vertices of the cells. In the FEM, the elements are usually triangles or quadrilaterals in 2-D, and tetrahedra or hexahedral bricks in 3-D, and are of appropriate sizes—most likely varying throughout the mesh. If elements of uniform size were to be used throughout the mesh, one would have to choose a size small enough to guarantee sufficient accuracy in the most demanding portion of the problem domain, and would thereby incur excessively large computational demands. The FEM employs a node at every element vertex (and sometimes at other locations); each node is typically shared among several elements. The collection of nodes and elements is called a finite element mesh. 2- and 3-D finite element meshes are illustrated in Figure 12.12.

In practice, *curved* boundaries—such as apply in intracardiac flow problems—can often be approximated by piecewise linear boundaries, so theoretical mesh generation algorithms are often based upon the idealized assumption that the input geometry is piecewise linear, i.e., composed without curves. Because elements have simple shapes, it is easy to approximate the behavior of partial differential equations, such as the Navier–Stokes equations, on each element. By accumulating these effects over all the elements, one derives a system of equations whose solution approximates a set of physical quantities such as the velocity at each node. Solution methods that employ finite element or "boundary-fitted coordinates" generate a solution grid that conforms to the geometry of the flow region. For increased accuracy, it is advantageous to have coordinate lines running parallel to a particular boundary or flow direction.

Subdivision of constituent elements for refinement of volumetric grids can be accomplished by various volumetric subdivision schemes. Consider, for illustrative purposes, linear subdivision on a mesh of tetrahedra: we can define a split on a single tetrahedron, which can then be applied to all the tetrahedra in the grid. Taking one tetrahedron, we insert new vertices at the midpoints of each edge and connect the vertices together to form four new tetrahedra, at the corners of the original tetrahedron. Chopping in our mind these four offspring off the corners of the parent tetrahedron, leaves an octahedron, as is indicated pictorially in Figure 12.13 Ia. Consequently, the subdivision scheme becomes a tetrahedral/octahedral subdivision scheme, and not simply a tetrahedral subdivision process. This calls for a refinement rule for octahedra. We insert vertices at the midpoints of each edge on the octahedron and at the centroid of the octahedron, which is formed by averaging all of its vertices together. Next, we connect the vertices together to form six new octahedra, corresponding to the six vertices of the original octahedron, and eight new tetrahedra, corresponding to the eight faces of the original octahedron. The octahedral subdivision scheme is illustrated in Figure 12.13 Ib.

It is noteworthy that performing the corner-chopping procedure on a triangle yields a triangle, making linear subdivision for triangular meshes covering a *surface* much easier than linear subdivision on a *volumetric* grid of tetrahedra.

Clearly, it is a nontrivial task to generate these grids with acceptable element sizes and shapes for accurate numerical approximations. Even when automatic grid generating software is employed, there are requirements for users to supply dynamic geometric data for the beating heart chambers, to control the number and type of finite elements, their connectivity, aspect ratios and other features. The computational geometry-conforming grid must not only fill the intracardiac flow field but must also conform closely to its boundaries. In complicated cases this type of grid generation may consume a significant amount of time and effort. Some programs attempt to eliminate this gridding problem by using only rectangular grid elements.

An important limitation of rectangular elements, however, is that the geometric flow boundaries are usually approximated by blocking out entire cells, which leads to serrated

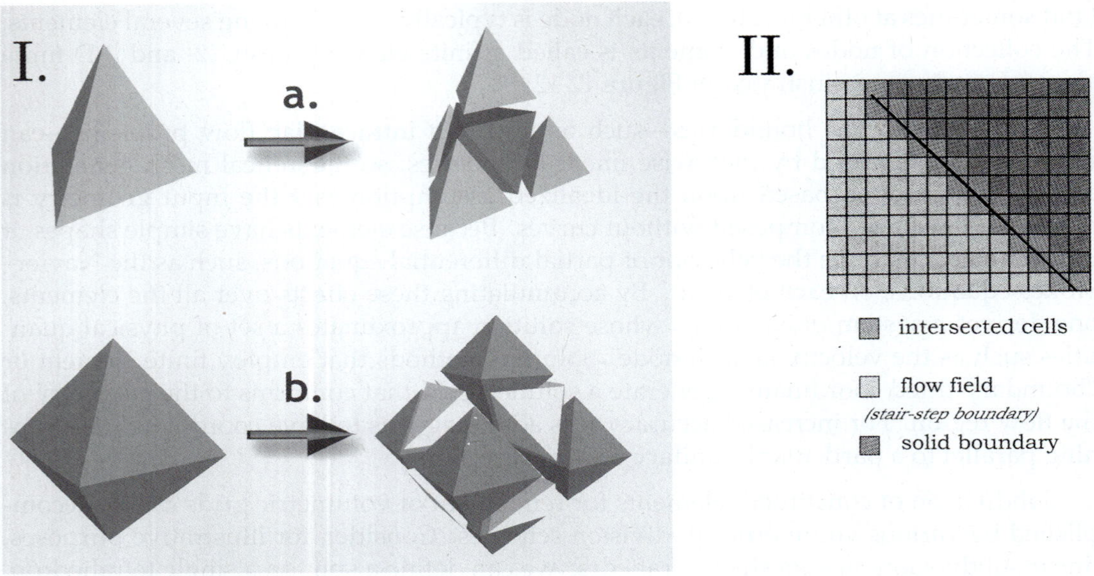

Figure 12.13: I. a. Linear subdivision splits a tetrahedron into four tetrahedra and an octahedron. b. An octahedron is then split into six octahedra and eight tetrahedra. II.–When solid flow boundaries are approximated by blocking out entire intersected cells, stair-step boundaries result with discrete steps, instead of smooth surfaces.

boundaries with discrete steps, instead of smooth surfaces (see Fig. 12.13 II.). These unrealistic "stair-step" boundaries can alter flow features and can significantly overestimate the inner surface areas of the cardiac chambers, which obviously has objectionable consequences.

The optimal choice for a grid system depends on several considerations: convenience in generation, memory requirements, numerical accuracy, flexibility to conform to complex geometries and to accommodate localized regions of higher or lower resolution. For complex intracardiac flow domains with curved, moving boundaries, and with embedded subregions that require higher resolution than the remainder of the flow field, grid generation can be a formidable task.

12.6.1 Structured and unstructured grids

Simple rectangular boundaries are never encountered in intracardiac blood flow-field simulations; indeed, nearly all boundaries are irregular.[8] Irregular boundaries create enormous difficulties in implementation of the boundary conditions. Various procedures are available to treat irregular boundaries. A popular approach is *grid generation*. Broadly

[8] Some problems of classical engineering interest have nice rectangular boundaries, on which a computational grid system can be readily superimposed.

speaking, grid generation schemes can be categorized into two groupings: the so-called structured and unstructured grids. Thus, when faced with the problem of fitting a grid to an intrinsically complex cardiac chamber geometry, we have the two alternatives [15,41]: (a) to partition the domain into "convenient" elements (e.g., triangular, quadrilateral or other exotic elements), or (b) to decompose the domain into regular subdomains (e.g., blocks which can be mapped, conformally or otherwise, into squares or cubes). The first approach summarizes the geometry-based gridding method and leads to generally unstructured grids [32,33], while the second leads to structured grids.

A *structured* grid means that the volume elements are well ordered, and a simple scheme (e.g., $i-j-k$ indices) can be used to label elements and identify neighbors. In unstructured grids, volume elements can be joined in any manner, and special lists must be kept to identify the neighboring elements. Structured grids come in several classes, depending on the shape of their elements. The simplest grid is generated from a rectangular box by subdividing it into a set of rectangular elements with faces parallel to the sides of the box. Most often the elements are arranged by counting in the x-, then in the y-, and lastly in the z-direction, so that grid element (i, j, k) would be the *ith* element in the x-direction, etc.

Grids composed of regular brick elements have the simplest structure, since it is only necessary to define three 1-D arrays for the x-, y-, and z-values of the surfaces defining the cell surfaces. If I, J and K are the maximum indices in the x-, y-, and z-directions, then the total number of values needed to define the rectangular grid is $I \times J \times K$. Rectangular grids with slowly varying element sizes also demonstrate a geometric regularity, which contributes toward maintenance of numerical accuracy. Any grid cell distortion will reduce numerical accuracy because numerical approximations are no longer centered (or symmetric) about the centroid of the distorted cell. Accordingly, a consequence of cell distortion is that, to maintain accuracy, numerical approximations must become more complicated. To overcome this problem efficiently, a mathematical transformation—from the irregularly shaped *physical domain* to a regular *computational domain*—is introduced.

For structured grids, a transformation from the physical space to the computational domain is performed as is exemplified schematically in Figures 12.14 and 12.15, in two and three dimensions, respectively. There are several different types of transformations that will map the nonrectangular, nonuniform grid of the physical domain to a rectangular grid with regular grid spacing in the computational domain. By deformation of the physical domain, i.e., appropriate stretching and twisting, the irregular physical domain is transformed into the rectangular regular computational domain.

In general, there are two classes of methods for numerical 3-D structured grid generation: (a) grid generation by solving partial differential equations (almost invariably using elliptic equations), and (b) by algebraic interpolation. From a practical standpoint, a mixture of elliptic solvers and algebraic interpolation techniques is typically the best solution in optimizing the gridding. The former contribute to mesh smoothness while the latter give better control of grid resolution. Commonly, an algebraic method gives the initial guess for the grid, while the final grid comes as a result of solving an elliptic partial differential equation. The flow-field governing equations are subsequently solved

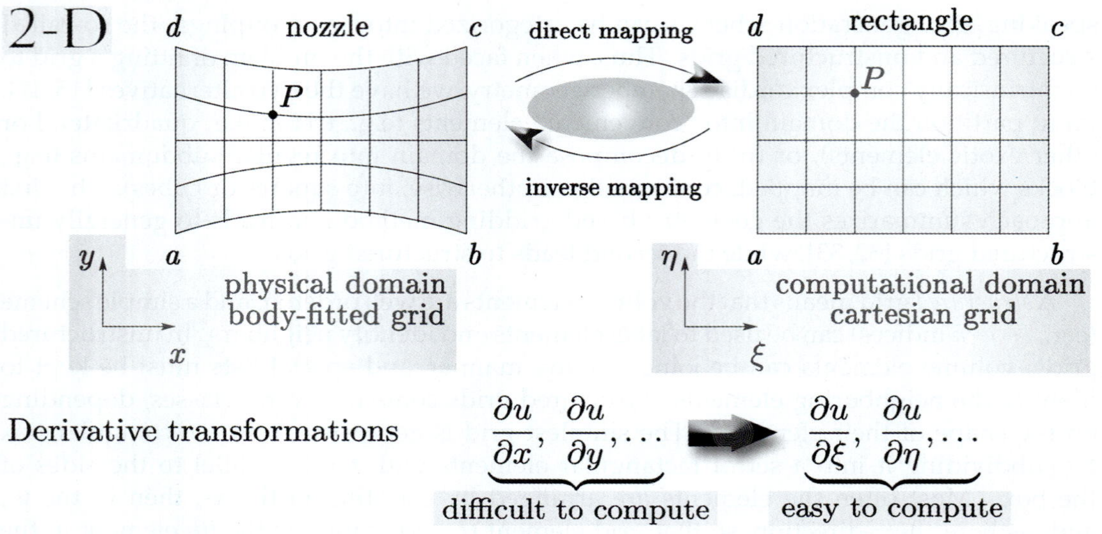

Figure 12.14: Grid transformations are needed in order to provide a simple treatment of curvilinear boundaries with improved solution accuracy. The irregular physical domain (x, y) is transformed into the rectangular computational domain (ξ, η), which has a uniform grid distribution with equidistant nodes. The original flow-field partial differential equations must be rewritten in terms of (ξ, η), instead of (x, y) and must be discretized in the computational domain rather than the physical one.

numerically in the computational domain. The solution of the equation system is iterative; for large grids the computing time is considerable. Finally, the computed field-variables information can be transformed back to the physical domain by applying the one-to-one mapping correspondence of grid points in the two domains. In conclusion, this approach enables us to perform all integration operations over a computational domain with regular geometry, and to then map the results into the physiologically meaningful physical domain. *Unstructured* grids are easier to generate and the process can be automated. They have the advantage of generality in that they can be made to conform to nearly any applying geometry. The grid generation process, however, is not completely automatic and may require substantial user interaction, to produce grids with acceptable levels of local resolution while concurrently maintaining a minimum of element distortion.

The process of solving the linear or nonlinear systems of equations yielded by the FEM and its brethren is, in fact, simpler and faster on structured meshes, because of the ease of determining each node's neighbors. Because unstructured grids necessitate the storage of pointers to each node's neighbors, their demands on storage space and memory traffic are greater. Unstructured grids not only require more information (namely, the generally extensive neighbor connectivity list) to be stored and recovered than structured grids, but changing element types and sizes can increase numerical approximation errors too. Furthermore, the regularity of structured meshes makes it straightforward to

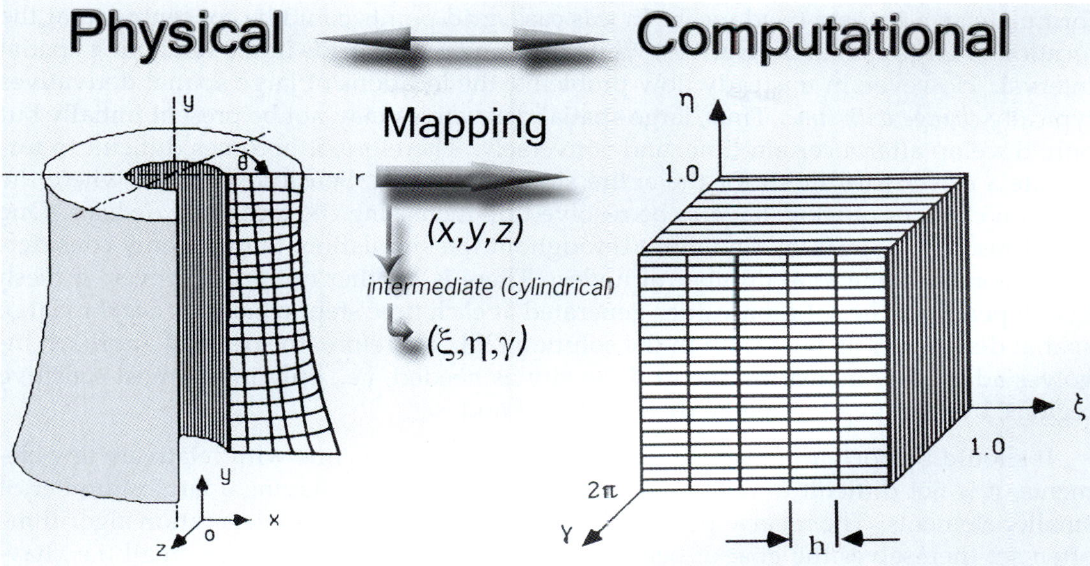

Figure 12.15: By deformation of the physical domain, i.e., appropriate stretching and twisting of the grid coordinates, the irregular physical domain (x, y, z) is transformed into the rectangular computational domain (ξ, η, ζ), which has a uniform grid distribution with equidistant nodes. (Adapted and modified from Georgiadis, Wang, and Pasipoularides [15], by kind permission of the Biomedical Engineering Society and Springer.)

parallelize computations upon them, whereas unstructured meshes engender the need for sophisticated partitioning algorithms and parallel unstructured solvers.

In addition, unstructured grids introduce severe complications during the solution of the field equations which are discretized on them; one difficulty is that the resulting linear systems have nonsparse matrices and are therefore unwieldy. Accordingly, the solvers for algebraic equation systems of unstructured grids are generally slower than those for structured grids. In contrast, structured grids allow the implementation of more efficient CFD flow solvers [54]. The trade-off is that the governing equation is mapped into the local coordinate system and therefore it becomes more complicated. The approach followed depends on one's philosophy and specifically on the answer that is selected to the question whether it is is better to solve difficult field equations in regular domains or to solve simple equations in physically complicated domains [15].

Numerical accuracy considerations impose certain quality criteria to a successful numerical grid: high resolution, smoothness, uniformity, and reduction of skewness (i.e., small deviations from orthogonality). Grid generation is an *iterative* (see Fig. 12.18, on p. 659), adaptive process since it is not possible to optimize nodal density independently of the numerical solution algorithm. The corresponding spatial mesh must be quite fine in regions where the derivative is large to resolve the solution correctly. If the regions of large derivative remained stationary with respect to time, it would be straightforward to formulate an adequate fixed mesh. In this case, grid points could be concentrated at the location of large spatial derivatives, while choosing coarse grids in the remaining spatial interval. However, in unsteady flow problems, the locations of large spatial derivatives typically *change with time*. Thus, large spatial derivatives may not be present initially but only develop after a certain time, and conversely. Therefore, it becomes difficult to formulate a clever *fixed* mesh for the entire simulation time. Sensitive regions, where the solution changes quickly, have to be resolved by increasing the local grid density. One might resort to a uniform, fine mesh throughout the simulation, but economy considerations constrain the total number of nodes. There is another option, however: a mesh that depends on the solution values generated at each time step, which can *adapt* to large spatial derivatives as they form in the solution [25]. Therefore, the optimal approach involves adaptively increasing the grid density as needed, i.e., only in the most sensitive regions, by changing the spatial distribution of nodes.

It should be born in mind that given a coarse mesh, i.e., one with relatively few elements, it is not difficult to refine it to produce another mesh having a larger number of smaller elements. The reverse process is not so easy. Hence, mesh generation algorithms often set themselves the goal of being able, in principle, to generate as small (i.e., having as few elements as possible) a mesh as is feasible. They typically offer the option to refine *portions* of the mesh whose elements are not small enough to yield the required numerical solution accuracy.

12.6.2 The need for boundary-fitted coordinate systems

When a finite difference scheme is employed in the numerical solution of partial differential equations, it is necessary to make use of a rectangular grid system for the discretization of the solution domain. If the domain happens to be of rectangular shape, then it is straightforward to create a uniform rectangular grid system. However, most intracardiac blood flow applications of computational fluid dynamics involve solution domains that have complex shapes. When such domains are discretized using a rectangular grid system, some *incomplete cells* are created, which have some of their defining nodes outside of the solution domain and others inside the domain, as is exemplified by the endocardial boundary cells in the case of the nonboundary-fitted grid in Figure 12.17, on p. 656. As a rule, such incomplete cells appear at the boundary of the flow domain. The existence of incomplete cells makes the implementation of boundary conditions a difficult task. Although the use of interpolation schemes may resolve the implementation issue, the solution accuracy will likely suffer from the application of lower order approximations.

Another problem associated with the incomplete cells relates to numerical stability. Whenever explicit schemes are used to solve a time-dependent system of equations, it is well known (see Section 12.8.2, on pp. 665 ff.) that, in order for the numerical scheme to be stable, the temporal step size (Δt) and spatial step size (Δx) must satisfy the Courant–Friedrichs–Lewy (CFL) condition given by Equation 12.1, on p. 665. In other words, for the solution to be stable over the entire flow region, Δt must be chosen such that Equation 12.1 is satisfied, even for the minimum Δx.

As can be seen from Equation 12.1, the smaller the minimum Δx happens to be, the smaller must be the corresponding Δt allowed. In cases that involve incomplete cells, the minimum Δx can be very small. Accordingly, the allowed Δt is required to assume minuscule values in order to fulfill Equation 12.1. Thus, with incomplete boundary cells, the stability requirement renders explicit solution schemes very inefficient. The aforementioned reasons motivate CFD schemes utilizing boundary-fitted coordinate systems.

With boundary fitted coordinate systems, a virtual space, the *computational space*, is introduced. A mapping between the physical space and this computational space is defined, such that the generally nonrectangular domain in the physical space is mapped onto a rectangular domain in the computational space. The term "boundary-fitted coordinate system" reflects the fact that the boundary of the physical domain corresponds to the boundary of the computational domain that is aligned to the computational coordinate system. When rectangular discretization is performed in the computational domain, the corresponding physical domain is also discretized in such a way that no incomplete cells are generated [15]. Furthermore, it is also possible to set up the mapping such that the computational coordinate lines are orthogonal at the boundaries. In this manner, the imposition of the boundary conditions, especially those involving derivatives, becomes much easier, because no interpolation is necessary.

The governing equations, with physical spatial coordinates as independent variables, also need to be represented in the computational domain, with the computational spatial coordinates as independent variables. These transformed equations contain certain coefficients that describe the mapping relation between physical and computational spatial coordinates. These coefficients are termed *transformation metrics*, and are in the form of derivatives, $\partial\xi/\partial x$, where ξ is the computational coordinate and x is the physical coordinate [15]. The numerical evaluation of these coefficients may be a source of error in the computational solution of the flow-governing equations.

The boundary fitted coordinate system is very useful when dealing with flow problems involving moving boundaries, as in the simulation of intracardiac flows. In this situation, the mapping between computational domain and physical domain is a time-dependent function, and the grid system in physical space needs to be reconstructed for every time step. Despite the additional transformation metrics in the governing equations, the implementation of the boundary conditions is as simple as for the situation involving stationary boundaries.[9] Thus, the use of a time-dependent boundary-fitted coordinate system simplifies the implementation of the boundary conditions, at the expense of requiring that the grid be regenerated at every time step.

Special care needs to be taken when using the boundary-fitted coordinate system. First, as pointed out by Fletcher [14], the smoothness of the boundary fitted coordinate system plays a vital role in the accuracy and efficiency of the numerical solution, especially when second order partial differential equations, such as the Navier–Stokes equations, are considered. As a rule of thumb, the variation of dimensions between neighboring cells

[9] In contrast, the immersed boundary method of Peskin, which will be discussed in the next chapter is essentially a time-dependent method utilizing a Cartesian grid with incomplete cells and, as discussed above, requires a time-dependent interpolation for imposition of the boundary conditions.

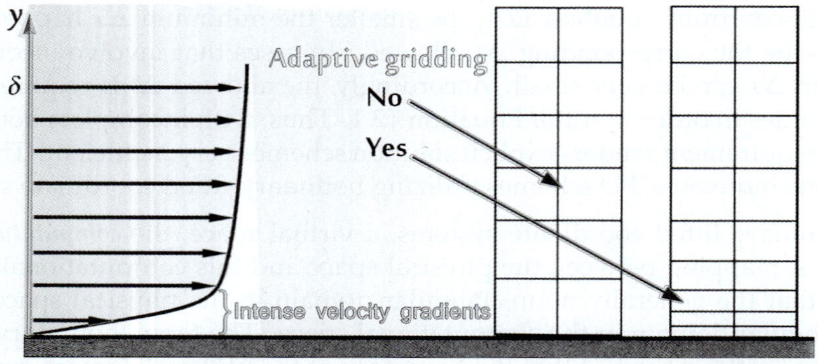

Figure 12.16: Adaptive gridding results in higher grid resolution only in regions of the flow field where the velocity gradients are high, e.g., across more or less of the thickness (δ) of a boundary layer.

should be of order 1, i.e., $\Delta x_2 = [1 + O(\Delta x)] \cdot \Delta x_1$. Secondly, when numerically evaluating metric coefficients in the governing equations, it is recommended that, as a rule, the same discretizing formula be used as used in the discretization of the derivatives of the dependent variables [14]. This leads to cancellation of a major portion of the truncation error and thus achieves smaller solution errors. Violation of this rule may result in a loss of the conservative property in the discretized version of the flow-governing equations.

12.6.3 Adaptive and moving grids

A major CFD challenge when coping with real-world problems is that of accuracy. Ideally, the higher the spatial resolution of the flow-field grid, the more accurate will be the result. However, in the application of a numerical solution scheme, a grid system with high resolution throughout the physical domain may not be necessary. For example, for a viscous flow over a flat surface, it is necessary to have higher resolution only across the *boundary layer* (see Section 4.9 on pp. 197 ff.), where the velocity gradients are high; for the areas far away from the solid surface it is still feasible to use a coarser grid, because not much cross-stream (transverse) velocity and pressure nonuniformity is manifest there (see Fig. 12.16).

Hence, for an optimal usage of computational resources, a flow-field dependent gridding scheme is a reasonable approach. However, the costs associated with the procedure for regridding must be balanced by the savings accruing by reducing the total number of computational grid points, while maintaining a comparable spatial accuracy level where it matters. Thus a *trade-off* exists between the expense for regridding and the benefit from reducing the total number of grid points. Typically, elliptic and parabolic partial differential equation solution methods are used for implementing the regridding. Such approaches provide an efficient way for an adaptive grid regeneration while tracking the temporal evolution of the flow field.

Adaptive methods in CFD are generally based on a simple idea: when the error in a computation is too large, change the structure of the approximation (the mesh size, the location of grid points, the order of the approximation, etc.) in order to reduce it. Interest in such procedures has grown gradually with the realization that they may embody ways to *optimize* computations—to deliver the best answers in some sense for the least effort. Adaptive gridding techniques fall into two broad groupings, adaptive mesh *redistribution* and adaptive mesh *refinement*, both encompassed by the acronym AMR. Adaptive mesh redistribution continuously *repositions* a fixed number of cells, and so it improves the resolution in particular locations of the computational domain, as called for by the solution [33].

Stationary grids may be used as the initial grids for time-varying grid problems, such as moving boundary or flow-adaptive grid simulations, or for use in fixed grid problems with steady and unsteady flows. The concept of solution-adaptive grid-generation can be applied to steady as well as unsteady flow problems. For steady flow fields, a progressive improvement of the grid as well as the flow solution can be achieved iteratively and the result is a more efficient deployment of the grid points. For unsteady flow fields, the grid-clustering region(s) should develop in a synchronized manner with the evolving critical flow regimes that give rise to regions with high spatial gradients in the dependent flow variables, if a superior spatial resolution is to be achieved. Such adaptive schemes can apply to both stationary grid and moving grid problems.

It is very important to have sufficient nodal density, or domain resolution, in regions where dependent variables have steep gradients. For example, the velocity, vorticity and pressure may have large gradients in regions near walls, inlets and outlets, bends, and shear layers. Shear in the fluid, for example, generally steepens gradients and generates more fine-scale structure as time advances. Adaptive mesh refinement *adds* new cells as required and *deletes* other cells that are no longer required. Because of the great potential of AMR algorithms for reducing computational costs without reducing the overall level of accuracy, they are an intensive area of research in CFD.

The computation of real intracardiac flow fields using 3-D digital imaging data falls within a class of problems where numerical grid generation is crucial. 3-D boundary-fitted grids consist of rows and columns of finite elements or "cells." Unlike Cartesian grids, which consist of cells that are aligned with a conventional coordinate system, the cells in boundary-fitted grids can have any quadrilateral shape and therefore are not necessarily aligned with the conventional coordinate directions. Because of this, the grid better fits the boundary of the intracardiac flow field. As an example, the solution of the flow-governing equations in the ejecting left ventricular chamber requires the generation of boundary-fitted composite grids [15]. Boundary-fitted grids are superior compared to non-boundary-fitted grids, as we have already noted in Section 12.5, on pp. 638 ff. in this chapter.

Figure 12.17 depicts the gridding of a cross-section of the left ventricular chamber using two different grids, (a) a simple Cartesian grid superimposed on the physical domain and (b) a boundary-fitted grid. Given the curved and complex shape of the ventricular cavity, the boundary-fitted grid is preferred for two reasons: (a) the implementation of

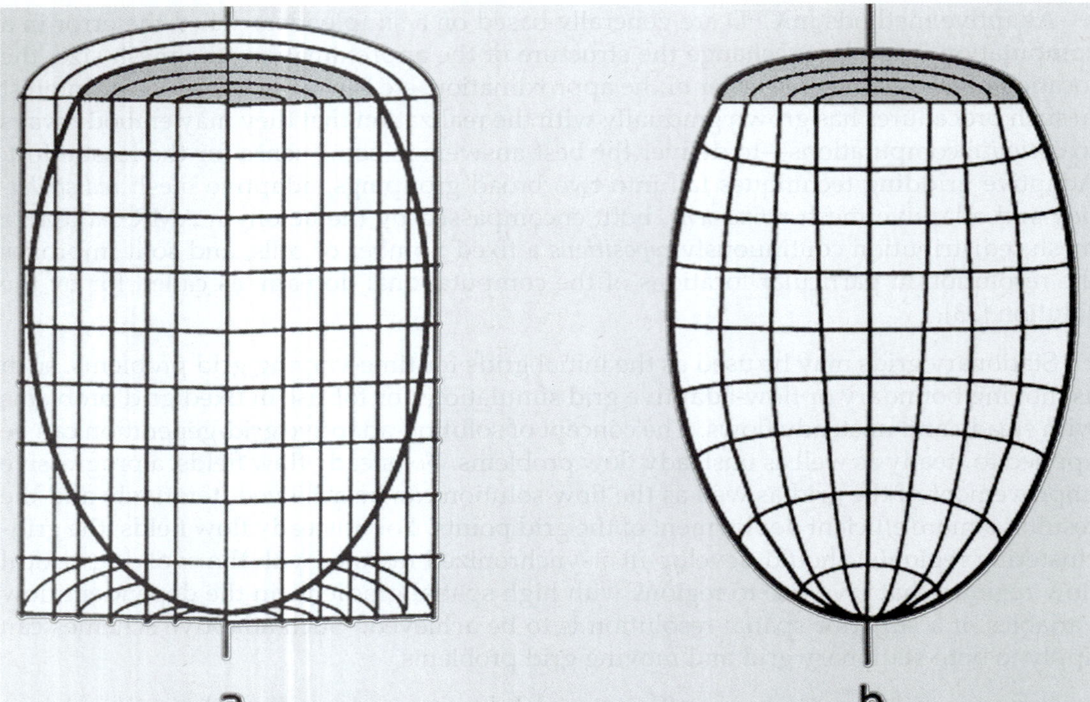

Figure 12.17: Two structured gridding schemes applied to an ellipsoidal LV chamber during ejection. a. Cylindrical coordinate system with a Cartesian grid on the cross-section of the chamber. b. Curvilinear coordinate system. Based on whether or not the grid conforms to the boundaries of the flow field, the former represents a nonboundary-fitted grid; the latter, a boundary-fitted grid. Note that only in the boundary-fitted coordinate system do the grid points fall on the endocardial contour of the LV chamber; the endocardial boundary cells in the case of the nonboundary-fitted grid represent incomplete cells. (Adapted from Georgiadis, Wang, and Pasipoularides [15], by kind permission of the Biomedical Engineering Society and Springer.)

boundary conditions is simpler since the boundary coincides with grid lines and (b) the boundary layer near the cavity wall can be resolved by increasing the local grid node density in a straightforward manner. After a grid has been set up, additional software tools can be used to manipulate individual cells, and to define the appropriate boundary conditions, as is indicated pictorially (arrows) for the nodes of the septal portion of the inner chamber surface in the instantaneous RV grid depicted in Figure 12.10, on p. 642. The discretized flow field is then saved and available for the simulation process.

In realistic, patient-specific, simulations of intraventricular flow fields, a moving-grid capability is an indispensable requirement. It should utilize as input the dynamically changing endocardial surface contours of the cardiac chambers obtained by suitable digital imaging modalities; together with a grid-smoothing algorithm, it should be able to propagate the boundary movements of the endocardial chamber surface through the CFD mesh. This is an example of a so-called "fluid–structure interaction" (sometimes referred to as *FSI*) problem [11, 52, 63, 67]. For instance, the intraventricular diastolic inflow field depends on the dynamic chamber geometry, and the deformation of the expanding ventricular walls depends on the blood inflow.

The interaction of the pulsating walls with the inflowing liquid that they surround gives rise to a rich variety of physical phenomena, as we shall see in subsequent chapters. Here, we simply note that the deformation of the filling chamber is not small, and the intraventricular inflow-field phenomena will therefore dynamically change. This means that any change in the bounding wall *structure* is coupled back to the *fluid dynamics*. As the chamber boundaries undergo large movements during most phases of the cardiac cycle, a fixed mesh structure will lead to badly distorted elements. This means that a sequence of at least partial regenerations of the computational domain will be required. The idea is to regenerate the whole computational domain *adaptively*, taking into consideration the current flow-field solution. When movement of the contracting or filling chamber geometry becomes too large to allow the original topology to be kept, adaptive remeshing together with a second-order solution interpolation must be used, before the solution continues. A significant speed-up can be achieved by first generating a coarser, but stretched mesh, and then refining globally this mesh. Such geometric adjustments may be called for repeatedly, after every 2–3 successive timesteps, in the course of an intracardiac flow-field simulation [41–43].

12.7 Iterative solution of the discretized flow-field equations

On the mesh, the discretized Navier–Stokes equations take the form of a large system of nonlinear equations [2, 3]; thus, transforming the partial differential equations of intracardiac flow into a finite number of algebraic relations produces a set of equations that can he written, manipulated, and analyzed in matrix form—with every row representing a separate equation and every column representing a specific variable. This process of going from the continuum to the discrete set of equations is a problem that combines both physics and numerical analysis [14, 15, 23, 41]. For example, it is important to maintain conservation of mass in the discrete equations. At every node in the mesh, several variables are associated: the pressure, the three velocity components, etc. Furthermore, capturing physically important phenomena, such as vortices or flow disturbances, may require extremely fine meshes in parts of the physical domain. Currently, meshes with millions of nodes are typical in simulations of right ventricular inflow-field phenomena (see Chapter 14), leading to systems with up to 100,000,000 unknowns.

Explicit and implicit methods [14, 47, 60] are approaches for the mathematical simulation of intracardiac flow processes involving partial differential equations. Explicit methods calculate the state of a flow field at a *later* time from the state of the field at the *current* time, while an implicit method finds it by solving an equation involving *both* the current state of the field and the later one. Implicit methods require extra computation and they can be much harder to implement. However, they are used to advantage because many intracardiac flow problems are *stiff*,[10] for which the use of an explicit method requires impractically small timesteps (Δt) to keep the error in the result bounded. For such problems, to achieve given accuracy, it may require much less computational time to use an implicit method with *larger* (and thus *fewer*) timesteps, even though each timestep takes more computation.

Solution of the system of nonlinear equations is typically by a Newton-like iterative method (see Fig. 12.18, on p. 659), which in turn requires solving in a coupled manner a large, sparse system of equations, on each step. Sparsity, here, means that the matrix of coefficients for the system consists mainly of zeros, with relatively few nonzero entries. Storing the coefficients requires development of efficient data structures that require little overhead storage but allow efficient performance of the necessary manipulations. Methods for solving large sparse systems of equations are an area of intense research right now [10], since that is often the most time-consuming part of the program, and because the ability to solve them is the limiting factor in the size of problem that is tractable, and thus in the complexity of the flow characteristics that can be simulated.

Direct methods, which factor the matrices, require more computer storage than is permissible for all but the smallest problems. Iterative methods use less storage but they often fail to converge. The way out is to use *preconditioning*; that is, to pre-multiply the system by some matrix that makes it easier for the iterative method to converge [58]. Moreover, segregated solvers can substantially reduce disk storage requirements compared to fully coupled solvers. The savings in storage become greater as the size of the problem increases. This solution technique, designed for large-scale simulations, avoids the direct formulation of a global system matrix. Instead, there is matrix decomposition into smaller submatrices, each governing the nodal unknowns associated with only one conservation equation. The storage requirements for the individual submatrices are considerably less than would be needed to store the global matrix. This solution technique is usually the most effective for intracardiac flow problems.

CFD problems are at the limits of computational power [10], so parallel programming methods are used. This brings in the research problem of how to partition the data to assign parts of it to different processors; usually domain decomposition methods are applied (see Fig. 12.19, on p. 660), and the subdomains are mapped onto the individual processors of a parallel system. In general, the number of subdomains is set to equal the number of processors in a parallel system. Domain decomposition is a partitioning problem, namely finding a minimum edge cut partitioning of the discrete mesh, with roughly the same number of nodes in each partition set. An additional problem with parallel programming is that the better methods for solving the resultant linear systems often have inherently sequential characteristics, while parallel solution methods are not robust enough.

[10] A stiff equation is a differential equation for which numerical solution methods are numerically unstable, unless the step size is taken to be extremely small.

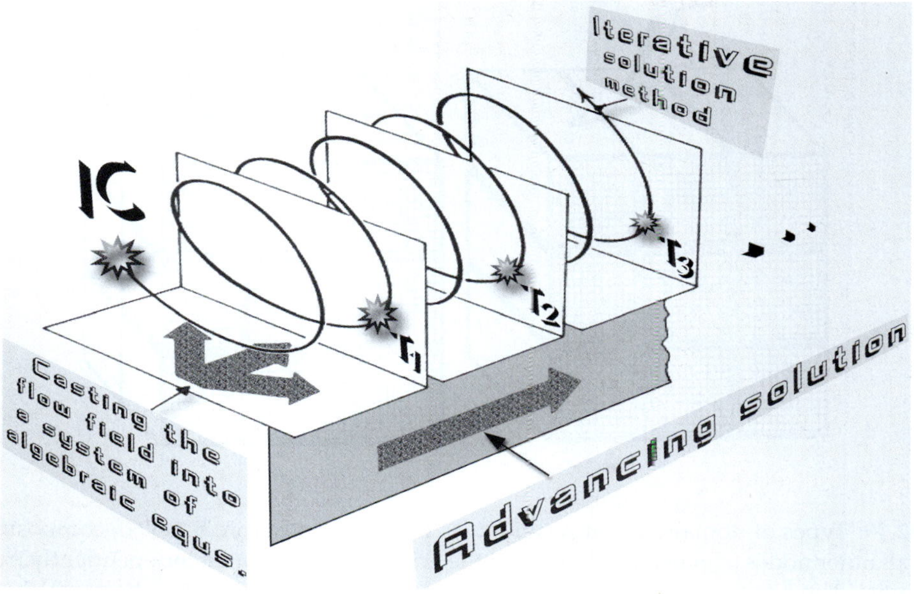

Figure 12.18: An iterative method advances the solution to a problem [e.g., the system of discretized flow-field governing equations with appropriate boundary and initial (IC) conditions] by finding, through a sequence of repeating-step loops, successively closer approximations to the *"exact"* solution at successive instants of time (T_1, T_2, ...), starting from an initial guess. In each loop, the current values of every unknown flow field variable are used to determine new values, which are then substituted in the next iteration for the old values.

To ensure convergence of the computation, an intermittent exchange of relevant data between processors treating adjacent subdomains is necessary. Generally, it is critical that only the indispensable data be exchanged in as few communication steps as possible, because establishing a connection between processors and exchanging data, requires an enormous amount of time, compared to that required for arithmetic operations on most parallel computers. The increased communication requirements of a parallelized CFD algorithm may reduce, to a greater or lesser extent, the gain in speed imparted by the parallelization of the computations.

12.7.1 Convergence

Implicit methods for nonlinear and coupled equations require iterative solution methods. Iterative solution methods calculate a sequence of approximations that converge to the solution. We expect the corresponding numerical solutions to converge and become better representations of the continuous flow-field variables as the size of the cells and timesteps becomes smaller and smaller, and the granularity of the grid of finite elements becomes finer. Convergence is the tendency for the numerical solution to approach the exact solution as the solution domain becomes more refined [30]. Equivalently, we say that

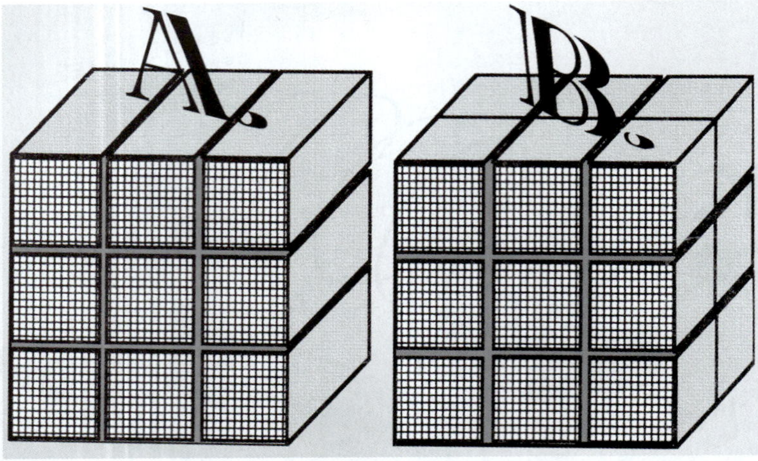

Figure 12.19: Types of domain decomposition: A. 2-D decomposition; B. 3-D decomposition. Notice that all inner nodes of every subdomain of the grid can be calculated independently from other subdomains. The border and corner nodes of every subdomain must then be correctly updated after every timestep using reciprocal interprocessor communication to exchange information with the adjoining subdomains.

a numerical scheme or algorithm converges when successively reducing the grid spacing Δx and the time step Δt produces correspondingly more accurate answers. The convergence rate is the speed at which the numerical solution approaches the true solution. It is necessary to check the residuals, relative solution changes and other indicators to make sure that the iterations converge.

Because of the nonlinearity of the equation set being solved, it is necessary to control the change of the solution variable. *Under-relaxation* is a constraint on the change of a dependent or auxiliary variable from one solution iteration to the next. It is required in order to maintain the stability of the coupled, nonlinear system of the flow-field equations. This benevolent effect of under-relaxation is accomplished by reducing the computed change in the solution variable produced by each iteration within each cell, by an under-relaxation factor, α; this leads to smaller steps toward convergence but with a lesser tendency toward unstable oscillations in the iterative solution process.

Every numerical solution contains errors [50]. The key is to understand how large those errors are, relatively speaking, and whether their level is acceptable in a particular application. A common convergence criterion is to require that the absolute values in the changes of the solution variables at each node be smaller than a preset tolerance. One encounters terms such as "orders of magnitude," "percent error," or "significant digits." They can all be related to one another, as one order of magnitude is similar to 10% error and similar to one significant digit, two orders of magnitude is similar to 1% error and two significant digits, etc. A general rule of thumb is that 3–5 orders of magnitude of convergence is a good objective. Therefore, although the "exact" solution is not obtained, one

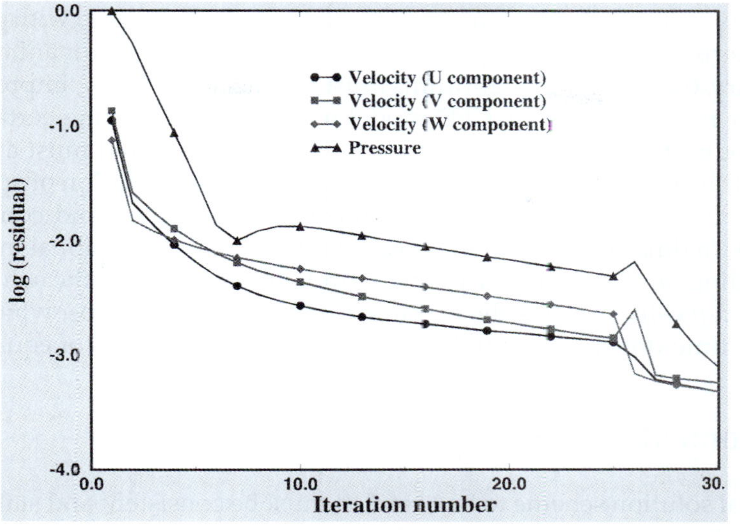

Figure 12.20: Representative rate of convergence of the solution for the flow-field variables at a given timestep, from a typical simulation of the intraventricular diastolic RV inflow field [41–43]. The computer-generated plot shows the natural logarithm of the residuals against the iteration number. Convergence is reached when the residuals of all variables become less than a preselected threshold value, here set at 0.1%. In this case, thirty iterations were required before attaining convergence. Note that individual variables have distinct rates of convergence, and have different residuals at the time of convergence. Moreover, the residuals for individual variables do not necessarily show a monotonic decrease. (A typical single-timestep iteration required 10–20 *min* of CPU time on a CRAY T-90 supercomputer.)

stops calculating when either the difference between successive iterates, or the residuals, are acceptably small.[11] In common practice, a solution converges when two successive iterations do not differ by more than 0.01% in any solution variable. It is often the case that certain quantities may reach convergence at a different rate than other variables (cf. Fig. 12.20). Moreover, the variable values will approach their final converged value at different rates depending upon where they lie within the flow field. Generally, the *smallest* flow patterns and flow structures are the *slowest* to converge. Obviously, a less strict convergence criterion implies that the solution should be achieved quicker, but perhaps with a lower accuracy than a stricter convergence criterion.

Although a particular solution may converge, the flow field to which it converges may not be the physiologically correct one. This might happen because of too coarse a mesh, computational errors, inappropriate boundary conditions, or invalid assumptions about the flow. Accordingly, the CFD user should have a good qualitative understanding of the fluid dynamic phenomena, which pertain to the flow that is being modeled, as is discussed

[11] Solver *residuals* represent the absolute error in the solution of a particular variable. The CFD "solver" program sums the absolute value of this error over all the cells in the simulation and presents that information for every solution variable, for each iteration, in the *residuals file*.

in the Appendix. Ultimately, the computed results must be compared with general flow behavior characteristics known from pertinent clinical measurements or animal experiments and, if necessary, the numerical algorithms must be adjusted (by, e.g., improved discretization via higher resolution) or the CFD model modified by adjusting certain parameters, or even by modifying some of the equations. The discrete model must approximate the continuous intracardiac flow field well. The required high resolution of space by discrete points invariably leads to great demands on computer memory and computation time, in particular with time-dependent processes in three-space dimensional intracardiac flow fields. Depending on the particular problem under consideration, the solution of the discrete problem typically requires the execution of many nested loops, which may involve nonlinearities, time-dependence, and the solution of large systems of equations.

12.7.2 Consistency and stability

For a numerical solution scheme to be useful, it must be consistent and stable. *Consistency* simply means that, as Δx and Δt are made progressively smaller, the corresponding iterations of the solution of the discretized governing equations must satisfy the numerical scheme with errors that also tend to vanish. The difference between the discretized equation and the exact one is called the truncation error. For a CFD method to be *consistent*, the truncation error must become zero when the grid spacing $\Delta x \longrightarrow 0$. The truncation error is usually proportional to a power of the grid spacing Δx or of the time step Δt. If the most important term is proportional to $(\Delta x)^n$ or $(\Delta t)^n$, we call the method an *nth order approximation*; $n > 0$ is required for consistency. Ideally, all terms should be discretized with approximations of the same order of accuracy; nevertheless, some terms may be dominant in a particular flow situation, and it may then be reasonable to treat them with more accuracy than the others. Consistency guarantees that the scheme *truly* approximates the equations we intend to solve with it.

Stability simply means that the scheme does not amplify errors. Obviously, this is very important, since errors are impossible to avoid in any numerical calculation. In fact, even in the ideal case of infinite precision, we still have to deal with discretization errors. A numerical solution method is characterized as *stable* if it does not magnify errors. For temporal problems, stability guarantees that the method produces a bounded solution whenever the solution of the exact equation itself is bounded. For iterative nethods, a stable method is one that does not diverge. Clearly, if errors are amplified, soon they will dominate any computation and render it useless. In practise, consistency and stability yield convergence.

12.7.3 Conservation

Since the flow-governing equations to be solved are conservation laws, the numerical scheme should also—on both a local and a global basis—respect these laws. Nonconservative terms are equivalent to *sources* or *sinks* (see Section 2.6.1, on pp. 55 ff.). The treatment of these terms should be consistent, so that the total source or sink in the flow domain is equal to the flux of the conserved quantity through the domain boundaries. In an incompressible steady flow regime, the density is constant. Thus, fluid entering a cell cannot accumulate within it; everything that comes in has to come out again. This is the continuity equation.

The Navier–Stokes equations can be applied to find the relationships between the forces at the edges of every grid cell. First, though, it is necessary to find expressions for the acceleration of the fluid, taking into account the fact that the velocity components may vary with both time and displacement. When this total acceleration is multiplied by the mass, the result is the force acting in one direction, e.g., the x-direction. This is defined by Newton's second law of motion. The force in the x-direction is a combination of normal stress and tangential shear components acting on the four sides of the cell. Combining these mathematically with the pressure, viscosity and density gives the conservation of momentum, or Navier–Stokes, equations. All the preceding equations are partial differential equations. Since computers can only work in binary, all the equations need to be transformed into equations containing only numbers. The system of converting a partial differential to its numerical analogue is the *numerical discretization*. The resulting continuity and momentum equations work well for most intracardiac flows, but the addition of complicated secondary flows, highly disturbed flows and, possibly, turbulence leads to requirements for greater processing power from the computer and the solutions can take longer to obtain.

High performance computers are invaluable, in that greater memory resources, greater computational power, and faster speed of computation allow, *ceteris paribus*, for finer finite element grids, a larger number of elements, and more accurate CFD solutions. After successful convergence, analyzing, validating, and presenting the solution calls into play visualization and graphics techniques. Those techniques are useful for more than just viewing the computed flow field. Visualization can help with understanding the nature of the phenomena and their interactions with cellular and organ physiology (cf. Sections 1.10 and 14.15, on pp. 23 ff. and 791 ff., respectively).

12.8 Computational costs of realistic chamber geometries

Intracardiac flow fields often have complicated dynamic geometries. In principle, larger, faster computers can solve the spatial, temporal, and computational problems associated with modeling complicated geometry. Visualizing solutions in complex geometry is also more difficult, time consuming and costly than with simpler flows. It takes more time to program a system with complex time-dependent geometry than one with simple steady geometry, and there is more computer code to go awry. Even if the program runs properly the first time, it will take longer to run and more time to get to the point where there are worthwhile results. It will require more computer storage, and the output will be harder to interpret.

Geometric complexity requires increased dimensionality and boundary conditions that are more complex. For example, an axisymmetric LV chamber model has been found adequate for simulations of the left ventricular systolic ejection flow field under most physiologic states and many pathologic conditions [15, 21, 22]. However, realistic geometric complications force many intracardiac flow problems to be formulated in three dimensions. For instance, simulations of the right ventricular diastolic flow field generally involve multidimensional effects such as separating flow and formation of vortices and require nonaxisymmetric 3-D fluid dynamics [41, 42]. What can be achieved with patient-specific *detailed* 3-D models is still limited, as regards routine clinical studies, by computer time and memory requirements and the associated costs.

Another related computational cost of intracardiac flow-field complexity is the increase in the time required to gather input data [41], and to write and debug the more complicated numerical algorithms. At times, the accuracy in the input data is not sufficient for the level of accuracy that may be expected from the simulation. If the input dynamic geometric data have errors, the accuracy and level of detail asked of the simulation may be unreasonable. A much less expensive computation with lower resolution might do as well.

12.8.1 Spatial and temporal resolution

The spatial and temporal resolutions required depend upon the dynamic geometric flow boundary details. The spatial resolution relates to the smallest volume that can be resolved by the particular imaging modality within the region of interest. This is dictated by the dimensions of the region, the resolution of the imager (the number of pixels in the array), and the thickness and spacing of the imaged planes. The parameter that dictates the temporal resolution of the system as a whole is the time to perform a complete volume scan, namely, the duration of one complete timestep. This relates to how well the volume is "frozen," or specifically, to the motion and spatial evolution of the dynamic pattern between and during successive imaging volume scans. In particular, the spatial resolution of a stack of 2-D images is dependent on several parameters. The spatial resolution of each image in the stack depends on the dimensions of the region of interest, the resolving power of the imager (pixel array size) and the imaging modality employed (see Chapters 5, 10 and 11). In addition, imaging any slice in the stack performs a "visual" integration over the thickness of the individual slice. It is therefore desirable to use the thinnest slices practicable. The spacing of the slices introduces another restriction on the spatial resolution along the axis normal to the slices.

The spatial and temporal resolution achieved by a 3-D scanning system, such as MRI, represents a compromise between competing factors. Reducing the number of slices without changing the spacing in order to speed up volume acquisition and improve time resolution, reduces the spatial extent of the volume. On the other hand, increasing the size of the volume by spacing the slices further apart—leaving unscanned volume between the slices—decreases the spatial resolution in the direction normal to the slice. Consequently, it will usually require the use of an interpolation scheme to "fill-in" the missing information. In a related vein, when scanning intracardiac flow fields directly (rather than the dynamic cardiac chamber geometry for determination of flow boundary conditions), the method of scanning is also important as it relates to convection of the flow during the imaging of each image plane. The retrace time also influences the time resolution as it represents a time delay between individual sweeps or between successive volume scans.

In order to match a 3-D imaging system to a given intracardiac flow, the temporal and spatial resolution requirements must be established. For example, for a system to resolve large-scale features of the flow, the field of view must encompass the largest length scale within the flow. The time between volumes must also be sufficiently smaller than the relevant flow time scale—e.g., filling-vortex formation time. In practice, the Nyquist criterion (see Section 2.17, on pp. 72 ff.) requires that the timestep be substantially less than half of the relevant flow time scale in order to acquire unambiguous observations.

12.8.2 Spatiotemporal accuracy constraints and the Courant condition

Physically important spatiotemporal scales of intracardiac pulsatile flow patterns can range over several orders of magnitude. Limitations in spatiotemporal accuracy in intracardiac flow-field simulations typically arise from restrictions in the corresponding resolutions of the imaging modalities used for deriving dynamic cardiac chamber geometries. As long as the relevant time scales can be resolved by the numerical method used, obtaining the desired simulation accuracy is not necessarily a limitation. Computing for more timesteps takes longer, but does not cause the problem to exceed the computer memory. Cost, however, can grow rapidly. In general, we seek numerical methods that maximize accuracy with a minimum number of grid points. When large spatial gradients are present, greater accuracy comes with finer resolution in both space and time. If we want to calculate the behavior of a small region in the flow with even moderate accuracy, we must have a minimum of *several* computational cells traversing it. If steep spatial gradients in a flow variable are present, more cells will normally be required. Because the computational cells have a finite size, there is uncertainty exactly where in the cell a smaller feature of the flow actually lies. This kind of uncertainty diminishes with improved spatial resolution.

Improvements in spatial resolution may actually complicate matters, because *the size of the computational cells imposes a computational constraint on the timestep* that is needed to maintain a stable and accurate solution. The reason that this is so can be readily appreciated intuitively: The timestep must be small enough so that the distinct components of the convective fluxes into and out of each cell do not *change* the properties of a cell appreciably during the timestep. Theoretical analysis has shown that, for a simulation to be stable, it must comply with the Courant—or Courant–Friedrichs–Lewy (CFL)—condition [7]:

$$\alpha \equiv \frac{v \cdot \Delta t}{\Delta x} \leq 1, \tag{12.1}$$

where, α signifies the Courant number and v an effective local fluid velocity magnitude. Obviously, the smaller the grid cell size and Δx, the smaller the timestep, Δt, needed in order to keep the simulation stable.

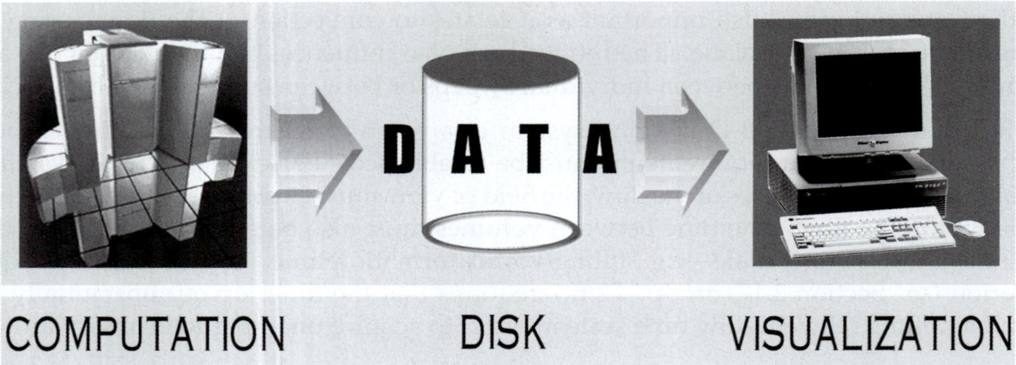

Figure 12.21: Postprocessing data visualization. After a computational run has been completed, the results are saved to disk, and visualization work can be performed on the dataset. In all but the simplest intraventricular CFD flow simulations the user does not have interactive control of the computation, because the calculations are so demanding that interactivity, in the sense of concurrent computation and visualization, is not a reasonable possibility, at present.

When the grid point separation is reduced to improve the accuracy of the simulation results, the upper limit for the timestep also decreases. Some reflection leads one to the understanding that the Courant condition on the timestep is set by the assumption that each grid-cell interacts only with its direct neighbors: the domain of influence of any individual cell should not reach cells beyond its immediate neighbors. After having defined a certain α and having determined the effective grid cell dimension Δx, we can decide on the Δt to use. It should be noted that this timestep denotes the maximum *internal timestep* that the CFD solver may take during the time integration and is not necessarily the same as the *external* timestep of the simulation.

The Courant constraint on the timestep is determined by the ratio of the mesh spacing and the magnitude of the velocity. In a variety of interesting situations, specifically in the simulation of intracardiac blood flows, the magnitude of v and the grid spacing can vary substantially throughout the computational domain. In these situations, where the grid spacing is nonuniform, *local* Courant time-stepping is feasible and can result in substantial savings in computation time. This saving in computational demands is very useful, as can be appreciated by considering that, e.g., in a 1-D calculation, doubling the spatial resolution usually requires a *fourfold* increase in computation to "integrate," or "advance" the solution over a given length of time—one factor of two comes from the additional "cells," while another factor of two is caused by the halved timestep required, by the Courant constraint, to integrate the equations using the smaller "cells." Similarly, doubling the resolution in two dimensions requires a factor of *eight* times as much work to advance the calculation the same physical time. In three dimensions, a factor of *sixteen* times as much work is required. Repeating this process one more time would increase the computational work, in three dimensions, by a factor of $(16 \times 16) = 256$ compared to the original grid size!

Obviously, geometries that are irreducibly 3-D, such as that of the right ventricular chamber, are a lot more demanding computationally than might be anticipated without knowledge of the Courant computational constraint. The maximum timestep is not fixed, but depends on the conditions on the grid, and it must, therefore, be recalculated every timestep. When the regional demands for higher resolution differ greatly within the flow field, adaptive gridding methods may be used to provide higher spatial resolution only *when and where* it is needed. The fundamental timestep is determined through the finest computational cells—those with the lowest volume/surface ratio in the entire grid. Implicit solution methods allow much larger Courant numbers than explicit methods (see Section 12.7 on p. 657), but they are not unconditionally stable, and using too large an α value can lead to loss of numerical accuracy.

12.9 Postprocessing and scientific visualization

Imagine trying to understand intraventricular velocities during diastolic filling from juxtaposed columns of numbers in reams and reams of computer printout. Visual images convey qualitative information about flow phenomena with greater understanding than lists of numbers. Therefore, postprocessing uses computer graphics to transform such columns of data into images, as is indicated in Figure 12.21, on p. 666. This imagery enables us to assimilate the enormous amount of data required in some scientific investigations. The size and complexity of the flow data obtained by CFD may otherwise make it difficult or impossible to understand the solution even at a single timestep. In addition, the data is generated at successive times during the period encompassed by the simulation and understanding how the data varies with time by direct inspection may be difficult, e.g., when investigating the evolution of intracardiac flow.

Postprocessing and visualization (see tabulation on next page) can help with these difficulties by representing the data so that we may view it in its entirety. It allows us to transform massive amounts of data into a variety of XY, 2- and 3-D spatial plots [65]. In the case of time varying data, we can create animations as well, showing the evolution of the flow in a natural way [38, 53]. Such techniques allow us to better understand our *spatiotemporal* 4-D data (see Section 12.9.1, which follows). For instance, viewing the data in this way can quickly draw attention to interesting or abnormal portions of the flow field.

Through the availability of increasingly powerful computers with growing amounts of internal and external memory, it is possible to investigate incredibly complex intracardiac flow phenomena by means of ever more realistic simulations. However, this brings with it vast amounts of simulated flow-field data. The ability to simulate different intracardiac flow fields on a computer is almost useless if the results cannot be "seen." To analyze these multi-dimensional, information-rich datasets, it is imperative to have software tools that can visualize them. Such visualization software is incorporated into high performance applications, so that the investigator can envision the phenomena that are being simulated. It is clear that visualization of intracardiac CFD data is invaluable, yet difficult.

Postprocessing and analysis

Postprocessing of the simulation results is carried out in order to extract the desired information from the computed flow field, and entails:

- Calculation of derived quantities (streamfunction, vorticity)
- Calculation of integral parameters (volumetric inflow, outflow)
- Visualization (representation of numbers as images)
  - 1D data: function values connected by straight-line segments
  - 2D data: streamlines, contour levels, color diagrams
  - 3D data: cutlines, cutplanes, isosurfaces, isovolumes
  - arrow plots, particle tracing, animations . . .
- Systematic data analysis by means of statistical tools
- Debugging, verification, and validation of the CFD model.

For complicated, time-dependent simulations, the running of the simulation may involve the calculation of many (*external*) timesteps, which requires a substantial amount of CPU time, and since memory resources are still relatively limited, one cannot save the results of every timestep. Hence, it is often necessary to visualize and store the results selectively in real time, so as not to have to recompute the dynamics to see the same scene again [41–43]. "Real time" means that the selected timestep is visualized as soon as its computation has been completed in the course of the simulation.

12.9.1 Scientific visualization

Scientific visualization[12] is a relatively new computer-based field concerned with techniques that allow graphical representations from the results of computations and *simulations* (cf. Fig. 12.21, on p. 666). Scientific visualization is a very effective tool both for interpreting image data and for generating images from complex, multidimensional datasets [5, 13]. It embraces both image understanding and image synthesis. The data generation step is not part of the scientific visualization process itself. Accordingly, its tools are also available for analysis of *experimental* and *clinical diagnostic imaging* data.

[12] There are, in principle, three levels of visualizing numerical simulation data: postprocessing, tracking, and steering. Whereas *postprocessing* refers to portraying the data after the numerical simulation is complete, *tracking* provides *real-time* displays, allowing termination of a faulty simulation. *Steering* actually permits *interaction* with the computation; simulation parameter values can be altered midstream and the computation continued. To date, most efforts in cardiological applications deal with techniques for effective postprocessing.

Experimental and clinical measurement datasets are also growing in size as new methods of collecting intracardiac flow data are becoming established, such as velocity encoded MRI. 3-D imaging techniques, such as 3-D magnetic resonance velocity mapping, or particle trace flow visualization using time-resolved 3-D phase-contrast MRI, can deliver quantitative visualization of intracardiac velocity fields. In fact, any imaging techniques that can be applied on an individual plane can he used to obtain volumetric information using multiple-slice aquisition.

Whether the flow-field data comes from simulations, diagnostic imaging or experiments, scientific visualization can be exploited to show the trends, the anomalies, and the physics in the data, to best advantage. Like good writing, good graphical displays of data communicate ideas with efficiency, clarity, and precision. Visualization generally starts with the retrieval of the dataset from a storing device such as a disc or digital tape. Its goal is to assist in developing a deeper understanding of the dataset under investigation, and to provide new insights relying on the human's powerful visual cognitive abilities. In the initial stages, the visualization process of a newly simulated flow field clearly benefits from the added value of an interactive postprocessing environment.

The flow dataset contains an abundance of detailed information [38]. Interaction is necessary for gaining new insight in the nature of a simulated flow because it is not *a priori* known which spatiotemporal aspects of the flow will turn out to be most interesting fluid dynamically, physiologically, or clinically—e.g., will actually exhibit abnormal flow features. Interactive scientific visualization is analogous to trying to comprehend an abstract sculpture in a museum. One tends to walk around the sculpture, viewing it from many different angles.

Scientific visualization entails the creation of visual images of things that we are unable to see, and ways to display at a glance qualitative and quantitative attributes of information-rich datasets. To achieve this, scientific visualization utilizes techniques from computer graphics encompassing image processing, signal processing, and user-interface methodology [13,35,37]. However, there is a fine but crucial distinction between graphics processing and visualization:

- Graphics generation is utilized to *display accurate*—and realistic—*images*, which can vary with the viewpoint of the observer, the illumination pattern, and the like.
- The object of scientific visualization is the *perception of data*, and it uses graphics methods and tools in order to display *information*.

Advances in scientific computation are allowing CFD simulations to become increasingly complex and to generate tremendously large amounts of data, and the amounts of information produced by such simulations can be understood only when transformed into a visual representation. Visualization attempts to convey all this information in an effective manner using graphical representations [51]. Computer-generated images combined with human perceptive vision are the foundations of scientific visualization.

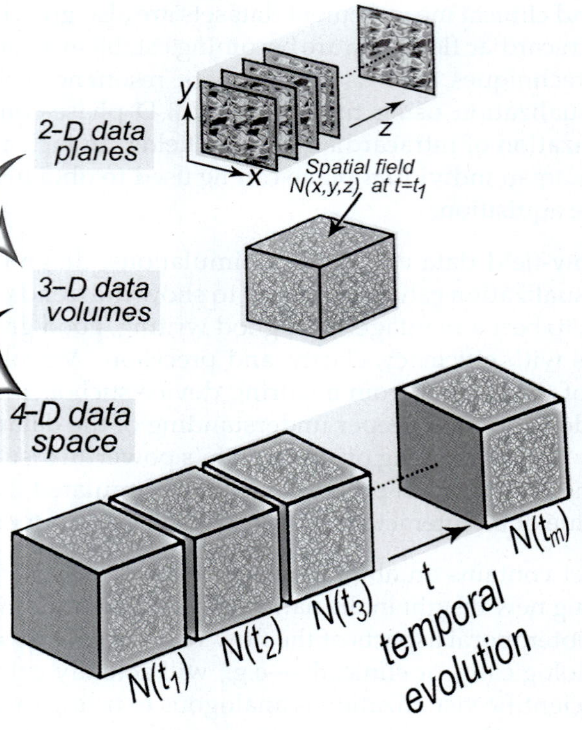

Figure 12.22: Structure of spatiotemporal 4-D data. The 3-D cube $N(x, y, z)$ is composed of a dense set of 2-D planar sections along the z-axis. Successive iterations of the process at times $t_1, t_2, t_3, \ldots, t_m$ make up the 4-D representation.

The process itself involves four steps:

1. **Data preparation:** Common operations that are applied in this stage are filtering, interpolation, and feature extraction and selection. The goal is to make the data suitable for the visualization technique, which we wish to apply. Often this means a reduction in the amount of data, for example by resampling the data at a lower resolution.

2. **Mapping:** In the mapping step numerical data is translated to graphics primitives. Even the most complex computer-generated graphic images are produced by a relatively small set of graphics primitives. The usual set of basic primitives is a single point, a line with given end-points, a polyline, i.e., a line joining a sequence of points, a filled polygonal area with given points as vertices, and text, including numbers. There may be additional, but not essential, primitives such as rectangles, circles, curves of various types, images, etc.

   Associated with each graphics primitive is a set of attributes. The attributes of a primitive determine its appearance on the output device. For example, a line commonly has attributes such as color, width, and style (full, dotted, dashed, etc.). There are many ways to map numerical information to attributes of graphical primitives. Often used techniques are volume rendering, i.e., a direct display of a sampled 3-D scalar field without first fitting geometric primitives to the samples, plots of isosurfaces and streamlines, and arrowhead vector plots. The choice of mapping depends on the type of data visualized, the available display algorithms, and personal preferences.

3. **Rendering:** In the rendering stage, the geometric primitives are traversed and an image is generated. An image is a 2-D raster of pixels each of which has a certain color or intensity value. Often the mapping assumes a 3-D space which is projected onto a plane, the "viewing plane," using a viewpoint and lighting conditions as input. Workstations equipped with special-purpose hardware allow rendering of complex images in only a fraction of a second.

4. **Display and communication:** The rendered image has to be presented on some display device; this is done in the display step. The most common device used for this purpose is a raster display (a CRT, LCD, or plasma display). Other media such as video may be used for presentation purposes. Devices such as printers or plotters can produce hard copy of the visualization. Image data need a large amount of storage and communication capacity; thus, image compression is essential for storage and communication of images.

At the present time, cardiac flow imaging in general is entering an era of "data wealth." The development of computer-aided modern imaging modalities and visualization technologies allows the transformation of wide ranges of intracardiac flow phenomena that vastly exceed all human perceptual capacities and their translation into visual forms. For example, now we are able to measure and cast in graphic form intracardiac velocity fields using noninvasive imaging modalities such as Doppler echocardiography and velocity encoded cardiac MRI. This capability will only *increase* in the future. Consequently, we are led to think of an intracardiac flow field as being given by an extensive digital data file, which might be either the output of a numerical CFD simulation [15,21,22,41–44], or the result of a noninvasive clinical, or experimental, measurement [39,49,64].

The visual representation of such data must clarify mutual relations, time dependencies, location and scale of interesting phenomena. Scientific visualization can compress a lot of data into one picture (data browsing), it can reveal correlations between flow-field variables in space and time, it can furnish new space-like structures beside the ones already known, and it opens up the possibility to view the data selectively and interactively in real time. By following the evolution in time—formation and dissipation—as well as the movements of intracardiac flow patterns, such as the diastolic intraventricular vortices, we gain deeper *insight* into their complicated dynamics. Such understanding can lead to better appreciation of pathophysiologic mechanisms, and to improved, more sensitive and less invasive diagnostic signs and indices.

It is during the postprocessing portion of the analysis, that we examine the results of the CFD simulation using scientific visualization. The postprocessing components

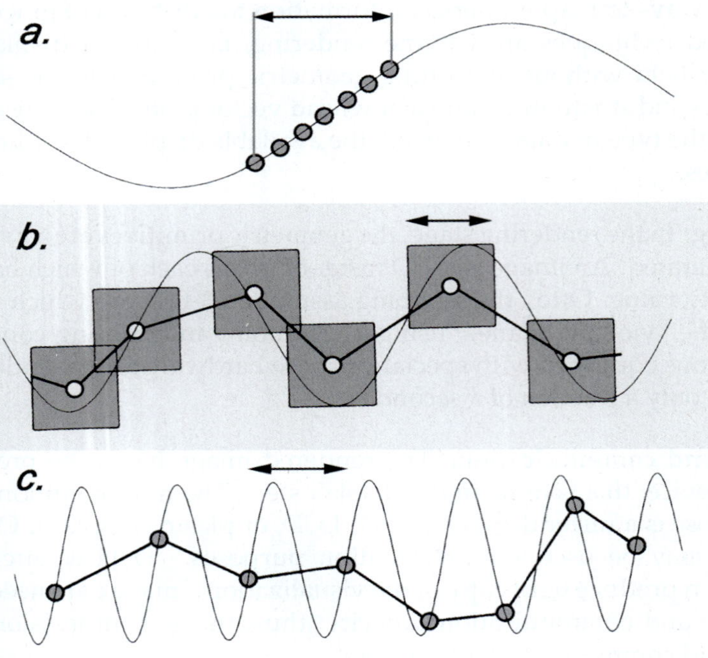

Figure 12.23: The effect of measurement scale properties on recovering the true underlying spatiotemporal pattern in measured data. The circles are the measurements and the thin line is the "true" underlying pattern. The squares quantify spatiotemporal resolution limits (see discussion in text).

of integrated CFD software packages can work on data in the form of a series of five-dimensional rectangles. That is, the data are real numbers at each point of a "grid" which spans three space dimensions, one time dimension, and one additional dimension for enumerating each of the individual flow-field variables (cf. Fig. 12.22, on p. 670). They have the capability of presenting the desired calculated quantities, such as intraventricular pressure and velocity, using relatively simple interactive commands and menus. Velocity field visualizations may involve velocity vector plots. Contour plots of the intraventricular pressure or velocity are also valuable.

Phenomena in intracardiac flow fields are characterized by flow patterns of widely varying spatial and temporal scales. In state of the art simulations, flow feature sizes may vary by one or more orders of magnitude. Visualization methods should be able to cope with these different levels of scale. This is much more satisfactorily accomplished by scientific visualization of CFD simulation data than of direct imaging modality measurements, which may have difficulties arising out of the three kinds of potential pitfalls that are exemplified in the three panels of Figure 12.23:

a. the data sample *window* may be be too narrow (in space or time) to capture the underlying true spatiotemporal pattern;

b. the spatiotemporal *resolution* may be too coarse to capture the fine details in the underlying spatiotemporal pattern;

c. the *sampling rate* may be too low, with overly long time or spatial intervals between successive samples to capture small-scale patterns, or high spatiotemporal frequency components, in the patterns.

In addition to the directly calculated dependent variables, derived quantities such as blood speed can be calculated and presented in terms of contour plots or profiles. There is also the capability of choosing arbitrary lines or planes or "cuts" in the flow field and plotting profiles or contours of any variable along these lines or planes. Hard copy printouts of the values of all flow variables at each point in the flow-field grid at any time are readily obtainable.

Images are powerful and can present a lot of data at the same time, but this is not necessarily what the clinician or the basic scientist are looking for. Visualization is an aid to *extract information* from data. It is a tool to look at data. Just like a microscope reveals things which are too small to be perceived with the unaided eye, visualization offers a view into the world of *numerical data*. This is achieved by mapping the data to visual parameters, such as shape, color and texture. However, a scientific visualization tool is just that, a tool. It is the trained investigator who must direct the orchestra of visualization methods and who must perform adjustments needed to discern interesting flow patterns. To get a useful visual representation, different settings and approaches must be tried, which requires informed interaction. More importantly, it is the trained *pluridisciplinary* investigator who can truly evaluate and fully appreciate the visual information with the critical hermeneutic vision of the expert. To the trained investigator, the various visualization techniques are useful for far more than just viewing a computed or directly imaged flow field.

With the great strides in imaging and CFD, it is becoming imperative to exploit the eye-brain system's great skill at distinguishing structure in a complicated medium like flowing intracardiac blood. Therefore we need to make noninvasive imaging, as well as CFD computer-output, visualizable and we need to quantify what we see, so that we are not mere passive onlookers but active collaborators with the computer. Scientific visualization can help with understanding the evolution of intracardiac flow-field phenomena and their interactions with cellular and organ physiology and pathology. In the final analysis, inspection of the computed field of a CFD simulation provides detailed insights into flow patterns and flow-field structure (cf. Sections 1.10 and 14.15, on pp. 23 ff. and 791 ff., respectively) in the same sense as a high-resolution imaging experiment. In this respect and others, CFD complemented by scientific visualization is *more akin to experiment* than to theory.

In the ensuing Chapters, I will present and validate results from the new paradigm of Functional Imaging, or *simulation-based intracardiac fluid dynamics*, which, by directly solving the flow field governing equations through computer simulation based on patient-specific cardiac imaging datasets, can digitize and visualize intracardiac blood flow patterns during ejection and filling, under normal and pathological conditions. We will see that this new paradigm can provide detailed information on physical variables such as intraventricular velocity and pressure distributions at macro- and "microscopic" levels of spatiotemporal resolution, and also on wall shear stress and mass transport phenomena that are important but cannot be measured directly by using imaging alone. Hence, it can give a more detailed, thorough, and multifaceted overall understanding of the interrelated *intracardiac blood flow phenomena* that are involved in ejection and filling. A baseline for this paradigm is an integrated computational system, involving a cardiac imaging component with a morphological modeling subsystem, a kinematic modeling subsystem, a CFD modeling subsystem, and a postprocessing subsystem for scientific visualization.

References and further reading

[1] Abbott, M.B., Basco, D.R. Computational fluid dynamics: an introduction for engineers. 1989, Harlow, Essex, England; New York: Longman Scientific & Technical; Wiley. xiv, 425 p.

[2] Anderson, J.D., Computational fluid dynamics: the basics with applications. 1994, New York: McGraw-Hill. xxiv, 547 p.

[3] Blazek, J., Computational fluid dynamics: principles and applications. 1st ed. 2001, Amsterdam; New York: Elsevier. xx, 440 p.

[4] Canny, J. A computational approach to edge detection. IEEE Trans. Pattern Anal. Machine Intell. 8: 679–98, 1986.

[5] Card, S.K., Mackinlay, J.D., Shneiderman, B. Readings in information visualization: using vision to think. 1st ed. 1999, San Francisco, CA: Morgan Kaufmann Publishers. xvii, 686 p.

[6] Cerqueira, M., Weissman, N., Dilsizian, V., Jacobs, A., Kaul, S., Laskey, W., Pennell, D., Rumberger, J., Ryan, T., Verina, M. Standardized myocardial segmentation and nomenclature for tomographic imaging of the heart. Circulation 105: 539–42, 2002.

[7] Courant, R., Friedrichs, K., Lewy, H. Über die partiellen Differenzengleichungen der mathematischen Physik. Mathematische Annalen 100: 32–74, 1928.

[8] Dale, N.B., Lewis, J. Computer science illuminated. 2002, Boston: Jones & Bartlett Publishers. xxvii, 656 p.

[9] Date, A.W. Introduction to computational fluid dynamics. 2005, New York: Cambridge University Press. xx, 377 p.

[10] Devlin, K.J., The millennium problems: the seven greatest unsolved mathematical puzzles of our time. 2002, New York: Basic Books. x, 237 p.

[11] Doyle, M.G., Vergniaud, J.-B., Tavoularis, S., Bourgault, Y. Numerical simulations of blood flow in artificial and natural hearts with fluid–structure interaction. Artif. Organs 32: 870–9, 2008.

[12] Drikakis, D., Rider, W. High-resolution methods for incompressible and low-speed flows. 2005, Berlin; New York: Springer-Verlag. xx, 622 p.

[13] Earnshaw, R.A., Wiseman, N. An introductory guide to scientific visualization. 1992, Berlin; New York: Springer-Verlag. xvi, 156 p.

[14] Fletcher, C.A.J., Srinivas, K. Computational techniques for fluid dynamics. 2nd ed. Springer series in computational physics. 1991, Berlin; New York: Springer-Verlag.

[15] Georgiadis, J.G., Wang, M., Pasipoularides, A. Computational fluid dynamics of left ventricular ejection. Ann. Biomed. Eng. 20: 81–97, 1992.

[16] Gonzalez, R.C., Woods, R.E. Digital image processing. 3rd ed. 2008, Upper Saddle River, N.J.: Prentice Hall. xxii, 954 p.

[17] Gresho, P.M., Sani, R.L., Engelman, M.S. Incompressible flow and the finite element method. 2000, Chichester [England]; New York: Wiley. 2 vols.

[18] Gunzburger, M.D., Nicolaides, R.A. [Eds.] Incompressible computational fluid dynamics: trends and advances. 1993, Cambridge; New York, UK: Cambridge University Press. xiii, 481 p.

[19] Gustafson, K.E., Abe, T., Kuwahara, K. Lectures on computational fluid dynamics, mathematical physics, and linear algebra. Singapore; River Edge, NJ: World Scientific, 1997.

[20] Hamming, R.W., Numerical methods for scientists and engineers. International series in pure and applied mathematics. 1962, New York: McGraw-Hill. 411 p.

[21] Hampton, T., Shim, Y., Straley, C., Pasipoularides, A. Finite element analysis of cardiac ejection dynamics: Ultrasonic implications. Am. Soc. Mechan. Engin., Bioengineering Division–BED, v 22, 1992 Advances in Bioengineering, 1992, pp. 371–4.

[22] Hampton, T., Shim, Y., Straley, C., Uppal, R., Smith, P.K., Glower, D., Pasipoularides, A. Computational fluid dynamics of ventricular ejection on the CRAY Y-MP. IEEE Proc. Comp. Cardiol. 19: 295–8, 1992.

[23] Hoffmann, K.A., Chiang, S.T. Computational fluid dynamics for engineers. 4th ed. 2000, Wichita, Kan: Engineering Education System. v2.

[24] Hooper, A., Makers of mathematics. 1948, New York: Random House. ix, 402 p.

[25] Huang, W., Ren, Y., Russell, R.D. Moving mesh methods based on moving mesh partial differential equations. J. Comput. Phys. 113: 279–90, 1994.

[26] Huang, X., Paragios, N., Metaxas, D. Establishing local correspondences towards compact representations of anatomical structures. Medical Image Computing and Computer-Assisted Intervention (MICCAI'03), Montreal, Canada, November, 2003. Lecture Notes in Computer Science 2879: pp. 926–34, Springer, 2003.

[27] Jones, T.N., Metaxas, D.N. Segmentation using deformable models with affinity-based localization. In: J. Troccaz, E. Grimson, R. Mosges [Eds.] Lecture Notes in Computer Science, Volume 1205: CVRMED '97, pp. 53–62. Springer, 1997.

[28] Kass, M., Witkin, A., Terzopoulos, D. Snakes: active contour models. Int. J. Comp. Vision 1: 321–31, 1988.

[29] Löhner, R. Applied computational fluid dynamics techniques: an introduction based on finite element methods. Chichester; New York: Wiley. x, 366 p.

[30] Lomax, H., Pulliam, T.H., Zingg, D.W. Fundamentals of computational fluid dynamics. 2001, Berlin; New York: Springer. xiv, 249 p.

[31] Marr, D.C., Hildreth, E.C. Theory of Edge Detection. Proc. Roy. Soc. Lond. Ser. B, 207: 187–217, 1980.

[32] Mavriplis, D.J. Multigrid solution of the 2-D Euler equations on unstructured triangular meshes. AIAA J. 26: 824–31, 1988.

[33] Mavriplis, D.J. Unstructured Grid Techniques. Ann. Rev. Fluid Mech. 29: 473–514, 1997.

[34] McInerney, T., Terzopoulos, D. Deformable models in medical image analysis: a survey. Med. Image Anal. 1: 91–108, 1996.

[35] Merzkirch, W., Flow visualization. 2nd ed. 1987, Orlando, FL: Academic Press. x, 260 p.

[36] Metaxas, D.N. Physics-based deformable models : applications to computer vision, graphics, and medical imaging (SECS 389). 1997, Boston, MA: Kluwer Academic Publishers. xiii, 308 p.

[37] Nakayama, Y., Nihon Kikai Gakkai. Visualized flow: fluid motion in basic and engineering situations revealed by flow visualization. 1st English ed. 1988, Oxford, UK; New York: Pergamon. xxiii, 137 p.

[38] Nieuwstadt, F.T.M., Flow visualization and image analysis. Fluid mechanics and its applications; v. 14. 1993, Dordrecht; Boston, MA: Kluwer Academic Publishers. vii, 271 p.

[39] Paelinck, B.P., Lamb, H.J., Bax, J.J., Van der Wall, E.E., de Roos, A. Assessment of diastolic function by cardiovascular magnetic resonance. Am. Heart J. 144: 198–205, 2002.

[40] Paragios, N. A variational approach for the segmentation of the left ventricle in cardiac image analysis. Int. J. Comp. Vision 50: 345–62, 2002.

[41] Pasipoularides, A.D., Shu, M., Womack, M.S., Shah, A., von Ramm, O., Glower, D.D. RV functional imaging: 3-D echo-derived dynamic geometry and flow field simulations. Am. J. Physiol. Heart Circ. Physiol. 284: H56–65, 2003.

[42] Pasipoularides, A.D., Shu, M., Shah, A., Womack, M.S., Glower, D.D. Diastolic right ventricular filling vortex in normal and volume overload states. Am. J. Physiol. Heart Circ. Physiol. 284: H1064–72, 2003.

[43] Pasipoularides, A., Shu, M., Shah, A., Tucconi, A., Glower, D.D. RV instantaneous intraventricular diastolic pressure and velocity distributions in normal and volume overload awake dog disease models. Am. J. Physiol. Heart Circ. Physiol. 285: H1956–65, 2003.

[44] Peskin, C.S. The fluid dynamics of heart valves: experimental, theoretical, and computational methods. Ann. Rev. Fluid Mech. 14: 235–59, 1982.

[45] Pozrikidis, C., Introduction to theoretical and computational fluid dynamics. 1997, New York: Oxford University Press. x, 675 p.

[46] Preparata, F.R., Shamos, M.I. Computational geometry: an introduction. New York: Springer-Verlag, 1985. xii, 390 p.

[47] Quartapelle, L., Numerical solution of the incompressible Navier–Stokes equations. 1993, Basel; Boston: Birkhèauser Verlag. xii, 291 p.

[48] Reilly, E.D. Concise encyclopedia of computer science. 2004, Chichester; Hoboken, NJ: J. Wiley. xxvi, 875 p.

[49] Reiser, M.F., Takahashi, M., Modic, M., Becker, C.R. [Eds.] Multislice CT. 2nd edn. 2004, Berlin; Heidelberg; New York: Springer-Verlag. x, 280 p.

[50] Roache, P.J. Fundamentals of computational fluid dynamics. 1998, Albuquerque, NM: Hermosa Publishers. xviii, 648 p.

[51] Samimy, M., Breuer, K.S.,. Leal, L.G, Steen, P.H. A gallery of fluid motion. 2003, Cambridge, UK; New York: Cambridge University Press. x, 118 p.

[52] Shyy, W., Udaykumar, H.S., Rao, M.M., Smith, R.W. Computational fluid dynamics with moving boundaries. 1996, Washington, D.C.: Taylor & Francis. xvii, 285 p.

[53] Smits, A.J., Lim, T.T. Flow visualization: techniques and examples. 2000, Singapore; River Edge, NJ: Imperial College Press. xii, 396.

[54] Staniforth, A. Review: Formulating efficient finite-element codes for flows in regular domains. Int. J. Num. Meth. Fluids. 7: 1–16, 1987.

[55] Stetten, G.D., Pizer, S.M. Medial-node models to identify and measure objects in real-time 3-D echocardiography. IEEE Trans. Med. Imag. 18: 1025–34, 1999.

[56] Stetten, G., Pizer, S.M. Automated identification and measurement of objects via populations of medial primitives, with application to real time 3D echocardiography. Information Processing in Medical Imaging (IPMI '99), Lecture Notes in Computer Science, Springer-Verlag 1613: pp. 84–97, 1999.

[57] Taron, M., Paragios, N., Jolly, M.-P. Border detection on short axis echocardiographic views using an ellipse driven region-based framework. Medical Image Computing and Computer Assisted Intervention (MICCAI'04), Saint-Malo, France, September, 2004. Lecture Notes in Computer Science 3216: pp. 443–50, Springer, 2004.

[58] Turkel, E. Review of preconditioning methods for fluid dynamics. Appl. Numer. Math. 12: 257–84, 1993.

[59] Visualization Society of Japan., Fantasy of flow: the world of fluid flow captured in photographs. 1993, Tokyo, Amsterdam; Washington: Ohmsha; IOS Press. 184 p.

[60] Warsi, Z.U.A. Fluid dynamics: theoretical and computational approaches. 2006, Boca Raton, FL: CRC Press/Taylor & Francis. 845 p.

[61] Wendt, J.F., Anderson, J.D., and von Karman Institute for Fluid Dynamics. Computational fluid dynamics: an introduction. 2nd ed. 1995, Berlin; New York: Springer. xii, 301 p.

[62] Wilkes, J.O. Fluid mechanics for chemical engineers with Microfluidics and CFD. 2006, Upper Saddle River, NJ: Prentice Hall Professional Technical Reference. xvii, 755 p.

[63] Wrobel, L. C., Sarler, B., Brebbia, C. A. [Eds.] Computational modelling of free and moving boundary problems III. 1995, Southampton; Boston, MA: Computational Mechanics Publications. 379 p.

[64] Yacoub, M.H., Cohn, L.H. Novel approaches to cardiac valve repair. From structure to function: Part I. Circulation 109: 942–50, 2004.

[65] Yang, W.-J., Computer-assisted flow visualization: second generation technology. 1994, Boca Raton, FL: CRC Press. vi, 342 p.

[66] Yang, J., Duncan, J.S. 3D image segmentation of deformable objects with joint shape-intensity prior models using level sets. Med. Image Anal. 8: 285–94, 2004.

[67] Zerroukat, M., Chatwin, C.R. Computational moving boundary problems. 1994, Taunton, Somerset, England; New York: Research Studies Press; Wiley. x, 212 p.

Chapter 13

CFD of Ventricular Ejection

All truths are easy to understand once they are discovered; the point is to discover them.

——Galileo Galilei (1564–1642)

Now with the advent of large computers, sophisticated graphical algorithms and interactive terminals, we can undertake large-scale numerical simulations of these systems and probe those regions of parameter space that are not easily accessible to the theorist/analyst or experimentalist. ... This is a new approach to understanding ... through formulating, exercising, comparing results and then improving mathematical models that we believe describe the real world.

——Norman Zabusky, 1973 [77].

VENTRICULAR SYSTOLIC EJECTION is a highly unsteady flow process in a chamber with complex geometry whose walls are compressed forcibly together by myocardial contraction. The present chapter is aimed at providing a conceptual framework for understanding ventricular ejection dynamics under normal and abnormal operating conditions, and with and without outflow obstruction. The ejection process involves negative feedback (see Section 2.23, on pp. 105 ff.) from hemodynamic loads opposing ventricular and myocardial shortening, which are discussed in Section 7.9, on pp. 369 ff. Admittedly, the complexity of the fluid dynamic and control problems encompassed by ejection creates serious analytic and computational difficulties.

Contemporary high-fidelity instantaneous measurements of rapidly varying pressures and flows, angiocardiographic, and noninvasive intracardiac flow visualization methods [4–6, 21, 26, 29, 36, 37, 39–43, 60, 63, 64, 72] offer investigators and clinicians the opportunity to assess ventricular function in a quantitative dynamic fashion. This allows subtle performance abnormalities to be identified or elicited *before* the usual clinical manifestations of overt cardiac muscle or pump failure. A more complete theoretic understanding is now necessary in order to fulfill the promise of this new era of advanced diagnostic capabilities. Indeed, the increasingly accurate, refined and exhaustive diagnostic measurements available in modern clinical practice incorporate intricate 3-D details of unsteady hemodynamic phenomena. Proper interpretation of the measurements rests on an understanding of such phenomena.

CFD simulations (see Fig. 13.1) can contribute knowledge and powerful insights to aid such interpretation. While clinical measurements and laboratory experiments are indispensable, CFD is currently finding increased acceptance as an intracardiac flow-field study tool. Another productive application of CFD simulations pertains to the development of artificial organs and devices such as artificial hearts, ventricular assist devices (VADs), vascular stents, and heart valves. Accurate quantification of blood flow patterns and fluid dynamics plays a crucial role in developing such devices. Thus, CFD simulation of blood flow in and over such devices has become a very important part of the design process. One pertinent example is the CFD-supported design of the DeBakey VAD, where

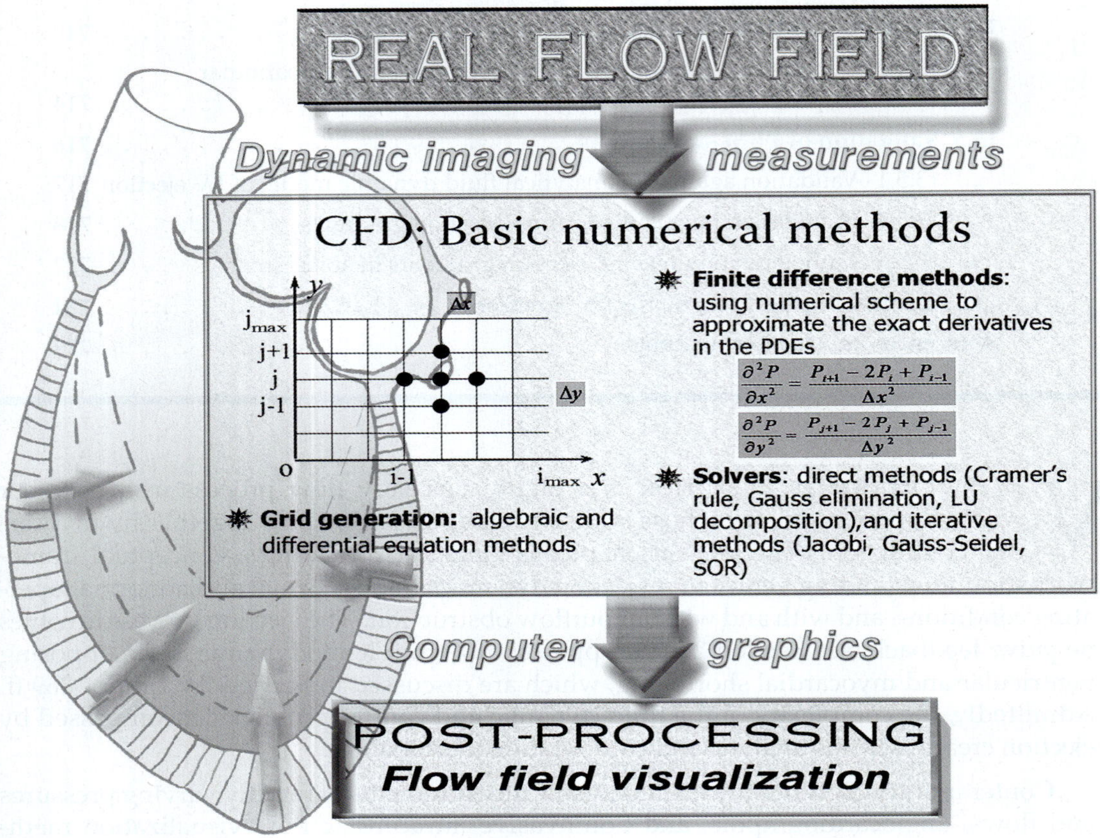

Figure 13.1: In modeling a real flow, CFD works by dividing the flow region of interest, into a large number of cells or volume elements, the *mesh* or *grid*. In each of the cells of the grid, the partial differential equations describing the fluid flow appear as nonlinear algebraic equations that relate flow-field variables, e.g., pressure, velocity, vorticity) to the values in the neighboring cells. Solution of the discretized flow-field equations proceeds on the grid by a selected numerical scheme, with suitable implementation specifications. This is followed by visualization, analysis, and interpretation of the CFD flow simulation results. (The CFD approach is considered in detail in Chapter 12.)

CFD-aided design *improvements* enabled human implantation by minimizing thrombus formation and lowering hemolysis to an acceptable level [27].

Numerical simulation is very important, for it is able to give the full picture of the flow field quantitatively, especially for complicated heart chamber geometries under pumping, pulsatile flow, conditions. In the past, most of the works done were 2-D, and were consequently misleading at times, mainly as a result of inadvertently underestimating by a great amount the magnitude of the applying convective acceleration effects. This generally unappreciated but critically important point of the much more pronounced convective acceleration effects under the actually applying 3-D flow circumstances, relative to 2-D oversimplified (and *inappropriate*) planar flow models, is discussed in Section 4.4.4, on pp. 179 ff., and is depicted pictorially in Figure 4.5, on p. 180. However, with cheaper and extremely powerful computers becoming available, 3-D simulations have been rendered feasible, and no plausible reason for any continued use of oversimplified planar (2-D rather than 3-D) flow models remains.

Today, exciting discoveries await clinical and basic investigators who can combine the new diagnostic technologies with a better grasp of the unsteady fluid dynamics of ventricular ejection. Because the measurements often entail expensive, tedious and sometimes hazardous diagnostic procedures, it is important to glean every useful insight from them. A case in point: the stationary flow model of the Gorlin formula and the theoretic understanding it calls for were well matched to the technology of the mid 1950s and the subsequent two or three decades (fluid-filled catheter-transducer systems, Fick or thermodilution cardiac output). They are grossly outmatched by the information content of the sophisticated diagnostic instrumentation of the past two decades, including the multisensor micromanometric/velocimetric catheter and Doppler or MRI velocimetry (see Sections 5.9 and 10.3, on pp. 280 ff. and 531 ff., respectively). Over that time span, observations derived using this instrumentation has allowed the formulation of a new integrative framework pertaining to ventricular function under normal and abnormal conditions.

Within this integrative framework there are innovative, clinically important, ideas. Several of these have been already introduced in Chapter 7, in discussing the cardiac cycle and the central pressure, flow and volume pulses. These new ideas include the concept of *complementarity and competitiveness* of the *intrinsic* and *extrinsic* components of the total ventricular systolic ejection load [36–38]; the concept of the diastolic *convective deceleration load* [38,46,47], which corresponds to the intrinsic component of the systolic ejection load and is an important determinant of diastolic inflow during the upstroke of the E-wave; and the correlate concepts of systolic [36–38] and diastolic [38,45–47] *ventriculoannular disproportion*. Their conception and formulation was predicated on the development of advanced catheterization instrumentation, and of analytical and computational methods for the detailed investigation of the unsteady pressure and velocity distributions within the ventricular flow fields during ejection and filling, in health and disease.

It may be instructive in this context to note that, as I emphasized in a survey published in the Journal of the American College of Cardiology in 1990 [36], dynamic intraventricular regional ejection pressure differences were, to my knowledge, first looked for, recorded in canine preparations and published by the pioneering Swiss hemodynamicists Laszt and Müller [28] in 1951! Important strides in understanding intracardiac fluid dynamics responsible for such intracardiac pressure gradients and other fascinating phenomena have been accomplished since then, and more recently by using CFD methodology.

In recent years, a confluence of conditions, including mathematical advances, progress in imaging and hemodynamic high-technology instrumentation and powerful computing capabilities, is leading to rapid progress in this field. In fact, we may now be seeing early signs (straws in the wind) that a new kind of quantitative cardiac fluid dynamics, not merely a more quantitative phase, is starting to impact academic cardiology [35]. Accordingly, we begin this chapter with a brief historical overview of these developments.

13.1 Brief historic survey of CFD approaches to intracardiac flow

There are two main methods that have been developed for the study of intracardiac blood flow problems by CFD: the Immersed Boundary method, and the Predetermined Boundary Motion method. Both methods require application of high performance computer hardware and software, and the Predetermined Boundary Motion method reqires, in addition, high spatiotemporal resolution cardiac digital imaging data from individual patients or experimental animals.

13.1.1 Immersed boundary method

The *Immersed Boundary (IB) method* was developed in the 1970s by Peskin and McQueen [30, 50, 51] to study flow patterns around heart valves, and in a highly schematized 2-D model of a canine heart. It is based on the viewpoint that heart tissues are effectively incompressible and exhibit an essentially uniform mass density; therefore, the flow-field equations for an incompressible fluid, suitably modified, can be applied to the four-chambered heart and great vessels. Then, the ensuing simulation can provide the coupled fluid-structure interactions of blood, wall and valve leaflet motions as functions of space and time.

The earlier Peskin models represent a 2-D section through a long axis plane of the heart, and portray blood flow in the heart and the movement of the atrial and ventricular boundaries and the flexible valve leaflets throughout a cardiac cycle. Atrial inflows and ventricular outflows are modeled by sources and sinks (cf. Fig. 13.2, on p. 688). In this context, a "source" is a mathematical point or region that produces fluid; a "sink" is a mathematical point or region at which fluid magically vanishes. At the aortic sink it is assumed that blood leaving the heart takes its momentum with it. At the atrial source it is assumed that blood enters the heart with no velocity, and thus with no momentum, and that the fluid is incompressible and homogeneous.

The IB model represents the tissues of the heart, such as active muscle or passive valve leaflets, as neutrally buoyant, infinitely thin, elastic boundaries that are totally immersed in blood (i.e., with blood on *both* sides). These boundaries exert force on the fluid and are themselves moved by it with the local fluid velocity. The beating of the model heart is induced by alternating contractions and relaxations of the elastic boundaries that represent cardiac muscles; these contractile actions are prescribed by simplified activation functions. It is these preselected activation functions which determine the time-course of contraction and relaxation of cardiac muscle. A 3-D model that uses the IB method to simulate blood flow in the left ventricle during part of systole was developed by Yoganathan et al. [74], who also presented some comparisons to experimental findings. This model was subsequently applied to a study of the systolic anterior mitral valve motion syndrome [75].

The Immersed Boundary method is special in the way it models the interaction between fluid flow and the tissues of the heart. Recently, Adeler and Jacobsen presented a 2-D IB model of blood flow in the human heart [1,22], obtained by modifying Peskin's model. Peskin's heart model has a simple outflow condition at the aorta and can float freely in the surrounding domain, conditions that distort the intracardiac flow patterns and render the model unsuitable for comparison with MRI measurements. The modifications that Adeler and Jacobsen made reflected common physiologic knowledge and human heart MRI measurements. They compared the modified model with human heart MRI measurements. Intraventricular flow patterns from their simulations and the MRI data showed a fair agreement. The flow pattern displayed the phases of the heart cycle, including aortic ejection phase outflow, and mitral early ($E-$) and late ($A-$) inflow waves. The axial velocity distributions over the mitral and aortic ring diameters from simulation and MRI measurements matched reasonably well, but the shape and peak values of both the ejection and the inflow velocity *vs.* time curves showed some discrepancies. The duration of ventricular systole, myocardial excitation and relaxation parameters, and muscle properties were adjustable IB model parameters of particular significance.

In my view, the approach of Adeler and Jacobsen is interesting and may render broader physiological relevance and clinical value to the IB method, in elucidating the influence of normal and abnormal *myocardial* properties and function on cardiac blood flow patterns. This will be all the more likely using a fully 3-D heart model, with more realistic geometric aspects. Nevertheless, the IB method, does not render itself to realistic, patient-specific simulations of clinically relevant intracardiac fluid dynamics problems.

13.1.2 Predetermined boundary motion method

To address such clinical and physiological issues, my coworkers and I developed, in the early 1990s, an alternative CFD approach to the study of intraventricular fluid dynamics during systolic ejection [17–19,36,37]. Adeler and Jacobsen have designated [1] our approach as the method of *Predetermined Boundary Motion, (PBM)*; in our PBM method, the movement of the endocardial chamber boundary is determined independently of the flow, which is *generated by* and *depends on* it. Only the resulting flow field of the intraventricular blood must be computed, by incorporating the uncoupled wall motion into the CFD. Using normal and pathologic velocimetric ejection patterns and reconstructed dynamic 3-D LV configurations obtained from angiocardiographic studies at catheterization, we simulated intraventricular flow fields and calculated representative normal and abnormal intraventricular ejection gradients.

These gradients were compared retrospectively with the corresponding gradients determined with multisensor (micromanometric and velocimetric) Millar catheters (see Section 5.2 on pp. 243 ff.) during our previously published left-heart *catheterization studies*

[4,20,21,36,37,39–43,63]. An assortment of left ventricular contracting ellipsoid geometries were simulated [17–19,36,37], conforming to angiocardiographic and echocardiographic determinations on patients with normal left ventricles, as well as with differing degrees of outflow orifice stenosis, chamber enlargement and *systolic ventriculoannular disproportion* [17,36,37], and with varying chamber eccentricities.

Following these clinically motivated, pioneering cardiac CFD studies of the ejection phase, we augmented the PBM method. We adapted it to utilize prospectively obtained combined real-time 3-D echocardiographic and sonomicrometric dynamic cardiac geometric data; these were applied as boundary conditions to a powerful Navier–Stokes based CFD solver,[1] in a finite element simulation model of right intraventricular flow during diastolic filling. We then examined (see Chapter 14) clinically important aspects of intracardiac fluid dynamics in conscious dogs, under normal and abnormal volume overload states, induced in surgical, chronic animal models of heart disease [45–47].[2]

Taylor and Yamaguchi [66,67] applied a variant of our PBM method, with an assumed realistic time-course for the movement of the wall, to a 3-D geometric model of a dog's left ventricle, conforming to a cast taken in the diastolic configuration, to evaluate intraventricular ejection fluid dynamics. Similarly, Ding and Schoephoerster [12] used cineangiograms to construct a 3-D model of the left ventricle during ejection, assuming circular short-axis cross-sections. Metaxas and his collaborators [23,34] applied the PBM method utilizing tagged MRI (MRI-SPAMM) data[3] as boundary conditions to a Navier–Stokes based solver in their CFD model of the left ventricle. Similarly, Saber et al. [62] obtained anatomical data by MRI scanning to construct a moving mesh model of the left ventricle, from time-resolved anatomical slices of the ventricular geometry. They simulated left ventricular blood flow during systolic ejection and early diastolic filling.

Redaelli and his collaborators [13,58] applied a variant of the PBM method to an axisymmetric model of the left ventricle in which the Navier–Stokes equations were solved by using a finite element CFD approach, similar to that of Hampton et al. [18,19]. To account for the inner surface movement of the LV chamber during the ejection phase, they assigned displacements and velocities to each moving boundary node through predetermined time functions. Redaelli et al.'s simulations showed the intraventricular ejection pressure gradient to be more sensitive to changes in *ventricular contractility* than the commonly used first time derivative of ventricular pressure [59], and indicated that the ventricular recoil during ejection affects the noninvasive estimation of the transvalvular pressure gradient using Doppler ultrasound [57]. Oertel and his coworkers [24,32,33] have developed an analogous heart model simulating flow in the left human ventricle and aorta, in which the flow calculation is performed with a finite volume method using MRI measurements.

---

[1] A "solver" is a computer program that performs the main body of CFD computations and produces numerical results. The results comprise long lists of numbers that represent computed flow-field variables, such as velocity, pressure, etc.

[2] These diastolic studies are presented in the next chapter.

[3] MRI-SPAMM allows tracking of material points on the heart, and provides an accurate representation of the left ventricular wall motion from end-diastole to end-diastole.

Most recently, Peng et al. [49] developed an ejection dynamics CFD model of the human left ventricle, similar to that of Georgiadis et al. [17]. The flow-field equations were expressed in a vorticity–streamfunction formulation, in a prolate spheroidal coordinate system. These equations were combined with boundary conditions derived from ultrasonographic measurements, and were numerically solved using an alternating-direction-implicit (ADI) algorithm (see Section 13.3.3, on pp. 703 ff.); the unsteady flow aspects of the ejection process were subsequently introduced into the numerical simulation. Their initial results agree with our early work [17] simulating the left ventricular ejection flow field.

13.1.3 Hybrid correlative imaging–CFD method

Song et al. [65] pioneered a hybrid imaging–CFD approach, which combines velocity measurements with a CFD solution based on the Navier–Stokes equations. They applied their method to demonstrate cardiac velocity fields and the corresponding relative cardiac pressure distributions, as derived from a sequence of ultrafast CT cardiac images (see Section 10.1.5, on pp. 498 ff.). The quality of the pressure field in that initial study was impaired by the limited accuracy of the measured cardiac velocity field. Subsequently, this method was used successfully to obtain the relative aortic pressure field from time-resolved phase-contrast MRI velocimetric data [69, 73]. 3-D flow and relative pressure fields within the human left ventricle were also investigated through such an approach by Ebbers et al. [14]. Using time-resolved 3-D phase-contrast MRI, they measured the velocity field throughout the left atrium and ventricle of a normal human subject; subsequently, the time-resolved 3-D relative pressure was calculated from this velocity field by a CFD method using the pressure Poisson equation [14].

Such a hybrid imaging–CFD approach was also utilized by Bermejo et al. [2, 76]; they adapted it to digital color Doppler M-mode echocardiograms, which were combined with a simplified CFD algorithm to compute intraventricular pressure gradients. Instantaneous blood velocity data were first fitted to a bivariate spatiotemporal tensor-product smoothing spline. This fitting process allowed subsequent application of the Euler equation to solve for the corresponding pressure gradients, and the computed pressure gradients could then be overlaid, as a color-coded planar representation, on the original color Doppler image. Curves of instantaneous pressure differences between selected intracardiac locations could then be derived by spatial integration. Because both the local inertial and the convective components of the total pressure gradients are measured, this method is generally accurate *when applied during ejection*, during which the flow is [17, 21, 36, 42] effectively inviscid and irrotational under most operating conditions.[4]

DeGroff et al. [9] combined digitized, calibrated 2-D cross-sectional sequential image sets from stage-10 and -11 early human embryo hearts, each stacked to define a 3-D blood-contacting tubular surface, and CFD methods for steady and pulsatile flow. Sections of

[4]In [2], this approach was also applied to intraventricular flow throughout diastolic filling; this is fluid dynamically inadmissible because, aside from the normal upstroke of the E-wave when the flow is indeed irrotational [45], intraventricular diastolic flow is rotational and vortical [46, 47]. In the diastolic flow field, vorticity is generated (and annihilated) by the action of nonconservative viscous forces; consequently, its simulation calls for the solution of the full Navier–Stokes equations, as we shall see in the next chapter.

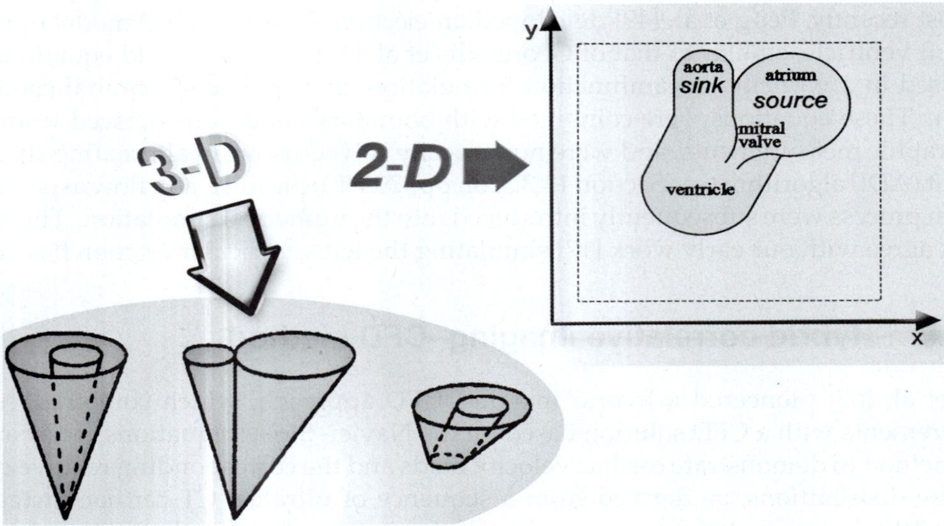

Figure 13.2: In the Immersed Boundary method, the basic heart geometry is idealized, being made up of straight-line segments and circular arcs in 2-D models, and correspondingly simple geometric solid constituents, e.g., cone and cylinder surfaces in 3-D models.

each embryonic heart were artificially reshaped. CFD flow solutions were obtained and surface stress changes analyzed. They demonstrated that streaming flow patterns exist in the early embryonic heart, and that fluid shear stresses change significantly with alterations in lumen shape.

13.2 Immersed Boundary (IB) method

The Immersed Boundary (IB) method was developed in the 1970s by Peskin and McQueen [30, 50, 51] to study flow patterns around heart valves, and in a highly schematized 2-D model of a canine heart (see Fig. 13.2). It represents the effects of a deformable bounding surface, or an immersed body, on the enclosed or surrounding flow, respectively, without using body-fitted grids (see Fig. 12.17, on p. 656). Other advantages beyond the use of simple Cartesian grids, include the relative ease with which moving boundary effects can be formulated, and the comparative simplicity with which it can be implemented into Navier–Stokes solvers. Therefore, it appears well suited for the study of physiologic flows that are generated by the movement of flexible boundaries, as prescribed by physiologic properties of various contractile cells or subcellular motile apparatuses. In the case of the pumping heart, the heart muscle relaxes and contracts according to prescribed myocardial dynamic properties [37], forcing the blood to flow through the heart.

In another setting, the IB method has been utilized to model platelet aggregation [71]. It has also been used to model the motion of the basilar membrane of the cochlea in the inner ear [3], bacterial swimming [10], and a biofilm in a porous medium [11]. What these problems have in common with the problem of blood flow in the heart is that they involve the motion of a viscous incompressible fluid, and the motion of one or more deformable elastic surfaces that bound the fluid, or that form deformable elastic objects immersed in the fluid. Because the objects or surfaces are deformable and elastic their motion is coupled to the fluid motion; i.e., the motion of the one affects the other. These features are shared to a greater or lesser extent by all biomedical fluid–structure interaction problems (cf. Section 12.6.3 on pp. 654 f.). Each of these applications involves a "coupled system"—the elastic boundary moves the fluid at the same time as the fluid pushes back against it.

The flow in such applications is an incompressible, viscous flow governed by the full Navier–Stokes equations. Because of the challenges involved in solving these equations even in the simplest of geometries, the IB method is attractive for some analyses because, to apply it, one only needs to include the boundary effects as external sources and sinks. No special discretizations are needed near the endocardial–blood interface, and in particular, one need not have detailed information about the geometry of the interface. The Navier–Stokes equations are discretized on a uniform Cartesian mesh and discretized delta functions—whose strength is specified by the forces exerted on the fluid by the flexible wall boundary—are included in the equations as a source term [50].

In the overall Immersed Boundary approach [52, 53], the configuration of the elastic structure is formulated in terms of Lagrangian variables (i.e., variables indexed by a coordinate system attached to the elastic structure), whereas the momentum, velocity, and incompressibility of the coupled fluid-structure system are formulated in terms of Eulerian variables (i.e., in reference to fixed physical coordinates)—see Figure 1.5, on p. 19, and the associated discussion in Section 1.8.

The basic idea is to consider the structure as a part of the fluid where additional forces are applied and additional mass is localized. The forces exerted by the structure on the fluid are taken into account as a source term in the Navier–Stokes equations and are mathematically described as a set of discrete delta-functions lying along the immersed structure. These delta-functions spread the entire force exerted by the immersed boundary to nearby fluid grid points, linking *Eulerian* (fluid) with *Lagrangian* (immersed boundary) variables (see Fig. 1.5, on p. 19). The boundary forces are then advected with the fluid and their location is updated at each timestep, as is summarized pictorially in Figure 13.3, on p. 690. Because the boundary action term only appears as a source term—the force density term in the fluid dynamics equations, which drives the fluid motion—the equations can be discretized on a uniform mesh using a simple Cartesian lattice.

13.2.1 Whole heart pumping dynamics by IB method

The original application of the Immersed Boundary method was a 2-D model of the left ventricle. The methodology has since been upgraded to a geometrically simplified but 3-D model in which all four heart chambers and their valves are considered, along with all the major arteries and veins leaving and entering the heart [52, 53]. Computation of

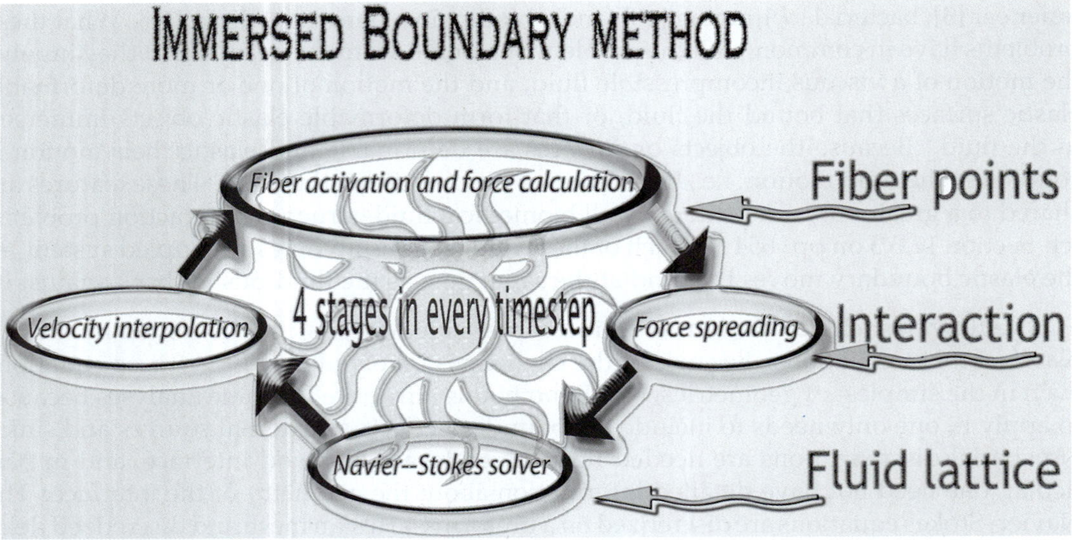

Figure 13.3: In the Immersed Boundary method, the sequence of computing myocardial forces and their spread, then fluid motion, and then new boundary velocities and location, is repeated *cyclically* in a time-stepping procedure with a suitably chosen timestep. In recent 3-D simulations on a $128 \times 128 \times 128$ grid, this sequential finite difference solution may be repeated nearly 60,000 times, in order to model a single complete heart beat.

blood flow in such a virtual heart[5] model requires specifying the initial geometry for the heart, stipulating the physiological, time-dependent, myocardial properties of the model fibers, including contractile patterns, and then the repeated application of the Immersed Boundary method (see Fig. 13.3). Such a computation requires hundreds of CPU hours on a large, shared-memory multiprocessor supercomputer. The IB method simultaneously computes the motion of the fluid and the motion of an elastic boundary that is immersed in and is interacting with that fluid.

In the IB method, Eulerian velocities and pressures that are stored on a regular 3-D computational lattice represent the fluid. The size of the heart chambers allows blood to be treated as a Newtonian fluid (see Section 4.6 on pp. 190 ff.). Fluid dynamics is computed by numerical solution of the Navier–Stokes equations (see Sections 4.6 on pp. 190 ff., 4.7, on pp. 191 f., and 12.7, on pp. 657 ff.), including a distributed force. Elastic structures that are free to move continuously in the space sampled by the computational lattice take the place of the myocardial boundary.

The CFD requirement to adapt the mesh *pari-passu* with the requirements of the advancing solution process is considerably difficult to implement and computer intensive for most intracardiac flow applications. In the IB method, the flow-bounding structures

[5]As used here, the term *virtual heart* signifies the computational model that is used as a substitute for a real heart.

are thought of as a part of the fluid where additional forces are applied, and where additional mass may be localized. Essentially, the IB method replaces the myocardial boundary by the forces that result from its active contractile dynamics or passive deformations. These forces are applied to the lattice in the neighborhood of the elastic boundary with the aid of a numerical approximation to the Dirac delta function. The fluid moves under the action of this distributed force. The numerical delta function is then used again, to interpolate the newly computed lattice velocities to the locations of the boundary, and then the boundary is moved at the *interpolated velocity* (satisfying the "no-slip" condition (cf. Section 4.12, on pp. 208 ff.) to a new location.

The sequence of computing myocardial forces, then fluid motion, and then new boundary location is repeated cyclically in a time-stepping procedure, with a suitably chosen timestep. Therefore, instead of separating the system in its two components coupled by interface conditions, the incompressible Navier–Stokes equations, with a nonuniform mass density and an applied elastic force density, are used to describe in a unified way the coupled motion of the *hydroelastic* system. The advantage of this method is that the fluid domain can have a simple shape, so that a simple, uniform and fixed, Cartesian structured grid can be used, together with a fluid solver. On the other hand, the immersed boundary is typically not aligned with the grid, and it is represented using Lagrangian variables, defined on a curvilinear mesh that is moving through the domain. Another fundamental assumption of the IB method is that the immersed boundary has a fiber-like 1-D structure, which may have a mass but occupies no volume in the fluid domain [51].

The only requirements for the application of this method are the physical properties of the fluid, the time-dependent elastic properties of the cardiac chamber boundaries, and the initial geometry of the virtual heart. Geometric parameters determine the size and shape of the model heart at the start of the simulation. Heart geometry is idealized, being made up of *straight-line* segments and *circular arcs* in 2-D models, and correspondingly simple *geometric solid* constituents in 3-D models (see Fig. 13.2, on p. 688). This geometry obviously changes during an evolving simulation of the cardiac cycle.

The immersed boundary points are joined by links representing muscle and connective tissues, which may be either active or passive. The link configuration, which defines the topology of the virtual heart, is adjusted throughout the cardiac cycle. The elastic properties of the immersed boundary links change with time according to preselected activation-relaxation patterns. During the active contraction of the cardiac muscle, modeled using a set of elastic links, the resting ("end-diastolic") lengths of the links would shorten at speeds that depend both on the time-course of the activation function and on the load (tension) that they sense. This implies that the myocardial wall movements at any instant depend on *what the fluid is doing* to the ends of the sets of links that simulate myocardial fibers. In turn, the force field that appears in the fluid equations depends on the boundary configuration. The situation exemplifies nicely a fully coupled fluid–structure interaction, or FSI, problem—see Section 12.6.3, on pp. 654 ff. The end product of the IB method is a prediction of dynamic flow patterns of blood throughout the virtual heart, and a *simultaneous* prediction of the motion of the heart walls and valve leaflets.

13.2.2 Limitations of the IB method in intracardiac flow simulations

In typical IB method formulations, a finite-difference scheme developed by Chorin [8], the classic Chorin's *projection method*, is applied in the computational solution of the Navier–Stokes equations, in order to treat the incompressibility condition. Overall, projection methods take into account fluid convection, viscous forces, and outside forces (i.e., the forces exerted by the flexible boundaries) to define an interim or provisional velocity field, which does not necessarily satisfy the incompressibility condition. Then, this provisional velocity is *projected* on the set of incompressible velocity fields, giving both the final velocity and the pressure at the end of the timestep at each point of the field. Finally, the condition of "no-slip" between a point of a viscous fluid and a point of the boundary immediately adjacent to it furnishes an equation of motion for each immersed boundary point: namely, the velocity of the immersed boundary point matches that of the fluid at the same location. Accordingly, the immersed boundary point location is adjusted by an amount equal to this velocity multiplied by the duration of the timestep.

To specify the elastic properties of the immersed boundaries, an energy function of the immersed boundary point coordinates is created for each entity, or subset of connected immersed boundary points, and the elastic forces that act on the immersed boundary points are calculated from the derivatives of this energy function. For each immersed boundary entity, the energy function comprises three contributions: energy from stretching springs, energy from bending the entity, and energy from moving the entity away from a specified location. One or more of these contributions may be zero for a given entity at a given time. Moreover, in modeling *myocardial contraction* using a set of elastic links, the resting lengths of the links is made to shorten at a prescribed speed during the active contraction of the muscle. Subroutines provide means for extracting immersed boundary point and spring data and implementing rules for dynamically changing the corresponding spring properties and tether-point locations.

Chorin's method was one of the first projection methods, and has some intrinsic limitations. These limitations have effectively restricted its application to only unphysiologically small, insofar as intracardiac flows are concerned, Reynolds numbers—lower than, 50, or so. Thus, in Peskin and McQueen's classic heart flow simulations [54] the blood viscosity had to be arbitrarily increased by a factor of 25, in order to effectively reduce the Reynolds number by the same factor. Smaller (less unphysiological) viscosity values could not have been used, because they would have required very fine computational meshes, at least near the boundary. The present form of the Immersed Boundary method uses a *uniform mesh*, which is therefore (see Section 12.6.3, on pp. 654 ff.) expensive to refine, but future research may make it possible to perform *local* mesh refinement, or to actually use a grid-free method that automatically concentrates the computational effort in flow-field regions of high vorticity. Even with uniform meshes, future progress in computer hardware could eventually make it feasible to use finer and finer lattices, and hence to reduce the simulated viscosity of blood toward more physiologic values. Efforts that are more recent aim to implement improved projection methods that should be able to handle intracardiac flows with more realistic—less subnormal—Reynolds numbers of up to about 1000.

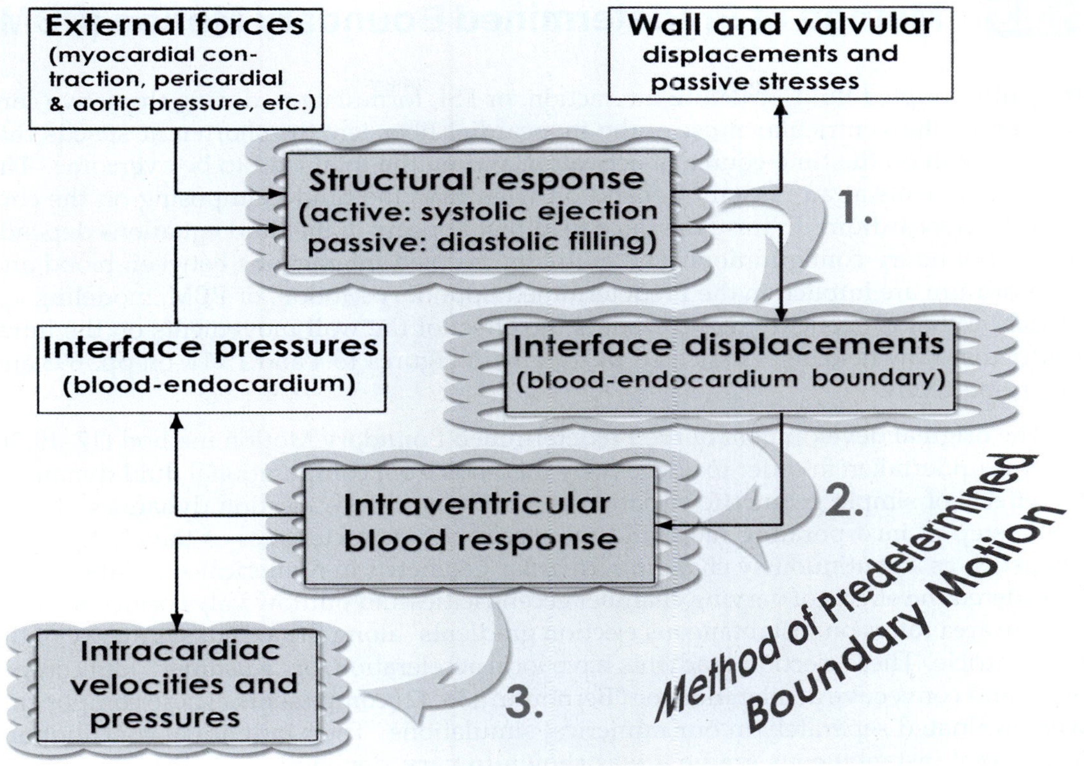

Figure 13.4: The niche of the method of Predetermined Boundary Motion (PBM) within the overall feedback loop in the FSI approach to intracardiac fluid dynamics. In the PBM method (gray-cloud shaded boxes), the movement of the endocardial chamber boundary is determined independently of the flow, which is generated by and depends on it. Consequently, Steps 2 and 3 are all that is recognized explicitly, whereas Step 1 is recognized only implicitly. Only the resulting flow field of the intraventricular blood must be computed, by incorporating the uncoupled wall motion into the CFD.

Furthermore, and because the IB method relies on discrete delta functions, its accuracy is limited to the accuracy of the driving force approximations effected by these functions, and their spacing along the boundary. Typically, with the *sharp* liquid-boundary interfaces of actual intracardiac flows, this accuracy corresponds to only a first-order approximation.[6] Another shortcoming of the IB method is that there is nothing to prevent fluid from passing between these singular forces, and hence through the irregular boundaries. This is a problem in intracardiac flow applications, since the endocardial boundaries should be impermeable, but ways have been developed [55] to cope with it.

[6] If a high-order polynomial approximation would be actually required to fit accurately multiple data points, a first-order approximation will be a *straight line* with a given slope. When a number is needed, an answer with only *one* significant figure is then all that is warranted.

13.3 Method of Predetermined Boundary Motion (PBM)

In a fully coupled fluid–structure interaction, or FSI, formulation, during the active contraction of the ventricular muscle, the myocardial fiber lengths shorten at speeds that depend both on the time-course of activation and on the total load to be overcome. The wall movements at any instant depend on what load the fluid is imposing on the contracting myocardium. In turn, the force field that appears in the fluid equations depends on the boundary configuration. The mutually coupled interactions between blood and myocardium are implicit in the Predetermined Boundary Motion, or PBM, modeling approach. What is explicitly recognized, is the effect of the wall movements on the intraventricular flow field, as is indicated pictorially in Figures 13.4 and 13.11, on pp. 693 and 711, respectively.

The original development of the Predetermined Boundary Motion method [17–19,36, 37] was undertaken in order to address, by methods from computational fluid dynamics, the effects of simple geometric variations on intraventricular ejection dynamics. It was a first step in incorporating more and more relevant characteristics of the ejection process, such as a continuously changing irregular geometry, in numerical simulations. We considered the effects of varying chamber eccentricities and outflow valve orifice-to-inner surface area ratios on instantaneous ejection gradients[7] along the axis of symmetry of the left ventricle. These ejection gradients have local acceleration, or "Rushmer" [36] components and convective acceleration, or "Bernoulli" [36,42] components. These components were evaluated separately in our numerical simulations. Their individual contributions to the total instantaneous gradient was shown to vary, depending on chamber outflow port area and eccentricity, both in absolute and in relative terms.

Numerical simulation of intraventricular flow dynamics during ejection involves the formulation and solution of mathematical model equations by computer. We begin by summarizing the basic steps of the traditional numerical solution methods.[8] The first step is *grid generation*, a finite grid is superimposed on the solution domain. Second, the flow-field governing equations are transformed from the physical to the computational domain and a *discretized* version of the equations is solved numerically. Such discrete systems can be obtained by approximating, for example, spatial derivatives with finite difference expressions between grid nodes, which leads to a whole class of finite-difference schemes. While the physical problem is posed in terms of a set of partial differential equations defined on a continuum, its numerical approximation consists of a system of algebraic equations defined on a finite number of grid *nodes*. The science and art of numerical analysis provide ways of ensuring that the solution of the discrete system converges to the solution of the continuum system as the grid is progressively refined.

[7]The terms "pressure drop" and "gradient" are used interchangeably in cardiology and hemodynamics. Although gradient refers to the rate of change of pressure with distance, both terms emphasize that, so far as the flow is concerned, it is *differences* in pressure that matter, not the pressure itself. Whereas pressure drop points in the direction of decreasing pressure, pressure gradient points in the direction of *increasing* pressure, by mathematical convention.

[8]To understand our solution, readers who are not familiar with computational fluid dynamics should refer to Chapter 12.

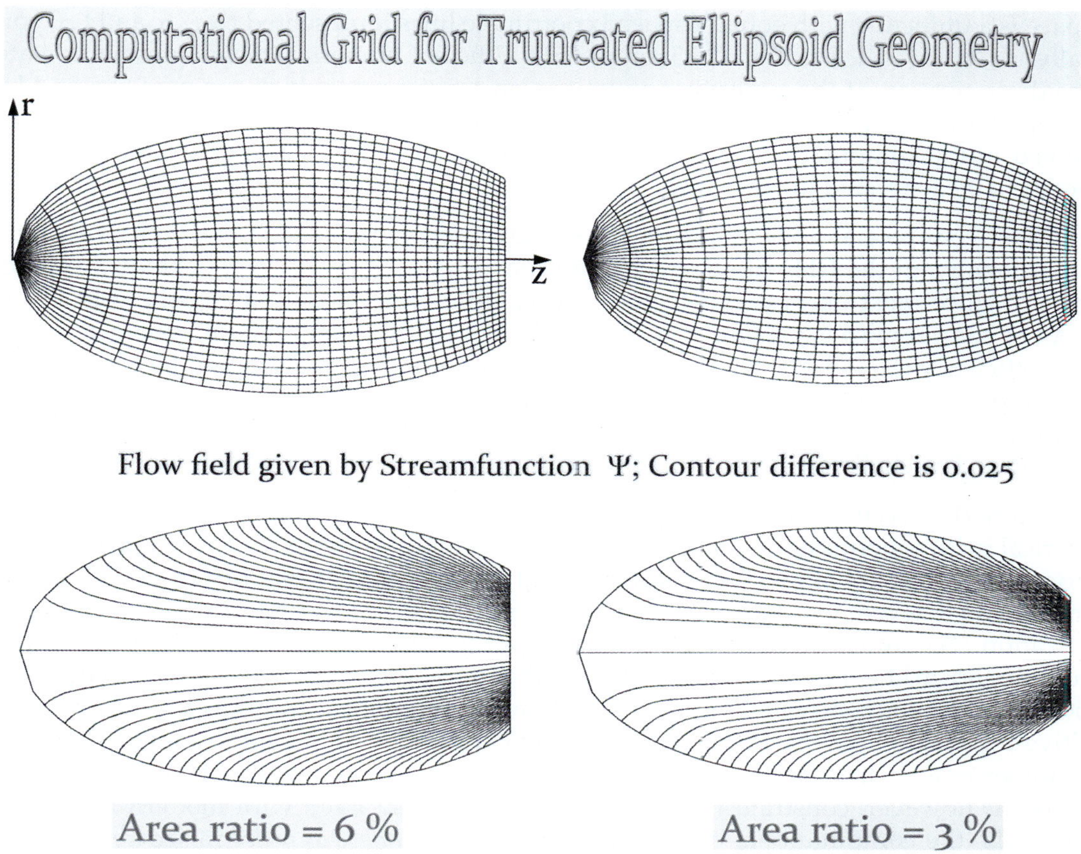

Figure 13.5: Computational fluid dynamic simulation of viscous flow in ellipsoidal ejecting LV chamber. Aortic ring cross-section to inner wall surface area ratios of 6% and 3% correspond to instantaneous Reynolds numbers of 4,100 and 6,000, respectively. Note the strong convective acceleration of the intraventricular flow, which is reflected in the convergence of the streamlines in the vicinity of the aortic ring and is intensified when there is ventriculoannular disproportion (left), as occurs with ventricular chamber enlargement, compared to normal (right). The intensified velocities in the vicinity of the aortic ring underlie the adaptive increase in grid density in this region, exemplified in the top panels. (Adapted from Georgiadis, Wang, and Pasipoularides [17], by kind permission of the Biomedical Engineering Society and Springer.)

13.3.1 Numerical grid generation

The actual flow domain represented by the ejecting left ventricle will be referred to as the physical space. It is the region where the blood flow is defined by the physical chamber boundaries and corresponding boundary conditions.[9] The computational, or logical,

[9]In general, intracardiac flow domains are categorized as convex because any two arbitrary points within can be connected by a single line segment that lies entirely within such domains; grid generation on convex domains is often less problematic than on nonconvex ones.

space is a unit cube with equally spaced coordinate lines represented by ξ, η, and ζ. Typically, $0 \leq \xi, \eta, \zeta \leq 1$ (see Fig. 12.15, on p. 651). Efficient numerical techniques necessitate the discretization of the governing equations on a finite grid which can conform and be mapped to the physical domain. The governing differential equations are discretized and solved in the computational space as functions of ξ, η, and ζ. The grid almost always needs to be generated numerically.

Most commercial CFD packages have a grid generator as part of "preprocessing." Occasionally, in the CFD literature, a compromise is sought between flexibility and accuracy, since most users prefer to invest very little time on optimizing the grid. This kind of compromise is generally unacceptable in scientific computation, where accuracy and efficiency are important. Recent advances in numerical analysis can be exploited in developing a quantitative tool for grid selection and optimization to suit any particular application. There is a plethora of gridding schemes that have been applied in simple domains. The challenge is to implement them in solving fields with realistic geometries.

Numerical accuracy considerations impose certain quality criteria to a successful numerical grid: smoothness, uniformity, and reduction of skewness, namely, small deviations from orthogonality. The gridding of all but the most trivial of physical domains introduces a severe overhead in terms of time expenditure during grid setup and optimization. As far as the time of total throughput is concerned, from project initiation to completion, grid generation necessitates another iteration process, because grid construction cannot be accomplished independently of the numerical solution algorithm. Sensitive regions, where the solution changes quickly, as the immediate vicinity of cardiac chamber *orifices*, have to be resolved by increasing the grid density. Economy considerations, however, constrain the total number of nodes. Even with modern numerical methods, the computational cost increases with the *number of nodes* raised to a power, which generally falls between 1 and 2 (see also Section 12.8.2, on pp. 665 ff.).

Adaptive methods are those where the grid is tailored according to geometric considerations or solution characteristics (see Section 12.6.3, on pp. 654 ff.). Geometric adaptation usually results in refining the grid near boundaries. It is a static adaptation, because the refinement is usually done prior to actually solving the governing differential equations on the generated grid. Solution adaptive techniques may be static or dynamic, in that the grid resolution may change as the solution evolves; an example would be where the grid refinement follows a changing chamber orifice diameter. The optimal approach involves increasing the grid density only in the most sensitive regions, by changing adaptively the spatial distribution of nodes; an example is provided in Figure 13.5, on p. 695.

The computation of flow in the beating heart chambers represents a class of problems where numerical grid generation [17,70] is crucial. In particular, the solution of the equations of fluid mechanics in the left ventricular chamber requires the generation of boundary-fitted composite grids. The superiority of boundary-fitted compared to nonfitted grids [17,68] is demonstrated in Figure 12.17, on p. 656 and was discussed at length in Sections 12.5 and 12.6, on pp. 638 ff. and 646 ff., in Chapter 12. As we saw in that chapter, numerical grid generation can be performed by solving partial differential equations, or

NOMENCLATURE

h	= grid size in computational domain	x, y	= radial, axial coordinate, respectively
J	= Jacobian of coordinate transformation	f_x	= $\partial f/\partial x$, partial derivative of f with respect to x
P, Q	= control function for grid generation	α	= $x_\eta^2 + y_\eta^2$
r	= radial coordinate ($r = x$)	β	= $x_\xi x_\eta + y_\xi y_\eta$
u	= velocity component in radial direction	γ	= $x_\xi^2 + y_\xi^2$
U	= average velocity	ξ, η	= coordinates in the computational domain
v	= velocity component in axial direction	Ψ	= stream function

by algebraic interpolation. In practice, a mixture of elliptic solvers and algebraic interpolation techniques is the best solution in optimizing the gridding. The former contribute to mesh smoothness while the latter give better control of grid resolution. In the present application [17], an algebraic method gave the initial guess for the grid, while the final grid came as a result of solving an elliptic partial differential equation. Computational fluid dynamics symbols and nomenclature are defined in the nearby Nomenclature tabulation.

A domain provides a logical representation of the input dataset involved in a computation. It gives meaning and logical structure to the dataset given. For example, a spatial domain indicates that the dataset is ordered in physical coordinates in space. Grid generation may be thought of as a transformation, or mapping, from the computational to the physical domain. Each node in the computational space, including boundary nodes, is mapped to a corresponding node in the physical space. The x, y, and z coordinates in the physical domain of a point with (ξ, η, ζ) coordinates in the computational space are given by coordinate functions $x(\xi, \eta, \zeta)$, $y(\xi, \eta, \zeta)$, and $z(\xi, \eta, \zeta)$, respectively. In the case of a 3-D computational space being mapped to a 3-D physical space, the transformation is given by three coordinate functions, each of which is a function of the three variables ξ, η, and ζ.

In mapping the computational to the physical domain, we require certain characteristics for our transformation: e.g., that the boundary of the computational space be mapped to the boundary of the physical domain. Such a coordinate mapping is called boundary conforming or boundary-fitted (see Fig. 12.10, on p. 642). Additionally, each node of the computational space must be mapped to a unique node in the physical space, and *vice versa*. Such a transformation is called a *homeomorphism* [7]. For the coordinate mapping to be smooth, the coordinate functions $x(\xi, \eta, \zeta)$, $y(\xi, \eta, \zeta)$, and $z(\xi, \eta, \zeta)$ must be differentiable with respect to ξ, η, and ζ. A smooth homeomorphism transformation is called a *diffeomorphism* [7]. When the coordinate mappings of a grid transformation are smooth, their partial derivatives with respect to ξ, η, and ζ are defined and continuous. Under these conditions, the Jacobian matrix, J, for the transformation from the computational to the physical space, becomes a very useful tool in coordinate generation [7, 16], as will be seen below.

In sum, the problem at hand represents computations characterized by an underlying system of flow-governing equations, simulating the behavior of intracardiac blood flow through discrete timesteps. There exists an intuitive algorithm that solves the problem in a single domain (usually the physical domain with discrete spatial coordinates), but this can result in high algorithmic complexity, inaccuracy, and instability. Such issues are reconciled by using special properties from the underlying equations to mathematically transform the problem space into a different domain that may be able to produce the solution in a more accurate and efficient manner. It is a convenient practice to perform the grid generation by seeking the *inverse transformation* from the computational to the physical domain. This simplifies the derivation of the transformed governing equations in the computational domain.

For axisymmetric flow, the transformation from the computational grid (ξ, η, ζ) coordinates to the physical Cartesian (x, y, z) coordinates is accomplished through an intermediate cylindrical coordinate system. The first step is to map the base of the cube, i.e., the ζ-equal-to-zero surface (see Fig. 12.15, on p. 651) onto the $y-r$ cross-sectional planar domain in the (x, y, z) space, which is defined by letting z equal to zero (crosshatched area in the left diagram of Fig. 12.15). Second, this planar geometry is rotated about the vertical y axis to form the axisymmetric physical domain which is occupied by the fluid. In the computational domain, this corresponds to a translation of the ζ-equal-to-zero surface in the ζ direction, which sweeps out a cube with a side that is 2π long. Expressed mathematically, the inverse transformation is:

$$
\begin{aligned}
y &= y(\xi, \eta), \\
r &= r(\xi, \eta), \\
\theta &= \zeta.
\end{aligned}
\tag{13.1}
$$

The second step involves a coordinate transformation based on the method developed by Thompson et al. [68]. This step concerns the gridding of the crosshatched area in Figure 12.15. The transformation from the computational (ξ, η) to the physical (x, y) space is given by the solution of the following elliptic[10] partial differential equations:

$$
\begin{aligned}
\alpha \frac{\partial^2 x}{\partial \xi^2} - 2\beta \frac{\partial^2 x}{\partial \xi \partial \eta} + \gamma \frac{\partial^2 x}{\partial \eta^2} &= -J^2 [\frac{\partial x}{\partial \xi} P(\xi, \eta) + \frac{\partial x}{\partial \eta} Q(\xi, \eta)], \\
\alpha \frac{\partial^2 y}{\partial \xi^2} - 2\beta \frac{\partial^2 y}{\partial \xi \partial \eta} + \gamma \frac{\partial^2 y}{\partial \eta^2} &= -J^2 [\frac{\partial y}{\partial \xi} P(\xi, \eta) + \frac{\partial y}{\partial \eta} Q(\xi, \eta)],
\end{aligned}
\tag{13.2}
$$

[10]These partial differential equations are called *elliptic* because of their similarity to the equation for an ellipse, in 2-D (or an ellipsoid, in 3-D). They are typified by the Laplace and Poisson equations and are used to describe time-independent, i.e., steady-state distribution, physical problems. There are also *parabolic* (typified by the Navier–Stokes equations) and *hyperbolic* (typified by the pulse wave propagation equations) partial differential equations, which remind us of corresponding parabolic and hyperbolic conic section forms, respectively.

where α, β, γ are defined as

$$\begin{aligned}\alpha &= \left(\frac{\partial x}{\partial \eta}\right)^2 + \left(\frac{\partial y}{\partial \eta}\right)^2, \\ \beta &= \frac{\partial x}{\partial \xi}\frac{\partial x}{\partial \eta} + \frac{\partial y}{\partial \xi}\frac{\partial y}{\partial \eta}, \\ \gamma &= \left(\frac{\partial x}{\partial \xi}\right)^2 + \left(\frac{\partial y}{\partial \xi}\right)^2 .\end{aligned} \tag{13.3}$$

P and Q are the control functions [17, 68] for adjusting the distribution of grid nodes, and x is identified with the radial coordinate, r. J denotes the derivative of the coordinate transformation, which is called the Jacobian of the transformation and is defined pictorially in Figure 13.6, on p. 700. As is shown there, the derivative of a coordinate transformation is the matrix of its partial derivatives. In the case of 3-D coordinate systems this is always a three-by-three matrix. As a transformation, in 2-D, the Jacobian maps tangent vectors to a curve C in the one coordinate plane to tangent vectors to the image of C in the other coordinate plane.[11] It follows that the determinant of the transformation closely scales the area of a small region in the computational plane to the area of the image of the region in the physical plane. In 3-D, the determinant of the Jacobian matrix measures how infinitesimal volumes change under the transformation [16]. For this reason, the Jacobian determinant is the *multiplicative factor* needed in order to adjust the differential volume form when changing coordinates.

13.3.2 Mathematical formulation of the flow field

To begin with, we consider the numerical simulation of a quasi-steady[12] incompressible and inviscid flow in an axisymmetric model of the left ventricular chamber using standard finite difference approximations. Then, we introduce the unsteady aspects of the ejection process to the numerical simulation. We envisage the flow in an axisymmetric chamber in the form of a truncated ellipsoid, as is shown in Figure 13.7, on p. 701. The chamber wall is collapsing at a uniform rate. For incompressible and irrotational flow [36] (see Section 9.3, on p. 448 ff.), the flow field satisfies Laplace's equation (cf. Section 2.11, on p. 62) for the streamfunction Ψ. For illustrative purposes, Figure 13.8, on p. 704, depicts the steps for deriving the governing equation for a simple 2-D flow field.

As we noted in Section 12.3, on pp. 633 ff., in addition to expressing the flow-field equations in terms of the so-called "primitive variables," namely, velocity and pressure,

[11] The Jacobian can be generally used to calculate derivatives for a function in one coordinate sytem from the derivatives of that same function in another coordinate system.

[12] The admissibility of this quasi-steady flow assumption will be explained shortly.

Curvilinear coordinate physical space		Cartesian computational space	Jacobian matrix of the transformation

$$\begin{bmatrix} \frac{\partial u}{\partial x} & \frac{\partial u}{\partial y} & \frac{\partial u}{\partial z} \\ \frac{\partial v}{\partial x} & \frac{\partial v}{\partial y} & \frac{\partial v}{\partial z} \\ \frac{\partial w}{\partial x} & \frac{\partial w}{\partial y} & \frac{\partial w}{\partial z} \end{bmatrix} = \begin{bmatrix} \frac{\partial u}{\partial \xi} & \frac{\partial u}{\partial \eta} & \frac{\partial u}{\partial \zeta} \\ \frac{\partial v}{\partial \xi} & \frac{\partial v}{\partial \eta} & \frac{\partial v}{\partial \zeta} \\ \frac{\partial w}{\partial \xi} & \frac{\partial w}{\partial \eta} & \frac{\partial w}{\partial \zeta} \end{bmatrix} \begin{bmatrix} \frac{\partial \xi}{\partial x} & \frac{\partial \xi}{\partial y} & \frac{\partial \xi}{\partial z} \\ \frac{\partial \eta}{\partial x} & \frac{\partial \eta}{\partial y} & \frac{\partial \eta}{\partial z} \\ \frac{\partial \zeta}{\partial x} & \frac{\partial \zeta}{\partial y} & \frac{\partial \zeta}{\partial z} \end{bmatrix}$$

Figure 13.6: Example illustrating how the Jacobian matrix serves in mapping flow-field variables from one coordinate system to another. The velocity gradient terms are transformed from physical to computational space, via the chain rule, where the Jacobian matrix of the transformation is given by the derivative of the coordinate transformation.

their representation with streamfunction and vorticity as the unknown flow-field quantities is also advantageous in some situations, particularly in 2-D and in axisymmetric 3-D flows. Detailed derivations of the 2- and 3-D streamfunction and vorticity equations are found in Fletcher's elegant treatise [16].

Expressing the Navier–Stokes equations using the streamfunction or the vorticity, in place of the primitive variables, accomplishes wittingly the *elimination of the pressure* from the flow-governing equations, thus yielding one dependent variable less.[13] Introducing the streamfunction also eliminates the need for explicit solution of the continuity equation. Thus, the governing equation for the axisymmetric 3-D intraventricular flow field in the flow under consideration is given parsimoniously by the single Laplace's equation for the streamfunction, Ψ, in cylindrical coordinates:

$$\left(\frac{\partial^2 \Psi}{\partial r^2} + \frac{1}{r}\frac{\partial \Psi}{\partial r} + \frac{\partial^2 \Psi}{\partial y^2} + \cancelto{0}{\frac{1}{r^2}\frac{\partial^2 \Psi}{\partial \theta^2}} \right) = 0.$$

The velocity components in the r and y directions at a given flow-field point are given by the partial derivatives of the stream function at that point. The partial derivatives with respect to the azimuthal coordinate, θ, reduce to zero because there is no azimuthal

[13]In *nonaxisymmetric* 3-D flows, however, this formulation leads to six unknowns rather than four (in primitive variables), which makes this approach less attractive for that case. Moreover, the treatment of the boundary conditions becomes more complicated in both 2- and 3-D situations.

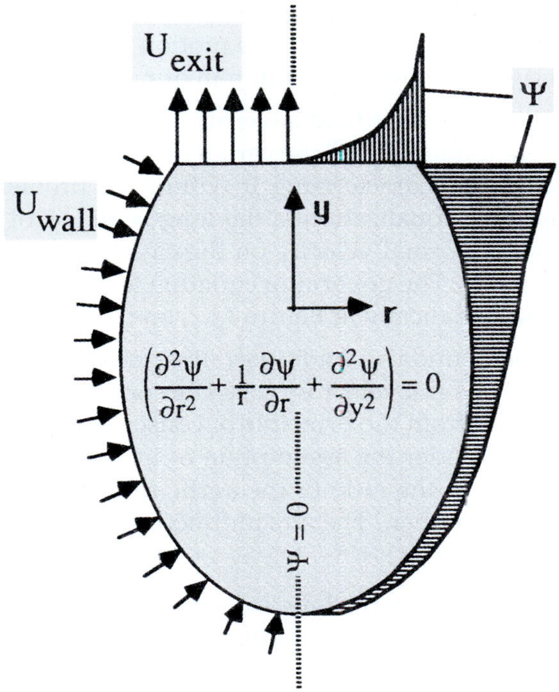

Figure 13.7: The left ventricular diametral plane section, which delineates the physical domain, is shown along with the imposed instantaneous hydrodynamic boundary conditions. On the left of the axis, is sketched the velocity distribution, which consists of two parts: an inward component normal to the inner surface of the chamber wall, associated with the wall contraction; and a blunt outflow velocity profile at the aortic ring. On the right side, the corresponding streamfunction distribution on the collapsing chamber boundary is also plotted; the slope of the streamfunction curve is proportional to the local velocity of the boundary. (Adapted, slightly modified, from Georgiadis, Wang, and Pasipoularides [17], by kind permission of the Biomedical Engineering Society and Springer.)

velocity component and the flow is axisymmetric; accordingly, the corresponding term drops off and the equation becomes:

$$\left(\frac{\partial^2\Psi}{\partial r^2}+\frac{1}{r}\frac{\partial\Psi}{\partial r}+\frac{\partial^2\Psi}{\partial y^2}\right)=0. \tag{13.4}$$

Any function that satisfies Laplace's equation is called *harmonic*. Laplace's equation is a 3-D second-order elliptic partial differential equation and in the present context it is an expression of the principle of mass conservation, or flow continuity, for an incompressible fluid. Although time does not come into view explicitly in this equation, the velocity field, and thus the streamfunction, will be time-dependent when the flow is unsteady, as it is in the ejecting ventricle. The absence of explicit time dependence renders the irrotational flow of an incompressible fluid a *quasi-steady* flow, meaning that the instantaneous structure of the flow field depends solely on the instantaneously applying boundary geometry and boundary conditions, and is independent of the motion at previous times [56], hence the admissibility of the *quasi-steady* flow assumption in our approach.

This Laplace's equation is the flow-field governing equation that needs to be discretized and solved on the computational grid. All the variables are nondimensionalized, by scaling each one of them by a value characterizing it within the problem. The characteristic length used in the nondimensionalization is the long semiaxis of the ellipsoid, and the characteristic velocity is the normal velocity on the cavity wall, i.e., the uniform rate of collapse of the chamber walls. The governing equation and the corresponding boundary conditions are depicted schematically in Figure 13.7, on p. 701.

The specification of the boundary conditions, illustrated in Figure 13.7, hinges on the definition of the instantaneous exit velocity, U_{exit}. The corresponding velocity of wall contraction, U_{wall} can be derived from the principle of conservation of fluid mass (*continuity*) for any given exit velocity. Under the assumption of incompressibility, this implies that the ratio U_{wall}/U_{exit} is equal to the ratio of the aortic ring cross-sectional area to the inner surface area of the LV chamber. The streamfunction boundary conditions are given below:

$$\Psi = 0, \quad \text{on the long axis of the ellipsoid;}$$
$$\Psi = \pi \cdot U_{\text{exit}} \cdot r^2, \quad \text{at the outflow orifice.}$$

The distribution of the streamfunction on the wall, which results from the condition on the ratio U_{wall}/U_{exit}, is too complicated to be expressed in closed form; it is represented pictorially in Figure 13.7.

In the curvilinear coordinate system of Equation 13.2, the governing Equation 13.4 assumes the following form [17]:

$$\frac{1}{rJ^2}\left[\alpha\frac{\partial^2\Psi}{\partial\xi^2} - 2\beta\frac{\partial^2\Psi}{\partial\xi\partial\eta} + \gamma\frac{\partial^2\Psi}{\partial\eta^2} + J^2P_1\frac{\partial\Psi}{\partial\xi} + J^2Q_1\frac{\partial\Psi}{\partial\eta}\right] = 0, \tag{13.5}$$

where, P_1 and Q_1 are defined by [17]:

$$P_1 = P(\xi,\eta) - \frac{1}{rJ}\frac{\partial y}{\partial\eta}, \qquad Q_1 = Q(\xi,\eta) + \frac{1}{rJ}\frac{\partial y}{\partial\xi}. \tag{13.6}$$

All the partial derivatives in Equations 13.2 and 13.5 are discretized using second-order finite difference approximations on a uniform (ξ, η) grid. This choice of uniform distribution of nodes in the computational domain greatly simplifies the finite difference expressions. For example, the finite difference approximation of a second derivative at the node (ξ_0, η_0) is

$$\frac{\partial^2 y}{\partial\xi^2} = \frac{y(\xi_0+h,\eta_0) - 2y(\xi_0,\eta_0) + y(\xi_0-h,\eta_0)}{h^2} + \text{(terms of order } h^2\text{)}, \tag{13.7}$$

where h is the grid "size," i.e., the distance between nodes. The two coupled partial differential Equations 13.2 were solved iteratively and a grid was produced inside the ellipsoidal LV chamber starting from a specified distribution of grid points on its boundaries. The method of solution is described in the following section.

13.3.3 Numerical solution scheme

The "workhorse" in our numerical solution of the equation of motion (13.5), as well as of the coordinate transformation equations (13.2), is the Alternating-Direction-Implicit, (ADI), algorithm. We adapted the conventional ADI method of Peaceman and Rachford [48], which is designed for 2-D problems. The method is parsimonious and can be expected to require about $(2 \log N)/N$ as many calculations as other, less efficient, iterative procedures for solving Laplace's equation, where N^2 is the number of points for which the solution is computed [48]. The partial differential equation is first split into two ordinary differential equations (corresponding to the two directions, ξ and η). The solution is obtained iteratively since the two split equations remain coupled (hence, the name "Implicit").

Each iteration involves two steps, corresponding to the solution of the two equations. Each of the split equations generates a tridiagonal linear system when discretized via second-order finite differences. Such systems are solved directly by exploiting a Lower–Upper (LU) decomposition of the tridiagonal linear algebraic system; this decomposition into the product of lower and upper triangular matrices is equivalent to Gauss elimination for solving linear systems of algebraic equations. The upper triangular matrix, $[U]$, is the one produced by the forward phase of Gauss elimination and the elements of the lower triangular matrix, $[L]$, are the factors used in the elimination process. The name Alternating-Direction method is derived from the observation that for the ξ-split equation, we solve along the ξ-grid lines, and then, for the η-split equation, along the η-grid lines.

At the start of the computation, the input to the code are the $x(\xi, \eta)$, $y(\xi, \eta)$ matrices which are obtained from the grid generation step. The correspondence between the computational domain and the physical domain in the form of $x(\xi, \eta)$, $y(\xi, \eta)$ matrices provides the metric tensor components (α, β, γ) in the equations of motion, as given by Equation 13.3. To start the iterative calculation of the streamfunction, Ψ, subject to the instantaneously applying boundary conditions, an initial guess of zero within the interior domain works as provided *initialization* input. With this initial guess, the streamfunction is then updated by solving Laplace's equation for Ψ iteratively, using ADI, with the specified boundary conditions that are depicted pictorially in Figure 13.7. The velocity field is subsequently computed from the converged streamfunction field, in principle according to the definitions given in Figure 13.8, on p. 704 (see also Section 4.2.2, on pp. 171 ff.).

13.3.4 Left ventricular ejection flow-field computation

In this and the ensuing sections of this chapter, we present and validate results from the new paradigm of the simulation-based intracardiac fluid dynamics, which—by directly solving the flow-field governing equations through computer simulation—can digitize and visualize intracardiac blood flow patterns during ejection, under normal and pathological conditions. Accordingly, this new paradigm can provide detailed information of physical variables such as intraventricular velocity and pressure distributions at

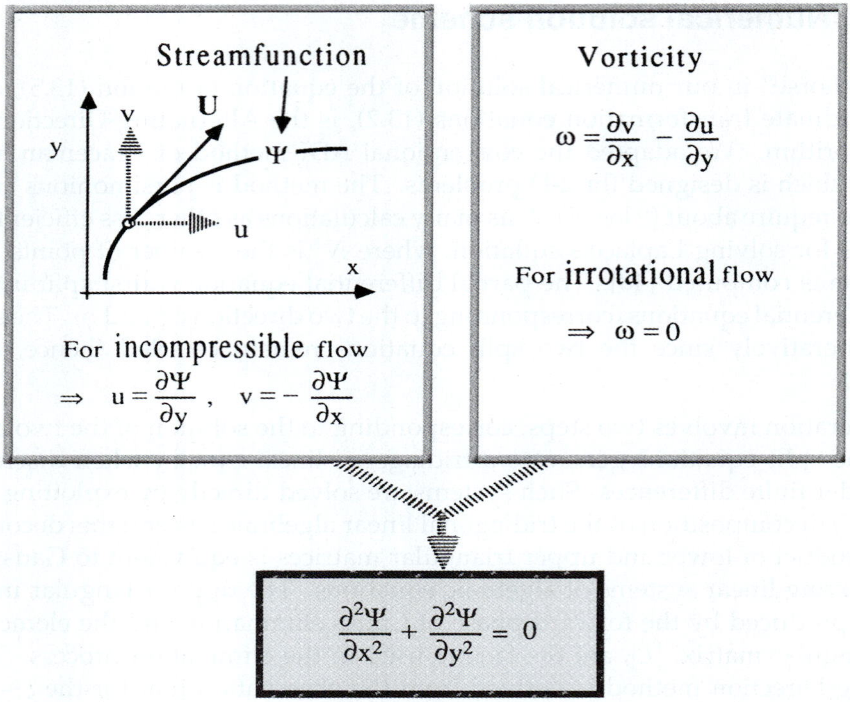

Figure 13.8: Pictorial outline of the derivation of the governing equation, in terms of the streamfunction Ψ, for an incompressible and irrotational 2-D flow. The upper left panel shows that the velocity is tangent to lines of constant streamfunction Ψ, which are called *streamlines* (cf. Fig. 4.3, on p. 172). The upper right panel shows the condition satisfied by the velocity components for an irrotational flow. Substituting from the left into the right upper panel, yields Laplace's equation for the streamfunction Ψ, which is shown in the lower panel. (Adapted from Georgiadis, Wang, and Pasipoularides [17], by kind permission of the Biomedical Engineering Society and Springer.)

macro- and micro-scopic levels, and hence it can give agreatly enhanced overall understanding of the physical phenomena involved in ejection under various applying operating conditions.

Because of the complicated dynamic cardiac chamber geometry and the high Reynolds numbers that apply in the vicinity of the outflow orifice of the LV (or RV) chamber through most of the ejection period, numerical solution of the Navier–Stokes equations by a finite difference based CFD method as the one developed above is a formidable, highly intensive computationally, task. A computational example of the intraventricular LV ejection flow field is shown in graphical form in Figure 13.5, on p. 695.

The LV chamber is modeled as an ellipsoid of revolution with an *aspect ratio* of 2 : 1, defined as major divided by minor axis. The chamber is truncated by a plane passing through the aortic anulus, in such a way that the cross-sectional area of the outflow section is 6% (left panels) or 3% (right panels) of the endocardial surface area of the truncated ellipsoid. The assumed instantaneous volumetric outflow rate is 360 cm^3/s for both cases and, using exit diameter and linear velocity in the calculation, the respective Reynolds numbers are 4,100 in the larger-orifice chamber and 6,000 in the smaller-orifice chamber, which exemplifies a systolic *ventriculoannular disproportion* [36]. The corresponding computational grids and streamline fields are depicted in the top and bottom panels of Figure 13.5.

It is noted in Figures 13.5 and 13.7, on pp. 695 and 701, that the cross-stream (transverse) gradient, $\partial\psi/\partial r$, of the stream function is increased greatly as the streamlines approach the aortic anulus. This reflects the strong convective acceleration of the flow and is much more *intense* when there is ventriculoannular disproportion, as occurs with ventricular chamber enlargement, than in the normal ventricle (Fig. 13.5).

It is important to observe in Figure 13.5 that all streamlines originate normal, i.e., perpendicularly, to the inner (endocardial) surface of the contracting chamber, because the underlying simulation pertains to viscous flow. Thus, there is no finite component of velocity in the tangential direction (Fig. 13.8, on p. 704) and the condition of "no slip" relative to the wall is satisfied (see Section 4.9 on pp. 197 ff., Section 4.10 on pp. 202 ff., Section 4.12 on pp. 208 ff., and Section 7.2.1 on pp. 327 f.). However, because of the great predominance of inertial effects in the ejection flow field [4, 17, 36, 42, 43], viscous effects are negligible throughout ejection within the contracting chamber, and are significant only within a thin, undeveloped unsteady *boundary layer* in the outflow tract and in the juxtaposed outflow trunk [36, 42, 43]. Accordingly, the intraventricular flow field calculated assuming inviscid dynamics is quite similar to the viscous field depicted in Figure 13.5. The notable difference is that the streamlines for the inviscid case are no longer originating normal to the endocardial surface of the ejecting ellipsoidal chamber—there is "slip" relative to the wall.

13.3.5 Pressure calculation in the *unsteady* intraventricular flow field

The relationship between the velocity and pressure fields in unsteady, irrotational flow of an incompressible fluid is given by the Euler equation

$$\frac{\partial \boldsymbol{U}}{\partial t} + \vec{\nabla}\left(\frac{\boldsymbol{U}\cdot\boldsymbol{U}}{2} + \frac{P - P_0}{\rho}\right) = 0, \tag{13.8}$$

where $\boldsymbol{U}$ is the velocity vector, P is the static pressure, P_0 a reference pressure value, and ρ blood's density; the arrow over ∇ is a reminder of the vectorial nature of the result of its operation on the terms within the parentheses. Given the velocity field, $\boldsymbol{U}$, and the local acceleration, $\partial \boldsymbol{U}/\partial t$, as functions of position, Equation 13.8 can be integrated to give the local pressure, P, at any point within the unsteady intraventricular flow field. It is simpler to perform this integration along the ellipsoidal LV chamber *axis* of symmetry, which is known a priori to be a streamline, and along which clinical and experimental intracardiac fluid dynamics measurements are obtained and available for *comparison* [4, 20, 21, 36, 37, 39–43, 63]. Equation 13.8 then yields:

$$\frac{\partial v}{\partial t} + \frac{\partial}{\partial s}\left(\frac{v^2}{2} + \frac{P_s - P_{\text{exit}}}{\rho}\right) = 0, \tag{13.9}$$

where v is the axial component of the velocity vector, s is the streamwise coordinate along the long axis of the chamber, and P_{exit} is the reference pressure at the outflow orifice.

It is also important to discuss the procedure for evaluating the local acceleration in Equation 13.9. The fundamental assumption is that the ventricular cavity remains similar to itself as it contracts. This simplifies the flow field: the ratio R of the velocities at two different points along the axis, e.g., $R = U_{exit}/U_s$, is constant with respect to time, i.e., the velocity field remains *self-similar* as the chamber contracts. This is possible only if the local acceleration field is *also self-similar*, and the following relation holds [36]:

$$R = \frac{U_{exit}}{U_s} = \frac{\left(\frac{\partial U_{exit}}{\partial t}\right)}{\left(\frac{\partial U_{exit}}{\partial t}\right)}. \tag{13.10}$$

Equations 13.9 and 13.10, in conjunction with U_{exit}, and $\partial U_{exit}/\partial t$ data are adequate to describe $P_s - P_{exit}$ on the *axis* of the LV chamber. Using the velocity data on the grid points along the axis, Equation 13.9 was integrated numerically with respect to the streamwise coordinate, s.

13.3.6 The effect of ventriculoannular disproportion on intraventricular flow dynamics

The effect of varying chamber outflow port area and ventriculoannular disproportion [36] on intraventricular LV ejection pressure gradients is displayed in Figure 13.9. The total chamber volume is fixed for all cases at $150\ cm^3$. The ratio of minor-to-major semiaxis is similarly fixed at 0.67 (an eccentricity of 0.75). The left panels correspond to boundary conditions of $250\ cm^3/s$ and $20{,}000\ cm^3/s^2$ for volumetric outflow rate and acceleration, respectively. Thus, they correspond to conditions early during the upstroke of the ejection velocity waveform. The right panels correspond to peak ejection, with the volumetric outflow rate set at $500\ cm^3/s$.

The top panels correspond to a normal outflow orifice area of $4.75\ cm^2$ and the bottom to an abnormally low orifice area of $1.0\ cm^2$, such as would be typical of aortic stenosis. The middle panels pertain to an orifice area of $2.75\ cm^2$, implying some ventriculoannular disproportion.

As is exemplified in Figure 13.9, outflow orifice stenosis is characterized by a strong augmentation of the convective acceleration, or *Bernoulli* gradient—the eponym needs no further elaboration. Its contribution in even moderately severe aortic stenosis (bottom panels) renders that of the local acceleration, or *Rushmer*, gradient totally negligible throughout ejection. This is to be contrasted to the normal situation (top panels), where the Rushmer gradient predominates in early (and late) ejection when velocities are low and local accelerations (decelerations) high. It should be noted, parenthetically, that in recognition of Rushmer's far-reaching influence in formulating a view of the impulsive nature of ventricular ejection, I have previously denoted [36] the impulse or local acceleration components of ejection gradients as "Rushmer gradients." All early investigations were

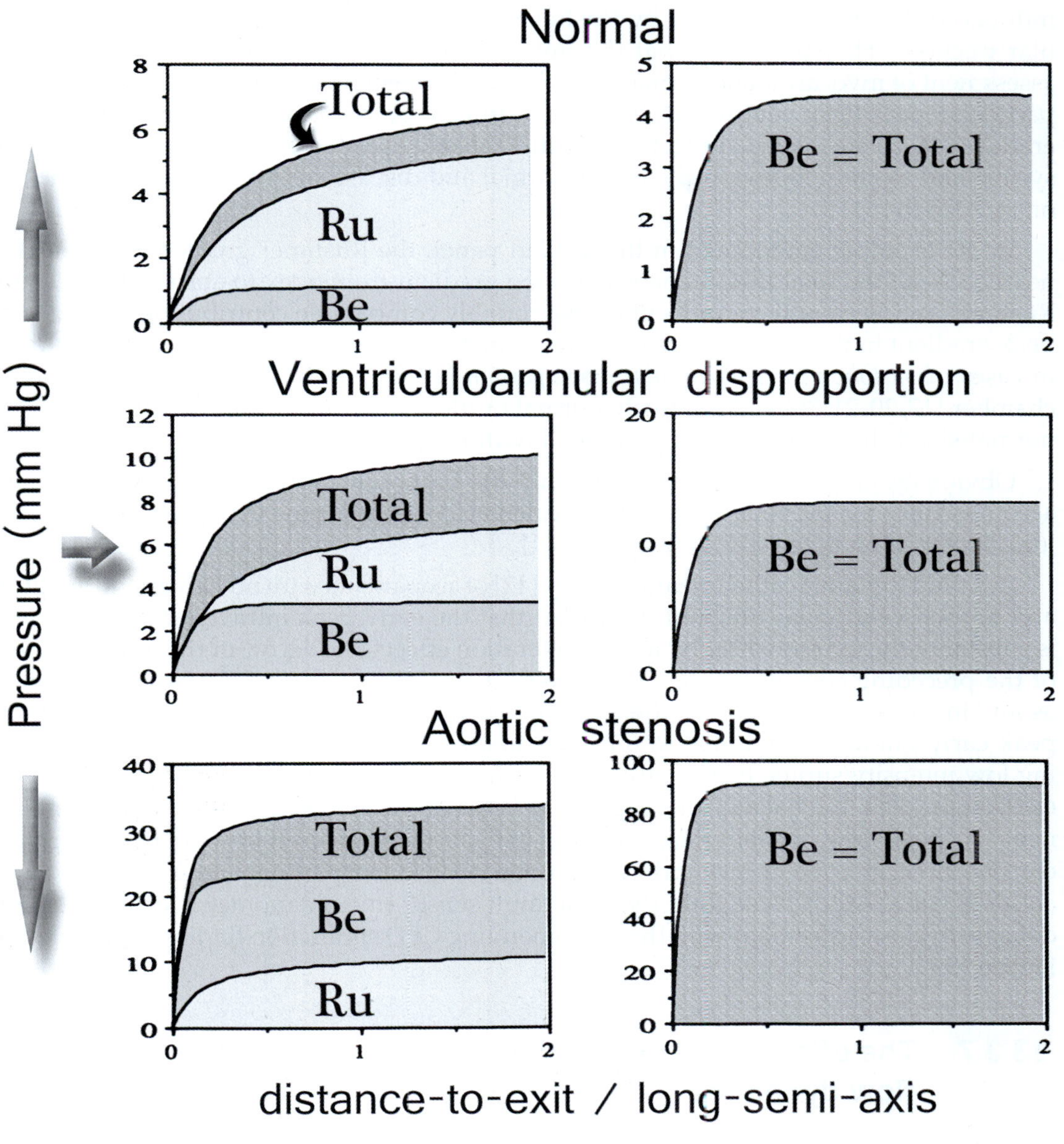

Figure 13.9: The effect of ventriculoannular disproportion and outflow orifice stenosis on the ejection pressure gradient distribution along the outflow axis of the left ventricle. The outflow orifice area decreases progressively from top to bottom. Pressure rises from its value at the outflow port (aortic anulus) of the chamber to higher values as the distance from the port increases along the axis. Note the sharp accentuation of the intraventricular gradients in the *immediate vicinity* of the outflow port. Be = Bernoulli, and Ru = Rushmer gradients. See discussion in text. (Adapted from Georgiadis, Wang, and Pasipoularides [17], by kind permission of the Biomed. Eng. Soc. and Springer.)

influenced directly or indirectly by Rushmer's view of the impulsive nature of ventricular ejection. His suggestion that the initial ventricular impulse may be a key to the assessment of myocardial performance [61] underlies several widely used indices [36]. In particular, peak deep ventricular dP/dt and aortic, or pulmonary arterial, root flow acceleration (dQ/dt) are taken to reflect myocardial forces generated during the initial stages of systole and ejection, respectively, under normal and disease conditions (see Section 7.11, on pp. 375 ff.).

In the example entertained in the top left panel, the Rushmer gradient accounts for nearly 85% of the total instantaneous ejection gradient from apex to aortic anulus. Both Rushmer and Bernoulli components make roughly comparable contributions to the total peak gradient in the intermediate case, illustrated in the left middle panel. This is typical in cases of *systolic ventriculoannular disproportion* [17, 36], such as occurs with a dilated chamber [17,20,21,36] and relatively normal outflow port (aortic anulus) area, or with a normal-sized chamber and relatively small outflow port area.

Obviously, at the time of peak flow only the Bernoulli component is operative, and accounts fully for the total measured or calculated ejection pressure gradient, since the local acceleration is zero [17,20,21,36,40–44].

In a fluid dynamic catheterization study [42] of six patients with no valve abnormalities and normal ventricular function, we found that the early peak intraventricular gradient is substantially accounted for by local acceleration effects ($85\% \pm 5\%$ of the total). In view of the preceding considerations, reference to the nonobstructive early ejection gradient as an "impulse or Rushmer gradient" seems justified. The mean (standard deviation) peak early gradient amounted to $6.7 \pm 1.9\ mm\ Hg$ at rest, and $13.0 \pm 2.3\ mm\ Hg$ during low intensity supine bicycle exercise. With the sharp increase in outflow velocity as ejection unfolds, the balance tilts rapidly in favor of the convective or Bernoulli component. At peak flow, the latter accounts for 100% of the measured intraventricular gradient ($5.4 \pm 1.7\ mm\ Hg$ at rest and $10.0 \pm 1.8\ mm\ Hg$ during submaximal exercise) since dQ/dt is zero. All of these fluid dynamic multisensor micromanometric catheterization data are in close agreement with the corresponding CFD simulation findings presented in Figure 13.9.

13.3.7 The effect of LV eccentricity on intraventricular flow dynamics

The effect of varying LV chamber eccentricity on intraventricular ejection pressure gradients is presented graphically in Figure 13.10. The total chamber volume is fixed for all cases at $150\ cm^3$. The cross-sectional area encompassed by the aortic anulus is similarly fixed at $5\ cm^2$. The left panels correspond to boundary conditions of $50\ cm/s$ and $2{,}000\ cm/s^2$ for aortic anulus velocity and acceleration, respectively. Thus, they represent conditions during the upstroke of the ejection velocity waveform. The right panels correspond to peak ejection, with the boundary condition for aortic anulus velocity set at $90\ cm/s$.

The middle panels apply for a ratio of minor-to-major semiaxis of 0.67 (an eccentricity of 0.75), i.e., for a representative normal chamber shape. The top panels correspond to a

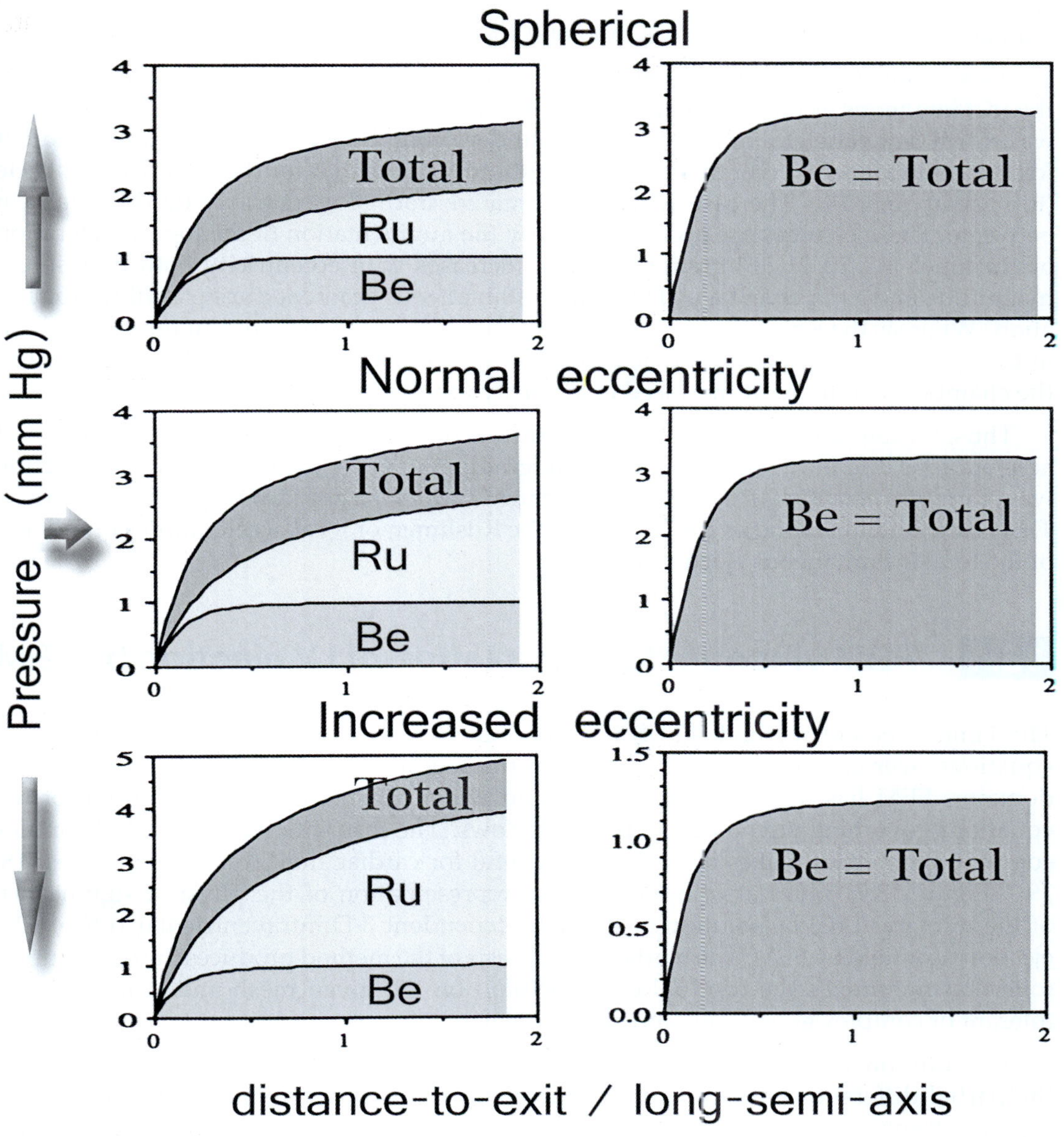

Figure 13.10: The effect of varying eccentricity on the ejection pressure gradient distribution along the outflow axis of the left ventricle. Eccentricity increases from top to bottom. Explanation of plots and abbreviations as in Figure 13.9, on p. 707. See discussion in text. (Adapted from Georgiadis, Wang, and Pasipoularides [17], by kind permission of the Biomedical Engineering Society and Springer.)

spherical ventricle, with zero eccentricity. The bottom panels pertain to a more ellipsoidal than normal chamber, with an axis ratio of 0.40 and eccentricity of 0.92.

As is shown in Figure 13.10, with an increase in eccentricity there is an *accentuation* of the instantaneous ejection pressure gradient during the upstroke of the ejection velocity waveform (left panels). For the assumed boundary conditions, the total pressure gradient for the chamber with eccentricity of 0.92 (bottom) *exceeds* that for the spherical ventricle (top) by about 35%. The case with representative normal eccentricity (middle) falls in between. These changes are accounted for by the augmentation of the local acceleration or Rushmer [17, 20, 21, 36] gradient, which increases with eccentricity both in absolute magnitude and as a percentage of the total instantaneous gradient during outflow acceleration. Whereas the Rushmer gradient accounts for 68% of the total instantaneous gradient in the spherical ventricle (top) it accounts for 80% of the total instantaneous gradient in the chamber with more pronounced eccentricity (bottom).

Thus, for the same chamber volumes, outflow orifice areas and ejection velocities and accelerations, the intraventricular pressure gradients during the upstroke of the ejection waveform are *accentuated* in the more eccentric and *minimized* in the spherical ventricle. This is attributable to the augmentation of the Rushmer, or local acceleration, component of the total instantaneous ejection gradient.

13.4 PBM viscous flow simulation of LV ejection by FEM

The Finite Element method (FEM) is a good choice for solving the full Navier–Stokes equations over complex domains, or when the required accuracy varies over the flow domain. FEM has found increasing use and wider acceptance for the solution of the equations governing viscous incompressible flows. The ease with which the FEM handles complex geometries makes it particularly useful for cardiac fluid dynamic analyses [18, 19]. Figure 13.11 gives a synoptic pictorial representation of the physical significance of the numerical (CFD) solution of the time-dependent 3-D intraventricular (LV or RV) ejection flow field by FEM. The mathematical basis of the method produces the *best* solution (one that minimizes the residual error *globally*) on the given mesh and is much more tolerant of complex geometries and skewed elements.

The solution approach for intracardiac unsteady flow problems is based on rendering the partial differential equations into equivalent ordinary differential equations, which are then transformed into finite difference algebraic equations and solved using standard techniques. In the finite differences method, the governing differential equations are approximated by having their derivatives replaced by different quotients involving solution values at discrete mesh points. In the FEM, a so-called "variational formulation" of the differential equations is used, in which the approximate solution is assumed to be a combination of appropriate *basis*, or *shape*, functions—in a sense, this is akin to the approximation of a time series by a Fourier sum of sinusoidal basis functions.

As is shown in Figure 13.12, there are two essential steps that one must take to solve, using the FEM, a boundary value problem (BVP).

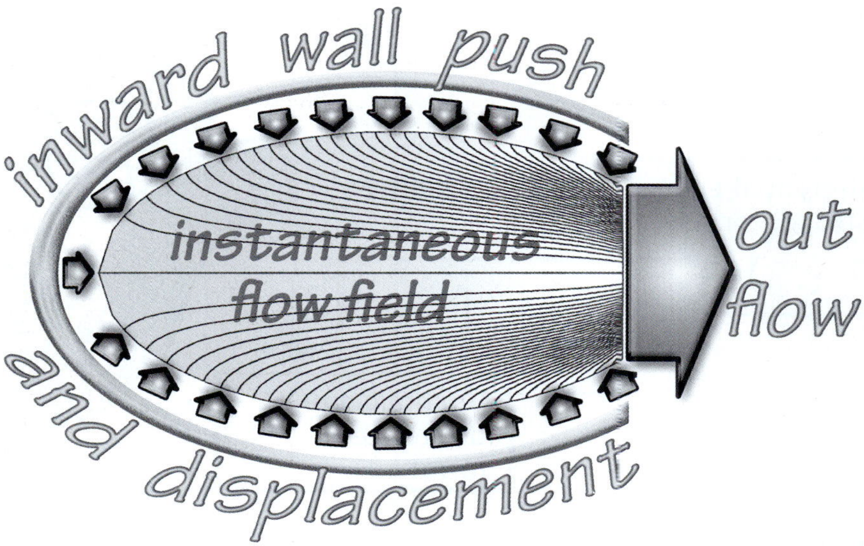

Figure 13.11: The physical significance of the numerical (CFD) solution of the time-dependent 3-D intraventricular (LV or RV) ejection flow field is as follows: the incompressible and irrotational flow within the chamber *connects*, in a manner compatible with the constraints imposed by the flow-governing equations (continuity, and Euler or Navier–Stokes), the instantaneous kinematic (velocities, accelerations) patterns of the *endocardial surface* of the ventricular walls to the resultant instantaneous volumetric outflow rate and acceleration at the *outflow valve ring* (aortic or pulmonic, respectively).

1. The BVP comprises the flow governing differential equations with the applying boundary and initial conditions, in the so-called "strong form" of the mathematical representation. In the first step, one *reformulates* the original strong form of the BVP into its "weak," or "variational" form, which involves integral equations. Little to no computation is usually required for this step, the transformation is done by paper and pencil.

2. The second step is the *discretization*, where the weak form is considered at only a finite number of selected nodal points in space and time. In this second step, we acquire particular formulas for a large but finite[14] dimensional problem whose solution, represented by a combination of sums of appropriate nodal basis functions, will approximately solve the original BVP. This finite dimensional nonlinear problem is then implemented on a high performance computer, and solved iteratively to the desired degree of accuracy.

The nonlinearity of the Navier–Stokes equations (NSE) that describe viscous flow demands sophisticated numerical techniques and large computational resources for their

[14]A number is *finite* if we do not have to do an *endless* sequence of operations on other numbers to generate it. Thus, a finite set of selected points means that no matter how many there are, given enough time, you can count them all.

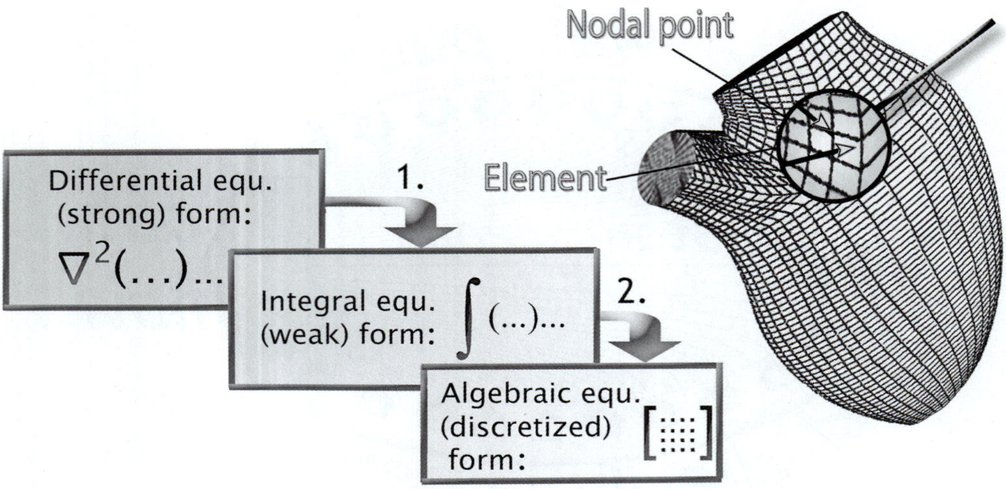

Figure 13.12: Diagrammatic representation of finite element discretization of the flow-field governing equations. In Step 1, the original governing differential equation, or *strong form*, is formulated as an integral variational *weak form* statement of the problem. This weak form is applied to the discretized domain through the introduction of a set of approximate nodal basis functions. In Step 2, this discretization of the weak form results in a discrete set of unknown coefficients that are related by a system of nonlinear algebraic equations, assembled in a matrix.

solution. The high Reynolds numbers applying during ejection require extremely fine 3-D computational grids. The strong time-dependence of ejection flow calls for high temporal resolution as well. Incorporation of detailed geometric data in the finite-element analysis can lead rapidly to inordinate computational costs. Increased storage and computing time requirements necessitate the use of a supercomputer and the adoption of special software for the solution of very large matrix equations.

The Fluid Dynamics Analysis Package (FIDAP™, Fluent Inc., Lebanon, NH) is one of the more popular available flow analysis commercial software packages, because of its ability to handle 3-D geometries. In studying LV fluid dynamics in the early 1990s, my pluridisciplinary Cardiac Function research group at the Duke ERC for Emerging Cardiovascular Technologies used FIDAP run on a supercomputer to generate numerical solutions for 3-D modeling of systolic ejection, in various configurations representing both normal and pathologic states. We considered the effects of outflow valve orifice to inner surface area ratios, and varying chamber eccentricities, on instantaneous ejection gradients along the outflow axis of the LV chamber. The local and convective acceleration components (*Rushmer* and *Bernoulli* components, see Section 13.3.6, on pp. 706 ff.) were evaluated separately in our CFD simulations. The individual absolute and relative contributions of these components to the total instantaneous LV intraventricular unsteady pressure gradient were found to vary very strongly depending on chamber outflow port area and eccentricity.

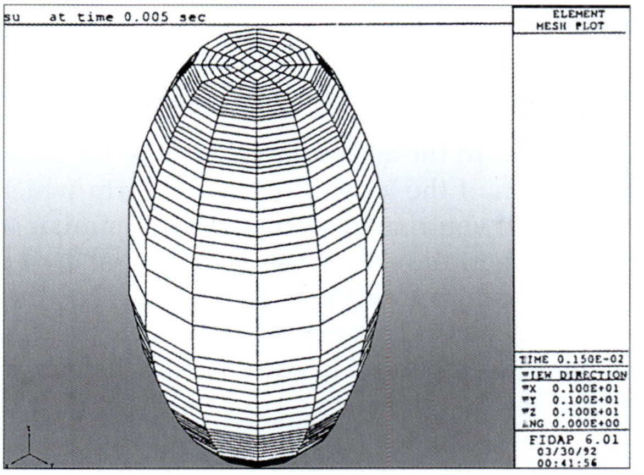

Figure 13.13: Boundary-fitted computational grid for a FIDAP model of the left ventricle. (Adapted from Hampton et al. [18], by kind permission of the American Society of Mechanical Engineers, Bioengineering Division.)

The complete Navier–Stokes equations have not been widely used in cardiac modeling because of the computational costs of their numerical solution. We obtained numerical solutions of the full NSE on a massively parallel processing supercomputer (CRAY Y-MP^{TM}, Cray Inc., Seattle, WA) using FIDAP coupled with our own custom software, written in FORTRAN [18, 19]. FIDAP is a general purpose code for simulating steady and transient flows of an incompressible viscous fluid in complex 2- or 3-D geometries. The flow governing equations are discretized on a grid of nodes and elements which conforms to the physical domain, i.e., the intraventricular LV flow field. FIDAP has a grid generator as part of its preprocessing capabilities. It also has a companion postprocessor program which has the capability of creating many types of desired flow-dataset information, including such graphical output as velocity-vector and pressure-contour plots.

Solution of the NSE for the LV ejection flow field requires the generation of *boundary-fitted* composite grids, because of the curved and complex shape of the LV cavity. Implementation of the applying boundary conditions is then simplified considerably, since the boundary coincides with the grid lines [17–19]. With FIDAP, it is possible to combine different elements within a given mesh, e.g., quadrilateral and triangular, to enable mesh discretization of complex geometries, such as that posed by the LV chamber. An example of a representative computational grid is shown in Figure 13.13. The chamber is modeled as a 3-D ellipsoid truncated by a plane passing through the aortic anulus. In the example shown, the mesh consists of 4,776 elements.

In considering the numerical simulation of an unsteady incompressible flow in an axisymmetric model of the LV chamber, we assumed blood to be a homogeneous, Newtonian fluid. As is implied by the diagram connecting wall velocities to instantaneous outflow velocity in Figure 13.11, on p. 711, the definition of the boundary conditions hinges on the definition of the instantaneous exit velocity, U_{exit}. The corresponding velocity of wall contraction, U_{wall}, was derived from the principle of conservation of fluid mass (continuity) for any given exit velocity. Under the assumption of incompressibility, this implies that the ratio of U_{wall}/U_{exit} is equal to the ratio of the outflow orifice cross-sectional area to the inner surface area of the LV chamber [36].

An important consideration in these simulations of the LV intraventricular flow field is the procedure for evaluation of the local acceleration term which appears in the NSE. Under the assumption that the ventricular cavity remains similar to itself as it contracts, the flow field is simplified: the ratio, R, of the velocities at two different points along the axis, e.g., $R = U_{\text{exit}}/U_s$, is constant with respect to time; i.e., the velocity field *remains self-similar* as the chamber contracts. This is possible only if the local acceleration field is *also self-similar*, and the relation embodied in equ. 13.10, which was developed in Section 13.3.5, on pp. 705 f., holds [36].

Our custom-made software was interfaced with FIDAP, in order to provide real-time analysis of the ejection process. A subroutine read a data file containing ejection velocity data digitized at either $200\ Hz$ or $500\ Hz$. Inputs to the program include the LV chamber volume at the onset of systole, the ratio of long to short axis, and aortic ring area. The output from the program is a series of FIDAP source files which define the ejection process, including all boundary and initial conditions representing wall velocities and accelerations.

13.4.1 Viscous flow simulation of the effects of ventriculoannular disproportion and varying LV chamber eccentricity

The effects of ventriculoannular disproportion (VAD), which in terms of the inviscid flow model simulation are summarized in Figure 13.9, on p. 707, were also investigated with this (*viscous*) computational model. Computer simulations of ejection were run on the CRAY Y-MP for chambers of various ratios of outflow orifice-to-inner surface area, and various chamber eccentricities. VAD was modeled by decreasing the chamber outflow orifice area. The simulation results are displayed in the left panel of Figure 13.14, on p. 715. The chamber volume was fixed for all cases at $150\ cm^3$. The ratio of long to short axis was fixed at 1.5. The volumetric outflow rate was set at $500\ cm^3/s$, representing conditions at peak ejection. The bottom curve corresponds to a normal outflow orifice area of $4.75\ cm^2$ (as do the top panels in Fig. 13.9) and the top curve to an abnormally low orifice area of $1.0\ cm^2$ (as the bottom panels in Fig. 13.9), such as would be encountered in moderately severe aortic stenosis. Mild stenosis, with a valve area of $2.75\ cm^2$ and an attendant VAD, is represented by the middle curve (cf. the bottom panels in Fig. 13.9).

At the time of peak flow, only the Bernoulli component is operative, and accounts fully for the total ejection pressure gradient, since the local acceleration is zero. However, increasing outflow orifice stenosis is characterized by a progressive augmentation of the Bernoulli gradient *throughout* ejection, rapidly rendering the Rushmer gradient negligible with severe or even moderate outflow orifice stenosis. This is to be contrasted to the normal situation (no ouflow valve stenosis or VAD), displayed in the right panel of

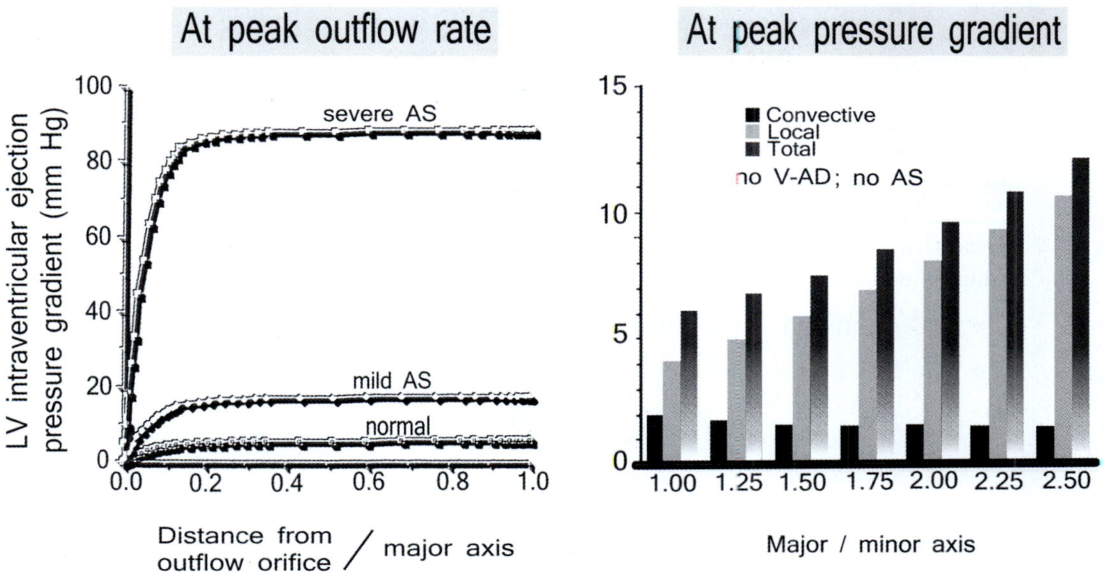

Figure 13.14: Left panel: The effect of stenosis of the outflow orifice area and of *ventriculoannular disproportion* on the intraventricular pressure gradient, at the time of peak LV outflow rate. Right panel: The relative contribution of local and convective components to the total instantaneous intraventricular pressure gradient as a function of *LV chamber eccentricity*, at the time of peak intraventricular pressure gradient in early ejection. (Adapted from Hampton, Shim, Straley, and Pasipoularides [18], by kind permission of the American Society of Mechanical Engineers, Bioengineering Division.)

Figure 13.14 where in early ejection, when velocities are low and the local accelerations high, the Rushmer gradient predominates.

These results, obtained using the complete NSE and the Finite Element method for viscous flow, *parallel* our previous findings summarized in Figures 13.9 and 13.10, on pp. 707 and 709, respectively, where a finite difference approach with an Alternating-Direction-Implicit (ADI) algorithm was implemented for an *inviscid* flow model. In particular, the strong accentuation of the axial pressure gradients, or slope of the total pressure versus distance from the outlet, in the *immediate vicinity* of the outlet, is striking with both approaches. Similarly, *both* computational approaches show the distribution of the local acceleration gradient to be much more uniform along the outflow axis than the convective component, and the striking augmentation of the convective acceleration component in the presence of ventriculoannular disproportion or organic outflow orifice stenosis.

For given chamber volume and outflow orifice area, a high chamber eccentricity requires higher intraventricular ejection pressure gradients for the same velocity and local acceleration values than do more spherical shapes. This finding agrees with the results of

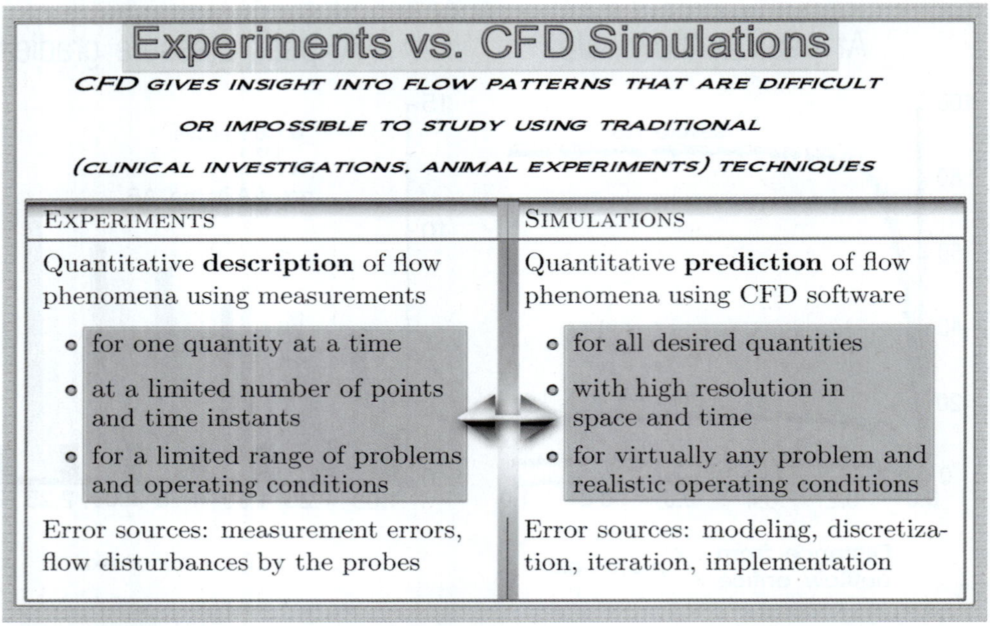

the inviscid finite difference approach, which are summarized in Figure 13.10. It is due to an enhancement of the local acceleration effects along the (longer) outflow axis. This is to be contrasted with the case of outflow orifice stenosis, in which the convective effects are shown by both approaches to be intensified strongly.

It should be noted that the finite element solution of the complete NSE yields results which are in excellent *qualitative* and *quantitative* agreement with the independent simulations employing the Euler (inviscid flow) finite difference model. These mutually independent CFD simulation results reflect accurately the fluid dynamics of the ejecting LV, as is verified by comparing them with the findings of numerous multisensor catheterization studies and analytical models of intraventricular flow [4,20,21,36,37,39–43,63].

13.5 Validation of PBM simulations

[15] During ejection, the unsteady intraventricular flow field is normally well behaved in its primary characteristics: unsteady streamlines originate in the endocardial surface of the LV chamber and converge onto the aortic anulus and into the root of the ascending aorta. By comparing measurements obtained at catheterization using high-fidelity multisensor catheters with the corresponding results obtained by CFD simulations of the ejection flow field, we can ascertain the validity and reliability of the CFD methodology. If the admittedly sparse quantitative micromanometric/velocimetric catheterization dataset is in

[15]See also the Appendix.

Verification of CFD codes

Verification amounts to looking for errors in the implementation of the models (loosely speaking, the question is: "are we solving the flow field governing equations right"?)

- Examine the computer programming by visually checking the source code, documenting it and testing the underlying subprograms individually
- Examine iterative convergence by monitoring the residuals, relative changes of integral quantities and checking if the prescribed tolerance is attained
- Examine consistency (check if relevant conservation principles are satisfied)
- Examine grid convergence: as the mesh and/or and the timestep are refined, the spatial and temporal discretization errors, respectively, should asymptotically approach zero (in the absence of round-off errors)

- Compare the computational results with analytical and numerical solutions for representative test cases.

good agreement with the corresponding CFD data *subset*, then one can accept the incomparably richer (see nearby tabular comparison of CFD simulations *vs.* measurements), in terms of spatial resolution, complete CFD simulation dataset with a high degree of confidence. The latter is strengthened further by qualitative and quantitative agreement of the CFD findings with findings obtained utilizing semiempirical correlation models, analytical fluid dynamic models, and noninvasive MRI PCVM and Doppler echocardiographic investigations of the intraventricular LV and RV ejection flow fields (see also the accompanying tabulation on this page).

13.5.1 Validation against an analytical fluid dynamic model of LV ejection

Figure 13.15, on p. 719, presents the output of a computerized analytical fluid dynamic model developed by Isaaz and Pasipoularides [21,36] for the instantaneous LV intraventricular ejection gradients in a normal human left ventricle. It shows the contributions by convective and local acceleration mechanisms to the total instantaneous pressure drop along the long axis of the chamber at three distinct instants of time during ejection.

Panel A represents conditions during the upstroke of ejection velocity measured by the catheter-mounted electromagnetic velocity sensor at the aortic ring. The striking augmentation of the total instantaneous pressure drop in the immediate vicinity of the aortic ring is underlain mainly by the convective acceleration effect. In contrast, beyond this portion of the field, the local acceleration effect is predominant and only a second-order convective acceleration effect is associated with the *collapse* of the walls of the chamber (see discussion on p. 65 of Section 2.13.) Panel B is representative of peak ejection when, because dQ/dt is zero, only convective inertial effects are operative and account fully for the total gradient. Panel C exemplifies conditions during the downstroke of the ejection flow. Now, the contribution of the local acceleration to the total instantaneous pressure drop is negative. Thus, it opposes the simultaneous effect of the convective opponent.

These results, obtained by an independent mathematical fluid dynamic model, are in agreement with the findings of the CFD simulations for inviscid and viscous flow employing finite difference and Finite Element methods, respectively, which we surveyed in Sections 13.3 and 13.4.

13.5.2 Catheterization results: normal ejection gradients

In considering findings from human cardiac catheterization studies of the fluid dynamics of ejection, which validate the results of CFD simulations using the Predetermined Boundary Motion method (PBM), the reader will find it instructive to begin by reviewing again Chapter 7, and particularly Section 7.5.8, on pp. 350 ff.

In a milestone study, simultaneous intraventricular pressure gradients and ejection flow patterns were measured by multisensor catheters in the Catheterization Laboratories at Brooke Army Medical Center [42]. The study group comprised six patients catheterized for evaluation of a chest pain syndrome. Biplane left ventriculography, proximal aortography, and routine hemodynamic measurements confirmed the precatheterization expectation on the basis of clinical examination, M-mode, and 2-D echocardiography that there was neither fixed nor dynamic outflow obstruction and no impairment of left ventricular (LV) function. All subjects were studied in a basal fasting state, and were unsedated or lightly premedicated with oral diazepam (10 mg) 1 hour before the procedure. The study was approved by the Clinical Investigation Department and the Human Use Committee at Brooke Army Medical Center [36,42].

A No. $7F$ or No. $8F$ (see Section 5.2, on pp. 243 ff.) Millar left heart multisensor catheter with 2 laterally mounted solid-state micromanometers, one at the tip and the second $5\ cm$ proximal, and an electromagnetic flow velocity probe at the level of the proximal (downstream) micromanometer (see top left panel in Fig. 13.16, on p. 721), was used for the fluid dynamic measurements. This retrograde catheter was manipulated so that the proximal sensors (pressure/velocity) were within the chamber as close as possible to the aortic ring, while the tip micromanometer was in the vicinity of the center of the chamber, as is illustrated in Figure 13.16. The velocity and pressure sensors (Mikro-Tip^{TM}, Millar Instruments, Inc., Houston, TX) and associated amplifiers were calibrated and pressure gain-settings were matched, as is described in Section 5.3, on pp. 247 ff. The flow velocity probe was energized using a sine wave flowmeter (model BL613, Biotronex, Silver Spring, MD.). The frequency response of the flow velocity measurements was determined primarily by the electronics with low-pass characteristics (see Section 2.17.1, on

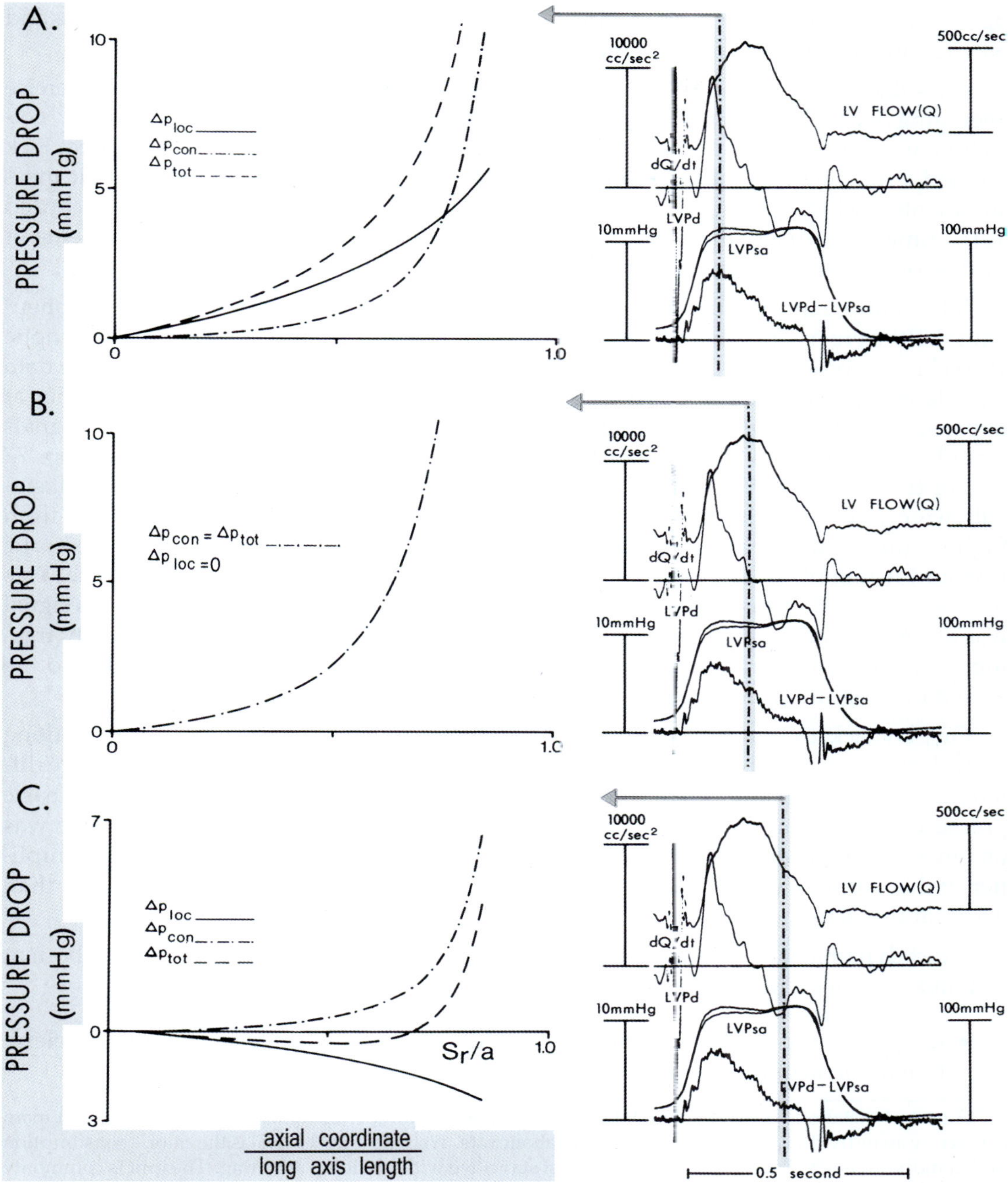

Figure 13.15: Output of a computerized analytical fluid dynamic model [21, 36] of normal LV ejection: contributions by convective and local acceleration mechanisms to the total instantaneous pressure drop along the long axis of the chamber, modeled as a truncated ellipsoid of revolution, at three distinct instants of time during ejection (arrows).

pp. 77 f.), down 3 dB at 100 *Hz*. A time delay of 5 *ms* was present at this filter setting and was accounted for in the measurements [42].

All subjects were studied at rest and during submaximal supine bicycle exercise averaging 3-4 METs[16], sustained at steady state over a 5-*min* period of Douglas bag[17] collection of expired air. Duplicate cardiac outputs were measured at rest by the direct Fick method,[18] and single determinations were made during exercise. All fluid dynamic measurements, including intraventricular pressure and flow velocity signals, were recorded at the time of cardiac output determination. Multiple thermodilution measurements of cardiac output were also obtained [15].

Intraventricular pressure and flow velocity, an ECG, and a respiratory signal (pneumatic belt) were recorded on a Honeywell 5600 analog tape recorder and an 1858 fiberoptic strip chart recorder (Test Instruments Division, Honeywell, Inc., Denver, CO.). The data were later replayed from the FM tape and displayed on the 1858 fiberoptic recorder at paper speeds of 200 *mm/s*; for all hemodynamic measurements, pressure and flow signals were low-pass filtered with corner frequencies at 100 *Hz* (see Section 2.17.1, on pp. 77 f.). For the representative hemodynamic signal *illustrations* shown in Figure 13.16 all signals were recorded with a lower filter setting of 20 *Hz*, to suppress any artifacts from high-frequency interference and noise. Because of the flat velocity profile at the aortic ring and negligible cyclic variations in the size of the ring, the flow velocity signal was used to represent instantaneous volumetric outflow. Volumetric calibration of this signal was accomplished by setting the systolic summated area under the ejection velocity tracing obtained by integration over 20 *beats* as equal to the outflow volume, scaled to the period of integration, determined from the simultaneous cardiac output value [42].

On playback, the left ventricular pressure and flow measurements were recorded along with electronically derived volumetric flow acceleration and intraventricular pressure difference signals, the latter displayed at a scale with 10 times the sensitivity of the basic pressures, as is shown in the top right panel of Figure 13.16. The flow derivative was obtained using an Accudata™132 (Honeywell, Inc., Denver, CO) differentiating amplifier with a corner frequency of 800 *Hz*; the time delay of the differentiator was less than 0.5 *ms* at this setting.

Fluid dynamic variables averaged from at least 10 steady-state cardiac cycles, both at rest and in exercise in each subject, were

- the peak intraventricular gradient and the volume flow velocity and flow acceleration at the instant at which the peak gradient occurred and

[16] A unit of metabolic equivalent, or MET, is defined as the number of calories consumed per min in an activity by an individual relative to the basal metabolic rate. A single unit (1 MET) is the caloric consumption of that individual while at complete rest, or to just stay alive without doing anything. The unit is commonly used in the context of physical exercise, to gauge its intensity. A workout of 2–4 METs is considered light, while intensive running (8 *min/mile*) can yield exercise intensities of 12 or more METs.

[17] A rubber-lined canvas bag for the collection of gas exhaled by a person, to be used to measure oxygen uptake during exercise. It is not as convenient to use as the newer Waters oximetry hood [25].

[18] A method for measuring cardiac output at steady-state in which the rate of oxygen uptake by the lungs is divided by the arteriovenous oxygen difference, to give the rate of blood flow across the pulmonary capillaries and the cardiac output.

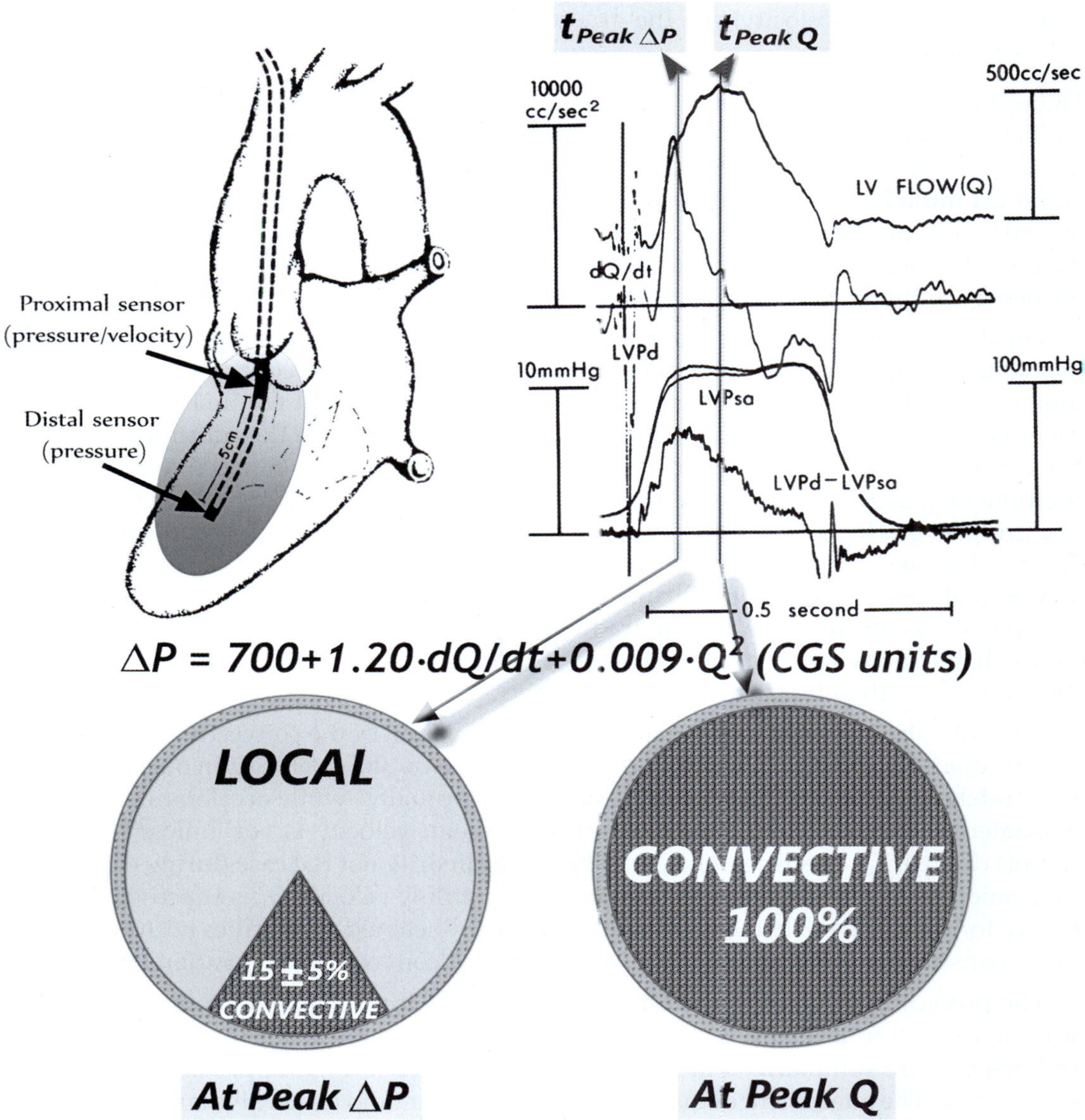

Figure 13.16: Top left: Multisensor catheter placement for measurement of intraventricular pressure gradients and outflow velocity. The distance between the two micromanometers is 5 *cm*; the velocity sensor is at the same site as the downstream micromanometer. Top right: Oscillographic recording illustrating the impulsive early systolic development of ejection flow acceleration and intraventricular pressure gradient. Bottom panel: Early in ejection, at peak pressure gradient, the local acceleration pressure gradient accounts for about 85% of the total inertial gradient. With the sharp rise in ejection velocity, the balance *tilts rapidly* in favor of the convective acceleration component. At peak flow, the latter accounts for 100% of the measured intraventricular pressure gradient. (Adapted from figures in Pasipoularides et al. [42], by kind permission of the AHA.)

- the peak flow velocity and the gradient at the instant at which the peak velocity occurred.

The unknown model parameters α and β of a semiempirical fluid dynamic model for the flow-associated local and convective LV intraventricular ejection pressure gradients (equation shown in Fig. 13.16) were estimated by standard formal identification technique via multivariate least-squares regression. The input dynamic measurements used were the volume flow velocity and acceleration at peak pressure gradient, and the output data was the peak intraventricular ejection gradient. Validation of the model was accomplished by numerical and statistical criteria arising from the least-squares procedure.

For the combined rest and exercise data, the local acceleration component was found to account for roughly 85% of the total peak inertial gradient. Its contribution tends to be somewhat higher at rest than during exercise, because dQ_r/dt at the time of peak gradient is not augmented as much as the outflow velocity and Q_r^2 in the transition from rest to exercise. At peak flow, the local acceleration is zero and the convective acceleration component accounts for 100% of the inertial intraventricular ejection gradient (Fig. 13.16). The impulse gradient associated with the local acceleration effect is proportional to the distance between upstream and downstream measurement sites [36, 42]. Since its contribution in absence of outflow obstruction amounts to roughly 85% of the total measured peak instantaneous intraventricular gradient, it follows that the values of the impulse gradients that actually apply across the *entire length* of the LV outflow axis should be considerably *higher* than those measured across the *5-cm length* of the multisensor catheter.

It should also be noted that the numerical formulation of the convective ejection pressure gradient component in terms of the square of the outflow velocity, in our semiempirical model equation, is somewhat misleading conceptually: while acceleration is always associated with a force and thus a pressure gradient, velocity is not, unless significant viscous dissipative effects are present, which is ordinarily not the case during ejection. In our semiempirical formulation, the square of the outflow velocity Q_r^2 is effectively used as a *proxy* for the *difference* between the squares of the linear axial velocities at the upstream and downstream measurement sites, which entails a convective acceleration process.

The preceding results obtained by an independent fluid dynamic method in absence of LV anatomic abnormalities or dysfunction are in harmony with the CFD simulation findings that are summarized in Figures 13.9, 13.10, and 13.14, on pp. 707, 709, and 715, respectively. The attainment of the peak intraventricular (and transvalvular) pressure gradient early in ejection, and well before the attainment of the peak flow rate, is the major distinguishing hallmark of the nonobstructive ejection pressure gradient. With tight or moderate outflow valvular stenosis, the intraventricular subvalvular and the transvalvular peak ejection pressure gradient are attained *later* in systole at the time of the *peak* ejection rate.

13.5.3 Catheterization results: ejection gradients in aortic stenosis

The total instantaneous intraventricular pressure drop can be measured by multisensor catheter across a 5 *cm* segment along the LV long axis. The intervening segment in

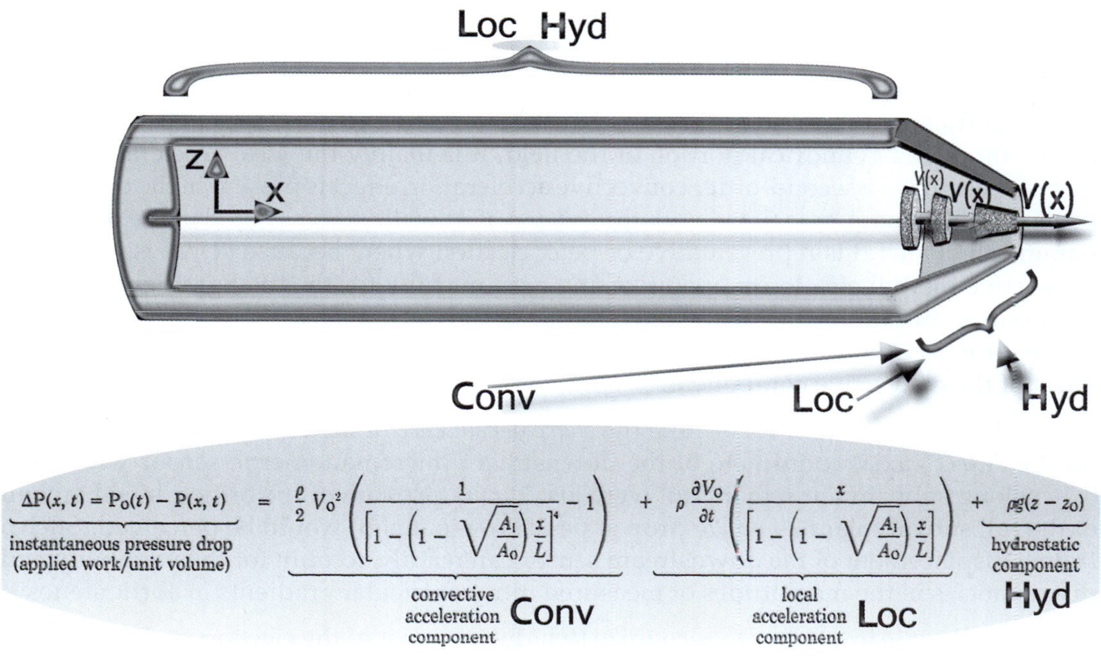

Figure 13.17: Top panel: Diagrammatic representation of a 5 *cm* segment (the distance between the micromanometers in the left-heart multisensor catheter) comprising a 4.5 *cm* cylindrical portion and a 0.5-*cm* long subvalvular tapering region. (Collage adapted from the model development in Pasipoularides et al. [43], by kind permission of the American Physiological Society.)

presence of aortic valvular stenosis can be modeled geometrically as comprising a 4.5 *cm* cylindrical portion and a 0.5-*cm* long subvalvular tapering region, as is shown in Figure 13.17. Across this segment arise the contributions by convective (Conv) and local (Loc) acceleration mechanisms, and possibly by coexisting hydrostatic (Hyd) effects, to the measurable total instantaneous pressure drop.

The equation for the apportionment of the instantaneous pressure drop between the upstream station (0) and any other station (x) along the tapering segment is given in the bottom panel of Figure 13.17. The first term on the right side corresponds to the applying convective acceleration effect; the second term corresponds to the local acceleration effect, and the last term to the hydrostatic effect. The latter can be eliminated altogether by choosing to impose a horizontal orientation on the tapering tract, which corresponds to the outflow axis of the LV chamber. Although a second-order convective acceleration effect is present in the cylindrical portion of the model, associated with the *collapse* of its walls (see discussion on p. 65 of Section 2.13.), it is negligible in comparison with the convective component in the 0.5-*cm* long subvalvular tapering region.

Figure 13.18, on p. 725, presents the output of a computerized fluid dynamic model developed by Pasipoularides et al. [36, 43] for the intraventricular pressure gradient in aortic stenosis. Panel A represents conditions during the upstroke of ejection velocity (V_0) at the aortic ring, just upstream of the short conical region, which represents the stenosed valve (see also Fig. 13.17). The striking augmentation of the total instantaneous pressure drop in aortic stenosis is underlain mainly by the convective acceleration effect. In contrast, in the untapered cylindrical portion of the field, it is mainly the local acceleration effect that is operative—a second-order convective acceleration effect is present in the cylindrical portion of the model, associated with the *collapse* of its walls, as was noted in the preceding paragraph. Panel B is representative of peak ejection when, because dQ/dt is zero, only convective inertial effects are operative and account fully for the total gradient. Panel C exemplifies conditions during the downstroke of the ejection flow. Now, the contribution of the local acceleration to the total drop is negative. Thus, it opposes the simultaneous effect of the convective component.

In all panels of Figure 13.18, note the *sharp dependence* of the convective pressure drop on the *"exact"* axial coordinate of the downstream micromanometric sensor within the 0.5-*cm* long subvalvular region; if it were just 1 *mm* upstream of the orifice, less than half of the full subvalvular 60-*mm Hg* drop at peak flow (panel B) would be perceived. Such a *trifling* displacement of the downstream sensor can readily account for the variability and discrepancies in the magnitudes of measured intraventricular gradients in aortic stenosis.

Clinically, it is important to recognize that during most of the ejection period, a lateral pressure measurement made *just upstream* of the stenosed orifice is apt to underestimate elevated wall and cavity pressures throughout *most* of the left ventricle. Such a situation would also complicate evaluation of the patient with low gradient aortic stenosis (LGAS), which constitutes an infrequent but not rare challenging situation for clinical decision making. Similarly, transvalvular decreases could be underestimated considerably if the upstream micromanometric sensor happens to be within the tapering subvalvular region rather than deep in the chamber. Such potential pitfalls for micromanometric gradient and pressure determination are usually not encountered with the standard fluid-filled systems using multiple side holes. Obviously, however, any information about subvalvular gradients is completely lacking with the crude standard technique.

These results, obtained by an independent mathematical fluid dynamic model, are again in agreement with the findings of the CFD simulations of LV *intraventricular* ejection pressure gradients in the presence of outflow valve stenosis for inviscid and viscous flow, employing finite difference and Finite Element methods, which were surveyed in Sections 13.3 and 13.4, respectively.

13.6 Clinical implications of ejection gradients

Because intraventricular flows are generally dominated by inertial rather than viscous forces, ejection gradients go mostly into local and convective accelerations. These impulsive gradients bring about a briskly accelerated expulsion of blood into the root of the aorta (and pulmonary artery) and then reverse direction and decelerate the flow to bring ejection to a rapid end. In absence of outflow obstruction, it is the maximal outflow

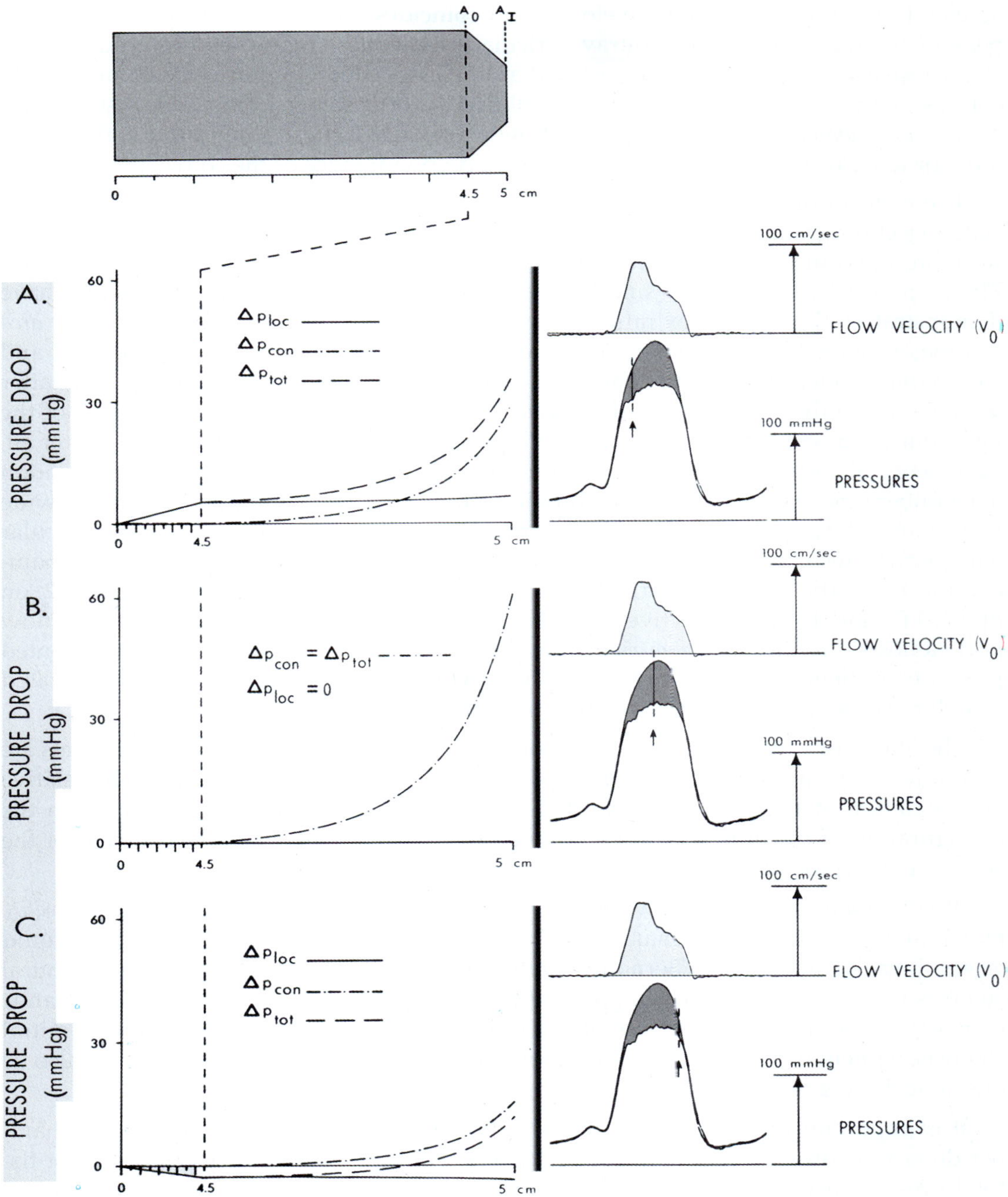

Figure 13.18: Output of a computerized analytical fluid dynamic model of intraventricular gradients in aortic stenosis (cf. Fig. 13.15). (Reproduced, slightly modified, from Pasipoularides et al. [43], by kind permission of the American Physiological Society.)

acceleration rather than ejection velocity that coincides with the attainment of the early peak of the transvalvular and intraventricular gradients. These pressure gradients are characteristically even more *asymmetric* than the associated ejection velocity signals. In contrast, large obstructive gradients exemplified in aortic stenosis tend to be distinctively *rounded and symmetric*, as do also the outflow waveforms, whose configuration they track more or less closely, depending on the relative preponderance of the convective effects.

The concept of *ventriculoannular disproportion* in the dilated ventricle, and the associated ejection gradient characteristics referable to enhanced convective inertial effects, were brought out distinctly in the CFD results (see Figs. 13.9 and 13.14, on pp. 707 and 715, respectively. As the CFD simulations of the ejection flow field in this chapter have demonstrated, the area index ratio of *aortic anulus cross-section*-to-*inner-wall surface area* is a major geometric determinant of intraventricular ejection gradients. Both local and convective acceleration components of the pressure gradient are accentuated, the latter more so, when this area index is depressed. In view of the discussion of the CFD of the intraventricular ejection flow field in aortic stenosis, this makes intuitive sense. After all, the essence of aortic stenosis is the diminution of the size of the outflow orifice in relation to chamber size. As seen in diverse chronic volume overload conditions, including wide aortic valvular regurgitation, and in the various dilated cardiomyopathies, left ventricular enlargement results in a relative disproportion between the size of the globular chamber and the aortic ring—a ventriculoannular disproportion (see Sections 7.9 and 8.2, on pp. 369 ff. and 410 ff., respectively), which is *functionally equivalent* to a relative outflow port stenosis. Accordingly, ventriculoannular disproportion can account for augmented pressure gradients in the enlarged ventricle, which may not be accompanied by elevated velocities of circumferential fiber contraction, or dR/dt.

The effects of ventriculoannular disproportion on impulse and Bernoulli gradients are exemplified further in Figure 8.2, on p. 415, and the associated discussion. The relative augmentation of the convective effects is responsible for characteristic changes in the configuration of ejection pressure gradients, which are qualitatively reminiscent of the pattern that typifies aortic valve stenosis.

A *reduction* in chamber size would increase the *area index* (ratio of aortic ring, or *orifice* in valvular stenosis, to inner chamber surface area). Such a chamber size reduction would *depress* impulse and *a fortiori* Bernoulli coefficients in aortic stenosis coexisting with mitral stenosis from levels that would apply with a larger ventricle. This is the fluid dynamic explanation for the occasional *"masking"* of coexisting aortic stenosis in the setting of mitral stenosis, a phenomenon described in classic textbooks of cardiology [36]. It could also be one contributing factor in the syndrome of *"low gradient aortic stenosis."*

It is important to bear in mind that the dynamics of flow within the ejecting chamber determine only the instantaneous *gradients* of intraventricular pressure and not the total pressure itself (see Section 7.9, on pp. 369 ff.). The systolic portion of the lateral pressure waveform at the aortic root contributes a very large additional component that acts uniformly throughout the collapsing chamber and over its entire shrinking inner surface. The aortic root pressure waveform embodies the interactive coupling between ejection kinematic patterns and the systemic arterial input impedance. Thus, the total ventricular (pressure) load comprises both *extrinsic* and *intrinsic* dynamic components [36]; total muscle (wall stress) load comprises corresponding fractions. Intrinsic and extrinsic components are in a dynamic interplay in the course of every ejecting beat, and their interaction is *complementary* and *competitive* [36] (see Sections 7.9 and 8.2, on pp. 369 ff. and 410 ff., respectively). Similar considerations apply for the right heart and pulmonary arterial root; the only difference being that, in view of the much lower normally applying levels of the outflow trunk pressure, the intrinsic component represents a *much larger* portion of the systolic total right ventricular (pressure) load than on the systemic side.

At present, contributions to our understanding of ejection dynamics come from many directions and sources: from both fundamental and clinical studies of ventricular pumping and myocardial contractile behavior; from use of multisensor catheterization and digital angiocardiographic techniques; from detailed Doppler echocardiographic and color flow mapping measurements and quantitative magnetic resonance velocity imaging and mappings; and from simulations based on computerized analytic and CFD approaches to the unsteady intraventricular ejection flow equations. The more sophisticated of these approaches, both instrumentational and theoretic, have developed rapidly over the last few years. They are now defining ejection flow-field characteristics at a level of detail *unimagined* less than a generation ago. (However, we should acknowledge that key pioneers in this area of cardiac research, such as Rushmer, identified major features of the local acceleration component of normal ejection dynamics nearly half-a-century ago [61].)

As advances have occurred in instrumentation and measurement techniques, so accurate instantaneous dynamic data can be and are routinely collected in invasive and noninvasive diagnostic studies combined with patient-specific CFD simulations. The importance of such studies stems from the opportunity they offer to assess ejection dynamics in a quantitative dynamic fashion, such that abnormalities in contraction may be elicited *before* the manifestation of overt heart muscle or pump failure. Several areas of research are emerging (see also Chapter 16):

Ventricular ejection flow-field dynamics: What is important here is how normal and abnormal geometric details, including regional contraction abnormalities, affect ejection velocity and pressure distributions. Critical questions are: Can characteristics, at rest and with provocation, of intraventricular gradients be used to assess ventricular pumping and myocardial contractile performance? Can abnormal geometry or contraction patterns, or both, induce valve leaflet dysfunction (aortic preclosure, mitral systolic anterior motion) and how? A related interesting issue is whether typical distortions in multigated 3-D Doppler and 3-D velocity-encoded MRI velocity profiles in the aortic root, without or with provocation, map out *specific regional patterns* of asynergy, asynchronism or hyper- and hypocontractility. To incorporate all relevant phenomena of the ejection process and the continuously changing irregular geometry, methods from computational fluid dynamics will need to be employed. Ejection flows pose a challenging problem for CFD. Their high Reynolds numbers require extremely fine 3-D computational grids, and their strong time dependence calls for high temporal resolution as well.[19] Results of the CFD research reviewed in this chapter are encouraging.

Quantitation of Rushmer (local) and Bernoulli (convective) pressure gradients with and without outflow obstruction: In coming years, the old familiar paradigms of (mean) pressure overload and (mean flow) volume overload will be supplemented or *superceded* by new cardiodynamic concepts. These will pertain to *phasic* ejection variables and their characteristics in health and disease. The essential questions here are: What are the relative intensities, waveshapes of and phase relations between the local and convective acceleration contributions to the total ejection pressure gradients and systolic ventricular load? How do they change with time, pharmacologic agents (afterload reducing, inotropic) or interventions (valvuloplasty, surgery)? How are they modified, in view of complementarity and competitiveness between intrinsic and extrinsic load components, by coexisting arterial hypertension? The ultimate questions are: How do the relative preponderance of Rushmer (proportional to myocardial fiber acceleration) and Bernoulli (proportional to myofiber velocity squared) components of the intrinsic load influence the evolution of muscle stresses and global and regional kinematics? How does this relative preponderance influence physiologic adaptations and pathologic processes involving the myocardium over the long term? Integration of such quantitative information into a coherent framework will require sophisticated mathematic modeling involving adaptive control systems theory, entailing control parameters that can be modified as needed, in order to adapt ejection dynamics to changing (patho)physiologic conditions and demands. A basic relevant fact is that the heart compensates very well, e.g., for the presence of even severe muscle damage, and this fact demonstrates the effectiveness of the feedback mechanisms that can be brought into play, adaptive mechanisms that are by no means fully understood.

Over the coming years, a confluence of intellectual advances, progress in imaging and hemodynamic high technology instrumentation, and powerful computing capabilities and CFD and visualization software, will shape a new model of what diagnostic and interventional cardiology are and what clinical hemodynamicists do. The limits of past static concepts and ideas will need to be extended to encompass the true dynamic behavior of the ejection process, in health and disease. This underlines the growing need for clinicians and basic scientists alike to keep their intellectual muscles in good trim to cope with the demands of the growing spectrum of quantitative imaging and CFD evaluation approaches and, above all, with the implications of the information that they can provide.

---

[19]Bear in mind also that, as we have discussed at some length in Sections 12.6.2 and 12.8.2, on pp. 652 ff. and 665 ff., respectively, for a simulation to be stable, it must comply with the Courant–Friedrichs–Lewy (CFL) condition given by Equation 12.1, on p. 665. See also related discussion on pp. 761 f.

References and further reading

[1] Adeler, P.T., Jacobsen, J.M. Blood flow in the heart. In: Ottesen, J.T., Olufsen, M.S., Larsen, J.K. [Eds.] Applied mathematical models in human physiology. 2004, Philadelphia: Society for Industrial and Applied Mathematics. xiii, 298 p.

[2] Bermejo, J., Antoranz, J.C., Yotti, R., Moreno, M., Garciá-Fernández, M.A. Spatio-temporal mapping of intracardiac pressure gradients A solution to Euler's equation from digital postprocessing of color Doppler M-mode echocardiograms. Ultrasound Med. Biol. 27: 621–30, 2001.

[3] Beyer, R.P. A computational model of the cochlea using the immersed boundary method. J. Comput. Phys. 98: 145–62, 1992.

[4] Bird, J.J., Murgo, J.P., Pasipoularides, A. Fluid dynamics of aortic stenosis: subvalvular gradients without subvalvular obstruction. Circulation 66: 835–40, 1982.

[5] Caiani, E.G., Corsi, C., Sugeng, L., MacEneaney, P., Weinert, L., Mor-Avi, V., Lang, R.M. Improved quantification of left ventricular mass based on endocardial and epicardial surface detection with real time three-dimensional echocardiography. Heart 92: 213–9, 2006.

[6] Caiani, E.G., Corsi, C., Zamorano, J., Sugeng, L., MacEneaney, P., Weinert, L., Battani, R., Gutierrez, J.L., Koch, R., De Isla, L.P., Mor-Avi, V., Lang, R.M. Improved semiautomated quantification of left ventricular volumes and ejection fraction using 3-dimensional echocardiography with a full matrix-array transducer: comparison with magnetic resonance imaging. J. Am. Soc. Echocard. 18: 779–88, 2005.

[7] Chen, C.J. Finite analytic method in flows and heat transfer. 2000, New York: Taylor & Francis. xix, 332 p.

[8] Chorin, A.J. Numerical solution of the Navier–Stokes equations. Math. Comput. 22: 745–62, 1968.

[9] DeGroff, C.G., Thornburg, B.L., Pentecost, J.O., Thornburg, K.L., Gharib, M., Sahn, D.J., Baptista, A. Flow in the early embryonic human heart: a numerical study. Pediatr. Cardiol. 24: 375–80, 2003.

[10] Dillon, R., Fauci, L., Gayer, D. A microscale model of bacterial swimming, chemotaxis and substrate transport. J. Theor. Biol. 177: 325–40, 1995.

[11] Dillon, R., Fauci, L., Fogelson, A., Gayer, D. Modeling biofilm processes using the immersed boundary method. J. Comput. Phys. 129: 57–73, 1996.

[12] Ding, T., Schoephoerster, R. Evaluation of global left ventricular function based on simulated flow dynamics computed from regional wall motion. Am. Soc. Mechan. Engin., Bioengin. Div.(ASME BED) Adv. Bioengin. 35: 193–4, 1997.

[13] Dubini, G., Redaelli, A. Different finite element approaches to fluid-structure interaction problems in biofluid mechanics. Ann. Biomed. Eng. 25: 218–31, 1997.

[14] Ebbers, T., Wigström, L., Bolger, A.F., Engvall, J., Karlsson, M. Estimation of relative cardiovascular pressures using time-resolved three-dimensional phase contrast MRI. Magn. Reson. Med. 45: 872–9, 2001.

[15] Espersen, K., Jensen, E.W., Rosenborg, D., Thomsen, J.K., Eliasen, K., Olsen, N.V., Kanstrup, I.L. Comparison of cardiac output measurement techniques: thermodilution, doppler, CO2-rebreathing, and the direct Fick method. Acta Anaesthesiol. Scand. 39: 245–51, 1995.

[16] Fletcher, C.A.J., Srinivas, K. Computational techniques for fluid dynamics, 3 Vols. [v. 1. Fundamental and general techniques – v. 2. Specific techniques for different flow categories – v. 3. A solutions manual.], 2nd ed. 1991, Berlin; New York: Springer-Verlag.

[17] Georgiadis, J.G., Wang, M., Pasipoularides, A. Computational fluid dynamics of left ventricular ejection. Ann. Biomed. Eng. 20: 81–97, 1992.

[18] Hampton, T., Shim, Y., Straley, C., Pasipoularides, A. Finite element analysis of cardiac ejection dynamics: Ultrasonic implications. Am. Soc. Mechan. Engin., Bioengin. Div.(ASME BED) Adv. Bioengin. 22: 371–4, 1992.

[19] Hampton, T., Shim, Y., Straley, C., Uppal, R., Smith, P.K., Glower, D., Pasipoularides, A. Computational fluid dynamics of ventricular ejection on the CRAY Y-MP. IEEE Proc. Comp. Cardiol. 19: 295–8, 1992.

[20] Hoadley, S.D., Pasipoularides, A. Are ejection phase Doppler/echo indices sensitive markers of con-tractile dysfunction in cardiomyopathy? Role of afterload mismatch. Circulation 76: Suppl. IV-404, 1987.

[21] Isaaz, K., Pasipoularides, A. Noninvasive assessment of intrinsic ventricular load dynamics in dilated cardiomyopathy. J. Am. Coll. Cardiol. 17: 112–21, 1991.

[22] Jacobsen, J., Adeler, P.T., Kim, W., Houlind, K., Pedersen, E., and Larsen, J. Evaluation of a 2D heart model against magnetic resonance velocity mapping. Cardiovasc. Eng. 1: 59–76, 2001.

[23] Jones, T.N., Metaxas, D.N. Patient-specific analysis of left ventricular blood flow, Medical Image Computing and Computer-Assisted Intervention (MICCAI'98), Cambridge, MA, October, 1998. Lecture Notes in Computer Science 1496: pp. 156–66, Springer, 1998.

[24] Keber, R. Simulation der Strömung im linken Ventrikel eines menschlichen Herzens. Universität Karlsruhe, Fak. f. Maschinenbau. Diss. v. 22.07.2003.

[25] Kern, M.J. The Cardiac Catheterization Handbook. 4th ed. 2003, Philadelphia, PA: Mosby. xx, 650 p.

[26] Kim, W.Y., Walker, P.G., Pedersen, E.M., Poulsen, J.K., Oyre, S., Houlind, K., Yoganathan, A.P. Left ventricular blood flow patterns in normal subjects: a quantitative analysis by three-dimensional magnetic resonance velocity mapping. J. Am. Coll. Cardiol., 26: 224–38, 1995.

[27] Kiris, C., Kwak, D., Benkowski, R. Incompressible Navier–Stokes calculations for the development of a ventricular assist device. Comput. Fluids 27: 709–19, 1998.

[28] Laszt, L., Müller, A. Über den Druckverlauf im linken Ventrikel und Vorhof und in der Aorta ascendens. Helv. Physiol. Acta 9: 55–73, 1951.

[29] Lotz, J., Meier, C., Leppert, A., Galanski, M. Cardiovascular flow measurement with phase-contrast MR imaging: basic facts and implementation. RadioGraphics 22: 651–71, 2002.

[30] McQueen, D.M., Peskin, C.S. Shared-memory parallel vector implementation of the immersed boundary method for the computation of blood flow in the beating mammalian heart. J. Supercomput. 11: 213–36, 1997.

[31] McQueen D.M., Peskin C.S. A three-dimensional computer model of the human heart for studying cardiac fluid dynamics. Comput. Graph. 34: 56–60, 2000.

[32] Oertel jr, H. [Ed.] In: Prandtl – Führer durch die Strömungslehre. Grundlagen und Phänomene. 11th ed. 2002, Braunschweig, Wiesbaden: Vieweg Verlag. xi, 718 p.

[33] Oertel, H. Modelling the human cardiac fluid mechanics. 2005, Karlsruhe: Univ.-Verl. iv, 49 p.

[34] Park, J., Metaxas, D.N., Axel, L. Analysis of left ventricular wall motion based on volumetric deformable models and MRI-SPAMM. Med. Image Anal. 1: 53–71, 1996.

[35] Pasipoularides, A., McElhaney, J.H. Introduction. In: Pasipoularides, A., McElhaney, J.H. [Eds.] Special Issue: Hemodynamics. Ann. Biomed. Eng. 20: 1–2, 1992.

[36] Pasipoularides, A. Clinical assessment of ventricular ejection dynamics with and without outflow obstruction. J. Am. Coll. Cardiol. 15: 859–82, 1990.

[37] Pasipoularides, A. Cardiac mechanics: basic and clinical contemporary research. Ann. Biomed. Eng. 20: 3–17, 1992.

[38] Pasipoularides, A. Complementarity and competitiveness of the intrinsic and extrinsic components of the total ventricular load: Demonstration after valve replacement in aortic stenosis [Editorial]. Am. Heart J. 153: 4–6, 2007.

[39] Pasipoularides, A., Kussmaul, W.G., Myers, B.S., Doherty, B.J., Stoughton, T.L., Laskey, W.K. Phasic characteristics of transaortic pressure gradients in valvular stenosis. J. Am. Coll. Cardiol. 17: 254A, 1991.

[40] Pasipoularides, A., Miller, J., Rubal, B.J., Murgo, J.P. Left ventricular ejection dynamics in normal man. In: Melbin, J., Noordergraaf, A. [Eds.] Proceedings of the Vlth International Conference and Workshop of the Cardiovascular System Dynamics Society. Philadelphia, PA: University of Pennsylvania, 1984: pp. 45–8.

[41] Pasipoularides, A., Murgo, J.P. Ejection dynamics in man with and without outflow obstruction. In: Proceedings of the 20th Annual Meeting of the Association for the Advancement of Medical Instrumentation. 1985, Boston: AAMI. p. 68.

[42] Pasipoularides, A., Murgo, J.P., Miller, J.W., Craig, W.E. Nonobstructive left ventricular ejection pressure gradients in man. Circ. Res. 61: 220–7, 1987.

[43] Pasipoularides, A., Murgo, J.P., Bird, J.J., Craig, W.E. Fluid dynamics of aortic stenosis: Mechanisms for the presence of subvalvular pressure gradients. Am. J. Physiol. 246: H542–50, 1984.

[44] Pasipoularides, A., Murgo, J.P., Bird, J.J., Craig, W.E. Fluid dynamics of aortic stenosis: Mechanisms of subvalvular gradient generation. In: Proceedings of the Sixth Annual Conference of the American Society of Biomechanics. 1982, Seattle: ASB. p. 5.

[45] Pasipoularides, A.D., Shu, M., Womack, M.S., Shah, A., von Ramm, O., Glower, D.D. RV functional imaging: 3-D echo-derived dynamic geometry and flow field simulations. Am. J. Physiol. Heart Circ. Physiol. 284: H56–65, 2003.

[46] Pasipoularides, A.D., Shu, M., Shah, A., Womack, M.S., Glower, D.D. Diastolic right ventricular filling vortex in normal and volume overload states. Am. J. Physiol. Heart Circ. Physiol. 284: H1064–72, 2003.

[47] Pasipoularides, A., Shu, M., Shah, A., Tucconi, A., Glower, D.D. RV instantaneous intraventricular diastolic pressure and velocity distributions in normal and volume overload awake dog disease models. Am. J. Physiol. Heart Circ. Physiol. 285: H1956–65, 2003.

[48] Peaceman, D.W., Rachford, H.H., Jr. The numerical solution of parabolic and elliptic differential equations. J. Soc. Indust. Appl. Math. 3: 28–41, 1955.

[49] Peng, Y., Wu, S., Geng, S., Liepsch, D., Liao, D., Qiao, A., Zeng, Y. Theoretical approach to blood ejection from the human left ventricle. Biorheology 42: 271–81, 2005.

[50] Peskin, C.S. Numerical analysis of blood flow in the heart. J. Comput. Phys. 25: 220–52, 1977.

[51] Peskin, C.S. The immersed boundary method. Acta Numer. 11: 479–517, 2002.

[52] Peskin, C.S., McQueen, D.M. A three-dimensional computational method for blood flow in the heart: I Immersed elastic fibers in an incompressible fluid. J. Comput. Phys. 81: 372–405, 1989.

[53] Peskin, C.S., McQueen, D.M. A three-dimensional computational method for blood flow in the heart: II Contractile fibers. J. Comput. Phys. 82, 289–98, 1989.

[54] Peskin, C.S., McQueen, D.M. A general method for the computer simulation of biological systems interacting with fluids. Symp. Soc. Exp. Biol. 49: 265–76, 1995.

[55] Peskin, C.S., Printz, B.F. Improved volume conservation in the computation of flows with immersed elastic boundaries. J. Comput. Phys. 105 33–46, 1993.

[56] Pozrikidis, C. Fluid dynamics: theory, computation, and numerical simulation: accompanied by the software library FDLIB. 2001, Boston: Kluwer Academic Publishers. x, 675 p.

[57] Redaelli, A., Maisano, F., Schreuder, J.J., Montevecchi, F.M. Ventricular motion during the ejection phase: a computational analysis. J. Appl. Physiol. 89: 314–22, 2000.

[58] Redaelli, A., Montevecchi, F.M. Computational evaluation of intraventricular pressure gradients based on a fluid-structure approach. J. Biomech. Eng. 118: 529–37, 1996.

[59] Redaelli, A., Montevecchi, F.M. Intraventricular pressure gradients dp/dx and aortic blood acceleration df/dt as indexes of cardiac inotropy: a comparison with dp/dt based on computer fluid dynamics. Med. Eng. Phys. 20: 231–41, 1998.

[60] Rebergen, S.A., van der Wall, E.E., Doornbos, J., de Roos, A. Magnetic resonance measurement of velocity and flow: technique, validation, and cardiovascular applications. Am. Heart J. 126: 1439–56, 1993.

[61] Rushmer, R.F. Initial ventricular impulse: a potential key to cardiac evaluation. Circulation 29: 268–83, 1964.

[62] Saber, N.R., Gosman, A.D., Wood, N.B., Kilner, P.J., Charrier, C.L., Firmin, D.N. Computational flow modeling of the left ventricle based on in vivo MRI data: initial experience. Ann. Biomed. Eng. 29: 275–83, 2001.

[63] Shim, Y., Hampton, T.G., Straley, C.A., Harrison, J.K., Spero, L.A., Bashore, T.M., Pasipoularides, A.D. Ejection load changes in aortic stenosis. Observations made after balloon aortic valvuloplasty. Circ. Res. 71: 1174–84, 1992.

[64] Sondergaard, L., Stahlberg, F., Thomsen, C. (1999) Magnetic resonance imaging of valvular heart disease. J. Mag. Res. Imag. 10: 627–38, 1999.

[65] Song, S.M., Leahy, R.M., Boyd, D.P., Brundage, B.H., Napel, S. Determining cardiac velocity fields and intraventricular pressure distribution from a sequence of ultrafast ct cardiac images. IEEE Trans. Med. Imag. 13: 386–97, 1994.

[66] Taylor, T., Yamaguchi, T. Flow patterns in three-dimensional left ventricular systolic and diastolic flows determined from computational fluid dynamics. Biorheol. 32: 61–71, 1995.

[67] Taylor, T., Yamaguchi, T. Realistic three-dimensional left ventricular ejection determined from computational fluid dynamics, Med. Eng. Phys. 17: 602–8, 1995.

[68] Thompson, J.F., Warsi, Z.U.A., Mastin, C.W. Boundary-fitted coordinate systems for numerical solutions of partial differential equations. A review. J. Comp. Phys. 47: 1–108, 1982.

[69] Tyszka, J.M., Laidlaw, D.H., Asa, J.W., Silverman, J.M. Three-dimensional, time-resolved (4D) relative pressure mapping using magnetic resonance imaging. J. Mag. Res. Imag. 2000 12: 321–9, 2000.

[70] Wang, M., Georgiadis, J.G. Controlled grid generation on PC and workstation for heat transfer. Am. Soc. Mechan. Engin., Heat Transfer Div. (ASME HTD) 185: pp. 67–74, New York, 1991.

[71] Wang, N.T., Fogelson, A.L. Computational methods for continuum models of platelet aggregation. J. Comput. Phys. 151: 649–75, 1999.

[72] Wang, X-F., Deng, Y-B., Nanda, N.C., Deng, J., Miller, A.P., Xie, M-X. Live three-dimensional echocardiography: imaging principles and clinical application. Echocardiography 20: 593–604, 2003.

[73] Yang, G.Z., Kilner, P.J., Wood, N.B., Underwood, S.R., Firmin, D.N. Computation of flow pressure fields from magnetic resonance velocity mapping. Magn. Reson. Med. 36: 520–6, 1996.

[74] Yoganathan, A.P., Lemmon, J.D., Kim, Y.H., Walker, P.G., Levine, R.A., Vesier, C.C. A computational study of a thin-walled three-dimensional left ventricle during early systole, J. Biomech. Eng. 116: 307–14, 1994.

[75] Yoganathan, A.P., Lemmon, J.D., Kim, Y.H., Levine, R.A., Vesier, C.C. A three-dimensional computer investigation of intraventricular fluid dynamics: examination into the initiation of systolic anterior motion of the mitral valve leaflets. J. Biomech. Eng. 117: 94–102, 1995.

[76] Yotti, R., Bermejo, J., Antoranz, J.C., Rojo-Álvarez, J.L., Allue, C., Silva, J., Desco, M.M., Moreno, M., Garciá-Fernández, M.A. Noninvasive assessment of ejection intraventricular pressure gradients. J. Am. Coll. Cardiol. 43: 1654–62, 2004.

[77] Zabusky, N.J. Solitons and energy transport in nonlinear lattices. Comput. Phys. Comm. 5: 1–10, 1973.

Chapter 14

CFD of Ventricular Filling: Heart's Vortex

...tous les mouvements qui se font au Monde sont en quelque façon circulaires... [All movements that take place in the World are in some fashion circular.]—Descartes (1596–1650).

——René Descartes: Oeuvres Philosophiques, ed. Ferdinand Alquié (Paris, 1963), I, 332.

VENTRICULAR DIASTOLIC FILLING is a highly unsteady flow process in a chamber with complex and time-dependent geometry; as such, its quantitative fluid dynamic analysis in health and disease is fraught with extreme mathematical difficulties. Nonetheless, ventricular diastolic filling abnormalities, and diastolic cardiac dysfunction as an important component of congestive heart failure, are now sufficiently recognized as to be a new part of coding for congestive heart failure in the Tenth Revision of the International Classification of Diseases (ICD-10, codes I50.30-33). This World Health Organization recognition of diastole has come on the heels of forward strides in the assessment of diastolic function [3,4,65,120,121], as technology has progressed beyond multisensor cardiac catheterization to new digital noninvasive imaging modalities. It is now widely appreciated that enhancing diastolic filling has clinical merit and that the clinical significance of diastolic dysfunction is far reaching [89].

The fact that diastolic ventricular filling is dependent on a large number of factors and interactions (see Fig. 7.13, on p. 344) has frustrated investigators and clinicians for decades. At present, characterization of ventricular diastolic function remains one of the great challenges in cardiology. In this chapter, we will focus on some recent research findings and cardiodynamic concepts regarding interactions of formative fluid dynamic mechanisms with intracardiac filling patterns and diastolic function changes accompanying ventricular enlargement and dilatation [78–80]. The underlying research aimed at a better understanding of right ventricular (RV) diastolic myocardial properties and mechanics utilizing chronically instrumented animal models of RV disease [81,82]. The concepts regarding interactions of fluid dynamic mechanisms with intracardiac diastolic flow phenomena are general, however, and should apply in the *left heart* too.

14.1 Myocardial diastolic function

The initial phase of the research which brought about the viewpoints presented here involved baseline and longitudinal studies [81,82] on surgical canine models of RV volume overload, pressure overload and myocardial ischemia, utilizing right-heart multisensor Millar catheters and specially designed pulse-transit ultrasonic dimension transducers. Only chronically instrumented conscious dogs were studied, because of the important, multifaceted limitations of acute studies under conditions of anesthesia, recent surgery, and open-chest [51,81].

As far as RV diastolic myocardial function is concerned, in contrast to the results obtained for RV pressure overload and myocardial ischemia, no significant change from control was found with volume overload in the RV time constant of relaxation, tau (τ). The only significant change in volume overload was a raised RV diastolic pressure asymptote, reflecting increased diastolic pericardial constraint from elevated right heart volumes [25,42,65]. These results suggest that the relaxation mechanism is unimpaired in subacute-to-chronic RV volume overload.

A new *sigmoidal* model for passive filling pressure *vs.* volume relations and resultant RV myocardial compliance formulations was developed and used, along with the conventional exponential approach. The sigmoidal model is more sensitive to changes in the pressure-volume curve than the exponential; it showed that the passive diastolic properties of the RV muscle changed significantly from control with RV pressure overload, ischemia and volume overload [82]. The maximum RV myocardial compliance, which is attained during early filling, was reduced significantly from control with pressure overload and ischemia but not with volume overload [82]. The passive filling pressure at which maximum compliance is reached was higher in pressure overload than at control.

As noted above, in contrast to pressure overload, in volume overload the pressure-volume relationship shifts downward in the early portion of the filling process [82]. In pressure overload, the RV end-diastolic pressure was greatly elevated but the decrease in the end diastolic RV myocardial compliance did not attain statistical significance. In RV ischemia, no significant change was seen in either end-diastolic myocardial compliance or end-diastolic pressure. End-diastolic myocardial compliance actually increased in volume overload compared to control, while end-diastolic pressure was unchanged [82]. Because of this diastolic compliance rise, in RV volume overload, there is less of a tendency to elevate central venous pressure than in RV pressure overload or myocardial ischemia. In volume overload by tricuspid regurgitation it is the regurgitant flow surge (v-wave, see Fig. 14.6 B.a., on p. 749) itself that can *directly* elevate central venous pressure.

The above findings regarding myocardial relaxation and diastolic compliance properties correlate with familiar clinical observations that the right ventricle, as a thin-walled, low-pressure system (see Section 7.1, on pp. 325 ff.), tolerates increases in the *preload* better than increases in the *afterload*. This may partly explain why, e.g., acute RV failure after cardiac transplantation occurs commonly due to high pulmonary vascular resistance in the transplant recipient, while patients with congenital heart disease or rheumatic

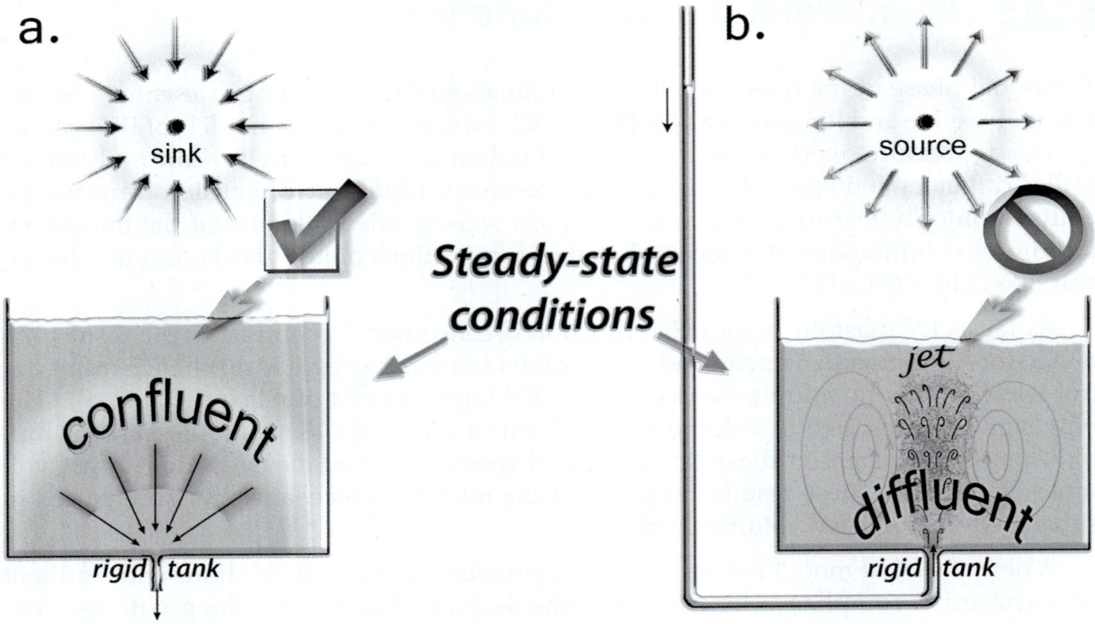

Figure 14.1: Left panels: The upper half of the *"point sink"* flow of the top left panel *can* be used, as shown in the bottom panel, to model the flow pattern developed within a large tank emptying through an outflow orifice in its flat bottom. Right panels: The upper half of the *"point source"* flow of the top right panel *cannot* be used to model the flow pattern developed within a large tank being filled through an inflow orifice. As is shown in the bottom right panel, the flow pattern fails to even approximately follow in reverse the streamlines of the bottom left panel; rather, it separates from the boundary and forms a central jet that is surrounded by a prominent large scale vortex. This is a much more complicated flow behavior than that applying to the emptying process. Such a *nonsymmetric behavior* is typical with nonlinear processes, entailing convective acceleration and deceleration (cf. Section 9.2, on pp. 444 ff).

heart disease can tolerate tricuspid regurgitation and pulmonary valvular regurgitation for decades.

14.2 Fluid dynamic underpinnings of diastolic function changes with chamber dilatation

The most provocative aspect of the findings of the preceding cardiac mechanics investigations is that RV volume overload resulted in minimal abnormalities relative to control in the RV myocardial properties compared to the other RV disease models [81,82]. Since RV size in RV volume overload ($60 \pm 29\ mL$) increased greatly ($P < 0.05$) from control

($45 \pm\ 21\ mL$), reflecting myocardial creep and remodeling, it was hypothesized that it might be responsible for heretofore unrecognized dynamic filling changes relative to control. Therefore, it became apparent that a fuller understanding of integrative RV diastolic mechanics would only be obtained by expanding the scope of the diastolic function investigations beyond the studies of RV myocardial dynamics, including myocardial relaxation and myocardial compliance. A comprehensive examination of the *fluid dynamic* aspects of ventricular loading during filling [78–80] thus came about.

The ensuing fluid dynamic studies of filling in the normal and the volume overloaded right ventricle confirmed the existence of important and until then *unrecognized* mechanisms, responsible for the filling impairment in the volume-overloaded, dilated chamber. These underlying mechanisms were revealed and investigated through a new Functional Imaging (FI) method [78], which is a particular implementation to animal- or patient-specific data of the Predetermined Boundary Motion method (see Sections 10.5, 13.1.2, and 13.3, on pp. 566 ff., 685 ff., and 694 ff., respectively).

In FI, an integrated software system can accept data from real-time 3-D echocardiographic (RT3D) and other digital imaging sources, such as computed tomography or magnetic resonance imaging, to generate dynamic geometric reconstructions of the cardiac chambers, which are then passed on to an automatic finite element mesh generator and a CFD finite element solver (see Chapters 12 and 13).

Following computational solution of the flow-governing field equations with appropriate boundary and initial conditions, the flow fields of interest are displayed using scientific visualization techniques, as explained in Chapters 12 and 13. The FI method yields values of velocity and pressure at literally scores of thousands of discrete points in space and time within each cardiac flow field simulated. From these *"high-density of information"* datasets, interactive graphic modules can extract high-resolution scientific visualization plots of instantaneous intraventricular flow velocity and pressure distributions.

14.3 Disparate patterns of confluent and diffluent flows

The nature of the mathematical difficulties that the study of ventricular filling entails can be appreciated intuitively by considering Figure 14.1, on p. 738. The top left panel of Figure 14.1 depicts a mathematically hypothesized "point flow-sink," where fluid is being removed at a certain volumetric flow rate, Q. The flow into a flow-sink is spherically symmetric, since removal of fluid at the sink draws more fluid toward it equally from all directions in the main body of fluid.

The magnitude of the linear velocity, v, of inward radial flow across any spherical surface at distance r from the point sink, with area $4\pi r^2$, is clearly

$$v = Q/(4\pi r^2)\,, \tag{14.1}$$

if the volume flow across the surface is to balance the rate, Q, of fluid removal at the sink. Thus, the velocity is increasing as r decreases, and the flow is accelerating convectively,

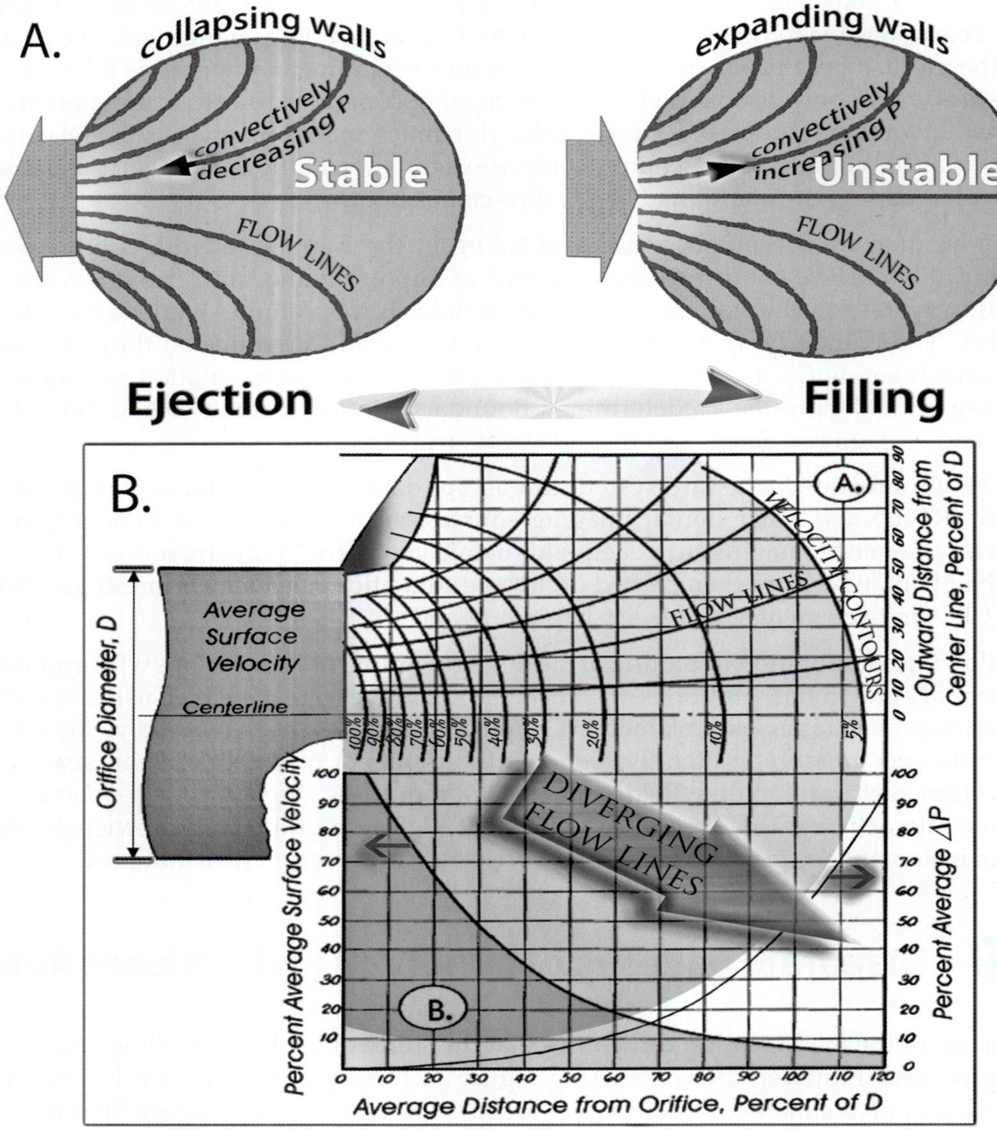

Figure 14.2: **A.** In diastole, the reversal of flow direction from the *outflow sense* applying for systole to the *inflow sense* applying for diastole should produce a *diffluent* flow that is faced with an *adverse* convective pressure gradient and is, therefore, not capable of persisting. **B.** Schematic representation of the *Bernoulli-induced* pressure changes (ΔP) associated with the convectively produced accelerations (*converging flow lines*) and decelerations (*diverging flow lines*) in an ellipsoidal chamber. Note the decreasing average surface velocities applying at successive velocity contour surfaces that are at increasing distances from the chamber (*inflow*) orifice. The associated *Bernoulli-induced* pressure increase (ΔP) is striking.

as it moves radially inwardly. There is consequently no tendency toward any disturbance and a radial, confluent, streamline pattern can prevail.

The same general tendency is exemplified by a confluent, radially accelerating, flow into an outflow orifice at the bottom of a tank, as in the lower left panel of Figure 14.1; there is no tendency toward boundary layer separation as the fluid flows along the solid internal surface of the bottom of the tank, as is discussed in Section 4.12.1, on p. 209 f. The intraventricular flow field during ejection exemplifies an analogous behavior, with confluent streamlines spanning the contracting space between the collapsing walls of the chamber and the outflow valve orifice (see top panel of Fig. 7.2, on p. 328).

We now consider the situation with reversed flow direction where fluid is being introduced into the tank at a steady volumetric flow rate, Q. We encounter what on the face of it is startling to anyone familiar only with linear dynamics where, if we were to *change the sign* of a velocity solution we would obtain a *reversed field of motion*, namely, the "point flow-source," identical with that of the sink but with the direction of flow reversed on each streamline, as shown in the top right panel of Figure 14.1—see also Sections 2.6 and 4.4.2, on pp. 53 ff. and 176 f., respectively. At the flow-source, fluid is appearing at the steady volumetric flow rate Q. The question of whether this flow can persist as a steady pattern of fluid motion with solid boundaries depends on rules which are embodied by the nonlinear Navier–Stokes equations (NSE) of motion. There is actually no reason whatsoever why the *reversal* of the flow direction applying in the bottom left panel should produce an *enduring* flow pattern.

Indeed, plain experience bears out the fact that fluid emerging from a pipe into a fluid-filled tank with the geometry of the lower panels of Figure 14.1 shows no persisting tendency to follow the streamlines of the left panel in reverse, spreading out in all radial directions. Instead, the fluid forms a *jet* and the flow goes through a massive boundary layer separation at the orifice itself. This is because, along the solid surface, the flow would entail a radially outward motion of speed $Q/(4\pi r^2)$, which decreases *extremely abruptly* as r increases, implying a strong *convective deceleration* and an *adverse pressure gradient* by the Bernoulli theorem (see Section 4.4.6, on pp. 182 ff.). This adverse pressure gradient induces boundary layer separation at the orifice, and generates the large-scale toroidal vortex that encircles the jet-type flow within the central core. Thus, the motion in the lower left panel is not "reversible." In fact, steady flow into a large tank through an orifice in its flat bottom fails even approximately to follow in reverse the simple confluent radial streamlines suggested in the lower left panel of Figure 14.1; rather, it exhibits a *complex pattern*, as is suggested in the juxtaposed lower right panel.

The foregoing considerations have implications of fundamental importance for the fluid dynamics of ventricular filling, as is summarized pictorially in Figure 14.2, on p. 740. The ejection flow with streamlines directed radially inward from the collapsing walls of the ventricular chamber toward the "sink" at the outflow orifice proceeds down the pressure gradient of a convectively *accelerating* flow field, and is *stable*. On the contrary, the diastolic filling flow with streamlines directed radially outward from the "source" at the inflow orifice toward the expanding walls must proceed *against* the adverse pressure gradient of a convectively *decelerating* flow field, and is consequently *unstable*.

14.4 The role of high-pass filters

It should be emphasized, at this juncture, that high-pass filters (see Section 2.17.1, on pp. 77 ff.) commonly referred to as *"wall filters,"* are used routinely to remove from the Doppler cardiac flow datasets signals corresponding to frequencies (velocities) that are below a threshold frequency (see Section 5.9, on pp. 280 ff.). In some cases, the operator has control over the threshold frequency and can adjust it up or down; usually, however, the wall filter is set automatically by the anatomic configuration for which the scanner is set. Accordingly, in situations where the flow velocities are very low, as near the expanding walls of a filling ventricular chamber during the *upstroke* of the E-wave, a wall filter set with too high a threshold inadvertently removes these Doppler shift frequencies (see Section 5.9.3, on pp. 282 ff., and Fig. 5.33, on p. 285). As a result of this, the corresponding intense convective decelerations *fail to be noted* by clinicians and technicians alike.

Intraventricular flow field investigators must pay attention to ensure that the proper instrument configuration is used when exploring the spatiotemporal evolution of the intraventricular flow field, especially during the *upstrokes* of the E- and A-waves. It is nevertheless impossible to adjust the angle of insonation to maximize the obtainable Doppler shifts for complex unsteady fields with multidirectional instantaneous velocities, as those characterizing vortical filling patterns.

14.5 Overview of the CFD challenge

In view of the preceding considerations, it is to be expected that the CFD of ventricular filling presents great challenges.[1] Extreme mathematical difficulties are encountered in the dynamic mesh generation process involving the time-dependent, complicated geometry of the cardiac chambers, especially for the right ventricle (see Fig. 14.5, on p. 747). Because of its particularly complicated dynamic geometry, the fluid dynamics of diastolic filling had remained essentially unexplored for the right ventricle [65,74], until the publication of our CFD investigations [78–80], although in the relatively simpler case of the left ventricle CFD had been shown to hold great importance in the investigation of ventricular function [59,72,88,92]. The strong velocity fluctuations, which occur in the form of the E- and A-wave ventricular inflow surges, require high temporal and spatial resolutions for direct numerical simulation, such that can be implemented only on the most powerful of currently available computing machines. Presently available numerical solutions of the NSE, implemented on high-performance computers, enable the simulation of 3-D, highly time-dependent, incompressible diastolic filling flows for (patho)physiologically encountered Reynolds numbers.

Because of the large storage capacities required, parallel vector computers are preferred for intensive diastolic flow-field simulations. The domain of integration is divided into several subdomains (cf. Fig. 12.19, on p. 660) with each of them assigned to a processor of a parallel vector computer. Such parallelization necessitates the exchange of

[1]See also the Appendix.

data across the boundaries of the computational subdomains, and special communication procedures have to be implemented to guarantee computationally effective simulations. Moreover, the numerical simulation of flows containing vortices requires the flow field to be resolved with fine grid-spacing so that the details of the motion of the vortices and their interactions with anatomic structures, such as atrioventricular valve leaflets, can be adequately described.

Two other problems that need to be mentioned here are the analysis and the presentation of the computed *flow-field data*. Because of the great quantity of data to be handled, parallel computers may also be necessary for the scientific visualization of the results. Since time-dependent flows are considered, time dependent visualization techniques should also be brought into play; the evolution of flow-field characteristics can be depicted by, e.g., showing particle traces, streak lines, streamlines, or vortex lines, as *functions of time* in the course of diastole. Such representations require specific methods of data handling, which can be rather time-consuming if large amounts of data have to be sent across the boundaries of flow-field subdomains (see Section 12.7, on pp. 657 ff.). However, the presently available computers offer the possibility of capturing large diastolic intraventricular vortex structures with good accuracy [96,118]. To indicate the magnitude of the visualization task, we note that closed or spiraling streamlines must be computed for *identifying* the vortex cores. This can be done in the following way: the velocity field is first obtained for a specified time level by numerical integration of the unsteady flow-field governing Navier–Stokes equations. Then the velocity vectors are projected on a plane, chosen with an orientation such that the axes of the vortical structures expected to intersect the plane do so, if possible, at a right angle. In the next step, elements of the streamline projections in the chosen plane are pieced together from the projections of the velocity vectors with the aid of the discretized differential equation for the streamlines. Subsequently, the process is repeated for subsequent time levels of interest in the course of the simulation of the evolution of the diastolic filling process.

Direct quantitative comparison of flow simulations with animal experiments or clinical measurements for intraventricular flow fields remains impracticable. Therefore, qualitative comparisons of flow-field patterns derived by imaging methods, including color flow mapping and 3-D Doppler and magnetic resonance velocity mapping, as well as quantitative comparisons with fluid dynamic data subsets gained by multisensor catheterization and angiography, are used for validation of the CFD methodologies and verification of the simulation results. Although the predictions cannot quantitatively be validated in the "native" *spatiotemporal detail* of the CFD simulations, a better understanding of flow phenomena in the cardiac chambers in health and disease can be obtained, which is crucial for future developments in pathophysiology, diagnosis and management.

Transvalvular right-sided pressure differences can be identified and measured under experimental (hyperdynamic) conditions and demonstrate dynamic characteristics, including timing relative to inflow velocity, similar to those reported by Isaaz [52] for the left-sided atrioventricular transvalvular pressure drop. On the other hand, right-sided instantaneous intraventricular diastolic pressure gradients are smaller [80] than their left-sided counterparts are, and generally do not render themselves to reliable micromanometric multisensor catheter measurement.

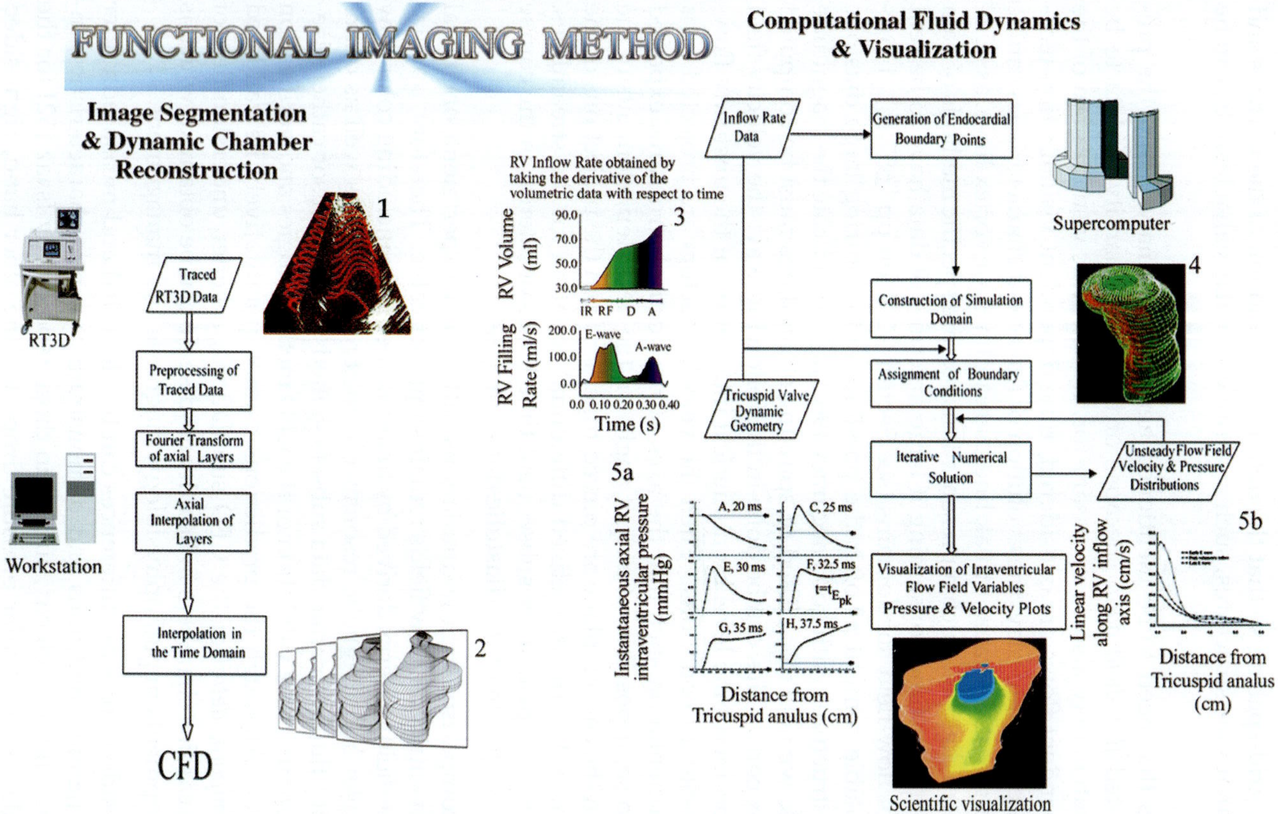

Figure 14.3: Functional Imaging (FI) comprises three parts. First, a semiautomated segmentation aided by intraluminal contrast medium locates the RV endocardial surface. Second, a geometric scheme for dynamic RV chamber reconstruction applies a time interpolation procedure to the RT3D data to quantify wall geometry and motion at 400 Hz. Finally, the RV endocardial border motion information is used for mesh generation on a computational fluid dynamics (CFD) solver to simulate development of the early RV diastolic inflow field. Boundary conditions (tessellated endocardial surface nodal velocities) for the solver are directly derived from the endocardial geometry and motion information. Postprocessing visualization provides flow field dynamic plots and graphic renderings of pressure and velocity. (Adapted from pictorial representations in refs. [78–80], by permission of the American Physiological Society.)

High-resolution dynamic pressure and velocity spatiotemporal distributions of the intraventricular RV flow field obtained by the Functional Imaging method revealed time-dependent, remarkable interactions [80] between intraventricular local acceleration and convective pressure gradients. Not only does the smallness of the normal early diastolic intraventricular pressure gradients render their measurement by catheter unreliable, but, until the CFD studies on which we are focusing in this chapter, this smallness also concealed the important fluid dynamic mechanisms which underlie them. These mechanisms entail, as we shall see shortly, an interplay between convective and local acceleration effects.

14.5.1 Validation of simulated velocity fields using MR measurements

Quantitative validation of velocity field simulations by means of high-quality phase-contrast MRI is not a trivial undertaking even for simple velocity fields, because of MRI's lower temporal resolution, because velocity accuracy and precision are highly dependent on acquisition parameters, and because MR voxel shapes and dimensions *do not* coincide with those of the CFD grid cells. A thorough review is available [62] regarding accuracy of phase-contrast measurements with regard to MR image acquisition parameters and data processing. Moreover, spatial resolution has been shown to have a considerable effect on the accuracy of MRI velocity data [46]. In any case, the velocity fields obtained in the CFD simulation studies should *replicate* those measured by MRI, at least in coarse magnitude, qualitative flow patterns and complexity, and temporal variation. Here, MRI flow visualization is in the *supporting* role (CFD code validation), computer simulation in the *leading* (quantitative) role.

When comparing CFD-derived unsteady velocity fields to results acquired by MR velocity measurements, one should be aware that in MR flow imaging a *phase difference threshold* [90] is commonly used (see Section 14.4, on pp. 742, and Section 5.9.3, on pp. 282 ff.), vitiating detection of *low-velocity regions* in convectively decelerated diastolic fields. Moreover, nonperiodic flow phenomena will not be captured because MR velocity fields are periodic as a result of *temporal averaging*. In any event, one can perform consistency checks by means of so-called convergence studies, looking at the effect of increased or decreased spatial and temporal resolution of the computational grid on the velocity field data, to gain some insight into the validity of any particular CFD simulation (see Appendix).

14.6 The Functional Imaging (FI) method in RV filling simulations

Because of the complicated dynamic RV geometry, our investigations of RV filling dynamics required application of the Functional Imaging method (see also Section 10.5, on pp. 566 ff.), which comprises real-time, 3-D cardiac imaging, and computational fluid dynamics (CFD), as is indicated in Figure 2.38, on p. 103. Figure 14.3, on p. 744, summarizes pictorially the main steps of this method, which has been detailed in several publications

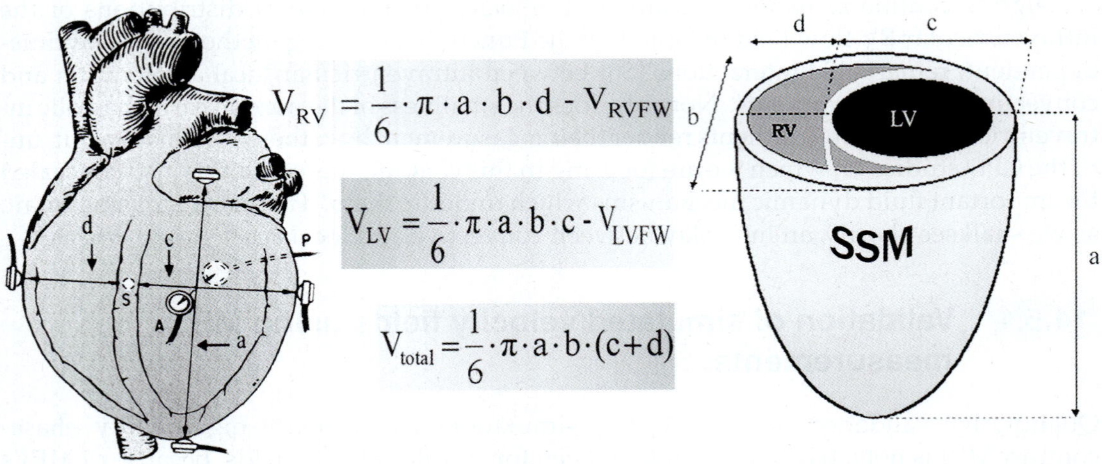

Figure 14.4: Diagram of the instrumented canine heart demonstrating the sonomicrometric implanted sensors (left) and measured dimensions needed for application of the Duke shell subtraction model (right). V_{RVFW} denotes the right ventricular (RV) free wall (FW) volume, determined by water displacement during autopsy. LV, left ventricular; V_{total}, total volume. (Slightly modified from Pasipoularides et al. [82], by kind permission of the American Physiological Society.)

from our laboratory [78–80]. Geometric fidelity between the actual dynamic geometry of the RV chamber and its computational reconstruction is crucial to obtaining accurate CFD results. The FI method has been experimentally validated [78] both under control and volume overload conditions. It has been shown under both conditions to yield RV diastolic flow-field spatiotemporal velocity and pressure distribution patterns [78–80] that are in complete agreement with the available left-sided experimental and clinical findings [9, 10, 91, 101, 109].

14.6.1 Experimental animals and procedures

Experiments were performed on seven 20- to 30-kg dogs. The dogs were premedicated with cefazolin (500 mg) and anesthetized with intravenous pentobarbital (20 mg/kg) and succinylcholine (1 mg/kg). They were ventilated with a respirator (MA 1TM, Puritan-Bennett; Los Angeles, CA). Sonomicrometric transducers were sewn, as indicated in Figure 14.4, across the base-apex, anterior-posterior, and septal-free wall axes of the LV, and across the RV septal-free wall axis for volume measurements, and for the validation of the RT3D-derived dynamic RV chamber reconstruction [35, 41, 78] using the Duke shell subtraction (SSM) model [35, 41, 64, 82, 94], both under control conditions and during subacute, surgically induced, volume overload.

Each experimental animal recovered for 7–10 days before being subjected to control data acquisition in a lightly sedated (morphine 0.7 mg/kg), awake state. Control data

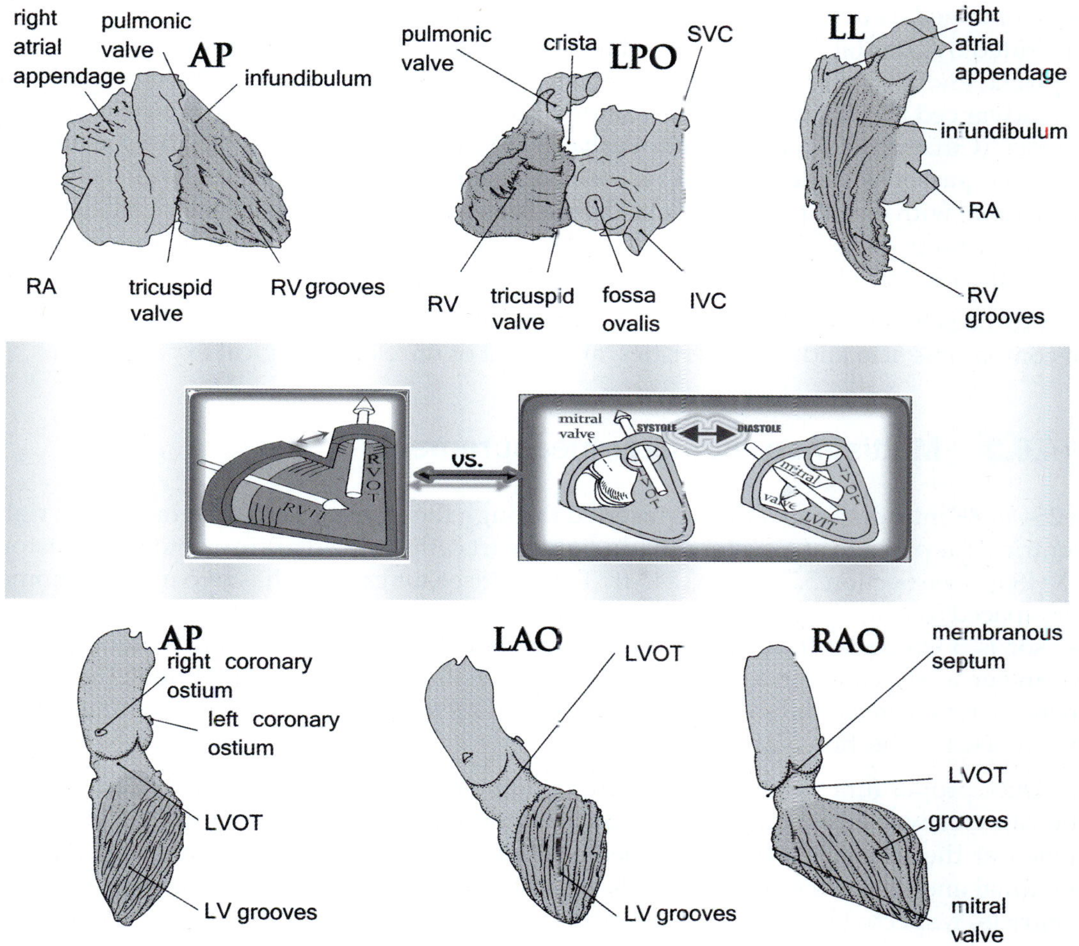

Figure 14.5: Top panels: Different views of a plastic cast of the right heart of a dog demonstrating the complex anatomy of the right ventricle (RV) and its *distinct* inflow (RVIT) and outflow (RVOT) tracts, as highlighted in the inset (middle panels). The inlet chamber is closer to the apex than the outlet. Ridges in all the casts correspond to blood-conducting grooves in the chamber walls; note the curved trajectory of the blood from the apex to the outlet. Bottom panels: Different views of a cast of the left heart. As in the right ventricle, the blood grooves from the inlet to the apex of the left ventricle (LV) are again short and straight; along the outflow tract (LVOT) from the apex to the aortic outlet the grooves follow a curved pathway and are longer. The functional significance of this particular architecture has not been established. We may assume that the grooves act as blood channels. Conceivably, the viscoelastic myocardial ridges dampen vibrations of the blood over certain frequencies. Developmental reasons, as well as the existence of the papillary muscles may also be responsible for this configuration. As shown in the inset, inlet and outlet long axes are separated by around 90°in the right ventricle; in the left, the corresponding angle amounts to about 30°. AP = anteroposterior view, LL = left lateral; LAO = left anterior oblique; LPO = left posterior oblique; RAO = right anterior oblique; SVC = superior vena cava; IVC = inferior vena cava.

were obtained as described in the following Sections. Subsequently, *volume overload* was instituted by chordal rupture-induced tricuspid regurgitation. The right jugular vein was exposed, and an 8F (French size, see Section 5.2, on pp. 243 ff.) 25-cm introducer sheath was advanced into the right ventricle under fluoroscopic guidance. A 6F urological biopsy forceps (Circon Instruments; Santa Barbara, CA) was then inserted via the sheath, and multiple passes were taken to sever chordae until 3–4 + regurgitation was developed [78,81,82], with elevation of right atrial pressures assessed micromanometrically (see Fig. 14.6 B., a, on p. 749). The vein was ligated and the wound closed. Volume overload data were taken 2–3 weeks later in a similar manner to control.

Cardiac chamber casts (see Fig. 14.5, on p. 747) were obtained in another eight dogs of comparable size and characteristics, at the end of unrelated surgical experiments.

14.6.2 Multisensor catheter measurements

A 25-cm 8F introducer sheath was inserted through the exterior jugular vein into the right ventricle for passage of a custom-made right heart catheter (Millar Instruments; Houston, TX) [80]—see Section 5.2, on pp. 243 ff. The multisensor catheter has two micromanometers spaced 5 cm apart; the distal micromanometer is at the tip, and a Doppler velocimeter sensor is 3 cm away from the distal micromanometer. The micromanometers and velocimeter were soaked in a saline bath at $36-38°C$ for a minimum of 3 hours; the micromanometers were simultaneously balanced, and all sensors were calibrated immediately before use (see Section 5.2, on pp. 243 ff.).

Once proper functioning of the micromanometers and velocimeter had been verified, the catheter was advanced and guided by fluoroscopy until the velocimeter was positioned at the tricuspid orifice. Proper positioning of the velocimeter ensured that the proximal and distal micromanometers were located inside the right atrium and the right ventricle, respectively. In a steady physiological state, right atrial and ventricular pressures and linear tricuspid inflow velocity were obtained and digitized at 400 Hz (see Fig. 14.6 B., on p. 749).

As we will see later, in comparing FI with multisensor catheterization, reliable multisensor catheter measurements of pressure gradients in the RV diastolic intraventricular flow field are not ordinarily possible, *inter alia*, because of their smallness. *Transvalvular* (see Fig. 14.6 A.) atrioventricular pressure differences such as those presented in Figure 14.6 B., b, are, in fact, indicative of the best that is achievable by direct multisensor ("high-fidelity") catheter measurement.

14.6.3 3-D real-time echocardiography and image segmentation

Real-time 3-D images of the RV were obtained using the Duke RT3D ultrasound scanner (Volumetrics Medical Imaging; Durham, NC)—see Section 10.4, on pp. 547 ff. The scanner was initially set to the multiple-scanning mode, enabling observation of images on two mutually orthogonal B-mode scans as well as several parallel horizontal C-scan planes

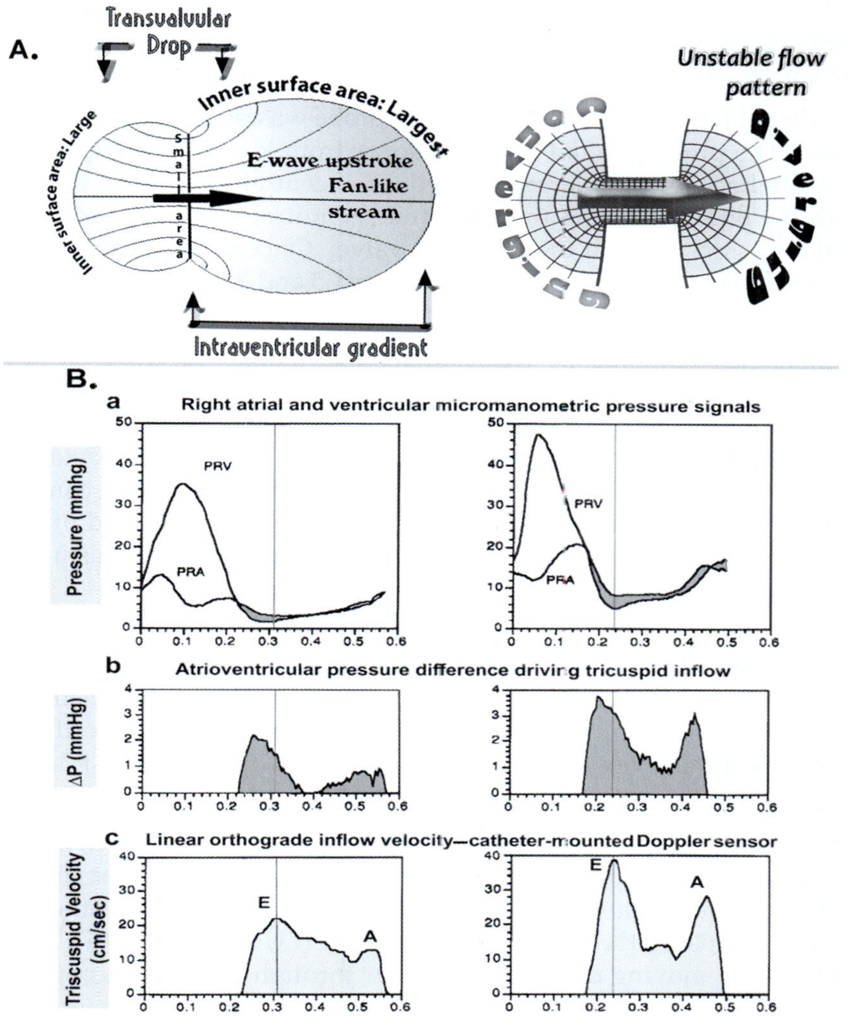

Figure 14.6: **A.** During the E-wave upstroke, flow is *confluent* between atrial endocardium and tricuspid orifice and *diffluent* between the latter and the ventricular walls. There is convective acceleration up to the orifice and convective deceleration beyond it, where the *diverging* streamlines imply an unstable flow regime. Transvalvular pressure drops embody convective *acceleration*, whereas intraventricular pressure gradients convective *deceleration* that *counterbalances* the local acceleration gradient during the E-wave upstoke. **B.** Right-sided transvalvular atrioventricular pressures and tricuspid inflow velocity, measured by multisensor catheter, approximately 0.5 hour (left) after induced tricuspid regurgitation and 1 week later (right). Note the pressure levels and the atrial *"cannon v-wave."* As shown by the vertical hairlines, at the time of peak tricuspid inflow velocity, the atrioventricular transvalvular pressure difference, ΔP, has already declined markedly from its peak value. E and A denote the E- and A-waves of diastolic inflow. PRA = right atrial pressure; PRV = right ventricular pressure. (Slightly modified, from Pasipoularides et al. [80].)

(see Fig. 10.40, on p. 555). The maximum depth of scanning was set at either 12 or 14 cm, depending on thoracic size and geometry. At these settings, framing rate was 22 or 19 $frames/s$, respectively, axial resolution $1-1.5$ mm, and lateral resolution $1.5-2$ mm.

With the dog at left decubitus, the scanning probe was positioned at the point of maximal impulse. The probe pointed into the thorax from lower left to upper right and an apical four-chamber view was first obtained. The central axis of the scan was initially aligned with the line connecting the apex and the mitral valve. It was then shifted *in-parallel* until it passed through the tricuspid valve. Once the right ventricle was maximally visualized, recording loops lasting between 1.5 and 2.5 s were captured and stored in memory.

The number of instantaneous RV chamber 3-D images included in any loop varied from 29 to 50, encompassing 2–5 complete cycles. The loops were immediately replayed to ensure image quality. Once satisfactory loops were acquired, after intravenous contrast injection of an agitated air microbubble mixture in bacteriostatic saline [71,78], the positions of the RV apex and the tricuspid valve along the scanning axis were recorded. The positions of the mutually orthogonal B-mode scans and of the successive short-axis C scans were similarly recorded. These landmarks served as important references during the endocardial border detection.

Endocardial border detection involved proprietary software, which displayed one RV 3-D frame at a time. The software displays all horizontal cross-sections in an apex-to-base order, along with the two mutually orthogonal B-mode images. With the use of the reference record taken during the experiment, as described in the preceding paragraph, the cross-sections at the levels of the tricuspid valve and apex were first determined.

A "2-D Swath" algorithm [78, 105, 106] located the most likely position of the endocardial border. The putative border is represented by a moving stack of contours in a set of 2-D slices. An operator initiates the moving endocardial border stack by entering a rough initial contour on a single slice. This contour then adapts automatically to the endocardial border using the 2-D Swath algorithm [71, 78, 98, 105–107]. The Swath algorithm follows the moving endocardial border through all the slices of the frame (see Fig. 14.12A., on p. 760), as well as through the successive time frames. Each contour in the moving stack is then converted to its elliptical Fourier series allowing for evenly spaced endocardial border coordinates.

The elliptical Fourier series is useful in representing cardiac chamber shapes and in automated methods for finding boundaries [103, 105]. These representations provide a frequency-based decomposition of an object and describe its overall shape efficiently using relatively few harmonic coefficients. With the use of a desired number of harmonics, evenly spaced, smoothed endocardial points can be regenerated from the Fourier transformations. The individual points were converted into 3-D Cartesian coordinates and stored in a file. Each file was a 4-D matrix containing a sequence of 3-D RV chamber *volumetric* datasets ordered *chronologically* (cf. Figs. 10.35 and 12.22, on p. 544 and 670, respectively). Each "volume" was a *succession* of instantaneous *endocardial border layers* from apex to base (see Figs. 14.3, inset 1, and 14.12A., on pp. 744 and 760, respectively).

14.6.4 Reconstruction of endocardial border points

The data representing the extracted endocardial edges were in layered form and were further processed to generate the desired coordinates in 3-D. To obtain RV diastolic flow-field simulations at a temporal resolution of 400 Hz, it was necessary to approximate the 3-D RV geometry at time instants between successive RT3D images. Under steady-state conditions, RV geometry was calculated at these instants as a quadratic weighted average of the dynamic geometry in contiguous RT3D frames [78]. Typical RV reconstructions are shown in Figures 14.3, inset 2, and 14.12B., on pp. 744 and 760. The dynamic RV chamber volume, using the *shell subtraction model* and *sonomicrometric dimensions*, and its time derivative or "inflow rate" were also calculated and compared with those obtained by our volumetric *"Prism Method,"* using *RT3D data* (cf. Fig. 14.3, inset 3, and 14.12C.).

The volumetric inflow rate through the tricuspid orifice can be obtained digitally as the time derivative of the RV chamber volume, by using the central difference method. The calculated rate of volume change over time (dV/dt) signal was smoothed using the first 20 harmonics of its Fourier decomposition, and tricuspid inflow rate values were sampled at 800 Hz; representative tracings of RV chamber volume and its time derivative signal obtained in this way are presented in Figure 14.12C., on p. 760. In this figure, the adjusted volume points corresponding to the original RT3D data, and the associated dV/dt values are superposed on the SSM-derived tracings of RV chamber volume and its time derivative. This procedure allowed adjusting the instantaneous volume and velocity boundary conditions in the computational fluid dynamic (CFD) simulations of the flow field, as needed in order to satisfy the conditions of *mass conservation* and *incompressibility* of blood, according to a rigorous computational scheme presented in a detailed paper on the method [78]. The final set of endocardial border points served as input for the generation of the *instantaneous computational grids* for the time-dependent diastolic RV flow field.

14.6.5 Model of the tricuspid orifice

A model of the tricuspid orifice was constructed using realistic geometry and dimensions observed during the animal experiments. Published M-mode and 2-D echocardiographic studies [65,69] show that the tricuspid valve leaflets open fully during the early ascending phase of the E-wave. Based on our own empirical observations on dog hearts [85], we constructed an elliptical tricuspid orifice with a fully open area of approximately 5 cm^2. During the descending phase of the E-wave, we simulated the motions of the tricuspid leaflets and their geometric role in preventing regurgitant flow through the tricuspid orifice, by selectively blocking portions of the tricuspid orifice as a function of time.

In order to obtain an intraventricular flow behavior that approximates closely the actually applying flow patterns, it seemed to be more important to simulate the change in the size of the opening of the tricuspid inflow orifice than the (unmeasurable) detailed dynamic motions of the short leaflets, or of the overall tricuspid valvular apparatus. Accordingly, we modeled the tricuspid valve by opening and closing an inflow orifice corresponding to the tricuspid anulus. We also carried out simulations of the intraventricular

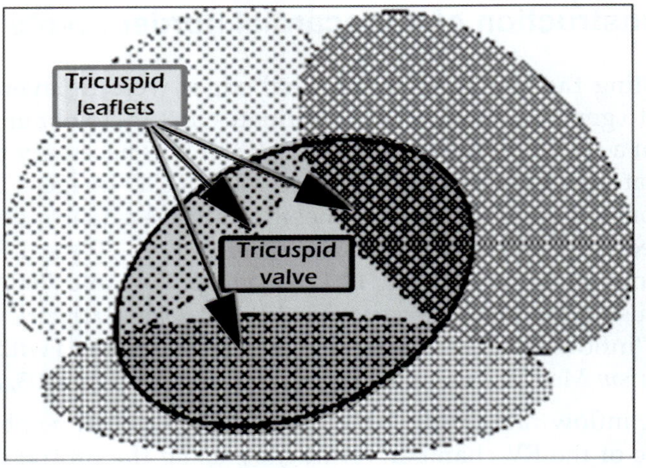

Figure 14.7: Illustration of the analytical geometric method devised to vary the patent area of the orifice of the tricuspid valve during diastolic filling in the CFD simulations (see discussion in text).

flow using an RV chamber model *without* this geometric valve-closure analog and found that *large regurgitation* then occurred at the entrance of the chamber. Thus, having an anatomically not very realistic but *functionally effective* variable area gate-like tricuspid valvular mechanism was useful for preventing the occurrence of excessive regurgitation.

We modeled the geometry of each leaflet of the tricuspid valve using the intersection between the ellipse that represents the fully opened tricuspid orifice and another ellipse. The instantaneous locations for the foci of the ellipses (representing each valve leaflet) and their radii were varied parametrically, as functions of time, depending on the size of the tricuspid orifice remaining open for inflow, which we determined using results from our 2- and 3-D ultrasonic imaging studies [77,78,87,99,100]. The *decreasing orifice size* during the downstroke of the E-wave *contributes* to the *narrowing* of the central blood core that is surrounded by the *expanding filling vortex*, which squeezes it centrally (see Fig. 14.17, on p. 774, and the associated discussion in Section 14.7.3, on pp. 771 ff.). A schematic diagram for the tricuspid orifice at one instant during the downstroke of the E-wave is shown in Figure 14.7.

14.6.6 Volumetric Prism Method

To calculate the chamber volume encompassed by the endocardial border, a volumetric *"Prism Method"* was developed, which represents an adaptation of the Archimedean[2] *method of exhaustion* for computing areas and volumes of various geometric objects [49,78].

[2]The method was actually introduced by the earlier Greek mathematician, Eudoxus (ca. 365–300 B.C.E.) [2]. Archimedes employed it to approximate the value of π. He did this by drawing a larger polygon outside a circle and a smaller polygon inside the circle. As the number of sides of such polygons increases, they become more accurate approximations of a circle. When the polygons had 96 sides each, he calculated

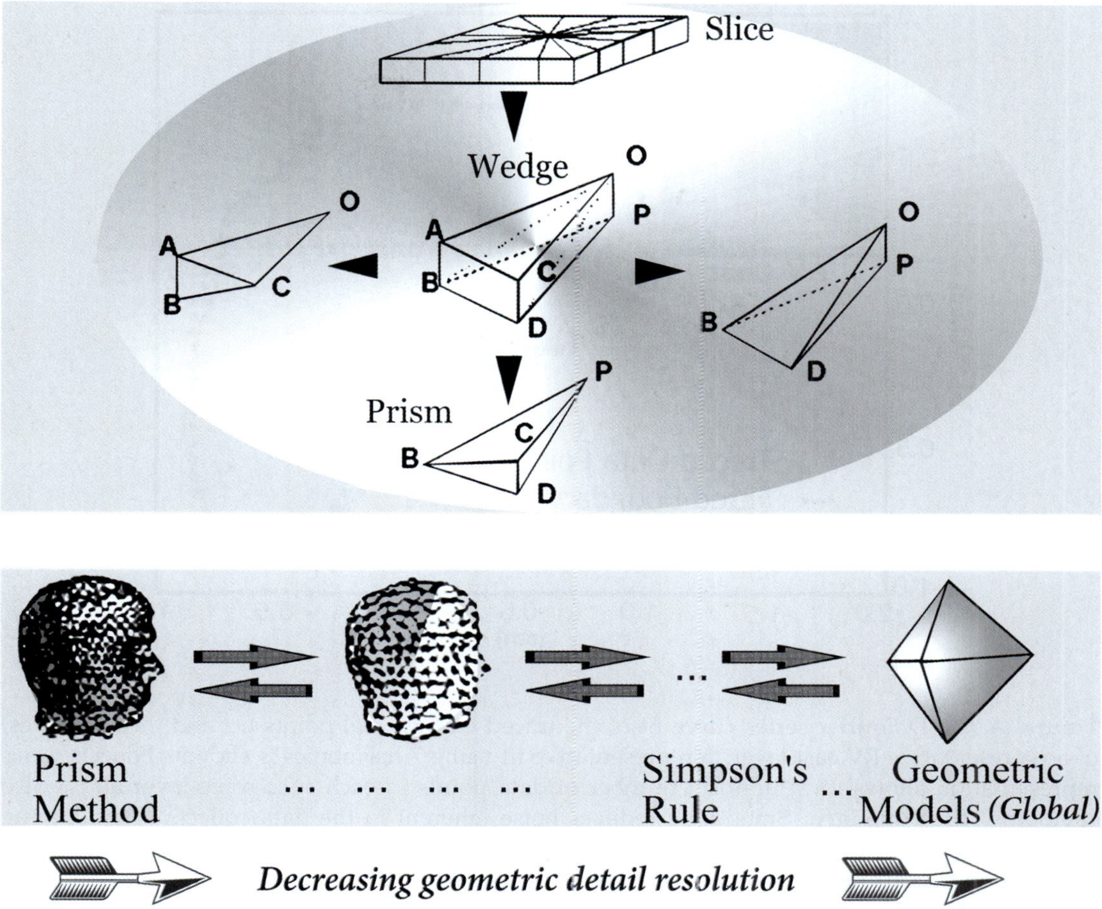

Figure 14.8: Schematic diagram illustrating the volumetric Prism Method. The algorithm is an adaptation of the "Archimedean method of exhaustion" for computing volumes of various geometric objects. Unlike abstract geometric solids and "disk summation" using Simpson's or other integral algorithms, the vertices of the tetrahedral tessellation can accurately follow endocardial surface details corresponding to local "features" (bottom). (Adapted, slightly modified, from Pasipoularides et al. [78] by kind permission of the American Physiological Society.)

Advantages of the prism method are that its individual steps can be easily automated, and, unlike "disk summation" using Simpson's or other integral algorithms, the vertices of the tetrahedral tessellation (see Section 11.6.1, on pp. 610 f.) can accurately follow endocardial surface details corresponding to local *"features"* (see Fig. 14.8, bottom), such as *papillary muscles*.

the lengths of their sides and showed that the value of π lay between $3 + 1/7$ ($\approx$ 3.1429) and $3 + 10/71$ ($\approx$3.1408). He also proved that the area of a circle is equal to π multiplied by the square of its radius.

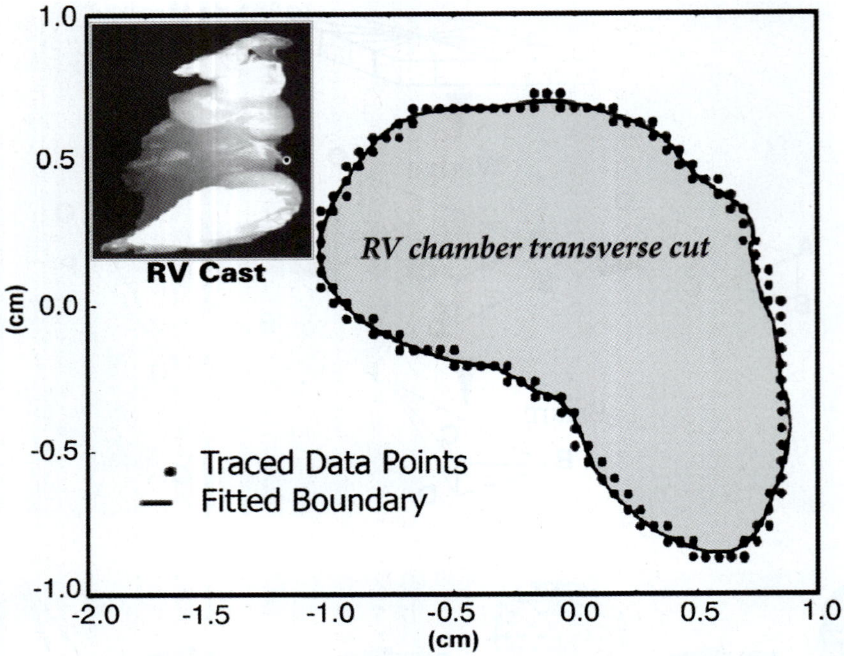

Figure 14.9: 2-D Fourier series curve fit of the traced endocardial points (x- and y-coordinates) of a representative RV cast layer: a representative fit using 7 harmonics is shown. Fourier series representation allows for a uniform number of data points in each successive layer and it also "smooths" the boundary. Smoothing reduces noise inherent in the data collection and tracing process. Inset: typical RV cast obtained using custom designed apparatus; the cast reveals precise information concerning tricuspid (and pulmonic) valve ring location and orientation. (Adapted, slightly modified, from Pasipoularides et al. [78], by kind permission of the APS.)

The primary steps are shown graphically in Figure 14.8, on p. 753, and include the following: (1) Connect the corresponding points of adjacent layers, forming a slice. (2) With the use of the *"pseudocenters"* defined by the means of the x- and y-coordinates separately for the points of the top and bottom layers, divide each slice into n wedges, where n is the number of points within each layer. (3) Decompose each wedge into three tetrahedra in the manner illustrated in Figure 14.8. (4) For an arbitrary tetrahedron with vertices O, A, B, and C, calculate its volume using the scalar triple product (see Section 2.2.3, on p. 43)

$$Volume_{OABC} = (1/6) \mid \overrightarrow{OA} \cdot (\overrightarrow{OB} \times \overrightarrow{OC}) \mid . \tag{14.2}$$

(5) Obtain the volume of each wedge as the sum of the volumes of its three tetrahedra, that of each slice by summing its wedges, and that of the RV chamber by summing all slices.

The volumetric Prism Method was itself validated first on RV chamber casts. At the end of unrelated surgical experiments, eight dogs (comparable in size and characteristics to the chronically instrumented animals) were euthanized with intravenous KCl $(1-2\ mmol/kg)$ to result in cardiac *diastolic arrest*. The heart was quickly excised with the stumps of the great vessels. After being thoroughly cleaned, cardiac chamber casts were immediately prepared under physiological diastolic hydrostatic loading [85]. Left and right ventricles, in that order, were filled with molten paraffin retrogradely through the aorta and pulmonary artery. Paraffins with a low melting point $(115°F)$ were employed to *minimize heat introduction*. Once set, the casts were removed, and surface points corresponding to *endocardial landmarks* were noted. A representative RV cast is shown in Figure 14.9, inset.

The volume of each RV chamber cast was measured by direct water displacement, and the mean of three independent measurements was recorded. A 2-D digitization technique was used to obtain the endocardial border coordinates for each cast [85]. First, a z-axis was established corresponding to a line extending from the apex to base. The casts were then mechanically sectioned into 1- to 5-mm thick sections perpendicular to the z-axis. These sections, with their z-coordinates recorded, were subjected to individual 2-D analysis. Reference markings were applied to each cast to ensure proper section alignment. Each section was photographed, and the images were filtered and enlarged (200%) to optimize outline digitization by using a Summagraphics™ digitizing tablet (Summagraphics; Seymour, CT) and SigmaScan™ software (HALLoGRAM Pub; Aurora, CO). With these digitized data as input, custom software then reconstructed the successive *planar arrays* of x- and y-coordinates for ascending z-axis values.

Fixing the number of layers along the z-axis of each RV chamber cast to 25, we first assessed the impact of varying the number of Fourier harmonics representing the endocardial border of a 2-D layer on the accuracy of the geometric reconstruction for the 3-D chamber. Each layer outline was fitted with 3, 5, 7, and 10 harmonics. A representative fit using 7 harmonics is shown in Figure 14.9, on p. 754. Analysis of variance (ANOVA) and standard statistical procedures were performed by using SAS™ (SAS; Cary, NC) and Statgraphics Plus™ (Manugistics Group; Rockville, MD). ANOVA showed no statistically significant difference among the volumes measured ($F = 0.01$, $P = 0.99$). When the statistical linear regression model was used for calibrating each prism method calculation against direct water displacement, on the basis of standard error of estimate (SEE) and root mean square (RMS) error of the residuals, the best fit was obtained using five harmonics.

A possible relationship between the number of successive 2-D layers interpolated along the z-axis, and the accuracy of the geometric reconstruction was then explored. Each layer was represented using five harmonics. Accuracy tests were performed for 10, 15, 25, 35, and 50 layers along the z-axis. The volumes of all eight RV casts obtained by the prism method for each of these numbers of z-axis layers were compared with the volumes obtained by water displacement. Again, ANOVA showed no significant difference between the six sets (*viz.*, the *computed* 10, 15, 25, 35, and 50 axial layer volumes and direct *water displacement* volume), and linear calibrations versus water displacement showed no significant differences in SEE and RMS error.

Bland and Altman's [13,14] approach was applied to assess statistically the agreement between *measurement modalities* [78]. The mean of the methods is treated as the best estimate

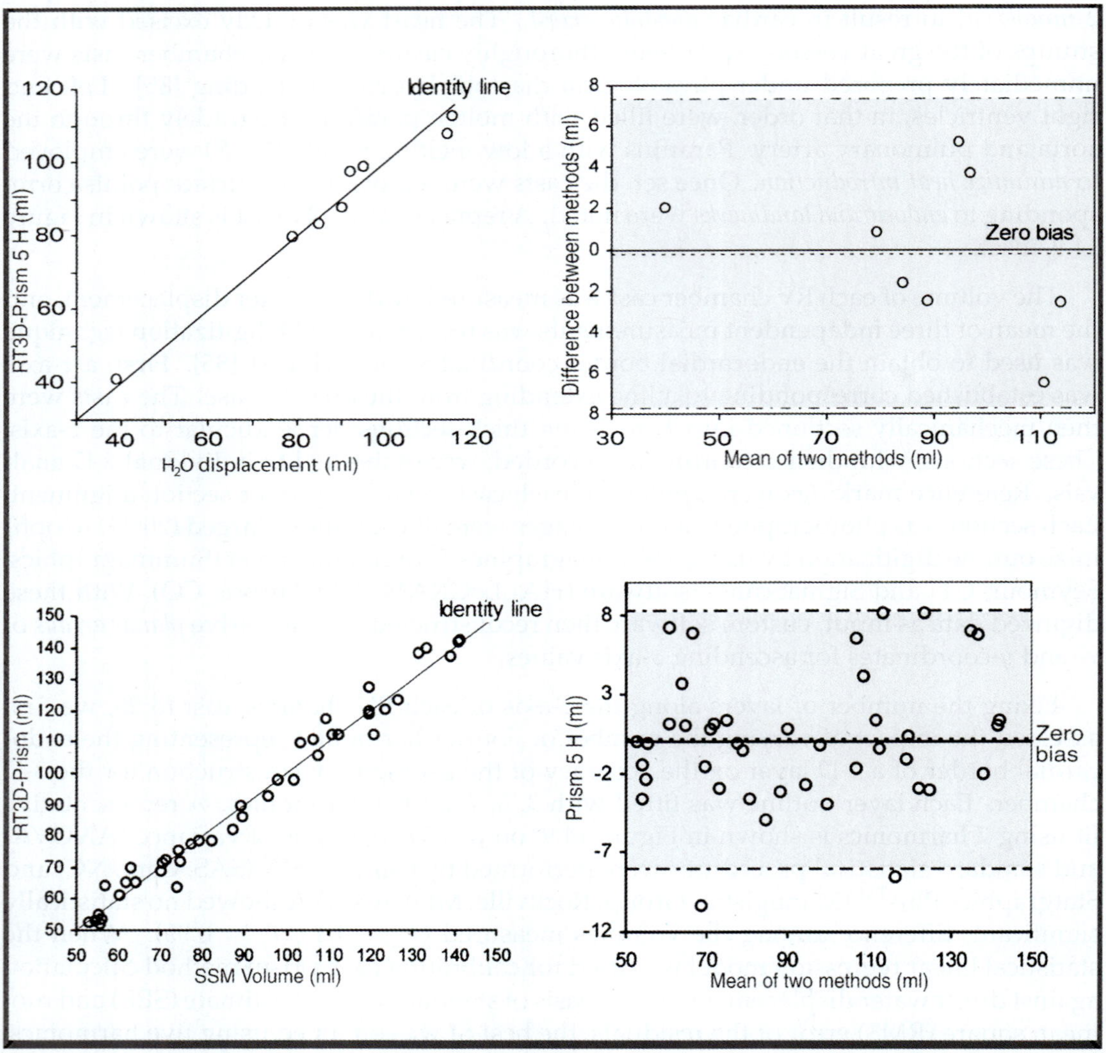

Figure 14.10: Top: Bland–Altman plots demonstrating agreement (left) between volumes obtained by the prism method on geometric reconstructions of RV chamber casts and direct water displacement. Note closeness of data points to the identity line and the near zero bias and narrow 95% confidence interval bounds, in gray (right). Bottom: Bland-Altman plots showing close agreement (left) between the dynamic RV chamber volumes (prism method) reconstructed using RT3D data and the SSM volumes in awake dogs (pooled control and volume overload data). Note closeness of data points to the identity line and the near-zero bias with tight 95% confidence intervals, in gray (right). (Adapted, slightly modified, from Pasipoularides et al. [78], by kind permission of the American Physiological Society.)

of true value [13]. Alternate methods were visually compared for agreement, any bias due to systematic error, and to spot any possible relationship between imprecision and chamber size. The agreement between the prism method, using the first 5 harmonics for 2-D smoothing and 25 z-axis layers, and water displacement is demonstrated in Figure 14.10. As is shown in this figure, the measurement points follow the identity line very closely (top left). The difference plot (Fig. 14.10, top right) shows the variance of the observations to be small and constant across the sampling range and the lack of bias or systematic error in the prism calculations. The bias was -0.19%, so on average volumes of the RV geometric reconstructions were -0.19% lower than the direct measurements of cast volume by *water displacement*.

The panel labeled as control conditions (CL) in Figure 14.11, on p. 758, shows a representative comparison of instantaneous RV chamber volumes, obtained in an awake chronically instrumented dog heart by using SSM, with simultaneous volumes calculated by applying the prism method to the RT3D imaging data under the control condition. The panel labeled volume overload (VO) is similar but under conditions of volume overload, which produced considerable increases in operating RV chamber volume levels. A *comparison* of the instantaneous RV volumes using SSM with those computed by the prism method from the RT3D imaging reconstructions was performed by using pooled data from four dogs under control and volume overload. The experimental determinations involved in validating RT3D volumes against simultaneous sonomicrometric volumes using SSM are exceedingly complex and resource demanding, both in the stage of the *simultaneous* data acquisition in the animal lab and in their *computational* phase.

These four out of the seven dogs were examined in the validation studies because they exhibited diastolic paradoxical septal motion (PSM) and thus afforded a more severe test, while providing more than ample data points for a thorough comparison. Figure 14.10, bottom, illustrates the agreement between the prism method using RT3D data and SSM. Notable on the left panel of Figure 14.10 is how closely the measurement points follow the identity line. The difference plot similarly shows the variance of the observations to be small and constant across the entire volume range and lack of bias of the prism method compared with SSM. The bias was $0.18\ mL$; accordingly, RV chamber reconstructions from noninvasive RT3D data had volumes $0.18\,mL$ (0.2%) higher on average than corresponding SSM measurements.

The Prism Method can be used with other noninvasive digital imaging modalities, including MRI (see Section 10.2, on pp. 505 ff.) and CT scanning (see Section 10.1, on pp. 484 ff.), in addition to 3-D echocardiography. Advantages of the prism method are that its individual steps can be easily automated and that, as already pointed out, unlike "disk summation" using Simpson's or other integral algorithms, the vertices of the tetrahedral tessellation can accurately follow endocardial surface details corresponding to local "features" (see Fig. 14.8, on p. 753), such as papillary muscles. Because it remains difficult to extract the RV chamber directly by automated endocardial border recognition from RT3D frames, it is currently more appropriate to segment the chamber slice-by-slice, isolating the endocardium, and to then tessellate the surface from the layered 2-D contour stack. On the basis of our dog heart findings, it is recommended to use five to seven harmonic

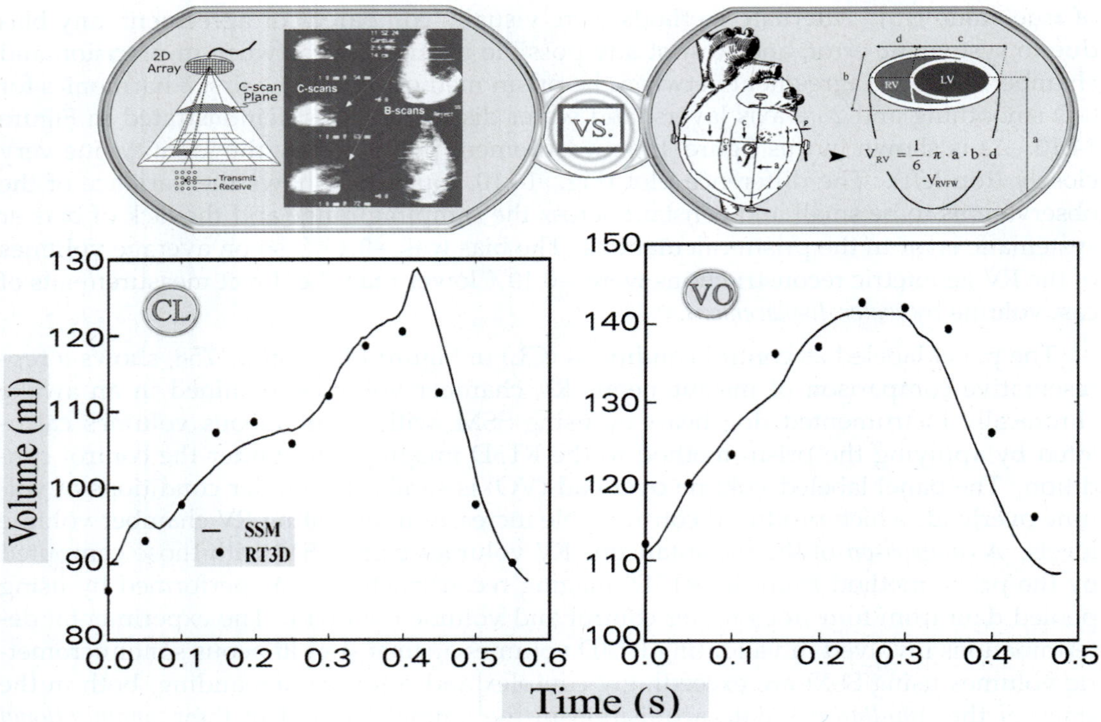

Figure 14.11: RV instantaneous volumes calculated noninvasively by the prism model for chamber geometric reconstructions using RT3D serial chamber reconstructions (top left) agree closely with those using the SSM (top right), under control conditions (CL) and chronic volume overload (VO) (bottom). Note the instrumentation and measurements needed for application of the SSM; VRVFW is the RV free wall volume determined by water displacement during autopsy. (Adapted, slightly modified, from Pasipoularides et al. [78], by kind permission of the American Physiological Society.)

2-D layer Fourier representations and no more than 25 z-axis layers. This represents the best balance between the tightness of fit of each 2-D layer, the smoothness of each regenerated layer, and the accuracy of the geometric reconstruction.

With continuing advances in *spatiotemporal resolution* and *accuracy* of imaging technologies, however, it should become possible to extract the chamber *automatically* from the imaging dataset and to then obtain the Fourier transform to the volume image (constructed of *voxels* instead of *pixels*) in the 3-D frequency space directly [78].

14.6.7 Mesh generation and determination of boundary conditions

A combination of FIDAP (cf. Section 13.4, on pp. 710 ff.) and custom software [78] generated the mesh representing the 3-D domain for simulation of RV intraventricular diastolic flow (see Figs. 14.3, inset 4, on p. 744, and 14.13, top, on p. 766). To satisfy the requirements of continuity and incompressibility of blood, the following equation must apply:

$$V_{i+1} = V_i + \Delta t \cdot \frac{dV_i}{dt}, \tag{14.3}$$

where, V_i and V_{i+1} are the RV chamber mesh volumes at instants i and $i+1$, Δt is the time increment (2.5 ms) between these two instants, and dV/dt is the rate of change of volume at $t + 1.25\ ms$.

For RT3D-derived meshes of which the instantaneous volume differed from that calculated using the previous equation, a uniform expansion/contraction method [78] was applied to obtain a mesh with the desired volume while preserving the geometric similarity. For an arbitrary boundary point $(x_0,\ y_0,\ z_0)$ in the *original mesh*, the coordinates of its corresponding point $(x,\ y,\ z)$ in the *adjusted mesh* were

$$x - x_c = (x_0 - x_c) \cdot \sqrt[3]{\frac{V}{V_0}}, \quad y - y_c = (y_0 - y_c) \cdot \sqrt[3]{\frac{V}{V_0}}, \quad z = z_0 \cdot \sqrt[3]{\frac{V}{V_0}}, \tag{14.4}$$

where the subscript c denotes the *"pseudocenter"* of each endocardial contour defined by the means of x- and y-coordinates of its points.

Results of this procedure for echocardiographic RV instantaneous chamber volume adjustment are illustrated in Figure 14.12C., on p. 760. The instantaneous geometry defined the external nodal points of the mesh, to which were assigned boundary conditions, i.e., nodal velocity vectors describing direction and speed of instantaneous motion, as is exemplified in Figures 14.3, inset 4, and 14.13, top, on pp. 744 and 766, respectively—see also Figure 12.10, on p. 642.

14.6.8 Reynolds number, adaptive gridding and the Courant condition

The local Reynolds number, $Re \propto D \cdot v$, of the RV diastolic inflow field [43,47,73,79] constitutes a very important parameter in our computational fluid dynamics analysis. The characteristic length, D, in Re is proportional to the square root of flow cross-sectional area, whereas the velocity, v, in a diverging flow field decreases rapidly as the area increases—see Figure 14.2B., on p. 740. Because the RV endocardial surface area is much larger than the tricuspid orifice area (*area of walls/ area of orifice* ≥ 10), blood entering the chamber during the *upstroke* of the E-wave (*before* the flow breaks down into the *vortical pattern*, see Fig. 14.15, on p. 770) experiences powerful *convective deceleration* [75,76,78–80]. The net effect of a rapidly decreasing velocity v and a slowly increasing characteristic length D is a decrease in Re away from the orifice along the flow lines (see Fig. 14.2B.). The drop in Re is proportional to the square root of upstream to downstream flow cross-sectional areas. The local Re is therefore highest near the tricuspid orifice.

The large velocities of flow combined with the asymmetric 3-D nature of the complex dynamic RV geometry call for the use of a large number of finite element nodes for numerical stability and convergence of the simulations. The number of nodes along each

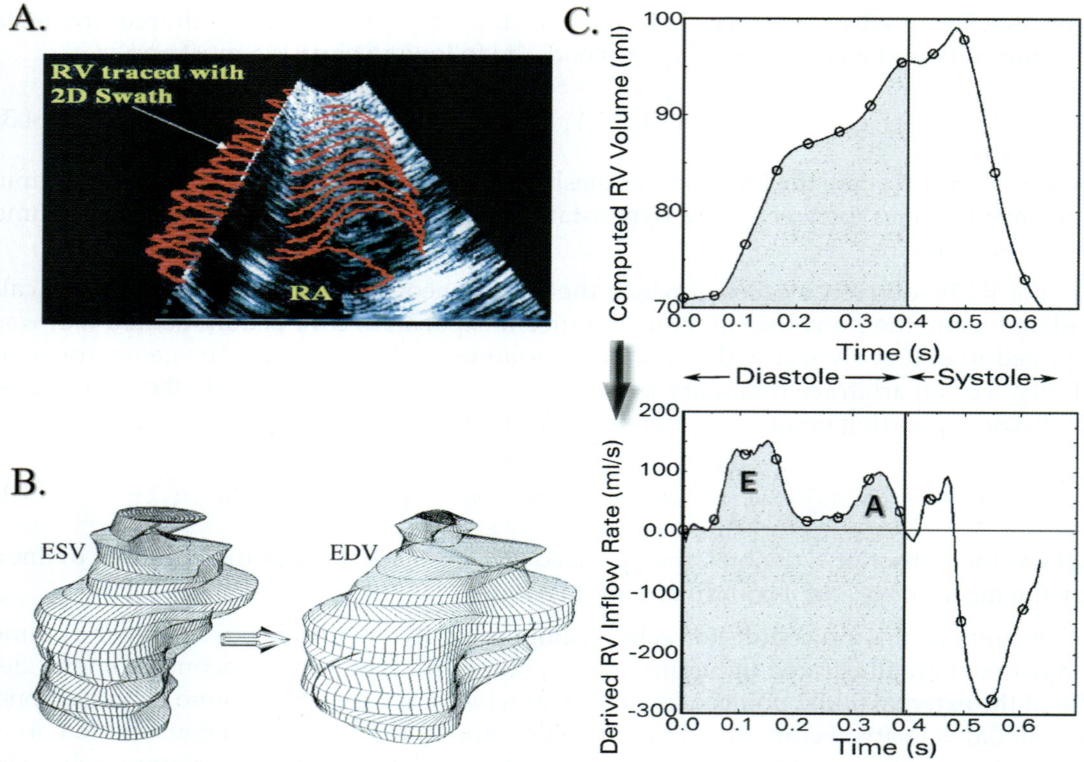

Figure 14.12: **A.** RV endocardial border of each C-mode slice is traced manually as a closed loop representing an initial guess. "2-D Swath" border detection algorithm then adjusts the initial guess so that the border falls on the "most likely position" and allows visualization of the stack of 2-D contours of each RT3D frame using the B-mode, as pictured. **B.** representative end-systolic (ESV) and end-diastolic (EDV) RV chamber reconstructions. **C.** Continuous line tracings of instantaneous RV chamber volume (top) by shell subtraction model (SSM) using sonomicrometric measurements, and its digitally obtained time derivative signal (bottom). These instantaneous values were used for adjusting the RT3D-derived volume and velocity boundary conditions in successive $2.5\ ms$ intervals before their use in the CFD simulations of the RV diastolic flow field. Representative adjusted points corresponding to the original RT3D data, and the associated rate of volume change (dV/dt) values are superposed (open circles) on the SSM-derived tracings of RV chamber volume and its time derivative. (Adapted, slightly modified, from Pasipoularides et al. [78], by kind permission of the American Physiological Society.)

axis must be of the order of the maximum Re in order to ensure *numerical stability* (see Section 12.7.2, on pp. 662 f.). The highest nodal densities are thus reserved for regions with the highest Re (near the inflow orifice). Consequently, to keep the problem tractable we used [43, 78–80] *adaptive gridding* (see section 12.6.3, on pp. 654 ff.): the *nodal density* near the inflow orifice varied from 6 to 10 times that in the apical region.

Such required improvements in spatial resolution complicate matters, because the size of the computational cells imposes a computational constraint on the timestep that is needed to maintain a stable and accurate solution. The timestep must be *small enough* so that the distinct components of the convective fluxes into and out of each cell do not change the properties of a cell appreciably *during* the timestep.

As we have discussed at some length in Sections 12.6.2 and 12.8.2, on pp. 652 ff. and 665 ff., respectively, for a simulation to be stable, it must comply with the Courant–Friedrichs–Lewy (CFL) condition given by Equation 12.1, on p. 665. In other words, for the solution to be stable over the entire flow region, Δt must be chosen such that Equation 12.1 is satisfied, even for the minimum Δx. Obviously, *the smaller the grid cell size* and Δx, *the smaller the timestep* Δt needed in order to keep the simulation stable. When the grid point separation is reduced to improve the accuracy of the simulation results, the upper limit for the timestep *also* decreases *pari-passu*. It should be noted that this timestep denotes the maximum internal timestep that the CFD solver may take during the time integration and is *not the same* as the timestep of the simulation.

The Courant constraint on the timestep is determined by the ratio of the mesh spacing and the magnitude of the velocity, which can vary substantially throughout the computational domain. In the situation at hand, where the grid-spacing is in fact strongly nonuniform, *local* Courant time-stepping was feasible and resulted in substantial savings in computation time (see Section 12.8.2, on pp. 665 ff.).

14.6.9 Computer simulations and flow visualization

With the use of the prism model with RT3D data, RV chamber dynamic geometry and boundary conditions (RV endocardial velocities) were obtained for solution of the flow-governing equations by CFD methods. We used a combination of custom software [78–80] and FIDAP™ (Fluid Dynamics International; Evanston, IL) to perform the computations involved in solving the NSE, which govern the evolution of the RV diastolic filling flow field (cf. Section 13.4, on pp. 710 ff.). We carried out the numerical simulations of the flow field under normal and abnormal operating conditions, associated with subacute-to-chronic surgically induced volume overload, on the CRAY T-90 supercomputer running FIDAP on the UNICOS™ operating system (Cray; Mendota Heights, MN) at the North Carolina Supercomputing Center (Research Triangle Park, NC).

As we have already learned (cf. Section 13.4, on pp. 710 ff.), FIDAP is a general-purpose computer program that uses the finite element method (FEM) to simulate fluid flows. Furthermore, as we have seen in Chapters 12 and 13, in applying FEM the flow domain represented by the filling RV chamber is tessellated into small "finite elements," forming a mesh. The definition of the elements is accomplished by identifying the locations of the *element corners* in space. These identified points are called "nodes," or *nodal points* (see Fig. 13.12, on p. 712). The partial differential Navier–Stokes equations covering the flow domain as a whole are replaced by ordinary differential equations for the unsteady flow analyses at hand. The resulting system of equations has matrix coefficients that are derived by approximating the continuum equations on each element.

The boundary condition assigned to each external nodal point was the time-dependent velocity vector describing the direction of instantaneous motion of the nodal point (see Fig. 14.13, top, on p. 766). This nonlinear system of equations was solved by numerical techniques to determine velocity distributions at each node in every element throughout the "discretized" flow field.

The computational steps of the overall approach [78–80] are summarized schematically in the main right portion of Figure 14.3, on p. 744. The unsteady flow-field simulations had to be completed through consecutive runs, each advancing the solution by two to four 2.5–*ms* timesteps. Blood was assumed to be a Newtonian, incompressible fluid with a kinematic viscosity of $0.04\ Stokes$ and a mass density of $1.05\ g/cm^3$.

Our custom software package was responsible for the reconstruction and the final generation of the moving endocardial border points, for the calculation of the unsteady initial/boundary conditions, and for generating FIDAP-readable commands for mesh generation and boundary condition assignments. FIDAP executed these commands to generate the time-dependent 3-D mesh for the right ventricle as outlined by the moving endocardial border points, assigned the initial and the boundary conditions, and performed the numerical computations involved in solving the NSE. All other computational work was performed on the local area networks at Duke University, equipped with the SUN Ultra workstations.

The arrangement described above allowed for optimal distribution of workload across the resources. The CRAY T-90 can reach a peak speed of $7.28\ GFLOPS$—see Section 12.1, on pp. 626 ff. It is therefore well suited to carry out the numerical simulation step, which is highly intensive computationally. Running on a batch mode, a typical timestep (2.5 *ms*) of simulation was usually completed within 2–4 *hours* of CPU time. Each SUN Ultra workstation runs on a 400 *MHz* RISC microprocessor.[3] It was used to complete all tasks other than the numerical simulation, as is represented pictorially in the left main right portion of Figure 14.3. The more computationally intensive steps among them, such as the mesh generation and the boundary condition assignments, required 4–6 *min* to complete for a typical timestep. For these tasks, the SUN workstation, which runs on an *interactive* mode, has a significant advantage over the CRAY T-90 in that it provides maximum flexibility in terms of *"on-the-fly"* adjustments and corrections.

Given the size of this problem, all practical numerical solution schemes employed are *iterative* in nature—see Section 12.7, on pp. 657 ff. All iterative algorithms require initialization values, which serve as an initial guess, starting from which the numerical solver software can seek the "true" solution. The initial condition for the very first timestep of each flow simulation was the so-called *Stokes solution*, which neglects the nonlinear convective acceleration terms. When successive timesteps were distributed in separate runs,

[3]RISC, or Reduced Instruction Set Computer, is a type of processor architecture that utilizes a small, highly-optimized set of instructions. Certain design features characterize most RISC processors: one-cycle execution time, pipelining and multiple registers. RISC processors have a CPI (clock per instruction) of one cycle; this is due to the optimization of each instruction on the CPU and a technique called pipelining. Pipelining allows for simultaneous execution of parts, or stages, of instructions in order to more efficiently process instructions. Large numbers of registers generally prevent substantial amounts of interactions with memory.

the geometric domain used for the simulation often changed. In this case, the FICONV module of FIDAP was used to interpolate the solution to conform to the geometry of the new simulation domain.

Both the successive substitution and the segregated solver (see p. 658) techniques were used for the solution. The advantage of the *successive substitution* algorithm is that it has relatively high tolerance for errors in the initial guess. Hence, the solver may converge even with a relatively inaccurate initial guess; however, the rate of convergence is slow. On the other hand, the *segregated solver* has a significantly shorter convergence time, but its requirement for accuracy in the initial guess is higher. Accordingly, the successive substitution method was employed at the *beginning* of our simulations to provide solutions of relatively high accuracy even with relatively poor initialization values. Once such a solution had been obtained which could function as the initial guess, the segregated solver was *then* used. It is very useful also to always remember that the converged *("true")* solution for any given timestep can be used as the *initial guess* for the subsequent timestep. Experience is required optimally to control the solution procedure to achieve convergence for each given simulation.

Convergence is a major issue when using CFD software. CFD software simulates nonlinear processes and it is *not* guaranteed that there will be a "converged" solution to a problem. The CFD iterative process successively improves a solution, until convergence is attained. It is clear that the iterative solution will not be a good approximation to the exact solution if the iterations are stopped too early. On the other hand, since discretization errors exist a priori, a highly accurate iterative solution may require *too many* iterations and simply waste computation time without enhancing the overall solution qualities.

It is clear, therefore, that an important aspect of any iterative method is to determine when the iterations should be stopped. The exact solution to the iterative problem is unknown, but we want to be sufficiently close to the solution for a particular required level of accuracy. To assert convergence is to claim the existence of a limit, which may itself be unknown. For any fixed standard of accuracy, we can always be sure to be within it, provided we have *gone far enough*. As this definition indicates, the exact solution to the iterative problem is unknown, but we want to be sufficiently close to the solution for a *particular* required level of *accuracy*.

Convergence criteria for the iterative solution process were established according to the discussion in Section 12.7.1, on pp. 659 ff. Figure 12.20, on p. 661, is an typical plot of the natural logarithm[4] of the residuals against iteration number from one of the RV diastolic flow-field simulations under discussion. Convergence is reached when the residuals of all variables become less than an upper *threshold* value, which in the case illustrated in Figure 12.20 was set at 0.1%. As is shown in that figure, individual variables have, in general, distinct rates of convergence, and have nominally different residuals at the time of convergence. It should further be noted that in a convergent case the residuals for individual variables do not necessarily show a monotonic decrease. Thus, in the example at hand, both the *V component* of the velocity and the pressure have circumscribed regions of transient small increases in their residuals between successive iterations.

[4] In logarithmic transformations, we are interested in the *relative* change in the plotted variable.

14.6.10 Flow visualization and Functional Imaging

After the CFD simulation for any particular flow field of interest has been obtained, the flow field can be visualized using FIPOST, FIDAP's postprocessing module. FIPOST allows the user to define an arbitrary plane within the pressure and velocity fields by specifying the Cartesian coordinates of *three points* within the plane. Once the plane is thus defined, FIPOST extracts the flow-field variables of interest *on this plane*. The selected image can subsequently be further enhanced with various commercial graphic software packages, such as Adobe *Creative Suite*™, MathWorks *Matlab*™, Microsoft *PowerPoint*™, and Advanced Visual Systems *AVS/Express*™. The vital area of scientific visualization is presented in Sections 1.11, 2.22.2, 3.12, 10.5, and 12.9, on pp. 26 ff., 101 ff., 154 ff., 566 ff., and 667 ff., respectively.

The growth of digital graphic imaging techniques and software and their adoption in research and clinical cardiac applications of CFD are accompanied by an increasing usage of image manipulation tools, providing for more elaborate FI analyses and measurements. As we will see in the sections that follow, the emerging quantitative FI evaluations lead to more refined diagnostic accuracy and may possibly reveal *warning signs* of diseases not yet overt. They can provide *deeper pathophysiologic understanding* than could ever be gleaned from visual interpretation of static or dynamic anatomic datasets alone. Moreover, complex mathematical procedures are being used to localize and highlight important alterations in cardiac function that are reflected in subtle *intracardiac flow phenomena* changes although they cannot be visually detected or inferred directly from the original anatomic images.

With the *concurrent* development of high-performance computers and analytical CFD software, the new Functional Imaging discipline is now evolving within Cardiology [78–80]. It is geared toward the creation of physiological *intracardiac blood flow* images that are the result of a mathematical simulation derived from a set of *dynamic anatomic images*. As opposed to structural anatomic imaging, Functional Imaging centers on revealing physiological and pathophysiological flow patterns within the cardiac chambers by employing modern digital imaging modalities. Such Functional Imaging will allow visualization and understanding of the evolution of any time-dependent process of interest (*filling, ejection*) within the heart. It is in the *cross-roads* of many basic sciences impacting Cardiology. Accordingly, it should allow better insights into cardiac development and physiology, as well as pathophysiology, including cardiac phenotypic plasticity, adaptations and transition to disease, as well as possible avenues to reversal and regression of pathology (see discussions in Sections 1.9 and 1.10, on pp. 20 ff., on p. 569, and in Section 15.6, on pp. 835 ff.).

In using modern imaging modalities, it should be born in mind that cardiac CT and cardiac MR imaging each present potential *patient safety* issues. Cardiac CT safety issues are related to radiation exposure and to administration of intravascular contrast media. The safety concerns for cardiac MR imaging are primarily related to the strong magnetic field and its potential effect on implanted devices, but MR imaging contrast agents and patient sedation also present potential safety issues. In addition, pharmacologic agents may be administered for either CT or MR imaging examinations. Thus, the possibility of extracting the *maximum amount* of helpful *diagnostic and pathophysiologic* information by applying FI is of great clinical as well as investigative value and interest.

14.7 Diastolic RV flow fields in individual animal hearts

Simulations using the FI method [75,76,78–80] have yielded important information about the detailed diastolic RV flow fields in individual animal hearts in lightly sedated, awake dogs under control and volume overload conditions associated with surgically induced experimental chronic tricuspid insufficiency. All seven experimental dogs exhibited normal wall motion (NWM) at control; three had normal and four had diastolic paradoxical septal motion (PSM) in volume overload (*vide infra* and cf. Fig. 14.25, on p. 792). This research produced for the first time finite element CFD recreations of spatiotemporal diastolic blood flow patterns within the RV chamber.

Using *in vivo*, real-time 3-D dynamic RV geometric data, simulations of the evolution of the RV diastolic flow field through the entire duration of the E-wave have allowed us to demonstrate the existence of large-scale 3-D vortical motions, which develop inside the RV chamber during diastole both at control and under volume overload conditions [77–80]. These simulations have also provided strong and important evidence regarding the impact of the applying *chamber size* and *wall motion patterns* on the development of the RV *velocity field* during *diastole*. In the following sections, we examine throughout the entire E-wave illustrative RV intraventricular pressure and velocity distributions, obtained by the FI method in individual dog hearts exhibiting NWM at control and PSM in volume overload.

The differences between volume-overloaded and normal-sized chambers illustrated in the accompanying graphic plots are for the most part quantitative, i.e., they pertain to *degree* or *intensity* rather than to qualitatively different phenomena (see exception in Section 14.7.1). The FI approach is by no means limited to the right ventricle but can also be used to study the flow field in the *left ventricle*. Moreover, the concepts regarding interactions of fluid dynamic mechanisms with right-sided intracardiac diastolic flow phenomena and loading are general and should apply *in the left heart* too—initial proof of this has been provided in subsequent clinical corroborative studies [61].

14.7.1 Onset of *E*-wave upstroke

Figure 14.13, on p. 766, shows representative FI simulation results (*comparative fluid dynamics*) of the commencing diastolic RV inflow field under control and volume overload conditions. The left panels exemplify normal wall size and motion conditions (NWM), in which the septum moves toward the RV free wall; the right panels exemplify volume overload with diastolic paradoxical septal motion (PSM), in which the septum moves toward the left ventricle. The flow fields are illustrated at instants just after the onset of the upstroke of the E-wave at which the average inflow velocities were comparable. Major differences between the two simulations were the *direction* of the interventricular septal motion, as is shown in Figure 14.13, top, and the *magnitude* of RV free wall velocity.

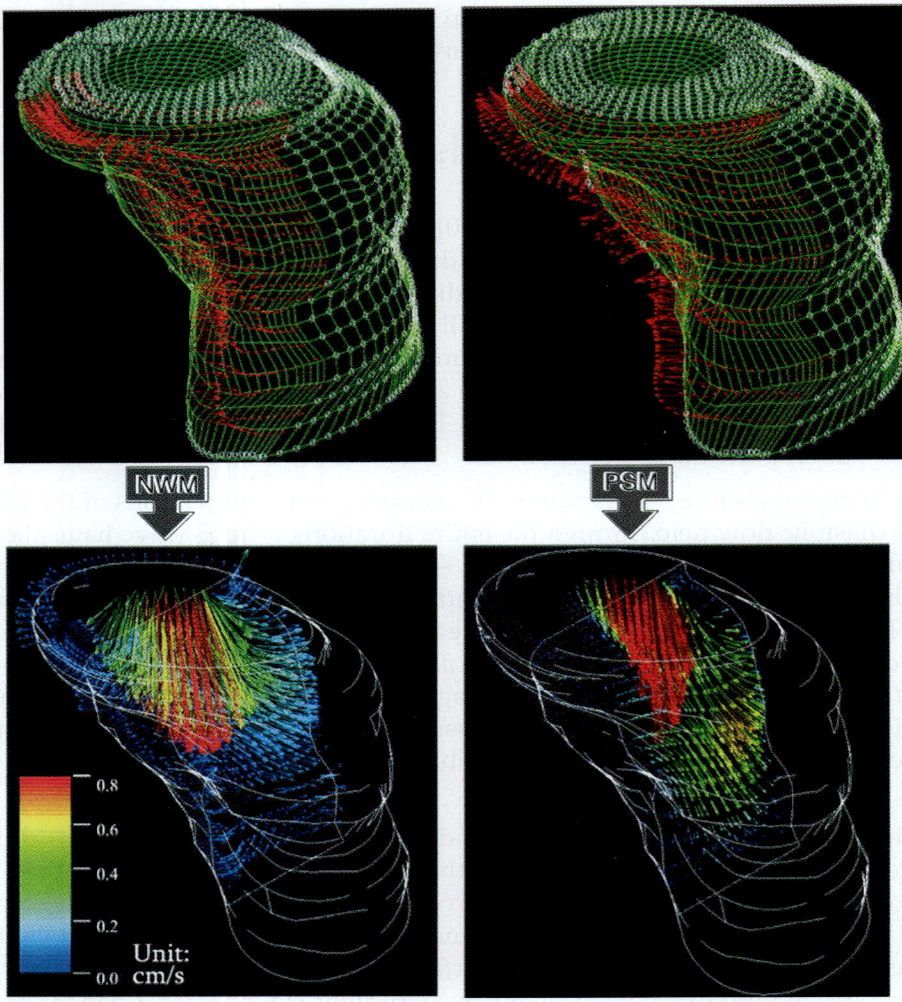

Figure 14.13: Functional Imaging of commencing RV inflow using RT3D imaging data, under normal wall motion (NWM) conditions and during volume overload with paradoxic diastolic septal motion (PSM). *Top*: external (endocardial) surface nodes of instantaneous computational meshes and application of boundary conditions (red velocity vectors on endocardial surface nodes). Only velocity vectors on the septal border of each RV mesh are shown to avoid clutter. Septal nodal velocity vectors (red) point *toward RV chamber and free wall* in the normal case but *toward the left ventricle* with PSM. *Bottom*: median sagittal (anteroposterior) plane *"cuts"* of the resulting velocity fields at the very start ($\approx$10 *ms* from onset) of the *E*-wave. With NWM there is blood flow toward the free wall in the septal region, whereas with PSM there is very little blood flow in that region. Note the *different* velocity profiles at the tricuspid orifice, and the *abrupt* transition (*signifying strong deceleration*) from red-yellow-green to black in the dilated chamber (PSM) compared with the more *gradual* transition through blue hues in the normal. (Adapted from Pasipoularides et al. [78], by kind permission of the American Physiological Society.)

Accordingly, the early inflow field with normal wall motion exhibits blood velocities toward the free wall in the septal region, whereas with diastolic paradoxical septal motion no flow is seen in this region (Fig. 14.13, bottom panels).

Compared with normal wall motion, volume overload with diastolic paradoxical septal motion yields conspicuously different velocity profiles at the tricuspid anulus. In both cases, the highest velocities are concentrated in the *vicinity of the inflow orifice*. The magnitude of blood velocities below the inflow orifice falls off more gradually in the normal case, as is revealed by the step-by-step transition in blue color hues of the velocity vectors; the blue hues light up a large area of the plane of the "cut." In the volume-overloaded ventricle, the transition from higher (red/yellow) through low (blue) flow velocities is abrupt; most of the "cut" beyond the immediate locality of the orifice is black.

The comparative fluid dynamics of the commencing diastolic RV inflow field that are displayed in Figure 14.13, are interesting. The PSM case exhibits a flow field that is qualitatively different from that of NWM: with NWM there is blood flow *toward the free wall* in the septal region, whereas with PSM there is *very little blood flow* in that region. Compared with normal, wall motion abnormalities in volume overload yield conspicuously different velocity profiles at the tricuspid anulus. This result suggests that presence of subtle diastolic *wall motion abnormalities* may be detected by clinical Doppler evaluation of diastolic *inflow velocity profiles* in the earliest stage of diastolic inflow.

At that earliest stage, the flow field is *irrotational* [43,53,73,74,78]. From the fluid dynamic standpoint, irrotational flow patterns in regions such as the ventricular chamber (*"simply connected"*) are exclusively dependent on the instantaneous velocity of the flow-field boundary (see Sections 13.3.2 and 13.3.5, on pp. 699 ff. and 705 ff., respectively). Alternatively, *different patterns* of motion by the endocardial surface (including the interventricular septum) are transmitted *instantaneously throughout* the flow field, including at the tricuspid orifice. In both cases, highest velocities are concentrated in the vicinity of the inflow orifice. This reflects the strong convective deceleration ensuing as blood moves from the orifice to the periphery of the chamber (cf. Fig. 14.2, on p. 740). It is *analogous* and *exactly the converse* of the strong convective acceleration of the intraventricular ejection flow in the immediate vicinity of the *outflow orifice*, which has previously been demonstrated in cardiac catheterization and CFD studies that were discussed in Chapter 13 (see also [12,43,47,48,73,74,83,84]).

In the time-varying and nonuniform intraventricular diastolic flow field, the velocity is a function of both time and space. Generally, there can be acceleration of fluid passing through a point even when the velocity at the given point is constant, i.e., even if the local acceleration is zero [73,78]. Streamlines connect velocity vectors in a flow field at a given instant. Juxtaposed streamlines outline fluid layers, or laminae, in motion. When successive laminae are at distances of equal volumetric flux, the resulting picture gives information about regions of high and low velocities. Closely spaced streamlines indicate relatively high linear velocities, and *vice-versa*. Converging streamlines in a flow region imply convective acceleration; diverging streamlines, convective deceleration.

Because the RV endocardial surface area is much larger than the tricuspid orifice area (*endocardial surface/orifice area* ≥ 10), blood entering the irrotational flow field of early

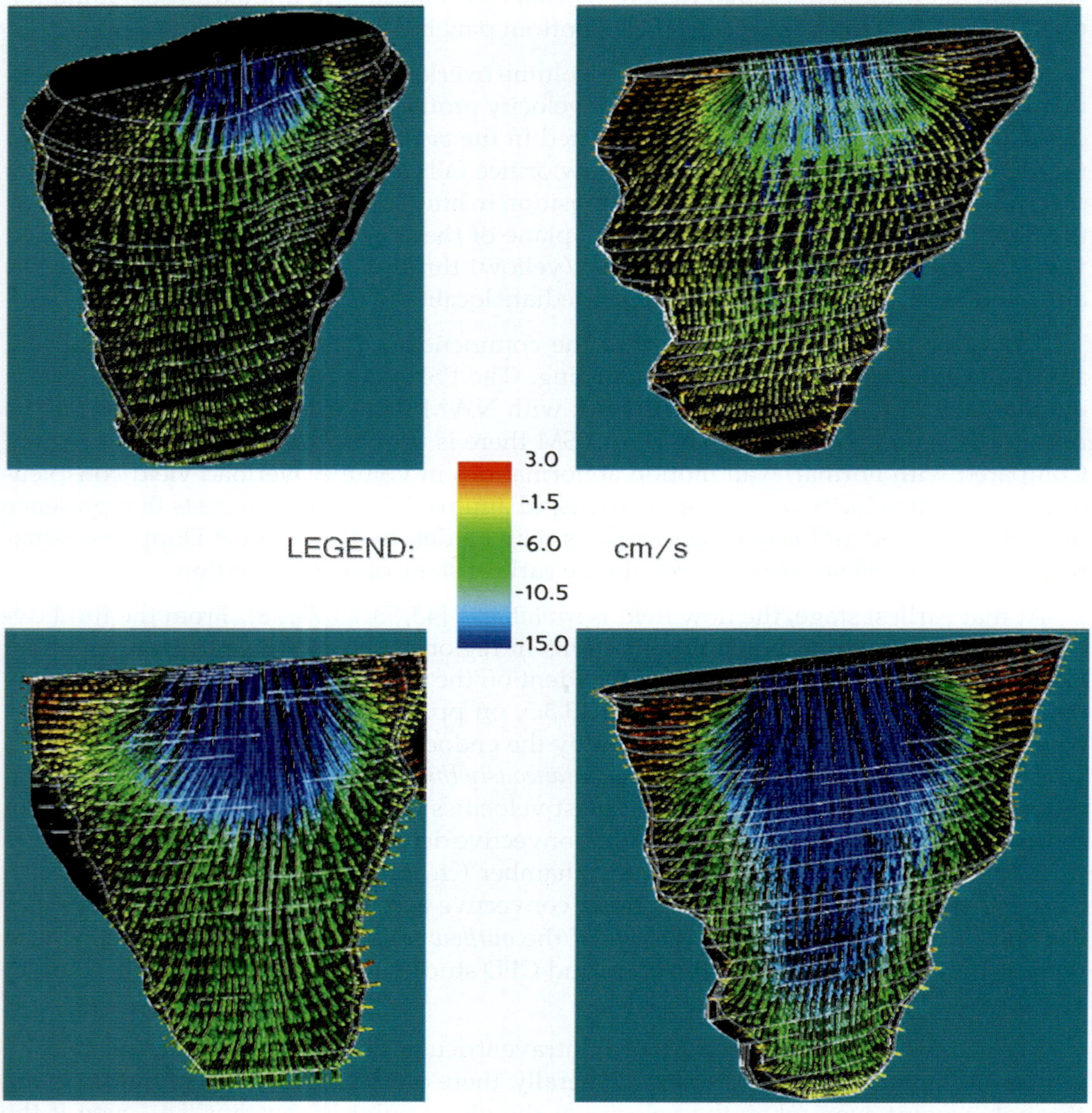

Figure 14.14: Representative fan-like frontal plane RV flow velocity fields during early stage of filling (*top*) and at E-wave peak volumetric inflow rate 136 cm^3/s for normal wall motion (NWM) and 216 cm^3/s for paradoxical septal motion (PSM) (*bottom*). *Left*, NWM; *right*, chamber dilatation with PSM in the same dog. (Adapted from Pasipoularides et al. [79], by kind permission of the American Physiological Society.)

diastole experiences convective deceleration (see Figs. 14.2 and 14.6, on p. 740 and p. 749, respectively). The magnitude of blood velocities below the inflow orifice falls off more gradually in the normal case reflecting a lower convective deceleration than in the volume-overloaded ventricle with diastolic paradoxical septal motion, where the transition from higher to lower flow velocities is more abrupt.

The *larger* the endsystolic size of the chamber relative to the inflow valve anulus, the *higher* is the diastolic convective deceleration. This reveals a subtle but important influence on filling dynamics of an *"inflow, or diastolic, ventriculoannular disproportion,"* [75,78–80] ensuing with chamber dilatation in volume overload. The concept is the counterpart of the *"outflow, or systolic, ventriculoannular disproportion,"* which was introduced and elaborated in earlier publications [43, 48, 73–75] and is discussed in Chapters 7, 8 and 13. The rise in downstream pressure underlying the diastolic convective deceleration load is *proportional* to the *square* of the applying velocities, e.g., at the tricuspid anulus. From this *quadratic* relationship, we may conclude that in early diastole, when ventricular filling is overlapping ventricular relaxation, as the inflow velocity rises to the peak of the E-wave, the much larger becomes the convective deceleration load, and the more difficult the inflow.

14.7.2 Upstroke through the peak of the *E*-wave

Figure 14.14, on p. 768, illustrates typical RV flow fields developing during the early upstroke of the E-wave, soon after the onset of filling (top), and at peak volumetric inflow rate (bottom). The left panels show the flow fields applying at control with NWM and the right panels show the fields applying under conditions of RV dilatation with PSM in the same animal. The velocity fields are visualized on an RV coronal (frontal) plane. The arrows indicate both direction and magnitude of the flow velocity at each *depicted* (a minute fraction of the *actual* node number in the simulations) node within the plane. Such arrow maps are effective in revealing the *spatial organization* of flow within the entire flow field. Flow velocity is encoded in the length of an arrow, whereas its color is assigned according to the z-component of the velocity vector. A negative z-component (i.e., the blue-green region of the spectrum) maps flow toward the apex, whereas a positive one (red-orange region) represents a velocity pointing toward the RV base (see color scale inset in Fig. 14.14).

Figure 14.14, top, shows that the computed flow fields on an RV frontal plane were quite similar for both wall motion patterns. In both, the inflow velocities in the region of the tricuspid anulus and below have a balanced distribution, being directed approximately *equally* in each of the following directions: the anterior wall, the apex, and the posterior wall. Essentially all inflow velocity vectors are directed in a *fan-like* pattern toward the chamber walls, which they meet *perpendicularly*, satisfying the *no slip* condition—see Section 4.12, on pp. 208 ff. This fan-like pattern is consistent with the motion of intraventricular blood similar to displacement of a laminar telescoping fluid trunk peeling off successive layers that *flare out laterally* and meet the *receding endocardium* at *right angles*; this pattern is depicted schematically in Figure 14.15.

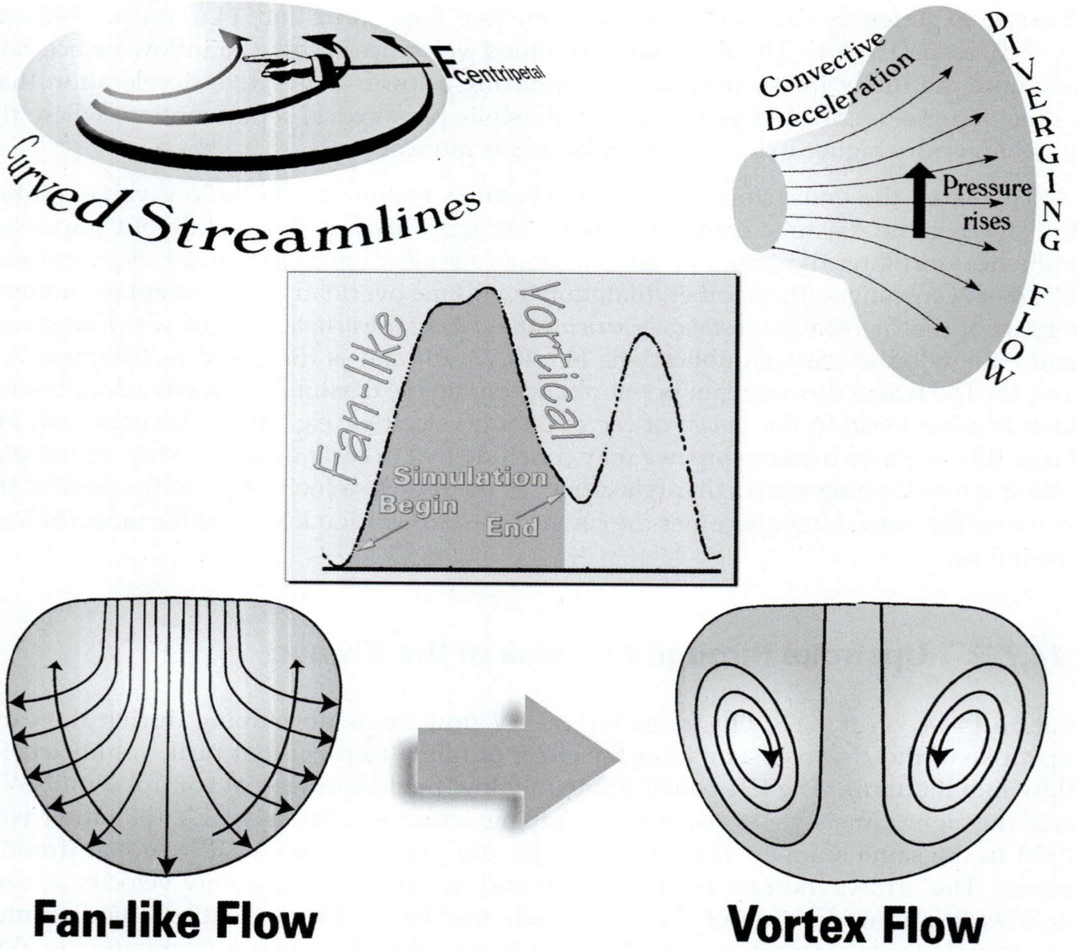

Figure 14.15: As blood fans away from the central stream toward the endocardial walls, the convective deceleration effect tends, by the Bernoulli mechanism, to elevate downstream pressure opposing ventricular inflow (*top right*). There is an additional convective pressure decrease normal to the curved fanning streamlines (*top left*), which tends to decrease pressure in the direction of the chamber's base and away from the endocardial walls (long arrows crossing streamlines, *lower left*). During the upstroke of the E-wave, these combined adverse convective pressure effects are opposed by the local acceleration gradient, which favors forward flow. During the E-wave downstroke, they are joined in sense and augmented by the local deceleration gradient and can now reverse the flow. This leads to disruption of the boundary between oncoming blood and endocardial walls, or "flow separation," and to the formation of a toroidal vortex that surrounds the central core. *Center inset*, volumetric filling rate calculated by numerical differentiation of RV chamber volume obtained from dynamic representations using real-time 3-D echocardiographic measurements; small arrows point to representative beginning and ending points of the simulations. (Adapted, somewhat modified, from Pasipoularides et al. [79], by kind permission of the American Physiological Society.)

On the other hand, NWM and PSM exhibited *dissimilar* flow fields in the (median) sagittal plane: blood velocities were slanted toward the RV *free wall* in the NWM model and toward the *septum* in the PSM model, as previously described [78,79].

The bottom panels in Figure 14.14 pertain to peak volumetric inflow rate: the peak volumetric inflow velocity was 136 cm^3/s for NWM and 216 cm^3/s for PSM. Because of the higher inflow rates compared with the earlier inflow stage depicted in the top panels, stronger velocity fields are observed with both NWM and PSM. The magnitudes of the axial (z-components) of the velocity vectors were predictably larger (dark blue) in PSM than NWM because of the much higher peak volumetric inflow rate in the volume overloaded (tricuspid regurgitation) condition. As earlier in the E-wave, NWM and PSM yield fundamentally similar fan-shaped flow velocity fields in the coronal (frontal) plane. The inflow velocity profiles in the region of the tricuspid orifice remain balanced. In a sagittal plane, with NWM the motion of the septum induced strong flow velocities toward the RV free wall, whereas with PSM the septal motion away from the RV free wall caused the individual velocity vectors to be slanted in the *reverse direction*, toward the septum and the left ventricle.

14.7.3 Downstroke of the *E*-wave

Figure 14.16, *top*, on p. 772, illustrates representative simulation plots of velocity vectors in the frontal plane. These results were obtained in the same dog as those in Figure 14.14 but at instants *close to the end* of the E-wave. The left panels show the flow field applying at control with NWM; the right panels show the field applying under conditions of RV dilatation with PSM. The instantaneous volumetric inflow velocity was 39 cm^3/s at control (NWM) and 71 cm^3/s in the dilated chamber.

The most distinct feature of both flow fields at this later stage of the E-wave is the existence of large-scale vortical motions [79,80]. In both the NWM and the PSM situations, streams roll up from regions near the apex toward the base. These streams are directed toward the plane of the inflow orifice, and some regurgitant flow was present under both control and volume overload conditions. In addition, the streams directed toward the inflow orifice interact with the incoming flow directed toward the apex. This interaction results in strong swirling motions, visualized nicely in Figure 14.16.

The extent of vortex formation appears to be stronger for the NWM case. Surprisingly, although the applying instantaneous volumetric inflow rate in NWM was *much smaller* than in PSM, *higher* (dark blue) velocity vector magnitudes are present within the control (NWM) flow field than in the dilated ventricle. The reason for this is going to be discussed shortly.

The formation of large-scale vortices results in a highly complex flow field. The general characteristics of the velocity field are better revealed using color mapping as is shown in Figure 14.16, *middle* and *bottom* panels. These panels show color maps of the velocity fields at the same instants as the corresponding velocity plots of the top panels. Such mappings are *familiar to echocardiographers* and suitable for revealing the *global* organization of the flow field. The regions with red and orange colors represent blood

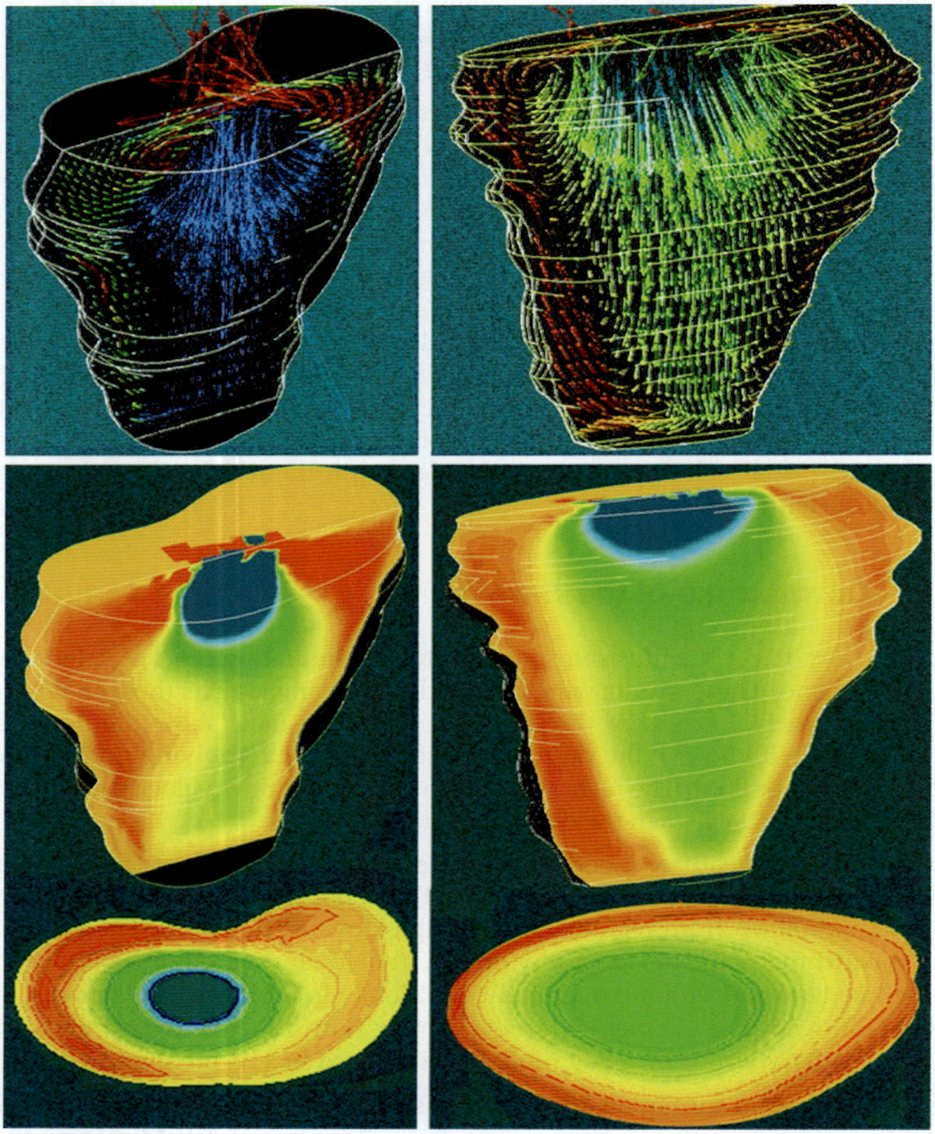

Figure 14.16: Frontal plane RV flow velocity fields (*top*), and color maps (*middle*) near end of *E*-wave, from same dog as Figure 14.14, on p. 768. Instantaneous inflow rate was 39 cm^3/s for NWM (*left*) and 71 cm^3/s for PSM (*right*). Both visualization planes and color coding are identical to those in Figure 14.14. *Bottom*, simultaneous transverse "cut" color maps in a plane 2.5 cm below the inflow orifice show to advantage the higher axial core velocities in the normal and the larger core cross-sectional area in the volume-overloaded chamber—cf. Fig. 14.17. (Adapted, slightly modified, from Pasipoularides et al. [79], by kind permission of the American Physiological Society.)

flow toward the base of the right ventricle, whereas regions with blue and green colors represent blood flow toward the apex.

Comparison between NWM and PSM simulations showed that the vortical motion was *stronger* in the former, with a high intensity in the region surrounding the main incoming stream below the inflow orifice [79,80]. This effectively *encroaches* on the available *central core area* beyond the inflow orifice that is *available for flow* toward the apex, as is shown schematically in Figure 14.17, on p. 774. The encroaching effect was *more pronounced* in the simulations under *control conditions* than in the dilated volume-overloaded ventricles (cf. Fig. 14.17). This is responsible for the *higher* velocity vector magnitudes present within the normal flow field, referred to in a preceding paragraph.

As is illustrated in the representative case shown in Figure 14.16, the vortical motion generated in the dilated ventricles with PSM had a more even spatial distribution than was prevalent under normal operating conditions. In addition, the space available for flow toward the apex, marked by the blue, green, and yellow zones, was significantly greater for the volume-overloaded situation (see also discussion pertaining to Fig. 14.21, on p. 783).

As we saw in Section 2.8, on pp. 59 f., by Newton' s Second Law of motion, the angular acceleration of a rotating object or medium is directly proportional to the net force acting on it and inversely proportional to its *moment of inertia*, the rotational analog of mass for linear motion. It depends, most importantly, on how the mass of the rotating medium is distributed with respect to the rotational axis. When the rotating mass is distributed at larger distances from the axis of rotation (*dilated* chamber), the rotational inertia is greater and the vortex strength *smaller*.

14.8 Doppler echocardiographic implications

Previous papers, discussed by Isaaz [52], had demonstrated that Doppler echocardiography using the simplified Bernoulli equation is not accurate for calculating the transvalvular pressure drop across a normal mitral valve, and had emphasized the contribution by local acceleration to diastolic transvalvular pressure differences across a nonobstructive mitral valve. However, the work under consideration [77–80] was the first to distinguish the *mutually opposed* effects of the local acceleration and convective deceleration during the upstroke of the E-wave on the *intraventricular—RV, LV—flow-field dynamics*.

The findings surveyed in the preceding Sections demonstrate that application of the simplified Bernoulli equation even at the time of the peak of the E-wave, when local acceleration vanishes, to calculate an intraventricular pressure decrease makes no sense. Rather than a convective *decrease*, at the E-wave peak there is actually a convective *increase* in the intraventricular pressure away from the tricuspid (mitral) anulus, and flow persists under its previously built-up momentum.

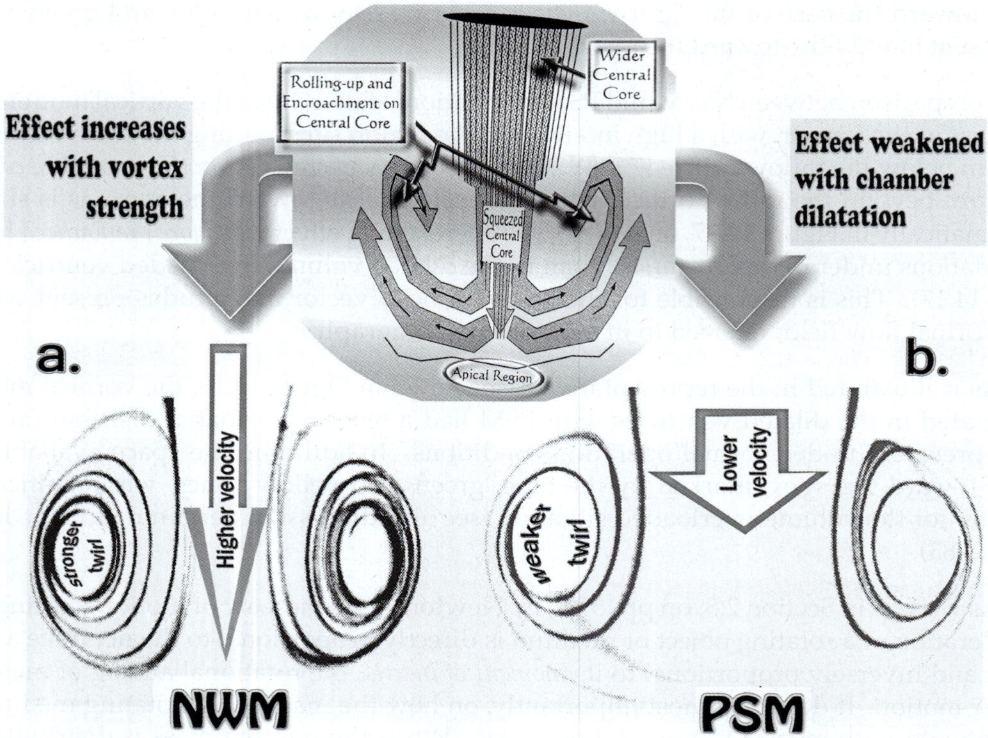

Figure 14.17: The high-intensity vortical motion in the region surrounding the main incoming stream effectively encroaches on the available central core area beyond the inflow orifice that is available for flow toward the apex. This explains how, although applying instantaneous volumetric inflow rate at control was much smaller than with volume overload, *higher* core velocities were present in the control flow field after vortex development. Visualization of simulation results from NWM and PSM (cf. Fig. 14.16) showed that the vortical motion was stronger in the former. Vortex ring encroaches on the available central core area for flow toward the apex: more substantially so in NWM (*a.*) than in the dilated ventricle (*b.*). Width of each white arrow is proportional to the central core area beyond the inflow orifice that is available for flow toward the apex; the length, to linear inflow velocity in the central core—see also Figure 14.25, on p. 792. (The lower panels (*a.* & *b.*) are adapted, slightly modified, from Pasipoularides et al. [79], by kind permission of the American Physiological Society.)

14.9 Functional imaging *vs.* multisensor catheterization

Multisensor catheters can derive pressure and velocity satisfactorily in many applications, especially involving the stable, "irrotational" (see Section 9.3, on pp. 448 ff.) intraventricular field of ejection [12, 73, 74, 83, 84, 97]. However, catheters inside the flow field can directly disturb it. In the case of the intraventricular RV inflow field, detailed, accurate catheter measurements are not practicable. It is impossible to obtain intraventricular pressure and velocity distributions, as those shown in Figures 14.21–14.24, through multisensor catheters. Unavoidable motions of any catheter buffeted by onrushing and whirling flow, global motions of the heart, and, in the case of pressure, attendant hydrostatic effects on the micromanometric sensors vitiate any attempt to measure along the inflow axis *instantaneous high axial resolution distributions* of pressure and velocity.

It is likewise impossible to obtain by catheter high-information-density data series in successive "snapshots," as in Figures 14.22 and 14.23, on pp. 785 and 786. Transvalvular atrioventricular pressure differences such as those presented in Figure 14.6B., b, exemplify what is *at best achievable* by direct multisensor catheter measurement; the sensors on the catheter are not really fixed *along the inflow axis* throughout the measurement process.

Functional Imaging results are in harmony with fundamental fluid dynamics theory and with the experimental in vitro findings on mechanical left heart models by Bellhouse [8–10] affirming that dilatation decreases vortex strength in the mechanical left ventricular chamber. Moreover, FIDAP™ results [47, 48] agreed closely, as is detailed in Chapter 13, with a proprietary CFD code developed in our laboratory [43] and with analytic [53, 84], semiempirical correlation [83], and similarity [73] solutions in our investigations of the intraventricular left ventricular *ejection flow field*, under diverse clinical conditions.

Though still in its relative infancy, image-based CFD simulations encompassed in Functional Imaging show immense promise as a viable means for *elucidating intracardiac blood flows* in individual subjects in health and disease. Whether particular fluid dynamic *indicators*, derived from Functional Imaging, patient-specific simulations, are sufficiently *accurate and precise*, particularly in the context of normal physiological variability, remains to be seen in the absence of tests for hemodynamic significance. Nevertheless, previously inaccessible subtleties [65, 74] in the dynamics of the RV diastolic flow field can now be investigated by FI, and important but formerly unrecognized aspects of pressure and flow dynamics during ventricular filling can be examined. As shown in Figures 14.21–14.24, on pp. 783—788, inspection of the time-dependent distributions of flow-field variables provides a detailed insight into filling dynamics, akin to an ideal *high-resolution catheterization experiment*.

The work under discussion here was the first to properly recognize, characterize, and distinguish the complex contributions by local and convective acceleration gradients to diastolic instantaneous intraventricular pressure and velocity distributions in normal and dilated diseased ventricles. It has shown that the smallness of normal (nonobstructive) early RV diastolic intraventricular pressure gradients for inflow is referable to the partially *counterbalancing* actions of convective deceleration and local acceleration components working *concurrently* during the upstroke of the E-wave. The same mechanism should account for the small *left* ventricular intraventricular gradients. Detailed dynamic intraventricular pressure and axial velocity distribution patterns have corroborated the concepts [79, 80] of a convective deceleration load and the useful role of the diastolic ventricular vortex in promoting filling.

Acquisition and interpretations of Doppler and catheterization measurements should consider such effects more closely than in the past. The utility and applicability of

Functional Imaging will surely increase rapidly in the near future, with forthcoming further advances in digital imaging modalities, computing, and scientific visualization.

14.10 The RV diastolic vortex

In all FI simulations conducted in the seven dog hearts under control and volume overload conditions, development of large-scale vortical motions was observed during the downstroke of the E-wave [79, 80]. During this period, inflow velocity decreases while the pressure level rises within the flow field. As one moves away from the central stream toward the endocardial wall, convective pressure rise by the Bernoulli mechanism (see Sections 4.4.6 and 4.5, on pp. 182 ff. and 187 ff.) raises the pressure energy opposing ventricular inflow along any streamline. An adverse convective pressure gradient develops, and this is augmented [79, 80] by the local deceleration gradient during the downstroke of the E-wave.

As is shown diagrammatically in Figure 14.15, on p. 770, *bottom left*, the fanning streamlines are *curved*. This implies that the streaming blood is acted upon by a *centripetal* force and that the convective pressure gradient has also a component that is normal to the *concave streamlines* and that tends to drive the onrushing blood *toward the base* of the chamber (see Fig. 14.15). Ultimately, the combined adverse pressure gradient forces arrest forward flow and deflect the direction of blood near the endocardial surface toward the base, leading to *flow separation*, roll up, and recirculating *vortical motions* within the chamber. Large-scale vortices form, as shown in Figures 14.15 and 14.16—cf. also Figures 14.1 and 14.2, on pp. 738 and 740, respectively.

To look now, from a somewhat different than the preceding viewpoint, at why a vortex display comes about, we can also invoke the Theory of Dissipative Structures, formulated by Nicolis and Prigogine [68, 86] (see Sections 1.5 and 9.2.1, on pp. 10 ff. and 445 f.). Because of the movement and exchange of energy, when the simple fan-like pattern breaks down, the flow is likely to reorganize itself in a more complex interactive form and achieves coherence in the vortical arrangement. Blood moves *through* the filling vortex and *forms it* at the same time. Energy moves likewise through the vortical structure and the latter embodies the energy, highly organized and in motion, as *rotational kinetic energy* of the vortex.

A heretofore unsuspected but extremely important physiological role of the ventricular filling vortex has emerged out of these detailed investigations of the diastolic intraventricular flow field: it is *indispensable* in promoting diastolic filling. The pressure and velocity data surveyed and discussed at length in the present chapter corroborate the hypothesis [79, 80] that the dissipative vortical structures facilitate filling and attainment of higher volumes (larger endocardial surface areas) by robbing kinetic energy that would otherwise contribute to the convective pressure rise representing what I have denoted as a *convective deceleration load*—see Section 14.15.1, on pp. 795 ff. Thus, the diastolic vortex facilitates, indeed *allows*, higher diastolic filling and stroke volume maintenance.

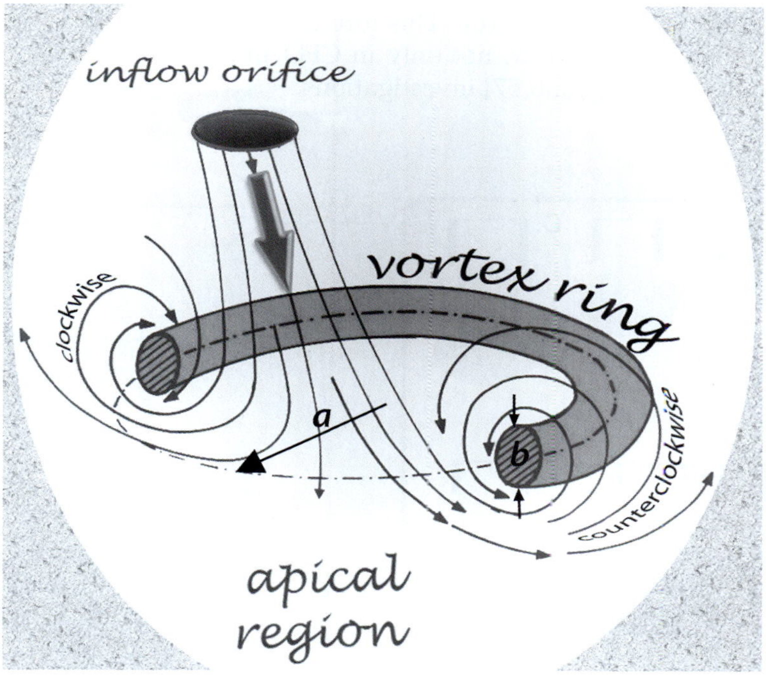

Figure 14.18: On a long axis "cut," the toroidal LV filling vortex appears as two 2-D vortices, on the anterior and posterior sides of the inflow jet, with clockwise and counterclockwise flow, respectively. a = radius of the vortical ring; b = vortex core diameter.

14.11 The LV diastolic vortex

The physiologic and pathophysiologic fluid dynamic mechanisms (convective deceleration load, diastolic ventriculoannular disproportion, etc.) that were found to apply to RV filling dynamics in health and disease [75,76,78–80], apply also to the left ventricle, because *fundamentally the two ventricles in diastole share common fluid dynamic characteristics* and operating conditions [65,74].

In early diastole, during the upstroke of the E-wave, the laminar inflow jet is wide and occupies the whole LV region. In the vicinity of the expanding LV chamber walls, the kinetic energy of the fluid particles is reduced by a *very substantial* amount from that of fluid particles in the region of the mitral anulus and the mainstream inflow; thus, the motion in the periphery is very susceptible to the influence of the convective pressure rise and to a consequent flow reversal. Thus, the adverse pressure gradient after the E-wave peak provokes the formation of a zone of recirculating flow, which expands laterally and grows rapidly in a direction normal to the walls during the downstroke of the E-wave. It forms a large toroidal filling vortex within the expanding chamber (see Fig. 14.18). On a long axis visualization plane, this is depicted as two vortices, on the anterior and posterior sides of the inflow jet, with clockwise and counterclockwise flow, respectively [1,5,20,31,50,58,66,92,93,116]. This toroidal filling vortex is a key feature of the LV intraventricular diastolic flow, not only in CFD simulations but also in experimental [8–10,104] and clinical [33,56,57] investigations.

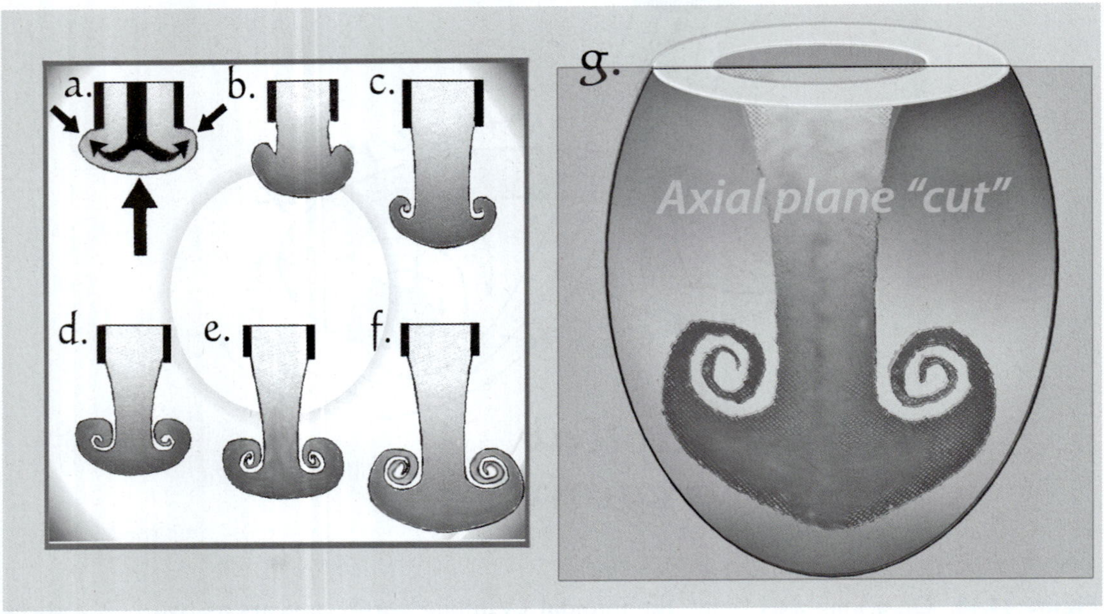

Figure 14.19: Due to shear between the forward edge of the onrushing E-wave column and the intraventricular endsystolic blood volume, a toroidal circulation may develop, giving rise to a toroidal vortex with a familiar *"mushroom shape"*; its *"stem"* increases in length with time, as the *"cap"* travels toward the ventricular apex, passing through the successive states (a–g).

In CFD simulations encompassing the atrial contraction phase, a similar but relatively weaker vortex ring forms and grows during the downstroke of the A-wave. This vortex is wider behind the posterolateral leaflet of the mitral valve. The swirling motion is more vigorous behind the anterior cusp because of the *smaller* space between it and the wall; this is just a manifestation of the conservation of angular momentum, which is proportional to a fluid particle's tangential velocity and to its distance from the center of rotation, and of the *(near)* constancy of circulation in a *(nearly)* irrotational flow (see Section 9.3, on pp. 448 ff.). As we saw in Section 3.3, on pp. 119 ff., Leonardo da Vinci anticipated this key concept of modern hydrodynamics, that is, the notion of *circulation* (circular path times fluid particle velocity), and aptly ascertained that in an irrotational flow this quantity is invariant with radial distance from the axis of the circulatory motion. Since the thrust exerted by the vortex on the anterior cusp is greater than that exerted on the posterior one, the anterior cusp is pushed toward the closed position *earlier and faster* than the posterior—see Section 7.13.3, on pp. 388 ff., for the role of the vortex thrust in mitral valve leaflet closure.

The CFD simulations of Nakamura et al. [67] on the entire cardiac cycle have shown that the LV diastolic vortex structure is highly stretched during systole, and that it is ejected or dissipated almost completely before the next diastole begins. The vorticity remaining from the previous cycle is, commonly, extremely weak at the onset of diastolic filling; thus, the simulated LV vortex structure was shown [67] to be affected only weakly by flow *disturbances remaining* at the onset of diastole.

When fluid is forced through an orifice (a model for the *mitral anulus*) into a cylindrical container (a model for the *left ventricle*), the spatial velocity profile is blunt. The cross-sectional average of the outflow velocity magnitude at the orifice is U. Consider an injection which is uniform in time and is started and stopped abruptly, so that the mass of the injected fluid, m, is equal to $\rho\pi R^2 L$ with ρ the density of the fluid, R the radius of the orifice, and L the injection length, defined as the product of injection velocity and injection time ($L = Ut$). As fluid particles flow within the *"atrial"* container and past the orifice, *vorticity* is created within the undeveloped, thin boundary layer. At the orifice, this vortex sheet is shed into the receiving container, *viz.*, LV chamber. Downstream of the orifice, the vortex sheet rolls up and changes considerably, but its strength is conserved. This vortex strength, Γ, is by definition the circulation of the velocity (see Equation 9.3, on p. 452) taken along any circuit around the sheet. Bot and his coworkers [15] studied thoroughly the conditions necessary for the creation and for the downstream propagation of such a vortex ring, applying sound fluid dynamic theory, experiments, and computational methods.

Their analytical and experimental findings [15] show that the radius of the generated vortex ring is determined solely by the inflow orifice radius and is independent of the injection speed; it is roughly 40% larger than the orifice radius. Moreover, their computational results indicate that a vortex ring will continue to move forward only if its diameter is less than about 50% or 60% of that of the cylindrical container, *viz.*, LV chamber. The vortex speed W for downstream *("apical")* travel is proportional to the injection velocity, but it depends also on b/a (see Fig. 14.18, on p. 777), which depends, in turn, on L/R. For a given orifice radius, this *("propagation speed")* increases with L. Qualitatively, their experiments confirmed their analytical fluid dynamic expectation that the *close proximity of the wall* of the containing chamber will lead to the disappearance of a generated vortex, or will *impede the generation* of a vortex by such a mechanism. Applying this to the left ventricle, they demonstrated that vortices will be arrested, or will not develop in the first place, if the orifice to cylinder diameter is larger than 0.6. Experimentally, it has been independently corroborated that vortices do develop by such a mechanism in *some dilated left ventricles*, but certainly *not under normal operating conditions* [27].

The normal end-diastolic left ventricular diameter lies in a range from 35 to 56 *mm* [26,34], suggesting the midvalue of this range, 45 *mm*, as a typical value for a normal short-axis ventricular diameter. Dilatation of the left ventricle in congestive cardiomyopathy or secondary to myocardial infarction leads to values of the end-diastolic inner diameter of the sphericalized ventricle ranging from 57 to 83 *mm* [23,26], yielding a value of 70 *mm*, in the middle of this range, as typical under conditions of LV chamber enlargement. The findings of Bot et al. [15] demonstrate that the ratio of *mitral orifice-to-LV chamber radius* in LV dilatation is small enough to admit vortex generation by this mechanism, while for a normal left ventricle the conditions are such that it is most likely that vortices will *not* be generated in such a fashion.

In some patients with severely impaired left ventricular function and chamber dilatation, the pulsed-Doppler transmitral flow pattern can be *"normalized"* (pseudonormalization) by an increased atrioventricular pressure gradient. Formation and propagation of a mushroom-shaped vortex during the acceleration of early filling has been reported [54] in the abnormally enlarged left ventricle with a pseudonormalized filling pattern. In the presence of a well developed mushroom-shaped vortex, the blood within the filling flow front moves in a circular pattern into the vortex, instead of fanning out toward the expanding walls and traveling toward the apex. This can result in an *apical filling delay* by color M-mode Doppler in the left ventricle with a pseudonormalized filling, although the mitral inflow velocity by pulsed-Doppler appears to be normal.

The ratio between the mitral valve orifice diameter and the ventricular diameter is therefore a paramount factor for the generation of vortices in ventricles by vortex sheet shedding from the mitral anulus. Creation by vortex sheet shedding with downstream propagation of LV vortex rings toward the apex, as some investigators have proposed [22, 28, 55], does not seem likely unless the short axis diameter of the chamber is about three times the diameter of the mitral anulus, which is about *double* the normally applying value. The *tricuspid orifice-to-chamber radius* pertaining to the right ventricle makes vortex formation by such a mechanism *very unlikely* not only under normal conditions but *also under RV chamber enlargement states*; the septal-to-free wall RV dimensions are *smaller* than corresponding LV short-axis diameters, while the effective diameter of the tricuspid anulus is *at least* 20% *greater* than that of the mitral anulus, implying that the tricuspid anulus area normally exceeds the mitral by about 50% [16, 39, 70].

The normal tricuspid anulus has a nonplanar or 3-D structure; a similar, but more planar, 3-D shape is prevalent in patients with functional tricuspid regurgitation and RV enlargement. In patients with functional tricuspid regurgitation, the tricuspid anulus is dilated in the septal-to-lateral direction, resulting in a more circular shape and larger anteroseptal dimension than in healthy subjects. Both the maximum (7.5 ± 2.1 *vs.* 5.6 ± 1.0 cm^2/m^2 BSA) and the minimum (5.7 ± 1.3 *vs.* 3.9 ± 0.8 cm^2/m^2 BSA) tricuspid anulus area index (area divided by body surface area, BSA) in tricuspid regurgitation are larger than normal (both $P < 0.01$) [39].

14.12 Color M-mode Doppler echocardiograms and the intraventricular vortex

Color M-mode Doppler (CMD) echocardiography of the left ventricle scans the distribution of the diastolic inflow velocity in the direction of an ultrasound beam, transmitted along the long axis of the LV chamber, as a function of time [11]. It provides this inflow velocity distribution as a *spatiotemporal map* in which the inflow linear velocity magnitude is conveyed by color and brightness as is demonstrated in Figure 14.20, on p. 781. The two phases of early filling denoted by Steen and Steen [104] as Phase I., or *"column propagation,"* and Phase II., or *"vortex propagation,"* are indicated. As shown in the inset of Figure 14.20, Phase I. is actually the *"fan-like flow"* phase, which was introduced in Section 14.7.2, on pp. 769 ff., and Phase II is the ensuing *"vortical flow"* phase, which was introduced in Section 14.7.3, on pp. 771 ff.

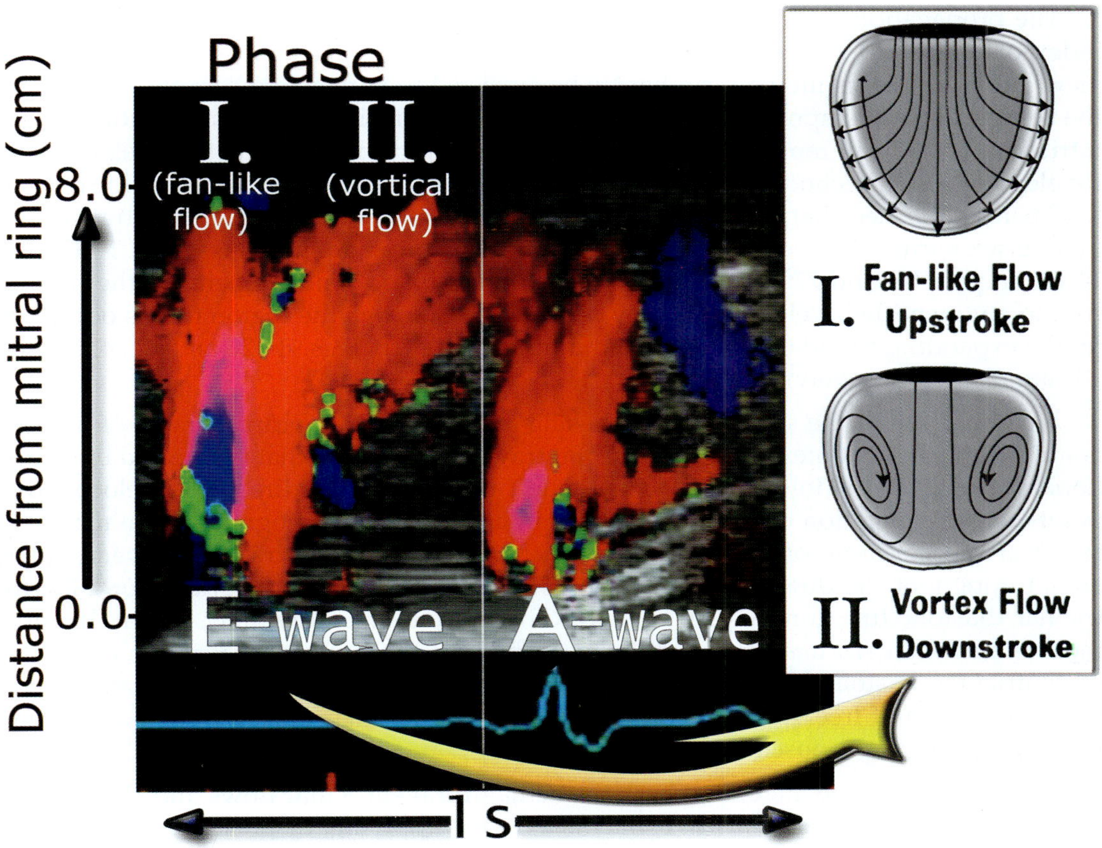

Figure 14.20: Normal color M-mode LV echocardiogram. The main panel shows the early filling E-wave and the atrial systolic A-wave. The two phases of early filling denoted by Steen and Steen [104] as Phase I., or *"column propagation,"* and Phase II., or *"vortex propagation,"* are indicated. As shown in the inset on the right, Phase I. is actually the *"fan-like flow"* phase in which blood flow proceeds along streamtubes extending between the atrioventricular valve anulus and the endocardial surface of the expanding chamber, and Phase II. is the ensuing *"vortical flow"* phase (see discussion in text).

Using CMD echocardiography, one can measure the times at which the peak inflow velocity appears at successive levels, from the mitral anulus plane[5] to the apex, as well as

[5]The mitral anulus is not, strictly speaking, planar; it is actually "saddle-shaped."

the propagation velocity of the inflow velocity maximum from the center of the entrance of the left ventricle to the ventricular apex. Numerous methods are employed in the estimation of various propagation velocities from the CMD echocardiogram [6,17,32,45, 109–112].

The propagation velocity of the inflow velocity maximum has been proposed as an index of diastolic LV function [17, 32, 45, 109, 110, 112]. Clearly, however, the *ice pick* view afforded by this method can hardly be expected to survey and sample adequately the complex spatiotemporal patterns of diastolic intraventricular flow as a whole, or the intricacies of LV wall motion abnormalities. Accordingly, many deductions relating the topology of a CMD echocardiogram to ventricular diastolic function remain uncertain. It has been established that the toroidal, i.e., ellipsoidal ring-shaped, diastolic intraventricular vortex narrows the central passageway available for blood inflow (see Fig. 14.17 and 14.16, on pp. 774 and 772, respectively). This forces blood fluid elements in the central core to augment their velocities as they pass *into and through* the region that is occupied by the expanding toroidal vortex surrounding the core (cf. Figs. 14.21 and 14.24, on pp. 783 and 788, respectively).

A comparison of the shapes of the aliasing area in CMD echocardiograms of the left ventricle and the spatiotemporal pattern of intraventricular flow that is revealed by Functional Imaging methodology applied to the left ventricle, or by direct MRI velocimetry, points to the elongation of the aliasing area in a CMD echocardiogram as the manifestation of the *expansion* of the toroidal vortex, and its *migration* toward the ventricular apex throughout the downstroke of the E-wave. Thus, the clinical evaluation of ventricular diastolic function by CMD echocardiography may, in my view, reveal, mainly, the *evolution of the size and shape* and, only secondarily, the shifting localization of the intraventricular diastolic filling vortex with progressive ventricular expansion, rather than the propagation of free vortex ring(s) through intraventricular quiescent blood as some investigators have proposed [22,28,55].

Suffice it to observe, here, that both the actual intraventricular flows and their simulation using CFD are very sensitive, *inter alia*, to the applying, or prescribed, geometric boundary conditions. Consider now that, e.g., a 50-*gallon* water tank [22], and a 13 *cm* (width) by 13 *cm* (depth) by 13–20 *cm* (height) Plexiglas box [55], were used to represent the *left ventricle* in conjunction with properly sized inflow (*"mitral"*) orifices, around an inch (2.54 *cm*) in diameter. Is it surprising then that creation and travel of *free vortex rings* akin to those released into quiescent air from an experienced smoker's lips were observed in such studies?

14.13 Evolution of axial velocities and pressures throughout the *E*-wave

The spatial distribution of the time-varying intraventricular pressure values, obtained by the CFD simulations during the filling process, determines the instantaneous force acting on flowing blood particles within the filling chamber. The assemblage of the un-

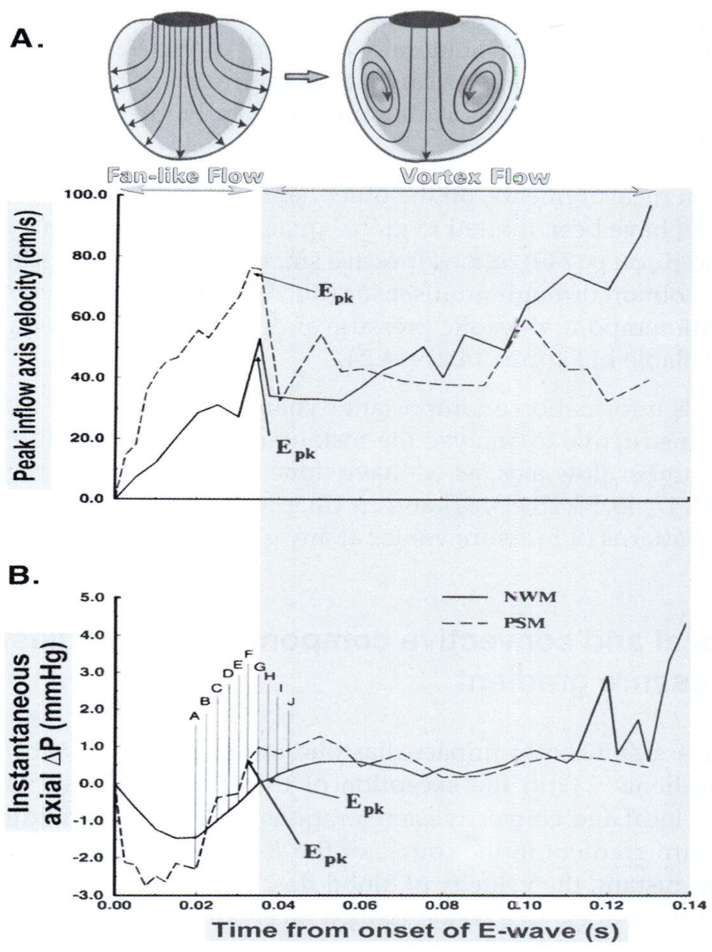

Figure 14.21: **A:** peak linear velocity along the RV inflow axis (V_{max}) through the E-wave for NWM and volume overload with PSM. Note that with NWM, V_{max} continues to rise late in the E-wave although the volumetric inflow rate is actually decreasing (cf. Fig. 14.17). **B:** development of the axial RV intraventricular pressure gradient (ΔP = apical pressure – tricuspid anulus pressure) throughout the E-wave. ΔP inverts from negative (*favorable*) to positive (*adverse*) around the time of peak volumetric inflow velocity (E_{pk}) and remains positive throughout the remainder of the E-wave. Note that more prominent fluctuations in the magnitude of the pressure gradient occur after E_{pk} with NWM than under volume overload with PSM. Such fluctuations are indicative of strong large-scale vortical motions. The axial pressure distributions that correspond to *instants* A–J are discussed in detail in the text and in Figures 14.22 and 14.23. (Adapted, slightly modified, from Pasipoularides et al. [80], by permission of the American Physiological Society.)

steady pressure values on all of the intraventricular flow-field points is the instantaneous pressure field. A major advantage of the Functional Imaging method is that much more extensive information can be extracted compared with experimental measurements; it yields values of the field variables at literally *thousands of discrete points* in space and time. From this *high-density information*, we can extract informative *snapshots* of instantaneous *velocity and pressure distributions*, as is demonstrated in Figures 14.13, 14.14, 14.16, and 14.21–14.24.

Catheterization measurements, on the other hand, traditionally [8–10, 21, 24, 60, 65, 74, 91, 97, 101, 102, 109] have been limited to global quantities (cf. chamber "pressure" values in Fig. 14.6 A. and B., on p. 749) or to values at a small number of points in space and time. It is impossible to obtain through multisensor (micromanometric/velocimetric) catheters high-density spatiotemporal diastolic pressure and velocity distribution values, such as those that are available in Figures 14.21–14.24.

Thus, FI reveals information on important dynamic flow behavior that was *previously inaccessible*. It is instructive to analyze the instantaneous distribution of pressure along the line of the chamber flow axis, as we have done in our studies of the fluid dynamics of ejection [12, 43, 47, 48, 53, 73, 83, 84] and in Chapter 13. Discrete points along the axis exhibit different patterns of pressure values at any given time during filling.

14.13.1 Local and convective components of the diastolic pressure gradient

Convective effects significantly impact diastolic intraventricular velocity distributions and pressure gradients. With the exception of the instant of peak volumetric inflow ($dQ/dt = 0$), both local and convective accelerations make their individual contributions to the total pressure gradient in the course of the E-wave. Our FI findings demonstrate that, at any given instant, the velocity of blood flow tends to decrease away from the inflow orifice toward the apex; this is exemplified nicely in Figure 14.24, on p. 788. Because acceleration is associated with a drop in pressure in the flow direction, the local acceleration ($\partial v/\partial t$) component causes a pressure decrease from the orifice to the apex during the upstroke of the E-wave. The total intraventricular pressure gradient is then the *algebraic sum* of the pressure *decrease* contributed by the local acceleration and the pressure *rise* contributed by the convective deceleration.

The convective intraventricular pressure *rise* demonstrated in Figures 14.22 and 14.23, reproduced from Pasipoularides et al. [80] on pp. 785 and 786, during the upstroke of the E-wave had previously never been commented upon or demonstrated. It has *crucial implications* for diastolic fluid dynamics. During the E-wave upstroke, the total pressure gradient along intraventricular flow is the algebraic sum of a pressure decrease contributed by local acceleration, and a pressure rise contributed by a convective deceleration that counterbalances partially the local acceleration gradient. This *counteracting action* [80] is what underlies the peculiar *smallness* of early diastolic intraventricular pressure gradients. During ejection, on the other hand, throughout the upstroke of the ejection

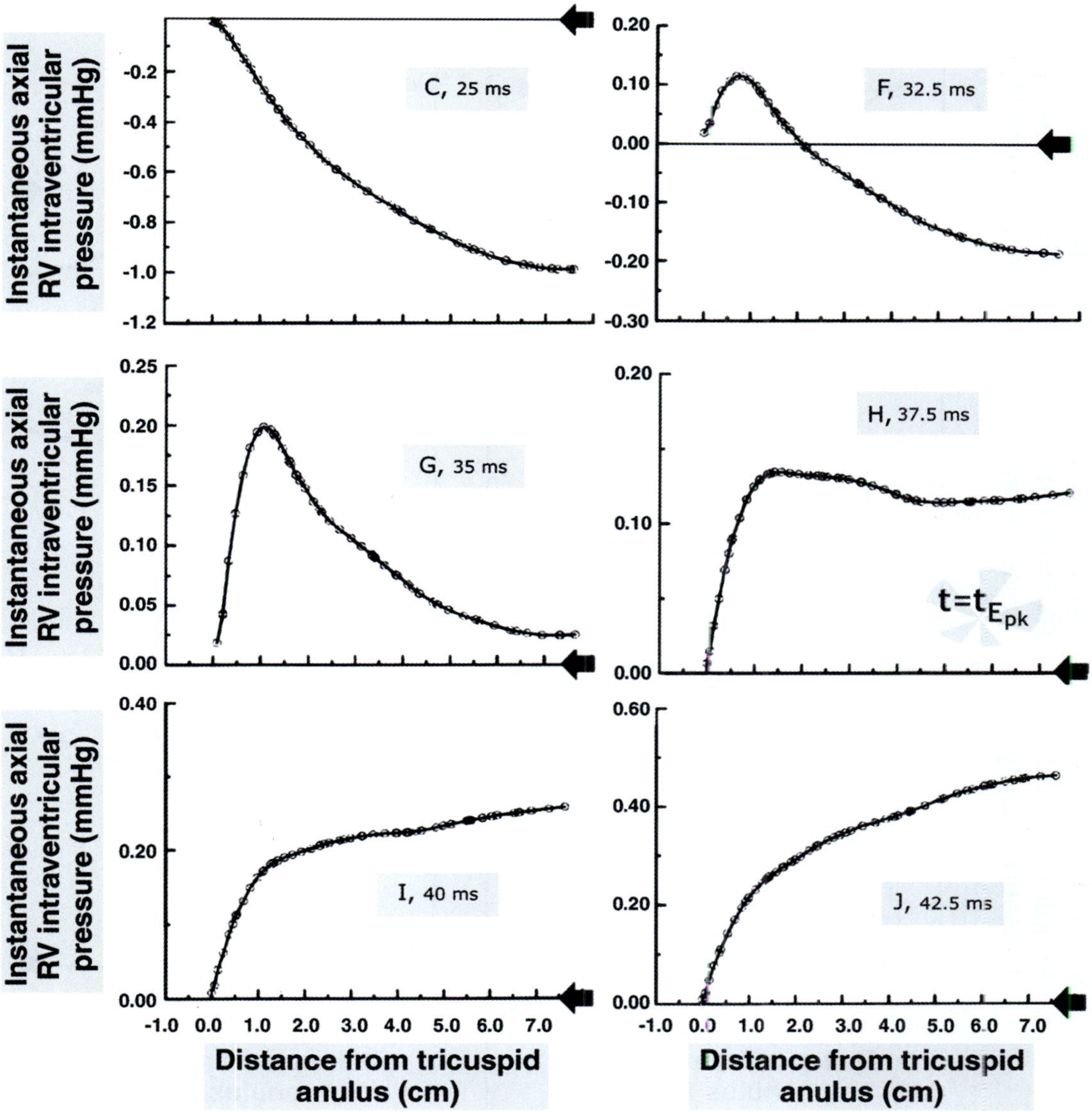

Figure 14.22: Normal wall motion. Apportionment of the instantaneous axial pressure gradient along the main inflow axis of the RV chamber around the time of the peak of the E-wave. *Instants C–J*: pressures computed at the successive instants of time labeled in Figure 14.21B. Note that at the time of peak volumetric inflow rate *(instant H, $t = t_{E_{pk}}$)*, the pressure distribution is transformed from a predominantly favorable (accelerating) to a predominantly adverse (decelerating) axial pressure gradient, in reference to apically directed flow. Arrowheads at the right margin of each panel indicate the zero pressure level with reference to tricuspid anulus pressure. (Adapted, slightly modified, from Pasipoularides et al. [80], by kind permission of the American Physiological Society.)

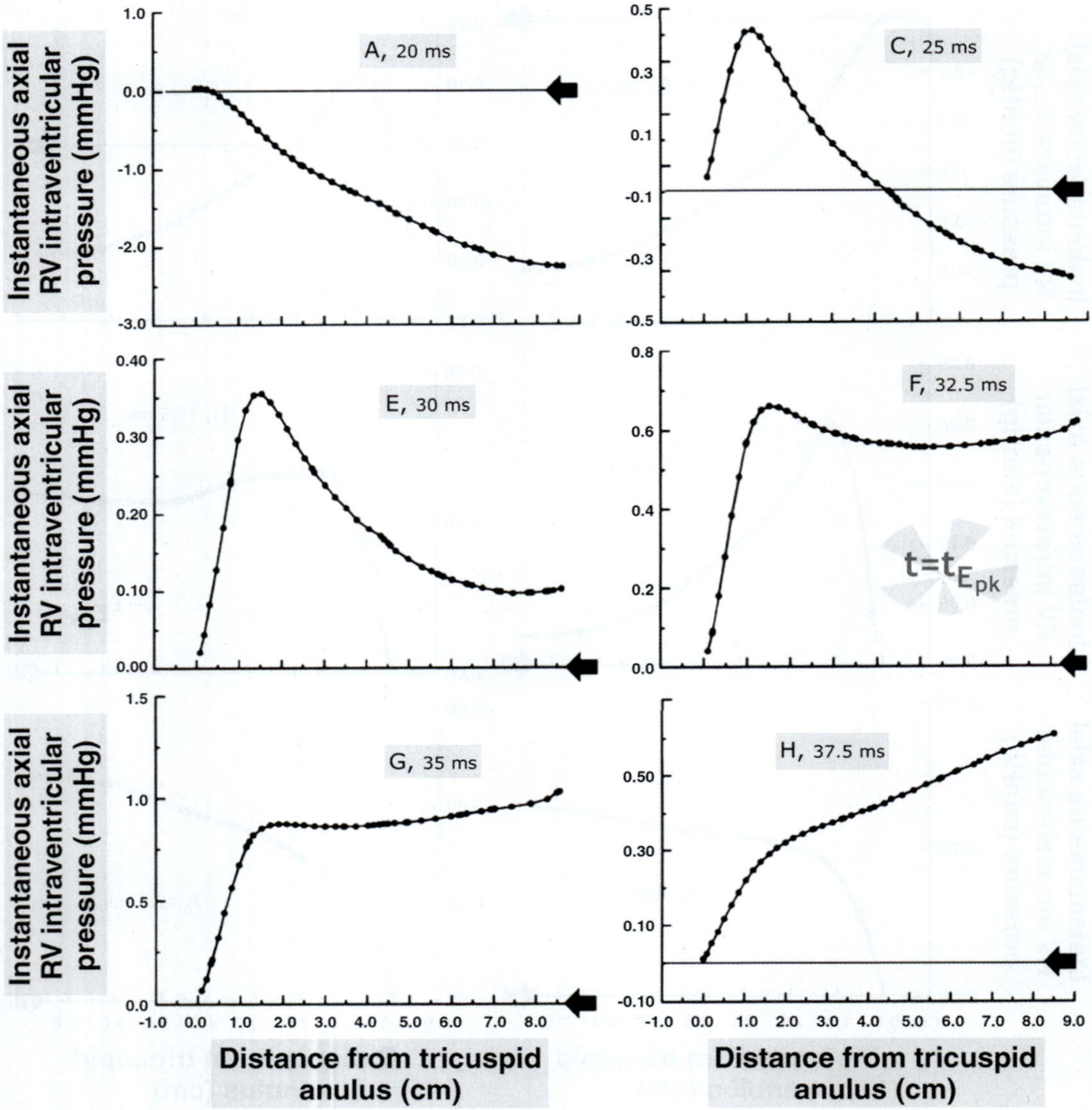

Figure 14.23: Volume overload with PSM. Apportionment of the instantaneous axial pressure gradient along the main inflow axis of the RV chamber during the E-wave. *Instants A–H*: pressures computed at the successive instants of time labeled in Figure 14.21B. Pressure distribution at the time of peak volumetric inflow rate *(instant F,* $t = t_{E_{pk}}$*)*, has the same characteristics as that of *instant H* in Figure 14.22. Note the sharper, compared with normal (cf. Fig. 14.22), convective accentuation of the pressure gradient near the inflow orifice, which is a hallmark of *ventriculoannular disproportion*. Arrowheads at the right margin of each panel indicate the zero pressure level with reference to tricuspid anulus pressure. (Adapted, slightly modified, from Pasipoulardes et al. [80], by kind permission of the American Physiological Society.)

outflow waveform convective and local acceleration effects act in the *same sense*, actually *reinforcing each other* [73]. These *contrasting dynamics* of the two components of the diastolic pressure gradient underscore the *more prominent* total (*viz.*, measured by multisensor catheter) intraventricular gradient during the upstroke of the ejection waveform than the upstroke of the E-wave, especially under hyperdynamic conditions, such as during exercise when both convective and local acceleration components are augmented.

At E_{pk} the local acceleration component vanishes, and the total pressure gradient is convective. In the E-wave downstroke, the strongly adverse pressure gradient is the sum of pressure augmentations along the flow path from *both* local and convective *decelerations*. Soon after the onset of the downstroke of the E-wave, the overall adverse pressure gradient causes flow separation and inception of *recirculation* with a vortical motion surrounding the central inflowing stream [79, 80], as is shown in Figure 14.17, on p. 774. Subsequent interaction of the central stream with the expanding vortex, which *encroaches* on it, is responsible for the *continuous rise* of the peak RV axis velocity throughout the downstroke of the E-wave that is typical under normal conditions (NWM) and was demonstrated for the first time, to my knowledge, in Figure 14.21 [80].

14.13.2 Interplay of convective with local acceleration effects

An interplay of convective with local acceleration effects underlies a nonuniformity in the spatiotemporal characteristics of the distribution of the pressure gradient along the chamber axis. The monotonic decrease in pressure along the inflow axis epitomized in Figure 14.22, instant C, reveals that the local acceleration effect completely dominates the convective during the first 25 *ms* of the upstroke of the E-wave. During the subsequent interval up to E_{pk}, the impact of an intense convective deceleration becomes prominent in the segment of the axis immediately beneath the tricuspid orifice.

During this interval, although the volumetric inflow rate continues to accelerate toward its peak, the acceleration magnitude has begun to diminish. Hence, the favorable *(negative)* pressure gradient contributed by the local acceleration is being reduced in magnitude. On the other hand, the magnitude of the inflow velocity near the tricuspid orifice has risen to higher levels. Consequently, the adverse pressure gradient contributed by the convective deceleration now overpowers in the first 1–2 *cm* of the inflow axis the favorable pressure gradient contributed by the local acceleration. This explains why pressure is rising in the first 1–1.5 *cm* of the axis and decreasing in the remaining $6.5-7$ *cm* (Fig. 14.22, instants F and G). The reduction in velocity, because of the intense convective deceleration in the *immediate vicinity* of the tricuspid orifice (cf. Fig. 14.24, on p. 788), allows the local acceleration to regain its dominance, generating a pressure *drop* in the remaining segment of the inflow axis, after the initial 1–2 *cm*.

Because at the instant of the peak volumetric inflow the local acceleration vanishes, the convective deceleration contributes exclusively to the total pressure gradient, resulting in a predominantly monotonic pressure rise along the inflow axis (Fig. 14.22, instant H). The sharp rise in the magnitude of the adverse pressure gradient near the tricuspid inflow orifice is notable. During the downstroke of the E-wave, the local acceleration turns into

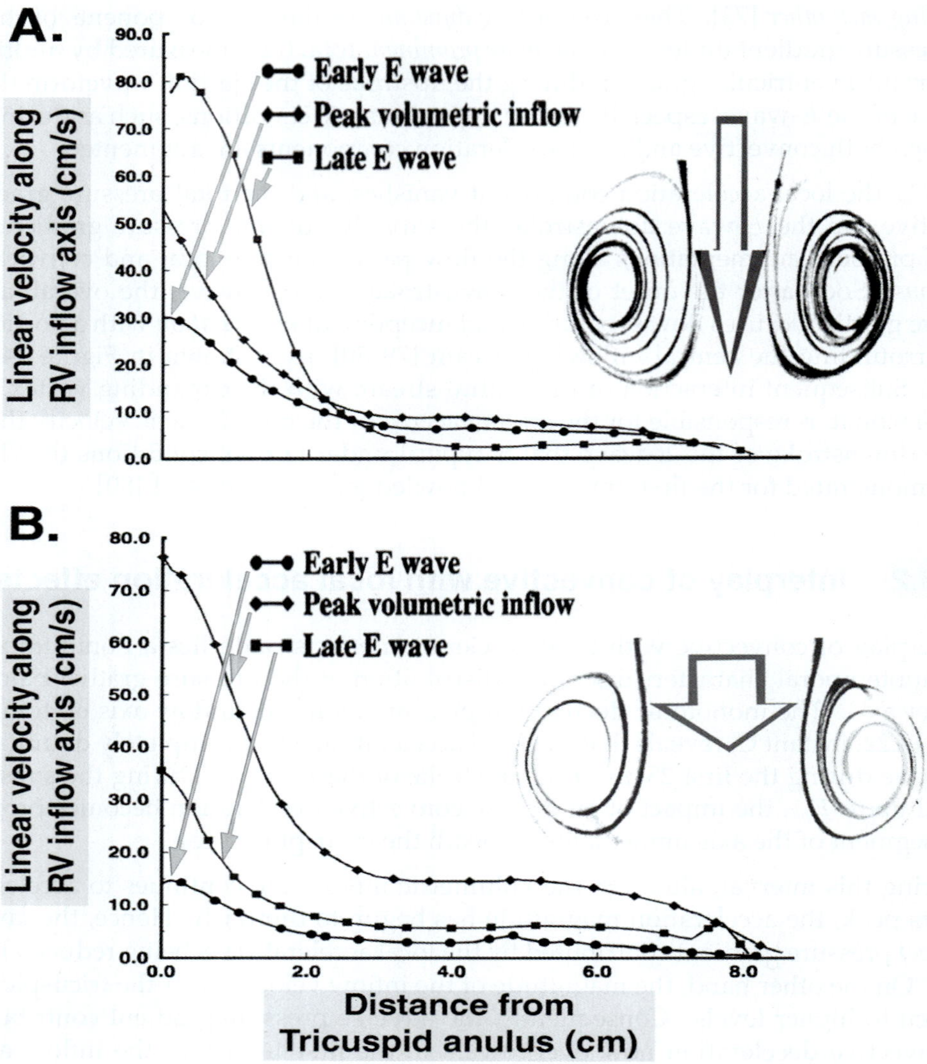

Figure 14.24: Velocity distributions along the main inflow axis of the RV chamber. **A.** Results from Functional Imaging simulations under control conditions (NWM). **B.** Results from simulations under volume overload with PSM. Note that under control conditions, the velocities along the axis in the basal region of the RV chamber are substantially higher late in the E-wave than their levels at the time of peak volumetric inflow rate, E_{pk}, although the *volumetric* inflow rate is then *much lower*. It is a corollary of conservation of mass or "continuity of flow" and is graphically explained by the insets accompanying the velocity distribution plots. The length of the arrows is proportional to linear velocity; their width, to volumetric inflow rate. (Adapted, slightly modified, from Pasipoularides et al. [80], by kind permission of the American Physiological Society.)

local deceleration. The local and the convective components now *both add to the total* pressure gradient. As the rate of deceleration increases, so does the magnitude of the pressure rise, as seen in Figure 14.22, instants I and J, and this leads to subsequent flow separation and *vortex formation* (cf. color maps in Fig. 14.16, on p. 772).

The *rise* in the linear inflow velocity within the basal region of the chamber during the *downstroke* of the E-wave under control conditions had been an unrecognized phenomenon until the publication of our work [80], which includes the figures under discussion. It is a corollary of the large-scale vortical motion (see Fig. 14.17, on p. 774), which develops within the chamber and is intense at control but diminishes in strength and extent with chamber dilatation. The greater filling vortex strength at control manifests itself dynamically in the more prominent pressure fluctuations late in the E-wave in Figure 14.21, on p. 783. Figure 14.23, on p. 786, shows a qualitatively similar spatiotemporal development pattern of the pressure gradient along the inflow axis in volume overload with PSM. For instance, the pressure distribution at the time of E_{pk} (Fig. 14.23, instant F) has the same characteristics as that of Figure 14.22, instant H (E_{pk} panel). In the dilated chamber there is, however, a *much sharper accentuation* of the pressure gradient near the inflow orifice, a result of *diastolic ventriculoannular disproportion* [75,78–80].

Analogous distributions demonstrating that the overwhelming proportion of the intraventricular convective acceleration occurs in the immediate vicinity of the outflow orifice were also found in studies of the intraventricular ejection flow field [43,47,48,53,73,83,84]. The magnitude of the sharp intensification of the convective acceleration (deceleration) in the immediate neighborhood of the outflow (inflow) orifice of the spheroidal 3-D chamber is inadvertently *underestimated* by looking at standardized 2-D streamline representations. Flow that is generated by the inward collapse of the entire inner *spheroidal* surface of the 3-D chamber must exit through the 2-D surface of its circular outflow orifice during ejection; analogous considerations apply, conversely, for the fan-like inflow streamlines during the *upstroke* of the E-wave during filling—cf. Figures 4.5, 14.2, and 14.15, on pp. 180, 740, and 770, respectively.

14.14 Physiological significance of the filling vortex: to facilitate diastolic filling

With the use of Functional Imaging [78], these investigations [79,80] were the first to show the existence of vortical motion inside the right ventricle. The physiological repercussions of the vortical motion are most intriguing for both ventricles. Bellhouse [9,10], who conducted experimental studies on the LV diastolic vortex in the context of cardiac physiology in the early 1970s, proposed that vortical motion might assist in valve closure, a notion traceable back to Leonardo da Vinci (see Section 3.3, on pp. 119 ff.). Therefore, any chamber dilatation that reduces the vortex strength behind the mitral cusps, will cause the valve to no longer be almost fully closed before the onset of the ensuing ventricular contraction: a functional mitral insufficiency of variable degree can then result, as is described in Section 7.15.1, on pp. 393 f.

Others [56, 113] have suggested that the presence of chirally asymmetric LV diastolic vortical motions helps in the ensuing process of ejection, by conversion of vortex kinetic energy into kinetic energy of LV outflow after aortic valve opening. According to this view, the filling vortex within the ventricle would act as an energy-preserving flow structure [40]. This vortex persisting throughout the whole diastole would serve as a storage place for the kinetic energy of the incoming blood, reducing the work necessary for the acceleration of blood toward the outflow tract. The rotating stream of blood in the larger lobe of the persisting chirally asymmetric LV vortex would then leave the chamber in a tangential direction when ventricular contraction started.

It is well known in fluid mechanics, however, that large vortices and rotational fluid flow structures *never unwind smoothly*. Instead, they break up into smaller eddies, and this process is continued, until the vortices are reduced to micron-size eddies and at that level *(Kolmogorov "microscale")* they dissipate under the action of viscous forces [95]. The process is known as the vortical cascade mechanism (see Section 4.14.4, on pp. 217 ff.). This implies that vortices are essentially *"traps"* or *"sinks"* of energy [79]. Whatever kinetic energy is trapped in the recirculating motion of a vortex is bound to be converted into heat, as is shown pictorially in Figure 4.21, on p. 218. It is bound to be lost from the motion and therefore cannot, in fact, aid ejection.

Vortical energy dissipation can occur both within the ventricles and within their outflow trunks and beyond. Virtually all of the *diastolic vortex* energy extraction is expected [29, 30] to occur as a result of interactions with smaller eddies that are at least one order of magnitude smaller than it. This is in contrast to the possibility that the energy might be *deposited* directly from the large, energy-containing vortices into the small Kolmogorov microscale eddies. The dissipation of vortical structures in the flow at scales appreciably larger than the Kolmogorov microscale is sufficiently strong that little structure actually survives to reach these highly dissipative scales.

Recently, Japanese investigators [117] developed a multiscale, multiphysics heart simulation model, based on the finite element method, and compared the hemodynamics of ventricles with physiological and nonphysiological diastolic vortical flow paths. In this model, the molecular mechanism of excitation-contraction coupling implemented in each element is activated by the propagation of excitation. In their simulations, the equations governing the dynamics of the fluid (blood) and the structure (LV wall) were solved by a strong coupling method [119], and they could obtain detailed information regarding the spatiotemporal distributions of LV chamber velocities and pressures, as well as the stress-strain relationships in the LV wall, which are necessary for energetics considerations.

Taking advantage of this model, they examined the effects of the inflow direction in the left ventricle on its performance under conditions where other experimental variables, including ventricular morphology, myocardial properties, and pre- and afterloads, were completely matched. Such a controlled study is only possible with this kind of *in silico* experiment. They found that the physiological vortical flow path did not have *any energy-saving* effect. The *stroke work* performed by the LV wall was comparable at both slower and faster heart rates (physiological *vs.* nonphysiological, 0.864 *vs.* 0.874 *J*, at a heart rate of ≈ 60 *beats/min*; and 0.599 *vs.* 0.590 *J*, at a heart rate of ≈ 100 *beats/min*), indicating that chiral asymmetry of the flow paths in the mammalian heart has minimal, if any, energetic functional merit.

This thorough and meticulously documented investigation has totally contradicted the view of an energy-saving, fluidic effect of cardiac looping [56] and diastolic vortex motions [40, 113], and clinical observations support its results. Maire, et al. [63] compared two groups of patients with either physiological (parallel flow; clockwise vortex) or nonphysiological (cross flow; counterclockwise vortex) LV diastolic flow patterns, brought on by differences in the orientation of prosthetic mitral valves. They found no differences between the morphologies, hemodynamics, or exercise capacities, other than a larger atrial size in the nonphysiological group. Since that study was performed *more than five years* after the mitral valve replacement in each patient, had even a small functional difference existed between the two intraventricular flow patterns, it would have accumulated and would have brought about notable (deleterious) clinical consequences in the *nonphysiological* group.

In view of the important findings of our FI studies of the diastolic intraventricular flow field that are detailed in the preceding Sections, I have advanced a new hypothesis concerning the useful role played by the vortices in overall diastolic function [75, 76, 79, 80]. According to the hypothesis, the difference between the inflow orifice area (A_i) and the endocardial surface area (A_{endo}) is responsible for generating strong convective deceleration before transition to vortical flow in diastole (cf. Figs. 14.2, 14.6, and 14.15, on pp. 740, 749, and 770, respectively). The diastolic intraventricular pressure gradient resulting from this convective deceleration, termed [75, 78–80] *"convective deceleration load,"* adversely impacts diastolic inflow. This adverse impact is amplified in the presence of ventricular dilatation with attendant *diastolic ventriculoannular disproportion*, as has been already emphasized in Section 14.7.1, on pp. 765 f.

The key to the proposed useful physiological role of the diastolic filling vortex lies in its *impounding* of a certain amount of energy, and this becomes manifest as a decrease in the pressure energy of the inflowing blood. By *shunting* the inflow work and kinetic energy, which would otherwise contribute an inflow-impeding *pressure-rise* between inflow orifice and the endocardial surface of the expanding chamber, into the *kinetic energy of the vortical motion* (Figs. 14.15 and 14.17) that is destined to be *dissipated as heat*, the diastolic vortex actually *facilitates filling* and the attainment of higher end-diastolic volume.

14.15 Clinical impact of chamber size and wall motion patterns

Using Functional Imaging [78], we have demonstrated [79, 80] that not just quantitative but qualitative important alterations in the intraventricular velocity field result from changes in applying RV dynamic geometry and wall motion patterns. As shown by the results presented in the preceding sections, the impact of abnormal chamber dilatation and wall motion patterns on RV flow is manifested throughout the entire E-wave, and

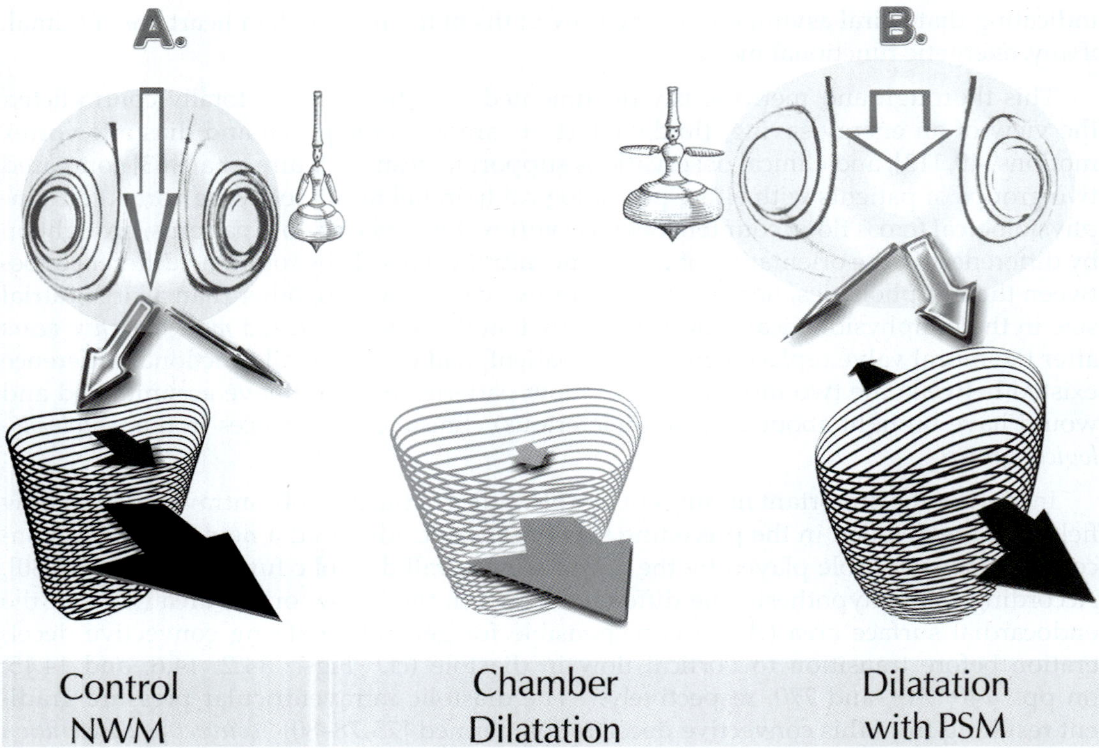

Figure 14.25: Under control conditions of normal wall motion (NWM), filling is accompanied by anterior-directed motion of both the free and septal right ventricular (RV) walls (*black* arrows, **A.**). In chamber dilatation with paradoxic septal motion (PSM), the septal motion is directed toward the left ventricle (back-pointing *black* arrow, **B.**). Interposed is the intermediate pattern of dilatation with normal motion (*gray* arrows). By increasing both intraventricular mass and effective rotation radii, an increased chamber size leads to smaller effective recirculating velocities and vortex strength, as the "whirling dervish" tops suggest: with a wider girth and arms extended, spinning is slower in **B.** than **A.**—see discussion in Section 2.8, on pp. 59 f. Although instantaneous volumetric inflow rates at control were smaller than with volume overload, after vortex development higher linear core velocities were present at control than with chamber dilatation. The more intense vortex ring squeezes the central core area more in **A.** The width of each *white* arrow in the top panels is proportional to central core area; the length, to linear velocity. (Adapted, somewhat modified, from Pasipoularides et al. [80], by permission of the American Physiological Society.)

we have been able to characterize extensively the resultant alterations of the diastolic intraventricular flow field. Our Functional Imaging simulation findings are in agreement with the classic studies of Brian Bellhouse [8–10], who reported reduced vortex strength and extent in dilated ventricles.

When the *vorticity* of intraventricular blood flow is intense, there are strong velocity gradients transverse to the local direction of the fluid motion (see Fig. 4.13, on p. 201,

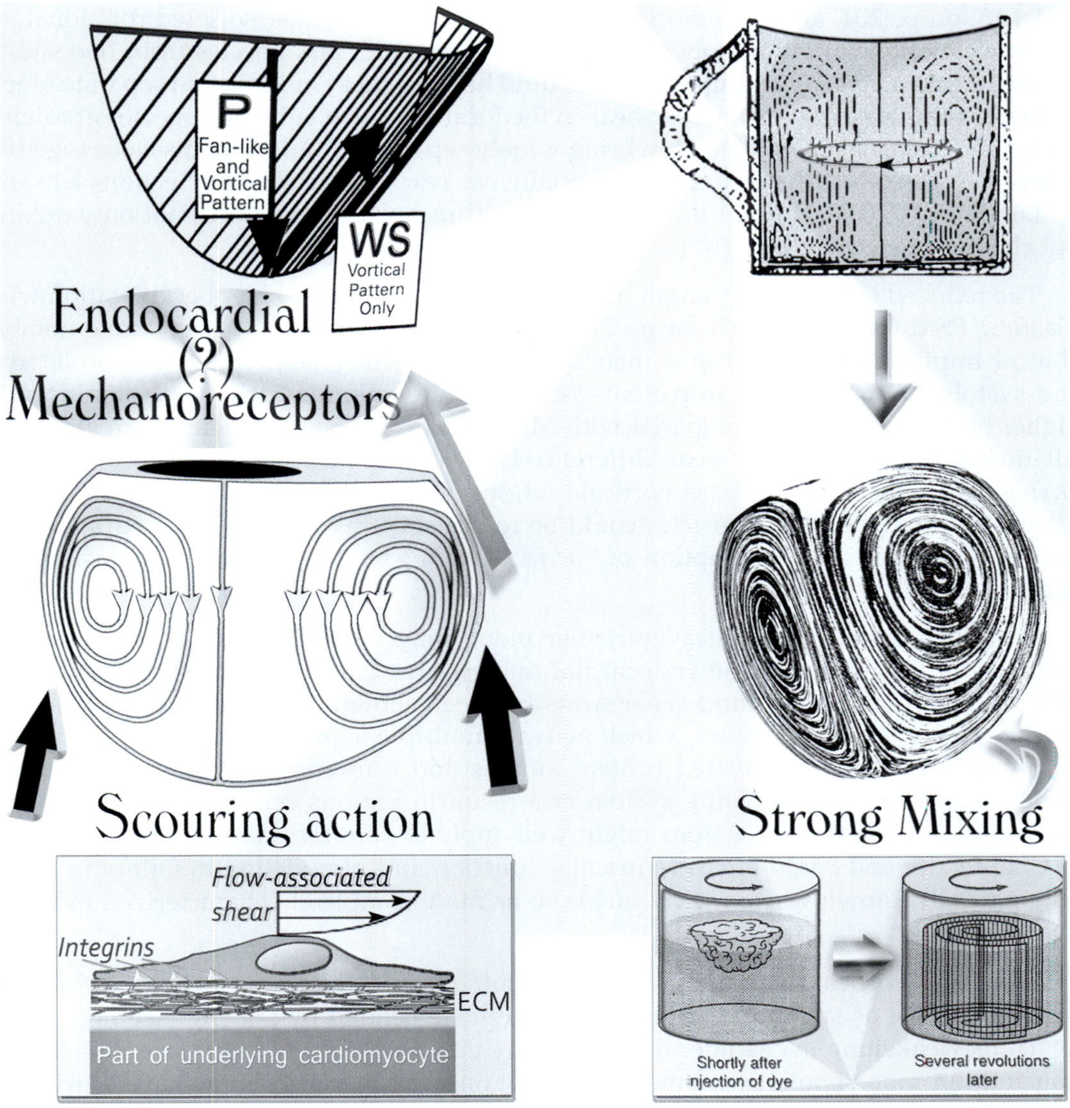

Figure 14.26: Rotation in the intraventricular blood stream may naturally encourage a gentle scouring (shear) of the endocardial lining of the chamber (left); vortical spinning may promote chemical mixing and keep formed and unformed blood elements suspended as sugar and tea leaves are kept suspended by vigorous stirring, which sets up secondary vortical motions in a tea cup (right). The lower right inset shows how a blob of dye released in a rapidly rotating fluid (before solid body rotation is reached) is deformed into spiral twirling sheets with enormously expanded areas for diffusive mixing. P, pressure: acts *perpendicularly*; WS, wall shear: acts *tangentially* on the endocardial lining. The lower left inset is explained further in Figures 15.14 and 15.15, on pp. 838 and 839, and the related discussions. (Adapted, in part, from Pasipoularides et al. [79], by kind permission of the American Physiological Society.)

and 4.15, on p. 204, and the associated discussion in text). The associated rotational, or shearing, motions allow dissolved or suspended particles and species from one site to penetrate and convectively mix with other fluid because these motions can separate blood elements that were initially close. Shear in the local flow also enhances species gradients and causes faster *mixing*, which can bring widely separated fluid elements close together where they can mix diffusively and, potentially, can react chemically (see Sections 4.13 and 4.14.6, on pp. 210 ff. and 224 ff., respectively). Thus vorticity enhances not only mixing but chemical reactivity too.

The reduced extent and strength of the diastolic vortex in RV chamber dilatation with diastolic PSM (cf. Fig. 14.17, on p. 774, and Fig. 14.25, on p. 792) may have notable clinical implications. Thus, in a meticulous clinical study [44], RV end-diastolic and end-systolic volume indices in patients with dilated cardiomyopathy were significantly higher by thermodilution compared with MRI, and exclusion of patients with atrial fibrillation did not reduce the mean difference between both methods. *Impaired* indicator *mixing* associated with *weakened* vortical motions (see Fig. 14.26, *right*, on p. 793) in the dilated cardiomyopathic ventricles could be responsible, by introducing a strong violation of the underlying assumption of *"perfect mixing"* between injection and sampling sites.

Vortical rotation in the intraventricular blood may naturally encourage gentle tangential *scouring* (shear) of the endocardial lining of the chamber (Fig. 14.26, *left*, on p. 793). In endothelial cells, fluid shear stress has been shown to activate cytoskeletal and biochemical mechanoreceptors, which activate multiple signal transduction pathways, involving sequentially activated protein kinases and transcription factors that form a highly interconnected signaling system and result in various cellular physiological responses [114, 115]. Similar actions might well apply to endocardial cells, as we shall see in Chapter 15, and could affect ventricular function and remodeling in failure in as yet only partially known ways, which remain to be more completely characterized in future investigations.

Moreover, vortical rotation may maintain both formed and unformed blood elements suspended, just as sugar and tea leaves are kept suspended by stirring (see Fig. 14.26, *right*). Its weakening in chamber dilatation may therefore contribute to thrombus formation and thromboembolic phenomena [79]. Not only might vortical flow have bearing on the avoidance of thrombosis, but also, by being responsible for the swirling flow (augmented shear) arriving at the nearby pulmonary arterial branches in the ensuing ejection, it might be a factor contributing to the well-known *avoidance of atherogenicity* in the pulmonary arterial system.

This avoidance would be a corollary of the notion formulated by Friedman [36–38] that a fluid dynamic wall shear near zero for an appreciable part of the pulsatile cycle favors atherogenicity. Friedman and coworkers used 2-D CFD models of a symmetric aorto-iliac bifurcation to demonstrate the "considerable spatial and temporal variations" in wall shear stress and their effect on transport into the vessel wall. Caro and colleagues had also suggested that low wall shear favors the adhesion and infiltration of macromolecules and/or blood born cells into the vessel wall [18, 19], based on the observation that the distribution of early atherosclerotic lesions is coincident with regions of low shear.

14.15.1 Convective deceleration load and diastolic ventriculoannular disproportion

The dynamic pressure and velocity distributions revealed by FI [80], some of which are displayed in Figures 14.21–14.24, corroborate flow visualization findings that led me to formulate the diastolic *"convective deceleration load" (CDL)* mechanism [78–80], as an important determinant of diastolic inflow. The magnitude of CDL affects strongly peak E-wave velocities. The larger the ventricle, the larger is the CDL. To be more precise, the greater the discrepancy, or *"diastolic ventriculoannular disproportion" (DVAD)* between the sizes of the endocardial surface and the inflow orifice, the larger is the CDL (see Fig. 14.27). The rise in pressure representing CDL is proportional to the *square* of applying velocities. From this, a larger ventricle in early diastole engenders a disproportionate increase of CDL and a much more difficult inflow. Matters should be worsened with tachycardia, which accompanies heart failure. Such augmentation of CDL may contribute to depressed E-wave amplitude and E–to–A ratio abnormalities in acute or chronic chamber dilatation. Ensuing atrial overload (active support of filling) may account for the association of atrial fibrillation with clinical ventricular enlargement *in absence* of coronary disease [80].

14.16 Conclusions

In conclusion, our findings regarding the intraventricular diastolic flow field should improve application and interpretation of diagnostic studies and measurements and lead to improved understanding of the flow-pattern-associated implications of ventricular dilatation and failure on the energetics of diastolic filling.

We recognize now that conditions leading to eccentric hypertrophy, and the mechanical remodeling with chamber enlargement seen in congestive heart failure, should increase the diastolic CDL and at the same time reduce the intensity of the filling vortex that normally facilitates filling. The converse applies for interventions reducing the size of dilated ventricles, such as cardiac resynchronization therapy [108] and the Battista procedure [7] (partial left ventriculectomy, or *"cardioreduction"*—see Fig. 14.28) [7], which reverse the mechanical remodeling seen in congestive heart failure. Such interventions should decrease the diastolic CDL by diminishing diastolic ventriculoannular disproportion, as well as by promoting stronger diastolic intraventricular vortical motions. Diastolic ventriculoannular disproportion and convective deceleration load may also be greater than before after tricuspid annuloplasty or tricuspid valve replacement for tricuspid regurgitation; each of these procedures will tend to decrease effective tricuspid orifice area relative to right ventricular volume.

The important findings and innovative concepts developed in this chapter should also stimulate further work leading to improved recognition of subtle flow-associated ab-

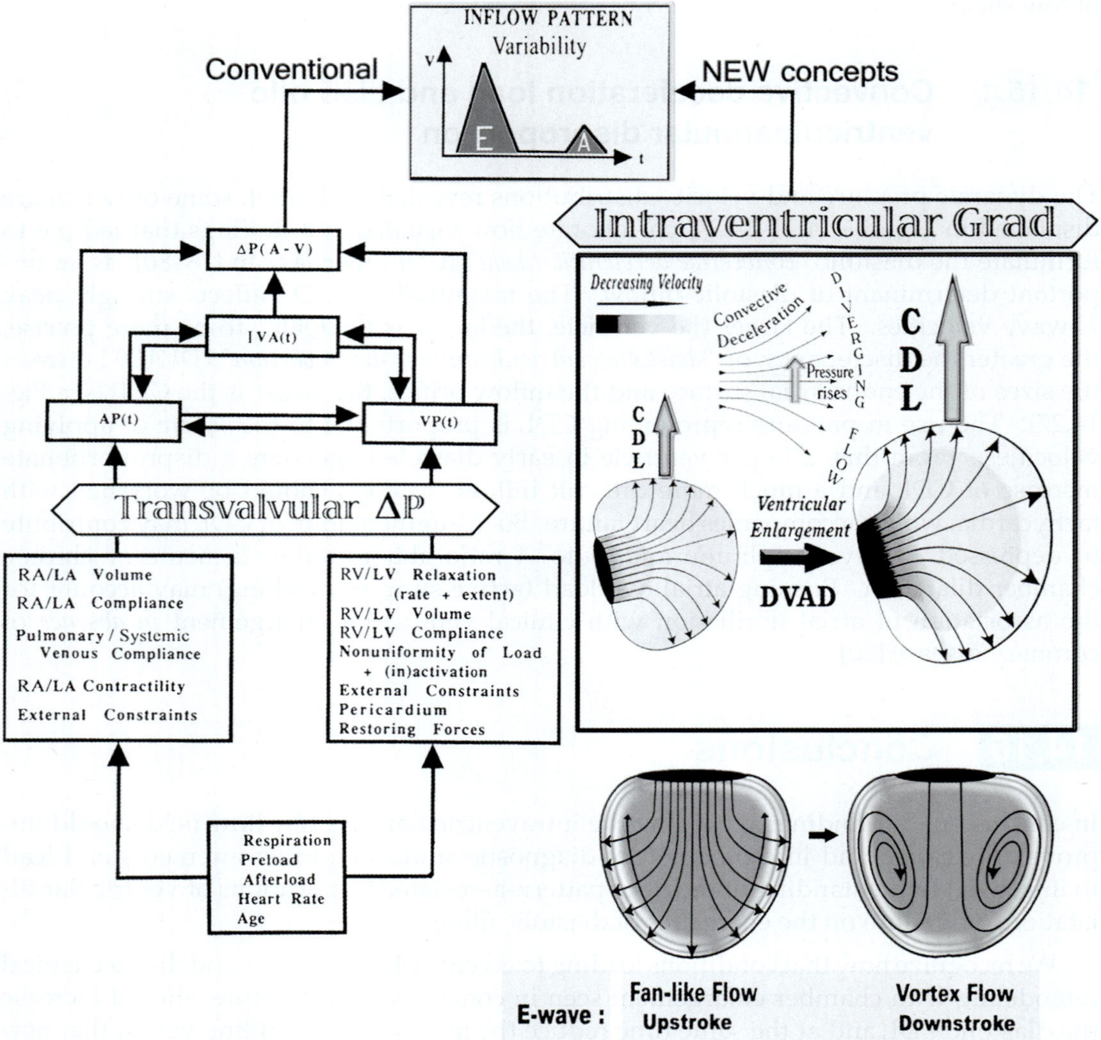

Figure 14.27: The determinants of ventricular inflow patterns and diastolic filling include factors intrinsic and extrinsic to the ventricle—see also Fig. 7.13, on p. 344. The new diastolic function paradigm (on right) complements and acts in parallel with the traditional one (on left): Changes in RV size, diastolic myocardial dynamics, and wall motion patterns cause concomitant changes in the magnitude of the convective deceleration load (CDL) and the properties of the inflow vortex, which affect inflow patterns and ventricular filling. A = atrial; V = ventricular; IVA = inflow valve area; P = pressure; t = time; DVAD = diastolic ventriculoannular disproportion; Grad = P gradient. (Collage adapted, somewhat modified, from Pasipoularides [74] and Pasipoularides et al. [80], by permission of the Biomedical Engineering Society and of the American Physiological Society.)

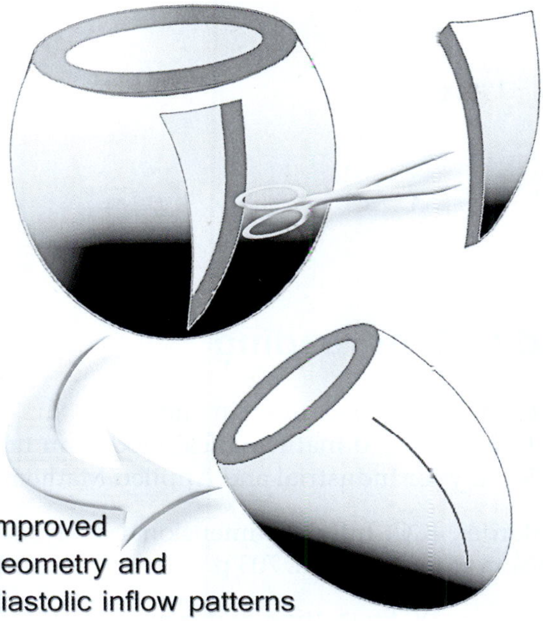

Figure 14.28: The Battista procedure or partial left ventriculectomy consists of a resection of a segment of the lateral wall of the left ventricle. The edges are then reapproximated, accomplishing the goals of decreasing the chamber size and increasing chamber eccentricity.

normalities and their multifaceted sequelae in dilatation. Future clinical Functional Imaging studies should provide further insights useful in the diagnosis and management of filling abnormalities associated with diverse types of ventricular dysfunction. Developments in computer software and hardware and in imaging will undoubtedly accelerate such contributions to the understanding and management of ventricular dysfunction and failure.

References and further reading

[1] Adeler, P.T., Jacobsen, J.M. Blood flow in the heart. In: Ottesen, J.T., Olufsen, M.S., Larsen, J.K. [Eds.] Applied mathematical models in human physiology. 2004, Philadelphia, PA: Society for Industrial and Applied Mathematics. xiii, 298 p.

[2] Aliprantis, C.D., Border, K.C. Infinite dimensional analysis: a hitchhiker's guide. 2006, Berlin; New York: Springer. xxii, 703 p.

[3] Angeja, B.G., Grossman, W. Evaluation and management of diastolic heart failure (Clinician Update). Circulation 107: 659–63, 2003.

[4] Aurigemma, G.P. Diastolic heart failure—a common and lethal condition by any name. N. Engl. J. Med. 355: 308–10, 2006.

[5] Baccani, B., Domenichini, F., Pedrizzetti, G. Vortex dynamics in a left ventricle during filling. Eur. J. Mech. B/Fluids, 21: 527–43, 2002.

[6] Baccani, B., Domenichini, F., Pedrizzetti, G. Model and influence of mitral valve opening during the left ventricular filling. J. Biomech. 36: 355–61, 2003.

[7] Batista, R.J., Verde, J., Nery, P., Bocchino, L., Takeshita, N., Bhayana, J.N., et al. Partial left ventriculectomy to treat end-stage heart disease. Ann. Thorac. Surg. 64: 634–8, 1997.

[8] Bellhouse, B.J. Fluid mechanics of model aortic and mitral valves. Proc. Roy. Soc. Med. 63: 996–1013, 1970.

[9] Bellhouse, B.J. Fluid mechanics of a model mitral valve and left ventricle. Cardiovasc. Res. 6: 199–210, 1972.

[10] Bellhouse, B.J. Bellhouse, F.H. Fluid mechanics of the mitral valve. Nature 224: 615–6, 1969.

[11] Bermejo, J., Antoranz, J.C., Yotti, R., Moreno, M., Garciá-Fernández, M.A. Spatio-temporal mapping of intracardiac pressure gradients. A solution to Euler's equation from digital postprocessing of color Doppler M-mode echocardiograms. Ultrasound Med. Biol. 27: 621–30, 2001.

[12] Bird, J.J., Murgo, J.P., Pasipoularides, A. Fluid dynamics of aortic stenosis: subvalvular gradients without subvalvular obstruction. Circulation 66: 835–40, 1982.

[13] Bland, J.M., Altman, D.G. Comparing methods of measurement: why plotting difference against standard method is misleading. Lancet 346: 1085–7, 1995.

[14] Bland, J.M., Altman, D.G. Measuring agreement in method comparison studies. Stat. Meth. Med. Res. 8: 135–60, 1999.

[15] Bot, H., Verburg, J., Delemarre, B.J., Strackee, J. Determinants of the occurrence of vortex rings in the left ventricle during diastole. J. Biomech. 23: 607–15, 1990.

[16] Bowman, A.W., Frihauf, P.A., Kovacs, S.J. Time-varying effective mitral valve area: prediction and validation using cardiac MRI and Doppler echocardiography in normal subjects. Am. J. Physiol. Heart Circ. Physiol. 287: H1650–7, 2004.

[17] Brun, P., Tribouilloy, C., Duval, A.M., Iserin, L., Meguira, A., Pelle, G., Dubois-Rande, J.L. Left ventricular flow propagation during early filling is related to wall relaxation: a color M-mode Doppler analysis. J. Am. Coll. Cardiol. 20: 420–32, 1992.

[18] Caro, C.G., Fitz-Gerald, J.M., Schroter, R.C. Atheroma and arterial wall shear. Observation, correlation and proposal of a shear dependent mass transfer mechanism for atherogenesis. Proc. Roy. Soc. Lond. B. Biol. Sci. 177: 109–59, 1971.

[19] Caro, C.G., Fitz-Gerald, J.M., Schroter, R.C. Arterial wall shear and distribution of early atheroma in man. Nature 223: 1159–60, 1969.

[20] Cheng, Y., Oertel, H., Schenkel, T. Fluid-structure coupled CFD simulation of the left ventricular flow during filling phase. Ann. Biomed. Eng. 33: 567–76, 2005.

[21] Condos, W.R., Latham, R.D., Hoadley, S.D., Pasipoularides, A. Hemodynamic effects of the Mueller maneuver by simultaneous right and left heart micromanometry. Circulation 76: 1020–8, 1987.

[22] Cooke J., Hertzberg J., Boardman M., Shandas R. Characterizing vortex ring behavior during ventricular filling with Doppler echocardiography: an in vitro study. Ann. Biomed. Eng. 32: 245–56, 2004.

[23] Corya, B.C., Feigenbaum, H., Rasmussen, S., Black, M.J. Echocardiographic features of congestive cardiomyopathy compared with normal subjects and patients with coronary artery disease. Circulation 49: 1153–9, 1974.

[24] Courtois M, Barzilai B, Gutierrez F, and Ludbrook P. Characterization of regional diastolic pressure gradients in the right ventricle. Circulation 82: 1413–23, 1990.

[25] Craig, W.E., Murgo, J.P., Pasipoularides, A. Calculation of the time constant of relaxation. In: Grossman, W., Lorell, B. [Eds.] Diastolic relaxation of the heart. 1987, The Hague: Martinus Nijhoff. pp. 125–32.

[26] Curtius, J.M., Freimuth, M., Kuhn, H., Köhler, E., Loogen, F. Belastungsechokardiographie bei dilatativer Kardiomyopathie. [Exercise echocardiography in dilatative cardiomyopathy]. Z. Kardiol. 71: 727–35, 1982.

[27] Delemarre, B.J., Bot, H., Pearlman, A.S., Visser, C.A., Dunning, M. Diastolic flow characteristics of severely impaired left ventricles: a pulsed Doppler ultrasound study, J. Clin. Ultrasound 15: 115–19, 1987.

[28] De Mey, S., De Sutter, J., Vierendeels, J., Verdonck, P. Diastolic filling and pressure imaging: taking advantage of the information in a colour M-mode Doppler image. Eur. J. Echocardiol. 12: 219–33, 2001.

[29] Domaradzki, J.A. Analysis of subgrid-scale eddy viscosity with the use of the results from direct numerical simulations. Phys. Fluids A 4: 2037–45, 1992.

[30] Domaradzki. J.A., Metcalfe, R.W., Rogallo, R.S., Riley, J.J. Analysis of subgrid-scale eddy viscosity with the use of the results from direct numerical simulations. Phys. Rev. Lett. 58: 547–50, 1987.

[31] Domenichini, F., Pedrizzetti, G., Baccani, B. Three-dimensional filling flow into a model left ventricle. J. Fluid Mech. 539: 179–98, 2005.

[32] Duval-Moulin, A.M., Dupouy, P., Brun, P., Zhuang, F., Pelle, G., Perez, Y., Teiger, E., Castaigne, A., Gueret, P., Dubois-Rande, J.L. Alteration of left ventricular diastolic function during coronary angioplasty-induced ischemia: a color M-mode Doppler study. J. Am. Coll. Cardiol. 29: 1246–55, 1997.

[33] Ebbers, T., Wigstrom, L., Bolger, A.F., Wranne, B., M. Karlsson, M. Noninvasive measurement of time-varying three-dimensional relative pressure fields within the human heart. J. Biomech. Eng. 124: 288–93, 2002.

[34] Feigenbaum, H., Armstrong, W.F., Ryan, T. Feigenbaum's echocardiography. 6th ed. 2005, Philadelphia, PA: Lippincott Williams & Wilkins. xv, 790 p.

[35] Feneley, M.P., Elbeery, J.R., Gaynor, J.W., Gall, S.A., Davis, J.W., Rankin, J.S. Ellipsoidal shell subtraction model of right ventricular volume. Comparison with regional free wall dimensions as indexes of right ventricular function. Circ. Res. 67: 1427–36, 1990.

[36] Friedman, M.H., Brinkman, A.M., Qin, J.J., Seed, W.A. Relation between coronary artery geometry and the distribution of early sudanophilic lesions. Atherosclerosis 98: 193–9, 1993.

[37] Friedman, M.H., Ehrlich, L.W. Effect of spatial variations in shear on diffusion at the wall of an arterial branch. Circ. Res. 37: 446–54, 1975.

[38] Friedman, M.H., O'Brien, V., Ehrlich, L.W. Calculations of pulsatile flow through a branch: implications for the hemodynamics of atherogenesis. Circ. Res. 36: 277–85, 1975.

[39] Fukuda, S., Saracino, G., Matsumura, Y., Daimon, M., Tran, H., Greenberg, N.L., Hozumi, T., Yoshikawa, J., Thomas, J.D., Shiota, T. Three-dimensional geometry of the tricuspid annulus in healthy subjects and in patients with functional tricuspid regurgitation: a real-time, 3-dimensional echocardiographic study. Circulation 114 (1 Suppl): I-492–8, 2006.

[40] Fyrenius, A., Wigström, L., Ebbers, T., Karlsson, M., Engvall, J., Bolger, A.F. Three dimensional flow in the human left atrium. Heart 86: 448–55, 2001.

[41] Gaynor, J.W., Feneley, M.P., Gall, S.A., Maier, G.W., Kisslo, J.A., Davis, J.W., Rankin, J.S., and Glower, D.D. Measurement of left ventricular volume in normal and volume-overloaded canine hearts. Am. J. Physiol. Heart Circ. Physiol. 266: H329–40, 1994.

[42] Gelpi, R.J., Pasipoularides, A., Lader, A.S., Patric, T.A., Chase, N., Hittinger, L., Shannon, R.P., Bishop, S.P., Vatner, S.F. Changes in diastolic cardiac function in developing and stable perinephritic hypertension in conscious dogs. Circ. Res. 68: 555–67, 1991.

[43] Georgiadis, J.G., Wang, M., Pasipoularides, A. Computational fluid dynamics of left ventricular ejection. Ann. Biomed. Eng. 20: 81–97, 1992.

[44] Globits, S., Pacher, R., Frank, H., Pacher, B., Mayr, H., Neuhold, A., and Glogar, D. Comparative assessment of right ventricular volumes and ejection fraction by thermodilution and magnetic resonance imaging in dilated cardiomyopathy. Cardiology 86: 67–72, 1995.

[45] Greenberg, N.L., Vandervoort, P.M., Thomas, J.D. Instantaneous diastolic transmitral pressure difference from color Doppler M-mode echocardiography. Am. J. Physiol. Heart Circ. Physiol. 271: H1267–76, 1996.

[46] Greil, G., Geva, T., Maier, S., Powell, A. Effect of acquisition parameters on the accuracy of velocity encoded cine magnetic resonance imaging blood flow measurements. J. Magn. Reson. Imag. 15: 47–54, 2002.

[47] Hampton, T., Shim, Y., Straley, C., Pasipoularides, A. Finite element analysis of cardiac ejection dynamics: Ultrasonic implications. Am. Soc. Mechan. Engin., Bioengin. Div. (ASME BED) Adv. Bioengin. 22: 371–4, 1992.

[48] Hampton, T., Shim, Y., Straley, C., Uppal, R., Smith, P.K., Glower, D., Pasipoularides, A. Computational fluid dynamics of ventricular ejection on the CRAY Y-MP. IEEE Proc. Comp. Cardiol. 19: 295–8, 1992.

[49] Heath, T.L. The Works of Archimedes. New York: Dover, date unknown, pp. 107–9, 176–82.

[50] Hellevik, L.R., Dahl, S.K., Skallerud, B. A first-approach towards patient-specific 2D FSI-simulation of mitral valve dynamics during diastolic filling. In: Skallerud, B.,

Andersson, H.I. [Eds.] MekIT-07, Fourth national conference on Computational Mechanics. 2007, Trondheim (Norway): Tapir Academic Press. pp. 175–84.

[51] Ihara, T., Shannon, R.P., Komamura, K., Pasipoularides, A.D., Patrick, T., Shen, S., Vatner, S.F. Effects of anaesthesia and recent surgery on diastolic function. Cardiovasc. Res. 28: 325–36, 1994.

[52] Isaaz K. A theoretical model for the noninvasive assessment of the transmitral pressure-flow relation. J. Biomech. 25: 581–90, 1992.

[53] Isaaz, K., Pasipoularides, A. Noninvasive assessment of intrinsic ventricular load dynamics in dilated cardiomyopathy. J. Am. Coll. Cardiol. 17: 112–21, 1991.

[54] Ishizu, T., Seo, Y., Ishimitsu, T., Obara, K., Moriyama, N., Kawano, S., Watanabe, S., Yamaguchi, I. The wake of a large vortex is associated with intraventricular filling delay in impaired left ventricles with a pseudonormalized transmitral flow pattern. Echocardiography 23: 369–75, 2006.

[55] Kheradvar, A., Gharib, M. Influence of ventricular pressure drop on mitral annulus dynamics through the process of vortex ring formation. Ann. Biomed. Eng. 35: 2050–64, 2007.

[56] Kilner, P.J., Yang, G.Z., Wilkes, A.J., Mohiaddin, R. H., Firmin, D.N., Yacoub, M.H. Asymmetric redirection of flow through the heart. Nature 404: 759–61, 2000.

[57] Kim, W.Y., Walker, P.G., Pedersen, E.M., Poulsen, J.K., Oyre, S., Houlind, K., Yoganathan, A.P. Left ventricular blood flow patterns in normal subjects: a quantitative analysis by three-dimensional magnetic resonance velocity mapping. J. Am. Coll. Cardiol. 26: 224–38, 1995.

[58] Lemmon, J.D., Yoganathan, A.P. Three-dimensional computational model of left heart diastolic function with fluid–structure interaction. J. Biomech. Eng. 122: 109–17, 2000.

[59] Lemmon, J.D., Yoganathan, A.P. Computational modeling of left heart diastolic function: examination of ventricular dysfunction. J. Biomech. Eng. 122: 297–303, 2000.

[60] Ling, D., Rankin, J.S., Edwards, C.H., McHale, P.A., Anderson, R.W. Regional diastolic mechanics of the left ventricle in the conscious dog. Am. J. Physiol. Heart Circ. Physiol. 236: H323–30, 1979.

[61] Little, W.C. Diastolic dysfunction beyond distensibility: adverse effects of ventricular dilatation. Circulation 112: 2888–90, 2005.

[62] Lotz, J., Meier, C., Leppert, A., Galanski, M. Cardiovascular flow measurement with phase-contrast MR imaging: basic facts and implementation. RadioGraphics 22: 651–71, 2002.

[63] Maire, R., Ikram, S., Odemuyiwa, O., Groves, P.H., Lo, S.V., Banning, A.P., Hall, R.J. Abnormalities of left ventricular flow following mitral valve replacement: a colour flow Doppler study. Eur. Heart J. 15: 293–302, 1994.

[64] Mirsky, I., Pasipoularides, A. Elastic properties of normal and hypertrophied cardiac muscle. Fed. Proc. 39: 156–61, 1980.

[65] Mirsky, I., Pasipoularides, A. Clinical assessment of diastolic function. Prog. Cardiovasc. Dis. 32: 291–318, 1990.

[66] Nakamura, M., Wada, S., Mikami, T., Kitabatake, A., Karino, T. Computational study on the evolution of a vortical flow in a human left ventricle during early diastole. Biomech. Model. Mechanobiol. 2: 59–72, 2003.

[67] Nakamura, M., Wada, S., Mikami, T., Kitabatake, A., Karino, T., Yamaguchi, T. Effect of flow disturbances remaining at the beginning of diastole on intraventricular diastolic flow and colour M-mode Doppler echocardiograms. Med. Biol. Eng. Comput. 42: 509–15, 2004.

[68] Nicolis, G., Prigogine, I. Self-organization in nonequilibrium systems: from dissipative structures to order through fluctuations. 1977, New York: Wiley. xii, 491 p.

[69] Nishimura, R.A., Tajik, AJ. Quantitative hemodynamics by Doppler echocardiography: a noninvasive alternative to cardiac catheterization. Prog. Cardiovasc. Dis. 36: 309–42, 1994.

[70] Ormiston, J.A., Shah, P.M., Tei, C., Wong. M. Size and motion of the mitral valve annulus in man. A two-dimensional echocardiographic method and findings in normal subjects. Circulation 64: 113–20, 1981.

[71] Ota, T., Fleishman, C.E., Strub, M., Stetten, G., Ohazama, C.J., von Ramm, O.T., Kisslo, J. Real-time, three-dimensional echocardiography: feasibility of dynamic right ventricular volume measurement with saline contrast. Am. Heart J. 137: 958–66, 1999.

[72] Owen, A. A numerical model of early diastolic filling: importance of intraventricular pressure wave propagation. Cardiovasc. Res. 27: 255–61, 1993.

[73] Pasipoularides, A. Clinical assessment of ventricular ejection dynamics with and without outflow obstruction. J. Am. Coll. Cardiol. 15: 859–82, 1990.

[74] Pasipoularides, A. Cardiac mechanics: basic and clinical contemporary research. Ann. Biomed. Eng. 20: 3–17, 1992.

[75] Pasipoularides, A. Complementarity and competitiveness of the intrinsic and extrinsic components of the total ventricular load: Demonstration after valve replacement in aortic stenosis [Editorial] Am. Heart J. 153: 4–6, 2007.

[76] Pasipoularides, A. Invited commentary: Functional imaging (FI) combines imaging datasets and computational fluid dynamics to simulate cardiac flows. J. Appl. Physiol. 105: 1015, 2008.

[77] Pasipoularides A.D., Shu, M., Shah, A., Womack, M.S., Adkins, Z., Stetten, G.D., Rednam, S., von Ramm, O., Smith, P.K., Glower, D.D. Diastolic right ventricular vortical flow field: increased symmetry in volume overload with paradoxic septal motion. Circulation (Suppl.) 98: I-844, 1998.

[78] Pasipoularides, A.D., Shu, M., Womack, M.S., Shah, A., von Ramm, O., Glower, D.D. RV functional imaging: 3-D echo-derived dynamic geometry and flow field simulations. Am. J. Physiol. Heart Circ. Physiol. 284: H56–65, 2003.

[79] Pasipoularides, A., Shu, M., Shah, A., Womack, M.S., Glower, D.D. Diastolic right ventricular filling vortex in normal and volume overload states. Am. J. Physiol. Heart Circ. Physiol. 284: H1064–72, 2003.

[80] Pasipoularides, A., Shu, M., Shah, A., Tucconi, A., Glower, D.D. RV instantaneous intraventricular diastolic pressure and velocity distributions in normal and volume overload awake dog disease models. Am. J. Physiol. Heart Circ. Physiol. 285: H1956–65, 2003.

[81] Pasipoularides, A.D., Shu, M., Shah, A., Glower, D.D. Right ventricular diastolic relaxation in conscious dog models of pressure overload, volume overload and ischemia. J. Thorac. Cardiovasc. Surg. 124: 964–72, 2002.

[82] Pasipoularides, A., Shu, M., Shah, A., Silvestry, S., Glower, D.D. Right ventricular diastolic function in canine models of pressure overload, volume overload and ischemia. Am. J. Physiol. Heart Circ. Physiol. 283: H2140–50, 2002.

[83] Pasipoularides, A., Murgo, J.P., Miller, J.W., Craig, W.E. Nonobstructive left ventricular ejection pressure gradients in man. Circ. Res. 61: 220–7, 1987.

[84] Pasipoularides, A., Murgo, J.P., Bird, J.J., Craig, W.E. Fluid dynamics of aortic stenosis: Mechanisms for the presence of subvalvular pressure gradients. Am. J. Physiol. 246: H542–50, 1984.

[85] Pennington, P.T., Bischoff, J.E., Kypson, A., Shu, M., Ramaswami, B., Pasipoularides, A.D. Diastolic ventricular morphometry: analysis of polymeric and paraffin casting. J. Cardiovasc. Diag. Proc. 13: 285, 1996.

[86] Prigogine I. Time, structure, and fluctuations (Nobel Lecture Chemistry). Science 201: 777–85, 1978.

[87] Ramaswami, B., Shu, M., Pennington, P.T., Bischoff, J.E., Glower, D.D., Pasipoularides, A.D. Geometric modeling of the right ventricle and CFD simulation of the early diastolic inflow. J. Cardiovasc. Diag. Proc. 13: 296, 1996.

[88] Redaelli, A., Montevecchi, F.M. Computational evaluation of intraventricular pressure gradients based on a fluid-structure approach. J. Biomech. Eng. (ASME) 118: 529–37, 1996.

[89] Redfield, M.M., Jacobsen, S.J., Burnett, J.C. Jr., Mahoney, D.W., Bailey, K.R., Rodeheffer, R.J. Burden of systolic and diastolic ventricular dysfunction in the community: appreciating the scope of the heart failure epidemic. JAMA 289: 194–202, 2003.

[90] Riederer, S.J., Wright, R.C., Ehman, R.L., Rossman, P.J., Holsinger-Bampton, A.E., Hangiandreou, N.J., Grimm, R.C. Real-time interactive color flow MR imaging. Radiology 181: 33–9, 1991.

[91] Rodevand, O., Bjornerheim, R., Edvardsen, T., Smiseth, O.A., Ihlen, H. Diastolic flow pattern in the normal left ventricle. J. Am. Soc. Echocardiogr. 12: 500–7, 1999.

[92] Saber, N.R., Gosman, A.D., Wood, N.B., Kilner, P.J., Charrier, C., Firmin, D.N. Computational flow modeling of the left ventricle based on in vivo MRI data–initial experience. Ann. Biomed. Eng. 29: 275–83, 2001.

[93] Saber, N.R., Wood, N.B., Gosman, A.D., Merrifield, R.D., Yang, G.-Z., Charrier, C.L., Gatehouse, P.D., Firmin, D.N. Progress towards patient-specific computational flow modeling of the left heart via combination of magnetic resonance imaging with computational fluid dynamics, Ann. Biomed. Eng. 31: 42–52, 2003.

[94] Shah, A.S., Atkins, B.Z., Hata, J.A., Tai, O., Kypson, A.P., Lilly, R.E., Koch, W.J., Glower, D.D. Early effects of right ventricular volume overload on ventricular performance and β-adrenergic signaling. J. Thorac. Cardiovasc. Surg. 120: 342–9, 2000.

[95] She, Z.S., Waymire, E.C. Quantized energy cascade and Log-Poisson statistics in fully developed turbulence. Phys. Rev. Lett. 74: 262–5, 1995.

[96] Shen, H.-W., Li, G.-S., Bordoloi, U.D. Interactive visualization of three-dimensional vector fields with flexible appearance control. IEEE Trans. Visualiz. Comp. Graph. 10: 434–45, 2004.

[97] Shim, Y., Hampton, T.G., Straley, C.A., Harrison, J.K., Spero, L.A., Bashore, T.M., Pasipoularides, A.D. Ejection load changes in aortic stenosis. Observations made after balloon aortic valvuloplasty. Circ. Res. 71: 1174–84, 1992.

[98] Shiota, T., Jones, M., Chikada, M., Fleishman, C.E., Castellucci, J.B., Cotter, B., DeMaria, A.N., von Ramm, O.T., Kisslo, J., Ryan, T., Sahn, D.J. Real-time three-dimensional echocardiography for determining right ventricular stroke volume in an animal model of chronic right ventricular volume overload. Circulation 97: 1897–900, 1998.

[99] Shu, M., Ramaswami, B., Shah, S., Fleishman, C.E., Ota, T., Pennington, P.T., Bischoff, J.E., Stetten, G., von Ramm, O.T., Pasipoularides, A.D. Tricuspid velocity profiles reflect right ventricular diastolic wall motion abnormalities: Real-time 3D echocardiography and computational fluid dynamics. Circulation (Suppl.) 95: I-534, 1997.

[100] Shu, M, Stetten, GD, Ohazama, CJ, Bischoff, JE, Fleishman, C, Ota, T, Ramaswami, B, von Ramm, OT, Pasipoularides, AD. Digital geometric models using biventricular real-time 3D ultrasonography. Circulation (Suppl.) 94: I211–12, 1996.

[101] Smiseth, O.A., Steine, K., Sandbaek, G., Stugaard, M., Gjølberg, T. Mechanics of intraventricular filling: study of LV early diastolic pressure gradients and flow velocities. Am. J. Physiol. Heart Circ. Physiol. 275: H1062–9, 1998.

[102] Smiseth, O.A., Thompson, C.R. Atrioventricular filling dynamics, diastolic function and dysfunction. Heart Fail. Rev. 5: 291–9, 2000.

[103] Staib, L.H., Duncan, J.S. Boundary finding with parametrically deformable models. IEEE Pattern Anal. Mach. Intell. 14: 1061–75, 1992.

[104] Steen, T., Steen, S. Filling of a model left ventricle studied by colour M-mode Doppler. Cardiovasc. Res. 28: 1821–7, 1994.

[105] Stetten G.D., Drezek, R. Active Fourier contour applied to real time 3D ultrasound of the heart. Int. J. Imag. Graph. 1: 647–58, 2001.

[106] Stetten, G., Morris, R. Shape recognition with the flow integration transform. Information Sci. 85: 203–21, 1995.

[107] Stetten, G., Ota, T., Ohazama, C., Fleishman, C., Castelucci, J., Oxaal, J., Ryan, T., Kisslo, J., von Ramm O.T. Real-time 3D ultrasound: a new look at the heart. J. Cardiovasc. Diagn. Procedures 15: 73–84, 1998.

[108] St. John Sutton, M.G., Plappert, T., Abraham, W.T., Smith, A.L., DeLurgio, D.B., Leon, A.R., Loh, E., Kocovic, D.Z., Fisher, W.G., Ellestad, M., Messenger, J., Kruger, K., Hilpisch, K.E., Hill, M.R. Effect of cardiac resynchronization therapy on left ventricular size and function in chronic heart failure. Circulation 107: 1985–90, 2003.

[109] Stugaard, M., Risøe, C., Ihlen, H., Smiseth, O.A. Intracavitary filling pattern in the failing left ventricle assessed by color M-mode Doppler echocardiography. J. Am. Coll. Cardiol. 24: 663–70, 1994.

[110] Stugaard, M., Smiseth, O.A., Risøe, C., Ihlen, H. Intraventricular early diastolic filling during acute myocardial ischemia: assessment by multigated color M-mode Doppler echocardiography. Circulation 88: 2705–13, 1993.

[111] Stugaard, M., Greenberg, N.L., Zhou, J., Thomas, J.D. Automated eigenvector analysis for quantification of color M-mode Doppler filling patterns of the left ventricle in an ischemic canine model. IEEE Proc. Comp. Cardiol. 24: 61–4, 1997.

[112] Takatsuji, H., Mikami, T., Urasawa, K., Teranishi, J., Onozuka, H., Takagi, C., Makita, Y., Matsuo, H., Kusuoka, H., Kitabatake, A. A new approach for evaluation of left ventriculax diastolic function: spatial and temporal analysis of left ventriculax filling flow propagation by color M-mode Doppler echocaxdiography. J. Am. Coll. Cardiol. 27: 365–71, 1996.

[113] Taylor, T.W., Yamaguchi T. Flow patterns in three-dimensional left ventricular systolic and diastolic flows determined from computational fluid dynamics. Biorheology 32: 61–71, 1995.

[114] Tseng, H., Peterson, T.E., and Berk, B.C. Fluid shear stress stimulates mitogen-activated protein kinase in endothelial cells. Circ. Res. 77: 869–78, 1995.

[115] Ueba, H., Kawakami, M., and Yaginuma, T. Shear stress as an inhibitor of vascular smooth muscle cell proliferation: role of transforming growth factor-b1 and tissue type plasminogen activator. Arterioscler. Thromb. Vasc. Biol. 17: 1512–6, 1997.

[116] Vierendeels, J.A., Riemslagh, K., Dick, E., Verdonck, P.R. Computer simulation of intraventricular flow and pressure gradients during diastole. J. Biomech. Eng. (ASME) 122: 667–74, 2000.

[117] Watanabe, H., Sugiura, S., Hisada, T. The looped heart does not save energy by maintaining the momentum of blood flowing in the ventricle. Am. J. Physiol. Heart Circ. Physiol. 294: H2191–6, 2008.

[118] Wigström, L., Ebbers, T., Fyrenius, A., Karlsson, M., Engvall, J., Wranne, B., Bolger, A.F. Particle trace visualization of intracardiac flow using time resolved 3D phase contrast MRI. Magn. Reson. Med. 41: 793–9, 1999.

[119] Zhang, Q., Hisada, T. Analysis of fluid–structure interaction problems with structural buckig and large domain changes by ALE finite element method. Comput. Meth. Appl. Mech. Eng. 190: 6341–57, 2001.

[120] Zile, M.R., Brutsaert, D.L. New concepts in diastolic dysfunction and diastolic heart failure: Part I: diagnosis, prognosis, and measurements of diastolic function. Circulation 105: 1387–93, 2002.

[121] Zile, M.R., Baicu, C.F., Gaasch, W.H. Diastolic heart failure–abnormalities in active relaxation and passive stiffness of the left ventricle. N. Engl. J. Med. 350: 1953–9, 2004.

Chapter 15

Fluid Dynamic Epigenetic Factors in Cardiogenesis and Remodeling

The rapid motion of fluids will etch canals between delicate tissues. Soon their flow will begin to vary, leading to the emergence of distinct organs. The fluids themselves, now more elaborate, will become more complex, engendering a greater variety of secretions and substances composing the organs.

——M. le Chevalier De Lamarck (1744–1829), in *Histoire naturelle des animaux sans vertèbres* [71].

That form ever follows function. This is the law.

——Horatio Greenough (1805–52), American sculptor, architect and essayist, [34].

The form, then, of any portion of matter, whether it be living or dead, and the changes of form which are apparent in its movements and in its growth, may in all cases alike be described as due to the action of force. In short, the form of an object is a "diagram of forces," in this sense, at least, that from it we can judge of or deduce the forces that are acting or have acted upon it.

——D'Arcy Wentworth Thompson (1860–1948), in *On Growth and Form* [129].

THE CARDIOVASCULAR SYSTEM IS THE FIRST SYSTEM [20] to function in the developing embryo. It is functioning by the end of the third week of gestation. The heart is a highly modified muscular vessel (see Fig. 6.2, on p. 302). Heart development encompasses four consecutive stages: (*i*) heart tube formation, (*ii*) looping, (*iii*) chamber formation, and (*iv*) valve formation [87]. During embryonic development, the heart is the first organ to form, and peristaltic contractions begin as soon as a primitive tubular structure and vasculature are in evidence. The subsequent morphogenetic progressions that give rise to the four-chambered organ are the product of both embryonic and local patterning systems [38], and of a feed-forward circuitry that links form with function [117]. The result is a pulsating structure in which orthograde flow into and between adjacent chambers occurs in an elegant *"sling-like"* way [65]. Figure 15.1, on p. 810, summarizes the timing of human cardiogenesis[1] according to *Larsen's Human Embryology* [115], which should be consulted for a comprehensive, modern, descriptive treatment of the subject, replete with insightful illustrations. As is shown in this figure, between weeks 4 and 8 post conception, the primitive tubular heart undergoes a process of lengthening and looping, remodeling, realignment, and septation that converts its single lumen into the four chambers of the definitive organ.

15.1 The heart tube

The first sign of heart development is the formation of cardiogenic plates or cords (see Fig. 15.2); these are canalized to form two endocardial conduits that fuse to make one *heart tube*, through which blood eventually flows in a cranial direction. The heart tube pushes into the dorsal wall of the empty pericardial sac during development, and it becomes surrounded

[1]From the Greek words kardia ($\kappa\alpha\rho\delta\iota\alpha$) = heart and genesis ($\gamma\epsilon\nu\epsilon\sigma\iota\varsigma$) = creation, origin).

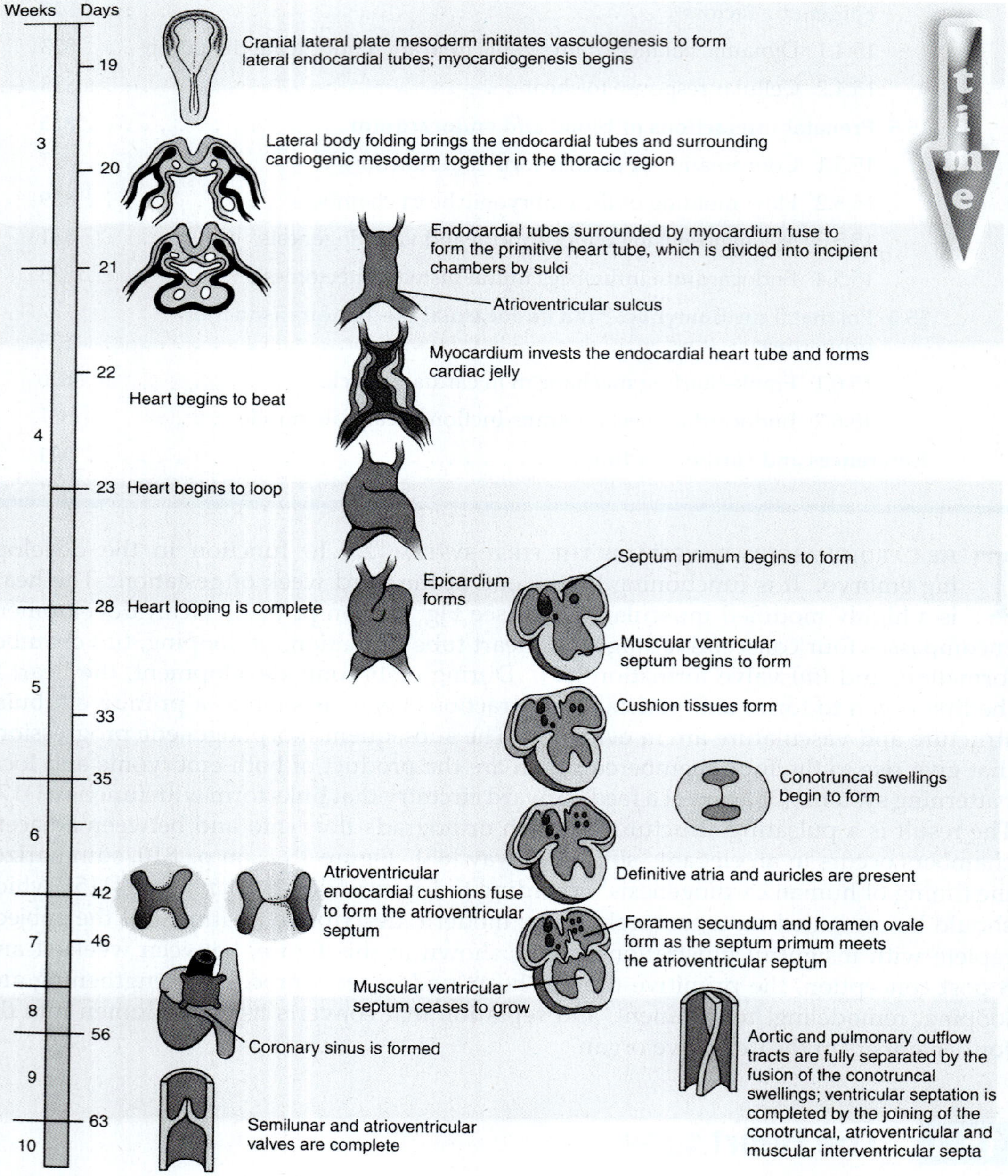

Figure 15.1: The timing of human cardiac development. Note the nonuniform time-axis and that cardiac development is essentially complete within 10 weeks from conception. (Slightly modified from *Larsen's Human Embryology* [115], by permission of Churchill Livingstone/Elsevier.)

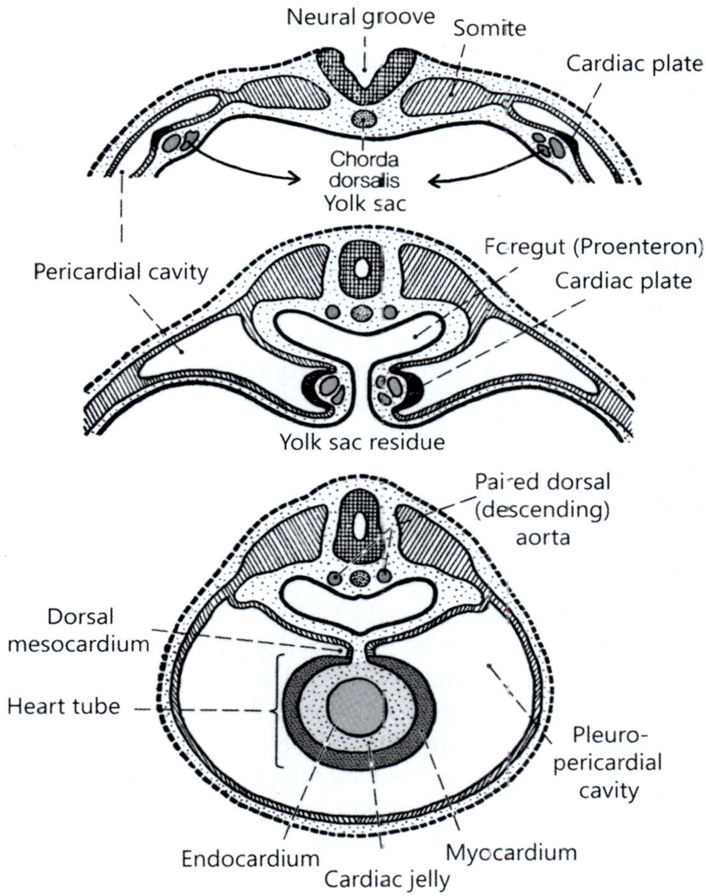

Figure 15.2: The bilateral cardiogenic plates are canalized and migrate centrally, where they fuse to form one *heart tube.*

by it to such a degree that two sides of the invaginating visceral layer of pericardium become apposed and are given the name, the *dorsal mesocardium* (see Fig. 15.2). The dorsal mesocardium suspends the heart tube at the back for a time, but it soon breaks down leaving the heart tube suspended at its cranial and caudal extremities, or poles, but not in between [126]. The heart tissue is still encased by the visceral layer of pericardium and the parietal layer surrounds it, defining a lubricating *potential space.*

The tissues surrounding the lumen of the heart tube (see Fig. 15.2) condense to form the myoepicardial mantle, the future *myocardium*. Gelatinous connective tissue, called *cardiac jelly*, separates this mantle from the endothelial heart tube, the future *endocardium*. At the time that the paired endocardial canals fuse to form a single tubular heart, several dilatations are becoming defined by interposed constrictions (or *"sulci"*), which demarcate the boundaries of future regions of the definitive heart (see Fig. 15.3, on p. 813). These divisions, from entrance of the veins in the caudal aspect of the heart tube to the cranially located aortic roots, are the *sinus venosus*, into which flow the developing common cardinal veins, venous tributaries of the embryo, the vitelline veins, draining the yolk sac, and the umbilical veins from the placenta; the primitive *common atrium*; the *primitive ventricle*; and the *bulbus cordis* with the heart tube's outflow tract.

It is actually the inferior portion of the bulbus cordis that gives rise to much of the right ventricle, whereas the primitive ventricle will form the left ventricle. The superior portion of the bulbus will form an outflow channel called the *conotruncus*; this will give rise to the more proximal *conus arteriosus*, and the more distal *truncus arteriosus*. Both of these then split in a spiral fashion (cf. Fig. 15.5, on p. 817) to become the outflow regions of the two ventricles and the ascending aorta and pulmonary trunk. The human heart is beating at Day 22 (see Fig. 15.1). Contractions are of intrinsic myocardial origin. Several processes that do not pertain to the heart proper continue to occur during this time and have a great influence on heart development: embryonic head folding, embryonic lateral folding, and *elongation* of the heart tube in an increasingly *confining* space within the pericardial cavity. Accordingly, the tube divisions are accentuated further by the heart tube bending upon itself, the looping of the heart tube.

The *looping of the heart tube* occurs between Days 23 and 28. The formation of the cardiac loop is facilitated further by the disappearance of the dorsal mesocardium thereby leaving all parts of the heart *free* in the pericardial cavity except at its two extremities, i.e., where the veins enter and the arteries leave. The tube, as it grows, cannot be accommodated within the pericardial cavity and undergoes bending. Looping of the heart tube is usually held to be the first visual evidence of asymmetry within the embryo [86]. The primitive atrium loops up behind and above the primitive ventricle and behind and to the left of the bulbus cordis. Blood begins to circulate through the human embryo by Day 24. The looping process brings the primitive areas of the heart into the proper spatial relationship for development of the adult heart (see Fig. 6.3, on p. 303).

As a result of asymmetrical continuing rapid growth and bending, the tubular heart is thrown into an S-shape with the primary flexure shifted to the right at the bulboventricular junction (see Fig. 15.3). A secondary flexure results in shifting of the atrium and the sinus venosus to a dorsal and more cephalic position from the rest of the heart. That portion of the pericardial cavity between the arterial and venous attachments of the heart will persist as the definitive transverse sinus of the adult.

With the continued growth of the bulboventricular loop, the adjacent walls of the bulbus cordis and ventricle at the bulboventricular groove regress in their development and, eventually, disappear. This results in the incorporation of the caudal part of the bulbus cavity into the formation of the *primitive ventricle*. The cephalic portion of the bulbus (truncus arteriosus) remains relatively unchanged at this time. The rapidly growing atrium is restricted between the pharynx dorsally and the bulbus cordis ventrally. Hence, it has enlarged greatly in its *lateral* extents; the outpouchings thus formed will turn into the future right and left atria (see Fig. 15.4A.). Although the cavities of these two lateral expansions are continuous, the site of the future interatrial partitioning is represented externally by the interatrial sulcus. The atria are delimited from the ventricle by the deep

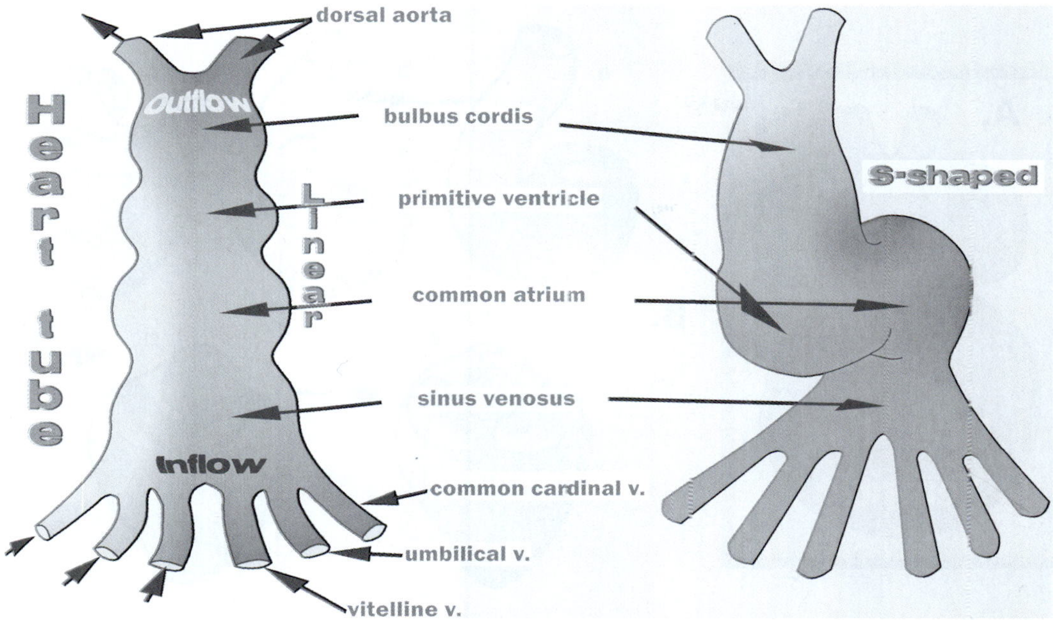

Figure 15.3: *Left*: A series of constrictions (sulci) divide the heart tube into several interposed dilated sections; the *sinus venosus*, into which the common cardinal veins, the umbilical veins and the vitelline veins drain; the primitive *common atrium*; the *primitive ventricle*; and the *bulbus cordis*, through which blood flows to the paired dorsal aortas. *Right*: Note that with the rightward bending of the tube, the primitive atrium loops up behind and above the primitive ventricle and behind and to the left of the bulbus cordis; thus, the atrium is now dorsal and the loop formed by the ventricle and the bulbus cordis *(bulbo-ventricular loop)* is ventral.

atrioventricular groove, the future *coronary sulcus*. As the heart continues to grow, the right side of the sinus venosus is incorporated into the right side of the primitive atrium.

By the end of the first month of development, the major regional divisions of the heart are recognizable externally. The internal chambers, however, are still *undivided*. Thus, at this stage blood enters the sinus venosus, passes into the common atrial chamber through its right dorsal wall, is pumped through the atrioventricular canal, which at this stage has significant length [86], to the ventricle and out through the bulbus cordis.

15.2 Formation of heart chambers

During the second month of growth, important changes in the internal configuration of the developing heart occur [72], which lead to formation of the definitive four-chambered organ (see Fig. 15.4B., on p. 814). Among these developments are the establishment of *endocardial cushions*, septa, and valves. The endocardial cushions begin the separation of

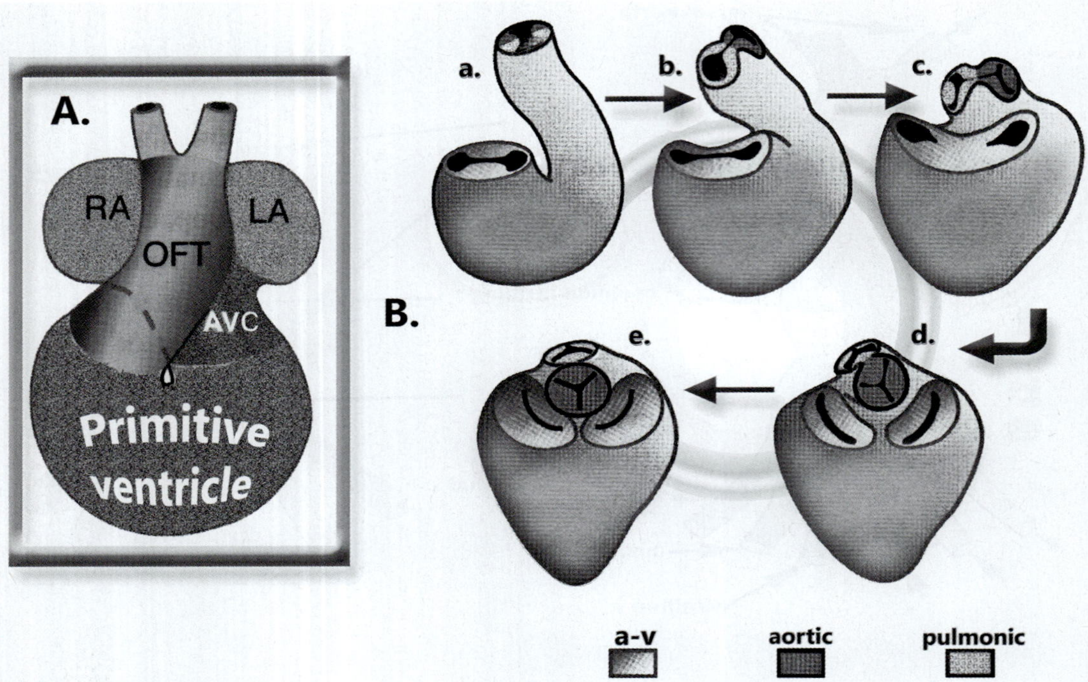

Figure 15.4: **A.** Convergence of the *outflow* (OFT, outflow tract and truncus arteriosus) and *inflow* (RA, right atrium, LA, left atrium, and AVC, atrioventricular canal) portions of the developing heart, viewed from the front. **B.** Development of *endocardial cushions* (a., b., c.) and formation of *valves* (d., e.).

the heart into upper and lower, right and left, chambers, which will become the atria and ventricles; while the endocardial cushions continue to develop, the atrial and ventricular septa begin to form.

All these formations are necessary for the partitioning of the common primitive chamber into right and left sides, and for the delineation of the ventricles from the atria and the outflow arterial trunks. In addition, the sinus venosus is absorbed into the right atrium, and the truncus arteriosus is divided into the pulmonary trunk and the aorta.

15.2.1 Right atrium

The sinus venosus undergoes early structural and positional changes. With the establishment of a venous shunt through the liver, much of the blood returning to the heart is directed to the right horn of the sinus venosus. Under this influence, the right horn of the sinus venosus enlarges, whereas the left one is reduced in size. As a result of this, the sinus venosus becomes incorporated in the dorsal wall of the prospective right atrium. The primitive atrial wall is pushed ventrally, eventually becoming the right auricle. The superior and inferior venae cavae and the coronary sinus, which developed from veins initially opening into the sinus venosus, now enter independently into the right atrium. In the adult heart, the right auricle contains *pectinate* muscle derived from the primitive atrium, whereas the sinus venarum is derived from the sinus venosus and is, therefore, *smooth-walled*.

15.2.2 Left atrium

The pulmonary veins, unlike the veins entering the right side of the heart, do not develop from the conversion of old vascular conduits. The left side of the primitive atrium sprouts a pulmonary vein, which branches and sends two veins toward each of the developing lungs. The trunk of this pulmonary vein is incorporated into the left side of the primitive atrium, forming the smooth wall of the adult left atrium. The left side of the primitive atrium is pushed forward and eventually becomes the *trabeculated* left auricle. Part of the initial atrioventricular canal becomes incorporated into the definitive left and right atrium as the vestibule of the mitral and tricuspid valve.

15.2.3 Interatrial septum

The interatrial septum in the adult heart is formed by the combination of two embryonic septa: the *septum primum*, and the *septum secundum* [1]. The *septum primum* grows along the midsagittal plane like a waxing moon toward the atrioventricular canal. This septum separates the two atria, except for a temporary space at the posteroinferior edge of the septum primum called the *foramen primum* which permits a right-to-left shunt of fetal blood. Blood is not oxygenated at the lungs but at the placenta instead; oxygenated blood is brought in by the umbilical vein into the right atrium of the heart (see Fig. 15.7, on p. 821). Therefore, there must be an opening between the right and left atrium of the heart, to ensure blood passes from the left atrium to the left ventricle for circulation.

At the superior edge of the septum primum clefts begin to form that provide a second opening, the *foramen secundum*. There must always be a right to left passage, since fetal lungs are developing and *atelectatic*, and consequently, blood from the right side of the heart has nowhere to go and needs to be "shunted" to the left! The foramen secundum provides an alternate right-to-left shunt, and the foramen primum closes. During this process a second, partial septum, the *septum secundum*, also begins to grow down from the roof of the right atrium, just lateral to the septum primum [2, 3, 72]. The septum secundum is thicker and more muscular than the membranous septum primum and permits the right-to-left shunt of blood through an opening called the *foramen ovale*. Fetal blood is shunted from the right atrium to the left atrium through the foramen ovale and the foramen secundum. The septum secundum eventually fuses inferiorly, but the foramen ovale stays patent, thus enabling the shunting of blood from the right to the left side of the heart.

Before birth, the vascular resistance is so much greater in the atelectatic pulmonary vasculature than in the systemic circulation that most of the flow is diverted around the lungs. The *foramen ovale* and *ductus arteriosus* act as bypasses permitting blood from the systemic veins to enter the systemic circulation without passing through the lungs (see Fig. 15.7, on p. 821). After birth, when pulmonary venous return increases blood pressure in the left atrium, the membranous septum primum is pressed against the septum secundum. They eventually fuse and block the right-to-left shunt of blood. If there is no orifice in the interatrial septum, LV output is restricted to the amount of blood flowing through the lungs. Under these conditions, the left ventricle pumps abnormally small amounts and may not develop normally, remaining *"hypoplastic."*

The output of the right and left ventricles is *balanced* by variations in the quantity of blood bypassing the lungs through the orifices which persist in the interatrial septum and through the ductus arteriosus. The flow of blood from the right into the left atrium and from the pulmonary artery into the aorta provides a fluid dynamic demonstration of the fact that pressures in the right atrium, right ventricle and pulmonary artery exceed the pressures in the corresponding channels on the left. This condition is, of course, the *reverse* of that which applies shortly after birth.

15.2.4 Interventricular septum

Two thickenings of embryonic connective tissue, called endocardial cushions, arise from the dorsal and ventral walls of the atrioventricular canal. During the sixth week, the dorsal and ventral endocardial cushions fuse to form a mass of tissue separating the common canal into right and left atrioventricular canals (see Fig. 15.4B., on p. 814). The ventricles also undergo their development while the atrial transformations are taking place.

The left ventricle is formed primarily from the primitive ventricle [1]. The right ventricle is formed primarily from the bulbus cordis. The superior portion of the bulbus cordis becomes the *conus arteriosus* and the *truncus arteriosus*. At the end of the fourth week, a sagittal muscular interventricular septum begins to develop superiorly from the ventricular floor between the presumptive right and left ventricles. This interventricular septum grows toward the endocardial cushions, and becomes more prominent by the enlargement of the prospective right and left halves of the common ventricle [2,3,72]. This septum stops short of the atrioventricular canal, leaving a space called the *interventricular foramen*, which permits blood from both ventricles to exit via the conus arteriosus.

The interventricular foramen is usually completely closed by week seven of gestation. Closure is accomplished by growth of membranous tissue derived from the endocardial cushions, the interventricular septum and from the conus ridges formed within the truncus and extending to the interventricular septum.

As the common ventricular chamber is being partitioned into right and left ventricles, an anatomically and functionally significant structure arising in the bulbus cordis leads to the formation of the ascending aorta and pulmonary trunk [38,72]. Within the conus arteriosus, i.e., the cephalad portion of the bulbus, two ridges of endocardial and subendocardial tissue grow toward each other from opposite walls of the lumen. Partitioning unfolds from the bottom to the top in a helix because the ridges grow spatially in a rotational shift.

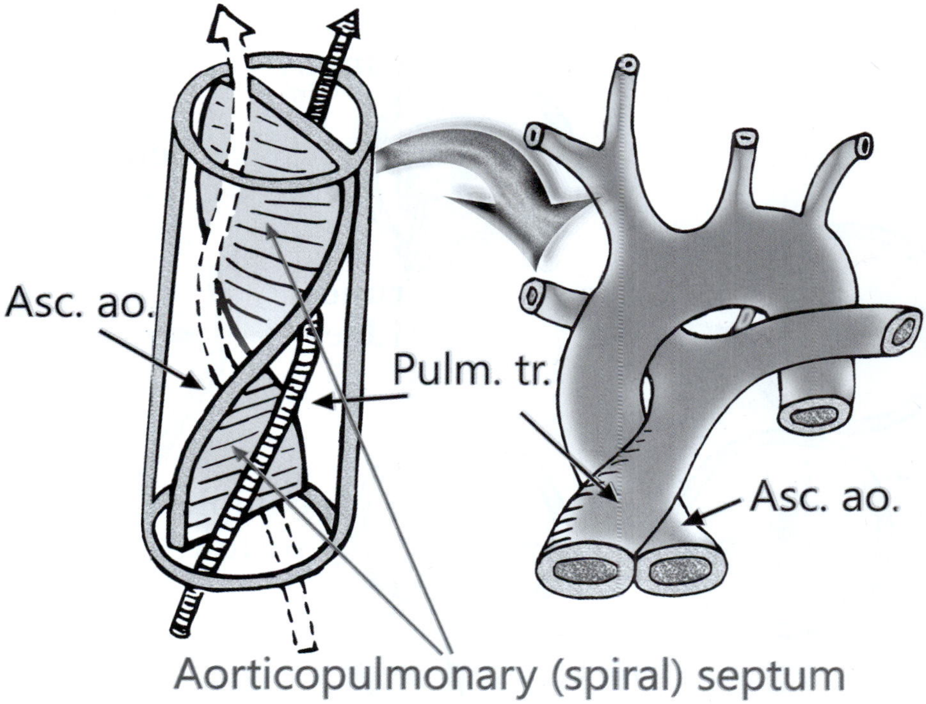

Figure 15.5: The spiral configuration of the interbulbar *aorticopulmonary septum* accounts for the way in which the ascending aorta and the pulmonary trunk *twist* around each other and communicate with the left and the right ventricle, respectively.

The fact that these ridges pursue a counterclockwise course as they spiral caudally in the bulbus has paramount importance (see Fig. 15.5) When they meet they form an interbulbar septum which separates the bulbus into the ascending aorta and the pulmonary trunk [72]. The spiral *aorticopulmonary septum* divides the conus in half, creating outflow tracts for the right and left ventricles and, extending inferiorly, fuses with and completes the *interventricular septum*. The spiral configuration of the interbulbar septum accounts for the way in which the aorta and the pulmonary trunk twist around each other and communicate with the left and the right ventricle, respectively.

The development of the aorticopulmonary septum is complex, and disorders of its development are associated with several congenital heart defects, including: persistent truncus arteriosus, when there has been improper formation of the truncal ridges and the aorticopulmonary septum such that the aorta and the pulmonary trunk are not fully divided; double outlet right ventricle, a form of ventriculoarterial connection in which both great arteries arise completely, or predominantly, from the morphologic right ventricle—since both great arteries arise from the right ventricle, a ventricular septal defect, or "VSD," is almost always present to allow egress of blood flow from the left ventricle, otherwise it would have *no outlet* to empty through; transposition of the great arteries, when there

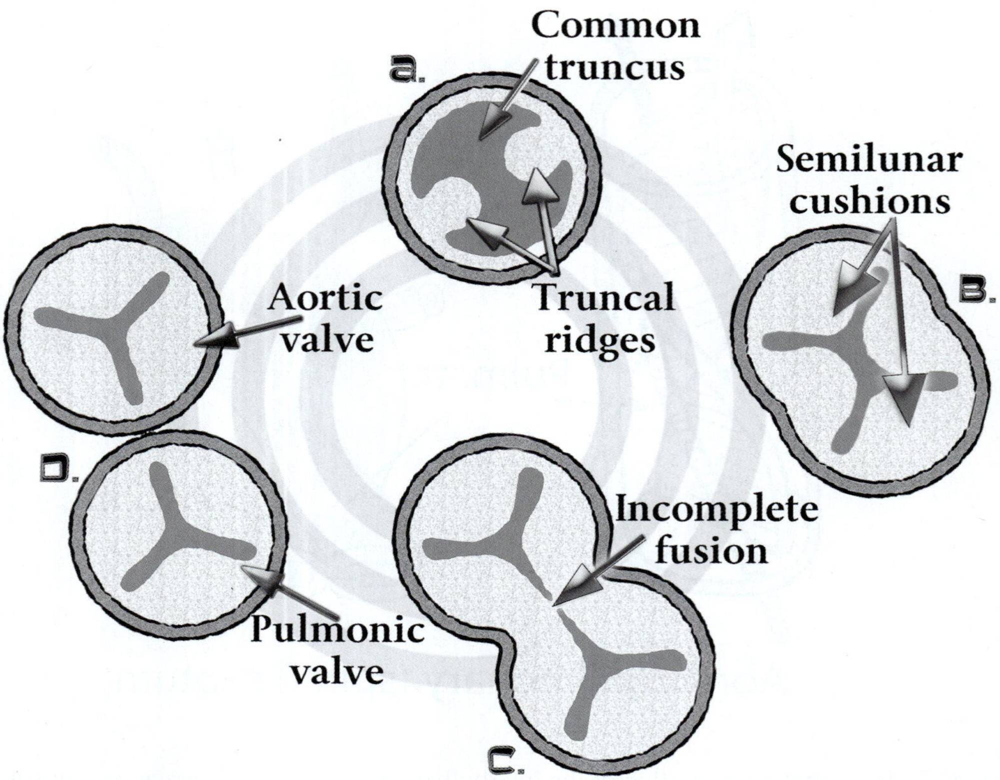

Figure 15.6: Formation of the aortic and pulmonary semilunar valves. (Adapted, modified, from a figure copyrighted by the Texas Heart Institute in Angelini [3], with their kind permission.)

has been failure of the aorticopulmonary septum to take a *spiraling* course; tetralogy of Fallot; and, Eisenmenger's syndrome.

Tetralogy of Fallot results from the asymmetric division of the aorticopulmonary septum. The result is a stenosed pulmonary artery and a VSD. The VSD arises from the deviation of the aorticopulmonary septum from the midline. The aorta thus overrides the VSD, allowing a left-to-right shunt of blood. Accordingly, the tetralogy comprises the following four defects: pulmonary artery/valve stenosis, ventricular septal defect, an overriding aorta, and right ventricular hypertrophy, which results from the increased right ventricular pressure levels and causes a characteristic boot-shaped (classic *"coeur-en-sabot"* sign) appearance as seen by chest x-ray.[2] Tetralogy of Fallot results in low oxygenation of blood due to the mixing of oxygenated and deoxygenated blood in the left ventricle via the VSD and the preferential flow of the mixed blood from both ventricles

[2]Congenital heart defects are now diagnosed with echocardiography, which involves no radiation, is very specific, and can be done *prenatally*.

through the aorta (a *right-to-left shunt*), because of the obstruction to flow through the stenotic pulmonary valve and artery.

Eisenmenger's syndrome is a related abnormality, which arises from the persistence of the truncus arteriosus. Failure of fusion between components of the membranous (cephalic) portion of the interventricular septum allows blood flow between chambers and recirculation of *oxygenated* blood back into the right ventricle and the lungs instead of orthograde flow out of the left ventricle to the systemic circulation. Over time, this extra blood flow to the lungs damages their vessels, causing pulmonary hypertension. The increased pressure levels in the right ventricle cause RV hypertrophy and eventually a reversed flow of blood, right-to-left shunt, so that the *deoxygenated* blood goes out to the rest of the body. Eisenmenger's syndrome refers to this combination of pulmonary hypertension with right-to-left shunt, which results in cyanosis. In Eisenmenger's syndrome, the division between the ascending aorta and the pulmonary artery are roughly equal. The position of the truncus directly above the VSD is referred to as an overriding truncus.

15.2.5 Semilunar and atrioventricular valves

In addition to the swellings (truncal ridges) that create the interbulbar *aorticopulmonary* septum, two other thickenings (semilunar cushions) occur in the anterior and posterior walls of the bulbus [2,3]. These four endocardial thickenings indicate the location of the future aortic and pulmonary *semilunar valves* (see Fig. 15.4B., on p. 814). The anterior thickening gives rise to the anterior semilunar valve of the pulmonary trunk, and the posterior develops into the posterior semilunar valve of the aorta. The halves of each truncal ridge, which persist in the aorta and the pulmonary trunk at this level, become converted into the right and left semilunar valves of each vessel (see Fig. 15.6, on p. 818).

The *atrioventricular valves* also develop from subendocardial tissue [3,63,72]. Proliferations of this tissue arise from the outer walls and the endocardial cushion lining the atrioventricular canals and project toward the cavities of the ventricles (see Fig. 15.4B.). Endocardial cushions represent areas of the fibrous skeleton forming between the right and left atrium and the primitive ventricle and serve two important functions: a.) they form a partition in the heart tube between the atria and the primitive ventricle, known as the AV canal; the resulting two channels represent sites for the future tricuspid and bicuspid valves, and b.) they provide a "scaffold" to which the interatrial septa and the interventricular septum will grow toward and fuse with.

Three endocardial cushion projections are formed on the right side and two on the left. The ventricular faces of these blunt projections are invaded by muscular tissue which is in direct contiguity with that lining the ventricular walls. As differentiation progresses, the size of the valve leaflets is increased by an undercutting, or excavating, process; this leads also to a thinning out of the muscle tissue attaching the cusps to the ventricular walls. Eventually, these muscular cords become partially tendinous and are transformed into *chordae tendineae* and *papillary muscles*. Valvular defects can arise if endocardial cushion fusion does not partition the AV canal evenly.

In the early tubular heart the myocardium is continuous throughout its extent [72]. Later on, the muscle in the region of the atrioventricular canal degenerates and is replaced by dense connective tissue, constituting the *anuli fibrosi* in the adult heart. Consequently, the myocardium of the atria and ventricles becomes essentially discontinuous in the region of the *atrioventricular groove*. A small bundle of specialized muscle tissue persists, however, dorsal to the atrioventricular endocardial cushion. This bridge between the right atrium and the top of the interventricular septum becomes the *electric impulse-conducting* atrioventricular bundle of His [3].

By the eleventh week of gestation, the heart of a human embryo has been fashioned into a four-chambered organ with the corresponding arterial trunks. Thus, over a relatively short period during gestation, the precociously developing heart has been transformed from a simple tubular structure to a complicated organ. Many of these transformations are, as we have seen, concerned with the development of certain portions of the endocardium and their muscular invasion. Other structural alterations are accompanied by many histogenetic modifications in the primitive epicardium and myocardium. The morphologic and circulatory patterns established at this time persist throughout the remainder of fetal development.

15.3 Fetal circulation

The developing circulatory system acts to bring oxygenated blood from the placenta through the umbilicus, distribute it throughout the fetal system, and return oxygen-depleted blood to the placenta. After birth, portions of this path become obsolete, but the obliterated vessels remain apparent in the adult body as thickened strands of connective tissue, or ligaments.

From the *placenta*, oxygenated blood and nutrients are carried through the *umbilical vein* to the liver. There, in the *ductus venosus*, this blood mixes with some deoxygenated blood from the portal vein (draining the gut) and then exits via the *inferior vena cava*. In the IVC the blood mixes with more deoxygenated blood returning from the legs and trunk and is carried to the *right atrium*. The basic difference between the postnatal and the developing and fetal circulations is that fetal lungs are nonfunctional and collapsed. Effectively, blood from the right side of the heart has nowhere to go and needs to be "shunted" to the left. Such a shunting passage exists between the right and the left atria.

In the right atrium the partially oxygenated blood (62–67%) is mostly shunted through the *foramen ovale* to the *left atrium* where it mixes with a very small amount of deoxygenated blood from the lungs. From the left atrium, the blood flows into the *left ventricle* and is pumped out the *ascending aorta*, delivering partially oxygenated blood to the head and arms and to the descending aorta. However, if no blood flowed through the right ventricle, that chamber would fail to develop. Thus, some blood does pass to the right ventricle.

Deoxygenated blood returning to the right atrium from the *superior vena cava* (draining head and arms) flows mostly into the right ventricle and it is pumped out the *pulmonary*

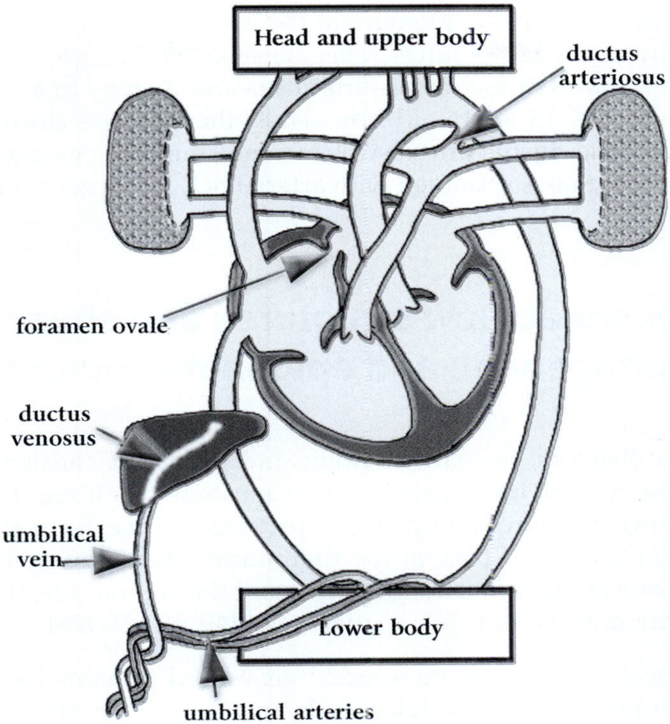

Figure 15.7: The fetal circulation.

trunk. From the pulmonary trunk, it needs to be shunted again, this time to the aorta. The *ductus arteriosus* shunts much of this blood from the pulmonary trunk to the descending aorta where it mixes with the blood that did not enter the arteries to the head and arms. The *descending aorta* carries semi-oxygenated blood (57%) to the gut and lower extremities, with a branch to the *umbilical arteries* that deliver the poorly oxygenated blood to the *placenta* for oxygenation.

At birth, with the activation of breathing, the alveoli fill with air, the pulmonary vessels including the alveolar capillary network expand, and the pressure in the pulmonary system drops as its flow impedance falls drastically. The greatly increased pulmonary venous return raises blood pressure levels in the left atrium. As an important outcome of these changes, the right atrial pressure levels sink in comparison to the left. This *flipping over* of the atrial pressure levels causes the septum primum to be pressed against the septum secundum and, as was already mentioned above, the foramen secundum becomes functionally closed. At the same time, spontaneous constriction (or clamping) of the umbilical vessels cuts off the exchange of blood with the placenta. As the low-resistance placental region disappears, the peripheral resistance increases in the systemic circulation. The pressure in the aorta is now higher than that in the pulmonary trunk and the *right-to-left* shunt via the ductus arteriosus that is present before birth is turned around into a *left-to-right* shunt. The pO_2 pressure in the aorta increases since the blood is now oxygenated directly in the baby's lungs. This increased pO_2 triggers a contraction of the smooth muscle in the wall of the ductus arteriosus and thereby to a functional shutting down, usually within 10–15 hours of birth. Thus, there ensues closure of both the interatrial septum and the ductus arteriosus, since no shunting passages are needed any longer, and only blood that is saturated with arterial pO_2 levels gets into the aorta.[3]

15.4 Intracardiac flow structures and shear as prenatal morphogenetic and epigenetic factors

In this and earlier chapters, histoarchitectonic and geometric cardiac form and movements have been seen to be interrelated with evanescent, albeit regularly repeating, intracardiac blood flow structures and pulsatile patterns; cardiac form and blood flow are brought together in space and time in the rhythmical cardiac pumping process. From the earliest embryonic stages of its development and throughout life, the heart integrates structure and function across multiple spatial scales [49, 91, 121, 136].

The physiological functions of myocardial genes and proteins have been shown to undergo endocardium-mediated modulations by mechanical "environmental factors." As I have pointed out in the Introduction, whose Sections 1.9 and 1.10, on pp. 20 ff., can be reviewed to good advantage at this juncture, mechanical stresses [48], or lack thereof, may act as important *epigenetic factors*[4] in cardiovascular development, adaptation, and disease. Shear stress, in particular, is the drag force (cf. Section 4.6, on pp. 190 ff.) that is imposed on endothelial cells by the viscous blood and acts on the endothelium in parallel to the blood flow.

Although the genetics of cardiogenesis are being analyzed intensively [11,22,26,85,123], inquiries into the influence of blood flow patterns as epigenetic factors in heart development have advanced more slowly, due to the technical difficulties [77] in mapping early embryonic intracardiac flow fields *in vivo*. Nevertheless, it appears that embryonic cardiogenesis is regulated by the harmonized *interplay* between a genetic program, fluid mechanical epigenetic stimuli, and the inter- and intra-cellular signals that link them [126–128]. Cardiac flow patterns change as the heart *loops*, its atrial and ventricular chambers form by a *ballooning process* (see Fig. 15.8, on p. 828), and the *endocardial cushions* begin to *expand*. Such changes in the flow boundaries cause temporal and spatial variations in *shear stress* along the endocardial lining of the primitive heart.

[3]There is normally some anatomic shunting, amounting to no more than 2–5% of the cardiac output; it comprises venous blood entering the systemic circulation directly without first passing through the alveolar capillaries. Such blood comes from some bronchial and pleural veins, and from the Thebesian veins, which allow a direct connection other than through the capillaries between the coronary arteries and the chambers of the heart.

[4] See footnote on p. 21.

15.4.1 Dynamic balance of myogenic tone and endothelial dilatation

Myogenic pressure-induced tone is a characteristic of muscular arterial resistance vessels and of some veins [23]. It is opposed by the *endothelial* flow-induced dilatation [54,74]. Mechanotransduction of shear stress has been shown to involve extracellular matrix and cell structure proteins [24,53–55]. The *dynamic balance* of these two mechanisms results in a constant basal tone in resistance arteries and allows a prompt adaptation to changes in flow and pressure. Myogenic tone develops upon stretch of the vascular wall, does not require a high level of intracellular calcium [40], and is largely independent of endothelial factors [23]. On the other hand, the endothelial mechanotransduction of shear that triggers dilatation involves the extracellular matrix and endothelial structural proteins. This flow-induced dilatation is, in part, dependent on the paracrine release of nitric oxide (NO) by the endothelium [24]. Nitric oxide synthase (NOS) inhibitors induce significant vasoconstriction, suggesting an indispensable role of NO as a local vasodilator. This is due mainly to its effects on the smooth muscle of large arterioles [108], which significantly control arterial conductance while scarcely being regulated by metabolites. The *endothelial cytoskeleton* (see Fig. 1.6, on p. 24) has a selective role in the mechanotransduction leading to flow-induced NO release [50].

Another interesting finding pertains to adrenomedullin (AM), an *antiproliferative* factor of vascular smooth muscle cells, which has potent vasorelaxant activity [57,92]. Both gene transcription and production of AM in human aortic endothelial cells are down-regulated by fluid shear stress in a time- and magnitude-dependent manner [119]. AM is a 52-amino acid peptide synthesized and secreted by endothelial cells [125]. It is a shear stress responsive element (SSRE), and *suppresses cell proliferation* in vascular smooth muscle [61]. Thus, its down-regulation by fluid shear stress elevations allows for proliferation of vascular smooth muscle and long-term increases in *luminal size*.

15.4.2 Cellular response to shear

The need to understand the role of fluid shear stress in endothelial cell function has led to a major new area of research of the cellular response to shear [41,46,78,82,103,107,109,127], as was noted in the Introduction—see Section 1.10, on p. 23. From early embryonic development onward through life, different operating levels and spatiotemporal patterns of mechanical factors such as fluid flow-associated shear stress, or pressure, or myocardial strain, may initiate or modulate signal transduction cascades and other cellular processes that underlie cardiac morphogenesis, adaptations, remodeling, and transition to pathology, which may be more or less reversible. Here we are focusing on *shear stress*—and its normal and abnormal variations—as a morphogenetic intracardiac blood flow-associated factor modulating cardiac development, adaptations and remodeling [40,106,126].

Laminar and disturbed flows produce different shear stress patterns that, in turn, should have disparate effects on endothelial cells and on prenatal heart development. Oscillatory shear stresses [95] induced by *vortical motions* [101] correlate with augmented cell proliferation [17]. Both the magnitude of shear stress and local fluctuations in shear stress may be important *mechanosensory signals* [17]. Diameter adaptation to maintain mean wall shear stress within limits also holds for changes in blood viscosity [81]. Such studies support the paradigm that alteration in fluid dynamic loading is a mechanism that can induce changes in *cardiac function* and *structure*.

A large number of endothelial mechanotransduction[5] responses to shear stress have been documented, since the early studies by Dewey et al. [28], examining the realignment of endothelial cells and their actin filaments caused by fluid shear. A host of other responses have been investigated, including the intracellular release of Ca^{++} ions and a variety of second messengers, and the shear-induced activation of various membrane receptor proteins [134]. There is no one molecular or anatomical structure that drives all mechanotransduction responses. There are numerous different cellular responses to mechanotransduced forces, and many special mechanisms by which such responses are mediated, too many to enumerate here—they are reviewed in depth by Orr et al. [94]. Perhaps the best described subcellular sites for sensing mechanical forces are primary cilia, the cytoskeleton, the nucleus, and stretch-modulated ion channels and focal adhesions of the cell membrane. However, the mechanisms responsible for converting frictional shear forces into multiple specific signaling responses remain incompletely characterized [74,78,82,103,107].

As we saw in the Introduction, the cells lining cardiovascular organs have *autocrine* and *paracrine* hormonal mechanisms[6] enabling them to respond immediately to local hemodynamic changes involving not only intramural stresses, which rise with actively generated or passive distending pressure, but also *shear stress*, which increases in intensity with flow velocity. The cells lining the developing cardiovascular system are equipped with numerous receptors that allow them to detect and respond to the mechanical forces generated by shear stress [73,74].

The cytoskeleton and other structural components of endothelial cells have an established role in mechanotransduction, being able to transmit and modulate tension within the cell via focal adhesion sites, integrins, cellular junctions and the extracellular matrix [53–55,113,116,120]. *Integrins* are part of a large family of cell adhesion-receptor proteins, involved in cell–extracellular matrix and cell–cell interactions [116] (see Fig. 15.14a, on p. 838). Consider, e.g., the example that we examined in Section 1.9.1, on pp. 22 f.: vascular tone is modified to compensate almost immediately for variations in endothelial shear accompanying flow changes and, ordinarily, this efficiently restores mechanical forces to normal levels. Continuing with this example, sometimes, the variations in vasomotor tone do not suffice to compensate, and the gene expression, or *phenotype*, of the vascular cells is altered, causing local adaptive adjustments, which also tend to restore mechanical forces to physiological levels. Many intracellular mechanotransduction cascades are activated by flow-induced shear and initiate, via sequential phosphorylation pathways, the activation of transcription factors and subsequent gene expression [75].

[5]Cellular mechanotransduction may be characterized as the biochemical response of cells to mechanical stimulation. Although the mechanisms of mechanotransduction remain incompletely delineated, it is obvious that it plays a major role in maintaining proper functioning of mechanically active tissues, like the myocardium, which must respond to diverse mechanical demands.

[6]See footnote on p. 23.

Vascular *remodeling* ensues; similar short-, intermediate-, and long-term adaptations are also operative both in the embryonic [35,36,82] and in the adult [56,95–97,101] heart.

Sometimes the adaptating organs undergo not simply quantitative but also qualitative changes and there is transition to disease that may or may not be reversible, or compatible with prenatal or longer term postnatal survival. Many receptors present on the surface of cells lining cardiovascular organs allow them to detect subtle changes in their physical environment, rendering them capable of a true autonomic regulation, which enables them to adapt to their mechanical environment. Although the initial interaction between the surface shear force and the cell occurs at the luminal surface, intracellular elements that connect to that surface provide continuity of structure and mechanics that extend to *other parts* of the cell; inside the cells, cytoskeletal proteins transmit and modulate mechanical forces (cf. Fig. 1.6, on p. 24). For that reason, mechanotransduction sites are not necessarily restricted to the cell surface.

The cell junctions, the nucleus, and focal adhesions are highly responsive to luminal shear stress. The pivotal apparatus linking all of these sites to the cell surface and with one another is, in fact, the cytoskeleton, which is a key component of endothelial and endocardial mechanotransduction [21,70]. In addition to *structural* modifications, shear forces may induce changes in the *ionic composition* of the cells, mediated by membrane ion channels [30], may stimulate various membrane receptors, and may induce complex biochemical cascades [73–75].

Mechanosensitive endothelial and endocardial membrane channels are *pores* lined by helicoidal proteins; they are specialized in the sense that they recognize mechanical deformation as a meaningful physiological signal and can vary, sometimes by orders of magnitude, their probability of being *open* depending on, e.g., the shear stress applied on their luminal surface [4,47,111,112]. Opening of the mechanosensitive channel is facilitated by an *iris-like* rotation and tilt of the pore-lining helicoidal protein macromolecules [80]. Evolving understanding of genetic factors relating to blood flow in the developing heart could eventually be used in early surgical correction of, or even genetic intervention in, prenatal heart disease. Moreover, the same responses to shear forces that normally shape the developing heart may also contribute to *later–onset* abnormalities and disease processes.

15.5 Prenatal interactions of blood and endocardium

Moving liquids, including primal blood in the developing heart, are inseparable from bounding surfaces. They both influence surfaces over which they flow and are influenced by them, impelled to create stream surfaces within their own volume. Moreover, because of the fundamental role of the heart in generating flow, the regulation of developmental and adult cardiac *phenotype* by the input parameters of *flow-associated* forces makes intuitive sense. In the human heart, *form and function* are interrelated via multifactorial epigenetic adaptive mechanisms (cf. *volume* vs. *pressure* overload states), under normal and abnormal operating conditions. Since from its earliest tubular stage the embryonic heart develops in the presence of flow-related forces and stimuli, the question comes up whether its structure influences its function, or, then again, whether the flows and flow-associated forces sustained by its walls influence its form [6,7,46].

Beginning as a linear tube in which the ventricular precursors are downstream of the future atria (cf. Fig. 6.3, on p. 303, and Figs. 15.3 and 15.4, on pp. 813 and 814), the primitive heart tube twists *dextrally*, i.e., undergoes *rightward* looping, to change from an anterior/posterior polarity to a left/right polarity. The outflow region bends caudally and to the right, while the atrial region moves dorsocranially and to the left. The tube loops around, fuses, and reconnects itself—all while continuing to function as a pump [5]. *Looping* causes the heart to fold in such a manner that the atria, ventricles, and outflow tract assume their adult position but remain unseptated. Heart formation, or *cardiogenesis*, requires complex interactions involving cells of multiple embryonic origins.

Recent investigations have begun to reveal the genetic pathways that control cardiac morphogenesis [87]. Many of the genes within these pathways are conserved across vast phylogenetic distances, which has allowed heart development to be dissected in organisms ranging from flies to mammals. As is true of many physiologic processes, many steps in cardiac morphogenesis can be viewed as an integrated feedback loop: alterations in flow-conduit or chamber shape change heart function, which changes the forces experienced by the cardiac cells, stimulating them to modify heart function both by secreting matrix and by continuing to change myofiber shape and arrangement in the walls, and the overall *heart shape* [12,103].

Capturing these *structure–function* relationships is an emerging challenge in clinical and investigative cardiology and basic research (cf. Section 1.10, on pp. 23 ff.). In view of the difficulty of effectively unlinking embryonic cardiac function and blood flow, sophisticated and carefully designed systematic studies are called for to elucidate the interacting contributions of myocardial function and endothelial shear stress on cardiac morphogenesis. In this context, it is inspiring to note that the striking spiral histoarchitectonic arrangements of the myocardial fibers in the heart walls bring to mind images of the archetypical pulsating spiral flow patterns that are exemplified in the diastolic filling vortices and in secondary flows (cf. Figs. 9.14 and 9.15, on pp. 470 and 471), as is suggested by the schematic drawings of LV myofibers and spiral flow (*inset* a.) in Figure 15.13, on p. 834.

Because of the smallness of tissues and organs in the embryo and fetus and the rapidity of successive changes in their structure, function and properties, there has been much more limited consideration of flow shear effects during prenatal development compared with studies during postnatal growth, adulthood and aging. Fortunately, however, technological advances are nowadays allowing this important aspect of biofluid dynamics to be studied experimentally in animals [44,69,105,110]. The need for such research is great. Recently, there has been a heightened interest in the relationships between *blood flow* and *cardiac embryology* and morphogenetic development. Evidence has been accumulating [46] that the creation of a normal heart involves *intricate interactions* between a genetic program, mechanical stimuli, and the cellular processes that link them, but the influence of factors such as blood flow [16] on heart development has been unclear.

It is noteworthy also that during embryogenesis, shear stress levels are rather uniform along the arterial tree in the developing arterial system, down to a luminal diameter of about 40 μm [76]. This suggests that during development arterial segments *adapt* their luminal diameters to the flow to be carried. Intriguingly, at the stage of development studied, a vessel wall *tunica media*, with differentiated vascular smooth muscle cells and active regulation of myogenic tone, is still lacking. Therefore, even in the absence of vascular smooth muscle, embryonic arteries can adapt their lumen size to shear stress, a process that is probably controlled by *endothelial cells* [76].

15.5.1 Coordination of cardiac form and function

Intravitally stained (using blood component staining methods *compatible* with life) flows are generally analyzed by tracking the positions of native particles in the flow or by seeding the flow with highly contrasting or fluorescent tracer particles. Measurements are then made by comparing two or more video frames captured in very quick succession, using specialized software (cf. Section 2.5.2, on pp. 52 f., and Fig. 2.12, on p. 53). Particle shifts between images yield information about the direction and magnitude of the flow velocities within the field being evaluated, akin to ultrasound speckle velocimetry [114]. Particle tracking velocimetry, or PTV, utilizes large native or injected tracer particles to give crude estimates of fluid velocity but does not allow accurate evaluation of shear stress. Digital particle image velocimetry (DPIV) uses smaller, more densely concentrated particles to better represent the microscale features of the flow field

Combined with special optics and custom defocusing software, DPIV allows extraction of the 3-D positions of tracer particles from single-plane images in a spatiotemporal imaging technique called 4-D-DPIV, where the fourth dimension is time. These techniques were used by Hove et al. [44–46], to elucidate intracardiac blood flow fields in zebrafish (*danio rerio*) embryos. To characterize accurately embryonic intracardiac flow and fluid forces, they used high-speed cine imaging at $440–1,000$ *frames/s* and DPIV [46, 135]. High framing rates allow the course of small groups of erythrocytes to be followed through the beating heart. DPIV revealed the intracardiac velocity vector field by means of vectors, superimposed on the micrographs, indicating the directionality and relative velocity (encoded in different colors) at successive instants of interest through the heart cycle.

Erythrocytes flowing through the constriction produced by the atrioventricular valve endocardial cushion that surrounds the atrioventricular canal reached velocities of at least 0.5 *cm/s* during diastole; comparable velocities during ventricular systole were associated with the constriction produced by the conotruncal (semilunar valve) endocardial cushion (see Fig. 15.8 a., on p. 828). For technical reasons [44–46], such intracardiac linear velocities of around 0.5 *cm/s* should be taken as lower (conservative) limits of the actual velocities.

Flow through the microscale cardiac structures of zebrafish embryos is highly viscous (Reynolds numbers $\ll 1$) implying that these relatively high-speed flows generate *enormous* physiological *wall shear stresses* (with $Re = 0.02$, shear stress $> 75\ dyn \cdot cm^{-2}$) in the endocardial cushion passageways. Endocardial shear stresses in these regions of the heart

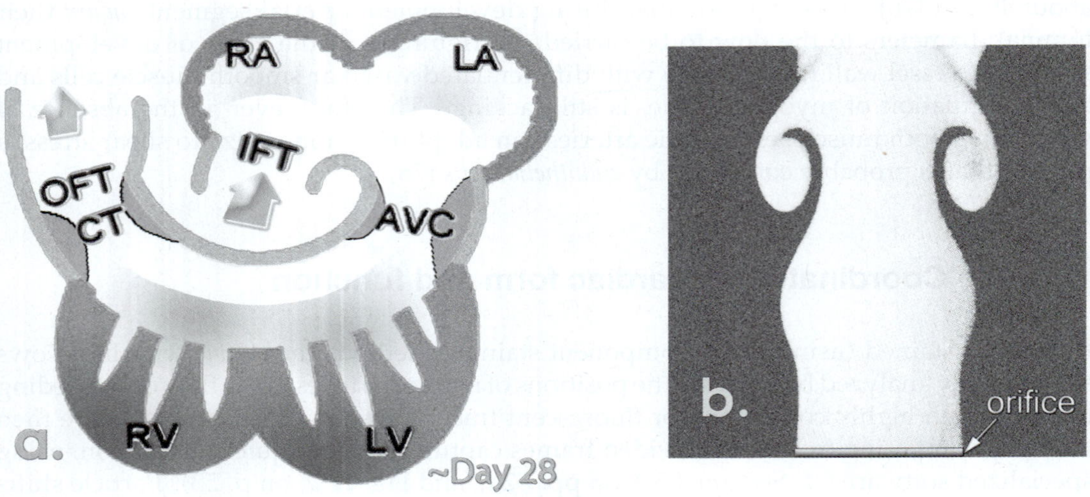

Figure 15.8: **a.** Chamber-specific ballooning is initially restricted to the ventral side of the linear tubular heart and the outer curvature of the looped tube. Thus, the right (RV) and left (LV) ventricular chambers balloon out from the primary heart tube. Distinct left (LA) and right (RA) atria bulge out more caudally on laterodorsal surfaces. The diagram corresponds approximately to the 28th day of human embryonic development. AVC, atrioventricular canal surrounded by atrioventricular valve endocardial cushion; IFT, inflow tract; OFT, outflow tract with CT, the conotruncal (semilunar valve) endocardial cushion. (Adapted, modified, from Christoffels et al. [18], by permission of Elsevier.) **b.** Flow pattern created by blowing chemical smoke (glycol and glycerol in deionized water) at the same temperature as the contiguous air through a smooth orifice. The first bulge is strongly reminiscent of the root of the aorta and pulmonary artery, and indicates the kind of molding forces at work during the prenatal formation of the aortic and pulmonic roots.

are amplified due to the convectively increased blood velocities. As a result, the endocardial cells overlying the developing endocardial cushions and the neighboring upstream region of intensely *confluent flow* (see Figs. 7.2, on p. 328, 7.9, on p. 339, 13.5, on p. 695 , 14.1, on p. 738, and 14.2, on p. 740) align themselves with and become elongated (*spindle-shaped*) along the flow direction, as has been shown by scanning electron microscopy of excised hearts [51,52]. Furthermore, changes in the expression patterns of several genes have been induced by embryonic vessel ligation [35,36], suggesting that endocardial cells can *sense* localized changes in fluid dynamics and respond with *transcriptional* changes. To place these findings in proper perspective, consider that shear forces $< 1\ dyn \cdot cm^{-2}$ are detectable by endocardial cells *in vitro*, and can result in *up-* or *down*-regulation of gene expression [93]; larger shear forces, on the order of $8-15\ dyn \cdot cm^{-2}$, have been shown to cause cytoskeletal rearrangements [25].

Through further investigations, Hove and his coworkers showed that the intracardiac flow-associated stresses are *essential* for normal heart looping and for chamber and valve development in early embryonic stages [46]. During early embryonic development, experimental interventions *reducing* the shear stress that is normally exerted by the flowing blood on endothelial and adjacent cells cause the growing heart to develop abnormally. In their elegant studies in zebrafish embryos, embryos with impaired cardiac flow demonstrated three dramatic phenotypes: first, their hearts did not form the bulbus cordis; secondly, they lacked heart looping, the normal process resulting in the repositioning of the ventricle and atrium from a cephalo-caudal into a side-by-side arrangement; finally, the walls of the inflow and outflow tracts collapsed and fused. Their meticulous studies strongly suggest that *structure and function* in the embryonic heart are linked by *hemodynamics*.

15.5.2 Flow molding of the embryonic heart chambers

Flow-associated structures appear to influence the formation of the cardiac chambers and of the outflow trunks of the great vessels. Figure 15.8 b. shows vortical bulges formed immediately downstream from a smooth orifice in a rising wide jet of chemical smoke. The resemblance to the shape of the aortic and pulmonary trunks immediately upstream from the ventricular outflow orifices is more than a fortuitous coincidence; the forces which produce the vortical bulges (cf. Fig. 14.19, on p. 778) are the same as those that mold epigenetically the outflow trunks. (By the way, similar vortical forces also produce widening and deepening in a river immediately below a waterfall.)

The bulging roots of the outflow trunks have a purpose, as is detailed in Section 7.13.2, on pp. 385 ff. During ejection the valve leaflets, pushed straight upwards, "hang" in the space of the bulges, the sinuses of Valsalva, being prevented from flattening back against the concavity of the outflow trunk walls by the vortices that are trapped in the sinuses (see Figs. 7.35 and 7.36, on pp. 386 and 387, respectively). Furthermore, the vortices that are trapped in the sinuses normally prevent the outflow from aspirating blood out of the coronary arteries as in a perfume spray where the air, rushing over an orifice, aspirates and entrains the perfume (see Fig. 7.36).

Interestingly, during systole, DPIV in zebrafish embryos has revealed [44–46] a vortex pair just downstream of the the conotruncal (semilunar valve) endocardial cushion, accompanying the blood influx from the ventricle into the bulbus arteriosus (outflow tract) during ventricular contraction (see Fig. 15.8 a., on p. 828). Moreover, during the diastolic phase of the heart cycle, vortices were shown [44–46] to be present behind the AVC constriction (see Fig. 15.8 a.) within the developing ventricle.

In Figure 15.9, I present a rudimentary model of incipient chamber development under the action of epigenetic flow-associated forces in the embryonic heart. Vortices, such as those forming beyond a constriction (cf. the endocardial cushion in the atrioventricular canal, (AVC, in Fig. 15.8 a.), exert a thrust *pushing outward* the flexible part of the wall and fostering *epigenetically* the development of the *incipient ventricular chamber*. Thus, fluid dynamic transitions such as the formation of vortices can signal cardiac *morphogenesis* through endocardial mechanotransduction dependent epigenetic processes. The end-result of the particular illustrative example at hand is the evolution of *chamber pumps* from

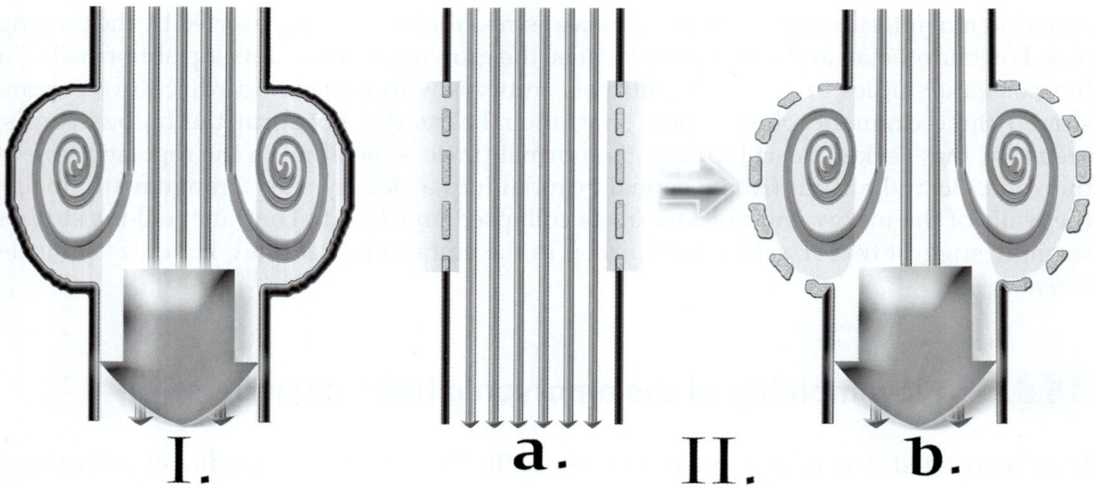

Figure 15.9: I. Rigid tube with vortices forming in a localized dilatation (bulges). II.**a.** Rigid tube with a distensible portion which can bulge out under the action of flow-associated forces to form a chamber. **b.** Vortical thrust pushes outward the distensible portion of the tube, bringing about a localized "ballooning" of the wall, and eventually leading by activation of epigenetic mechanisms to chamber development (cf. Fig. 15.8, on p. 828).

peristaltic tubular hearts (see Fig. 15.10, on p. 831). Peristaltic hearts exist in primitive circulatory systems—some worms, the *annelida*, have them, as do a curious group of sea creatures called sea squirts, or *tunicates*.[7] However, they are relatively inefficient in terms of their energetics [132].

Although the specific roles of epigenetic factors continue to be debated [6, 12, 103], it seems clear that many steps in cardiogenesis can be viewed as an integrated feedback loop: alterations in shape change heart function, which changes the forces experienced by the cells, stimulating them to modify heart function by continuing to change the developing cardiac shape. In our present context, during embryonic development the changing intracardiac flow patterns are associated with dynamic molding forces, which can give rise to *phenotypic variation* in conjunction with *genetic plasticity*. Accordingly, embryonic intracardiac *flow patterns* are intricately involved in *cardiogenesis*, as is summarized in Figure 15.12, on p. 833, and their derangements can be responsible for various congenital defects, which may be incompatible with prolonged survival. Even simple diagrams (see Figs. 6.3, 15.3, 15.4, on pp. 303, 813, and 814, respectively) of the heart tube and early embryonic heart, looping as it elongates within the constraining pericardial space, reveal the intraluminal blood flow kinematics to which its form is so perfectly adapted. The

[7]The tunicate heart is a long V-shaped tube with a pacemaker at each end. Pumping action is generated by a peristaltic wave starting at one end and traveling to the other. The direction of peristalsis *reverses* every minute or two, changing the direction of blood flow through the *valveless* vascular tree [68].

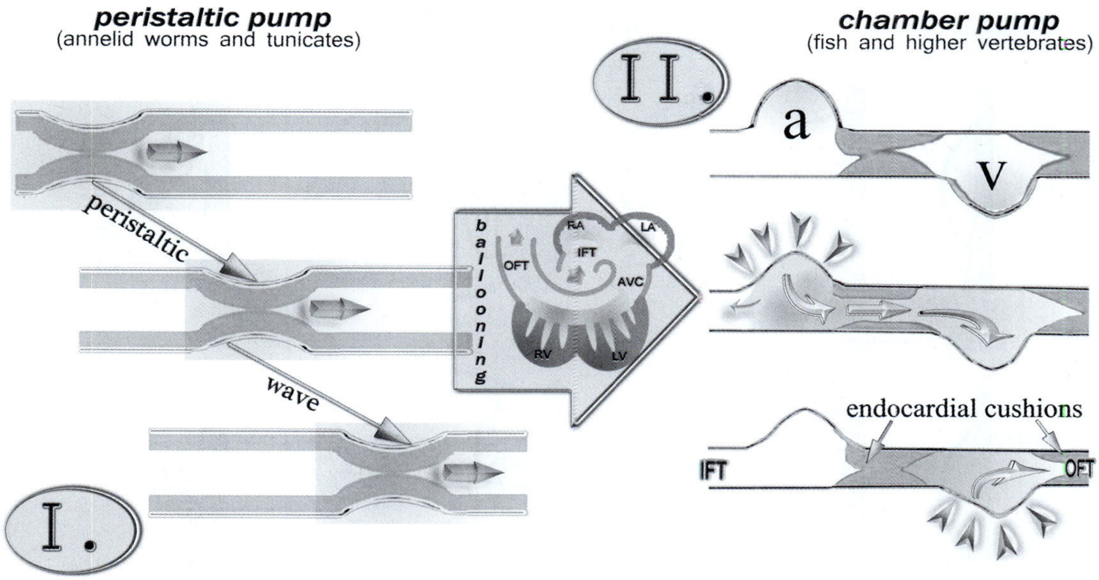

Figure 15.10: I. In the early stages of development, the heart acts as a peristaltic pump. II. At later stages, the embryonic heart develops into a two–chambered pump. Alternating contractions of the atrium and the ventricle pump the blood. (Adapted, modified, from Moorman et al. [88], by permission of the authors and the N. Y. Acad. Sci.)

pattern resembles that made when a stream of water flows into a confined cavity and is forced to describe sinuous trajectories and vortical patterns.

15.5.3 Mechanosensing endocardium and valvulogenesis

In Section 15.2.5, on pp. 819 f., I described some aspects of embryonic valvulogenesis. The embryonic heart is lined continuously with *mechanosensing* endocardium that *responds* to changing flow-associated forces. A vitally important endocardially mediated phenomenon is the development of the heart valves, which raises the question: Do fluid flow-associated forces regulate valvulogenesis? I have already discussed the seminal work of Hove and his coworkers, which showed that occlusion of the primitive cardiac tube at the inlet or outlet, with wall shear stresses just about 10-fold lower than normal, results in *disrupted valvulogenesis* and cardiac dysfunction [44–46]. The formation of both the atrioventricular and the semilunar valves progresses along parallel paths, as is shown in Figure 15.11, on p. 832.

Initiating the transformation of the early endocardial cushions into valve structures, there is initially a mesenchymal transformation of the endocardial cells (EMT, in Fig. 15.11) of the atrioventricular canal and the distal outflow tract cushions. However, the atrioventricular canal cushions subsequently *delaminate* from the underlying muscular walls, whereas the distal outflow tract cushions become *excavated* from the aortic side

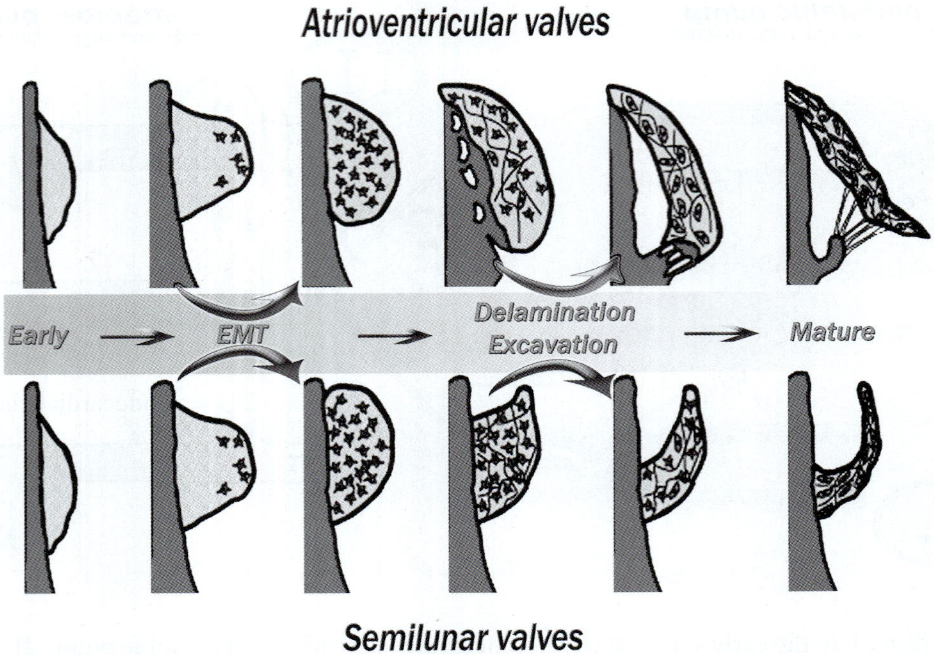

Figure 15.11: Successive stages in the parallel pathways of atrioventricular and semilunar valve development. (Adapted, modified, from J.T. Butcher and R.R. Markwald [14], by kind permission of the Royal Society of London.)

inward, as is shown in Figure 15.11. Many of the signaling proteins, or growth factors[8] (VEGF, BMP, TGF-b, NOTCH), which are responsible for the initiation of mesenchymal transformation have been demonstrated to be regulated by both shear stress and mechanical strain [13] in adult endothelial cells. This suggests that both endocardial cell strain and fluid shear stress have the capability to induce the expression of factors leading to mesenchymal transformation.

Flow-associated forces may also play a role in the remodeling of the primitive valvular cushions into fibrous leaflets. Endothelial changes with the formation of the semilunar valves show striking correlation to changes in local fluid dynamics, suggesting that flow-associated forces may regulate the *excavation* of these cushions [19]. Fluid dynamic changes associated with conotruncal banding in chick embryos result in persistent right atrioventricular cushions, suggesting impaired myocardialization of these cushions [117]. Mechanical inhibition of the impalement of the outflow tract into the interventricular groove results in hyperplastic inflow as well as outflow valve cushions [19]. These findings

[8]These signaling proteins commonly sit like triggers spanning the cell membrane, with a portion of them inside and a portion outside. Initiating factors, such as shear stress, acting on the extracellular domain induce proteolytic cleavage and release of the intracellular portion, which enters the cell nucleus to *alter gene expression* [89].

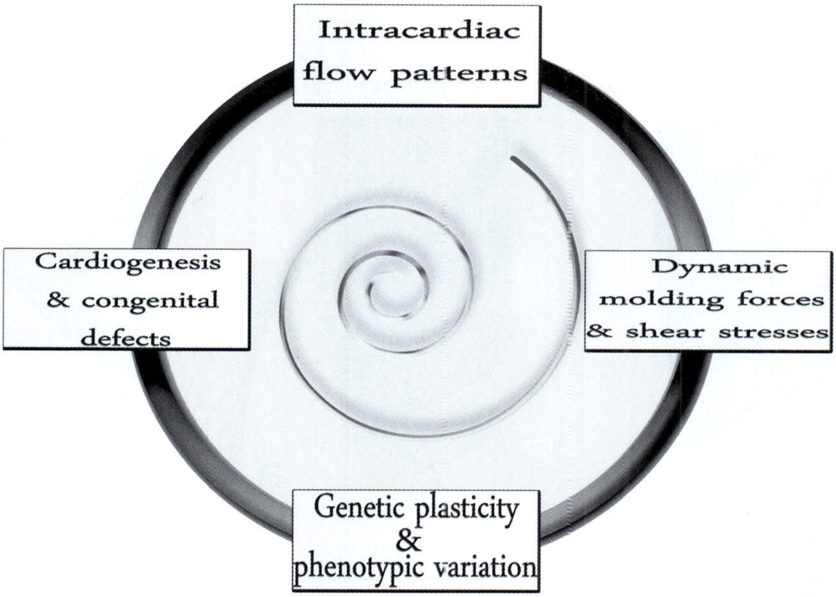

Figure 15.12: A circular regulatory pathway exists during cardiogenesis between the intracardiac flow patterns and associated force transmission to the walls, epigenetically influenced gene expression, and changes in the morphology of the developing embryonic heart.

demonstrate that flow-associated forces play an essential, albeit as of now incompletely characterized, role in valvulogenesis. Future studies will help to better elucidate these essential morphogenetic effects of intracardiac flow phenomena during the embryonic development of the heart.

15.5.4 Endocardium influences mural histoarchitectonics

The anatomy and histoarchitectonics of the adult human heart are detailed in Chapter 6. The left ventricle has the approximate form of a hemiellipsoid or an inverted asymmetric cone, the outer wall of which consists of fibers lying in a left-handed vortex passing steeply from the base to the apex, as is illustrated in Figures 7.22 and 6.2, on pp. 359 and 302, respectively, and in Figure 15.13, on p. 834. According to the Scottish anatomist J. B. Pettigrew [104], the wall of the LV chamber is formed of seven interconnected layers, as is depicted in Figure 15.13.

The myofibers of each successive layer spiral left-handedly downward, but at a progressively less steep pitch. The fourth, mid-wall, layer is distinctive, in that in it the myofibers run *horizontally* around the chamber. The fifth layer is similar to the third, with the fibers running at about the same pitch or steepness, but now the vortex is *right-handed*, going *upward* against the *downward* of the third layer. Similarly, the sixth layer is approximately a right-handed reflection of the second, and the seventh of the first (see Fig. 15.13).

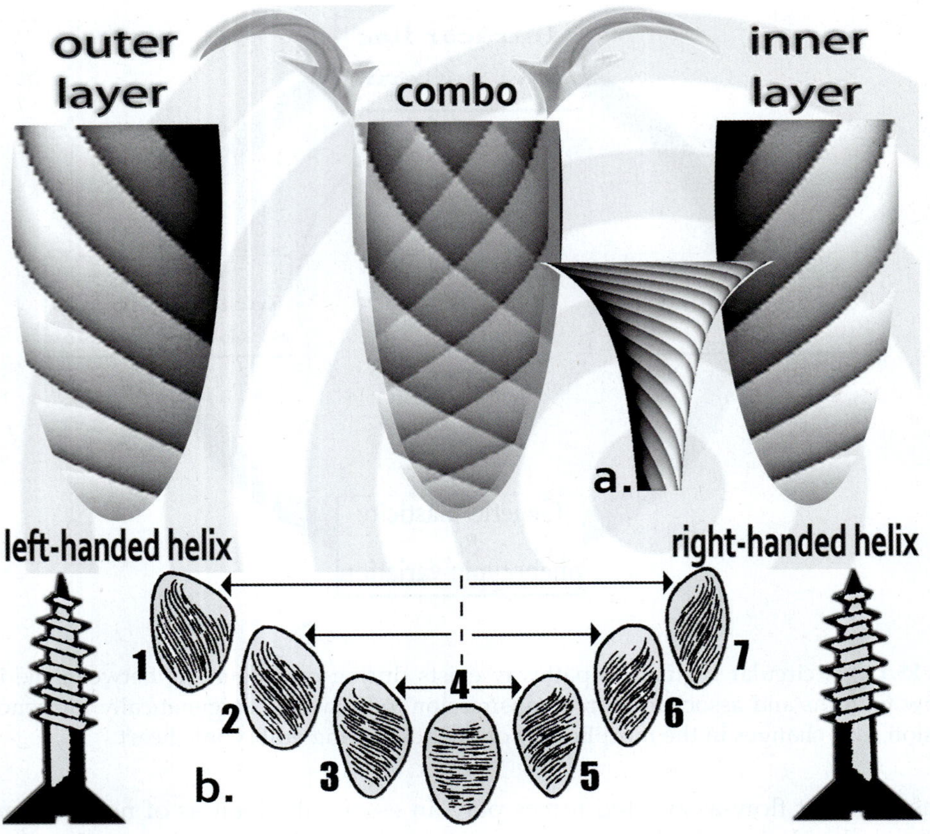

Figure 15.13: The spiral trajectories of myocardial fibers invoke images of *spiral flows* (cf. *inset* a.), which occur in the developing heart and are exemplified in the diastolic filling vortices in the adult. As far as the spiraling myofibers in the wall of the left ventricle are concerned, the circumferential mid-wall layer, whose fibers run more or less horizontally, may be construed to act as a *mirror* that reflects the outer into the inner layers of the wall (cf. *inset* b.). The mathematical transformation of *mirror-reflection* is, in fact, the only one which can change *left*-handedness into *right*-handedness. (These schematic diagrams do not follow *exact* forms and dimensions.)

Clearly, cardiogenesis requires the precise arrangement of numerous cells into a specific 3-D architecture that is essential for effective organ function, and involves a series of morphogenetic steps that must be carefully orchestrated. Recent work by Glickman Holtzman et al. [31–33] has utilized the zebrafish as a model system, and integrated cell biology, embryology, genetics, time-lapse video microscopy and computer-based cell movement analysis to elucidate coordinated cellular movements, cell shape changes, and cellular interactions during cardiogenesis. This ground-breaking work has provided initial evidence for the regulation of mural cardiomyocyte arrangement in the developing heart by the endocardium, revealing a dynamic cellular mechanism by which two cellular populations *interact* to create the foundation for an embryonic organ.

Two pivotal roles for the endocardium in regulating mural myocardial cell disposition in the developing heart have been demonstrated [31]: the endocardium actively provokes critical transitions in *cardiomyocyte movements*, and it also actively dictates the *angular direction* of cardiomyocyte movement within the cardiac walls during cardiogenesis. The findings of this work hold great interest for us in the present context, because they provide a *connection* between the *sinuous flowing movements* within the lumen of the forming heart and the *intertwining, spiraling myocardial fibers* and *surfaces* within its developing walls!

Flow-induced shear on the endocardial surfaces is likely to be the underlying mechanism for this beautiful example of adaptation and coordination of *form with function*. In other words, the endocardium intermediates the way fluid forces constrain and shape cardiac design and histoarchitectonics. The molecular mechanisms by which the endocardium stimulates and orients cardiomyocyte movement and mural histoarchitectonic disposition remain to be explored. The endocardium might communicate with the myocardium via direct cell-cell contacts, or via secreted paracrine cues.[9] In future work, it will be interesting to evaluate whether any of these signaling pathways are crucial for the myocardial-endocardial interactions that coordinate heart tube assembly. Alternatively, the endocardium might also play a less direct role, perhaps contributing to the local deposition of extracellular matrix components [131] in a way that affects the *available routes* for mural cardiomyocyte movement.

The focus of future work should be to investigate the developmental significance of fluid dynamic forces and to understand how fluid forces act as a regulator for cardiogenesis. To study these problems, a *three-pronged* approach should be used, encompassing measurements of morphology and kinematics, the use of physical models to measure flow velocities and shear forces, and CFD simulations casting light into the fluid dynamics of embryonic systems that are difficult to approach experimentally. These approaches compliment each other in a variety of ways. Measurements of morphology and kinematics are indispensable in setting appropriate parameter values both for CFD simulations and for physical models. In some situations, physical models can be used to study a wide range of parameter values that would be difficult to investigate using computational fluid dynamics. CFD simulations can be used to explore and to obtain spatiotemporally detailed descriptions of dynamic flow fields in complicated, evolving, embryonic systems [27].

15.6 Postnatal cardiomyocyte and endocardial mechanotransduction properties

The *postnatal* heart continues to have a vital ability to react to mechanical stimuli and the contractile performance of cardiac myocytes can respond properly to wide-ranging cardiac pumping demands. In addition to being an efficient pump, the fully developed heart is a mechanosensory organ, since the myocardial cells have the capacity to react to mechanical stimuli, such as cardiac chamber distention [133].

---

[9]See footnote on p. 23.

15.6.1 Frank–Starling mechanism in cardiac muscle

It should come as no surprise that mechanical motors including cardiac myocytes require mechanosensitive regulatory input, if they are to be utilized successfully in targeted blood pumping activity. Interestingly, the ventricular pressure–volume loops of the developing chick embryo also show an active response to increasing preload as the early myocardium organizes [64]. Quick adjustments in cardiomyocyte performance are mediated by controls in calcium release and reuptake, while longer-term adaptations require structural remodeling in the myocardium.

In classic papillary muscle preparations and in modern isolated single-cell ventricular myocyte investigations [90], it has been established that cardiomyocytes are mainly sensitive to axial stretch (i.e., stretch along their long axis). Through physiological research and clinical investigations over the last century, pumping myocardium has been shown to possess an intrinsic ability to sense its *filling state* and react to its variations, independently of any cardiac innervation that may, to some extent, subserve the same regulatory functions. This ability is codified in the *Frank–Starling* law of the heart, which is discussed in Chapter 3, on pp. 143 f., and in numerous other places in this book; for a recent review, see Katz [62].

The Frank–Starling law is a particular manifestation of the multifaceted mechanism of *mechanotransduction*. The ability of cardiac cells to sense the filling state of the cardiac chambers may be viewed, in the present context, as a process where a mechanical stimulus is transformed into a change in the myocardial cell's functions [15], such as the force of contraction, membrane voltage, ion balance, or in gene expression. Cardiac myocytes have at least one quite sensitive *length transducer*: the sarcomere. The Frank–Starling mechanism in cardiac muscle is generally attributed to *length-dependent activation*, a process by which the sarcomere can detect increases in its resting length and, at least within normal bounds, elicit the appropriate response, namely, a correspondingly increased contractile force [29, 66, 122]. Despite the depth of research into this field [37, 67, 118], the detailed subcellular mechanisms responsible remain not fully understood.

The Frank–Starling law has paramount clinical implications because it is connected with disturbances that may arise if a sustained abnormal mechanical loading of the cardiac myocytes changes their function. This generally leads to compensatory *epigenetic growth* of the heart muscle. It can also usher in serious maladaptive abnormalities, like excessive ventricular myocardial hypertrophy and dilatation, and eventual heart failure.

Consider, for instance, chronic increases in the total ventricular systolic load, commonly designated as volume or pressure overload.[10] Despite this straightforward distinction, improved insight into cardiomyocyte mechanosensing in the working heart is really challenging, because the globally homogeneous action of pressure and volume loading builds upon, and necessarily requires, internal inhomogeneity at the cellular and subcellular levels [124]. Pressure and volume overloads are mechanotransduced by cardiomyocytes: elevation of peak systolic stress with pressure overload stimulates compensatory *concentric* hypertrophy without dilatation (replication of sarcomeres *in-parallel*); elevation

[10]See Sections 7.1, 7.12, 13.6, and 14.1, on pp. 325 f., 380 f., 724 ff., and 737 f., respectively.

of end-diastolic wall stress with volume overload stimulates *eccentric* cardiac chamber enlargement (replication of sarcomeres *in-series*); persisting chronic chamber dilatation also induces a parallel replication of sarcomeres, accounting for an increase in wall thickness sufficient to return [83] systolic wall stresses resulting from chamber enlargement to normal. Chronic compensated pressure and volume overloads, if not corrected, usually progress to subendocardial fibrosis, myocardial fiber slippage and creep, and to dysfunction and heart failure [83, 84, 95–99].

One reason for decompensation and failure is that myocardial hypertrophy itself can actually *destabilize* local mechanics because hypertrophic myocardium has altered contractile (active) and relaxation (passive) properties. This complicating derangement introduces functional *disparities* [83] between myocardial load and performance. Furthermore, it appears that the same molecular responses that initiate the compensatory hypertrophy can lead to the reactivation of genes normally expressed in *embryonic* myocardium, altering the cellular phenotype and resulting in myocardial structural disarray, altered calcium kinetics, and increased interstitial collagen deposition [79].

Clearly, mechanically induced alterations in the local "environment" of the heart may have serious pathophysiological and clinical consequences following their mechanotransduction by myocardial, endocardial (see the next section), or even autonomic neural cells. There are various mechanisms through which mechanotransduction integrates cardiac function; it initiates time–related changes, as well as geometrical ones [70]. As is true of other homeostatic mechanisms, it can be treated as a feedback control system (see Section 2.23, on pp. 105 ff.). Finally, it also has vital *clinical relevance* because it demonstrates nonlinear complexity, as is to be expected with an integrative system, and thus it can either *stabilize* or *destabilize* the system.

15.6.2 Endocardial mechanotransduction in cardiac muscle

In Section 15.4.1, on p. 823, we saw how the dynamic balance of pressure-induced myogenic tone and endothelial flow-induced dilatation results in an appropriate *basal tone* in resistance arteries and allows *adaptations* of vessel diameter to changes in flow and pressure. In the preceding Section, we saw how the ability of cardiomyocytes to sense the filling state of the cardiac chambers may be viewed as a process whereby a mechanical stimulus elicits changes not only in cardiomyocyte functions, such as the force of contraction via the Frank–Starling mechanism, but also in *gene expression* and phenotype. In view of these intriguing findings, it appears likely that the response of cardiomyocytes to endocardial shear stress levels may tend to counteract the effects of the mural stresses both during normal operating conditions and in the course of compensatory adaptations to pathologic states. Such pathologic states are, in fact, characterized not only by abnormal conventional ventricular loading (systolic and diastolic myocardial stresses in "pressure" and/or "volume" overload) [83, 84, 95–99], but also by abnormal intracardiac flow-associated forces, particularly *endocardial shear* stresses [101, 102].

Such considerations, and the finding of reduced ventricular diastolic vortex strength in LV and RV chamber dilatation [8, 9, 101, 102], led me to propose [101] that altered

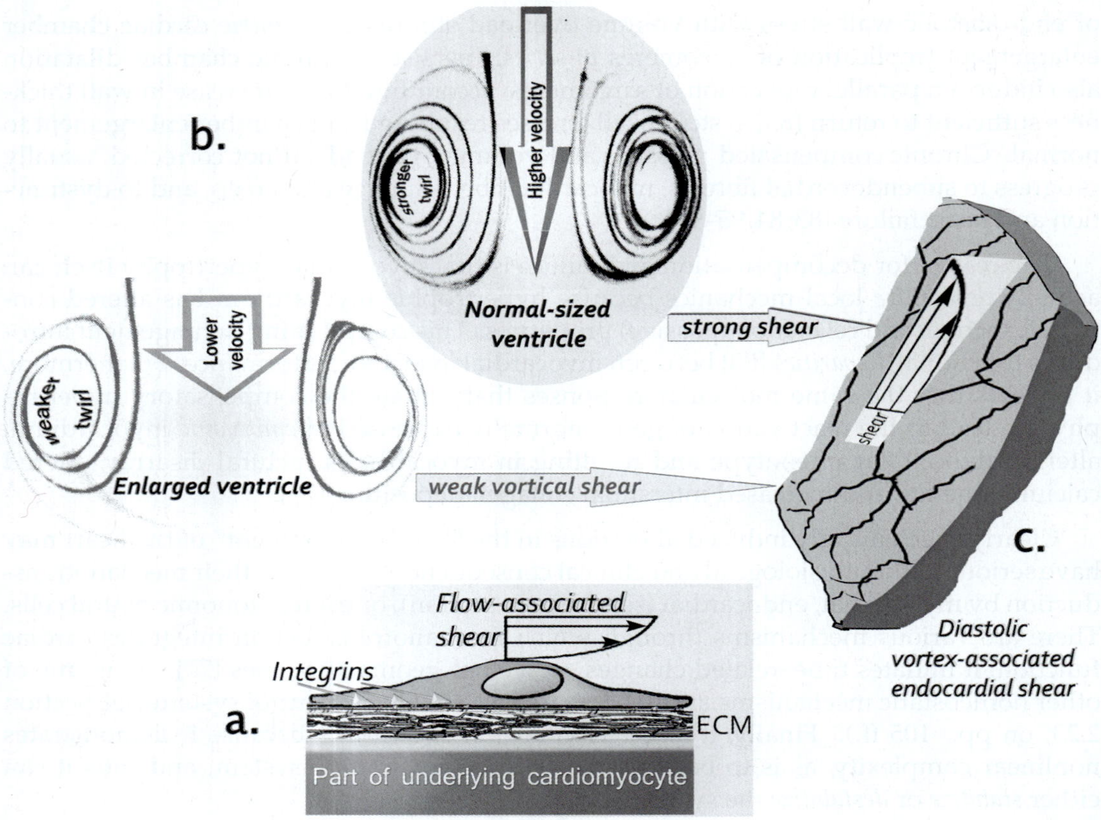

Figure 15.14: **a.** Endocardial cells are exposed to shear forces through blood flow over their luminal surface. Integrins are part of a large family of cell adhesion–receptor proteins, involved in cell–extracellular matrix and cell–cell interactions. They help transmit shear-induced signals from the endocardium to underlying cardiomyocytes, in parallel with endocardial paracrine shear stress responsive element release. **b.** Ventricular dilatation is associated with *depressed* ventricular filling vortex strength. **c.** Vortical intraventricular rotation of blood exerts shear stresses on the endocardium, whose intensity *depends on the strength* of the diastolic vortex. (Panel b. is adapted, strongly modified, from Pasipoularides et al. [101], by kind permission of the APS.)

intraventricular diastolic flow patterns in dilatation and failure might beget further dilatation and detrimental remodeling, by the *activation* or *inhibition* of endocardial shear stress responsive elements. Strong diastolic vortical rotation in the intraventricular blood normally engenders vigorous shearing (tangential surface *scouring* [101]) of the endocardial lining of the chamber.

As we have seen in this chapter, fluid shear stress acting on endothelial and endocardial cells lining the prenatal and postnatal heart and blood vessels activates cytoskeletal and biochemical mechanoreceptors. These, in turn, activate multiple signal transduction pathways, involving sequentially activated protein kinases and transcription factors that

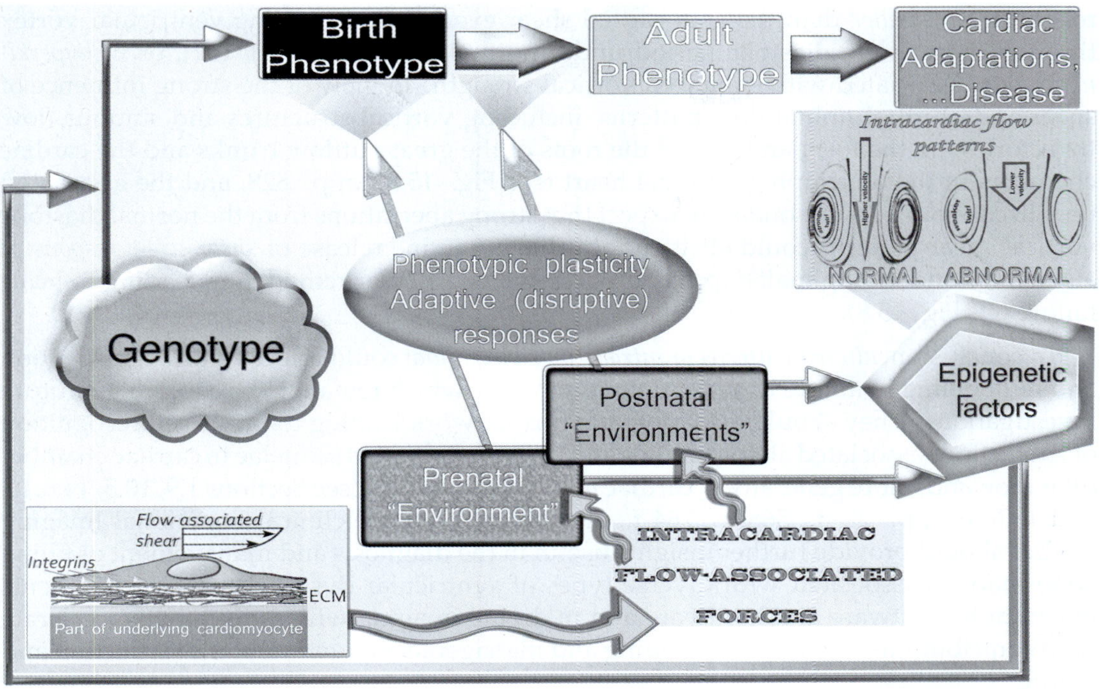

Figure 15.15: A circular regulatory pathway exists during cardiogenesis and in pre- and postnatal life between the intracardiac flow patterns and associated force transmission to the walls, epigenetically influenced gene expression, and changes in the morphology of the developing prenatal or in the phenotype of the adapting postnatal heart. Phenotypic plasticity can, in conjunction with pre- and postnatal operating "environmental" conditions, lead not only to adaptive but also to disruptive (*maladaptive*) responses, disease and decompensation.

form a highly interconnected signaling system and result in various cellular physiological responses. Similar actions might well apply to the postnatal heart's endocardial cells lining the cardiac chambers, and could affect ventricular function and remodeling. Moreover, as we saw in Chapter 14, which should be reviewed to good advantage at this juncture, the reduced intraventricular vortex strength [101,102] demonstrated by Functional Imaging [100] to ensue with chamber dilatation is associated with a great reduction in the shear stresses exerted on the endocardial cells over most of the diastolic filling period (see Figs. 14.17, on p. 774, 14.21, on p. 783, 14.24, on p. 788, 14.25, on p. 792, and 14.26, on p. 793).

Figure 15.14, on p. 838, summarizes pictorially the state of affairs that I envision; it should stimulate further work leading to improved recognition of more or less subtle intracardiac flow-associated abnormalities and their multifaceted sequelae in heart chamber dilatation and failure. On the basis of experiments subjecting vascular endothelial surface cells to tangential flow in vitro, it has been established [10] that signal transduction cascades regulating gene expression are transiently activated by shear stress levels at least as low as 0.5 dyn/cm^2; such shear stress levels are no less than by one order of magnitude[11] *smaller* than the endocardial shear exerted by the filling ventricular vortex through most of the diastolic period under normal conditions [101, 102], or in *hyperkinetic states* associated with enhanced vortical strength. In view of the strong influence of shear and of intraluminal flow patterns, including vortical structures and sinuous flow trajectories, on the form and size of the roots of the great outflow trunks and the cardiac chambers in the developing prenatal heart (see Fig. 15.8, on p. 828, and the associated text discussion), it is reasonable to expect that strong aberrations from the normal diastolic vortical shear patterns could elicit endocardial paracrine release of *shear stress responsive* element(s) underlying maladaptive, progressive ventricular remodeling leading to heart failure (cf. Fig. 15.8).

In conclusion, *altered patterns of intracardiac blood flow* could affect ventricular function and remodeling in failure in as yet unknown ways, which remain to be explored in future investigations. They should also motivate further work leading to improved recognition of subtle flow-associated abnormalities and their multifaceted sequelae in cardiac chamber dilatation and, more generally in cardiac *phenotypic plasticity* (see Sections 1.9, 10.5, 14.6.10, and 16.6, on pp. 20 ff., 566 ff., 764 f., and 874 ff.). Future clinical Functional Imaging studies should provide further insights useful in the diagnosis and management of filling abnormalities associated with diverse types of ventricular dysfunction. Developments in computer software and hardware and in digital imaging will undoubtedly accelerate such contributions to the understanding and management of ventricular dysfunction and failure.

[11]See footnote on p. 284.

References and further reading

[1] Anderson, R.H., Webb, S., Brown, N.A., Lamers, W.H., Moorman, A. Development of the heart: (2) Septation of the atriums and ventricles. Heart 89: 949–58, 2003.

[2] Anderson, R.H., Webb, S., Brown, N.A., Lamers, W.H., Moorman, A. Development of the heart: (3) formation of the ventricular outflow tracts, arterial valves, and intrapericardial arterial trunks. Heart 89: 1110–8, 2003.

[3] Angelini, P. Embryology and congenital heart disease. Tex. Heart Inst. J. 22: 1–12, 1995.

[4] Ashcroft, F.M. From molecule to malady. Nature 440: 440–7, 2006.

[5] Bartman, T., Hove, J. Mechanics and function in heart morphogenesis. Dev. Dyn. 233: 373–81, 2005.

[6] Bartman, T., Walsh, E.C., Wen, K.K, McKane, M., Ren, J., Alexander, J., Rubenstein, P.A., Stainier, D.Y. Early myocardial function affects endocardial cushion development in zebrafish. Public Library of Science-Biology 2: E129, 2004.

[7] Beis, D., Bartman, T., Jin, S.W., Scott, I.C., D'Amico, L.A., Ober, E.A., Verkade, H., Frantsve, J., Field, H.A., Wehman, A., Baier, H., Tallafuss, A., Bally-Cuif, L., Chen, J.N., Stainier, D.Y., Jungblut, B. Genetic and cellular analyses of zebrafish atrioventricular cushion and valve development. Development 132: 4193–204, 2005.

[8] Bellhouse, B.J. Fluid mechanics of a model mitral valve and left ventricle. Cardiovasc. Res. 6: 199–210, 1972.

[9] Bellhouse, B.J. Bellhouse, F.H. Fluid mechanics of the mitral valve. Nature 224: 615–16, 1969.

[10] Braddock, M., Schwachtgen, J.L., Houston, P., Dickson, M.C., Lee, M.J., Campbell, C.J. Fluid shear stress modulation of gene expression in endothelial cells. News Physiol. Sci. 13: 241–6, 1998.

[11] Bruneau, B.G. The developing heart and congenital heart defects: a make or break situation. Clin. Genet. 63: 252–61, 2003.

[12] Butcher, J.T., McQuinn, T.C., Sedmera, D., Turner, D., Markwald, R.R. Transitions in early embryonic atrioventricular valvular function correspond with changes in cushion biomechanics that are predictable by tissue composition. Circ. Res. 100: 1503–11, 2007.

[13] Butcher, J.T., Nerem, R.M. Valvular endothelial cells and the mechanoregulation of valvular pathology. Phil. Trans. Roy. Soc. B. 362: 1445–57, 2007.

[14] Butcher, J.T., Markwald, R.R. Valvulogenesis: the moving target. Phil. Trans. Roy. Soc. B 362: 1489–1503, 2007.

[15] Calaghan, S.C., White, E. The role of calcium in the response of cardiac muscle to stretch. Prog. Biophys. Mol. Biol. 71: 59–90, 1999.

[16] Cartwright, J.H., Piro, O., Tuval, I. Fluid-dynamical basis of the embryonic development of left-right asymmetry in vertebrates. Proc. Natl. Acad. Sci. USA 101: 7234–9, 2004.

[17] Chiu, J.J., Wang, D.L., Chien, S., Skalak, R., Usami, S. Effects of disturbed flow on endothelial cells. J. Biomech. Eng. 120: 2–8, 1998.

[18] Christoffels, V.M., Habets, P.E., Franco, D., Campione, M., de Jong, F., Lamers, W.H., Bao, Z.Z., Palmer, S., Biben, C., Harvey, R.P., Moorman, A.F. Chamber formation and morphogenesis in the developing mammalian heart. Dev. Biol. 223: 266–78, 2000.

[19] Colvee, E., Hurle, J.M. Malformations of the semilunar valves produced in chick embryos by mechanical interference with cardiogenesis. An experimental approach to the role of hemodynamics in valvular development. Anat. Embryol. (Berl.) 168: 59–71, 1983.

[20] Copp, A.J. Death before birth: clues from gene knockouts and mutations. Trends Genet. 11: 7–93, 1995.

[21] Dahl, K.N., Ribeiro, A.J.S., Lammerding, J. Nuclear shape, mechanics, and mechanotransduction. Circ. Res. 102: 1307–18, 2008.

[22] Dahme, T., Katus, H.A., Rottbauer, W. Fishing for the genetic basis of cardiovascular disease. Dis. Model Mech. 2: 18–22, 2009.

[23] D'Angelo, G., Meininger, G.A. Transduction mechanisms involved in the regulation of myogenic tone activity. Hypertension 23: 1096–105, 1994.

[24] Davies, P.F. Flow-mediated endothelial mechanotransduction. Physiol. Rev. 75: 519–59, 1995.

[25] Davies, P.F., Remuzzi, A., Gordon, E.J., Dewey, Jr. C.F., Gimbrone, M.A. Turbulent fluid shear stress induces vascular endothelium cell turnover in utero. Proc. Natl. Acad. Sci. USA 83: 2114–17, 1986.

[26] Davis, J., Westfall, M.V., Townsend, D., Blankinship, M., Herron, T.J., Guerrero-Serna, G., Wang, W., Devaney, E., Metzger, J.M. Designing heart performance by gene transfer. Physiol. Rev. 88: 1567–651, 2008.

[27] DeGroff, C.G., Thornburg, B.L., Pentecost, J.O., Thornburg, K.L., Gharib, M., Sahn, D.J., Baptista, A. Flow in the early embryonic human heart: a numerical study. Pediatr. Cardiol. 24: 375–80, 2003.

[28] Dewey, C.F., Bussolari, S.R., Gimbrone, M.A., Jr., Davies, P.F. Dynamic response of vascular endothelial cells to fluid shear stress. J. Biomech. Eng. (ASME) 103: 177–85, 1981.

[29] dos Remedios, C.G. The regulation of muscle contraction: as in life, it keeps getting more complex. Biophys. J. 93: 4097–8, 2007.

[30] Folgering, J.H.A., Sharif-Naeini, R., Dedman, A., Patel, A., Delmas, P., Honoré, E. Molecular basis of the mammalian pressure-sensitive ion channels: focus on vascular mechanotransduction. Prog. Biophys. Mol. Biol. 97: 180–95, 2008.

[31] Glickman Holtzman, N., Schoenebeck, J.J., Tsai, H.J., Yelon, D. Endocardium is necessary for cardiomyocyte movement during heart tube assembly. Development 134: 2379–86, 2007.

[32] Glickman, N.S., Yelon, D. Coordinating morphogenesis: epithelial integrity during heart tube assembly. Dev. Cell. 6: 311–12, 2004.

[33] Glickman, N.S., Yelon, D. Cardiac development in zebrafish: coordination of form and function. Semin. Cell. Dev. Biol. 13: 507–13, 2002.

[34] Greenough, H., Small, H.A. Form and function; remarks on art. 1947, Berkeley: University of California Press. xxi, 148 p.

[35] Groenendijk, B.C., Hierck, B.P., Vrolijk, J., Baiker, M., Pourquie, M.J., Gittenberger-de-Groot, A.C., Poelmann, R.E. Changes in shear stress-related gene expression after experimentally altered venous return in the chicken embryo. Circ. Res. 96: 1291–8, 2005.

[36] Groenendijk, B.C.W., Van der Heiden, K., Hierck, B.P., Poelmann, R.E. The role of shear stress on ET-1, KLF2, and NOS-3 expression in the developing cardiovascular system of chicken embryos in a venous ligation model. Physiology 22: 380–9, 2007.

[37] Hanft, L.M., Korte, F.S., McDonald, K.S. Cardiac function and modulation of sarcomeric function by length. Cardiovasc. Res. 77: 627–636, 2008.

[38] Harvey, R.P. Patterning the vertebrate heart. Nature Rev. Genet. 3: 544–56, 2002.

[39] Henrion, D., Laher, I., Bevan, J.A. Intraluminal flow increases vascular tone and $^{45}Ca^{2+}$ influx in the rabbit facial vein. Circ. Res. 71: 339–45, 1992.

[40] Hierck, B.P., Van der Heiden, K., Alkemade, F.E., Van de Pas, S., Van Thienen, J.V., Groenendijk, B.C., Bax, W.H., Van der Laarse, A., Deruiter, M.C., Horrevoets, A.J., Poelmann, R.E. Primary cilia sensitize endothelial cells for fluid shear stress. Dev. Dyn. 237: 725–35, 2008.

[41] Hierck, B.P., Van der Heiden, K., Poelma, C., Westerweel, J., Poelmann, R.E. Fluid shear stress and inner curvature remodeling of the embryonic heart. Choosing the right lane! Scientific World J. 8: 212–22, 2008.

[42] Hogers, B., DeRuiter, M.C., Gittenberger-deGroot, A.C., Poelmam, R.E. Unilateral vitelline vein ligation alters intracardiac blood flow patterns and morphogenesis in the chick embryo. Circ. Res. 80: 473–81, 1997.

[43] Hogers, B., DeRuiter, M.C., Gittenberger-de Groot, A.C., Poelman, R.E. Extraembryonic venous obstructions lead to cardiovascular malformations and can be embryolethal. Cardiovasc. Res. 41: 87–99, 1999.

[44] Hove, J.R. In vivo biofluid dynamic imaging in the developing zebrafish. Birth Defects Res. (Part C) 72: 277–289, 2004.

[45] Hove, J.R. Quantifying cardiovascular flow dynamics during early development. Pediatr. Res. 60: 6–13, 2006.

[46] Hove, J.R., Köster, R.W., Forouhar, A.S., Acevedo-Bolton, G., Fraser, S.E., Gharib, M. Intracardiac fluid forces are an essential epigenetic factor for embryonic cardiogenesis. Nature 421: 172–7, 2003.

[47] Hu, H., Sachs, F. Single-channel and whole-cell studies of mechanosensitive currents in chick heart. J. Memb. Biol. 154: 205–16, 1996.

[48] Humphrey, J.D. Cardiovascular solid mechanics: cells, tissues, and organs. 2002, New York: Springer. xvi, 757 p.

[49] Hunter, P., Nielsen, P. A strategy for integrative computational physiology. Physiology 20: 316–25, 2005.

[50] Hutcheson, I.R., Griffith,T.M. Mechanotransduction through the endothelial cytoskeleton: mediation of flow- but not agonist-induced EDRF release. Br. J. Pharmacol. 118: 720–26, 1996.

[51] Icardo, J.M., Colvee, E. Atrioventricular valves of the mouse: III. Collagenous skeleton and myotendinous junction. Anat. Rec. 243: 367–75, 1995.

[52] Icardo, J.M. Endocardial cell arrangement: role of hemodynamics. Anat. Rec. 225: 150–5, 1989.

[53] Ingber, D.E. Tensegrity-based mechanosensing from macro to micro. Prog. Biophys. Mol. Biol. 97: 163–79, 2008.

[54] Ingber, D.E. Cellular mechanotransduction: putting all the pieces together again. FASEB J. 20: 811–27, 2006.

[55] Ingber, D.E. Tensegrity: the architectural basis of cellular mechanotransduction. Annu. Rev. Physiol. 59: 575–99, 1997.

[56] Isaaz, K., Pasipoularides, A. Noninvasive assessment of intrinsic ventricular load dynamics in dilated cardiomopathy. J. Am. Coll. Cardiol. 17: 112–21, 1991.

[57] Ishiyama, Y., Kitamura, K., Ichiki, Y., Nakamura, S., Kida, O., Kangawa, K., Eto, T. Hemodynamic effects of a novel hypotensive peptide, human adrenomedullin in rats. Eur. J. Pharmacol. 241: 271–3, 1993.

[58] Janmey, P.A., McCulloch, C.A. Cell mechanics: integrating cell responses to mechanical stimuli. Annu. Rev. Biomed. Eng. 9: 1–34, 2007.

[59] Jones, E.A.V., Baron, M.H., Fraser, S.E., Dickinson, M.E. Measuring hemodynamic changes during mammalian development. Am. J. Physiol. Heart Circ. Physiol. 287: H1561–9, 2004.

[60] Johnson, C.P., Tang, H.Y., Carag, C., Speicher, D.W., Discher, D.E. Forced unfolding of proteins within cells. Science 317: 663–6, 2007.

[61] Kano, H., Kohno, M., Yasunari, K., Yokokawa, K., Horio, T., Ikeda, M., Minami, M., Hanehira, T., Takeda, T.,Yoshikawa, J. Adrenomedullin as a novel antiproliferative factor of vascular smooth muscle cells. J. Hypertension 14: 209–13, 1996.

[62] Katz, A.M. Ernest Henry Starling, his predecessors, and the "Law of the Heart." Circulation 106: 2986–92, 2002.

[63] Kanani, M., Moorman, A.F.M., Cook, A.C., Webb, S., Brown, N.A., Lamers, W.H., Anderson, R.H. Development of the atrioventricular valves: clinicomorphological correlations. Ann. Thorac. Surg. 79: 1797–804, 2005.

[64] Keller, B.B., Hu, N., Tinney, J.P. Embryonic ventricular diastolic and systolic pressure-volume relation. Cardiology 4: 19–27, 1994.

[65] Kilner, P.J., Yang, G.Z., Wilkes, A.J., Mohiaddin, R.H., Firmin, D.N., Yacoub, M.H. Asymmetric redirection of flow through the heart. Nature 404: 759–61, 2000.

[66] Konhilas, J.P., Irving, T.C, de Tombe, P.P. Frank–Starling law of the heart and the cellular mechanisms of length-dependent activation. Pflügers Arch. 445: 305–10, 2002.

[67] Konhilas, J.P., Irving, T.C., de Tombe, P.P. Myofilament calcium sensitivity in skinned rat cardiac trabeculae. Role of interfilament spacing. Circ. Res. 90: 59–65, 2002.

[68] Kriebel, M.E. Studies on cardiovascular physiology of tunicates. Biol. Bull. 134: 434–55, 1968.

[69] Kulesa, P.M. Developmental imaging: insights into the avian embryo. Birth Defects Res. (Part C) 72: 260–6, 2004.

[70] Lab, M.J. Mechanosensitivity as an integrative system in the heart: an audit. Prog. Biophys. Mol. Biol. 71: 7–27, 1999.

[71] Lamarck, J.B.P.A.d.M.d. Histoire naturelle des animaux sans vertèbres, les caractères généraux et particuliers de ces animaux, leur distribution, leurs classes, leurs familles, leurs genres, et la citation des principales espèces qui s'y rapportent; précédée d'une introduction offrant la détermination des caractères essentiels de l'animal, sa distinction du végétal et des autres corps naturels, enfin, l'exposition des principes fondamentaux de la zoologie. 1815, Paris: Verdière. 7 v. in 8.

[72] Lamers, W.H., Moorman, A.F.M. Cardiac septation. A late contribution of the embryonic primary myocardium to heart morphogenesis. Circ. Res. 91: 93–103, 2002.

[73] Lehoux, S., Castier, Y., Tedgui, A. Molecular mechanisms of the vascular responses to haemodynamic forces. J. Intern. Med. 259: 381–92, 2006.

[74] Lehoux, S., Tedgui, A. Shear and signal transduction in the endothelial cell. Med. Sci. 20: 551–6, 2004.

[75] Lehoux, S., Tedgui, A. Cellular mechanics and gene expression in blood vessels. J. Biomech. 36: 631–43, 2003.

[76] le Noble, F., Fleury, V., Pries, A., Corvol, P., Eichmann, A., Reneman, R.S. Control of arterial branching morphogenesis in embryogenesis: go with the flow. Cardiovasc. Res. 65: 619–28, 2005.

[77] Liebling, M., Forouhar, A.S., Wolleschensky, R., Zimmermann, B., Ankerhold, R., Fraser, S.E., Gharib, M., Dickinson, M.E. Rapid three-dimensional imaging and analysis of the beating embryonic heart reveals functional changes during development. Dev. Dyn. 235: 2940–8, 2006.

[78] Malek, A.M., Izumo, S. Control of endothelial cell gene expression by flow. J. Biomech. 28: 1515–28, 1995.

[79] Marian, A.J. Pathogenesis of diverse clinical and pathological phenotypes in hypertrophic cardiomyopathy. Lancet 355: 58–60, 2000.

[80] Martinac, B. Structural plasticity in MS channels. Nature Struct. Molec. Biol. 12: 104–5, 2005.

[81] Melkumyants, A.M., Balashov, S.A., Khayutin V.M. Control of arterial lumen by shear stress on endothelium. News Physiol. Sci. 10: 204–10, 1995.

[82] Mironov, V., Visconti, R.P., Markwald, R.R. On the role of shear stress in cardiogenesis. Endothelium 12: 259–61, 2005.

[83] Mirsky, I., Pasipoularides, A. Elastic properties of normal and hypertrophied cardiac muscle. Fed. Proc. 39: 156–61, 1980.

[84] Mirsky I., Pasipoularides A. Clinical assessment of diastolic function. Prog. Cardiovas. Dis. 32: 291–318, 1990.

[85] Moga, M.A., Nakamura, T., Robbins, J. Genetic approaches for changing the heart and dissecting complex syndromes. J. Mol. Cell. Cardiol. 45: 148–55, 2008.

[86] Moorman, A., Webb, S., Brown, N.A., Lamers, W., Anderson, R.H. Development of the heart: (1) formation of the cardiac chambers and arterial trunks. Heart 89: 806–14, 2003.

[87] Moorman, A.F., Christoffels, V.M. Cardiac chamber formation: development, genes, and evolution. Physiol. Rev. 83: 1223–67, 2003.

[88] Moorman, A.F.M., Soufan, A.T., Hagoort, J., De Boer, P.A.J., Christoffels, V.M. Development of the building plan of the heart. Ann. N.Y. Acad. Sci. 1015: 171–81, 2004.

[89] Morrow, D., Guha, S., Sweeney, C., Birney, Y., Walshe, T., O'Brien, C., Walls, D., Redmond, E.M., Cahill, P.A. Notch and vascular smooth muscle cell phenotype. Circ. Res. 103: 1370–82, 2008.

[90] Nishimura, S., Seo, K., Nagasaki, M., Hosoya, Y., Yamashita, H., Fujita, H., Nagai, R., Sugiura, S. Responses of single ventricular myocytes to dynamic axial stretching. Prog. Biophys. Mol. Biol. 97, 282–97, 2008

[91] Noble, D. Modeling the heart: from genes to cells to the whole organ. Science 295: 1678–82, 2002.

[92] Nuki, C., Kawasaki, H., Kitamura, K., Takenaga, M., Kangawa, K., Eto, T., Wada, A. Vasodilator effect of adrenomedullin and calcitonin gene-related peptide receptors in rat mesenteric vascular beds. Biochem. Biophys. Res. Commun. 96: 245–51, 1993.

[93] Olesen, S.P., Clapham, D.E., Davies, P.F. Haemodynamic shear stress activates a K^+ current in vascular endothelial cells. Nature 331(6152): 168–170, 1988.

[94] Orr, A.W., Helmke, B.P., Blackman, B.R., Schwartz, M.A. Mechanisms of mechanotransduction. Dev. Cell 10: 11–20, 2006.

[95] Pasipoularides, A. Clinical assessment of ventricular ejection dynamics with and without outflow obstruction. J. Am. Coll. Cardiol. 15: 859–82, 1990.

[96] Pasipoularides, A. Cardiac mechanics: basic and clinical contemporary research. Ann. Biomed. Eng. 20: 3–17, 1992.

[97] Pasipoularides, A. Complementarity and competitiveness of the intrinsic and extrinsic components of the total ventricular load: Demonstration after valve replacement in aortic stenosis [Editorial]. Am. Heart J. 153: 4–6, 2007.

[98] Pasipoularides, A.D., Shu, M., Shah, A., Glower, D.D. Right ventricular diastolic relaxation in conscious dog models of pressure overload, volume overload and ischemia. J. Thorac. Cardiovasc. Surg. 124: 964–72, 2002.

[99] Pasipoularides, A., Shu, M., Shah, A., Silvestry, S., Glower, D.D. Right ventricular diastolic function in canine models of pressure overload, volume overload and ischemia. Am. J. Physiol. Heart Circ. Physiol. 283: H2140–50, 2002.

[100] Pasipoularides, A.D., Shu, M., Womack, M.S., Shah, A., von Ramm, O., Glower, D.D. RV functional imaging: 3-D echo-derived dynamic geometry and flow field simulations. Am. J. Physiol. Heart Circ. Physiol. 284: H56–65, 2003.

[101] Pasipoularides, A., Shu, M., Shah, A., Womack, M.S., Glower, D.D. Diastolic right ventricular filling vortex in normal and volume overload states. Am. J. Physiol. Heart Circ. Physiol. 284: H1064–72, 2003.

[102] Pasipoularides, A., Shu, M., Shah, A., Tucconi, A., Glower, D.D. RV instantaneous intraventricular diastolic pressure and velocity distributions in normal and volume overload awake dog disease models. Am. J. Physiol. Heart Circ. Physiol. 285: H1956–65, 2003.

[103] Patwari P., Lee R.T. Mechanical control of tissue morphogenesis. Circ. Res. 103: 234–43, 2008.

[104] Pettigrew, J.B. Design in nature, illustrated by spiral and other arrangements in the inorganic and organic kingdoms as exemplified in matter, force, life, growth, rhythms, etc., especially in crystals, plants, and animals. With examples selected from the reproductive, alimentary, respiratory, circulatory, nervous, muscular, osseous, locomotory, and other systems of animals. 1908, London, New York: Longmans, Green, and Co. 3 v.

[105] Phoon, C.K.L., Turnbull, D.H. Ultrasound biomicroscopy-Doppler in mouse cardiovascular development. Physiol. Genom. 14: 3–15, 2003.

[106] Poelmann, R.E., Gittenberger-de Groot, A.C., Hierck, B.P. The development of the heart and microcirculation: role of shear stress. Med. Biol. Eng. Comput. 46: 479–84, 2008.

[107] Poelmann, R.E., Van der Heiden, K., Gittenberger-de Groot, A.C., Hierck, B.P. Deciphering the endothelial shear stress sensor. Circulation 117: 1124–6, 2008.

[108] Pohl, U., de Wit, C. A unique role of NO in the control of blood flow. News Physiol. Sci. 14: 74–80, 1999.

[109] Resnick, N., Yahav, H., Shay-Salit, A., Shushy, M., Schubert, S., Zilberman, L.C., Wofovitz, E. Fluid shear stress and the vascular endothelium: for better and for worse. Prog. Biophys. Mol. Biol. 81: 177–99, 2003.

[110] Ruijter, J.M., Soufan, A.T., Hagoort, J., Moorman, A.F. Molecular imaging of the embryonic heart: fables and facts on 3D imaging of gene expression patterns. Birth Defects Res. (Part C) 72: 224–40, 2004.

[111] Sachs, F., Morris, C. E. Mechanosensitive ion channels in nonspecialized cells. Rev. Physiol. Biochem. Pharm. 132: 1–77, 1998.

[112] Sackin, H. Mechanosensitive channels. Ann. Rev. Physiol. 57: 333–53, 1995.

[113] Sadoshima, J., Izumo, S. The cellular and molecular response of cardiac myocytes to mechanical stress. Ann. Rev. Physiol. 59: 551–71, 1997.

[114] Sandrin, L., Manneville, S., Fink, M. Ultrafast two-dimensional ultrasonic speckle velocimetry: a tool in flow imaging. Appl. Physics Lett. 78: 1155–7, 2001.

[115] Schoenwolf, G.C., Larsen, W.J. Larsen's human embryology. 4th ed. 2009, Philadelphia, PA: Churchill Livingstone/Elsevier. xix, 687 p.

[116] Schwartz, M.A., Schaller, M.D., Ginsberg, M.H. Integrins: emerging paradigms of signal transduction. Ann. Rev. Cell Dev. Biol. 11: 549–99, 1995.

[117] Sedmera, D., Pexieder, T., Rychterova, V., Hu, N., and Clark, E.B. Remodelling of chick embryonic ventricular myoarchitecture under experimentally changed loading conditions. Anat. Rec. 254: 238–52, 1999.

[118] Shiels, H.A., White, E. The Frank–Starling mechanism in vertebrate cardiac myocytes. J. Exp. Biol. 211: 2005–13, 2008.

[119] Shinoki, N., Kawasaki, T., Minamino, N., Okahara, K., Ogawa, A., Ariyoshi, H., Sakon, M., Kambayashi, J., Kangawa, K., Monden, M. Shear stress down-regulates gene transcription and production of adrenomedullin in human aortic endothelial cells. J. Cell. Biochem. 71: 109–15, 1998.

[120] Simpson, D.G., Terracio, L., Terracio, M., Price, R.L., Turner, D.C., Borg, T.K. Modulation of cardiac myocyte phenotype in vitro by the composition and orientation of the extracellular matrix. J. Cell. Physiol. 161: 89–105, 1994.

[121] Smith, N.P., Mulquiney, P.J., Nash, M.P., Bradley, C.P., Nickerson, D.P., Hunter, P.J. Mathematical modelling of the heart: cell to organ. Chaos, Solitons and Fractals 13: 1613–21, 2002.

[122] Solaro , R.J. Mechanisms of the Frank-Starling law of the heart: the beat goes on. Biophys. J. 93: 4095–6, 2007.

[123] Srivastava, D. Building a heart: implications for congenital heart disease. J. Nucl. Cardiol. 10: 63–70, 2003.

[124] Stones, R., Gilbert, S.H., Benoist, D., White, E. Inhomogeneity in the response to mechanical stimulation: cardiac muscle function and gene expression. Prog. Biophys. Mol. Biol. 97: 268–81, 2008.

[125] Sugo, S., Minamino, N., Kangawa, K., Miyamoto, K., Kitamura, K., Sakata, J., Eto, T., Matsuo, H. Endothelial cells actively synthesize and secrete adrenomedullin. Biochem. Biophys. Res. Commun. 201: 1160–6, 1994.

[126] Taber, L.A. Mechanical aspects of cardiac development. Prog. Biophys. Mol. Biol. 69: 237–55, 1998.

[127] Taber, L.A. Biomechanics of cardiovascular development. Annu. Rev. Biomed. Eng. 3: 1–25, 2001.

[128] Takahashi, M., Ishida, T., Traub, O., Corson, M.A., Berk, B.C. Mechanotransduction in endothelial cells: temporal signaling events in response to shear stress. J. Vasc. Res. 34: 212–19, 1997.

[129] Thompson, D.A.W., On growth and form. 2nd ed. 1963, Cambridge [England]: University Press. 2 v. viii, 1116 p.

[130] Topper, J.N. Gimbrone, M.A. Blood flow and vascular gene expression: fluid shear stress as a modulator of endothelial phenotype. Molec. Med. Today 5: 40–6, 1999.

[131] Trinh, L.A., Stainier, D.Y. Fibronectin regulates epithelial organization during myocardial migration in zebrafish. Dev. Cell 6: 371–82, 2004.

[132] Vogel, S. Vital circuits: on pumps, pipes, and the workings of circulatory systems. 1993, New York: Oxford University Press. x, 315 p.

[133] Ward, M.-L., Williams, I., Chu, Y., Cooper, P., Ju, Y.-K., Allen, D. Stretch-activated channels in the heart: contributions to length-dependence and to cardiomyopathy. Prog. Biophys. Mol. Biol. 97: 232–49, 2008.

[134] White, C.R., Frangos, J.A. The shear stress of it all: the cell membrane and mechanochemical transduction. Philos. Trans. Roy. Soc. Lond. B Biol. Sci. 362(1484): 1459–67, 2007.

[135] Willert, C.E., Gharib, M. Digital particle image velocimetry. Exp. Fluids 10: 181–93, 1991.

[136] Yoshida, H., Manasek, F., Arcilla, R.A. Intracardiac flow patterns in early embryonic life. A reexamination. Circ. Res. 53: 363–71, 1983.

Chapter 16

A Recapitulation with Clinical and Basic Science Perspectives: Directions of Future Research

Science is built up of facts, as a house is built of stones; but an accumulation of facts is no more a science than a heap of stones is a house.

——Henri Poincaré (1854–1912), in *Science and Hypothesis* [54].

The man of science who cannot formulate a hypothesis is only an accountant of phenomena.

——Lecomte du Noüy, P., French biophysicist (1883–1947), in *The road to reason* [35].

The heart of creatures is the foundation of life, the Prince of all, the Sun of their micro-cosmos from where all vigour and strength does flow.

——William Harvey (1628), in *de Motu Cordis* [22].

With the advent of multisensor micromanometric/velocimetric catheterization, which is discussed in Chapter 5, and powerful digital cardiac imaging modalities extensive fluid dynamic quantitation is now possible in cardiology. The cardiac imaging modalities have been examined in Chapters 5, 10, and 11; they include digital angiography, 2-D echocardiography, Doppler and color mapping velocimetry, 3-D live echocardiography and 3-D Doppler velocimetry, cardiac multidetector computed tomography, and cardiac magnetic resonance imaging and velocimetry.

The fusion of high-fidelity measurement modalities offers the clinician the prospect of identifying multifaceted changes in ventricular systolic ejection and diastolic filling dynamics that may disclose contraction, relaxation and ventricular compliance abnormalities before overt muscle or pump failure is manifested. Accordingly, building on the fundamental background of Part I, Part II of this book has provided the multidisciplinary background necessary for appreciating and for applying these measurements to Functional Imaging, which is developed at length in Chapters 12–14 and in the Appendix, and to the interpretation of intracardiac blood flow phenomena. In the process, we have developed new powerful conceptual frameworks for understanding ventricular *ejection* and *filling* dynamics in health and disease.

Recognizing the continuous spatiotemporal evolution of a succession of hemodynamic events and flow patterns from spatially or temporally discrete snapshots of information, as are provided by multisensor catheters or currently available digital imaging modalities, is something the human mind is especially good at. We may call it pattern recognition, or intuition, or perception, but I think that our natural skill has a lot to do with reading the

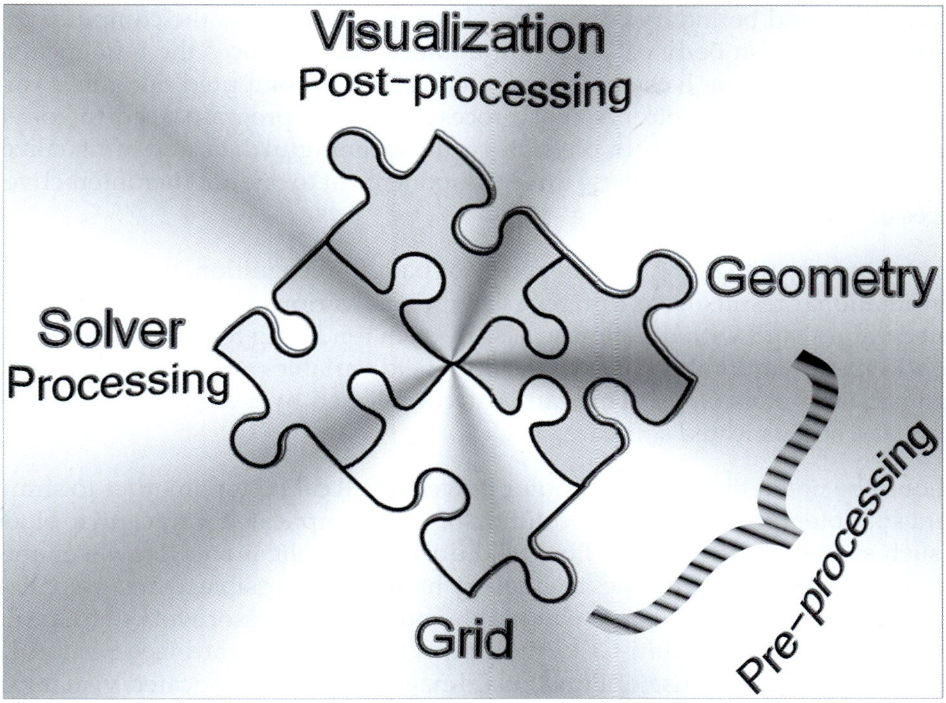

Figure 16.1: The components of a successful simulation are integrated interactively, like pieces in a jigsaw puzzle.

flows of events by expecting a *continuity* of spatiotemporal rates of change. In fact, one of the available "objective" methods for connecting discrete bits of data without any theory entails reading and *interpolating* the available data points of the flow-field variables (i.e., pressure, velocity, etc.). We do that as an essential step to rendering our discrete snapshots of a continuous flow field meaningful, and for recognizing when some single observation represents a change of direction in the whole and some *new origin* of events.

The Functional Imaging method (see Sections 10.5, 14.6, and 14.9, on pp. 566 ff., 745 ff., and 774 ff., respectively) can provide patient- or animal-specific simulations of the intracardiac flow field with extremely fine spatiotemporal resolutions. As we have seen in Part II of this book, based upon appropriate approximations and modeling, we formulate the flow-governing partial differential equations. Since the formulated partial differential equations are for continuous variables, we need to discretize the equations for numerical simulation on a digital computer (cf. Fig. 12.5 on p. 630).

In discretization, we utilize various numerical schemes. By these processes, we finally obtain algebraic equations which can be applied to reproduce numerically the flow field. A computer program called "preprocessor" is usually used to define the computational models for the dynamic geometry specified by the applying imaging dataset and to set the necessary initial and boundary conditions. Then, the "solver" is the computer program that performs the main body of CFD computations and produces the numerical results. The results comprise long lists of numbers that represent computed flow-field variables, such as velocity, pressure, etc. A "postprocessor" is the program used to convert the computed result into physically or physiologically meaningful data, and to visualize them. In a successful CFD simulation these three components fit to one another interactively, like the pieces of a jigsaw puzzle (see Fig. 16.1).

In order to fully utilize the human ability of pattern recognition, we need to visualize the computational results from different viewpoints, various thresholds of rendering of computed values, and with different scales. By such rendering techniques, we can depict even subtle spatiotemporal changes in the flow-field variables and can explore the underlying physics and physiology. This can be accomplished by a combination of powerful hardware and sophisticated software.

It should be noted that supercomputer power is still called for, in order to simulate in sufficient spatiotemporal detail the evolution of very complicated intracardiac blood flow fields, such as the intraventricular flow field during diastolic filling. However, the rapid advancement of computer graphics technology has made it possible to then visualize *interactively* complicated flow fields even by a high-end multiprocessor workstation equipped with a high-performance, multi-GPU, multipipe, 3-D graphics card (see Section 12.1, on pp. 626 ff.). Therefore the use of Functional Imaging with sophisticated visualization of the flow field should become a mandatory part of many clinical and basic science investigations relating fluid dynamic factors to normal and pathological behavior of cardiac cells and tissues.

Clearly, exciting discoveries await the clinical investigator, or basic medical science researcher, who can combine the new visualization technologies with a superior conceptual grasp of the pulsatile fluid dynamics of ventricular ejection and filling.

16.1 Normal ventricular ejection pressure gradients

In Chapters 7 and 13, we have developed conceptual frameworks for approaching ventricular ejection mechanics in light of new and emerging cardiovascular imaging instrumentation, and computational technologies. Myocardial contraction generates intense active stresses in the walls of the left ventricle. These stresses augment cavity pressures to ejection levels in an interplay with geometric and histoarchitectonic factors, as is described in Section 7.9, on pp. 369 ff. Despite the popular view, however, *"ventricular pressure"* is not distributed uniformly in the chamber, even during isovolumic contraction. During the ejection period, there are marked pressure variations with position within the chamber and around its contracting walls. The intraventricular ejection gradients are very real and significant, being associated with impulsive, inertia-dominated flow within the ventricular chambers.

16.1.1 Impulse and Bernoulli components

Because intraventricular flows are generally dominated by inertial rather than viscous forces (see Sections 4.1 and 4.4, on pp. 166 ff. and 174 ff., respectively), ejection gradients go mostly into *local* and *convective* accelerations. These impulsive gradients bring about a briskly accelerated expulsion of blood into the root of the aorta and pulmonary artery and then reverse direction and decelerate the flow to bring ejection to a rapid end (see Sections 4.2, 4.10 and 7.5.8, on pp. 170 ff., 202 ff. and 350 ff., respectively, along with Chapter 13). In absence of outflow obstruction, it is the *maximal outflow acceleration* rather than ejection *velocity* that coincides with the attainment of the early peak of the transvalvular and intraventricular pressure gradient (see Fig. 13.16, on p. 721).

With the onset of forward blood acceleration by the action of myocardial contraction, a velocity field ($v(s)$) is impulsively set up along the outflow axis, s, of the ejecting chamber (see Fig. 13.15, on p. 719). The early accelerating gradient ($-\partial p/\partial s$) is predominantly expended in overcoming blood's inertia to local acceleration ($\partial v/\partial t$), because the low levels of v and $\partial v/\partial s$ render the convective acceleration $v(\partial v/\partial s)$ negligibly small. The early intraventricular and transvalvular gradients can, therefore, be denoted as *"impulse gradients."*

At the time of peak ejection velocity, the intraventricular gradient ($-\partial p/\partial s$) is overcoming blood's inertia only to convective acceleration effects because $\partial v/\partial t$ is zero. In the context of ventricular contraction, we recognize two contributions to $v(\partial v/\partial s)$: 1) the predominant effect associated with the geometric constriction of the outflow tract, and 2) the usually subordinate effect of *wall collapse*, which by displacing a *sequentially increasing blood volume* from apex to aortic ring (cf. Fig. 8.3, on p. 418), necessitates an increase in v along the outflow axis *independently* of any coexisting geometric taper. Analogous but *opposite* considerations apply with *wall expansion* during ventricular *filling* (see Chapter 14). The intraventricular pressure drops associated solely (at peak ejection) with convective acceleration effects are proportional to the square of the applying flow rate or velocity, as expected from the familiar Bernoulli equation for steady flow. We, therefore, denote these pressure drops and the corresponding gradients *"Bernoulli gradients."*

Between these two extremes corresponding to the initial stage and peak of the ejection flow pulse, as well as during its downstroke, the unsteady Bernoulli equation (see Equation 4.13, on p. 187) describes the distribution of the intraventricular pressure drop in its two principal components. This elegant result, additively combining the expressions for local and convective components, is of the greatest conceptual value in understanding and quantifying ventricular ejection and systolic function with and without outflow obstruction.

16.1.2 Conditions with augmented nonobstructive ejection gradients

A wide array of conditions is commonly associated with an augmented nonobstructive ejection pressure gradient. Mathematic modeling (see Fig. 8.2, on p. 415) of the fluid dynamics of the ejecting chamber suggests that the instantaneous gradients are increased with the square of the applying rate of contraction $(dR/dt)^2$, of the effective chamber radius—Bernoulli component—and with the product ($R \cdot d^2R/dt^2$)—impulse component. Both components are accentuated, the Bernoulli component more so, with a lower ratio of aortic ring cross-section to inner wall surface areas, i.e., with a *ventriculoannular disproportion* (see below). For given chamber and outflow orifice areas and ejection velocity, the intraventricular gradients increase with higher chamber eccentricity—see Figs. 13.10 and 13.14 (right panel), on pp. 709 and 715, respectively. Left ventricular eccentricity has been shown to increase linearly with diminishing chamber volume by Olsen et al. [45].

Augmented physiologic intraventricular and transvalvular ejection gradients are generally associated with positive inotropic states, such as exercise (see Figs. 7.19 and 8.7, on pp. 353 and 423, respectively). The strong early systolic augmentation of the ejection pressure gradient during exercise is required by the increased ejection velocities and accelerations of exercise, because large impulsive forces (and the pressure gradient is *force per unit volume* of fluid—cf. Section 4.8, on pp. 193 ff.) can impart high velocities even when they act during relatively brief intervals (see Section 4.2.1, on p. 171).

Hemodynamic measurements in animals and humans at catheterization reveal intensified intraventricular nonobstructive ejection gradients not only with exercise [46, 52, 54, 56, 57], but also during the *positive inotropic states* induced by isoproterenol, norepinephrine and stellate ganglion stimulation [9, 15, 46, 80], and in beats following a long diastolic interval (*"compensatory pause"*), but *only* if ejection acceleration and velocity are enhanced [46], as is exemplified in Figure 4.23, on p. 222—cf. Figure 5.10, on p. 248, for a compensatory pause unaccompanied by augmented ejection velocity and gradient. Conversely, they are depressed during negative inotropic states, during premature ventricular contractions, acute coronary occlusion, and so on [46]. Inability to augment the ejection gradient with positive inotropic interventions might be an *early sign* of contraction abnormalities, elicited well in advance of overt muscle or pump failure [46]. After successful percutaneous *coronary transluminal angioplasty*, I have noted [46] that ejection gradients are frequently increased markedly. This may reflect recovery of "stunned myocardium." Thus, the nonobstructive ejection pressure gradient, a sign of changing ventricular impulse, may have significant diagnostic value in assessing the performance capability of the ventricle.

Hydrodynamic ejection pressure gradients can be greatly accentuated in conjunction with many clinical abnormalities. Moreover, there is a *qualitative* difference between impulse and Bernoulli gradients, just as there is a fundamental dissimilarity between accelerating a fluid by means of a *piston in a uniform tube* and accelerating it by means of a *luminal constriction*. Accordingly, proper interpretation of systolic gradients requires much more information than simply their magnitude. Because a considerable array of high fidelity clinical measurements are now available (multisensor heart catheters, cardiac dynamic anatomy and blood flow imaging datasets, and so on), better evaluation of ventricular systolic function and improved diagnostic insights are now within reach of the clinical hemodynamicist.

The nonobstructive, normal intraventricular and aortic transvalvular ejection pressure gradients are characteristically even more *asymmetric* than the associated ejection velocity signals, as is demonstrated in Figures 4.14, 7.19, 8.7 and 8.10, on pp. 203, 353, 423 and 426,

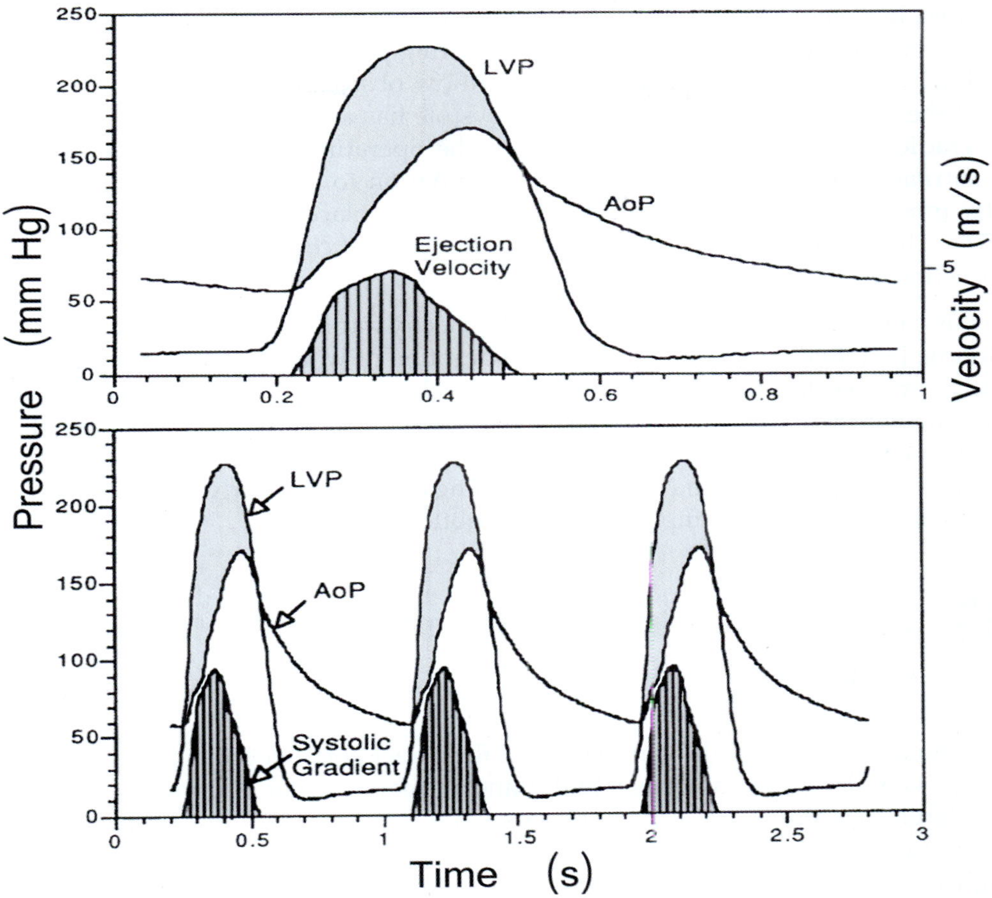

Figure 16.2: Computer plots showing multiple-beat ensemble averages of pressure waveforms, and the transvalvular pressure gradient and linear ejection velocity waveforms computed from them in aortic stenosis. LVP, left ventricular pressure; AoP, aortic pressure. LVP is greatly increased, and its waveform is symmetric and *bell-shaped*; peak AoP is attained in the latter part of ejection. The greatly increased transvalvular ejection pressure gradient (hatched area) is *symmetric* and *rounded*—cf. Figs. 7.19, 8.7 and 8.10, on pp. 353, 423 and 426, respectively.(Adapted, slightly modified, from Shim et al. [71], with kind permission from the American Heart Association).

respectively. In contrast [46], large obstructive gradients exemplified in aortic stenosis tend to be *distinctively rounded* and *symmetric*, as do also the outflow velocity waveforms whose configuration they track more or less closely, depending on the relative preponderance of convective effects, as is exemplified in Figures 16.2, 8.9 and 8.10, on this page and on pp. 425 and 426, respectively.

In closing this section, I will emphasize two points. First, during ordinary everyday activities when velocities and accelerations are *higher* than under *sedated, basal* catheterization conditions, intraventricular ejection pressure gradients can be expected to be *accentuated*. They will be even more accentuated not only during physical, but also during strenuous mental activity. Second, in the absence of outflow obstruction, the impulsive development of the ejection gradients very early in systole has an important corollary: because these gradients are attained at a time when the operating ventricular volume is *close to its maximal* (end-diastolic) levels, their contribution to the *total load* on the left ventricular muscle is *amplified* by consideration of the Laplace law (see also Fig. 7.27, on p. 370). Their action is *leveraged* greatly by the *maximal chamber radii* and *minimal wall thickness* that apply at that time.

In this context, it is provocative to recall the mostly forgotten finding in the early 1960s by Monroe [42], that 90% of the oxygen consumption of working myocardium occurs in the early part of systole during rapid pressure development and acceleration of blood. My own mathematical modeling of papillary muscle contractions [55] has also shown that the internally generated tension increases *explosively* to its peak very early in the twitch under a wide range of operating conditions. The loading dynamics in early ejection could affect myocardial performance in important, albeit subtle, ways.

16.2 Abnormal transvalvular and intraventricular ejection gradients

In the presence of left or right ventricular outflow tract obstruction, including aortic and pulmonic valvular stenosis, transvalvular and intraventricular ejection pressure gradients of large magnitude are typical [5, 46, 48, 53]. Augmented intraventricular gradients can also be demonstrated when blood is ejected rapidly from an enlarged chamber through a normal-sized outflow valve anulus [27,46] as in aortic regurgitation, an instance of systolic ventriculoannular disproportion [46], and in hypertrophic cardiomyopathy [46].

16.2.1 Transvalvular gradients in aortic stenosis

As aortic valvular stenosis develops, the maintenance of adequate levels of left ventricular output requires progressive obligatory increases in linear velocity through the narrowed valve. This is associated with greatly accentuated driving pressure gradients, as is indicated by the unsteady Bernoulli equation—see Section 4.5, on pp. 187 ff. The greatly increased intraventricular (subvalvular) and transvalvular pressure gradient is associated with a relatively low peak *volumetric* outflow rate recorded simultaneously at the aortic root. The obstructive micromanometric transaortic gradient tends to be quite symmetric and *rounded* and closely tracks the ejection waveform, as does the characteristic *crescendo-decrescendo* high frequency murmur (cf. Fig. 8.9, on p. 425).

It is the greatly augmented contribution of the convective acceleration, or "Bernoulli" component, to the systolic pressure gradient in aortic stenosis [46, 50, 53, 57] that causes it to be more *in phase* with the ejection velocity than is seen normally. This is equally as important a *fluid dynamic hallmark* of moderate or severe aortic stenosis as the augmentation of the magnitude of the driving pressure gradient. Moreover, it is only under conditions such that the Bernoulli component far outweighs the local acceleration component that the *time course* of the ejection pressure gradient can be obtained directly from noninvasive measurements of *Doppler* outflow velocities. This point [46,53,57], elegantly embodied in the Euler and unsteady Bernoulli equations (see Equations 4.10 and 4.13, on pp. 181 and 187, respectively), is sometimes overlooked, leading to erroneous estimates of the time course of the ejection pressure gradient using the so-called *simplified Bernoulli equation,* which allows only for *convective* acceleration effects and is not applicable in situations where the *local* acceleration gradient is not insignificant.

The sharp increase in convective acceleration effects renders local acceleration effects negligible in severe or moderate aortic stenosis and substantially alters left ventricular loading and ejection dynamics. Consequently, the *systolic time intervals* of flow and pressure deviate markedly from their normal ranges [43,46,57], both at rest and during exercise. Ejection flow time becomes greatly prolonged both at rest and during exercise, compensating for the depressed volumetric peak acceleration and outflow rates. The time to peak transvalvular gradient is extended, and the transvalvular gradient remains positive through nearly all of the ejection flow time (see Figs. 8.9 and 8.12, on pp. 425 and 428, respectively.). The peak transvalvular gradient tends to occur just after peak ejection; at this time, the convective acceleration effects are at, or near, maximal levels [46,53] while the intensity of turbulence beyond the stenosed orifice attains its peak [69,73,77].

Turbulent dissipative (frictional) mechanisms in the aortic root are responsible for a variable and only *incomplete recovery* of lateral pressure [46,53], as the jet that issues from the stenosed orifice reexpands, jet velocities decrease and flow reattachment to the ascending aortic walls ensues (see next section). Downstream from the stenotic orifice, turbulent shear regimes are induced locally by the jet confined within the large poststenotic trunk, and recognizable ejection velocity waveforms frequently cannot be recorded by a catheter-mounted electromagnetic velocity probe in the ascending aorta [5,46,53]. Here the sensor may be forced into the outer edge of the turbulent jet region, where the axial velocity cannot be expected to be large compared with radial components, and turbulent fluctuations are not small compared with the pulsatile velocity values of the ejection waveform. Thus, turbulent fluctuations may locally overpower the influence of the axial velocity on the microsensor, and its output may no longer be indicative of an average ejection waveform. Jet eccentricity must be taken into account because it affects the pressure gradient across the stenotic valve and, in turn, the relation between Doppler and catheter measurements [17,75].

Interaction of the bounded jet distal to the stenotic valve orifice with the adverse pressure gradient, which is associated with the abrupt increase in effective flow cross-section in the poststenotic dilatation of the ascending aorta, can induce a reverse flow (cf. Fig. 4.12, on p. 198) and a violently unstable swirling, or recirculating, motion. Such a swirling motion in the annular space between the outer edge of the usually eccentrically pointed expanding jet and the aortic walls, and the attendant vortex shedding, can frequently confound the axial velocity probe output beyond the stenosed valve. The methods of digital filtering and ensemble averaging (see Section 2.1, on pp. 37 ff.) offer means to relieve part of the problem, the latter by improving the signal to noise ratio in proportion to the *square root* of the number of ejection waveforms averaged. Thus, having decomposed the flow variables (velocity, pressure) into an ensemble average and a fluctuation from this average, we can characterize the dynamics of the complex unsteady flow downstream of the stenosis (cf. Fig. 16.2, on p. 857). The ensemble average includes the time-mean as well as the low-frequency portion of the variation, which is associated directly with the flow pulsation. On the other hand, the fluctuation from the ensemble average contains only the high-frequency content, which is characteristic of the nondeterministic, turbulence associated, variations in the flow. By averaging many beats, the random fluctuations, which are as likely to *add* as to *subtract* from the true underlying signal, cancel out (cf. the *signal-averaged* electrocardiogram).

16.2.2 Pressure loss recovery in aortic stenosis

Using solid-state multisensor catheters for simultaneous measurements of transvalvular pressure and aortic root electromagnetic flow velocity signals, along with continuous wave and pulsed Doppler velocimetry, my colleagues and I have examined pressure recovery in the ascending aorta of patients with aortic stenosis (see Section 13.5.3, on pp. 722 ff., and Figs. 8.8–8.12, starting on p. 424 in the *Gallery*). Such fluid dynamic clinical studies are technically difficult, especially in regard to derivations of adequate intravascular aortic velocimetric signals, for the reasons already discussed in the preceding paragraph. An intriguing phenomenon in aortic stenosis is *pressure loss recovery* [46, 47] in which some of the intrinsic LV load going into convective acceleration of the flow upstream of the stenosed orifice [53] is *regained* as a pressure rise, as the flow reexpands in the aortic root. *Aortic stiffness* may be an unrecognized determinant of this recovery [48], which was already mentioned in Section 7.9, on pp. 369 ff.

As has been noted in the international literature [34, 68], pressure loss recovery was a new and previously unreported catheterization finding at the time of publication of my survey on *Clinical Assessment of Ventricular Ejection Dynamics With and Without Outflow Obstruction* in *JACC* [46]. In that publication, I provided strong evidence that significant pressure loss recovery can occur in the ascending aorta of patients with aortic stenosis.

Figure 8.12, on p. 428, offers an example of a successful catheter pullback, demonstrating pressure loss recovery in the ascending aorta of an elderly patient with degenerative aortic stenosis. A left-heart catheter with two laterally mounted solid-state micromanometers, one at the catheter tip and the other $5\ cm$ proximally, was used; an electromagnetic velocity probe was mounted at the level of the proximal micromanometer. In the first panel, both micromanometers are deep in the chamber, and a barely discernible gradient is associated with the small, slowly rising, deep chamber velocity waveform. In the third beat of panel B. of Figure 8.12 (bottom), the downstream micromanometer and the velocimeter are in the vicinity of the stenosed orifice, and the measured gradient is increased along with the velocity.

Interestingly, the downstream pressure exhibits a prominent *mid-systolic dip* coincident with *peak velocity* in the third beat of the panel, where the velocity is highest. Such a *"dip"* requires meticulous effort to be demonstrated in aortic stenosis, although a large-scale counterpart is typically present in micromanometric recordings from the outflow tract or the aortic root in cases of *hypertrophic cardiomyopathy* with large dynamic systolic gradients (cf. Fig. 8.20, on p. 436). This is a *good example* of the important, albeit subtle, hemodynamic measurement findings and insights that are within the province of the cardiologist with requisite preparation in and understanding of cardiac fluid dynamics, while appearing to be "accidents" without apparent cause and void of any significance for the more casual observers.

As I have detailed in Section 8.2, on pp. 410 ff., it is my view, based on fluid dynamic analytic considerations and experience with micromanometric/velocimetric human catheterization data with and without outflow obstruction, that such a *"dip"* represents an unmistakable hallmark of *intensified convective acceleration* effects. In the aortic stenosis tracing in Figure 8.12, note that the instantaneous pressure gradient is maximum at the inscription of the mid-systolic dip, right at the time when the velocity and its square attain their *peak values*; this is exactly as required by a flow process dominated by convective acceleration effects according to the unsteady Bernoulli equation (Equation 4.13, on p. 187). Alternatively, the dip can be viewed as a reflection of the *transformation* of ventricular flow work or "pressure energy" into the kinetic energy of the flow through the converging field of the stenosed orifice (cf. Fig. 4.7, on p. 184).

In panel C. of Figure 8.12 (bottom), the proximal pressure sensor is lodged in the aortic root and records the characteristically slow-rising, highly asymmetric, aortic stenosis *pressure waveform* in *systole*. This sensor and its companion electromagnetic velocity probe are slightly downstream of the obstruction, within the jet issuing from it. *Highest velocity* signals are recorded along with *maximal peak instantaneous* and mean transvalvular *pressure gradients*. It is these maximal values of orifice velocity and pressure drops that should be used to assess effective *orifice area* by invasive and noninvasive methods.

In the last bottom panel of Figure 8.12, the downstream sensors for pressure and velocity are in the region of turbulent flow in the poststenotic dilatation of the ascending aorta. Note that the downstream pressure has *recovered* very markedly in conjunction with the *decrease* in the linear *velocity* and hence the *kinetic energy* of the flow, as required by the Bernoulli equation (cf. Fig. 4.7, on p. 184). Thus, although the upstream micromanometer still records deep left ventricular pressure levels unchanged from those of panels A., B., and C., the *downstream* one records *much higher* systolic pressures. In the case under consideration, the peak-to-peak pressure gradient is lower by about 20 *mm Hg* in panel D. than in panel C., as a result of the equal (20 *mm Hg*) *increase* in the peak downstream pressure.

Clearly, pressure recovery must be kept in mind in the catheterization laboratory, since the kinetic energy of blood accelerated through the stenotic orifice is *partially recovered* as pressure downstream in the aorta. It *reduces* the "wasted" power output of the left ventricle, which is proportional to the product of the applying transvalvular *pressure drop* by *flow rate*, and it effectively reduces the work load on the left ventricle. Moreover, it can cause substantial underestimation of the maximal values of the peak, the mean and the peak-to-peak transvalvular pressure drops that are correlated with *stenosis severity*. This is likely to occur if the downstream micromanometer is located well beyond the orifice in the poststenotic dilated aortic trunk, where incomplete but significant pressure recovery [46,48] is associated with the *flow deceleration* as the jet reexpands.

In fact, the pressure gradient measured by a "double-tip" micromanometric catheter withdrawn through the orifice will therefore progressively decrease over a few centimeters beyond the valve, as compared with that measured at the narrowest flow stream, or *vena contracta*—see Figure 8.12, and Section 4.4.7, on pp. 185 f. The aortic valve area calculated from these pressure gradients by the Gorlin equation will increase *pari-passu* to a downstream plateau. On the other hand, the Doppler-derived effective orifice area will be determined by the maximal velocity at the *vena contracta*; accordingly, it should agree with the catheter-derived area estimate only if the downstream sensor for the pressure gradient measurement were located directly at the *vena contracta*. The Gorlin area, typically derived from downstream pressure measurements, will therefore tend to exceed the Doppler value. Pressure gradient underestimations can be avoided by pulling the *multisensor* catheter back carefully and very slowly, so as not to miss the spot where highest gradient and velocity values are registered.

In the context of the preceding paragraph, it is imperative that, during the catheter pullaback procedure, one should keep in mind that if the upstream (intraventricular) micromanometer is located *within*, or even *very near*, the subvalvular region, the pressure gradient measured by a "double-tip" micromanometric catheter withdrawn through the orifice will progressively decrease not only because of the pressure loss recovery affecting the downstream micromanometer, but also because of *a fall in pressure* at the *upstream sensor*. This is a consequence of the fact that, as I have emphasized in earlier sections (see Figs. 7.21, 8.8, 8.12, 13.5, 13.15, 13.17, and 13.18, on pp. 357, 424, 428, 695, 719, 723, and 725, respectively, along with the associated discussions), most of the convective pressure drop occurs in the *subvalvular region*, where the convective acceleration effect during ejection is most intense [5,18,20,21,34,46,50,53,83].

Since the effective aortic (pulmonic) valve area is consistently overestimated by the area that is usually determined at cardiac catheterization, the severity of the aortic (pulmonic) valvular stenosis is consistently *underestimated* using the recovered pressure. The question, therefore, arises regarding the importance of these considerations for clinical decision making.

From a clinical viewpoint, it is unclear whether the maximum pressure drop at the *vena contracta* (cf. Fig. 4.8, on p. 186) or the net drop after pressure recovery best characterize the pathophysiologic relevance of the outflow valvular stenosis. There is a compelling argument for basing clinical decision-making on recovered pressure: the pressure that remains *after* pressure recovery has occurred determines the wasted work imposed on the pump, not the maximal pressure drop at the valve. On the other hand, the actual severity of the valvular disease is best reflected, with regard to clinical time course and consequences, by the effective *valve area* irrespective of the method of its assessment. However, the impact of pressure recovery may *outweigh* error ranges in aortic valve area calculations due to other factors; therefore pressure recovery should not be neglected in clinical practise.

The severity of aortic stenosis depends not only on the anatomic orifice area and the subvalvular geometry, which affects flow streamline convergence, and so the area of the *vena contracta*, but also on the ascending aortic geometry and wall stiffness [48]. Progression of hemodynamic stenosis severity might, consequently, not depend solely on progressive valvular disease alone, but also on an ensuing progressive *poststenotic aortic root dilatation* [46, 65, 66] and elevated aortic stiffness. Endothelial dysfunction, ischemia, and other factors might bring about the increased stiffness [2, 44]. As a result of these processes, a vicious cycle may come about: progressive poststenotic aortic dilatation caused by the valvular stenosis may, in itself, aggravate the hemodynamic severity of the lesion by minimizing pressure recovery and increasing turbulent energy dissipation. It would be useful to examine to what extent the natural history of aortic stenosis and rate of effective orifice area decline are influenced by the rate of development and the evolution of the poststenotic aortic root dilatation.

16.2.3 Apparent *"dynamic obstruction"* of the outflow tract post-AVR

In the rapidly tapering flow field upstream of a stenosed outflow orifice, the convective acceleration mechanism underlies the striking subvalvular pressure gradients in the streamwise direction. Turbulent mechanisms are set in motion downstream from the stenotic orifice and preclude complete recovery of static pressure. The observation of residual intraventricular and transvalvular gradients after aortic valve replacement (AVR) can be explained by applying fluid dynamic considerations.

It is implausible that aortic valve replacement could establish normal outflow orifice areas or subvalvular flow field tapering. It would surely not remove poststenotic aortic root dilatation, which is conducive to flow disturbance and turbulent pressure losses. Thus, residual subvalvular and transvalvular gradients post-AVR may be present *without* indicating a need for further surgical intervention. Lack of proper appreciation of this fact may contribute to some unnecessary myectomy–myotomy operations for relief of an apparent *"dynamic obstruction"* of the left ventricular outflow tract, developing after AVR for aortic stenosis [3, 6].

In fact, since ejection velocity patterns are heavily influenced by loading conditions and wall stresses (see Section 2.23, on pp. 105 ff., and Fig. 7.27, on p. 370), they will be changed post-AVR. In view of the inverse relationship between muscle shortening velocity and systolic load, wall collapse during ejection will be faster [27, 40, 47]. Faster patterns of wall collapse against the reduced component of the intrinsic load represented by the stenosed valvular orifice should strongly enhance ejection velocity and its time rate of change after valve replacement. These augmented velocities and accelerations, in turn, enhance measured ejection pressure gradients from the postoperative levels expected, *if preoperative contraction velocities still prevailed*. Accordingly, *"residual"* subvalvular and transvalvular gradients may be found in postoperative studies *without* necessarily implying the existence of a *subvalvular obstruction*. Only careful consideration of fluid dynamics including flow field geometry and ejection velocity patterns will permit correct delineation, surgical management, and follow-up of obstructive lesions [5, 46, 53].

16.2.4 The pressure gradients of hypertrophic cardiomyopathy

Somewhat more challenging, fluid dynamically, is the production of the LV intraventricular and aortic transvalvular pressure gradients in hypertrophic cardiomyopathy, as we have discussed at some length in Section 8.2, on pp. 410 ff. The *polymorphic* gradients of hypertrophic cardiomyopathy reflect dynamically *dissimilar* intraventricular flow regimes in early, mid and late systole. In early systole, the gradients are accounted for by local and convective inertial forces; in mid and late systole, viscous forces play a major role as well. The huge late systolic gradients are associated with progressive flow passage area shrinkage and sharp increases in convective acceleration and linear velocity despite a *volumetrically* diminutive outflow [46].

16.2.5 Ventriculoannular disproportion in the dilated ventricle

At the other cavity size extreme, the concept of ventriculoannular disproportion in the dilated ventricle was developed in Sections 7.9 and 8.2, on pp. 369 ff. and 410 ff., respectively, and the associated ejection gradient characteristics referable to enhanced convective inertial effects were considered. The *ratio* of aortic anulus cross section to inner wall surface area is a major geometric determinant of intraventricular ejection gradients [23,46,51]. Both *local* and *convective* components of intraventricular and transvalvular pressure gradients are accentuated, the latter more so, when this area index is depressed. In view of the fluid dynamics of ejection in aortic stenosis, this makes intuitive sense. After all, the essence of aortic stenosis is the diminution of the *size* of the outflow orifice in relation to chamber size. As seen in diverse chronic volume overload conditions, including wide aortic valvular regurgitation, and in the various dilated cardiomyopathies, left ventricular enlargement results in a relative disproportion between the size of the globular chamber and the aortic ring—a *systolic ventriculoannular disproportion*, which is functionally equivalent to a relative outflow port stenosis and is treated in Chapters 7, 8 and 13.

In aortic regurgitation, the effect of ventriculoannular disproportion in accentuating convective acceleration gradients may be amplified greatly by coexisting organic valvular stenosis. Indeed, it is well known that modest degrees of aortic stenosis can be associated with a very large transvalvular gradient in conjunction with significant aortic insufficiency. However, this has been accounted for solely by the fact that the total (forward plus regurgitant) stroke volume is larger and, thus, the ejection flow rate higher than would apply with a normal stroke volume. Undoubtedly, such flow rate-related considerations are important. However, my concept of ventriculoannular disproportion focuses on the consequences of the chamber enlargement *itself* on flow field geometry and fluid dynamics. Accordingly, ventriculoannular disproportion can account for augmented ejection pressure gradients in the enlarged ventricle, which are not necessarily accompanied by elevated velocities of circumferential fiber contraction, or dR/dt—cf. top panel of Figure 8.14, on p. 430, from a case of acute aortic insufficiency without any coexisting stenosis.

Conversely, a reduction in chamber size would increase the area index (ratio of outflow valve *ring*, or *orifice* in valvular stenosis, to inner chamber surface area). Such a chamber size reduction would depress impulse and Bernoulli coefficients and gradients in, e.g., aortic stenosis coexisting with mitral stenosis from levels that would apply with a larger ventricle. This is the fluid dynamic explanation for the occasional *"masking"* of aortic stenosis in the setting of mitral stenosis, a phenomenon described in classic textbooks of cardiology—see detailed treatment of this and related phenomena in Section 13.6, on pp. 724 ff.

16.3 Intrinsic and extrinsic components of ventricular load

The *ventricular* systolic ejection load represents pressure against which the walls contract and is to be distinguished from *myocardial loading* or wall stress, to which it is related by complex cardiomorphometric and histoarchitectonic factors [46–48]. The total ventricular systolic load, or afterload, determines the manner by which the mechanical energy generated by the actin–myosin interactions in the ventricular walls is converted to the work that pumps blood through the circulation. Under any given contractile state, increased afterload reduces ejection rate and stroke volume. Conversely, when afterload decreases, a larger volume is ejected at higher ejection velocities [5, 12, 27, 46–48]. These changes result from the inverse force–velocity relation of the working myocardium (see Fig. 2.40, on p. 107).

It is the interaction of the ejection flow patterns generated by the left (right) ventricle at the aortic (pulmonic) root with the systemic (pulmonary) input impedance [48,71,72] that gives rise to the *extrinsic component* of the total ventricular systolic load (see Section 7.9, on pp. 369 ff.). This view differs from the generally accepted and widely quoted formulation, by Milnor [39], of the arterial impedance as the complete representation of the ventricular afterload. First, Milnor's formulation neglects entirely the *intrinsic component* of systolic ventricular loading (i.e., the *intraventricular* flow-associated *pressure gradient*). Second, Milnor arrived at his conception that arterial impedance *per se* represents the systolic load because he felt that it would be wrong to conclude that the ventricle plays a part in determining its own afterload. However, invoking such a need is somewhat arbitrary [46]. It is tantamount to accepting that the load imposed on, e.g., the muscular system of a cross-country runner, is embodied solely in the terrain and not in the way (speed and acceleration patterns) in which he interacts with it.

In the 1980s and early 1990s, intensive catheterization and computer simulation studies of ejection were undertaken in patients evaluated for all kinds of heart disease and others found to have normal ventricular function [46, 48]. As we have seen in the pertinent sections of Chapters 4, 5, 7, 8, 12, and 13, these studies demonstrated the presence of intraventricular ejection gradients of *substantial magnitude* in the human left ventricle in the absence of any organic or dynamic outflow obstruction, and delineated characteristics distinguishing them from obstructive gradients and transvalvular pressure drops [18, 20, 21, 46–48, 71]. Larger intraventricular gradients can be demonstrated when blood is ejected rapidly from an enlarged chamber through a normal-sized aortic anulus [27, 46] as in aortic regurgitation, an instance of systolic ventriculoannular disproportion. In the presence of left (right) ventricular outflow tract obstruction, including aortic (pulmonic) valvular stenosis, intraventricular ejection gradients of large magnitude are typical.

Through the above-mentioned endeavors, the view was developed [46–48, 71] that total ventricular systolic load comprises both *extrinsic* (the aortic root ejection pressure waveform) and *intrinsic* (flow-associated intraventricular pressure gradients) components. The total ventricular systolic load, or afterload, determines the manner by which the mechanical energy generated by the actin–myosin interactions in the ventricular walls is converted to the work that pumps blood through the circulation. Figure 7.27, on p. 370, provides a conceptual framework for understanding systolic loading dynamics. A new concept was advanced of *complementarity* and *competitiveness* [46–48] in the dynamic interaction between the extrinsic and intrinsic components of the total systolic load under any given preload and contractility levels. A striking example of complementarity and competitiveness is provided in Figure 8.13, on p. 429, and the pertinent discussion in Section 7.9, on pp. 369 ff.

Needless to say, alterations in preload and contractility can *overpower* complementarity and competitiveness characteristics, so that both the intrinsic and extrinsic components of ventricular and myocardial loads *can change concordantly*. Moreover, many subtle but undoubtedly important aspects of the dynamic interplay between the two components remain to be characterized and quantified in physiologic and clinical contexts.

16.4 Implications for emerging research frontiers

It should be always born in mind that the dynamics of flow within the ejecting LV chamber determine only the instantaneous gradients of *intraventricular* pressure and not the *total* pressure itself. The systolic portion of the lateral pressure waveform at the aortic root contributes a *very large additional component* that acts uniformly throughout the collapsing chamber and over its entire shrinking inner surface. The aortic root pressure waveform embodies the interactive coupling between ejection kinematic patterns and the systemic arterial input impedance. Thus, the total ventricular (pressure) load comprises both *extrinsic* and *intrinsic* dynamic components; total muscle (wall stress) load comprises corresponding fractions.

Intrinsic and extrinsic components are in a dynamic interplay in the course of every ejecting beat, and their interaction is *complementary* and *competitive*. In view of the normally much lower pressure levels in the pulmonary arterial trunk than in the ascending aorta, which reflect mainly the lower pulmonary than systemic input impedance levels, the intrinsic component is a substantially greater percentage of the total systolic RV load than of the LV load.

At present, contributions to our understanding of ejection dynamics come from many directions and sources: from both fundamental and clinical studies of ventricular pumping and myocardial contractile behavior; from use of multisensor catheterization and digital angiocardiographic techniques and of noninvasive or minimally invasive imaging modalities for measurements of cardiac dynamic geometry and mappings of intracardiac flow fields; and from visualizations based on cardiac chamber dynamic geometry datasets combined with analytic solutions and computational fluid dynamic simulations of unsteady intraventricular flow fields. The more sophisticated of these approaches, both instrumentational and theoretic, have developed rapidly over the last few years. They are now defining ejection flow-field characteristics at a level of detail unimagined a generation ago.

As advances have occurred in instrumentation and in noninvasive, or minimally invasive, imaging technologies, so accurate instantaneous dynamic data can be and are collected in routine cardiac diagnostic studies. The importance of such high fidelity instantaneous measurements stems from the opportunity they offer to assess ejection dynamics in a quantitative dynamic fashion, such that abnormalities in contraction may be elicited before the manifestation of overt cardiac muscle or pump failure. Several areas of research are emerging.

16.4.1 Ventricular ejection flow-field dynamics

What is important here is how normal and abnormal geometric details, including regional contraction abnormalities, affect ejection velocity and pressure distributions. *Critical questions* are: Can characteristics, at rest and with provocation, of intraventricular gradients be used to assess ventricular pumping and myocardial contractile performance? Can abnormal geometry or contraction patterns, or both, induce valve leaflet dysfunction (aortic preclosure, mitral systolic anterior motion) and how? A related interesting issue is whether typical distortions in velocity profiles in the aortic root observed by multigated 3-D Doppler and cardiac MRA velocity mapping, without or with provocation, map out specific regional patterns of asynergy, asynchronism or hyper- and hypocontractility.

To incorporate all relevant phenomena of the ejection process and the continuously changing irregular geometry, methods from *computational fluid dynamics* will need to be employed. Ejection flows pose a challenging problem for computational fluid dynamics. Their high Reynolds numbers require extremely fine 3-D computational grids, and their strong time dependence calls for high temporal resolution as well. Nevertheless, patient-specific realistic computer simulations are at present feasible, as we saw in Chapter 13 thanks to advances in imaging, computer hardware and software, and scientific visualization methods (see Chapters 5, 10, 11, and 12), which provide the *"infrastructure,"* as it were, for the Functional Imaging method (see Sections 10.5, 14.6, and 14.9, on pp. 566 ff., 745 ff., and 774 ff., respectively, and Figs. 2.38 and 14.3, on pp. 103 and 744, respectively).

16.4.2 Quantitation of Rushmer and Bernoulli gradients with and without outflow obstruction

The *critical issues* here are: What are the relative intensities, waveshapes of and phase relations between the local and convective acceleration contributions to the total ejection gradients? How do they change with time, pharmacologic agents (afterload reducing, inotropic) or interventions (valvuloplasty, surgery)? How are they modified, in view of complementarity and competitiveness between intrinsic and extrinsic load components, by coexisting arterial hypertension? The ultimate questions are: How do the relative preponderance of Rushmer (proportional to myocardial fiber acceleration) and Bernoulli (proportional to myofiber velocity squared) components of the intrinsic load influence the evolution of muscle stresses and global and regional kinematics? How does this relative preponderance influence physiologic adaptations and pathologic processes involving the myocardium over the long term?

Integration of such quantitative information into a *coherent framework* will require sophisticated mathematic modeling involving adaptive control systems theory [10]. In the near future, the old familiar paradigms of (mean) *pressure overload* and (mean flow) *volume overload* will be supplemented or superceded by new cardiodynamic concepts. These will pertain to phasic ejection variables and their characteristics in health and disease.

Over the coming years, a confluence of intellectual advances, progress in digital imaging modalities and hemodynamic high technology instrumentation, and powerful computing capabilities will shape a new model of what diagnostic and interventional cardiology is and what clinical hemodynamicists and cardiac imaging specialists do. The limits of past static concepts and ideas will need to be extended to encompass the true dynamic behavior of the ejection process in health and disease.

16.5 Diastolic filling dynamics

Diastolic ventricular filling is dependent on a large number of factors and interactions (see Fig. 14.27, on p. 796) and had frustrated investigators and clinicians for decades. Even at present, characterization of ventricular diastolic function and of the diverse etiologies of its derangements remains one of the great challenges in cardiology. In Chapter 14, we focused on some recent findings and innovative concepts relating to interactions of formative fluid dynamic mechanisms with intracardiac filling patterns and diastolic function changes accompanying ventricular dilatation [58–60]. The underlying investigations aimed at a better understanding of right ventricular diastolic myocardial properties and mechanics utilizing chronically instrumented animal models of RV disease of diverse etiologies [61, 62]. We emphasized, however, that the cardiodynamic concepts regarding interactions of fluid dynamic mechanisms with intracardiac diastolic flow phenomena are general and should apply in the left heart too [59, 60]. Supporting evidence that this is indeed so has been accruing from subsequent corroborative studies by other investigative groups [37, 84].

An intriguing aspect of our findings was that RV volume overload resulted in the least impairment relative to control in RV passive myocardial compliance and active myocardial relaxation properties (arrows 1. and 2., respectively, in Fig. 16.3, on p. 872) compared to the other RV disease models (pressure overload and free wall ischemia) [61, 62]. It was nevertheless associated with strong filling abnormalities. Since RV size is greatly increased in RV volume overload (remodeling), it seemed that it was probably responsible, in some up until that time *unrecognized* way, for the filling difficulty relative to control. It became apparent that a fuller understanding of integrative RV diastolic mechanics would only be obtained by combining the studies of ventricular wall dynamics, including myocardial relaxation and compliance, with the *fluid dynamic* aspects of filling.

The ensuing fluid dynamic studies of filling in the normal and the volume overloaded RV confirmed the existence of two *previously-unrecognized* mechanisms for the filling impairment: First, the *"convective deceleration load" (CDL)*, which is important in early diastolic inflow dynamics. Its magnitude affects strongly the peak velocity of the E-wave in diastolic ventricular inflow velocity curves obtained, e.g., with Doppler echocardiography from the tricuspid (or mitral) valve. Second, the *reduction* in the diastolic *vortex strength* that was found to be common in the setting of *chamber dilatation*.

These mechanisms were revealed and investigated through the new Functional Imaging method (see Figs. 2.38 and 14.3, on pp. 103 and 744), which comprises 3-D, real-time echocardiographic and sonomicrometric measurements combined with computational fluid dynamics (CFD) flow field simulations and intracardiac flow field visualizations in individual dogs, at control and chronic RV volume overload.

16.5.1 Convective deceleration load and diastolic ventriculoannular disproportion

Figure 14.6, on p. 749, illustrates how, in combination, the local and convective acceleration terms of the Bernoulli equation lead to a first increasing and then decreasing favorable (accelerating) pressure gradient during the upstroke of the E-wave, as measured via multisensor right heart Millar catheters. High spatiotemporal resolution dynamic pressure and velocity distributions of the intraventricular RV flow field were obtained by Functional Imaging (see Section 14.9, on pp. 774 f.), which revealed the time-dependent, subtle interactions between the intraventricular local acceleration and convective pressure gradients.

The CFD simulations, which are detailed in Chapter 14, showed that up to the E-wave peak, instantaneous inflow streamlines extended from the tricuspid orifice to the RV endocardial surface in an expanding *fan-like* pattern (see Figs. 14.6, 14.14, 14.15, and 14.27, on pp. 749, 768, 770, and 796, respectively).

During the E-wave upstroke, the total pressure gradient along the fan-like inflow streamlines is the algebraic sum of a pressure decrease contributed by local acceleration, and a pressure rise contributed by a convective deceleration that counterbalances partially the local acceleration gradient (see Section 14.7.2, on pp. 769 ff.). This underlies the *smallness* of early diastolic intraventricular gradients. At peak volumetric inflow, local acceleration vanishes and the total adverse intraventricular gradient is convective.

The new mechanism of the *convective deceleration load*, or CDL, was shown [48,58–60] to be an important determinant of diastolic inflow (see Fig. 14.27). The magnitude of CDL affects strongly peak E-wave velocities. The larger the ventricle, the larger is the CDL. This gives rise to the concept of *"diastolic ventriculoannular disproportion" ("DVAD")* [48,58–60].

In conditions characterized by dilated chambers with low E-waves, interventions decreasing chamber size should lead to a reduced CDL during the upstroke of the E-wave and this should restore higher peak E-wave velocities. In this context, a ventricular myectomy (e.g., the Batista procedure, see Fig. 14.28, on p. 797, and associated discussion) would have a salutary *diastolic* effect by reducing chamber size and thus *diastolic ventriculoannular disproportion* and the convective deceleration load [48,49,58–60], *above and beyond* its well recognized *systolic* benefits.

Batista [4] invoked as the mechanism of cardiac improvement solely Laplace's law, whereby wall stresses are proportional to the effective ventricular chamber diameter. Accordingly, left ventricular wall stresses are decreased by reducing the effective diameter of the chamber and this brings about a systolic unloading. However, decreasing the end-diastolic volume by a cardioreduction procedure without an ensuing great *compensatory increase* in myocardial fiber shortening and EF will lead, because of simple *geometric* considerations,[1] to a deleterious fall in stroke volume. Thus, attributing clinical improvement accruing from cardioreduction solely to systolic effects overlooks the *tradeoff* between maximal cavity reduction in order to optimize geometry and the need for greatly increased fiber shortening in order to maintain stroke volume in the *smaller* ventricle.

Alternatively, a ventricular myectomy may act, at least in part, by *improving diastolic function*. This would occur as a result of a concomitant reduction of a diastolic ventriculoannular disproportion and CDL during the *upstroke* of the E-wave and an enhanced filling vortex strength *thereafter*. Therapeutic interventions (e.g., venodilators) that are used to improve early filling by reducing ventricular size and pericardial constraint, shifting the pressure-volume curve leftward and downward, may also act in part through a *concomitant reduction* of a diastolic ventriculoannular disproportion and CDL and an increased vortex strength. Similarly, agents (e.g., calcium channel blockers) thought to improve relaxation dynamics and hence early filling may act, in part, through such fluid dynamic mechanisms attendant to a reduction of diastolic operating ventricular *chamber size*, resulting from their venodilatory action.

In reviewing Section 14.13, on pp. 782 ff., and Figures 14.21–14.24, starting on p. 783 in that Section, which represent the CDL pictorially under conditions of *quiet recumbency*, it is important to bear in mind two pertinent considerations: a. during ordinary daily activities and, especially, under hyperdynamic circulatory conditions such as accompany physical and emotional exertion, inflow velocities through the upstroke of the E-wave and *a fortiori* the CDL, which depends on the *square* of these velocities (see Section 4.5, on pp. 187 ff.), increase substantially; and, b. in considering CDL levels amounting to a few *mm Hg*, it is noteworthy that in tricuspid stenosis we know that a pressure gradient of 5 *mm Hg* is associated with *systemic venous congestion*, and the diagnosis of tricuspid stenosis is done on the basis of an atrioventricular mean pressure gradient of only 2 *mm Hg* [8].

[1]This is readily quantifiable by considering that the rate of change of volume (V) with respect to radius (R) for, e.g., a sherical chamber is proportional to the square of the applying radius: $\frac{dV}{dR} = 4\pi R^2$.

During the E-wave *downstroke*, the strongly adverse gradient embodies the streamwise pressure augmentations from *both* local and convective decelerations. It induces flow separation and large-scale vortical motions, more forceful in the normal-sized chamber (see Figs. 14.15, and 14.16, on pp. 770, and 772). Their dynamic corollaries on intraventricular pressure and velocity distributions were ascertained; they are described in detail in Chapter 14. In the normal-sized chamber, the strong ring-like vortex surrounding the central core encroaches on the area available for flow toward the apex. This results in higher linear velocities later in the downstroke of the E-wave than at peak inflow rate, as is exemplified in Figures 14.21, and 14.24, on pp. 783, and 788, respectively.

16.5.2 Implications for invasive and noninvasive diastolic gradients

Clinical decisions in patients with valvular diseases, such as LV or RV atrioventricular valvular stenosis, are based on the evaluation of the severity of the stenosis. The evaluation is usually based on the estimation of the atrioventricular orifice area, which is derived from the pressure gradient across the stenosis. It should be noted that the geometric orifice area of a stenotic but pliable aortic valve may increase with flow rate; this flow dependence observed in clinical studies is likely a result of a variation of the valve inflow shape or of the geometric orifice area [46]. The usual evaluation of pressure gradient is performed by echo Doppler or by cardiac catheterization. The latter allows direct measurement of the atrial and ventricular pressures. In this case, the ventricular pressure measured embodies both the local acceleration gradient and the convective intraventricular pressure gradient.

The magnitude of the intraventricular gradient depends on the exact *positioning* of the micromanometers in the intraventricular pressure field (cf. the analogous ejection flow considerations that are exemplified in Figs. 13.15 and 13.18, on pp. 719 and 725, respectively). At the peak of the E-wave the local acceleration is zero. Accordingly, the pressure gradient from simultaneous recordings of atrial and ventricular sensors will be the *sum* (see panel A. *(top)* of Fig. 14.6, on p. 749) of a pressure *decline* between the atrium and the *vena contracta* (see Section 4.4.7, on pp. 185 f.) just distal to the orifice, plus a pressure *rise* between the *vena contracta* (orifice) and the ventricular endocardium.

The Doppler measurement of pressure gradient is based on the simplified Bernoulli equation (Equation 4.12, on p. 183). Therefore it is assumed that the blood always moves along a path where an accelerating pressure gradient exists. Because the continuous Doppler is usually employed, which measures all the velocities along a streamline, the output gives a spectrum whose border represents the maximum velocity along the streamline considered. Therefore by applying the simplified Bernoulli equation, what is obtained is the maximum pressure gradient, but this gradient is different from the gradient measured by cardiac catheterization. Indeed the maximum gradient measured by Doppler in assessing valvular stenosis is, in reality, the gradient between the atrium and the *vena contracta* just beyond the stenotic atrioventricular valve orifice. Yet the gradient measured by cardiac catheterization is an effective *atrioventricular* pressure gradient.

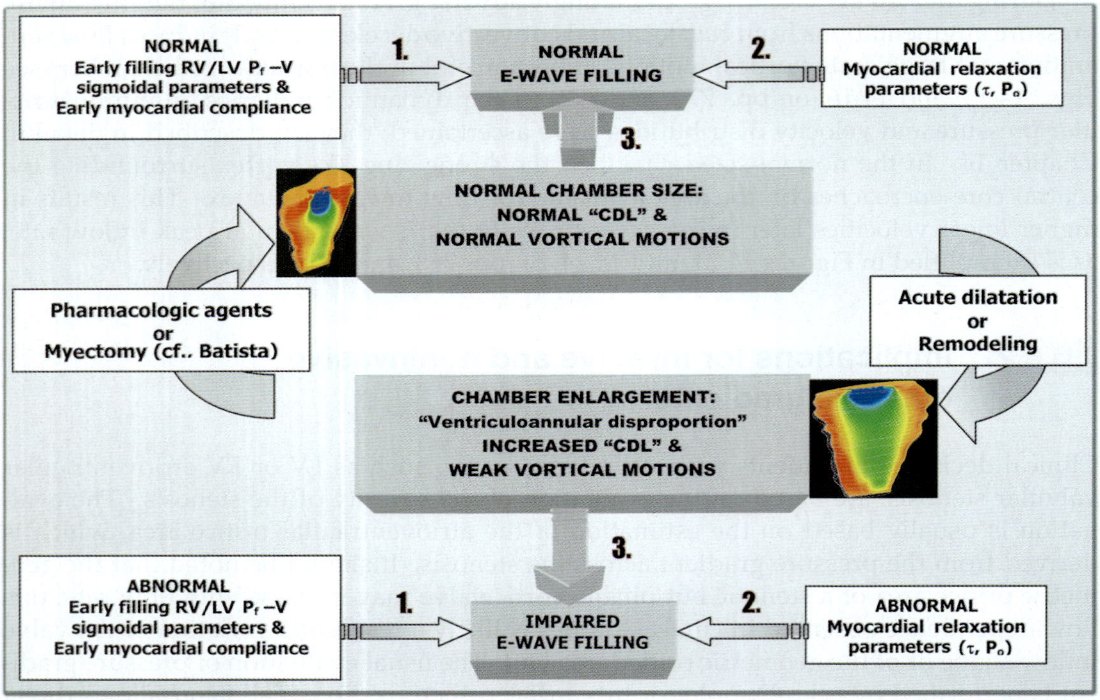

Figure 16.3: Intraventricular fluid dynamic phenomena [58–60], operating along with effective passive filling compliance properties (1.) and active myocardial relaxation (2.), are an important third underlying mechanism (3.), or determinant, of ventricular diastolic filling and its impairment. CDL = convective deceleration load; RV/LV $P_f - V$ = right/left ventricular passive filling pressure *vs.* volume diagram [62]; τ, P_o = active myocardial relaxation parameters [61].

16.5.3 Vortical motions facilitate diastolic filling by eliminating CDL

The extent and strength of the ring vortex surrounding the main stream are stronger under normal conditions (see Fig. 14.25, on p. 792). As is described in Section 14.14, on pp. 789 ff., I have advanced a hypothesis for a *facilitatory role* of the diastolic vortex for ventricular *filling*. Vortical motions facilitate diastolic filling by eliminating CDL to a variable degree, depending on their strength. Accordingly, the ventricular diastolic inflow vortex plays a substantial role in efficiently transferring atrial blood to the right and left ventricles.

By promoting the generation of stronger large vortical motions during the downstroke of the E-wave, medical and surgical interventions that decrease chamber size and increase linear inflow velocities augment filling. This can occur because vortical motions rob kinetic energy that would otherwise contribute to the pressure rise that represents

CDL. This mechanism represents a new useful role for the *diastolic ventricular vortex*, distinct from its role in valve closure, which was characterized in the pioneering studies of the LV by Bellhouse (see Section 7.13.3, on pp. 388 ff.).

Figure 16.3 offers a framework putting the roles of CDL, DVAD and vortical motions through the evolution of the E-wave in proper diastolic dynamics perspective. As it summarizes pictorially, chamber enlargement and the ensuing ventriculoannular disproportion increase the CDL during the upstroke and at the peak of the E-wave; moreover, chamber enlargement is responsible for weakened vortical motions during the downstroke of the E-wave. Similar effects are operative during the A-wave of ventricular diastolic filling. Thus, ventricular filling abnormalities associated with ventricular chamber enlargement have *fluid dynamic underpinnings*. Intraventricular fluid dynamic phenomena, operating along with effective passive filling compliance properties and active myocardial relaxation, have been shown conclusively [48, 49, 58–60] to be an important third underlying mechanism, or determinant, of ventricular filling.

Changes in RV size and diastolic wall motion patterns, which are influenced by passive diastolic ventricular compliance properties and active myocardial relaxation, cause concomitant changes in the magnitude of the CDL and the characteristics of the inflow vortex, which have strong effects on ventricular filling. The augmentation of CDL by ventriculoannular disproportion may contribute to E-wave and E/A-ratio depression with chamber dilatation. The basic information presented in Chapter 14 should improve application and interpretation of noninvasive (Doppler color flow mapping, velocity-encoded cine MR imaging, etc.) *diastolic diagnostic flow studies*, and lead to improved understanding, recognition and management of diastolic filling abnormalities.

Going forward, studies of ventricular wall dynamics, including myocardial relaxation and ventricular compliance [41], will be much more likely to lead to an innovative comprehensive understanding of *integrative* ventricular diastolic function only if they are combined with considerations of fluid dynamic aspects of the filling process [58–62].

16.5.4 Further clinical correlations of large vortical motions

The reduced extent and strength of the diastolic vortex in ventricular dilatation may have notable clinical implications. Thus, RV end-diastolic (EDVI) and end-systolic (ESVI) volume indices in patients with dilated cardiomyopathy are significantly higher when assessed by thermodilution compared to MRI, and exclusion of patients with atrial fibrillation does not reduce the mean difference between both methods [19]. Impaired indicator mixing associated with weakened vortical motions (see Fig. 14.26 [right panels], on p. 793) in the dilated cardiomyopathic ventricles could be responsible—by introducing a strong violation of the underlying assumption of *"perfect mixing"* between injection and sampling sites.

Similarly, the rotation in the intraventricular blood stream may naturally encourage a gentle *scouring* (shear) of the endocardial lining of the chamber (see Fig. 14.26 [left panels], on p. 793) and keep formed and unformed blood elements *suspended* as sugar and tea leaves are kept suspended by stirring (Fig. 14.26 [right panels]). Its weakening may therefore contribute to *thrombus formation* and thromboembolic phenomena. Not only might vortical flow have bearing on the avoidance of thrombosis, but also, by being responsible for *swirling flow* (augmented shear) arriving at the nearby pulmonary arterial branches in the ensuing ejection, it might be a factor contributing to the well known *avoidance of atherogenicity* in the pulmonary arterial system. This would be a corollary of the notion that a fluid dynamic wall shear near zero for an appreciable part of the pulsatile cycle favors atherogenicity.

16.6 Implications for emerging research frontiers

The combination of patient-specific dynamic cardiac anatomy datasets acquired by invasive or noninvasive digital imaging modalities [58,81], sophisticated hemodynamic measurements [41,46,57], and CFD models [18,20,21,58–60], is gaining growing importance in the development of diagnostic and management methods, as well as in the understanding of cardiac disease processes and pathophysiology [5,27,47,48,53,70]. Although clinical use is still held back by the complexity of the measurements and subsequent analyses, such methodological approaches are even being applied successfully to the investigation of the embryonic development of the heart [11,24–26,31,63,74,82], as is expounded in Chapter 15. Similar clinical research endeavors are related to ventricular wall motion and intracardiac flow patterns in the study of ventricular dysfunction of diverse etiologies and heart failure, and in the optimization of cardiac surgical procedures [38,78].

Recently, there has been recognition that the velocity field close to the cardiac chamber walls could exert an important influence on the biology of the cardiac muscle [21,28–30, 32,36,76]. As, for most purposes, intracardiac blood flow is dominated by inertial rather than viscous forces, the curvature of the cardiac chamber walls has a profound influence on the velocity fields within (see Sections 9.5.4–9.5.6, on pp. 463–472). This can give rise to a nonuniform changing pattern of endocardial wall shear. I have stressed the importance of rotational motions in the intracardiac diastolic blood stream, which encourage a gentle scouring of the endocardial lining [59,60].

The future bodes well for the emerging integrated imaging-CFD-hemodynamic approaches that utilize patient-specific dynamic anatomic datasets. Every component of the cardiovascular system, and especially the heart, shows very complex geometry. For instance, most of the inner surface of the heart is not smooth, but is covered by trabeculae. The pulmonary arterial and aortic trunks twist, branch, and distort to a large extent, with changes in their cross sectional contours. As we have seen, intracardiac flow patterns and their simulations are sensitive to applying dynamic geometry. Since the dynamic cardiac geometry is intricate and its influence cannot be faithfully reproduced nor evaluated in either experimental or analytical models, we need CFD methods. CFD methods can be applied to simplified models, but the complex geometric variability, which relates to genetics and phenotypic plasticity (see discussions in Sections 1.9 and 1.10, on pp. 20 ff., on p. 569, and in Section 15.6, on pp. 835 ff.), makes it necessary to describe dynamic cardiac geometry on a patient-specific basis.

Individual Functional Imaging (see Sections 10.5, 14.5, and 14.9, on pp. 566 ff., 745 ff., and 774 ff., respectively, and Figs. 2.38 and 14.3, on pp. 103 and 744) analyses can probably shed new light into the pathogenesis of some important cardiac disorders through analysis of the intracardiac and great vessel blood flow. However, we need to know detailed geometric information that is likely to be different from one person to another in order to evaluate, e.g., endocardial wall shear stress patterns. We must further recognize that the global configuration of the cardiac chambers determines only to a first-order[2] approximation the structure of the intracardiac flow field, and thus the distribution of the fluid dynamic parameters that may have an effect on pathophysiological phenomena. In this context, we do not know whether *instantaneous* or *long-term average* endocardial shear stress patterns actually govern aspects of the pathogenesis and progression of cardiac remodeling. This suggests that prediction, prevention and regression of intracardiac flow-pattern related abnormalities should be based on observations and follow-ups on a *very long time-scale*, and cardiac digital imaging–CFD applications should take this very long time-scale into account.

One should bear in mind that the disease process may not be clearly distinguishable from normal physiological alterations, such that the Functional Imaging analyses should be combined with an understanding of, most notably, the normal *aging* process. Aging is also accompanied by large-scale geometrical changes of the heart and great vessels, in the same way that growth in youth develops the whole structure of the adult body. Functional Imaging investigations of cardiac disease should allow for such considerations, and should be carried out paying proper attention to long-term phenomena. This is particularly true when we model ventricular function using modern imaging technology.

In a similar vein, the effects of *heart rate* have not been fully investigated in the context of computational fluid dynamics, but could be interesting when comprehensive evaluation of various physiological conditions is accumulated and convenient analysis tools are developed. It is known that tachycardia influences global and local flow patterns in the cardiovascular system. Other much longer time scales, however, have not received duly deserved attention. These are time scales related to growth and remodeling due to the organism's growth and aging process. In this context, the *"current"* construct of the cardiovascular system is a result of a multifaceted interplay between physiological and pathological processes of an extremely wide time-scale, from that of a *life-time* span to that of *beat-to-beat* fluctuations.

As we saw in Chapters 5 and *in primis* 10, various image-based technologies have been developed sufficiently to be suitable for the CFD analysis of intracardiac blood flow phenomena. They comprise digital angiography, computed tomography (CT), magnetic resonance imaging (MRI), and ultrasound methods. They will all continue to benefit from advances in image manipulation by computer. Among these digital imaging modalities, MRI approaches are most promising because of their inherently noninvasive nature, which allows for healthy subjects to be candidates for preventive and investigative examinations [7,16,79] . Methods utilizing x-rays, such as angiography and CT, are at a distinct disadvantage, in this regard, even though their resolution and reproducibility may be

[2]See the footnotes on pp. 497 and 693.

better than those of other methods. The trend in imaging is away from techniques which use ionizing radiation or require an invasive procedure. In any digital imaging modality, digital datasets containing pixel or voxel information of dynamic cardiac geometry can be obtained. Consequently, procedures for constructing computational models out of these datasets have been a focus of interest for several years, and many methods have been proposed, as we saw in Chapter 11.

The methodological approaches and the findings developed in Chapters 12–14 support the concept of combined CFD simulation and MR studies to investigate *patient-specific*, complex blood flow fields within the heart, and their interaction with the structure and function of the myocardium (see Chapters 6 and 7) and normal and abnormal valves. An alluring prospect for the future is the possible use of individualized 3-D simulation CFD models based on MRI datasets of basic heart morphology and dynamics. Such simulations could ultimately yield insights into the morphology and function of the heart in health and disease that *cannot even remotely* be provided by any direct analysis of acquired imaging datasets alone.

As a conclusion to this part of a computational mechanics approach to studies of intracardiac blood flow phenomena and fluid–solid interaction for the development of clinical applications, it is noteworthy to point out that many theoretical and fundamental questions are not yet solved. Massive computing power that is rapidly becoming available along with high spatiotemporal resolution cardiac imaging datasets will facilitate the undertaking of extremely large-scale computing problems. However, it is always necessary to keep in mind that the system we attempt to model is alive, with all the ramifications that this implies.

16.7 Modeling anatomic details of the cardiac chambers

There are a number of anatomical features of the right and left ventricles that have not been realistically modeled up until now but are expected to play a significant role in the development of intracardiac blood flow patterns. Chief among them are the cardiac valve leaflets and the limited extent and realism with which these important anatomical features are represented.

16.7.1 Valve leaflets and valve anulus orientation

The remarkably dynamic atrioventricular valve components (particularly, the longer mitral valve leaflets) efficiently control the flow of blood under a wide gamut of operating pressure, flow, and ventricular volume conditions and are, therefore, likely to make a considerable difference to the intracardiac flow simulations. This is likely to be more pronounced in the presence of valvular structural abnormalities, such as characterize mitral, or tricuspid, valvular stenosis.

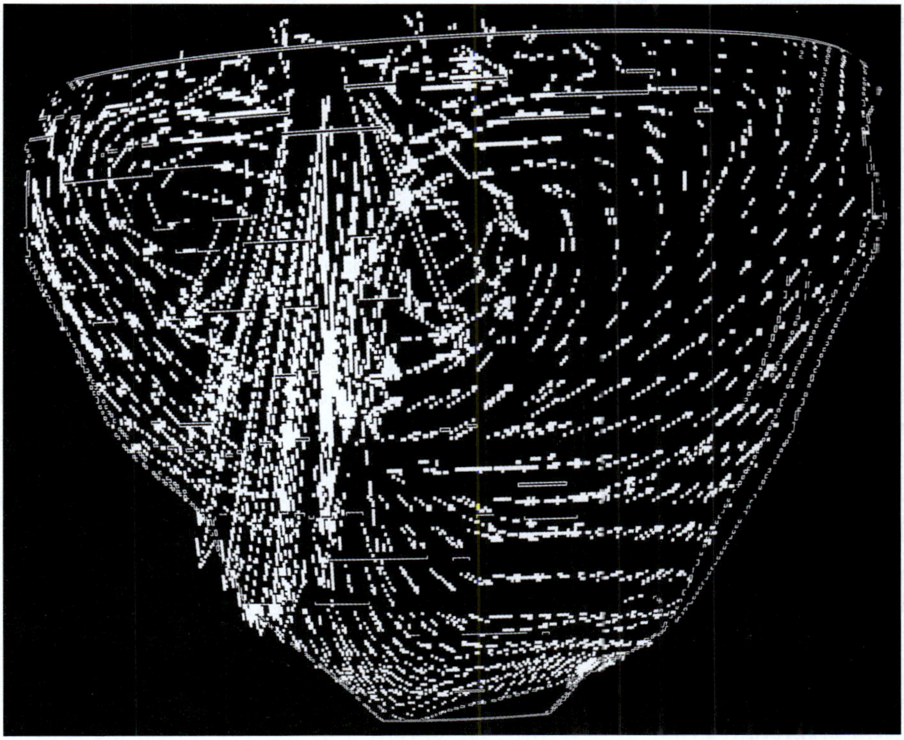

Figure 16.4: The orientation of the incoming blood stream affects strongly the patterns of intraventricular flow, as is readily ascertained by comparing this dog's chirally asymmetric RV diastolic vortical flow field with the symmetric RV vortical patterns exemplified by the animal in Figure 14.16, on p. 772, in which the inflow through the valve orifice is oriented axisymmetrically.

The necessity for the *approximate* handling of the valves in all extant Functional Imaging works stems, in large part, from the limited clarity of the dynamic imaging data pertaining to the valve regions, encompassing the semilunar valvular leaflets and atrioventricular valvular apparatuses, and impacting adversely the representation of the valve motions and pertinent flow boundary conditions (see Section 14 6.5, on p. 751 f., and Fig. 14.7, on p. 752). The complexities of the detailed valve motions present particularly difficult challenges. Such features can be represented in a CFD simulation; the limiting factor is how to *measure* them. Nevertheless, updating the valve leaflet position according to the measured dynamic valve leaflet configurations will increase memory usage and CPU-time requirements. In the near future, high-resolution MRI slice tracking should enable multidisciplinary research in this area to correctly define the size, instantaneous location, and transitory motion patterns of the valve leaflets in time.

The atrioventricular valve ring orientation influences on the whole the 3-D intraventricular flow patterns, as is ascertained by comparing the intraventricular vortical flow fields of the two different animals that are reproduced in Figures 16.4 and 14.16, on p. 772.

Accordingly, the interaction of the leaflets of the valve with the surrounding blood is also influenced. Furthermore, the movement of either one of the two ventricular valves will influence the motion of the other. Clinically, it is to be expected that the efficiency of the ventricle as a pump depends, in part, on the orientation of implantation of, e.g., a mitral valve prosthesis. Likewise, the orientation of an aortic valve prosthesis, including a *transcutaneous stent-valve*, with respect to the aortic root may well influence the motion of the valve leaflets, which could, in turn, have some bearing on ventricular pump function.

The valvular implant orientation will in all probability affect the optimal maximum opening angle, which could promote the entrainment of the valve leaflets in back-flow, promoting early valve closure and reducing the amount of valve regurgitation, while inducing less flow disturbance and transvalvular pressure loss. Since the *orientation* of a valve ring can affect strongly the blood velocity field, it should have an effect on the closure velocity of the valve leaflets and their loading at valve closure. The recognition and investigation of such fluid dynamic factors holds importance for the reconstructive technique of mitral *annuloplasty*, as well as for the design and implantation aspects of valve replacements that are conducive to better implant durability.

In view of the fact that the atrioventricular and semilunar valves are located side by side in the atrioventricular plane, an interdependence of the dynamic behavior of the two valves is to be expected, especially under hyperkinetic operating conditions. It should depend both on the applying flow rates and on atrioventricular valve ring orientation, and should be reflected in the pumping efficiency of the chamber. Thus, the interaction between the atrioventricular and semilunar valves and its repercussions on the related efficiency with which the heart can expel high cardiac outputs is another area in need of future Functional Imaging investigations.

16.7.2 Ventricular chamber wall twisting and untwisting

Myocardial contraction patterns combine with the LV fiber architecture to generate torsion (see also Chapters 6 and 7), wringing the ventricle in systole and storing energy that could be abruptly released in diastole, so as to contribute to vigorous LV filling, especially under conditions of high adrenergic drive and inotropy, efficiently and at low intracardiac pressures. Studies using myocardial markers have shown that LV torsion is proportional to contractility [33]. In recent years several key parameters of LV function, previously measurable only on experimental animals by invasive instrumentation, have become available by noninvasive means, including LV torsion and recoil. Magnetic resonance imaging can be used to track magnetically tagged myocardium, demonstrating distinct effects of preload, afterload, contractility and relaxation on LV *twisting* and *untwisting* [13, 14]. The twisting and untwisting motion of the LV endocardium may, in and by itself, generate secondary helical flow patterns during different phases of the cardiac cycle, and it would be interesting to see how they may affect or influence the intraventricular filling vortical motions. Rotational movements of the papillary muscles and of the large *trabeculae carneae* of the ventricular endocardial surface may have significant effects on intraventricular flow fields (see Section 16.7.4, below). Thus, it would be interesting to incorporate clinical data pertaining to these factors—acquired by using, e.g., MRI techniques employing magnetically tagged myocardium that can provide time-varying, 3-D imaging of ventricular chamber-wall twisting and untwisting—into future CFD computer simulations.

16.7.3 Incorporation of the correlate atrium and its inflow trunks

Another significant model improvement, for the simulation of ventricular filling dynamics, would be the incorporation of the correlate (left, right) atrium and its inflow venous trunks [67]. This would enable the inflow boundaries to be moved away from the ventricular chamber whose filling flow field is simulated. In the process, the flow of blood within the ventricle would become less sensitive to inaccuracies introduced by the imposed inflow boundary conditions.

On the other hand, as blood enters the atrium through its inflow trunks, a shear layer (see Section 9.5.1, on pp. 457 f., and Fig. 9.16, on p. 473) will develop between each incoming rapid stream and the more or less stationary blood within the atrial chamber; the surrounding fluid moves along with each inflow jet and some fluid is entrained. The inflow velocities will be slowed down due to momentum transfer in the entrainment process, and the streams will spread radially. Due to the confined space of the atrium while the atrioventricular valve is closed, the blood will have to move in *circular, swirling,* patterns. As the incoming streams issue into a relatively small chamber, and given that they have sufficient momentum, they should impinge on the distal atrial walls and this should result in an *azimuthal swirl. Mixing* is promoted by stretching and folding of fluid lumps in flows with vortices. The joint shears in both axial and azimuthal directions should accelerate a transition to small-scale vortical structures in the atrial flow, and thereby to a vigorous mixing.

Enhanced mixing, resulting from intraatrial swirling flows, should promote *dispersion* of erythrocyte rouleaux and of microthrombi (tiny aggregates of red cells, platelets and fibrin) that are continually formed and "lysed," i.e., dissolved; accordingly, it should oppose atrial clot formation and cerebrovascular emboli in atrial fibrillation. Complicated atrial flow patterns should also impact intaventricular inflow velocity field details, at least under some (hyperkinetic) operating conditions. Such issues merit future CFD studies.

16.7.4 Papillary muscles and the *trabeculae carneae*

The internal structure of the ventricle is significantly more complicated than the simplified geometry used in CFD studies. The papillary muscles and the *trabeculae carneae* form an intricate and dynamic set of structures that both obstruct and promote the flow of blood. The trabecular viscoelastic myocardial ridges may dampen vibrations of the blood and stabilize the flow during hyperdynamic ejection regimes (see Fig. 14.5, on p. 747). For the important role that the trabeculations play in allowing more complete chamber emptying and attainment of very low end-systolic volumes, see Section 7.8, on pp. 367 f., and Figure 7.26, on p. 368.

The network of helical trabeculations in the endocardium[3] may, in fact, act as flow-directing *minipaddles* that change reciprocally their orientation during the evolution of the cardiac cycle (see Section 16.7.2, above). However, as we have seen in Chapters 13 and 14, both during ejection and during Phase I., of *fan-like* inflow during diastolic filling, the blood velocity at the endocardium is normal to the surface, so that during those phases of the cardiac cycle it is important not to exaggerate the functional significance of these structures. During Phase II., of the large-scale diastolic vortical flow in diastole, on the other hand, they may subserve some heretofore unexplored, and possibly important role. It is necessary to investigate the detail with which these features must be modeled, such that the simulated flow fields are not significantly distorted from those that actually apply, under various operating conditions. Again, such geometric features can be represented in CFD simulations; the limiting factor is how to measure them with high spatiotemporal resolution.

16.8 Patient-specific predictive cardiology and surgery

As we have seen in Chapters 12–15, at the present time *pluridisciplinary* teams in many countries have taken the first steps in developing and implementing digital imaging-CFD systems able to model complex cardiovascular flows. The pertinent integrated software systems can assemble data from the cardiac imaging sources, such as cardiac computed tomography or magnetic resonance imaging, to generate dynamic geometric heart models, which are passed on to an automatic finite-element mesh generator, then to a finite-element CFD solver, with the results being ultimately displayed using modern scientific visualization methods.

Such simulations can in the near future yield important information about the effect of fluid dynamic factors on cardiac adaptations and disease, under realistic simulation conditions more complex than heretofore considered. More importantly, such work may lead to a new paradigm of predictive medicine, computer-aided surgical planning, in which the cardiologist-surgeon-CFD team utilize Functional Imaging-CFD tools to construct and evaluate a combined anatomical/physiological cardiac model to predict the outcomes of *alternative* treatment plans for an individual patient. Such developments will represent a fundamental *paradigm shift* in cardiology, as currently clinicians anticipate changes in blood flow *after* surgical interventions based, for the most part, on the *past experience* of themselves and others, and on the limited diagnostic data available for "that patient," whereas real intracardiac flows are far too complicated for their subjective predictions to succeed in detail without extensive *patient-specific* modeling of the flow.

Further rapid advances in cardiac imaging systems, in computing power (at increasingly lower cost), and in algorithmic grid generation, flow solver, and data visualization capabilities, will undoubtedly accelerate important major strides into predictive cardiology and surgery, thus enhancing the management of ventricular dysfunction and cardiac disease, in general. There is no doubt that prospects for Functional Imaging are bright

[3]See footnote on p. 369.

if one is willing to take advantage of the emerging clinical and investigative cardiology opportunities and tools, which are provided by a flourishing and growing technology.

References and further reading

[1] Arsenault, M., Masani, N., Magni, G., Yao, J., Deras, L., Pandian, N. Variation of anatomic valve area during ejection in patients with valvular aortic stenosis evaluated by two-dimensional echocardiographic planimetry comparison with traditional Doppler data. J. Am. Coll. Cardiol. 32: 1931–7, 1998.

[2] Barbetseas, J., Alexopoulos, N., Brili, S., Aggeli, C., Marinakis, N., Vlachopoulos, C., Vyssoulis, G., Stefanadis, C. Changes in aortic root function after valve replacement in patients with aortic stenosis. Int. J. Cardiol. 110: 74–9, 2006.

[3] Bartunek, J., Sys, S.U., Rodrigues, A.C., Schuerbeeck, E.V., Mortier, L., de Bruyne, B. Abnormal systolic intraventricular flow velocities after valve replacement for aortic stenosis. Mechanisms and prognostic significance. Circulation 93: 712–9, 1996.

[4] Batista, R.J., Verde, J., Nery, P., Bocchino, L., Takeshita, N., Bhayana, J.N., et al. Partial left ventriculectomy to treat end-stage heart disease. Ann. Thorac. Surg. 64: 634–8, 1997.

[5] Bird, J.J., Murgo, J.P., Pasipoularides, A. Fluid dynamics of aortic stenosis: Subvalvular gradients without subvalvular obstruction. Circulation 66: 835–40, 1982.

[6] Bloom, K.R., Meyer, R.A., Bove, K.E., Kaplan, S. The association of fixed and dynamic left ventricular outflow obstruction. Am. Heart J. 89: 586–90, 1975.

[7] Bolger, A.F., Heiberg, E., Karlsson, M., Wigström, L., Engvall, J., Sigfridsson, A., Ebbers, T., Kvitting, J.-P.E., Carlhäll, C.J., Wranne, B. Transit of blood flow through the human left ventricle mapped by cardiovascular magnetic resonance. J. Cardiovasc. Magn. Reson. 9: 741–7, 2007.

[8] Braunwald, E. Heart disease: a textbook of cardiovascular medicine. 1996, Philadelphia, PA: Saunders. 2 v (xxviii, lvi p.).

[9] Butler, C.K., Wong, A.Y.K., Armour, J.A. Systolic pressure gradients between the wall of the left ventricle, the left ventricular chamber, and the aorta during positive inotropic states: implications for left ventricular efficiency. Can. J. Physiol. Pharmacol. 66: 873–9, 1988.

[10] Cariani, P.A. The homeostat as embodiment of adaptive control. Int. J. Gen. Syst. 38: 139–54, 2009.

[11] DeGroff, C.G., Thornburg, B.L., Pentecost, J.O., Thornburg, K.L., Gharib, M., Sahn, D.J., Baptista, A. Flow in the early embryonic human heart: a numerical study. Pediatr. Cardiol. 24: 375–80, 2003.

[12] Devereux, R.B. Toward a more complete understanding of left ventricular afterload. J. Am. Coll. Cardiol. 17: 122–4, 1991.

[13] Dong, S.J., Hees, P.S., Huang, W.M., Buffer, S.A., Jr., Weiss, J.L., Shapiro, E.P. Independent effects of preload, afterload, and contractility on left ventricular torsion. Am. J. Physiol. Heart Circ. Physiol. 277: H1053-60, 1999.

[14] Dong, S.J., Hees, P.S., Siu, C.O., Weiss, J.L., Shapiro, E.P. MRI assessment of LV relaxation by untwisting rate: a new isovolumic phase measure of tau. Am. J. Physiol. Heart Circ. Physiol. 281: H2002–9, 2001.

[15] Falsetti, H.L., Verani, M.S., Chen, C.-J. Cramer, J.A. Regional pressure differences in the left ventricle. Cathet. Cardiovasc. Diagn. 6: 123–34, 1980.

[16] Finn, J.P., Nael, K., Deshpande, V., Ratib, O., Laub, G. Cardiac MR imaging: state of the technology. Radiology 241: 338–54, 2006.

[17] Garcia, D., Pibarot, P., Landry, C., Allard, A., Chayer, B., Dumesnil, J.G., Durand, L.G. Estimation of aortic valve effective orifice area by Doppler echocardiography: effects of valve inflow shape and flow rate. J. Am. Soc. Echocardiogr. 17: 756–65, 2004.

[18] Georgiadis, J.G., Wang, M., Pasipoularides, A. Computational fluid dynamics of left ventricular ejection. Ann. Biomed. Eng. 20: 81–97, 1992.

[19] Globits, S., Pacher, R., Frank, H., Pacher, B., Mayr, H., Neuhold, A., and Glogar, D. Comparative assessment of right ventricular volumes and ejection fraction by thermodilution and magnetic resonance imaging in dilated cardiomyopathy. Cardiology 86: 67–72, 1995.

[20] Hampton, T., Shim, Y., Straley, C., Pasipoularides, A. Finite element analysis of cardiac ejection dynamics: Ultrasonic implications. Am. Soc. Mechan. Engin., Bioengin. Div. (ASME BED) Adv. Bioengin. 22: 371–4, 1992.

[21] Hampton, T., Shim, Y., Straley, C., Uppal, R., Smith, P.K., Glower, D., Pasipoularides, A. Computational fluid dynamics of ventricular ejection on the CRAY Y-MP. IEEE Proc. Comp. Cardiol. 19: 295–8, 1992.

[22] Harvey, W. Exercitatio anatomica de motu cordis et sanguinis in animalibus (An anatomical disquisition on the motion of the heart and blood in animals). London, 1628. Translated by Robert Willis. Surrey, England: Barnes, 1847.

[23] Hoadley, S.D., Pasipoularides, A. Are ejection phase Doppler/echo indices sensitive markers of contractile dysfunction in cardiomyopathy: role of afterload mismatch. Circulation 76 (Suppl. IV): IV-404, 1987.

[24] Hogers, B., DeRuiter, M.C., Gittenberger-deGroot, A.C., Poelmam, R.E. Unilateral vitelline vein ligation alters intracardiac blood flow patterns and morphogenesis in the chick embryo. Circ. Res. 80: 473–81, 1997.

[25] Hogers, B., DeRuiter, M.C., Gittenberger-de Groot, A.C., Poelman, R.E. Extraembryonic venous obstructions lead to cardiovascular malformations and can be embryolethal. Cardiovasc. Res. 41: 87–99, 1999.

[26] Hove, J.R., Köster, R.W., Forouhar, A.S., Acevedo-Bolton, G., Fraser, S.E., Gharib, M. Intracardiac fluid forces are an essential epigenetic factor for embryonic cardiogenesis. Nature 421: 172–7, 2003.

[27] Isaaz, K., Pasipoularides, A. Noninvasive assessment of intrinsic ventricular load dynamics in dilated cardiomyopathy. J. Am. Coll. Cardiol. 17: 112–21, 1991.

[28] Ingber, D.E. Tensegrity: the architectural basis of cellular mechanotransduction. Annu. Rev. Physiol. 59: 575–99, 1997.

[29] Ingber, D.E. Cellular mechanotransduction: putting all the pieces together again. FASEB J. 20: 811–27, 2006.

[30] Janmey, P.A., McCulloch, C.A. Cell mechanics: integrating cell responses to mechanical stimuli. Annu. Rev. Biomed. Eng. 9: 1–34, 2007.

[31] Jones, E.A.V., Baron, M.H., Fraser, S.E., Dickinson, M.E. Measuring hemodynamic changes during mammalian development. Am. J. Physiol. Heart Circ. Physiol. 287: H1561–9, 2004.

[32] Johnson, C.P., Tang, H.Y., Carag, C., Speicher, D.W., Discher, D.E. Forced unfolding of proteins within cells. Science 317: 663–6, 2007.

[33] Knudtson, M.L., Galbraith, P.D., Hildebrand, K.L., Tyberg, J.V., Beyar, R. Dynamics of left ventricular apex rotation during angioplasty: a sensitive index of ischemic dysfunction. Circulation 96: 801–8, 1997.

[34] Laskey, W.K., Kussmaul, W.G. Subvalvular gradients in patients with valvular aortic stenosis: prevalence, magnitude, and physiological importance. Circulation 104: 1019–22, 2001.

[35] Lecomte du Noüy, P. The road to reason. 1948, New York: Longmans, Green. 254 p.

[36] Lehoux, S., Castier, Y., Tedgui, A. Molecular mechanisms of the vascular responses to haemodynamic forces. J. Intern. Med. 259: 381–92, 2006.

[37] Little, W.C. Diastolic dysfunction beyond distensibility: adverse effects of ventricular dilatation. Circulation 112: 2888–90, 2005.

[38] Liu, Y., Pekkan, K., Jones, C., Yoganathan, A.P. The effects of different mesh generation methods of fluid dynamic analysis and power loss in total cavopulmonary connection. J. Biomech. Engin. 126: 594–603, 2004.

[39] Milnor, W.R. Arterial impedance as ventricular afterload. Circ. Res. 36: 565–70, 1975.

[40] Mirsky, I., Pasipoularides, A. Elastic properties of normal and hypertrophied cardiac muscle. Fed. Proc. 39: 156, 1980.

[41] Mirsky, I., Pasipoularides, A. Clinical assessment of diastolic function. Prog. Cardiovas. Dis. 32: 291–318, 1990.

[42] Monroe, R.G. Myocardial oxygen consumption during ventricular contraction and relaxation. Circ. Res. 14: 294–300, 1964.

[43] Murgo, J.P., Altobelli, S.A., Dorethy, J.F., Logsdon, J.R., McGranahan, G.M. Normal ventricular ejection dynamics in man during rest and exercise. Am. Heart Assoc. Monogr. 46: 92–101, 1975.

[44] Nemes, A., Galema, T.W., Geleijnse, M.L., Soliman, O.I.I., Yap, S-C., Anwar, A.M., ten Cate, F.J. Aortic valve replacement for aortic stenosis is associated with improved aortic distensibility at longterm follow-up. Am. Heart J. 153: 147–51, 2007.

[45] Olsen, C.O., Van Trigt, P., Rankin, J.S. Dynamic geometry of the intact left ventricle. Fed. Proc. 40: 2023–30, 1981.

[46] Pasipoularides, A. Clinical assessment of ventricular ejection dynamics with and without outflow obstruction. J. Am. Coll. Cardiol. 15: 859–82, 1990.

[47] Pasipoularides, A. Cardiac mechanics: basic and clinical contemporary research. Ann. Biomed. Eng. 20: 3–17, 1992.

[48] Pasipoularides, A. Complementarity and competitiveness of the intrinsic and extrinsic components of the total ventricular load: Demonstration after valve replacement in aortic stenosis [Editorial]. Am. Heart J. 153: 4–6, 2007.

[49] Pasipoularides, A. Invited commentary: Functional imaging (FI) combines imaging datasets and computational fluid dynamics to simulate cardiac flows. J. Appl. Physiol. 105: 1015, 2008.

[50] Pasipoularides A, Murgo JP, Bird JJ, Craig WE. Fluid dynamics of aortic stenosis: mechanisms of subvalvular gradient generation. In: Proceedings of the Sixth Annual Conference of the American Society of Biomechanics. Seattle: ASB, 1982: p. 5.

[51] Pasipoularides, A., Murgo, J.P., Rubal, B.J. Left ventricular systolic dynamics and intrinsic hydrodynamic loading. Fed. Proc. 42: 763, 1983.

[52] Pasipoularides A, Miller J, Rubal BJ, Murgo JP. Left ventricular (LV) ejection pressure gradients in normal man are determined by geometry, wall kinematics and velocity patterns. Circulation 70 (Suppl. II): II-354, 1984.

[53] Pasipoularides, A., Murgo, J.P., Bird, J.J., Craig, W.E. Fluid dynamics of aortic stenosis: Mechanisms for the presence of subvalvular pressure gradients. Am. J. Physiol. 246: H542–50, 1984.

[54] Pasipoularides, A., Miller, J., Rubal, B.J., Murgo, J.P. Left ventricular ejection dynamics in normal man. In: Melbin, J., Noordergraaf, A. [Eds.] Proceedings of the VIth International Conference and Workshop of the Cardiovascular System Dynamics Society. 1984, Philadelphia, PA: University of Pennsylvania. pp. 45–8.

[55] Pasipoularides, A., Palacios, I., Frist, W., Rosenthal, S., Newell, J.B., Powell, W.J., Jr. Contribution of activation–inactivation dynamics to the impairment of relaxation in hypoxic cat papillary muscle. Am. J. Physiol. 248: R54–62, 1985.

[56] Pasipoularides, A., Murgo, J.P. Ejection dynamics in man with and without outflow obstruction. In: Proceedings of the 20th Annual Meeting of the Association for the Advancement of Medical Instrumentation. 1985, Boston, MA: AAMI. p. 68.

[57] Pasipoularides, A., Murgo, J.P., Miller, J.W., Craig, W.E. Nonobstructive left ventricular ejection pressure gradients in man. Circ. Res. 61: 220–7, 1987.

[58] Pasipoularides, A.D., Shu, M., Womack, M.S., Shah, A., von Ramm, O., Glower, D.D. RV functional imaging: 3-D echo-derived dynamic geometry and flow field simulations. Am. J. Physiol. Heart Circ. Physiol. 284: H56–65, 2003.

[59] Pasipoularides, A., Shu, M., Shah, A., Womack, M.S., Glower, D.D. Diastolic right ventricular filling vortex in normal and volume overload states. Am. J. Physiol. Heart Circ. Physiol. 284: H1064–72, 2003.

[60] Pasipoularides, A., Shu, M., Shah, A., Tucconi, A., Glower, D.D. RV instantaneous intraventricular diastolic pressure and velocity distributions in normal and volume overload awake dog disease models. Am. J. Physiol. Heart Circ. Physiol. 285: H1956–65, 2003.

[61] Pasipoularides, A.D., Shu, M., Shah, A., Glower, D.D. Right ventricular diastolic relaxation in conscious dog models of pressure overload, volume overload and ischemia. J. Thorac. Cardiovasc. Surg. 124: 964–72, 2002.

[62] Pasipoularides, A., Shu, M., Shah, A., Silvestry, S., Glower, D.D. Right ventricular diastolic function in canine models of pressure overload, volume overload and ischemia. Am. J. Physiol. Heart Circ. Physiol. 283: H2140–50, 2002.

[63] Poelmann, R.E., Gittenberger-de Groot, A.C., Hierck, B.P. The development of the heart and microcirculation: role of shear stress. Med. Biol. Eng. Comput. 46: 479–84, 2008.

[64] Poincaré, H. Science and hypothesis. 1905, London, New York: Scott. xxvii, 244 p.

[65] Roach, M.R. Biophysical analyses of blood vessel walls and blood flow. Annu. Rev. Physiol. 39: 51–71, 1977.

[66] Roach, M.R. Changes in arterial distensibility as a cause of poststenotic dilatation. Am. J. Cardiol. 12: 802–15, 1963.

[67] Rossi, A., Zardini, P., Marino, P. Modulation of left atrial function by ventricular filling impairment. Heart Fail. Rev. 5: 325–31, 2000.

[68] Schöbel, W.A., Voelker, W., Haase, K.K., Karsch, K.-R. Extent, determinants and clinical importance of pressure recovery in patients with aortic valve stenosis. Eur. Heart J. 20: 1355–63, 1999.

[69] Schultz, D.L., Tunstall Pedoe, D.S., Lee, G. de J., Gunning, A.J., Bellhouse, B.J. Velocity distribution and transition in the arterial system. In: Wolstenholme, G.E.W., Knight, J. [Eds.] Circulatory and Respiratory Mass Transport: A CIBA Foundation Symposium. 1969, London: Churchill. pp. 172–99.

[70] Sermesant, M., Peyrat, J.M., Chinchapatnam, P., Billet, F., Mansi, T., Rhode, K., Delingette, H., Razavi, R., Ayache, N. Toward patient-specific myocardial models of the heart. Heart Fail. Clin. 4: 289–301, 2008.

[71] Shim, Y., Hampton, T.G., Straley, C.A., Harrison, J.K., Spero, L.A., Bashore, T.M., Pasipoularides, A.D. Ejection load changes in aortic stenosis. Observations made after balloon aortic valvuloplasty. Circ. Res. 71: 1174–84, 1992.

[72] Shim, Y., Pasipoularides, A., Straley, C., Hampton, T.G., Soto, P., Owen, C., Davis, J.W., Glower, D.D. Arterial windkessel parameter estimation: a new time-domain method. Ann. Biomed. Eng. 22: 66–77, 1994.

[73] Stein, P.D., Sabbah, H.N. Turbulent blood flow in the ascending aorta of humans with normal and diseased aortic valves. Circ. Res. 39: 58–65, 1976.

[74] Topper, J.N. Gimbrone, M.A. Blood flow and vascular gene expression: fluid shear stress as a modulator of endothelial phenotype. Molec. Med. Today 5: 40–6, 1999.

[75] VanAuker, M.D., Chandra, M., Shirani, J., Strom, J.A. Jet eccentricity: a misleading source of agreement between Doppler/catheter pressure gradients in aortic stenosis. J. Am. Soc. Echocardiogr. 14: 853–62, 2001.

[76] Vogel, V., Sheetz, M. Local force and geometry sensing regulate cell functions. Nature Rev. Mol. Cell Biol. 7: 265–75, 2006.

[77] Walburn, F.J., Sabbah, H.N., Stein, P.D. An experimental evaluation of the use of an ensemble average for the calculation of turbulence in pulsatile flow. Ann. Biomed. Eng. 11: 385–99, 1983.

[78] Wang, C., Pekkan, K., de Zelicourt, D., Parihar, A., Kulkarni, A., Horner, M., Yoganathan, A.P. Progress in the CFD modeling of flow instability in anatomical total cavopulmonary connections. Ann. Biomed. Eng. 35: 1840–56, 2007.

[79] Westbrook, C. Handbook of MRI technique. 3rd ed. 2008, Oxford, UK; Malden, MA: Wiley-Blackwell. x, 414 p.

[80] White, R.I., Jr., Criley, J.M., Lewis, K.B., Ross, R.S. Experimental production of intracavity pressure differences: possible significance in the interpretation of human hemodynamic studies. Am. J. Cardiol. 19: 806–17, 1967.

[81] Young, A.A., Frangi, A.F. Computational cardiac atlases: from patient to population and back [Review]. Exp. Physiol. 94: 578–96, 2009.

[82] Yoshida, H., Manasek, F., Arcilla, R.A. Intracardiac flow patterns in early embryonic life. A reexamination. Circ. Res. 53: 363–71, 1983.

[83] Yotti, R., Bermejo, J., Antoranz, J.C., Rojo-Alvarez, J.L., Allue, C., Silva, J., Desco, M.M., Moreno, M., Garcia-Fernandez, M.A. Noninvasive assessment of ejection intraventricular pressure gradients. J. Am. Coll. Cardiol. 43: 1654–62, 2004.

[84] Yotti, R., Bermejo, J., Antoranz, J.C., Desco, M.M., Cortina, C., Rojo-Alvarez, J.L., Allue, C., Martin, L., Moreno, M., Serrano, J.A., Munoz, R., Garcia-Fernandez, M.A. A noninvasive method for assessing impaired diastolic suction in patients with dilated cardiomyopathy. Circulation 112: 2921–9, 2005.

Chapter 17

Epilogue

"MY OWN ORIGINAL INCLINATION WAS TOWARDS PHYSICS; external circumstance compelled me to commence the study of medicine, which was made possible to me by the liberal arrangements of this Institution. It had, however, been the custom of a former time to combine the study of medicine with that of the Natural Sciences, and whatever in this was compulsory I must consider fortunate; not merely that I entered medicine at a time in which anyone who was even moderately at home in physical considerations found a fruitful virgin soil for cultivation; but I consider the study of medicine to have been that training which preached more impressively and more convincingly than any other could have done, the everlasting principles of all scientific work; principles which are so simple and yet are ever forgotten again; so clear and yet always hidden by a deceptive veil.

Perhaps only he can appreciate the immense importance and the fearful practical scope of the problems of medical theory, who has watched the fading eye of approaching death, and witnessed the distracted grief of affection, and who has asked himself the solemn questions, Has all been done which could be done to ward off the dread event? Have all the resources and all the means which Science has accumulated become exhausted? ......

I rejoice, therefore, that I can once more address an assembly consisting almost exclusively of medical men who have gone through the same school. Medicine was once the intellectual home in which I grew up, and even the emigrant best understands and is best understood by his native land. If I am called upon to designate in one word the fundamental error of that former time, I should be inclined to say that it pursued a false ideal of science in a one-sided and erroneous reverence for the deductive method. Medicine, it is true, was not the only science which was involved in this error, but in no other science have the consequences been so glaring, or have so hindered progress, as in medicine. The history of this science claims, therefore, a special interest in the history of the development of the human mind. None other is, perhaps, more fitted to show that a true criticism of the sources of cognition is also practically an exceedingly important object of true philosophy. The proud word of Hippokrates, *ιατρος φιλοσοφος ισοθεος,*

"Godlike is the physician who is a philosopher," served, as it were, as a banner of the old deductive medicine. We may admit this if only we once agree what we are to understand as a philosopher. For the ancients, philosophy embraced all theoretical knowledge; their philosophers pursued Mathematics, Physics, Astronomy, Natural History, in close connection with true philosophical or metaphysical considerations. If, therefore, we are to understand the medical philosopher of Hippokrates to be a man who has a *perfected* insight into the causal connection of natural processes, we shall in fact be able to say with Hippokrates, Such a one can give help like a god.

Understood in this sense, the aphorism describes in three words the ideal which our science has to strive after. But who can allege that it will ever attain this ideal? ......

In order, finally, to conclude our consultation on the condition of Dame Medicine correctly with the epikrisis,[1] I think we have every reason to be content with the success of the treatment which the school of natural science has applied, and we can only recommend the younger generation to continue the same therapeutics.

———Excerpted from Hermann von Helmholtz: *On thought in Medicine*. In: Helmholtz, H. v., Atkinson, E. Popular lectures on scientific subjects. 1898, London; New York: Longmans, Green. vi, 291 p.—Footnote added.

[1]A critical study or evaluation; Gk. *επικρισις*, a *constructive criticism* or judgment.

Part III

Appendix

Functional Imaging as Numerical Flow Field Visualization, and Its Verification and Validation

As we have seen demonstrated abundantly in this book, the high-speed digital computer provides an additional and important tool, beyond the innovative digital imaging modalities (3-D Doppler and live echocardiography, multidetector cardiac CT, cardiac MRI and phase-contrast velocity mapping), which is available to clinicians and researchers alike in tackling complex intracardiac blood flow problems. Image processing, the extraction and evaluation of data from a visible pattern, is a powerful component of flow visualization that produces quantitative information from one or more recorded images or *video*-loop frames. It complements nicely the remarkable abilities of the human visual system; humans can easily discern and infer structural information in an image, but cannot readily make quantitative comparisons between brightness levels in different parts of the image, or assimilate vast reams of numerical computation outputs. Digital images, on the other hand, are processed pixel-by-pixel and precise comparisons between pixels are not complicated to perform on a digital computer, or to be discerned, in the form of pseudocolor mappings, by human examiners.

A.1 Functional Imaging is a numerical flow-field visualization

As is developed in Sections 10.5, on pp. 566 ff., 14.6, on pp. 745 ff., and 14.9, on pp. 774 ff., Functional Imaging (FI) is, effectively, *numerical* intracardiac flow field *visualization*, and can yield invaluable qualitative as well as quantitative information about the dynamics of a complex intracardiac flow. To recall briefly, FI uses quantitative methods of cardiac imaging dataset acquisition and postprocessing in combination with CFD simulation methods to provide animal- or patient-specific intracardiac flow field visualization [11–13]. Scientific visualization methods allow enhancement and feature extraction of digital images to assist data interpretation. With the recent availability of powerful computers, techniques for the measurements of instantaneous pressure, velocity and other intracardiac flow field variables, have become feasible. Intracardiac velocity field information, for instance, can be obtained from MR phase-contrast velocity mapping (PCVM), which permits quantitative calculation of intracardiac blood flow velocities in any spatial direction (see Section 10.3, on pp. 531 ff.). However, in investigations of intracardiac blood flow phenomena, it is impossible to extract *high spatiotemporal resolution* results from various catheter-mounted sensor measurements or even from the currently available imaging modalities, including live 3-D echocardiography and Doppler velocimetry, MRI, and multidetector CT. Accordingly, Functional Imaging—or, *numerical flow visualization*—represents an invaluable alternative.

Current advances in computer technology make the numerical integration of the complete Navier-Stokes equations (see Sections 2.22, on pp. 99 ff., 4.6, on pp. 190 ff., and 4.7, on pp. 191 ff., and numerous applications throughout this book) more feasible. Once the flow field is computed, contour plots of the instantaneous velocity, pressure, or wall shear can be readily created. Streaklines, or particle paths (see footnote on p. 200), can also be plotted by tracking passive particles released from a given location in the flow. Thousands of particles may be distributed and traced in three dimensions within the flow field. Flow paths can be obtained by numerical integration (see p. 625, and Section 14.5, on pp. 742 ff.) of particle velocity over time. The number of particles "seeded" in a cardiac chamber and remaining at the end of successive cardiac cycles, or cycle phases, can be plotted. Numerical-dye visualization methods are currently feasible and can be similarly applied to display computational data. *Cine-* or *video-*loops, as well as still frames, can be used to record and replay the resulting numerical visualizations.

When tracer substances are used to obtain quantitative velocity field information, the investigator must ensure that they are faithfully following the blood flow motions down to the finest flow structures to be resolved, and that they do not have undesirable cardiovascular actions. Unlike particles, or contrast media, or dye tracers released in analog or animal model experiments, or human diagnostic examinations, the *numerical markers* do not suffer any *inertial lag* or *mismatched diffusivity* effects. Moreover, the passive scalar introduction into the flowing blood does not cause any disturbance to the numerical flow field; the program is merely following selective fluid particles already existing within the computational domain. Finite difference, finite element, boundary element and spectral methods are among the numerical methods used to integrate the governing equations, as is developed in Chapters 12–14. In general, spectral methods are very accurate while finite-difference algorithms are more suited for complex geometries and are easier to set up. Once the specific intracardiac flow field of interest is obtained numerically, the digital data can then be processed straightforwardly with any of the image processing and computer graphics tools available for digital imaging datasets, as we have seen in many applications throughout this book. The most advanced (image synthesis, tomographic and gradient imaging) of the new image processing techniques used in flow visualization studies allow viewing of the flow field interior from different directions.

A.2 Error and uncertainty in Functional Imaging and verification and validation assessment activities

It is clear that different forms of error and uncertainty are introduced into a Functional Imaging application as data are acquired, transformed, and visualized. Starting with the *data acquisition* stage, nearly all datasets, whether they are derived from digital imaging of cardiac dynamic anatomy and intracardiac flow velocities or from multisensor catheterization measurements, have measurement error and uncertainty. With any kind of instrumentation there is measurement variability, whether the measurements are taken automatically by a machine or manually by a human operator [8]. If a measurement is taken multiple times, our confidence about its statistical distribution increases. In numerical CFD modeling, the computer model with its parameters have been decided by a CFD specialist, and it is inherently a simplification of the actual flow field that is being modeled. The next important source of uncertainty is in the *data transformation* stage [1]. In addition to model simplification and the sensitivity of simulation models to input parameters, boundary and initial conditions, numerical calculations performed on these models also introduce errors due to the integration algorithms and the limited precision of the computing machinery. Finally, uncertainty is also introduced in the *visualization stage* itself due to the errors and approximations associated with the postprocessing methods, the rendering models, and the algorithms employed in the rendering process [5]. In examining the results obtained through Functional Imaging, we face an essential issue: How should confidence in its multiple modeling and simulation components be critically assessed?

Verification and validation of computational simulations are the primary means for building and quantifying such confidence. These are the principal procedures for assessing the accuracy and reliability of any CFD simulations and, therefore, of Functional Imaging. Briefly, verification is the assessment of the accuracy of the solution to a computational model by comparison with known solutions. Validation is the assessment of the accuracy of a computational simulation by comparison with experimental or clinical data. In verification, the relationship of the simulation to the real world is *not* an issue. In validation, the relationship between computation and the real world, i.e., experimental or clinical data, *is* the issue. Stated in a different way, verification is primarily a mathematics

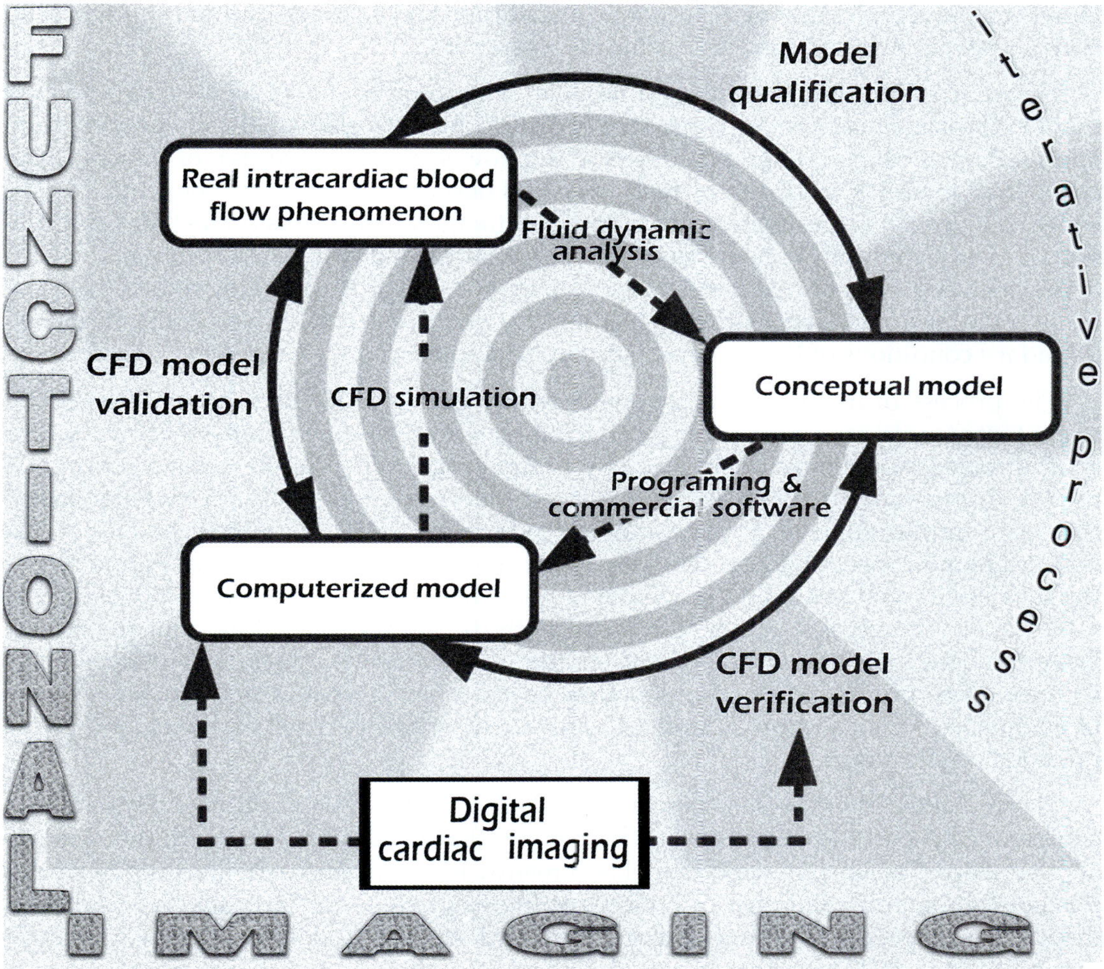

Figure A.1: Phases of cardiac imaging, modeling, and CFD simulation, and the role of verification and validation in assessing accuracy and reliability in Functional Imaging simulations.

issue; validation is primarily a physics issue [16]. According to Roache's succinct and pointed description [17], verification is "solving the equations right," whereas validation is "solving the right equations."

Admittedly, the prevalent method of qualitative graphical validation, i.e., comparison of high spatiotemporal resolution computational intracardiac flow field datasets with available (generally, sparse) experimental or clinical diagnostic graphed data, is imperfect. This limitation especially applies for complex flow fields, such as the diastolic intraventricular field, in whose case we rely heavily on computational simulation for understanding their detailed characteristics under normal and abnormal operating conditions.

However, the complexities of quantitative verification and validation are substantial, from both a research point of view and a clinical perspective.

Figure A.1 identifies two types of models: a conceptual model and a computerized model. The *conceptual model* is composed of all information, mathematical modeling data, and mathematical equations that describe the flow system, or process, of interest. The conceptual model is produced by analyzing and observing the flow system. In CFD, the conceptual model is dominated by the partial differential equations (PDEs) for conservation of mass (continuity), momentum (Navier–Stokes), and energy. In addition, the CFD model includes dynamic geometric data from diagnostic cardiac imaging modalities, auxiliary equations, such as constitutive relations for blood viscosity, and all of the initial and boundary conditions of the governing differential equations.

The process of model *verification* as used in Figure A.1, is the substantiation that a *computerized model* represents a conceptual model within specified limits of accuracy. The computerized model is an operational computer program that implements a conceptual model. Common terminology refers to the computerized model as the "computer code." The main implication is that the computer code must accurately mimic the model that was originally conceptualized. The process of model *validation* as used in Figure A.1, is the substantiation that a computerized model within its domain of applicability possesses a satisfactory range of accuracy, consistent with the intended application of the model. Both definitions contain an important feature: *substantiation*, which is evidence of correctness. The process of *model qualification* as used in Figure A.1, is the determination of adequacy of the conceptual model to provide an *acceptable* level of agreement for the intended application.

Figure A.1 clearly shows that verification deals with the relationship between the conceptual model and the computerized model and that validation deals with the relationship between the computerized model and reality. Rigorous and generalized procedures for verification and validation in Functional Imaging are in the early stages of development. These procedures should be directed toward increasing confidence in the predictive capability of the CFD model for any given levels of effort and cost expended on verification and validation activities. As is indicated on the diagram, the overall Functional Imaging approach and its components are *iterative* (see Fig. 12.18, on p. 659) in nature.

A.3 Verification assessment

The verification assessment activities under consideration apply to finite difference, finite element, and finite volume discretization procedures. Roache has treated the subject of verification extensively in his book [16], and a detailed description of verification methodology and procedures can be found there for the mathematically sophisticated. It is not my purpose here to review at length material that is otherwise available in that reference and others. Instead, I will summarize key features of verification assessment (see also Tabulation on p. 717, and the associated discussion) that serve to emphasize its role as an important partner with validation assessment.

Because of the *code-centric nature* of many verification activities, the terminology used in discussing verification often refers to computer code verification. What does this concept mean? To rigorously verify a computer code requires systematic proof that the computational implementation accurately represents the conceptual model and its solution. This, in turn, requires proof that the algorithms implemented in the computer code correctly approximate the underlying differential equations, along with the stated initial and boundary conditions. In addition, it must also be proven that the algorithms converge to the *correct solutions* of these equations in all circumstances under which the code will be applied. It is unlikely that such proofs will ever exist for any but the simplest CFD codes. The inability to offer proof of code verification in this regard is quite similar to the problems posed by validation. Verification, in a practical sense, then becomes the *absence of proof* that the code is *incorrect*. While it is possible to prove that a code is functioning incorrectly, it is effectively impossible to prove the opposite. Single examples suffice to demonstrate incorrect functioning, which is also a reason why testing occupies a large part of the verification effort.

Defining verification as the absence of proof that the code is wrong is unappealing from several viewpoints. For example, that situation could result, ostensibly, from lack of due diligence and inaction on the part of the code developers or the end-user community. An alternative definition that still captures the philosophical substance of the above argument is that verification of a CFD code is akin to the development of a *legal case*. Thus, verification assessment consists of accumulating evidence substantiating that the code does not have algorithmic or programming errors, that the code functions properly on specified hardware and operating system, and so on. This evidence needs to be documented, repeatable, accessible, and referenceable. The accumulation of such evidence also serves to reduce the regimes of operation of the code where one might possibly encounter such errors. Confidence in the verification status of the code then accrues from the accumulation of a sufficient mass of evidence, which is generally the case with most commercial codes, such as FIDAP™, FLUENT™(both, Fluent Inc., Lebanon, NH, U.S.A.), ANSYS CFX™(ANSYS, Canonsburg, PA, USA), and others, whose developers also gather evidence on the performance of their CFD codes from the end-user community.

The most accurate and traditional way to quantitatively measure the error in a computational solution is by comparing the computational solution to an available highly accurate solution. However, highly accurate solutions are known only for a relatively small number of simplified problems. They comprise analytical solutions and benchmark numerical solutions to the governing differential equations. Analytical solutions are closed-form solutions to special cases of the PDEs that are represented in the conceptual model. These closed-form solutions are commonly represented by infinite series, complex integrals, and asymptotic expansions [4, 10]. Numerical methods are usually used to compute the infinite series, complex integrals, and asymptotic expansions in order to obtain the solutions of interest. However, the accuracy of these solutions can be quantified much more rigorously than can the accuracy of the numerical solutions of the conceptual model. The most significant practical shortcoming of analytical solutions is that they exist only for very simplified physics and geometries.

The most important activity in verification testing of codes, and one that every user of commercial CFD codes should always apply him/herself, is the systematic refinement of the grid size and time step for specific problems. The discretization error should asymptotically approach zero as the grid size and time step approach zero, exclusive of computer round-off errors. If the order of accuracy is constant as the grid and time step are reduced beyond a specific threshold, we say that we are in the so-called *asymptotic region* of the discretization. It is essential to understand the influence of numerical issues, such as grid spacing and time step sizing, on simulation results before one can use the results obtained from a CFD flow model for clinical or research applications. One must resist the temptation to use physically realistic simulated results without quantitatively assessing grid dependence. This is true even when the objective is solely to understand *qualitatively* key flow features. It is plausible, in some cases, that a different grid spacing may show different key flow features. Occasionally, it is observed that computational results obtained with a specific grid show good agreement with the available data. This acceptable agreement can encourage immediate application of the CFD model to the problem being considered. It must be remembered, however, that no matter how good the agreement that one finds between available data and results simulated on a specific grid, if the solution is not grid independent, the agreement is probably an artefact of the specific grid size. It is, therefore, necessary to make an effort to obtain *grid-independent* results *before* they are used for clinical or research applications.

A.4 Validation assessment

The fundamental concept of *comparison and check of agreement* between Functional Imaging CFD results and pertinent (albeit typically sparse) measurement data (see Sections 13.5 and 14.5, on pp. 716 ff. and 742 ff., including all their subsections) is clearly consistent with the view of validation held by most investigators, which is necessitated by the lack of *in vivo* "gold standard" measurement techniques. Indeed, most postprocessors allow the user to import tabulated data for comparison with the simulation results. The fundamental reason that validation activities are difficult to conduct properly can be captured in the following two questions: "How is validation implemented?" and "What do model validation activities imply?" Concerning the first question, the approach to validation must be analogous to the strategy of verification discussed in Section A.3: validation of a model or code *cannot* be mathematically proven; validation can only be assessed for *individual realizations* of intracardiac flow fields of interest.

As to *what* model validation activities imply, only individual computational outcomes of a model are validated; codes are not validated [16]. This fundamental concept has been resolved philosophically [2, 14, 15], but commonly in the literature a favorable comparison of computational results and experimental or clinical data motivates the author to declare that the entire *computer model* is "validated." This view is not defensible in any meaningful way for complex flow processes. It seems that the more difficult of the two questions to answer is the second, which can be stated similarly as "What can be inferred when we make a prediction of some flow process with a CFD model that has completed some level of validation?" This question deserves our attention, because of the diverse views toward the meaning and processes of validation.

CFD simulation relies on the same logic as traditional science, but it also relies on many additional theoretical issues, e.g., discretization algorithms and grid quality, and practical issues, such as computer hardware, operating system software, source code reliability, and analyst skill, that are not present in classical science. One of the key classical theoretical issues is the state of knowledge of the process being modeled, i.e., the *complexity* of the process. For flow processes that are well understood both physically and mathematically, the inference from the comparison of the CFD simulation to the experimental realization can be quite strong. An example is laminar, incompressible, wall-bounded Newtonian flow. For a stationary geometry, i.e., fixed boundary conditions, there is only one nondimensional parameter appearing in the mathematical formulation: the *Reynolds number*. Even for such a simple flow, however, as the Reynolds number or geometry is changed, the flow can undergo *unanticipated* changes in character (for a thorough discussion of this important point, see Section 9.5.4, on pp. 463 ff.). Examples are: change from 2- to 3-D flow, and change from a steady flow to unsteady flow. The emphasis here is that the strength of the inference from the validation database becomes *weaker* as the complexity of the flow process of interest *increases*. A general mathematical method for determining how the inference value degrades as the physical process becomes more complex has not been formulated. For example, in a complex physical process how do you determine *"how nearby"* is the prediction case from cases in the validation database? Struggling with the strength or quantification of the inference in a flow field prediction is an important topic of CFD research .

It seems, to me, that now it can be argued that validation measurements and experiments actually constitute a new type of research activity that is ushered in by Functional Imaging as applied to clinical and animal experiment datasets. A validation experiment is conducted for the primary purpose of determining the validity, or predictive accuracy, of a CFD modeling and simulation procedure. In other words, a validation experiment is designed, executed, and analyzed for the purpose of quantitatively determining the ability of a mathematical model and its embodiment in a CFD code to simulate a well-characterized flow process. Thus, in a validation experiment "the code is the *customer*" or, if you like, "the CFD user is the *customer*." Only during the last 10–20 years has cardiovascular CFD simulation matured to the point where it could even be considered as a reason for experiments. As modern cardiology increasingly moves toward investigations of intracardiac flow fields based on Functional Imaging and visualization, so modeling and simulation itself will increasingly become the *customer* of experiments.

It should be noted that the *in vivo* validation of CFD simulations of complicated intracardiac 3-D vectorial velocity fields remains problematical at present, because there are no *in vivo* "gold standard" measurement techniques. A powerful instrument for *in vivo* validation investigations is a duplex ultrasound Doppler scanner, giving anatomical as well as flow field variable information from the investigated cardiac chamber(s). The acquired information is 2-D, but from this information a 3-D image can be reconstructed. A limitation with the ultrasound technique is the requirement of an "ultrasound window," without interposed bone or air. Another limitation is that the measured maximal flow velocities are limited by aliasing. The phase-encoded MRI is a more complex technique that also has the problem of velocity aliasing, but no "window" is needed. Validation of intracardiac velocity field simulations with time-resolved, phase-contrast velocity mapping MRI is not a straightforward task, primarily because velocity accuracy and precision are highly dependent on MR acquisition parameters. The velocity fields in the validation studies should replicate those being simulated, at least in magnitude, complexity, and temporal variation characteristics. Lotz et al. [9] presented a thorough review regarding accuracy of phase-contrast MRI measurements with regard to image acquisition parameters and data processing. Spatial resolution has a substantial effect on the accuracy of the velocity data [6]. When comparing MR velocity datasets to Functional Imaging results, one should keep in mind that MR voxels have finite dimensions that are typically larger than the grid size in the CFD simulations, and that nonperiodic flow phenomena will not be captured, because MR velocity fields are periodic as a result of temporal averaging.

A.5 Concluding remarks

Fundamental issues in systematic verification and validation are becoming important considerations in applying the Functional Imaging method to complex intracardiac blood flow field simulations. The fundamental strategy of verification is the identification and quantification of errors in the CFD model and its solution. In verification activities, the accuracy of a Functional Imaging computational solution can be measured relative to two types of highly accurate solutions that are usually available for some particular problems: analytical solutions, and highly accurate numerical solutions. Verification is, therefore, rooted in issues of mathematics and in the accuracy and correctness of complex computer codes and their execution; the importance of software testing during verification activities is obvious. Validation is deeply rooted in the question of how formal mathematical models of intracardiac flow phenomena can be tested by innovative digital imaging modality measurements, encompassing phase-contrast velocity MR mapping (see Section 10.3.2, on pp. 534 ff.) and 3-D Doppler echocardiography (see Section 10.4.4, on pp. 562 ff.).

MR 3-D velocity vector mapping is particularly well suited for studying spatiotemporal patterns of flow within the cardiac chambers. The robust detection of vortices and other salient flow features in the validating velocimetric intracardiac flow mappings can be made automatic by the use of the *phase portrait* method, widely used in exploring the properties of solutions of ordinary differential equations. This method, when applied to intracardiac flow pattern characterization [3, 7], allows us to evaluate the qualitative aspects of the flow field, i.e., its geometric properties, in particular the shape and stability of flow patterns and their relationship with the dynamic chamber geometry.

The renowned twentieth-century philosophers of science, Carnap [2] and Popper [14, 15], laid the foundation for our present-day concepts of validation. The fundamental strategy of validation is to assess how accurately the computational results compare with the *"real-world"* (experimental or clinical) data, with quantified error and uncertainty estimates. Validation assessment also encompasses a number of other important topics, including procedures for estimating experimental uncertainty referable to random and correlated bias errors in digital imaging and cardiac catheterization measurements. Since nondeterministic simulations are needed in many validation comparisons, statistical approaches are indicated for incorporating experimental uncertainties into the Functional Imaging analyses. As the complexity of a CFD model increases, its accuracy and range of applicability can become quite difficult to ascertain with confidence. Regardless of the difficulties and constraints, methods must continue to be perfected for measuring the accuracy of the CFD model for as many situations as the Functional Imaging method is deemed appropriate for.

References and further reading

[1] Buning, P.G. Sources of error in the graphical analysis of CFD results. J. Scient. Comput. 3: 149–64, 1988.

[2] Carnap, R. Testability and meaning. Philosophy of science, vol. III, 1963.

[3] Chong, M.S., Perry, A.E. A general classification of three-dimensional flow fields. Phys. Fluids A 2: 765–77, 1990.

[4] Ethier, C.R., Steinman, D.A. Exact fully 3D Navier–Stokes solutions for benchmarking. Int. J. Numer. Meth. Fluids 19: 369–75, 1994.

[5] Globus, A., Uselton, S. Evaluation of visualization software. ACM SIGGRAPH Comp. Graph. 29: 41–4, 1995.

[6] Greil, G., Geva, T., Maier, S., Powell, A. Effect of acquisition parameters on the accuracy of velocity encoded cine magnetic resonance imaging blood flow measurements. J. Magn. Reson. Imag. 15: 47–54, 2002.

[7] Helman, J., Hesselink, L. Representation and display of vector field topology in fluid flow data sets. IEEE Comp. 22: 27–36, 1989.

[8] Johnson, C.R., Allen, R. Sanderson, A. Next step: visualizing errors and uncertainty. IEEE Comp. Graph. Applic. 23: 6–10, 2003.

[9] Lotz, J., Meier, C., Leppert, A., Galanski, M. Cardiovascular flow measurement with phase-contrast MR imaging: basic facts and implementation. RadioGraphics 22: 651–71, 2002.

[10] Nayfeh, A.H. Perturbation methods. 1973, New York: Wiley.

[11] Pasipoularides, A.D., Shu, M., Womack, M.S., Shah, A., von Ramm, O., Glower, D.D. RV functional imaging: 3-D echo-derived dynamic geometry and flow field simulations. Am. J. Physiol. Heart Circ. Physiol. 284: H56–65, 2003.

[12] Pasipoularides, A., Shu, M., Shah, A., Womack, M.S., Glower, D.D. Diastolic right ventricular filling vortex in normal and volume overload states. Am. J. Physiol. Heart Circ. Physiol. 284: H1064–72, 2003.

[13] Pasipoularides, A., Shu, M., Shah, A., Tucconi, A., Glower, D.D. RV instantaneous intraventricular diastolic pressure and velocity distributions in normal and volume overload awake dog disease models. Am. J. Physiol. Heart Circ. Physiol. 285: H1956–65, 2003.

[14] Popper, K.R. The logic of scientific discovery. 1959, New York: Basic Books.

[15] Popper, K.R. Conjectures and refutations: the growth of scientific knowledge. 1969, London: Routledge and Kegan.

[16] Roache, P.J. Verification and validation in computational science and engineering. 1998, Albuquerque, NM: Hermosa Publishers.

[17] Roache, P.J. Quantification of uncertainty in computational fluid dynamics. Annu. Rev. Fluid Mech. 29: 123–60, 1997.

Index

Page numbers followed by an "f" indicate pages with figures.